Oxford Textbook of

Neuropsychiatry

OXFORD TEXTBOOKS IN PSYCHIATRY

Oxford Textbook of
Neuropsychiatry

EDITED BY

Niruj Agrawal

Department of Neuropsychiatry, St George's Hospital, London, UK

Rafey Faruqui

*University of Kent, and Kent & Medway NHS
and Social Care Partnership Trust, UK*

Mayur Bodani

*Department of Neuropsychiatry, Kent & Medway NHS
and Social Care Partnership Trust, UK*

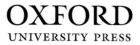

OXFORD
UNIVERSITY PRESS

OXFORD
UNIVERSITY PRESS

Great Clarendon Street, Oxford, OX2 6DP,
United Kingdom

Oxford University Press is a department of the University of Oxford.
It furthers the University's objective of excellence in research, scholarship,
and education by publishing worldwide. Oxford is a registered trade mark of
Oxford University Press in the UK and in certain other countries

First Edition published in 2020

Impression: 5

Published in the United States of America by Oxford University Press
198 Madison Avenue, New York, NY 10016, United States of America

British Library Cataloguing in Publication Data
Data available

Library of Congress Control Number: 2019955879

ISBN 978–0–19–875713–9

Printed and bound by
CPI Group (UK) Ltd, Croydon, CR0 4YY

Foreword

The *Oxford Textbook of Neuropsychiatry* is very timely. There is a growing awareness among psychiatrists and neurologists that the traditional Cartesian mind-brain dualism which fuelled division between their specialties is completely arbitrary and, in fact, contradicted by scientific research. Multidisciplinary team working has highlighted the extent of the overlap between psychiatric and neurological symptoms and disorders, as well as the implications for patients' functioning and quality of life. Indeed, the many disorders that do not fall neatly within the remit of either specialty need cross-disciplinary insights if they are to be fully understood and our patients are to receive the most appropriate care.

Neuropsychiatry is a well-recognized discipline in many countries, particularly those in which training in psychiatry and neurology has traditionally been combined. Elsewhere, there has been increasing interest in the subspecialty since the 1980s, witnessed by the establishment of national neuropsychiatric associations and the publication of specialized texts. Meanwhile, many countries have recognized the need to expand and improve upon the neuroscience knowledge base of psychiatry and neurology trainees through the modernization of training programmes. Advances in neuroscience research are appearing at an ever-faster rate and work in basic science is becoming increasingly 'translational', as scientists work to reduce the lag in transferring laboratory discoveries 'from bench to bedside'. If they are to keep up with the pace of progress, the next generation of clinicians must be 'neuroscientifically literate'. A deeper integration of neurosciences and neuropsychiatry in psychiatric and neurological training will better prepare trainees for the developments in diagnosis and treatment that stem from increased understanding of the brain in health and disease.

The practice of neuropsychiatry is driven by bringing together different perspectives and this comprehensive textbook includes contributions from renowned international experts in the neurological, psychiatric, psychological and neuroscientific fields from across the globe. The authors have kept in mind clinical relevance and an evidence-based approach to ensure that the book delivers exactly what its readers need. The different sections will be valuable to trainees and to established clinicians, to those who are moving into the subspecialty of neuropsychiatry and are looking for a thorough introduction, or for people seeking a detailed, up-to-date review of current understanding across the field.

This textbook is a considerable achievement and a very welcome resource.

Professor Wendy Burn
co-Chair, The Gatsby/Wellcome Neuroscience Project
President, Royal College of Psychiatrists

Preface

Neuropsychiatry is often misunderstood as a discipline and its definition and scope is interpreted differently across the world. However one looks at the scope of neuropsychiatry, its core identity lies at the interface between neurology and psychiatry. Traditional mind-brain dualism which fuelled division between neurology and psychiatry is now considered outdated and arbitrary. We are now increasingly aware of the extent of the overlap between neurological and psychiatric symptoms and disorders, and their implications on our patients' functioning and quality of life. This overlap ranges from common neurological disorders presenting with psychiatric symptoms; psychiatric conditions presenting with neurological symptoms; common neurological and psychiatric disorders co-existing by chance; or various brain disorders and syndromes which present with a range of neurological and psychiatric symptoms concomitantly. Effective and timely management of these conditions requires specific neuropsychiatric knowledge and experience brought together from a number of related fields including neurology, psychiatry, neuropsychology, neurophysiology and neuroradiology, along with a knowledge of basic neuroscience.

Popular psychiatric or neurological textbooks generally touch upon these neuropsychiatric conditions superficially, but do not do justice to the nature and complexity of these conditions and do not provide adequate information. Similar concerns are unfortunately also prevalent in the vast majority of neurology or psychiatry training programmes across the world. There are very few places at present with a formalized neuropsychiatry training programme globally. Despite this, patients with neuropsychiatric conditions commonly present in neurological and psychiatric clinical practice. This has led to an increasing recognition of the need to improve neuropsychiatric knowledge and skills of all neurology and psychiatry trainees that is long overdue. There has been a substantial global focus recently on more profound integration of neurosciences and neuropsychiatry in psychiatric training. Neuropsychiatry forms an important part of the psychiatric curriculum and is examined both in theory and in clinical exams. Similarly, neuropsychiatry is also of interest to neurology trainees, and it is increasingly recognized that all neurology trainees should have some knowledge and experience in neuropsychiatry.

The need for neuropsychiatric knowledge and skills is now recognized by trainees too. A survey of over 900 trainees at the Royal College of Psychiatrists (RCPsych) in the United Kingdom showed that over three-quarters of psychiatry trainees desired some knowledge and training in the field of neuropsychiatry. Most of these trainees, whilst they did not wish to specialize in neuropsychiatry, recognized the value of an understanding of neuropsychiatry in their preferred subspecialty as a career choice. There is currently a drive in a number of psychiatric programmes across the globe to improve exposure to basic and clinical neuroscience.

Currently, there are a small number of recognized textbooks of neuropsychiatry in the world. However, most of these are a bit old and are rather large reference works for specialists in this field. There is a dearth of neuropsychiatry textbooks which are pitched at the level of trainees and clinicians who are not specialists in the field. Hence this textbook is written in simple language, is clinically focused, is very comprehensive in its scope of topics, and covers a global perspective. We believe that the Oxford Textbook of Neuropsychiatry will help to bridge the gap between general psychiatric and neurology textbooks and neuropsychiatry reference books, and will become an essential training textbook for all psychiatry and neurology trainees worldwide.

This book is written by international experts, clinicians, and leaders in their field from a very large number of countries in the world and spanning several continents. They have taken an up-to-date evidence-based approach with clinical relevance in mind, taking a global perspective on neuropsychiatric problems and treatment. They come from primarily neurological, psychiatric, psychological, neuroscience, and neuropsychiatric backgrounds. This is truly a global multidisciplinary effort unlike any other neuropsychiatry textbook currently available.

This book is organized into four sections. The first section covers the foundation and basic skills, including basic science knowledge and clinical skills relevant to neuropsychiatry. The second section covers the details of a wide range of core neuropsychiatric conditions. The third section focuses on the principles of treatment in various modalities and neuropsychiatry service models and pathways. This section also covers the relevance of neuropsychiatry in criminal and civil courts. The last section is unique to this book and provides a snapshot of neuropsychiatry perspectives in various parts of the world. All chapters contain a number of key learning points at the end and key references.

We believe this book may also be of relevance to trainees in neurorehabilitation, allied professionals in neuroscience and mental health, in addition to neurology and psychiatry trainees and clinicians. It covers core knowledge and skills for training in neuropsychiatry but also covers the knowledge applicable to all neurology and psychiatry trainees. The book meets curriculum requirements for various international training programmes and examinations. We hope that you will enjoy reading this book as much as we have reading all the chapters.

We are most grateful to all our contributors internationally, many of whom are friends and colleagues. They have worked hard to simplify complex knowledge and distil a lifetime of experience concisely. It has been an honour and privilege to work with them.

We would also like to thank the Oxford University Press editorial team, Lauren Tilley, Karen Moore, Rachel Goldsworthy, and Pete Stevenson for their help and support at all the stages of this book's production.

Niruj Agrawal
Rafey Faruqui
Mayar Bodani

Contents

SECTION 3
Principles of treatment

SECTION 4
Perspectives of neuropsychiatry worldwide

Abbreviations

2-D	two-dimensional	AM	alpha mannosidosis
3-D	three-dimensional	AMP	amphetamine
μV	microvolt	AMPA R	AMPA receptor
A&E	accident and emergency	ANA	Asociación Neuropsiquiátrica Argentina (Neuropsychiatric Association of Argentina)
4AT	4As Test		
5HT	serotonin	aNMDARE	anti-NMDA receptor encephalitis
5CSRTT	5-choice serial reaction time task	APA	American Psychiatric Association
A	ampere	APOE	apolipoprotein E
AAN	American Academy of Neurology	ARAS	ascending reticular activating system
AASM	American Academy of Sleep Medicine	ARBD	alcohol-related brain damage; alcohol-related birth defects
ABI	acquired brain injury		
ABIBC	ABI Behaviour Consultancy	ARND	alcohol-related neurodevelopmental disorder
ABP	Associação Brasileira de Psiquiatria (Brazilian Psychiatric Association)	ART	antiretroviral therapy
		AS	Angelman syndrome
ABS	Agitated Behavior Scale	ASD	autism spectrum disorder
AC	anterior cingulum	ASV	adaptive servo-ventilation
ACC	anterior cingulate cortex	ATP	adenosine triphosphate
ACE	Addenbrooke's Cognitive Examination	ATX	atomoxetine
ACE-III	Addenbrooke's Cognitive Examination, third edition	BA	Brodmann area
		BADS	Behavioural Assessment of the Dysexecutive Syndrome
ACE-R	Addenbrooke's Cognitive Examination-Revised		
AChE	acetylcholinesterase	BASP1	brain abundant membrane-attached signal protein 1
ACT	Australian Capital Territory		
ACTH	adrenocorticotrophic hormone	BBB	blood–brain barrier
AD	Alzheimer's disease	BBI	blood–brain interface
ADC	apparent diffusion coefficient; AIDS dementia complex	BCAA	branched-chain amino acid
		BCI	brain–computer interface
ADEM	acute disseminated encephalomyelitis	BDI	Beck Depression Inventory
ADHD	attention-deficit/hyperactivity disorder	BDNF	brain-derived neurotrophic factor
ADL	activity of daily living	BED	binge eating disorder
AE	autoimmune encephalopathy	BETS	benign epileptic transients of sleep
AED	antiepileptic drug	BG	basal ganglion
AEN	Asociación Española de Neuropsiquiatría	BICAMS	Brief International Cognitive Assessment in multiple sclerosis
AES	Apathy Evaluation Scale		
agPPA	agrammatic variant primary progressive aphasia	BiPAP	bilevel positive airway pressure
		BIT	Behavioural Inattention Test
AHI	apnoea–hypopnoea index	BMI	body mass index
AHS	alien hand syndrome	BMPPS	Behaviour itself, Medical/organic issues, Person showing the behaviour, Psychiatric/psychological issues, and Social/occupational/personal issues
AI	artificial intelligence;		
AIDS	acquired immune deficiency syndrome		
AIE	autoimmune encephalopathy		
AIIMS	All India Institute of Medical Sciences	BN	behavioural neurology
AIP	acute intermittent porphyria	BN & NP	behavioural neurology and neuropsychiatry
ALA	amino-levulinic acid	BNS	Barbadian Nutritional Study
ALD	adrenoleukodystrophy	BPAD	bipolar affective disorder
ALS	amyotrophic lateral sclerosis	BPD	borderline personality disorder
ALSPAC	Avon Longitudinal Study of Parents and Children	BPS	behavioural and psychological symptoms

BPSD	behavioural and psychological symptoms of dementia
BRIEF	Behaviour Rating Inventory of Executive Functions
BRNB	Brief Repeatable Neuropsychological Battery
BSE	bovine spongiform encephalopathy
bvFTD	behavioural variant frontotemporal dementia
BVMT	Brief Visual Memory Test
CAA	cerebral amyloid angiopathy
CAD	coronary artery disease
CADASIL	cerebral autosomal dominant arteriopathy with subcortical infarcts and leukoencephalopathy
CAM	Confusion Assessment Method
CAMCOG	Cambridge Cognition Examination
CANS	childhood acute neuropsychiatric symptoms
CAP	Confusion Assessment Protocol
CARASIL	cerebral autosomal recessive arteriopathy with subcortical infarcts and leukoencephalopathy
CASPR2	contactin-associated protein-like 2
CAU	cognitive–anatomic unit
CBA	cell-based assay
CBD	corticobasal degeneration; cannabidiol
CBDATS	Community Brain Disorders Assessment and Treatment Service
CBF	cerebral blood flow
CBI	Cambridge Behavioural Inventory
CBIT	comprehensive behavioural intervention
CBS	corticobasal syndrome
CBT	cognitive behavioural therapy
CBTi	cognitive behavioural therapy for insomnia
CCAS	cerebellar cognitive affective syndrome
CD	conduct disorder
CDC	Centers for Disease Control and Prevention
CDR	Clinical Dementia Rating Scale
CDRH	Centre for Devices and Radiological Health
C-ECT	continuation electroconvulsive therapy
CENECON	Centro de Neuropsiquiatría y Neurología de la Conducta (Centre Neuropsychiatry and Behavioural Neurology)
CES	cranial electrical stimulation
CFD	cerebral folate deficiency
CFS	chronic fatigue syndrome
CFTD	cerebral folate transport deficiency
CGH	comparative genomic hybridization
ChEI	cholinesterase inhibitor
CI	confidence interval
CIA	chemiluminescence immunoassay
CIS	clinically isolated syndromes
CJD	Creutzfeldt–Jakob disease
cm	centimetre
CM	cerebellar mutism
CMR	cerebral metabolic rate
CMV	cytomegalovirus
CNP	Comprehensive Neuropsychiatry Programme
CNS	central nervous system
CNV	copy number variation
CoA	coenzyme A
COMT	catechol-O-methyltransferase
COWAT	Controlled Oral Word Association Test

CPAP	continuous positive airway pressure
CPR	Civil Procedure Rules
cps	cycles per second
CRH	corticotropin-releasing hormone
CRP	C-reactive protein
CRPS	complex regional pain syndrome
CRS	Coma Recovery Scale; chronic restraint stress; Catatonia Rating Scale
CRSD	circadian rhythm sleep disorder
CSA	central sleep apnoea
CSA/CSR	central sleep apnoea with Cheyne–Stokes respiration
CSE	Certificate of Secondary Education
CSF	cerebrospinal fluid
CSF-1	colony-stimulating factor-1
CSTC	cortico-striato-thalamo-cortical
CT	computed tomography
CTD	chronic tic disorder; Cognitive Test for Delirium
CTE	chronic traumatic encephalopathy
CTX	cerebrotendinous xanthomatosis
CUS	chronic unpredictable stress
CVLT	California Verbal Learning Test
CVS	caloric vestibular stimulation
DA	dopamine
DAIR	Dementia Apathy Interview and Rating
DAMP	damage-associated molecular pattern; deficits in attention, motor control, and perception
DAPI	4′,6-diamidino-2-phenylindole
DaT/DAT	dopamine transporter
DBS	deep brain simulation
DBT	dialectic behaviour therapy
ddNTP	dideoxynucleotide triphosphate
DEX	Dysexecutive Questionnaire
DGPPN	German Association for Psychiatry, Psychotherapy, and Psychosomatics
DHB	District Health Board
DHEA	dehydroepiandrosterone
DIDMOAD	diabetes insipidus, diabetes mellitus, optic atrophy, deafness
DIGE	difference-in-gel electrophoresis
DLB	dementia with Lewy bodies
DLBD	dementia with Lewy bodies disease
DLPFC	dorsolateral prefrontal cortex
DM	delirious mania
DMDD	disruptive mood dysregulation disorders
DMN	default mode network
DMS	delusional misidentification syndrome
DNA	deoxyribonucleic acid
DOC	disorders of consciousness
DOS	Delirium Observation Screening Scale
D2R	dopamine-2 receptor
DRG	dorsal root ganglion
DRPLA	dentatorubral-pallidoluysian atrophy
DRS	Delirium Rating Scale
DRS-R98	Delirium Rating Scale–Revised–98
dsDNA	double-stranded DNA
DSM-5	Diagnostic and Statistical Manual of Mental Disorders, fifth edition
DSPD	delayed sleep phase disorder

DT	distress thermometer	GC-MS	gas chromatography–mass spectroscopy
DTI	diffusion tensor imaging	GCS	Glasgow Coma Scale; Gudjonsson Compliance Scale
DVLA	Driver and Vehicle Licensing Agency	Gd	gadolinium
DWI	diffusion-weighted imaging	GDN	Gesellschaft Deutscher Nervenärzte
EBV	Ebstein–Barr virus	GDNP	Gesellschaft deutscher Neurologen und Psychiater
ECT	electroconvulsive therapy	GH	growth hormone
EDS	excessive daytime sleepiness	GHB	gamma-hydroxybutyric acid
EDSS	Expanded Disability Status Scale	GI	gastrointestinal
EEG	electroencephalogram	GOAT	Galveston Orientation and Amnesia Test
EFT	equivalent full-time	GP	globus pallidus
eGFR	estimated glomerular filtration rate	GPe	globus pallidus externa
EIA	enzyme immunoassay	GPi	globus pallidus interna
ELISA	enzyme-linked immunosorbent assay	GRE	gradient-recalled echo
EMDR	eye movement desensitization and reprocessing	GSS	Gerstmann–Sträussler–Scheinker (syndrome)
EMG	electromyography	GSS1	Gudjonsson Suggestibility Scale 1
EMR	electronic medical record	GSS2	Gudjonsson Suggestibility Scale 2
ENT	ear, nose, and throat	GVS	galvanic vestibular stimulation
EORTC	European Organisation for Research and Treatment of Cancer	GWAS	genome-wide association studies
		HAD	HIV-associated dementia
EPC	epilepsia partialis continua	HAD-S	Hospital and Anxiety Depression Scale (Anxiety sub-scale)
ERD	event-related desynchronization		
ERP	event-related potential	HAD-D	Hospital and Anxiety Depression Scale (Depression sub-scale)
ERS	event-related synchronization		
ESI	electrospray ionization	HADS	Hospital and Anxiety Depression Scale
FA	fractional anisotropy	HCN	hyperpolarization-gated cyclic nucleotide-gated
FAB	Frontal Assessment Battery	HCR-20	Historical Clinical Risk Management-20
FAS	fetal alcohol syndrome	HD	Huntington's disease
FASD	fetal alcohol spectrum disorders	HIV	human immunodeficiency virus
FBDS	faciobrachial dystonic seizures	HLA	human leucocyte antigen
FBI	Frontal Behavioral Inventory	HoNOS	Health of the Nation Outcome Scale
FBSS	failed back surgery syndrome	HPA	hypothalamic–pituitary–adrenal
FCD	functional cognitive disorder	HPPD	hallucinogen persisting perception disorder
FCSRT	Free and Cued Selective Reminding Test	HRQoL	health-related quality of life
FD	Fabry disease	HRT	habit reversal therapy
FDA	Food and Drug Administration	HSE	herpes simplex encephalitis
FDG	fludeoxyglucose	HSV	herpes simplex virus
FET	fluoroethyltyrosine	HSV-1	herpes simplex virus type 1
FFI	fatal familial insomnia	Htt	huntingtin protein
FIRDA	frontal intermittent rhythmic delta activity	Hz	hertz
FISH	fluorescence in situ hybridization	ICD	International Classification of Diseases
FLAIR	fluid-attenuated inversion recovery	iCJD	iatrogenic Creutzfeldt–Jakob disease
FMD	functional movement disorder; functional motor disorder	ICSD	International Classification of Sleep Disorders
		ICU	intensive care unit
FME	forensic medical examiner	ID	intellectual disability; iron deficiency
fMRI	functional magnetic resonance imaging	IDO	indoleamine 2,3-deoxygenase
FND	functional neurological disorder	IED	interictal epileptiform discharge; intermittent explosive disorder
FNEA	functional non-epileptic attack		
FRS	Functional Rating Scale	IEM	inborn error of metabolism
FrSBe	Frontal Systems Behaviour Scale	IFN-α	interferon-alpha
FSH	follicle-stimulating hormone	IFN-γ	interferon-gamma
FTA-Abs	fluorescent treponemal antibody absorption	IGF-1	insulin-like growth factor 1
FTD	frontotemporal dementia	IgG	immunoglobulin G
FXTAS	fragile X-associated tremor/ataxia syndrome	IgM	immunoglobulin M
GABA	gamma aminobutyric acid	IH	idiopathic hypersomnia; intermittent hypoxia
GABHS	group A β-haemolytic Streptococcus	IIS	Indian Institute of Science
GAD	generalized anxiety disorder	IL	interleukin
GAD-7	Generalized Anxiety Disorder-7 item	ILAE	International League Against Epilepsy
GBM	glioblastoma multiforme	ILF	inferior longitudinal fasciculus

IL-1ra	IL-1 receptor antagonist	MELAS	mitochondrial myopathy encephalopathy, lactic acidosis, and stroke-like episodes
IM	intramuscular	MENS	multiple endocrine neoplasia syndrome
IMP	iodoamphetamine	MEP	motor evoked potential
INA	International Neuropsychiatric Association	MERRF	myoclonic epilepsy with ragged red fibres
ION	International Organization of Neuropsychiatry	MET	methionine
IPA	International Psychoanalytic Association	MetS	metabolic syndrome
IPD	idiopathic Parkinson's disease	MFFT	Matching Familiar Figures Task
IQ	intelligence quotient	MHC	major histocompatibility complex
IRIS	immune reconstitution inflammatory syndrome	MHPG	3-methoxy-4-hydroxyphenylglycol
IST	Information Sampling Task	MINI	Mini-International Neuropsychiatric Interview
ISWRD	irregular sleep–wake rhythms disorder	MLD	metachromatic leukodystrophy
iTRAQ	isobaric tags for relative and absolute quantitation	MLPA	multiplex ligation-dependent probe amplification
ITU	intensive therapy unit	mm	millimetre
IV	intravenous	mmHg	millimetre of mercury
IVIG	intravenous immunoglobulin	MMPI	Minnesota Multiphasic Personality Inventory
JLD	jet-lag disorder	MMSE	Mini-Mental State Examination
JME	juvenile myoclonic epilepsy	MNC	Managed Clinical Network; Melbourne Neuropsychiatry Centre
JNA	Japanese Neuropsychiatric Association	MoCA	Montreal Cognitive Assessment
JSN	Japanese Society of Neurology	MPH	methylphenidate
JSPN	Japanese Society of Psychiatry and Neurology	MR	magnetic resonance
K+	potassium ion	MRI	magnetic resonance imaging
KS	Korsakoff's syndrome	mRNA	messenger ribonucleic acid
LACS	lacunar stroke	mRS	modified Rankin scale
LAMP	limbic system-associated membrane protein	MRS	magnetic resonance spectroscopy; Modified Rankin Scale
LARS	Lille Apathy Rating Scale	MS	mass spectrometry; multiple sclerosis
LART	left anterior right temporal	MSA	multiple (or multi-) system atrophy
LCA	latent class analysis	MSLT	multiple sleep latency test
LCECA	liquid chromatography electrochemical array	MSM	men who have sex with men
LC-MS	liquid chromatography–mass spectroscopy	MS-MLPA	methylation-specific MLPA
L-dopa	levodopa	MST	magnetic seizure therapy
LE	limbic encephalitis	MSUD	maple syrup urine disease
LGI1	leucine-rich glioma inactivated 1	mTBI	mild traumatic brain injury
LH	luteinizing hormone	mtDNA	mitochondrial DNA
LNAA	large neutral amino acid	MTHFR	methylenetetrahydrofolate reductase
LOC	loss of consciousness	mV	millivolt
LP	lumbar puncture	Na+	sodium ion
LPA	logopenic progressive aphasia	NA	noradrenaline
lPFC	lateral prefrontal cortex	NAcb	nucleus accumbens
LSD	lysergic acid diethylamide	NART	National Adult Reading Task
LTD	long-term depression	NBD	neurobehavioural disability
LTP	long-term potential	NBM	nucleus basalis of Meynert
m	metre	NbR	neurobehavioural rehabilitation
mA	milliampere	NBRC	National Brain Research Centre
MACFMS	Minimal Assessment of Cognitive Function in multiple sclerosis	NBSE	neurobehavioural status examination
MALDI	matrix-assisted laser desorption/ionization	NCBS	National Center for Biological Sciences
MAOI	monoamine oxidase inhibitor	nCPAP	nocturnal continuous positive airway pressure
MAST	Mississippi Aphasia Screening Test	NCSE	non-convulsive status epilepticus
MBD	Marchiafava–Bignami disease; minimal brain dysfunction	ND-PAE	Neurobehavioral Disorder Associated with Prenatal Alcohol Exposure
MBIA	microbead immunoassay	NEAD	non-epileptiform attack disorder
MBL	mannose-binding lectin	NES	Neurological Evaluation Scale
MCI	mild cognitive impairment	NET	neuro-electric therapy
MCS	minimally conscious state; motor cortex stimulation	NFT	neurofibrillary tangle
MDD	major depressive disorder	nfvPPA	non-fluent variant primary progressive aphasia
MDMA	3,4-methylenedioxymethamphetamine	NGO	non-governmental organization
MDT	multidisciplinary team		
MEG	magnetoencephalograpy		

NGS	next-generation sequencing		PBS	positive behaviour supports
NHI	Hospício Nacional dos Alienados Dom Pedro II (Dom Pedro II National Hospice for the Insane)		PCA	posterior cortical atrophy
			PCNSL	primary central nervous system lymphoma
NHS	National Health Service		PCR	polymerase chain reaction
NIBS	non-invasive brain stimulation		PCS	post-concussion syndrome
NICE	National Institute for Health and Care Excellence		PD	Parkinson's disease; personality disorder
NIHSS	National Institute of Health Stroke Scale		PDD	Parkinson's disease dementia
NIMH	National Institute of Mental Health		PEG	percutaneous endoscopic gastrostomy
NIMHANS	National Institute of Mental Health and Neurosciences		PET	positron emission tomography
			PF	posterior fossa
NK	natural killer		PFAS	partial fetal alcohol syndrome
NK1	neurokinin 1		PFC	prefrontal cortex
NLRP	NOD-like receptor protein		PFS	posterior fossa syndrome
nm	nanometre		PGD	pre-implantation genetic diagnosis
NMDA	N-methyl-D-aspartate		PGIMER	Post-Graduate Institue of Medical Sciences & Research
NMDAR	NMDA receptor			
NMO	neuromyelitis optica		Phe	phenylalanine
NMR	nuclear magnetic resonance		PHQ-9	Patient Health Questionnaire
NMS	neuroleptic malignant syndrome		PIT	psychodynamic interpersonal therapy
NNRTI	non-nucleoside reverse transcriptase inhibitor		PITAND	paediatric infection-triggered autoimmune neuropsychiatric disorders
NOD	nucleotide-binding oligomerization domain			
NOS	not otherwise specified		PIVC	parieto-insular vestibular cortex
NP	neuropsychiatry		PKAN	pantothenate kinase-associated neurodegeneration
NPC	Niemann–Pick disease type C			
NPH	normal pressure hydrocephalus		PKU	phenylketonuria
NPI	Neuropsychiatric Inventory; Neuropsychiatric Institute (Sydney)		PLACS	Pathologic Laughing and Crying Scale
			PLMD	periodic limb movement disorder
NREM	non-rapid eye movement		PLMS	periodic limb movements of sleep
NSAb	neuronal surface antibody		PMA	pre-market approval
NSW	New South Wales		PML	progressive multifocal leukoencephalopathy
N24SWD	non-24-hour sleep–wake rhythm disorder		PNES	psychogenic non-epileptic seizure
NT1	narcolepsy type 1		PNFA	progressive non-fluent aphasia
NTP	nucleotide triphosphate		PNS	peripheral nerve stimulation
OCD	obsessive–compulsive disorder		POCS	posterior circulation stroke syndrome
OCS	obsessive–compulsive symptoms		POMC	pro-opiomelanocortin
OCSP	Oxfordshire Community Stroke Project		POSTS	positive occipital sharp transients of sleep
ODD	oppositional defiant disorder		PPA	primary progressive aphasia
OFC	orbitofrontal cortex		PPAOS	primary progressive apraxia of speech
OHS	obesity hypoventilation syndrome		PPMS	primary progressive multiple sclerosis
O-log	Orientation Log		PRR	pattern recognition receptor
ONS	occipital nerve stimulation		PSD	post-synaptic density; post-stroke depression
OSAS	obstructive sleep apnoea syndrome		PSEN	presenilin
OT	occupational therapy		PSF	post-stroke fatigue
OTC	ornithine transcarbamylase deficiency		PSG	polysomnography
PA	propionic acidaemia		PSP	progressive supranuclear palsy
PACE	Police and Criminal Evidence Act 1984		PSWC	periodic sharp wave complex
PACS	partial anterior circulation syndrome		PT	physiotherapy
PAH	phenylalanine hydroxylase		PTA	post-traumatic amnesia
PAMP	pathogen-associated molecular pattern		PTCS	post-traumatic confusional state
PANDAS	paediatric autoimmune neuropsychiatric disorders associated with streptococcal infections		PTH	parathyroid hormone
			PTM	post-translational modification
PANS	paediatric acute-onset neuropsychiatric syndrome		PTSD	post-traumatic stress disorder
			PVS	persistent vegetative state
PANSS	Positive and Negative Syndrome Scale		PwMS	people with multiple sclerosis
PAR	Psychological Assessment Resources		PWS	Prader–Willi syndrome
PASAT	Paced Auditory Serial Addition Test		QIDS	Quick Inventory for Depressive Symptomatology
PBA	pseudobulbar affect		QoL	quality of life
PBG	porphobilinogen		QUIP	Questionnaire for Impulsive-Compulsive Disorders in Parkinson's disease
PBMC	peripheral blood mononuclear cell			

RAVLT	Rey Auditory Verbal Learning Test	SREAT	steroid-responsive encephalopathy associated with autoimmune thyroiditis
RBD	rapid eye movement sleep behaviour disorder; rapidly progressive dementia	SRED	sleep-related eating disorder
rCBF	regional cerebral blood flow	SRT	Selective Reminding Test
rCMR	regional cerebral metabolic rate	SSADH	succinic semi-aldehyde dehydrogenase deficiency
RCP	Royal College of Physicians	SSD	subsyndromal delirium
RCT	randomized controlled trial	SSEP	somatosensory evoked potential
RDoC	Research Domain Criteria	SSPE	subacute sclerosing panencephalitis
REM	rapid eye movement	SSRI	selective serotonin reuptake inhibitor
RESIS	Repetitive Transcranial Magnetic Stimulation for the Treatment of Negative Symptoms in Schizophrenia	SSRT	stop signal reaction time
		SST	Stop Signal Task
rIFC	right inferior frontal cortex	SSVD	subcortical small vessel disease
RLS	restless legs syndrome	STN	subthalamic nuclei
RMH	Royal Melbourne Hospital	STS	supraorbital transcutaneous stimulation
ROCF	Rey–Osterrieth Complex Figure Test	STXBP1	syntaxin-binding protein 1
RPR	rapid plasma reagin	SUS	Sistema Único de Saúde (Unified Health System)
R&R	reasoning and rehabilitation	SWD	shift-work disorder
RRMS	relapsing–remitting multiple sclerosis	SWI	susceptibility weighted imaging
rTMS	repetitive transcranial magnetic stimulation	SYDBAT	Sydney Language Battery
RT-QuiC	real-time quaking-induced conversion	tACS	transcranial alternating current stimulation
RVCL	retinal vasculopathy with cerebral leukodystrophy	TACS	total anterior circulation syndrome
s	second	TASIT	The Awareness of Social Inference Test
SCA	spinocerebellar ataxia	TAU	treatment-as-usual
SCAA	sulfur-containing amino acid	TB	tuberculosis
SCI	subjective cognitive impairment	TBI	traumatic brain injury
SCIA	Structured Clinical Interview for Apathy	TBM	tuberculous meningitis
SCID	Structured Clinical Interview for DSM-IV	TC	cytotoxic T-cells
sCJD	sporadic Creutzfeldt–Jakob disease	TCA	tricarboxylic acid
SCN	suprachiasmatic nuclei	TCET	transcerebral electrotherapy
SCS	spinal cord stimulation	tDCS	transcranial direct current stimulation
SD	standard deviation; semantic dementia	TDT	transdisciplinary team
SDMT	Symbol Digit Modalities Test	TEA	transient epileptic amnesia
SEGA	subependymal giant cell astrocytoma	TENS	transcutaneous electrical nerve stimulation
SELDI	surface-enhanced laser desorption/ionization	TES	transcranial electrical stimulation
SF-36	Short Form-36	TGA	transient global amnesia
SGA	second-generation antipsychotic	TGF-β	transforming growth factor-beta
SIADH	syndrome of inappropriate antidiuretic hormone secretion	TH	CD4+ helper T-cell
		THC	tetrahydrocannabinol
SIB	self-injurious behaviour	TIA	transient ischaemic attack
SIRS	Structured Inventory of Reported Symptoms	TIRDA	temporal intermittent rhythmic delta activity
SLE	systemic lupus erythematosus	TLE	temporal lobe epilepsy
SLF	superior longitudinal fasciculus	TLR	Toll-like receptor
SMA	supplementary motor area	TMS	transcranial magnetic stimulation
SMON	subacute myelino-optico-neuropathy	TNF	tumour necrosis factor
SNAps	synaptic and neuronal autoantibody-associated psychiatric syndromes	TOF	time-of-flight
		TOMM	Test of Memory Malingering
SNc	substantia nigra pars compacta	TOOTS	time-out-on-the-spot
SNr	substantia nigra	tPA	tissue plasminogen activator
SNRI	serotonin–noradrenaline reuptake inhibitor	tPCS	transcranial pulsed current stimulation
SOD	superoxide dismutase	TPHA	Treponema pallidum haemagglutination assay
SONS	supraorbital nerve stimulation	TPI	Treponema pallidum immobilization
SOREMP	sleep-onset REM period	TPPA	Treponema pallidum particle agglutination
SPECT	single-photon emission computed tomography	TRD	treatment-resistant depression
SPES	single pulse electrical stimulation	Treg	regulatory T-cells
SPMS	secondary progressive multiple sclerosis	tRNS	transcranial random noise stimulation
SPS	single prolonged stress	TROG	Test of Reception of Grammar
SRCA	synthetic cannabinoid receptor agonist	TRUST	toluidine red unheated serum test
		TS	Tourette syndrome

TSD	Tay–Sach's disease
TSH	thyroid-stimulating hormone
TSPO	translocator protein
TSS	toxic serotonin syndrome
TST	total sleep time
UCD	urea cycle disorder
UCNS	United Council for Neurologic Subspecialties
UPDRS	Unified Parkinson's Disease Rating Scale
UTR	untranslated region
UWS	unresponsive wakefulness syndrome
VAChT	vesicular acetylcholine transporter
VaD	vascular dementia
VBM	voxel-based morphometry
VCAT	Visual Cognitive Assessment Test
VCD	vascular cognitive disorder

vCJD	variant Creuztfeldt–Jakob disease
VDRL	Venereal Disease Research Laboratory
VGKC	voltage-gated potassium channel
VLCFA	very long-chain fatty acid
VNS	vagus nerve stimulation
VOR	vestibulo-ocular reflex
VOSP	Visual Object and Space Perception Battery
VS	vegetative state
VZV	varicella-zoster virus
WE	Wernicke's encephalopathy
WHO	World Health Organization
WK	Wernicke–Korsakoff's syndrome
WKS	Wernicke–Korsakoff syndrome
YOD	Younger Onset Dementia (Service)

Contributors

Dimitrios Adamis Sligo Mental Health Services, Ballytivan, Sligo, Ireland

Guleed Adan Clinical Research Fellow, University of Liverpool and Neurology Specialist Trainee, Walton Centre NHS Foundation Trust, Liverpool, UK

Niruj Agrawal Consultant Neuropsychiatrist and Honorary Senior Lecturer, St George's Hospital, London, UK

Nick Alderman Clinical Director, Neurobehavioural Rehabilitation Services, Elysium Neurological Services, Daventry, UK

Jonathan Bird Burden Centre for Neuropsychiatry, Neuropsychology and Epileptology, Frenchay Hospital, Bristol, UK

Sonja Blum NYU School of Medicine, New York City, New York, USA

Mayur Bodani Department of Neuropsychiatry, Kent & Medway NHS and Social Care Partnership Trust, Darent House, Sevenoaks, Kent, UK

Derek Bolton Professor of Philosophy & Psychopathology, King's College London, Institute of Psychiatry, UK

Borna Bonakdarpour Assistant Professor of Neurology, Mesulam Center for Cognitive Neurology and Alzheimer Disease, Ken and Ruth Davee Department of Neurology, Feinberg School of Medicine, Northwestern University, Chicago, Illinois, USA

Gilberto Slud Brofman Psychiatrist, Secretary of the International Neuropsychiatry Association, Former Director, Hospital Psiquiátrico São Pedro, Porto Alegre, Brazil

Stefania Bruno The Blackheath Brain Injury Rehabilitation Centre, The Huntercombe Group, London, UK

Luis Ignacio Brusco Professor of Psychiatry & Mental Health and Behavioural Neurology, School of Medicine, University of Buenos Aires, Buenos Aires, Argentina

Christine Burness Consultant Neurologist and Honorary Lecturer, Walton Centre NHS Foundation Trust, Liverpool, UK

James R. Burrell Concord General Hospital, Sydney, Australia

Alan Carson Consultant and Reader in Neuropsychiatry, Centre for Clinical Brain Sciences, University of Edinburgh, UK

Andrea E. Cavanna Department of Neuropsychiatry, BSMHFT and University of Birmingham, Birmingham, UK

Wai Chen School of Paediatrics, University of Western Australia (UWA); Graduate School of Education (UWA); Mental Health Service, Fiona Stanley Hospital, Perth (WA); Murdoch University (WA); School of Medicine, Fremantle, Notre Dame University (WA), Australia

Yvonne Chun Research Fellow in Geriatric Medicine, Centre for Clinical Brain Sciences, University of Edinburgh, UK

Jan A. Coebergh Consultant Neurologist, St George's University Hosptials NHS Foundation Trust, Chertsey, UK

Joseph J. Cooper Associate Professor of Clinical Psychiatry, University of Illinois at Chicago, Chicago, Illinois, USA

Sarah R. Cope Clinical Psychologist, South West London and St George's Mental Health NHS Trust, UK

Thomas E. Cope Department of Clinical Neuroscience, University of Cambridge, Cambridge, UK

Ester Coutinho Department of Basic and Clinical Neuroscience, Institute of Psychiatry, Psychology and Neuroscience, Maurice Wohl Clinical Neuroscience Institute, King's College London, UK

Cara Daly Graduate Entry Medical School, University of Limerick, Limerick, Ireland

Shoumitro (Shoumi) Deb Faculty of Medicine, Division of Brain Sciences, Imperial College London, London, UK

Tanya Deb Institute of Psychiatry, Psychology and Neuroscience, King's College London, London, UK

Nigel Eastman Emeritus Professor of Law and Ethics in Psychiatry, Honorary Consultant Forensic Psychiatrist, St George's University of London, London, UK

Mark Edwards St. George's Hospital, London, UK

George El-Nimr Consultant Neuropsychiatrist & Honorary Clinical Lecturer, North Staffordshire Combined Healthcare NHS Trust, UK

Rafey Faruqui Honorary Professor, University of Kent and Consultant Neuropsychiatrist, Kent & Medway NHS and Social Care Partnership Trust, UK

Anthony Feinstein Professor of Psychiatry, University of Toronto and Sunnybrook Health Sciences Centre, Toronto, Canada

Max Fink Professor of Psychiatry and Neurology Emeritus, State University of New York at Stony Brook, Long Island New York, USA

Greg Finucane Centre for Brain Research, University of Auckland, Auckland, New Zealand

Yulia Furlong Perth Children's Hospital, Perth, Western Australia, Australia

Alla Guekht Moscow Research and Clinical Center for Neuropsychiatry and Department of Neurology, Neurosurgery and Genetics, Russian National Research Medical University, Moscow, Russia

Neil A. Harrison Cardiff University Brain Research Imaging Centre (CUBRIC), Division of Psychological Medicine and Clinical Neurosciences, Cardiff, UK

John Hart Jr. School of Behavioral and Brain Sciences, The University of Texas at Dallas, Richardson, TX, USA

John R. Hodges Brain and Mind Centre, Sydney, Australia

Audrey Hopwood Clinical Nurse Specialist, University Hospitals Coventry and Warwickshire, UK

Robin A. Hurley Veterans Affairs Mid-Atlantic Mental Illness Research, Education, Salisbury, USA

Jeremy D. Isaacs Department of Neurology, Atkinson Morley Wing, St George's Hospital, Blackshaw Road, London, UK

Naga Kandasamy Consultant Neuroradiologist, Department of Neuroradiology, King's College Hospital, London, UK

Brian Kent Sleep Disorders Centre, Guy's Hospital, Guy's and St Thomas' NHS Foundation Trust, London, UK

Michael D. Kopelman Emeritus Professor of Neuropsychiatry, King's College London, Institute of Psychiatry, Psychology and Neuroscience, UK

Ennapadam S. Krishnamoorthy Neurokrish, The Neuropsychiatry Centre, Teynampet, Chennai, India

Nayana Lahiri St George's University, St George's University Hospitals NHS Foundation Trust, London, UK

Guy Leschziner Sleep Disorders Centre, Guy's Hospital, Guy's and St Thomas' NHS Foundation Trust, London, UK

David Linden School for Mental Health and Neuroscience, Faculty of Health, Medicine and Life Sciences, Maastricht University, Netherlands

Anne Lingford-Hughes Neuropsychopharmacology Unit, Division of Brain Sciences, Department of Medicine, Imperial College London, London, UK

Stefanos Maltezos South London and Maudsley NHS Foundation Trust, UK

Shane C. Masters Department of Radiology, Wake Forest School of Medicine, Winston-Salem, North Carolina, USA

Laura McWhirter Specialist Registrar in Neuropsychiatry, Centre for Clinical Brain Sciences, University of Edinburgh, UK

David Meagher Graduate Entry Medical School, University of Limerick, Ireland

Nick Medford Department of Neuropsychiatry, South London and Maudsley NHS Trust, London, UK

Vivek Misra Neurokrish, The Neuropsychiatry Centre, Teynampet, Chennai, India

Alex J. Mitchell Professor of Psycho-oncology, University of Leicester, Leicester, UK

Koho Miyoshi Jinmeikai Research Institute for Mental Health, Nishinomiya, Hyogo, Japan

Ramon Mocellin Neuropsychiatry Unit, Royal Melbourne Hospital, Melbourne, Australia

Adith Mohan Centre for Healthy Brain Ageing (CHeBA), School of Psychiatry, UNSW Medicine, University of New South Wales; Neuropsychiatric Institute, Prince of Wales Hospital, Sydney, Australia

Marco Mula Institute of Medical and Biomedical Education, St George's University of London and the Atkinson Morley Regional Neuroscience Centre, St George's University Hospitals NHS Foundation Trust, London, UK

Nandini Mullatti Consultant Clinical Neurophysiologist, Kings College Hospital, London, UK

Sam Nightingale Neurology Fellow at Groote Schuur Hospital and the University of Cape Town, South Africa

Dana Niry Department of Radiology, Tel Aviv Medical Centre, Sackler Faculty of Medicine, Tel Aviv University, Tel-Aviv, Israel

Fred Ovsiew Professor of Clinical Psychiatry and Behavioral Sciences, Feinberg School of Medicine, Northwestern University, Chicago, IL, USA

Jaime Pahissa Department of Psychiatry Instituto Universitario CEMIC, Buenos Aires, Argentina

Emma Palmer-Cooper Centre for Innovation in Mental Health, School of Psychology, University of Southampton, UK

Rachel Patel University of Oxford, Medical Sciences Division, John Radcliffe Hospital, Oxford, UK

Bennis Pavisian Sunnybrook Research Institute, Toronto, Canada

Olivier Piguet Brain and Mind Centre, Sydney, Australia

Thomas Pollak Nuffield Department of Clinical Neurosciences, University of Oxford, Oxford, UK

Norman A. Poole Consultant Neuropsychiatrist, South West London & St George's NHS Mental Health Trust, London, UK

Josef Priller Department of Neuropsychiatry, Charité –Universitätsmedizin Berlin, Germany

Suman Ray CSIR-National Institute of Science, Technology & Development Studies (NISTADS), Council of Scientific & Industrial Research (CSIR), New Delhi, India

Hugh Rickards Department of Neuropsychiatry, BSMHFT and University of Birmingham, Birmingham, UK

Keith Rix Honorary Consultant Forensic Psychiatrist, Norfolk and Suffolk NHS Foundation Trust, UK

Ivana Rosenzweig Sleep Disorders Centre, Guy's Hospital, Guy's and St Thomas' NHS Foundation Trust, London, UK

Perminder S. Sachdev Centre for Healthy Brain Ageing (CHeBA), School of Psychiatry, UNSW Medicine, University of New South Wales; Neuropsychiatric Institute, Prince of Wales Hospital, Sydney, Australia

Paul Shotbolt Clinical Senior Lecturer, Institute of Psychiatry, Psychology and Neuroscience; and Honorary Consultant Neuropsychiatrist, South London and Maudsley NHS Foundation Trust, London, UK

Jonathan Silver Clinical Professor, Department of Psychiatry, NYU School of Medicine, New York, USA

Elisaveta Sokolov Specialty Registrar in Clinical Neurophysiology, King's College Hospital, London, UK

Tom Solomon National Institute for Health Research Health Protection Research Unit in Emerging and Zoonotic Infections; Head of the Brain Infections Group; Professor of Neurological Science; Honorary Consultant Neurologist, Walton Centre NHS Foundation Trust and Royal Liverpool University Hospital, Liverpool, UK

Biba R. Stanton Consultant Neurologist, King's College Hospital, London, UK

Sergio Starkstein School of Psychiatry and Clinical Neurosciences University of Western Australia, Western Australia, Australia

Katherine H. Taber Veterans Affairs Mid-Atlantic Mental Illness Research, Education, Salisbury, USA

Michael Trimble Institute of Neurology, Queen Square, London, UK

Sam Turton Neuropsychopharmacology Unit, Division of Brain Sciences, Department of Medicine, Imperial College London, London, UK

Martín L. Vargas Pain Neuropsychiatry Program, Hospital Universitario Rio Hortega; Associate Professor of Psychiatry, University of Valladolid, Valladolid, Spain

Dennis Velakoulis Neuropsychiatry Unit, Royal Melbourne Hospital, Melbourne, Australia

Ashwin Venkataraman Neuropsychopharmacology Unit, Division of Brain Sciences,Department of Medicine, Imperial College London, London, UK

Angela Vincent Nuffield Department of Clinical Neurosciences, University of Oxford, Oxford, UK

Valerie Voon Department of Psychiatry, University of Cambridge, Addenbrooke's Hospital, Cambridge, UK

Mark Walterfang Neuropsychiatry Unit, Royal Melbourne Hospital, Melbourne, Australia

Susannah Whitwell South London and Maudsley NHS Foundation Trust, London, UK

David Wilkinson School of Psychology, University of Kent, Canterbury, UK

Ken Wilson Adult Cognitive Assessment Service, Stein Centre, St Catherine's Hospital, Wirral, UK

Roger L. Wood Psychology Department, Swansea University, Swansea, UK

Andrew Worthington Headwise, College of Medicine and College of Human and Health Sciences, Swansea University, Swansea, UK

Mahinda Yogarajah Atkinson Morley Regional Neuroscience Centre, St George's University Hospitals NHS Foundation Trust, London, UK

SECTION 1
Foundations and basic skills

The history and scope of neuropsychiatry

Michael Trimble

'Consciousness, then, does not appear to itself chopped up in bits. Such words as "chain" or "train" do not describe it fitly as it presents itself in the first instance. It is nothing jointed; it flows. A "river" or a "stream" are the metaphors by which it is most naturally described. *In talking of it hereafter, let us call it the stream of thought, of consciousness, or of subjective life.*'

William James, 1890

Introduction

On 23 June 1802, the fog which hung over Mount Chimborazo in the Andes lifted, and the young explorer Alexander von Humboldt (1769–1859) was enraptured by the great natural vision he beheld, witnessing, as he envisioned it, the great web of life, how everything was interwoven in what he sketched as *Naturgemälde*, an image of 'nature as a living whole' (Wulf, 2015, p. 88). At Lake Geneva, in June 1816, *Frankenstein* was born and his monster created by Mary Godwin (later Shelley 1797–1851) was given the spark of life with 'galvanism'. Humboldt had speculated before Darwin on a gradual transformation of the species, that things in nature were not fixed, but diverse and changing, and yet there was unity in diversity. The romantic revolution, interested in the forces of life, was quite under way, with its Gothic undertones, but with influence beyond literature. The Enlightenment enterprise of earlier generations was under pressure, academically and philosophically, but especially in neuroscience.

Where to begin?

As TS Eliot would have it, 'What we call the beginning is often the end. And to make an end is to make a beginning. The end is where we start from.' (Eliot, 1944). This chapter considers what I refer to as 'modern' neuropsychiatry. I wish to consider several historical epochs bridging key intellectual developments as the framework for a current understanding of neuropsychiatry. I opine that today's neuropsychiatry is neither an offshoot of neurology (associated with behavioural neurology) nor a branch of psychiatry, nor a bough of biological psychiatry, but is an independent discipline arising from a distinguished intellectual history, one which has been immersed and submerged within socio-cultural mists of Turneresque proportions, through which the sun rises through the vapour. The point

of view which has been expressed is that there can be no stable definition of neuropsychiatry and no identifiable conceptual core that may join up relevant historical periods (Berrios and Markova, 2002). This has implications, which have floundered on the rocks of criticism that, like psychiatry itself, neuropsychiatry is but a social creation set up to establish a power elite (doctors) to perform managerial and political duties, to the detriment of those whose behaviours are contrary to social norms.

Recent developments

'Neuropsychiatry' entered the English language in 1918, some 70 years after the word psychiatry. The *Weltanschauung* after the First World War dramatically altered perspectives, as the pre-War Victorian and Edwardian ideals were discarded, and to note Eliot again from the *Waste Land* (1922), there was left only a heap of broken images.

In the nineteenth century, psychopathologists were neuropathologists, and vice versa, and their interests were with the brain and its abnormalities linked with certain behaviour disorders. The early twentieth century saw a split between the developing brain-based neurology and psychological psychiatry which avoided flirting with neuroscience. Yet there were practitioners, especially in Europe and America, who were rescuing neuropsychiatry but were perhaps viewed as neither neurologists nor psychiatrists, but akin to a mythological chimera.

After the Second World War, the situation altered considerably for several reasons. The modern era of clinical texts devoted to neuropsychiatry perhaps began around the 1980s. My own *Neuropsychiatry* was published in 1981, and Jeff Cummings' *Clinical Neuropsychiatry* in 1985. The British Neuropsychiatric Association was established in 1987, the American Neuropsychiatric Association in 1988, and the Japanese Neuropsychiatric Association in 1996.

The International Neuropsychiatric Association was formed in 1998—neuropsychiatry is now a well-recognized discipline in many countries.

In my *Neuropsychiatry*, I had ventured the following definition—neuropsychiatry is a discipline which references certain disorders 'which, on account of their presentation and pathogenesis, do not fall neatly into one category, and require multidisciplinary ideas for their full understanding' (Trimble, 1981, p. xiv). Obviously, the definition bears heavily, but not exclusively, on what, at the time, was conventional neurology and psychiatry and covered a spectrum of disorders from epilepsy to conversion hysteria. Cummings and Hegarty in 1994 offered the following—'Neuropsychiatry is a clinical discipline devoted to understanding the neurobiological basis, optimal assessment, natural history, and most efficacious treatment of disorders of the nervous system with behavioural manifestations' (Cummings and Hegarty, 1994, p. 209). They emphasized that neuropsychiatry 'did not challenge the viability of psychiatry ... Neuropsychiatry, like neurology, is concerned with disorders of brain function and views behavioural abnormalities from a neurobiological perspective ... based on neuroanatomy and neurophysiology and attempts to understand the mechanisms of behaviour, whereas psychiatry integrates information from psychology, sociology and anthropology to grasp the motivation of behaviour'[1] (Cummings and Hegarty, 1994, p. 211).

Modern neuropsychiatry arose, in part, out of a clinical need. Many patients had conditions which were not well understood or managed by the structures of separated neurology and psychiatry as they had developed over the first 60 or so years in the last century. The specialty was catalysed by advances in neuroanatomy and neurophysiology, the use of newer methods of investigation of the brain, especially the electroencephalogram (EEG), and an awareness that a clinical understanding of the signs and symptoms of central nervous system (CNS) dysfunction could not be embraced by earlier neurological theories. Doctrines of psychoanalysis and behaviourist approaches rose and fell on fallow ground.

The first dawn

Hippocrates (460–370 BC) is usually the first person who comes to mind when a history of neuropsychiatry is written. His famous statement ' ... and men ought to know that from nothing else but thence (from the brain) comes joys, delights, laughter and sports, and sorrows, griefs, despondency and lamentations ... And by the same organ we become mad and delirious, and fears and terrors assail us ... ' puts the brain above the gods as responsible for such woes (Adams, 1939, p. 366).

Epilepsy (referred to as the sacred disease) was not sacred and was somehow related to the brain, yet the Greeks generally had little interest in the brain itself and were inclined to impute either the ventricles or the heart as central to our emotions.

Another epithet from the Hippocratic corpus which is often quoted is 'Most melancholics usually also become epileptics, and epileptics melancholics. One or the other (condition) prevails

according to where the disease leans: if towards the body, they become epileptics; if towards reason, melancholics' (Temkin, 1971, p. 55). This fascinating observation is a forerunner to an important biological link between seizures and mood, hardly discussed again until the twentieth century.

Hippocrates introduced the idea of disease having a longitudinal course. Static distinct entities were not his view, and he put emphasis on clinical examination and writing down his observations.

Any discussion of neuropsychiatry, ancient or modern, cannot escape the enigma of hysteria, first perhaps observed in Egyptian papyri, but the name derives from the Greek *hystera*, meaning uterus, found exclusively in women and due to a wandering womb which, frustrated by lack of proper use, leaves its anatomical position and travels around the body, causing pressure in anomalous places, and hence symptoms. On reflection, such ideas must have related to clinical observations, namely that of all the bodily organs, the uterus can be seen to move when prolapsed.

Perhaps the importance of these observations is that they remind us that disorders we recognize today were observed over 2000 years ago and in different cultures; there were then not any closed boundaries defining disorders of CNS function, and those who thought about them based their ideas on a palimpsest of philosophical ideas. These included the intellectual explorations of the pre-Socratic philosophers, asking questions about the existence and nature of things; water, air, fire, and earth featured prominently, as did the balance between them and the writings of Heraclitus who speculated on the unity of opposites and the idea that everything is in flux. There is a becoming and a change in all things, but a unity in duality. For Pythagoras, who believed in the migration of souls, numbers and mathematics were the key.

Heraclitus and Pythagoras had important influences on Plato, and hence Aristotle, the latter two philosophers whose antecedence underpins so much of Western thought, including neuroscience, even today. The philosophical traditions of idealism, empiricism, and dualism were founded in this era. Idealism holds that deduction was the way to understand the world, that knowledge is available only to the rational mind, and that the senses can only deceive. It was based on Plato's ideas of the existence of a timeless unchanging world of perfections, which he referred to as forms, which were accessible only to philosophers. The forms were mind-independent, eternally existent, and non-visible. In contrast, empiricism accepts as knowledge only that which can be derived from the senses, essentially visual. Dualism, the idea that body and soul were of differing substances, was one consequence of such theories. Along with idealism, dualism has been a main argument that has absorbed philosophers, scientists, and lay people since that time. Dualism, in particular, lies at the heart of the mind–brain problem.

In contrast to the Greeks, the Roman era added little to any understanding of the ideas discussed earlier. The most famous physician, whose books contributed so much that they remained quoted and in use for over 1000 years, was Galen (130–210 AD).

Using an Aristotlean approach, Galen described the cranial nerves, the elements of what became the sympathetic nervous system, and the ventricles. He disagreed with Aristotle, who championed the centrality of the heart, by placing the brain as central to the mind and emotions. He adhered to a system of spirits, which influenced bodily function, vital spirits being generated in the heart, which, in the brain, become animal spirits which were stored in the

[1] Reproduced with permission from Cummings J, Hegarty A. Neurology, Psychiatry, and Neuropsychiatry. *Neurology*, 44: 211. Copyright © 1994, American Academy of Neurology. DOI: https://doi.org/10.1212/WNL.44.2.209.

ventricles. The meaning and function of these various spirits are unclear to us, but they were associated with a kind of life force, which, via the nerves, regarded as hollow, initiating movement and sensation. The brain was the seat of voluntary power and sensation, and Galen identified the frontal areas as being the seat of the soul. He had no use for the cerebral convolutions, relegating them out of neurological history until prominence was given to them by the phrenologists at the beginning of the nineteenth century.

The circle of Willis

Thomas Willis (1621–1675), the man who gave us the word neurology (*Neurologie*), determinedly studied anatomy and took the brain out of the skull. He made the brain a visual object, an independent organ with separate parts, which could be preserved, cut into slices, viewed under a microscope, and with its blood vessels outlined. He illustrated the stria terminalis and the fornix, suggesting the latter was linked with the imagination, the first descriptions of what later became components of the limbic system.

Although what we refer to as the basal ganglia were outlined in the anatomical plates of Andreas Vesalius (1514–1564), it was Willis who gave the first detailed description of the *striate body*. He suggested it played a role in movement, via animal spirits traversing this area, and noted abnormalities at post-mortem in some who had died of long-term motor weakness. Willis was one of the first physicians to link pathology in death with signs and symptoms in life. He had extensive clinical experience with disorders of the brain, which included mental illness, providing perhaps the most extensive account of mental disorders that had appeared to his time. He was interested in 'psycheology' and introduced the concept of 'nerves' into our lexicon.

Interested in convulsions and hysteria, Willis attacked the long-standing uterine theories and placed their causes in 'the brain and nervous stock' (Hunter and MacAlpine, 1963, p. 190). Perhaps of importance was his recognition that males could be affected by the same symptoms and signs, even if women were more likely to suffer.

Willis and his collaborators were active at times of political upheaval. There was social unrest caused by the beheading of King Charles 1st and then later by the restoration of the monarchy (1660). Willis was a Royalist and, along with his views of social organization, he considered that there was a hierarchy embedded in the brain's organization. The cerebellum (cerebel) was under the control of the cerebral hemispheres; the rational soul was supreme. Such hierarchies, interlinked with brain anatomy, will appear again in the theories of anatomically interested neuroscientists.

This was an era following the contributions of Francis Bacon (1561–1626) who considered the advancement of science lay not in studying the Book of Revelation, but in studying the Book of Nature, forging a cleft between metaphysics and physics. Observation, recording of data, and seeking regularities which will reveal the laws of nature led him to seek causal, rather than teleological, explanations for his observations. The Royal Society was founded in 1660—Willis was a founding member.

This time also came after the speculations of René Descartes (1596–1650). Famous for his '*cogito ergo sum*' and his selection of the pineal gland as the seat of the soul, his broader scientific and philosophical scope is often ignored. He was after a new method of exploring the nature of knowledge, his solution contrasting totally that of Bacon. His method was to doubt everything since impressions could be deceiving, and how could he be certain that his daily experiences were not all dreams? What Descartes could not doubt was that he had conscious experiences, and therefore, he could not doubt that he existed.

For Descartes, the essence of matter was its extension in space, but thought was unrelated to matter—it was not extended and required no place to exist. Humans, he opined, are composed of two substances: *res cogitans* (thinking mind) and *res extensa* (the body). But he had a problem, referred to as Cartesian dualism, of how to join the soul to the body, hence the importance of the centrally located unpaired pineal gland.

One consequence was that Descartes liberated the body for physical science. He did much to explore the nature of the physical world, free from theological prohibition. Viewing the body as a machine, he studied anatomy and the nature of body–brain connections. The illustration in Fig. 1.1 prefigures the wiring diagrams of brain connections, which are still so popular today. His reflex arcs were to become central to neurophysiological understanding and to sadly naïve explanations of brain function. His drawings of the brain clearly show gyri and sulci, and he provided detailed descriptions of the eye. Later, Robert Whytt (1714–1766) made observations on spinal cord reflexes, which he referred to as involuntary motions, and he gave us the word 'nervous', which led to the term 'neurosis' and the adjective 'neurotic'.

Enlighted times

Classification of nervous disorders was proceeding at a pace through what may be referred to as the Enlightenment era. In part, this was supported by the philosophy of John Locke (1632–1734). His book *An Essay Concerning Human Understanding*, published in 1690, developed the view that the mind was a *tabula rasa* at birth and that all knowledge is founded on experience. The contents of our consciousness are derived from sense impressions, and simple impressions combine to make more complex ones. Locke's concept of the mind was that it required a passive vehicle in perception, but it possessed active properties, as 'ideas' are combined together, forming complex ones. This was a philosophy of an association of ideas, ideas keeping company as if they were one, but guided by reason.[2]

Medical ideas were separating from those of theology and philosophy, even though many wavered. Isaac Newton (1643–1727) conducted alchemical experiments and believed that he was working for the glory of God. Galileo, who rejected Aristotle, seems to have believed in Dante's descriptions of Hell in *Inferno* and set about estimating the height of Lucifer. Locke believed that man was made by God in His image and endowed with reason.

[2] It is not intended that references to historical epochs have any specific time intervals allocated to them, and most such designations are, of course, given retrospectively. Yet the contrast between the *Zeitgeist* of the Enlightenment thinkers differed radically from those of the later Romantic era.

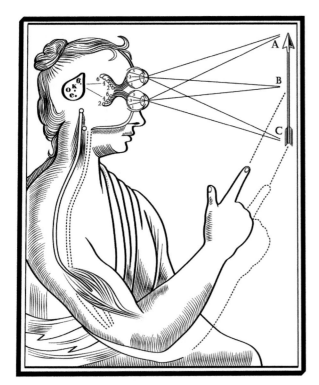

Fig. 1.1 Figure showing Descartes suggestions as to how the brain functions, the first example of a figure diagram showing reflex activity. Reproduced from *Treatise of Man*, Rene Descartes, 1664.

The Romantic brain

When and why the Romantic era unfolded when it did is a matter of much speculation. The Enlightenment period may be said to have continued through to around 1800, when a new spirit of understanding advanced social, artistic, and scientific developments. Minds, motivations, and memories of individuals became preoccupations of study, as there was a shift away from empirical philosophies towards idealism, even though the brain was, by now, an object of dissection and depiction as never before.

Although it may come as some surprise, the earliest of those who tried to understand links between the brain and the mind were poets, especially Samuel Taylor Coleridge (1772–1834), John Keats (1895–1821), and William Wordsworth (1770–1850). Several of the physicians writing at this time were also renowned poets such as Erasmus Darwin (1731–1802) and Humphry Davy (1778–1829).

Coleridge was influenced by German philosophy and could not accept that the mind was a *tabula rasa*; it was for him an active principal with powers to shape the world of individual experience. Going away from Descartes, he affirmed *sum quia sum* (I am because I affirm myself to be). He wrote that 'a sort of stomach sensation' was attached to all his thoughts. He introduced the English reader to the terms 'unconscious' and 'psychosomatic' and to the profoundly interesting notion that 'thought is *motion*' (Coleridge, 1956–71: p. 137).

The development of the ideas at this time, which remain so important for modern neurospychiatry, is brilliantly expounded in Alan Richardson's book *British Romanticism and the Science of the Mind* (Richardson, 2001). He discusses the origins of what he calls 'neural Romanticism', and the key scientific protagonists were Erasmus,

Darwin, Franz Gall (1758–1828), Pierre Cabanis (1757–1808), and Charles Bell (1774–1842).

Features of their developing theories were that the mind is embodied and that evolution was important to an understanding of brain–behaviour relationships (even if the ideas would now be referred to as based on Lamarckian principles, namely with the inheritance of acquired characteristics). They studied diseased brains, exploration of such phenomena as phantom limbs, and examination of emotional expressions (Bell, whose work influenced artists well beyond his time), and brain anatomy (Gall is of such importance as to what happened next).

Coming apart and putting it back together

Gall and his collaborator Johann Spurzheim (1776–1832) are most famous for the development of 'phrenology', although it was Spurzheim who most popularized phrenology, a word not used by Gall—organology, organoscopy, and cranioscopy were his preferred terms. Phrenology became a trivialized and much misused concept in the public eye but which profoundly altered neuroscience.

Gall was a comparative anatomist who examined the brains of animals, trying to understand the evolutionary development of brain shapes and sizes with differing naturalistic skills. He was impressed by the increasing complexity of the cerebral convolutions over evolutionary time, and in his own dissections, instead of looking at horizontal or vertical brain slices, he dissected along the lines of the white matter, showing that they issued from the grey matter, providing ideas of continuity and unity within the brain organization.

Gall elaborated five principles: (1) the brain is the organ of the mind; (2) the mind can be analysed into independent faculties; (3) these are innate and have their seat in the cortex of the brain; (4) the size of each cerebral organ is an indication of its functional capacity; and (5) the correspondence between the contour of the skull and the cortex of the brain such that the size of the organs and their potential role in the psychological make-up can be determined by inspection.

The cortex was no longer a disorganized mass but contained a subset of organs, which could be revealed by the shape of the head. As the historians Richard Hunter and Ida MacAlpine (1963) opined, this 'provided the first psychological framework within which mad-doctors struggling unguided with their patients could understand insane behaviour, and so gave a powerful fillip to the psychological approach. For the first time it became meaningful to get to know patients as persons, if only to be able to interpret bumps on their heads ...'[3] (Hunter and MacAlpine, 1963, p. 714). Richardson was even firmer on the importance of Gall's contributions stating that he was perhaps the most Romantic of the neuroscientists of this era, seeking to understand a unity of structure and function within diversity, not only from an evolutionary standpoint, but also within the individual brain.

Gall was interested in unconscious forces and the principles that united the faculties of the human brain. These were the

---

[3] Reproduced from Hunter R, MacAlpine I. *Three hundred Years of Psychiatry, 1535–1860*, 714. Oxford, UK: Oxford Universirty Press. Copyright © 1963, Oxford University Press.

preoccupations of neuroscientists of the Romantic era, which included dreams and transitory and transitional mental states, the effect of drugs on the mind, and some fundamental life force. Entered Luigi Galvani (1737–1798) who made frogs' legs twitch with electric sparks, and his nephew Giovanni Aldini (1762–1834) who showed in public demonstrations in London in 1803 that, with electricity, he could stimulate movements on the face and limbs of an executed criminal. Frankenstein; to give a 'spark' of life to the corpse of his monster using 'galvanism'—'spirits' were on their way out.

Irving Massey summarized the neuroscientific achievements of the Romantic era during the later eighteenth century. He noted that psychology moved from Cartesian mind–body dualism and a *tabula rasa* principle to 'arrive at what Richardson regards as a typically Romantic—and modern-view of the mind … (which) unites mind and body, operating as a single activity/entity in which affect and thought are one in their encounter with experience, so that, in a Wordsworthian phrase, we "half create" what we perceive, or, better still, in Shelley's terms, learn to imagine what we know'[4] (Massey, 2002, p. 78). The Romantic poets, but especially Coleridge, were exploring the creative mind in a post-Kantian enterprise which involved concessions to an unconscious edifice of uncertainty and an independence of the mind from conscious control, and which argued for an active and creative mind.

Towards the fin de siècle and onwards

The axis of the future development of neurospychiatry, for a while at least, revolved around Paris and the schools of psychiatry which first developed under Philippe Pinel (1745–1826) and later with Jean-Étienne Dominique Esquirol (1772–1840) and his circle, and then with Jean-Martin Charcot (1825–1893). Two disorders had a profound influence on the developing neuropsychiatry of the age, namely monomania and *dégénérescence* (degeneration). The former referred to a partial lesion of the intelligence, the mind of the afflicted being concerned mostly only with a single object, pursued contrary to any logic, and in the absence of fever. It was neither mania nor melancholia, but a partial 'delirium', an *idée fixe* with subtypes. It eventually accounted for some 10% of admissions to hospitals such as the Salpêtrière in Paris. Physicians by now were not only pursuing the classification of abnormal mental states, but also collecting statistics.

Daniel Pick referred to degeneration as a European disorder (Pick, 1989), which permeated all forms of life. Degeneration related not only to social groups and races, but also to families, bridging generations, as the sins of the forefathers are born by subsequent generations. Causation of these aberrances took on a biological imperative; they were not simply seen as the outcome of Rousseauean social pressures and chains. Bénédict Augustin Morel (1809–1873) thought the pathology related to hereditarily transmitted pathologies, following and influencing each other over a series of generations, leading finally to imbecility, idiocy, and cretinous degeneration. But, as the progeny dies out, there can be no more progression in that family line. Nature is restored to balance.

[4] Massey I. Review: *British Romanticism and the Science of the Mind*, Criticism 44.1 Wayne State University Press, 2002. (p 78)

> **Box 1.1** Hughlings Jackson's four principles of nervous action
> - Evolution of nervous functions
> - Hierarchy of those functions
> - Negative and positive symptoms of dissolution
> - Local and uniform dissolution

Degeneration became 'the condition of conditions, the ultimate signifier of pathology' (Pick, 1989, p. 8).

Charcot came to dominate late nineteenth-century clinical neurology in France, but he can be referred to as a neuropsychiatrist, especially through his considerable studies on hysteria. Further, in a well-known historical trail, he was very important in igniting the experimental neurologist Sigmund Freud's (1856–1939) ideas in the subject. The latter returned to Vienna to develop a psychologically based psychiatry, which literally lost sight of the brain. This incidentally is not to diminish the importance of Freud's ideas for neuropsychiatry, so often dismissed as good storytelling and poor science.

Of greater interest are the contributions of John Hughlings Jackson (1835–1911), one of the founders of modern neurospychiatry. Central to Hughlings Jackson's ideas are his four principles of nervous action and his four factors of insanity. These are shown in Boxes 1.1 and 1.2. Central to his conception of the development of the signs and symptoms of CNS disorders was their relation to the evolution of the human brain, which revealed hierarchies, with the cord, medulla, and pons being the lowest, the motor and sensory cortices and the basal ganglia being middle, and the frontal and posterior cortices being the highest. Damage to the brain led to both positive and negative effects, with damaged tissue taking away function (e.g. memory), while the remaining brain was related to positive symptoms. There was inhibition and release simultaneously, contributing to the clinical picture. Hughlings Jackson rejected the ideas of Paul Broca (1824–1880) on the localization of language to the anterior left hemisphere, was the first to champion the importance of the right hemisphere in our actions and emotions, and was very interested in the mind–brain problem, even if adopting a view that he referred to as the doctrine of concomitance, a parallelism of mental states and neural states, freeing neurology from the growing dominance of faculty psychology.

Hughlings Jackson's observations on epilepsy, and his description of 'dreamy states', however, led all the way to temporal lobe epilepsy. His works had a considerable impact on Freud, via the latter's book *On Aphasia*. In that book, we find ideas of 'dissolution' (the opposite to evolution) and hierarchies of neurological and psychological processes. The ability of higher aspects of psychological function to be overwhelmed by lower ones became the idea of regression, fundamental to psychoanalysis. Words such as 'overdetermination', 'projection', and 'representation' as physiological concepts appear, as does *Besetzung*, translated as cathexis

> **Box 1.2** Hughlings Jackson's four factors of insanities
> - The depth of the pathological process and dissolution
> - The person who has undergone dissolution
> - The rate of the dissolution
> - Influence of local bodily states and external circumstances

which became a central psychoanalytic theme for the way that the libido becomes invested in objects. Both Hughlings Jackson and Freud were interested in nervous functions as manifestations of nervous energies. Jacksonian neurodynamics were transformed into Freudian psychodynamics, and neuroses into psychoneuroses (Stengel, 1953).

The eclipse

In Vienna, Freud's split from neurology to develop his psychologically based psychiatry set him up against Julius Wagner–Jauregg (1857–1940). The latter had pursued physical treatments for psychiatric diseases and used blood from patients with tertian malaria to treat general paralysis of the insane, with apparent considerable success. Since such psychoses were considered incurable, the treatment was rapidly introduced internationally, and he was awarded the Nobel Prize for Medicine in 1927.

Wagner–Jauregg had with him a number of talented investigators who carried the mantle of neuropsychiatry through the first part of the twentieth century when the Freudian–Cartesian cataract was ever more forging ideas of a brainless mind on the general public and on developing clinical neuroscience.

A good deal of this occurred in America. Freud received an invitation from G Stanley Hall (1846–1924), President of Clark University in Worcester, Massachusetts, to go to America for a series of lectures. Hall founded the first American psychological laboratory at Johns Hopkins University in 1883 and had been teaching psychoanalysis. Freud was shown around the city by two psychoanalysts—Abraham Brill (1874–1948), founder of the New York Psychoanalytic Society (1911) and Ernest Jones (1879–1958) from Toronto. Freud also spent time with James Jackson Putnam (1846–1918) of Boston, the founder of both the American Psychoanalytic Association (1911) and the American Neurological Association (1874). Psychoanalysis was, in fact, supported by several of a neurological persuasion.

The total split of neurology and psychiatry in America was accelerated in the 1930s and 1940s when many European Jewish psychiatrists, steeped in Freudian and related therapeutic approaches, immigrated, often taking up senior academic posts. The theoretical boundaries of Freudian theories were soon breached by dissenters, such as Carl Jung (1875–1961) and Alfred Adler (1870–1937), and by the 'ego' psychologies and therapies. The situation became accentuated by Pavlovian ideas and learning theory, the ideas of John Watson (1878–1958), and the radical behaviourism of BF Skinner (1904–1990). In the lay mind, such therapists became identified with psychiatry, but to try and salvage the situation, somewhere along the way, in more recent times, the compromise nostrum 'biopsychosocial' has snaked into the psychiatry vocabulary, with arguable consequences (Ghaemi, 2012).

Hangers on

Hughlings Jackson shifted the narrow views of localization from strictly anatomical to physiological principles, and theories of holistic brain activity were pursued by several 'anti-localizers'. Constantin von Monokov (1853–1930), impressed by the recovery seen after cerebral lesions and the negative cases of cerebral

localization in which expected losses were not seen as expected, coined the term 'chronogenetic' localization, such that 'each nervous function is the result of a historical evolution … successive processes always involve the activity of several centres or mechanisms … early stages of nervous function are fragments of the finished one' (Riese, 1950, p. 92).

In America, at the Phipps Clinic in Baltimore, Adolf Meyer (1866–1950), who had a background in pathology was well acquainted with European ideas in neurology and psychiatry, had a considerable interest in patients' social surroundings and personalities, and developed his 'psychobiological' approach to mental illness.

Also from Wagner–Jauregg's group in Vienna was Paul Schilder (1886–1940) who went to America in 1929. He was an analyst well acquainted with the Viennese cultural and psychoanalytic movement. But he was interested in philosophy, childhood development, and language and wanted to write a book linking phenomenology, psychoanalysis, and neurology. In Baltimore, with Meyer at the Phipps Clinic, he wrote *Brain and Personality*. His most significant text *The Image and Appearance of the Human Body* (1935) should be revered as a neuropsychiatric classic.

Constantin von Economo (1876–1931) was also from Vienna. A brilliant neuroanatomist, he published one of the most important books of neuropsychiatry ever written. He studied cortical architecture, enumerating twice as many areas as Brodmann; nerve elements have become referred to as von Economo neurones, and towards the end of 1916, he reported many patients with an unusual variety of symptoms which followed an influenza-like prodrome. This disorder he called encephalitis lethargic (von Economo's disease today), recognized as an encephalitis secondary to the influenza pandemics which spread across Europe in the first few years of the twentieth century. Survivors had a variety of neuropsychiatric signs and symptoms, in which motor disorders were prominent. His own conclusions should be quoted frequently: 'The dialectic combinations and the psychological constructions of many ideologists will collapse like a pack of cards if they do not in future take into account these new basic facts. Every psychiatrist who wishes to probe into the phenomena of disturbed motility and changes of character, the psychological mechanism of mental inaccessibility, of the neuroses, etc., must be thoroughly acquainted with the experience gathered from encephalitis lethargic. Every psychologist who in the future attempts to deal with psychological phenomena such as will, temperament, and fundamentals of character, such as self-consciousness, the ego, etc., and is not well acquainted with the appropriate observations on encephalitic patients, and does not read the descriptions of the psychological causes in the many original papers recording the severe mental symptoms, will build on sand.'[5]

Some of the other talents to work with Wagner–Jauregg were Joseph Gerstmann (1887–1969; eponymous syndrome with key signs of agraphia, acalculia, finger agnosia, and right/left disorientation), Otto Kauders (1893–1949, who continued to study malarial therapy and encephalitis lethargica), and Erwin Stengel who became Professor of Psychiatry in Sheffield, (1902–1973). He described the condition of pain asymbolia and translated Freud's book on aphasia into English.

---

[5] von Economo 1931 p 167.

A now forgotten seminal text was Smithy Ely Jelliffe (1866–1945) and William White's (1870–1937) *Diseases of the Nervous System: A Text-Book of Neurology and Psychiatry* (1915) which provided a compendium of up-to-date information in neuropsychiatry and was continually revised.

The term 'integrated action' today is mostly associated with Sir Charles Sherrington (1857–1952), whose book *The Integrative Action of the Nervous System* emphasizes the body and mind as a unity implying the integration of all bodily organs, such that 'from such integrated organs the organism itself is in its turn integrated … integration by the nervous system is *Sui generis*' (Sherrington, 1940, p. 209).

The living brain

Hans Berger (1873–1941) at Jena discovered it was possible to record electrical potentials from the human brain from the surface of the skull. These findings, which later led to encephalography, changed everything. Examining brain function *in vivo* surpassed pathological inspections post-mortem, and the EEG was the technique which might be considered to be the foundation stone of modern neuropsychiatry.

Significant contributions of the EEG developed in America with Stanley Cobb (1887–1968), George Engel (1913–1999), and Fred (1903–1992) and Erna (1904–1987) Gibbs. Cobb's book, *Foundations of Neuropsychiatry* (1936) went to four editions, each one adding new information about brain anatomy and physiology, emphasizing the importance of maintaining integration between neurology and psychiatry since 'New points of view are continually emerging and disturbing the neurologist and the psychiatrist who had too soon settled themselves into orthodoxy'. He considered dichotomies between 'functional' and 'organic' to be simply misleading since the line between 'physical' and 'mental' was entirely arbitrary (Cobb, 1944, p. 1–4).

William Lennox (1884–1960) and the Gibbs made their first observations of epilepsy working with Cobb, and then, at the University of Illinois, the Gibbs did EEGs on psychiatric patients. Many were considered to have 'temporal lobe epilepsy', and they reported that anterior temporal lobe foci were associated with the highest frequency of psychiatric disorders, especially severe personality disorders and psychoses. In a summary of this work, Fred Gibbs and Stamps made a profoundly important statement which should have alerted anyone interested in the brain and behaviour instantly. Their conclusions were as follows: 'The patient's emotional reactions to his seizures, his family and to his social situation are less important determinants of psychiatric disorder than the site and type of the epileptic discharge' (Gibbs and Stamps, 1953, p. 78). But like von Economo's warnings, this made, for a while at least, little impression, especially amongst those dealing with epilepsy in America.

George Engel and John Romano (1908–1994) used the EEG to examine cerebral changes in patients with delirium, showing a close correlation between the degree of slowing on the EEG and the mental state. Their important observation that improvements or deteriorations of the latter could be followed by changes in the EEG receives so little interest today. But this still is a clinically very important investigation, e.g. in distinguishing states of delirium with minimal clouding of consciousness and hallucinations from schizophrenia, or the clouded mental states of hysterical pseudodementia from organic dementias. Psychiatrists soon lost all interest in the EEG, and in neurology, the possibility that it could be helpful in the differential diagnosis of the causes of an abnormal mental state was and is rarely heard, except from those who practice neuropsychiatry.

Perhaps Engel's most significant contributions, apart from the work on delirium, are his descriptions of the pain-prone patient (1959) and his book *Psychological Development in Health and Disease* (1964). These should be foundational reading for anyone interested in chronic pain (Engel, 1959).

The relevance of seizures for the brain and their clinical meaning moved ahead with the development of somatic therapies for psychiatric disorders. Manfred Sakel's (1900–1957) insulin therapy for psychiatric disorders, after much debate and falling out, led to the introduction of electroconvulsive therapy (ECT). Part of this story was the remarkable observation of Ladislas von Meduna (1896–1964) that histologically there were differences between the brain of patients with schizophrenia and the brain of those with epilepsy. In schizophrenia, there was loss of neurones and no glial reaction, while in epilepsy, he observed slight loss of neurones and massive glial reactions. He reasoned from these findings that the causes of epilepsy and schizophrenia were antagonistic and suggested inducing seizures as a treatment for schizophrenia. Complementary was the discovery of one of the most important neuropsychiatric syndromes of the last century from the Zurich epilepsy centre by Heinrich Landolt (1917–1971). He observed an antagonism between seizures and the mental state in some patients with epilepsy, which he called 'forced normalization'. The 'Landolt phenomenon' refers to the fact that during the behaviour disturbance, the EEG normalizes and that as the behaviour problems resolve, the EEG resorts to its abnormal configuration. His work went unnoticed in English-speaking countries by two generations of neurologists (Trimble and Schmitz, 1998).

On another front, Antonio Egan Moniz (1874–1955), a neurologist who studied psychoanalysis and hypnotism, developed the technique of cerebral angiography, which opened up possibilities for exploration of the brain without opening the skull. He developed the leucotome and initiated trials of leucotomy by cutting fibres between the frontal cortex and the thalamus, making him the founder of modern-day neurosurgery for psychiatric disorder, which he referred to as psychosurgery.

Important laboratory explorations of brain areas that were associated with emotional behaviour were carried out by Walter Hess (1881–1973) and Walter Cannon (1871–1945). Both worked on subcortical influences using animals with electrodes placed in the brain, a departure from the methods of British and American physiologists, who concerned themselves with fixed preparations of isolated segments of the nervous system.

This work was also quite neglected at the time. It was of no interest to psychiatrists and was quite in contrast to an alternative view of emotion, the James Lange theory of emotion, which was concerned with the peripheral nervous system as the prime generator of emotional feelings, as opposed to the CNS. These investigations heralded the start of a renewed paradigm of exploring brain–behaviour relationships that opened up a neuroanatomical focus upon which current neuropsychiatry is founded.

In 1937, James Papez (1883–1958) published a paper entitled *A Proposed Mechanism of Emotion*, outlining circuits which formed a 'harmonious mechanism which may elaborate the functions of central emotion as well as participate in emotional expression' (Papez, 1937, p. 743). In subsequent decades, neuroanatomists, such as Paul Yakovlev (1894–1983), Walle Nauta (1916–1994), Paul Maclean (1913–2007), and Lennart Heimer (1930–2007), and their numerous collaborators that included the neurologist, neurosurgeon, and psychiatrist Robert Heath (1915–1999), and the neuropsychiatrist Janice Stevens developed our understanding of the anatomical areas of the brain first named by Paul Broca as *le grande lobe limbique* in 1878.

Alongside these were developments understanding the relevance of areas of the frontal cortex, especially the prefrontal cortex, for the regulation of motor programmes and cognitive planning. In part, the effects were revealed by head injuries of the two World Wars, examined particularly by the German neuropsychiatrist Kurt Goldstein (1878–1965). He was much influenced by Gestalt psychology and, in part, by experimental observations on primates with brain lesions by Carlyle Jacobsen and John Fulton (1899–1960). These works were a delayed follow-up to the case history of Phineas Gage, who had his anterior frontal cortex damaged in an industrial accident, published in 1868 but which aroused little interest for nearly a century. Goldstein's book on the after-effects of head injury is another neuropsychiatric classic that should be on the shelf of every neuropsychiatrist (Goldstein, 1942).

Conclusion

von Humboldt became obsessed with galvanism and did over 4000 experiments, noting its effects on animals and on himself. He was a part of the scientific movement of the late seventeenth and early eighteenth centuries, which was seeking some underlying life force or principle which united natural things, including humans. Those involved were disenchanted with the growing tendency to split and classify (carve nature at the joints) and with Cartesian approaches to philosophy. Their interest was with individuality, emotions, and internal mental experiences. This was an anti-Enlightenment enterprise, within which echoed the contrasts between Aristotle and Plato and out of which Richardson's term neural Romanticism emerged.

As science of the nineteenth century progressed, the tensions with regard to understanding links between the brain and the mind were reflected in the eventual split between what became twentieth-century neurology and psychiatry. Many patients whose ailments slipped into the fissure between them, presenting with emotional and behavioural consequences of brain dysfunction and falling outside some committee-generated structure of a supposed diagnostic entity, were poorly served. Developmental and emotional disorders and psychoses, as long as they were not associated with neurological impediments, were accepted by psychiatry, and if associated with neurological illness, they were not for neurology.

Hence there was need for practitioners who were comfortable with a brain-based view of behavioural disorders, accepting the broad dimensions of human cultural and social impact on signs, symptoms, and the progression of illness, and understanding the difference between disease, as a somatically based change of tissue, and illness, with which patients present.

In this chapter, I have, in brief, highlighted several historical periods which have been important stepping stones on the way to the position of neuropsychiatry as I see the situation today. But stepping stones are liable to be washed away by the flow of river time, and some of the contributors discussed may be unfamiliar to those emulating to carry the moniker neuropsychiatrist. I have not been able here to go further into their backgrounds, nor discuss many others who have also been a part of the *Urgrund* of the developing discipline. Further, I have only been able to highlight a few staging points of considerable significance. Much more is covered in my book *The Intentional Brain: Motion, Emotion and the Development of Modern Neuropsychiatry* (Trimble, 2016). This also follows the shift of emphasis from a neurophilosophical perspective from considering the brain as a passive receptacle of sensory impressions, and the stark empiricism that went with this, to one in which the brain is seen as an acting, seeking, creative organ, with emotions embodied and enshrouding not only motion (*e-motion*), but also our thoughts, cognitions, and rationality.

From a neuroanatomical perspective, the elaboration of areas of the brain primarily linked with emotional feelings and expression (limbic has become a preferred term), which include their widespread connections to frontal and other cortical areas, provides the basic science substrate for an understanding of clinical neuropsychiatric presentations. From a neurophysiological perspective, the EEG and the discovery of what was referred to as 'psycho-motor' epilepsy, even with anatomical references in 'temporal lobe epilepsy', and the comorbid psychopathological associations gave modern neuropsychiatry one of its most important entrances to clinical necessity.

The interest and scope of neuropsychiatry have never been better. I recently attended three meetings devoted to the discipline: the International Neuropsychiatry meeting in India, the British Neuropsychiatry Association meeting in London, and the American Neuropsychiatry meeting in Boston. These were some of the finest meetings I have attended for some time, and the range of presentations and the number of young people attending the meetings was impressive. There is much scope for moving away from being shy about calling ourselves neuropsychiatrists. The demand for a sensitive approach to patients, adopting a phenomenological approach to understanding, and a feeling for how the brain is connected with the body and with the surrounding world, while not getting too overexcited about the latest technology are so important to embrace.

As of today, neuropsychiatry implies that its practitioners—neuropsychiatrists—are very familiar with neuroanatomy, neurochemistry, and neurophysiology, the signs and symptoms of a range of CNS disorders, and the psychology of human motivation and desire. Meyer, in a review of the Jelliffe and White's textbook stated: 'We want neuropsychiatrists—not merely neurologists and not merely psychologists, but primarily physicians able to study the entire organism and its functions and behaviour and more especially the shape of the nervous system and of the problems of adaptation' (Lief, 1948, p. 574). This is where modern neuropsychiatry starts from.

KEY LEARNING POINTS

- Hippocrates' original acknowledgement of the relation of the human brain to epilepsy is a starting point for the historical development of neuropsychiatry.
- The contrasting tensions between the philosophical and medical approaches to the discipline in the Enlightenment and Romantic eras are considered; conflicts which are still with us today.
- The growth of the field in the twentieth century, in spite of the rise of psychoanalysis and other psychological therapies, has been eclipsed by advances in neuroanatomy and neurophysiology, and the clinical need of patients served badly by historical legacies of the split between neurology and psychiatry.

REFERENCES

Adams F. *The Genuine Works of Hippocrates*. Williams and Wilkins, Baltimore, MD, 1939.

Berrios GE, Markova IS. The concept of neuropsychiatry: a historical overview. *Journal of Psychosomatic Research* 2002;53:629–38.

Cobb S. *Foundations of Neuropsychiatry*, third edition. Williams and Wilkins Company, Baltimore, MD, 1944.

Griggs EL, editor. *Collected Letters of Samuel Taylor Coleridge*, 6 volumes. Oxford University Press, Oxford, 1956.

Cummings J. *Clinical Neuropsychiatry*. Grune and Stratton, New York, NY, 1985.

Cummings J, Hegarty A. Neurology, Psychiatry, and Neuropsychiatry. *Neurology* 1994;44:209–13.

Eliot TS. Little Gidding. In: *Four Quartets*. Faber and Faber, London, 1944, p. 44.

Engel GL. 'Psychogenic' pain and the pain-prone patient. *American Journal of Medicine* 1959;26:899–918.

Ghaemi N. *The Rise and Fall of the Biopsychosocial Model: Reconciling Art and Science in Psychiatry*. The Johns Hopkins University Press, Baltimore, MD, 2012.

Gibbs FA, Stamps FW. *Epilepsy Handbook*. Charles C Thomas, Springfield, IL, 1953.

Goldstein K. *After Effects of Brain Injuries in War: Their Evaluation and Treatment*. William Heinemann, London, 1942.

Hunter R, MacAlpine I. *Three Hundred Years of Psychiatry*, 1535–1860. Oxford University Press, Oxford, 1963.

Lief A. *The Commonsense Psychiatry of Dr Adolf Meyer*. McGraw Hill, New York, NY, 1948.

Massey I. Review of British Romanticism and the Science of Mind. *Criticism* 2002;44:76–80.

Papez JW. A proposed mechanism of emotion. *Archives of Neurology and Psychiatry* 1937;38:725–43.

Pick D. *Faces of Degeneration: A European Disorder, c. 1848–1918*. Cambridge University Press, Cambridge, 1989.

Richardson A. *British Romanticism and the Science of the Mind*. Cambridge University Press, Cambridge, 2001.

Riese W. *Principles of Neurology: In the Light of History and Their Present Use*. Smith Ely Jelliffe Trust, New York, NY, 1950.

Sherrington C. *Man on his Nature*. Cambridge University Press, Cambridge, 1940.

Stengel E. *Aphasia: A Critical Study (1891)*. Trans. Stengel E. International Universities Press, New York, NY, 1953.

Temkin O. *The Falling Sickness*, second edition. The Johns Hopkins University Press, Baltimore, MD, 1971.

Trimble MR. *Neuropsychiatry*. J Wiley and Sons, Chichester, 1981.

Trimble MR. *The Intentional Brain: Motion, Emotion and the Development of Modern Neuropsychiatry*. The Johns Hopkins University Press, Baltimore, MD, 2016.

Trimble MR, Schmitz B. *Forced Normalisation and Alternative Psychoses of Epilepsy*. Wrightson Biomedical Publishing Ltd, Petersfield, 1998.

von Economo C. *Encephalitis Lethargica*. Trans Newman KO. Oxford University Press, Oxford, 1931.

Wulf A. *The Invention of Nature. The Adventures of Alexander von Humboldt*. John Murray, London, 2015.

2

Introduction to the neuropsychiatric examination

Jonathan Silver and Sonja Blum

Introduction

The field of behavioural neurology and neuropsychiatry (BN & NP) refers to a domain of practice that involves care of individuals with cognitive, emotional, and behavioural problems due to a recognized neurological disorder. In addition to any focal brain lesion, the commonest neurological disorders that lead to neuropsychiatric symptoms include traumatic brain injury (TBI), epilepsy, stroke/cerebrovascular diseases, autoimmune conditions (including multiple sclerosis, systemic lupus erythematosus, and antibody-mediated limbic encephalitides), neurodegenerative diseases, including fronto-temporal dementia (FTD), Alzheimer's disease (AD), Huntington's disease (HD), and developmental disorders such as autism spectrum disorders or inherited leukoencephalopathies. The common thread amongst the various aetiologies is either focal brain injury or disruption of cortico-cortical and cortical-subcortical circuits that support normal cognition and behaviour.

The presenting symptoms that are the primary focus of the neuropsychiatric assessment includes irritability, disturbance of mood and affect, anxiety, fatigue, sleep difficulty, problems with concentration and memory, disorders of arousal [e.g. coma, vegetative state (VS), minimal conscious state (MCS), etc.], disorders of perception (e.g. illusion, hallucinations, sensory impairments such as cortical blindness, etc.), disorders of attention (e.g. delirium, neglect, etc.), the various amnesias, aphasias, agnosias, apraxias, and disorders of motivation (e.g. apathy, abulia, akinetic mutism, etc.). Patients in an inpatient acute hospital setting and in inpatient acute rehabilitation tend to be more severely impaired than patients seen in an outpatient ambulatory setting. We find the difference in typical symptoms among inpatient versus outpatient patient populations useful, as it relates to structuring the neuropsychiatric examination. In this chapter, we will first focus on describing the neuropsychiatric examination applicable to patients with a milder spectrum of symptoms, typically seen in the outpatient setting, and followed by a description of the examination specific to patients who have severe disturbance of arousal, cognition, and/or behaviour and who are more often seen in the acute hospital or acute rehabilitation setting. Skills in performing the neuropsychiatric examination include adjusting the examination in a manner sensitive to the patient's presenting symptoms, abilities, or impairments, in order to facilitate a useful description of findings in patients who are unable to cooperate with any or all parts of a formal cognitive examination.

The examination begins with the initial observations upon meeting the patient and formally includes a detailed interview and history obtained from the patient, as well as from their family or close friends (collateral history), a formal mental status examination, and a brief neurological examination.

Initial observations can be quite informative, and skills should be honed in making these first observations. As the encounter begins, observe and listen. Note the overall demeanour, including the range of facial expressions, affect, speed, cadence, and fluency of speech, the pattern of thought content, the speed and pattern of movements, mannerisms, or tics. The patient may reveal reduced expressiveness of the face ('masked facies') or hypophonia of parkinsonism, grandiosity or flamboyance or pressured speech of mania, speech filled with neologisms of a thought disorder or aphasia, dishevelment of schizophrenia or dementia, or poor eye contact seen in autism spectrum disorders. Thought pattern and content can be observed for evidence of directed versus disorganized or concrete thoughts, as well as evidence of delusions or hallucinations that may be quite apparent without probing. Patterns of movement abnormality should be carefully observed while the patient is interacting with the examiner and may reveal evidence of a movement disorder such as dystonia, chorea, or tremor. Akinesia/poverty of movements or akathisia/motor restlessness may be seen. The gait may be suggestive of an extrapyramidal disorder, with smaller steps and poverty of accessory movements in parkinsonism.

Despite the utility of initial observations, a semi-structured interview and formal mental status and neurological examinations are valuable and provide more reliable clinical information. Non-structured interviews and examinations suffer from several inherent problems: (1) variance in information upon which a diagnosis is made (the diagnosis is based on different types and amounts of information about the patient); (2) variance in interpretation of information; and (3) use of different definitions of disorder, leading to different diagnoses. While a full structured psychiatric interview is not required, practitioners may choose to incorporate parts of a semi-structured interview, such as the Mini-International Neuropsychiatric Interview (MINI) (Sheehan et al., 1998).

The practice of neuropsychiatry requires a different set of skills to either psychiatry or neurology, although there is some overlap with each of these specialties. It requires the ability psychiatrists have in discussing emotional states with patients and the skills in observing and diagnosing mood, affect, and thought process disorders. It requires the knowledge neurologists have on neuroanatomy and localization of focal neurological symptoms and the comfort with diagnosis of classic neurological syndromes such as aphasia, neglect, and others. Neuropsychiatry also requires a separate skill set in evaluating patients with dementia, TBI, and their specific set of mental and physical findings, as well as variations in psychiatric presentation in patients who are suffering the consequences of stroke, TBI, neurodegenerative disease, or one of the myriad of other neurological conditions. Finally, neuropsychiatry also requires the knowledge of pharmacology of both neurology and psychiatry. The items needed to complete the examination include the usual note-taking equipment for the examiner and blank sheets of paper (usually use 8.5 × 11 in blank printer paper) and a pencil for the patient; printed forms for cognitive and behavioural scales you will use are helpful. In our experience, an initial evaluation of a neuropsychiatric patient takes 60–120 minutes.

In the United States, the field of BN & NP was formally recognized as a subspecialty by the United Council for Neurologic Subspecialties (UCNS) in 2004, with the aim of outlining more clearly a domain of clinical practice at the intersection of neurology and psychiatry (Silver, 2006).[1] With this in mind, a number of fellowships, accredited by the UCNS, exist where psychiatrists and neurologists can obtain further training specific to the practice of BN & NP.

The interview

The interview must elicit information about current symptoms and history of mood changes, including major depression, dysthymia, manic episodes or periods of hypomania (which is often missed), panic disorder, agoraphobia, substance use, and history of physical/emotional trauma/abuse. Inquiries about emotional state must be aimed at specifying the duration, variability, intensity, appropriateness, and degree of voluntary control over problems reported. For psychotic symptoms, we must inquire not only about the usual auditory and visual hallucinations, but also about olfactory ones, which may indicate partial seizures, and 'unusual experiences' such as déjà vu, jamais vu, derealization, and depersonalization.

Suicide attempts or plans, ideation, and risk factors (the MINI is excellent for covering these symptoms), as well as irritability and aggressive behaviour, must be queried. Input from family members about behaviours is invaluable. The Neuropsychiatric Inventory Questionnaire, which can be completed by a family member, can be helpful (https://download.lww.com/wolterskluwer_vitalstream_

com/PermaLink/CONT/A/CONT_21_3_2015_02_26_KAUFER_ 2015-10_SDC2.pdf). It is also imperative to obtain a list of all medications, including supplements, as these can impact behaviour, cognition, and emotion.

The interview must directly elicit information about cognition. Cognition is traditionally divided into domains of attention, executive function, memory, language, and visuospatial function. To probe about impairments in the various domains of cognition, inquire about real-life functions which relate to these domains: forgetfulness, misplacing items, leaving the stove on, missing appointments, forgetting movies seen or material read (books, newspapers), forgetting conversations or names, difficulty focusing or difficulty in sequencing and prioritizing a to-do list, difficulty with navigation in the community, or instances of getting lost.

Difficulties with sleep are common. Inquire about sleep pattern changes, abnormal or new movements in the night, acting out of dreams, vivid dreams, and difficulty with distinguishing sleep from awake state, all of which could suggest rapid eye movement (REM) sleep disorder which often tracks with synucleinopathies such as Parkinson's disease (PD) or dementia with Lewy bodies (DLB). Inquire about personality changes. This may be an early clue to FTD or HD, for example.

Directly inquire about perceptual disorders such as illusions, hallucinations, and delusions. Cultural factors may impact presenting symptoms (Laroi et al., 2014). We need to gain an understanding from family and friends about any cultural meaning of certain symptoms, in particular, as it relates to symptoms that may suggest psychosis. For example, in some cultures, it is accepted to speak with the dead, whereas in others, this may be considered a sign of psychosis. Aside from cultural sensitivity in interpreting certain neuropsychiatric symptoms, in particular hallucinations, which, in the right clinical setting, suggest psychosis, we must also be aware of 'benign' hallucinations, which also do not warrant a diagnosis of psychotic disorder. Many patients will experience 'benign' visual hallucinations or illusions, which must not be confused with psychotic disorder. For example, elderly patients with macular degeneration or other significant visual disturbance may experience visual hallucinations in dim light, typically reporting seeing animals or children (Charles Bonnet syndrome). These patients are not disturbed by the hallucinations and may even find them pleasant. They are also aware these images are not really there. We refer the reader to Oliver Sack's book *Hallucinations*, a wonderful and thorough resource describing variations of clinical presentation of hallucinations.

Questions about the past medical history should include eliciting relevant past neuropsychiatric history such as brain trauma, seizures/epilepsy, CNS infections, psychiatric admissions, personality changes, and prior medications for psychiatric conditions, as well as any significant medical conditions such as cancer (which can be associated with paraneoplastic syndromes of neuropsychiatric nature such as limbic encephalitis). Family history of neuropsychiatric illness, such as mood disorders, bipolar disorder, alcoholism, and dementia, should be elicited, and if several members of the family have a relevant history, a pedigree should be generated charting the genetic disorder in the family. Sometimes such a family history is not immediately apparent, so care should be taken to notice subtle signs of inherited neuropsychiatric disorders. For example, in HD, the family history may be not be entirely clear, but clues such as

---

[1] The UCNS was formed in 2001 to provide accreditation of fellowships and certification of practitioners in small neurologic subspecialties, in order to improve patient care and offer subspecialists a vehicle to enhance their fields of practice (refer to the UCNS site).

multiple family members with alcoholism and early death or some family members with 'strange movements' can give hints to this autosomal dominant disorder.

Collateral history is generally helpful and should be obtained whenever possible, even in cases when the patient seemingly is able to recount the details of the history of presenting symptoms, as it can help identify features relevant to the diagnosis such as lack of insight, poor judgement, personality change, aggression/agitation, or difficulty in functioning in activities of daily life. Collateral history must be obtained from family or friends whenever cognition is impaired to an extent that limits obtaining reliable information from the patient.

The mental status examination

A formal mental status examination is the next part of the examination, which will systematically probe the core domains of cognition, including attention, memory, language, visuospatial function, and executive function. The utility of this more formal aspect of the neuropsychiatric examination is to attempt to quantify the extent of the deficit, as well as to ensure that we do not miss an aspect of cognitive impairment, which may not have been apparent in the interview. The use of specific cognitive tests and/ or behavioural scales with recognized normative values can be invaluable, in particular in terms of inter-rater reliability and validity. The neuropsychiatrist can choose from the collection of cognitive and behavioural tests to create a patient-specific neurobehavioural status examination (NBSE). Formal measures are added to improve the reliability and validity of the clinical data. A recent report of the American Academy of Neurology (AAN) Behavioral Neurology Section Workgroup on improving clinical cognitive testing (Daffner et al., 2015a) identified frequently used single-domain cognitive tests that are suitable for an NBSE to help make informed choices about clinical cognitive assessment. Even when a neuropsychologist is available to perform formal neuropsychological testing services, the NBSE is still useful to the neuropsychiatrist during the initial assessment as an adjunct clinical tool or to help in determining whether more in-depth neuropsychological testing is needed. For detailed summary of tests, which can be used to probe each domain of cognition, please see the NBSE Evidence-Based Review: Test Summary Tables in Daffner et al. (2015b). As an additional resource for standardized brief cognitive and behavioural tests is the NIH Toolbox* (available at: http://www.nihtoolbox.org/Pages/default.aspx).

Measures typically address one or more or all of the aspects of cognition, behaviour, and mood. When choosing a measure, consider clinician time, patient time, and training requirements (training for interviewers and raters vary across measures—some require extensive training, while others require little or no training). The two principal psychometric properties of a measure are reliability and validity. We review only those psychometric measures that have good inter-rater reliability and normative data for adults across the life span. Some frequently used tests have limited normative data or have not been well studied in common neuropsychiatric disorders. We advise utilizing cognitive and behavioural tests with normative data based on the individual's age and educational level, which can enhance the rigour and utility of clinical cognitive

assessment. We are excluding tests that are not in the public domain and/or are copyright-restricted.

As a useful rule, attention should be tested first since impaired attention, as seen in delirium, for example, will confound the entire examination. To test attention, one can choose digit span forward and backward, the oral trail-making test and/or the written trail-making test, or serial 7s (start with 100 and go down by 7s) and/or spelling 'WORLD' backwards. Note that education is a confounding factor for interpretation of the mental status examination. If a patient is illiterate or partially literate and lacking mathematical skills, only gross assessments can be made. For executive function testing, the Frontal Assessment Battery (FAB) is a useful tool (Dubois et al., 2000). For language testing, one can use the Mississippi Aphasia Screening Test (MAST) (Nakase-Thompson et al., 2005). The Controlled Oral Word Association Test (COWAT)-FAS tests verbal fluency, which assesses both verbal ability and executive control. For memory, we suggest using the Rey Auditory Verbal Learning Test (RAVLT) (Strauss et al., 2006a). We discourage the use of the 3-word and 5-word recall tests, as there are limited normative data for these tests and their administration is not standardized (instructions given to patients vary and the actual time of testing recall at the bedside is notoriously variable). The recall of zero or one of three words presented may be a 'red flag' for memory impairment in adults aged 65–90 years, but up to 19% of older adults who recall only one word on a 3-word test perform normally on more detailed memory testing, suggesting that these simple tests may not accurately reflect a patient's memory function. For visuospatial function, line bisection, cancellation, cube copying, and intersecting pentagon copying are commonly used. The clock drawing test, which is commonly used to test visuospatial function, can be used as a global screening tool for dementia—this test has a relatively high sensitivity (~90%) in distinguishing older adults with normal cognition versus those with AD. The test has a much lower sensitivity in distinguishing mild cognitive impairment (MCI) from AD. We discourage interpretations of the clock drawing test for claims about performance in any specific domains of cognition, as the evidence does not support sufficient specificity or sensitivity to make such claims.

While the clinician has flexibility in choosing amongst the available brief tests to probe the individual domains of cognition, it is advisable to use at least one standardized global measure of cognition. There are many such tests, including the Mini-Mental State Examination (MMSE), the MoCA (Montreal Cognitive Assessment), and the Addenbrooke's Cognitive Examination (ACE) (for a review, see Martin, 1990 and Velayudhan, 2014). These brief cognitive tests (each <20 minutes to administer) differ in specificity and sensitivity for diagnosing different types of cognitive impairment. In addition to the above considerations, these tests differ in their copyright and accessibility of normative data.

The Folstein MMSE, which is the most widely used screening test for impairment of cognitive function, was developed by Marshal F Folstein and colleagues in 1975, in order to differentiate 'organic' from 'functional' psychiatric patients, and is a standard tool in screening for neurocognitive disorder (Folstein et al., 1975). The Folstein MMSE tests registration, attention and calculation, recall, language, the ability to follow simple commands, and orientation, and its administration takes between 5 and 10 minutes. Previously categorized into MCI and dementia, the *Diagnostic and Statistical Manual of Mental Disorders*, fifth edition (DSM-5) introduced a new terminology for the severity of cognitive dysfunction—minor and major neurocognitive disorder. A minor neurocognitive disorder is defined as a moderate cognitive decline which does not interfere with independence, and a major neurocognitive disorder is defined as severe cognitive decline which interferes with independence. Both diagnoses exclude delirium as a cause of cognitive impairment, as well as 'other mental disorders'. Folstein MMSE suggests a major neurocognitive disorder if the patient's score is two or more standard deviations (SDs) away from the mean for their age and education group. Mild neurocognitive disorder is diagnosed when the MMSE score is 1–2 SDs away from the mean. The normative data for the MMSE are presented in Crum et al. (1993). These data draw on MMSEs done on >18,000 community-dwelling individuals, ranging in age from 18 to >90 years and with a wide range of education levels. This normative data set represents the largest such set for any cognitive screening measure for civilians published to date and allows normative interpretation of performance in a manner consistent with the recommendations in the Neurocognitive Disorders section of the DSM-5.

It is important to note that, for 25 years, since its publication in 1975, the MMSE was widely distributed in textbooks and pocket guides and on the web. However, in 2000, the authors started to enforce copyright. A licensed version of the MMSE can now be purchased from Psychological Assessment Resources (PAR). The MMSE form is gradually disappearing from textbooks, websites, and clinical toolkits (Newman and Feldman, 2011).

The FAB is a brief battery of six neuropsychological tasks designed to assess frontal lobe function. The six FAB tasks probe conceptualization and abstract reasoning (via similarities), mental flexibility (via lexical fluency), executive control (via Luria sequencing motor task), resistance to interference (via conflicting instructions), inhibitory control (via go–no go), and environmental autonomy (via prehension behaviour). The FAB is particularly helpful in distinguishing frontal dysexecutive-type dementias and dementia of AD, although in our practice, we often use FAB to probe frontal functions in other patient populations, in particular those with TBI. A cut-off score of 12 on the FAB has a sensitivity of 77% and a specificity of 87% in differentiating between frontal dysexecutive-type dementias and AD.

The ACE is a short cognitive test sensitive for detection of early dementia, as well as for differentiation of dementia subtypes, including AD, FTD, Parkinson's disease dementia (PDD), and progressive supranuclear palsy (PSP) (Mathuranath et al., 2000; Reyes et al., 2009). The original ACE included the MMSE, but also frontal executive and more visuospatial items. The ACE was later modified to the ACE-R to account for cross-cultural sensitivity, and more recently to the ACE-III to optimize weaknesses of certain domains in the ACE-R such as repetition, comprehension, and visuospatial function testing. It was tested in 61 patients with dementia (FTD, $n = 33$, and AD, $n = 28$) and 25 controls. The ACE-III cognitive domains were found to correlate significantly with standardized neuropsychological tests used in the assessment of attention, language, verbal memory, and visuospatial function and also compared very favourably with its predecessor the ACE-R, with similar levels of sensitivity and specificity (Hsieh et al., 2013).

There is some recent evidence to suggest that although the ACE-III is a valid cognitive test for discriminating between AD and FTD,

the ACE-R yielded the highest level of evidence amongst the different versions in diagnostic accuracy sensitivity and specificity for differentiating early dementia, including AD, FTD, PDD, and PSP (Velayudhan et al., 2014). This is in contrast to the MMSE, which does not allow discrimination between types of cognitive disorders but rather is more sensitive to diagnosing major neurocognitive disorders. For a recent detailed review of brief cognitive tests applicable to patients with suspected major neurocognitive disorder, please see Velayudhan et al., 2014.

The MoCA is particularly well suited for those patients who fall into the mild neurocognitive disorder category (formerly MCI) on the MMSE (score of 26–30 on the MMSE) to help predict the onset of dementia (Smith et al., 2007). At 6-month follow-up, the MoCA detected mild dementia with 94% sensitivity and 50% specificity. The MoCA has excellent sensitivity (97%) for detecting MCI and MCI/AD combined, but poor specificity (35%) using a cut-off score of 26 or below (Luis et al., 2009). The MoCA is also accurate in PD, with cut-offs of 21/30 for PDD (sensitivity 81%; specificity 95%; negative predictive value 92%) (Dalrymple-Alford et al., 2010).

In our practice, we have traditionally started with the Folstein MMSE and the FAB.

Behavioural testing may be added to include measures of delirium or agitation, and mood scales for anxiety and depression can be useful. Some useful behaviour scales include the Delirium Rating Scale (DRS), the Agitated Behavior Scale (ABS), the Confusion Assessment Protocol (CAP), and the Pathologic Laughing and Crying Scale (PLACS). For example, in our practice, the ABS is often used in inpatients with TBI who are presenting with significant agitation. The ABS scale is useful in globally rating agitation, as well as providing information on the type of agitated behaviour—disinhibition, aggression, and impulsivity. It is easy to administer by a physician, nurse, or ancillary staff and can be done twice daily to track daytime and night-time agitation and help guide environmental and pharmacological interventions. As mentioned earlier in this chapter, the Neuropsychiatric Inventory is a useful tool for collateral history on behaviour and is filled by patient's family or cohabitant.

Formal measures of mood and anxiety can be helpful. The American Psychiatric Association (APA), in its practice guidelines for evaluation, offers a number of current and emerging measures for research and clinical evaluation (American Psychiatric Association, 2000). These are available for free and can be used for general screening or for specific syndromes (https://www.psychiatry.org/psychiatrists/practice/dsm/dsm-5/online-assessment-measures). Screening measures include the Patient Health Questionnaire (PHQ-9) (http://www.cqaimh.org/pdf/tool_phq9.pdf) (a score of >10 has a sensitivity and a specificity of 88% for major depression) and the Quick Inventory for Depressive Symptomatology (QIDS), a 16-item scale which can also be used to screen for somatic and mood symptoms of depression, focusing on the prior 7 days (https://www.mdcalc.com/quick-inventory-depressive-symptomatology-qids). Other measures include the Hamilton Depression Scale for patients who already carry the diagnosis of depression, the Beck Depression Inventory, and the Beck Anxiety Inventory (Beck et al., 1961 and 1988). A useful scale for post-traumatic stress disorder is Severity of Posttraumatic Stress Symptoms (APA_DSM5_Severity-of-Posttraumatic-Stress-Symptoms-Adult.pdf).

Neurological examination

A brief neurological examination should be performed to ensure there are no clear focal signs such as cranial nerve abnormalities, focal motor or sensory deficits, or a visual field cut, which can help localize a lesion in the nervous system. In addition to the brief standard cranial nerve, sensory, and motor examination, we highlight below some nuances in the neurological examination which can be added to shed light on neuropsychiatric diagnoses.

Examination of eye movements and vision can offer several insights into the functioning of the nervous system. Look for square wave jerks, broken saccades, broken smooth pursuit, or limitation in upgaze, which can suggest subcortical dementia and/or parkinsonism. The vestibulo-ocular reflex (VOR) often precipitates symptoms in individuals who have suffered concussions.

Olfactory examination is useful as many patients with inferior, even mild, TBI and without clear imaging abnormalities may have olfactory dysfunction, which may be a subtle sign of inferior frontal lobe injury. For testing, coffee beans and lavender essence are commonly used.

Observe for the presence of abnormal movements. Note the frequency and amplitude of tremor and whether it is present at rest, with posture and/or action. Note any involvement of the voice. Note hypophonia and test for micrographia, both of which may be subtle signs of a neurodegenerative process.

Check for frontal release signs and primitive reflexes (glabellar, snout, palmomental, grasp), as well as premotor function via praxis testing (ask the patient to show how they would light a match or brush their hair, etc.).

Useful diagnostic tests

Carefully chosen additional diagnostic tests, such as imaging and spinal fluid analysis, may be needed to clarify the diagnosis. Magnetic resonance imaging (MRI) of the brain, when available, is important in understanding the pattern of any focal atrophy and assessing for the presence of leukoencephalopathy. MRI sequences which should included are the standard T1 and T2 structural sequences, susceptibility weighted imaging (SWI) or gradient echo which will detect haemosiderin, and thus help in visualizing any evidence of prior haemorrhages, including microhaemorrhages seen in amyloid angiopathy, diffusion-weighted imaging (DWI) and apparent diffusion coefficient (ADC) sequences which will help rule out any ischaemic or other cytotoxic injury. Gadolinium MRI contrast is not necessary, unless a mass lesion or significant white matter disease is noted, which would benefit from contrast for clarification of the aetiology (to rule out active demyelination, for example, or better visualize a brain tumour or abscess). Softwares, such as NeuroQuant, now allow detailed automated structural and volumetric analysis of key brain regions for specific cognitive functions, such as the critical memory region the hippocampus, for which normative data are available, allowing comparison of patient total brain and hippocampal volumes to known norms for comparable age and education.

Positron emission tomography (PET) allows for metabolic assessment of the brain, most commonly using the fludeoxyglucose (FDG tracer). Single-photon emission computed tomography (SPECT) can also be used to obtain information about metabolism of the brain, based on observations of regional differences in blood flow. Ioflupane (iodine-123) injection for DaTScan, a contrast agent to be used with SPECT, can be used for detecting dopamine transporters (DaT) in suspected idiopathic PD. Emerging imaging modalities, including PET with amyloid tracers (e.g. Amyvid), sodium scans, large-scale intrinsic network analysis via functional MRI [default mode network (DMN), salience, etc.] are on the horizon as potentially useful clinical tools to help disentangle the aetiology of neuropsychiatric symptoms. These modalities at this time do not have normative data and are being used only in research setting.

Paroxysmal spells of behaviour should be evaluated by EEG. Seizures and interictal electrographic abnormalities can both present with agitation, psychosis, and behavioural disturbance, rather than with an overt movement disorder such as tonic–clonic movements characteristic of a generalized tonic–clonic seizure. There is little to no utility in performing a routine (brief 30–45 minutes) EEG to assess paroxysmal spells in a patient who is awake and alert at the time of examination. Whenever possible, at least 24-hour continuous EEG should be performed, preferably video EEG, but if not available or cost is too high, a Holter-type (ambulatory) EEG can be performed instead.

In a minority of patients, the only cause of a neurocognitive disorder is a sleep disorder such as obstructive sleep apnoea. Polysomnography should be strongly considered, especially if there is report of snoring or stopping breathing overnight.

Cerebrospinal fluid (CSF) analysis is needed to evaluate patients whose imaging or clinical examination/history suggest a possibility of infection or an inflammatory process. Patients with unexplained leukoencephalopathy should always have CSF analysis. CSF and serum samples can also be sent for a paraneoplastic autoimmune antibody panel. In a minority of patients presenting with neuropsychiatric symptoms, the underlying cause is antibody-mediated limbic encephalitis that requires immune therapy such as intravenous immunoglobulin (IVIG), plasmapheresis, or immune-suppressing medications (for review see Leypoldt et al., 2015).

Special considerations for patients in post-traumatic amnesia (PTA)/post-traumatic confusional state (PTCS) and disorders of consciousness (DOC)

The examination needs to be tailored to the level of arousal and the presence or absence of confusion and/or delirium (e.g. a patient recovering from moderate to severe TBI who is still in MCS will require a different clinical approach than an awake, alert patient who comes in for evaluation of mood disturbance). Whereas a full interview and the scales named earlier are appropriate in an awake, alert patient without severe cognitive impairment, patients recovering from severe TBI who are still in VS, MCS, or PTA/PTCS will require a tailored examination and different scales for assessment [i.e. the Coma Recovery Scale (CRS) for patients in VS and MCS; the Orientation Log (O-Log), the Galveston Orientation and Amnesia Test (GOAT), or the CAP for patients in PTA/PTCS].

Table 2.1 Assessment of patients with disorders of consciousness

	Purpose	References
Neurological examination	Integrity of brainstem reflexes, best motor response, monitoring for recovery of function (i.e. purposeful verbal, visual, motor behaviours) and neurological complications	Giacino et al., 2013
Standardized structured behavioural assessment	To mitigate the high misdiagnosis rate of unstructured bedside evaluation, which carries 30–40% risk of diagnostic error Example: CRS-R, SMART, DOCS, Western	Seel et al., 2010 Schnakers et al., 2009 Laureys et al., 2005 Majerus et al., 2005
Neuroimaging	Identify the type and extent of brain damage; especially important for assessment of cortical integrity—MRI more sensitive than CT in detecting cortical damage. MRI in patients with severe brain injury allows comprehensive assessment of the primary and secondary insult, thus giving an indicator of a possible long-term prognosis. Morphological images can now be coupled with metabolic analysis and white fibre track quantification, thus providing a more precise assessment of brain lesions	Torbey et al., 2000 Wijdicks et al., 2001 Lescot et al., 2009
EEG	To rule out non-convulsive seizures as the cause of DOC; to identify malignant EEG patterns consistent with poor outcome: generalized suppression, burst suppression with generalized epileptiform activity, and generalized periodic complexes on a flat background. Recommend 24-hour monitoring for non-coma, and 48 hours for coma	Claassen et al., 2004 Claassen et al., 2013 De Georgia and Raad 2012
Evoked potentials	To establish integrity of afferent sensory pathways, including the primary senses such as hearing, vision, and tactile sensation	Goldberg and Karazim 1998 De Georgia and Raad 2012

The neurobehavioural status examination may be limited to this in the initial stage of recovery due to patients' severely impaired attention and inability to participate in lengthy testing. The neurological examination and diagnostic tests used are as described earlier. The examination of patients in DOC, particularly as it relates to nuances between VS and MCS, is outlined in Table 2.1.

There are some specific considerations for examination of neuropsychiatric patients in different clinical settings. In the ambulatory (outpatient clinic) setting, the patients are generally functioning at a level consistent with living in the community (i.e. they are higher-functioning than hospital patients). The patient may come to see you alone and provide a full history. However, with the patient's permission, it is advisable to obtain a collateral history from a close relative or a close friend who may be able to provide useful observations that the patient may not be aware of due to their underlying neuropsychiatric condition This is fundamentally important in patients with frontal lobe disorders, with poor awareness and insight, those with memory dysfunction, and those with REM sleep disorders where only another person could report the observed symptoms. Whenever possible, collateral history is important. The ambulatory encounter consists of a formal interview lasting 30–60 minutes, followed by administration of a set of brief cognitive tests as part of the neurobehavioural examination. Finally, a brief neurological physical examination should be performed.

In the hospital setting, patients are typically quite impaired, limiting the ability to carry out an extensive interview, although patients at times are able to provide a useful history and this should always be attempted. However, more often than not, a collateral history from family or close friends is required for hospitalized neuropsychiatric patients. Patients are followed daily or at least several times per week while hospitalized, and the nature of the neuropsychiatric examination occurs on the initial day of the consult and over time. For a formal assessment, specific cognitive scales should be used when possible, e.g. for patients with recent TBI who are still in PTCS, the GOAT or the O-Log should be used daily to track their progress towards recovery. Delirium often confounds the mental status of hospitalized neuropsychiatric patients,

and detailed descriptive mental status examinations at this stage are important. Once patients demonstrate improvement, they are often transitioned to acute neurorehabilitation where the care shifts to implementing an aggressive recovery programme, including physical and cognitive rehabilitation. At this stage, the neuropsychiatrist will be particularly vigilant to diagnose and treat any complications from the underlying neurological condition such as seizures, infection, and sleep disorders. Targeted use of pharmacotherapy to optimize attention and initiation (methylphenidate, modafinil), help with arousal of patients in DOC (amantadine), and complement aphasia recovery (donepezil) may be used, as well as to optimize motor recovery after stroke (fluoxetine). Close collaboration with other professionals is needed to maximize positive outcomes at the stage of neurorehabilitation.

Formulation and diagnosis

Once data from the neuropsychiatric assessment are gathered, the clinician must integrate all the information acquired to formulate the differential diagnosis and plan of treatment. In this section, we highlight several clinical cases to illustrate examples of specific challenges to diagnosis and treatment in neuropsychiatric patients. These clinical cases also highlight the specific skill set of a neuropsychiatrist.

CASE STUDY 1

A 74-year-old woman with a past medical history notable for lifelong anxiety, in therapy once weekly for >20 years, now presents to our memory clinic with concerns for cognitive decline. She decided to come in after an event, which was very concerning for her—she went to her therapist's office very early in the morning at a time she was not scheduled for and ended up waiting there in the rain since dawn until her therapist arrived. The reason why this was so concerning for her is that she has come in to see this therapist for many years and had very set times, and it was terrifying to her that she showed up at the wrong time. Function is preserved, and except for this one episode, the patient does not mention any other significant memory lapses and she has never gotten lost or confused about directions. She makes it to her appointments on time, she pays her bills, cooks, and meets with friends. She is terrified of getting Alzheimer's disease. The patient is also terrified of ageing on the whole. She expresses concerns about death and decline of her body. She is single and has no children. She has many close friends who are supportive. Neurological examination is normal. She completed 16 years of education and got a score of 29/30 in the Folstein MMSE.

The patient presented with such a strong history of anxiety, and she appeared so anxious in the office that upon the initial clinical evaluation, we placed anxiety/somatic preoccupation related to ageing higher on the differential diagnosis than early stages of a neurodegenerative disorder. However, as part of the differential diagnosis, we included a mild neurocognitive disorder due to an underlying early neurodegenerative process such as Alzheimer's disease, due to the fact that the patient was reporting a memory problem and a cognitive decline.

Initial workup included neuropsychological testing and brain MRI. Neuropsychological testing revealed variable performance more consistent with anxiety, without a clear pattern of deficits to support an underlying neurodegenerative process. There was relative weakness in performance in memory domains but this did not meet statistically significant thresholds. Due to remaining questions about the diagnosis, we obtained an FDG-PET of the brain, which showed mild temporo-parietal hypometabolism. This supported a diagnosis of mild early AD pathology as the cause of her mild neurocognitive disorder.

The patient was started on the cholinesterase inhibitor donepezil at 5 mg daily. The focus of treatment otherwise remained her very significant anxiety disorder, which was paralysing and making the memory disorder symptomatically worse. Several anxiety medications were tried, including a selective serotonin reuptake inhibitor (SSRI) and a serotonin–noradrenaline reuptake inhibitor (SNRI); eventually, we achieved good anxiety control with buspirone and a small dose of quetiapine 12.5 mg in the morning, and 25 mg before bedtime. It is important to note that the choice of antipsychotics, including atypical antipsychotics, have a black box warning for patients with dementia, due to increased mortality with their use in this patient population (Rose and Kass, 2019). In this patient's case, she has mild neurocognitive disorder, not dementia, but regardless we reserve the use of antipsychotics to the last resort for cognitively impaired patients.

Learning points
1. PET brain can help reveal early metabolic changes suggestive of AD, when the diagnosis is not clear based on neuropsychological testing and structural imaging.
2. Treatment of psychiatric comorbidities remains a high priority to help maintain function, as well as because the cognitive disorder can be made symptomatically worse by undertreated anxiety and depression.
3. In choosing medications to treat psychiatric conditions in patients with an underlying neurocognitive disorder, it is imperative to be aware of considerations in medication choice specific to this patient population (https://www.fda.gov/drugs).

CASE STUDY 2

An 82-year-old patient with dementia and parkinsonism, now with hallucinations. At the time the patient presented to our office, he had been recently started on antipsychotics, which made his rigidity and gait worse.

Which medication would be the next best choice to treat hallucinations and agitation?

This patient most likely has DLB. Cholinesterase inhibitors have been shown to be useful in treating hallucinations in this patient population (Mori et al., 2012) and should be considered as first-line agents in patients with DLB or other synucleinopathies such as PD. The patient was started on donepezil 5 mg daily, which was increased after 1 week to 10 mg daily. Improvement in hallucinations was noted.

If cholinesterase inhibitors are not effective in treating hallucinations, we would consider pimavanserin, a selective 5HT2 reverse agonist recently approved by the US Food and Drug Administration (FDA) for treatment of psychosis in PD. The high cost of this new medication may be a limiting factor for many patients. If pimavanserin is not available or is not effective, or if the patient does not tolerate it, the atypical antipsychotic clozapine has the best side effect profile for patients with synucleinopathies, due to favourable minimal risk of extrapyramidal side effects, and should be the next in line as a choice. Clozapine does carry a risk of agranulocytosis; thus, close monitoring of serum white blood cell levels is required for the first year, then periodically after, as the risk of agranulocytosis falls to <0.01% per year after the first year. In regard to the use of antipsychotics in this elderly patient with dementia, there is a black box warning due to increased mortality with use of these agents in patients with dementia. Antipsychotics should be reserved as chemical restraint in extreme cases when the patient is at risk of harm to self or others and no alternative medication is working (see Case study 1).

Of note, not all hallucinations seen in patients with synucleinopathies indicate psychosis and not all should be treated equally. For example, some hallucinations will arise due to levodopa (L-dopa), and in that case, lowering the L-dopa dose would be a starting point for treatment.

Learning points
1. In patients with synucleinopathies, including DLB and PD, who are presenting with psychotic features, such as hallucinations, or presenting with agitation, antipsychotics pose a risk of worsening movement disorder/extrapyramidal side effects superimposed on underlying parkinsonism.
2. The first-line medications for psychosis in DLB are cholinesterase inhibitors.
3. The first-line antipsychotic in patients with synucleinopathies is clozapine or the newly FDA-approved selective 5HT2 reverse agonist pimavanserin.
4. Memantine, an NMDA antagonist, is FDA-approved for treatment of moderate to severe AD but is often used off-label in the same patient population to treat agitation.

CASE STUDY 3

A 67-year-old man, who is neurologically intact at baseline, fell downstairs and sustained large right temporal and frontal contusions. He had loss of consciousness for <30 minutes but remained disoriented and confused for several weeks. He was disoriented and not able to recall events in his life, to lay down new episodic memories, or to maintain continuous episodic memory function. His sleep–wake cycle was disrupted. He was at times combative and agitated. Overall his cognitive and behavioural symptoms fluctuated throughout the day during this period. This clinical presentation was consistent with PTA/PTCS, but we did ensure that there were no neurological complications contributing to the neuropsychiatric syndrome. A 24-hour EEG was normal, eliminating the diagnosis of seizures, and CT of the head revealed no ventriculomegaly that would be indicative of hydrocephalus. Supportive care was provided during the PTA/PTCS period. To manage his behaviour pharmacologically, we used valproic acid acutely for agitation and transitioned him to lamotrigine for longer-term treatment of post-TBI impulsivity and mood lability. We avoided antipsychotics, as following TBI, evidence suggests that a pro-dopaminergic state is favourable to recovery (for a review of treatment of behavioural disturbances in TBI, see Wortzel and Silver, 2019).

We tracked his mental status daily using the GOAT. GOAT scores of >75 on three consecutive days were considered an indication that the patient has emerged from PTA.

CASE STUDY 4

A 27-year-old right-handed woman, with normal development and no significant past medical or psychiatric history, sustained a TBI in the setting of a motor vehicle accident 7 years ago and has suffered a diverse set of neuropsychiatric symptoms since that time, which have impacted her function to a great degree.

She sustained right eye injury, a dislocated jaw, and multiple soft tissue injuries of the face, and lost consciousness for about 5–10 minutes. She was in PTA for ~24 hours. CT head did not reveal evidence of intracranial bleeding or other obvious injury and no skull fracture.

She has had numerous symptoms since the accident, including feeling like she has to exert extreme effort to achieve a basic level of normal functioning, leading to a constant state of physical and emotional exhaustion. Prominent symptoms include cognitive 'fog', unsteadiness, dizziness, visual disturbance characterized by difficulty focusing, headaches, and various somatic complaints. She exhibits a compulsion to record her symptoms, obsessively making lists and constantly noting down her many symptoms.

Over several years since her mild TBI, the patient's symptoms were attributed to anxiety and she was also given a diagnosis of depression. She was treated with oxycodone for leg discomfort and burning sensation, and various combinations of lorazepam, escitalopram, lamotrigine, bupropion, gabapentin, and trazodone for anxiety and depressed mood.

She was carefully weaned off medications which could be causing cognitive side effects, including benzodiazepines, opiates, and gabapentin. We treated her anxiety and obsessive–compulsive disorder (OCD) symptoms with the SSRI sertraline.

The patient improved with the above and treatment for concussion/mild TBI with simultaneous physical therapy and neuro-optometry-guided visual rehabilitation.

Learning points

1. Following TBI, PTA/PTCS are a common consequence, lasting from days to weeks. This is a condition characterized by fluctuation of cognition and behaviour throughout the day, and attention, memory, and orientation deficits.

2. Emergence from PTA/PTCS is typically tracked by one of several available standardized scales, including the GOAT, Westmead, or O-Log, amongst others. One scale should be used to track the patient until they meet the criteria for emergence from PTA/PTCS.

3. There is a need to identify and treat any active neurological complications contributing to cognitive and behavioural disturbance after TBI. The commonest such complications include seizures, hydrocephalus, and infection.

4. Limit the use of antipsychotics following TBI, as a pro-dopaminergic neurotransmitter state has been associated with better neuropsychiatric outcomes after TBI. We advise the use of mood stabilizers, valproic acid, or beta blockers as first line to help manage behaviour/agitation after TBI.

Conclusion

The neuropsychiatric assessment is aimed at diagnosis and formulation of treatment for the full spectrum of emotional, behavioural, and cognitive problems in the presence of a neurological disorder. The skill set of a neuropsychiatrist spans psychiatry, neurology, and the diagnosis and treatment of disorders which fall under the domain of this subspecialty.

It often takes a concerted effort of multiple practitioners to get the symptoms of neuropsychiatric patients under control. The team typically includes the neuropsychiatrist who makes the initial diagnosis and treatment plan, a collaborating psychiatrist or psychologist who performs supportive or other psychotherapy as needed, rehabilitation treatments including speech, occupational therapy (OT), physiotherapy (PT), and at times neuro-optometry.

Whenever possible, it is advisable that clinicians seeking the neuropsychiatry skill set spend a period of training at a specialized centre offering neuropsychiatry services, which would offer exposure to, and training in, the treatment of the relevant disorders. In the United States, training can be obtained through BN & NP fellowships certified by the UCNS.

REFERENCES

Beck AT, Epstein N, Brown G, Steer RA. (1988). An inventory for measuring clinical anxiety: Psychometric properties. *Journal of Consulting and Clinical Psychology* **56**:893–7.

Beck AT, Ward CH, Mendelson M, Mock J, Erbaugh J. (1961). An inventory for measuring depression. *Archives of General Psychiatry* **4**:561–71.

Claassen J, Mayer SA, Kowalski RG, et al. (2004). Detection of electrographic seizures with continuous EEG monitoring in critically ill patients. *Neurology* **62**:1743–48.

Claassen J, Taccone FS, Horn P, et al. (2013). Recommendations on the use of EEG monitoring in critically ill patients: consensus statement from the neurointensive care section of the ESICM. *Intensive Care Medicine* **39**:1337–51.

Crum RM, Anthony JC, Bassett SS, Folstein MF. (1993). Population-based norms for the Mini-Mental State Examination by age and educational level. *JAMA* **269**:2386–91.

Daffner KR, Gale SA, Barrett AM, et al. (2015a). Improving clinical cognitive testing: report of the AAN Behavioral Neurology Section Workgroup. *Neurology* **85**:910–18.

Daffner KR, Gale SA, Barrett AM, et al. (2015b). *NBSE Evidence-Based Review: Test Summary Tables* (supplemental material). Available from: http://www.neurology.org/content/suppl/2015/07/10/WNL.0000000000001763.DC1/Appendix_e-1.pdf

Dalrymple-Alford JC, MacAskill MR, Nakas CT, et al. (2010). The MoCA: well-suited screen for cognitive impairment in Parkinson disease. *Neurology* **75**:1717–25.

De Georgia M, Raad B. (2012). Prognosis of coma after cardiac arrest in the era of hypothermia. *Continuum (Minneap Minn)* **18**:515–31.

Dubois B, Slachevsky A, Litvan I, Pillon B. (2000). The FAB: a frontal assessment battery at bedside. *Neurology* **55**:1621–6.

Folstein MF, Folstein SE, McHugh PR. (1975). 'Mini-mental state': a practical method for grading the cognitive state of patients for the clinician. *Journal of Psychiatric Research* **12**:189–98.

Food and Drug Administration. (2016). *Atypical antipsychotic drugs information.* Available from: https://www.fda.gov/drugs/postmarket-drug-safety-information-patients-and-providers/atypical-antipsychotic-drugs-information

Giacino JT, Katz DI, Garber K, Schiff N. (2013). Assessment and rehabilitative management of individuals with disorders of consciousness. In: Zasler N, Katz D, Zafonte R (editors). *Brain Injury Medicine: Principles and Practice.* New York, NY: Demos Medical Publishing. pp. 517–35.

Goldberg G, Karazim E. (1998). Application of evoked potentials to the prediction of discharge status in minimally responsive patients: a pilot study. *Journal of Head Trauma Rehabilitation* **13**:51–68.

Hsieh S, Schubert S, Hoon C, Mioshi E, Hodges JR. (2013). Validation of the Addenbrooke's Cognitive Examination III in Frontotemporal Dementia and Alzheimer's Disease. *Dementia and Geriatric Cognitive Disorders* **36**:242–50.

Laroi F, Luhrmann TM, Bell V, et al. (2014). Culture and Hallucinations: Overview and Future Directions. *Schizohrenia Bulletin* **40**(Suppl 4):S213–20.

Laureys S, Perrind F, Schnakers C, et al. (2005). Residual cognitive function in comatose, vegetative and minimally conscious states. *Current Opinion of Neurology* **18**:726–33.

Lescot T, Galanaud D, Puybasset L. (2009). Exploring altered consciousness states by magnetic resonance imaging in brain injury. *Annals of the New York Academy of Sciences* **1157**:71–80.

Leypoldt F, Armangue T, Dalmau J. (2014). Autoimmune encephalopathies. *Annals of the New York Academy of Sciences* **1338**:94–114. doi: 10.1111/nyas.12553

Luis CA, Keegan AP, Mullan M. (2009). Cross validation of the Montreal Cognitive Assessment in community dwelling older adults residing in the Southeastern US. *International Journal of Geriatric Psychiatry* **24**:197–201.

Majerus S, Gill-Thwaites H, Andrews K, et al. (2005). Behavioral evaluation of consciousness in severe brain damage. *Progress in Brain Research* **150**:397–413.

Martin DC. (1990). The mental status examination. In: Walker HK, Hall WD, Hurst JW (editors). *Clinical Methods: The History, Physical, and Laboratory Examinations*, third edition. Boston, MA: Butterworths.

Mathuranath PS, Nestor PJ, Berrios GE, Rakowicz W, Hodges JR. (2000). A brief cognitive test battery to differentiate Alzheimer's disease and frontotemporal dementia. *Neurology.* **55**:1613–20.

Mori E, Ikeda M, Kosaka K; on behalf of the Donepezil-DLB Study Investigators. (2012). Donepezil for dementia with Lewy bodies: a randomized, placebo-controlled trial. *Annals of Neurology* **72**:41–52.

Nakase-Thompson R, Manning E, Sherer M, Yablon SA, Gontkovsky SL, Vickery C. (2005). Brief assessment of severe language impairments: initial validation of the Mississippi aphasia screening test. *Brain Injury* **19**:685–91.

Newman JC, Feldman R. (2011). Copyright and open access at the bedside. *New England Journal of Medicine* **365**:2447–9.

Reyes MA, Perez-Lloret S, Roldan Gerschcovich E, Martin ME, Leiguarda R, Merello M. (2009). Addenbrooke's Cognitive Examination validation in Parkinson's disease. *European Journal of Neurology* **16**:142–7.

Rose RV, Kass JS. (2019). Prescribing antipsychotic medications to patients with dementia: boxed warnings and mitigation of legal liability. *Continuum (Minneap Minn).* **25**(1):254–259.

Rush AJ; American Psychiatric Association and Task Force for the Handbook of Psychiatric Measures. (2000). *Handbook of Psychiatric Measures.* Washington, DC: American Psychiatric Association.

Schnakers C, Vanhaudenhuyse A, Giacino J, et al. (2009). Diagnostic accuracy of the vegetative and minimally conscious state: Clinical consensus versus standardized neurobehavioral assessment. *BMC Neurology* **9**:35.

Schneider LS, Dagerman KS, Insel P. (2005). Risk of death with atypical antipsychotic drug treatment for dementia: meta-analysis of randomized placebo-controlled trials. *JAMA* **294**:1934–43.

Seel R, Sherer M, Whyte J, et al. (2010). Assessment scales for disorders of consciousness: evidence-based recommendations for clinical practice and research. *Archives of Physical Medicine and Rehabilitation* **91**:1–19.

Silver JM. (2006). Behavioral neurology and neuropsychiatry *is* a subspecialty. Editorial. *Journal of Neuropsychiatry and Clinical Neurosciences* **18**:146–8.

Smith T, Gildeh N, Holmes C. (2007). The Montreal Cognitive Assessment: validity and utility in a memory clinic setting. *Canadian Journal of Psychiatry* **52**:329–32.

Strauss E, Sherman E, Spreen O. (2006b). *A Compendium of Neuropsychological Tests*, third edition. New York, NY: Oxford University Press .

Torbey MT, Selim M, Knorr J, et al. (2000). Quantitative analysis of the loss of distinction between gray and white matter in comatose patients after cardiac arrest. *Stroke* **31**:2163–7.

United Council of Neurological Subspecialties (UCNS). *Behavioral Neurology and Neuropsychiatry certification requirements and curriculum of fellowship*. Available from: https://www.ucns. org/Online/Initial_Certification/Behavioral_Neurology_ Neuropsychiatry/Online/Certification/Behavioral_Cert. aspx?hkey=0476b976-7a9c-49ec-adee-f1169c26ce08

Velayudhan L, Ryu S-H, Raczek M, et al. (2014). Review of brief cognitive tests for patients with suspected dementia. *International Psychogeriatrics* **26**:1247–62.

Wijdicks EF, Campeau NG, Miller GM. (2001). MR imaging in comatose survivors of cardiac resuscitation. *American Journal of Neuroradiology* **22**:1561–5.

Wortzel H, Silver JM. (2019). Behavioral dyscontrol. In: Silver JM, McAllister TW, Arciniegas DA (editors). *Textbook of Traumatic Brain Injury*, third edition. Washington, DC: American Psychiatric Publishing. pp. 395–412.

3

The neurological examination in neuropsychiatry

Jan A. Coebergh and Biba R. Stanton

Why and how do we examine patients?

Jaspers wrote that: 'The first and always most important method of examination is that of conversation with the patient … A physical examination is of course obligatory in all cases though it only rarely yields results which materially assist the assessment of the mental illness' (Jaspers et al., 1997).

The neurological examination in neuropsychiatry is an essential component of the assessment, diagnosis, and even treatment of neuropsychiatric disorders. Unfortunately few neurologists are trained in psychiatry, and vice versa, which can lead to 'mindless neurology, and brainless psychiatry' (Zeman, 2014). This chapter will discuss what is often called 'soft' neurological signs in psychiatry, but also 'hard' neurological signs in neuropsychiatry. It will describe the important role of the examination in functional neurological disorders, from diagnosis to treatment. It will discuss the value and validity of 'normal' and 'abnormal' and how the examination and diagnosis can change over time. It will discuss some scales used in the neurological examination in neuropsychiatry and their limitations. We refer only to adult neuropsychiatry; the neurological examination in children has many other dimensions like neurodevelopment that are not discussed here.

How a neurological examination should be performed depends on the setting, the experience of the examiner, and the clinical context. We need to ask ourselves the question 'exactly why am I trying to elicit this particular physical sign in this particular patient?' (Warlow, 2010). For a neurologist evaluating a patient with neurological symptoms, the primary purpose of the examination is to characterize any neurological deficit, localize the lesion, and help make a diagnosis. Using examination in this way requires neurological training. There are other purposes for examination that are perhaps more relevant to non-neurologists. We use it to evaluate function (e.g. walking) or change (are things getting better or worse?). Examination can identify avenues for treatment (e.g. spasticity or pain) (Wiles, 2013). It gives us time to think and look, allowing us to avoid unnecessary, expensive, and sometimes risky investigations. It can demonstrate understanding and relevance to the patient. The importance of ritual cannot be underestimated; examination is symbolic of 'I care about you and your problem' (Warlow, 2010).

A documented examination also helps when a complaint is made or if medicolegal action is taken against a healthcare professional. Finally, we should always be open to potentially changing our diagnosis. If your findings do not tally with a previous diagnosis, we might go down the route of 'undiagnosis', with all its implications (Coebergh et al., 2014), but a change in diagnosis does not necessarily mean you got it wrong first time around.

Knowing how to interpret the findings of a neurological examination requires more skill than simply performing it correctly. The more we examine, the more we know what is probably (ab-)normal (so we do not panic if the patient with functional symptoms says they feel less on the left side). It is important not to over-interpret equivocal positive signs (such as slightly brisk reflexes), particularly if they are inconsistent with the history. If in doubt, ask someone else or call it normal.

It is important to be aware of common cognitive biases that influence the way we interpret our examination findings. For example, 'availability errors' are defined as the tendency to judge the likelihood of explanation for an event by the ease with which relevant examples come to mind. This might be influenced by what we have encountered in recent times, individual memorable cases, or the setting. We may also apply the fallacy of logic (e.g. different tremors occur in Parkinson's disease, thereby not recognizing, for example, a functional tremor in someone with Parkinson's disease). In general, clinicians are over-confident in their diagnoses and tend to disregard uncertainty (e.g. a young woman with long-standing treatment-resistant depression and headaches who complains about her vision in whom papilloedema and an underlying large meningioma could be missed) (Groopman, 2009).

How to approach the neurological examination

In neuropsychiatry, we may pick up important signs from the general physical examination, as well as from the neurological examination (e.g evidence of self-harm/drug use, or high body mass index (BMI) in memory symptoms leading to consideration of sleep apnoea).

Neurologists 'never do a "full neurological examination" (whatever that is) in any one patient' (Allen, 2012). But, in some ways, doing a focused examination requires more skill (to know what is important) than a standardized examination. There have been attempts (using a Delphi method) to arrive at standard neurological examination that rules out significant disease (Moore and Chalk, 2009). (See Table 3.1.)

There is a YouTube instruction from the University of Birmingham (UK) available at https://www.youtube.com/watch?v=q56WgXvn0iU. This kind of examination can be done in about 5 minutes. Abnormalities should be interpreted in the context of the history and other examination findings, looking for patterns typical of a particular disease or anatomical localization. When an abnormality is seen later in the examination (e.g. gait), one might go back and re-examine an earlier part of the examination in more detail (e.g. Kayser–Fleischer ring for Wilson's disease).

Level of consciousness and the cognitive examination

The level of consciousness is generally obvious from conversation. The Glasgow Coma Scale (GCS) (Teasdale and Jennett, 1974) is often used and widely understood but was designed for trauma and has major limitations (e.g. in long-standing aphasia/dementia, closed eyes in dissociative seizure/psychogenic coma). The time course of changes in the GCS score can be extremely useful (e.g. recovery to maximum GCS score in 1 minute after a prolonged seizure is highly indicative of a dissociative seizure). Differentiating patients' responses into alert, verbal, (responsive to) pain, and unconscious often suffices.

When a more detailed cognitive assessment is needed, it is useful to do this early, as it will affect cooperation with the rest of the examination. There are more extensive introductions available (see especially Hodges, 2007). After Hodges, we have suggested a structured approach to examining distributed functions (attention, memory, and higher-order executive functions and social cognition), then localized functions—which, for the sake of simplicity, we have divided into dominant and non-dominant hemispheres (but, of course, are often the result of widespread network dysfunction).

CASE STUDY 1

A patient with severe depression had poor oral intake for a month and was sectioned and admitted to a mental hospital. Her consciousness levels fluctuated and she was perceived to be sleepy; by the time ophthalmoparesis was noted, her GCS was E4M4V1 and she was admitted to the intensive therapy unit (ITU). Only on day 2 was Wernicke suspected and treated. She was left with permanent severe disability.

Attention and concentration

It is important to describe attention in as much detail as possible, and at all times, avoid using the confusing word 'confusion'!

Table 3.1 High-rated elements of the neurologic examination

McGill neurologists	Canadian neurologists	McGill medical students
Visual fields*	Visual fields*	Visual fields
Fundoscopy	Fundoscopy	
Pupillary light reflex*	Pupillary light reflex*	Pupillary light reflex*
Pursuit EOM*	Pursuit EOM*	Pursuit EOM*
		Facial sensation*
Facial muscles*	Facial muscles*	Facial muscles*
		Sternocleidomastoid
Tongue	Tongue	Tongue
Gait*	Gait*	Gait*
Tandem gait	Tandem gait	
Pronator drift*	Pronator drift	Pronator drift*
RAM upper	RAM upper*	RAM upper*
Finger–nose*	Finger–nose*	Finger–nose
Tone arms*	Tone arms*	Tone arms
Tone legs*	Tone legs*	Tone legs
Power arms	Power arms*	Power arms*
Power legs	Power legs*	Power legs*
Biceps reflex"	Biceps reflex*	Biceps reflex*
Brachioradialis reflex*	Brachioradialis reflex*	Brachioradialis reflex*
Triceps reflex*	Triceps reflex*	Triceps reflex*
Patellar reflex*	Patellar reflex*	Patellar reflex*
Achilles reflex*	Achilles reflex*	Achilles reflex*
Plantar*	Plantar*	Plantar*
Light touch	N/A	
	Vibration	
	Pinprick*	
	Romberg	Romberg

EOM, extraocular eye movements; N/A, not available; RAM, rapid alternating movement.

All items shown had a mean score of 3 or greater. McGill students received the original version of the survey given to McGill neurologists, and therefore, light touch was not included.

* Mean score of 3.5 or greater.

Reproduced with permission from Moore, F.G.A. & Chalk, C. The essential neurologic examination: what should medical students be taught? *Neurology*, 72(23): 2020–3. Copyright © 2009, American Academy of Neurology. DOI: https://doi.org/10.1212/WNL.0b013e3181a92be6.

There is arousal (general wakefulness) and sustained attention (or vigilance). Other useful concepts are divided attention (ability to respond to multiple tasks at once—an aspect of executive function) and selective attention (ability to suppress awareness of competing stimuli). As described by Hodges, orientation, concentration, exploration, and vigilance are positive aspects of global attentive processes, while distractibility, impersistence, and fluctuating alertness reflect impaired attention (as seen typically in delirium).

Practical useful bedside tests are orientation in time and place, digit span (especially backwards), and, for example, serial 7s or months/days of the week in reverse order.

Memory

The assessment of memory is complex and can be confusing because of the differing nomenclature used by cognitive psychologists and clinicians. However, there are just a few key aspects that are important to assess in an everyday clinical setting.

Immediate memory (as assessed, for instance, by forward digit span) might also be seen as an aspect of attention. This is crucial to assess because if a patient is unable to register information due to attentional difficulties, they certainly will not be able to encode and remember it. This is relevant to patients with functional cognitive symptoms, whose perception of poor memory really reflects attentional difficulties. Working memory (the ability to manipulate information held in mind, e.g. backward digit span) is an aspect of executive function. New learning relies on the ability to encode information, store and consolidate it, and later retrieve it. Useful bedside tests of new learning include list-learning tasks (e.g. remembering 'apple, table, penny' in the MMSE (Folstein et al., 1975)) or learning a name and address (as in the ACE-III (Hsieh et al., 2013)). When performance is poor, cueing or tests of recognition memory (e.g. 'was one of the words apple or pear?') can be used to show whether the problem is with encoding and storage (not helped by cueing) or with retrieval (helped by cues). This allows us to differentiate true amnesia, usually arising from more medial temporal lobe pathology, from a failure of retrieval in a frontal–subcortical syndrome (where recognition will be preserved).

To fully assess non-dominant hemisphere function, analogous tests of visual memory should be performed, but these are done less often at the bedside. Assessment of memory for more remote personal events is rarely relevant, except in suspected transient epileptic amnesia where autobiographical memory deficits are a key feature. This is hard to test at the bedside, so it would usually be based on the patient's description or a more formal neuropsychological assessment.

The term 'semantic memory' refers to knowledge about the world. A deficit of semantic memory, as seen in semantic dementia, will often manifest primarily as a language disorder because of loss of concepts of object and word meanings.

Higher-order executive functions and social cognition

Executive functions cover a whole range of complex cognitive functions subserved by the frontal lobes, including working memory, planning and organization, shifting set, response inhibition, and abstract thinking. Useful bedside tests include the Luria motor sequence (asking the patient to make a repeating sequence of three hand gestures), go–no go tests (e.g. 'when I clap twice, you clap once; when I clap twice, you don't clap'), and phonemic verbal fluency (how many words beginning with F can be generated in 1 minute). Proverb interpretation, while often done, is probably less useful in practice because of cultural influences on performance. Neurologists also often look for so-called 'frontal release signs'—primitive reflexes that can re-emerge in the context of disease affecting the frontal lobes. These include the grasp reflex, palmomental reflex, and rooting reflex, but their sensitivity and specificity are limited (Schott, 2003).

Dominant hemisphere

Spoken language

By this point in the consultation, you will have had the opportunity to listen to the patient's spontaneous speech in conversation, which is the most useful way of assessing their language function. If there is evidence of dysphasia, the issues to think about are whether the speech is fluent or non-fluent and whether there are any paraphasias (phonemic or semantic). If the patient has difficulty in understanding language, you may wish to do further assessment of their receptive language function. More often, you might go on to test confrontation naming (using pictures in the ACE-III or objects at the bedside) and repetition of words and sentences.

Reading and writing

Further assessment of reading and writing is useful in patients who seem to have a language disorder. Asking them to read a passage of text that contains irregular words (e.g. yacht) and 'made-up' words than can be pronounced phonologically (e.g. the island of 'Scorba') will reveal evidence of any surface or deep dyslexia.

Calculation

Brief assessment of calculation skills is relevant when you wish to assess dominant parietal lobe function. Any mental arithmetic questions can be used, tailored to the educational level of the individual.

Praxis

At the bedside, the most commonly used methods to assess praxis are to ask the patient to copy meaningless hand gestures and asking them to 'mime' the performance of everyday tasks (e.g. using a hammer to bang in a nail, brushing their teeth). It is important to assess both hands, as dyspraxia is frequently asymmetric (as in corticobasal syndromes). It is also worth looking specifically for orofacial dyspraxia, perhaps by asking the patient to yawn or blow a kiss, as this is specifically associated with certain clinical syndromes (e.g. progressive non-fluent aphasia) (for further description, see, for example, Cassidy, 2016).

Non-dominant hemisphere

Spatially directed attention

The phenomenon of 'neglect' is a common and disabling cognitive consequence of non-dominant hemisphere pathology, often seen in the context of stroke. When severe, it can be obvious on informal observation that the patient tends to pay less attention to the (usually) left side. More formal tests include asking patients to bisect a line at the midpoint, cancellation tasks (e.g. drawing lots of lines all over a piece of paper and asking the patient to cross through all of them), or asking the patient to name things they see around the room. Neglect can also become obvious on a clock-drawing task, although this is primarily a test of visuospatial function.

Complex visuo-perceptual skills

These are hard to assess without test materials, but you could draw dots on a page and ask patients to count them without pointing. Another commonly used test (included in the ACE-III) is reading fragmented letters. These are particularly useful in patients with suspected posterior cortical atrophy.

Constructional abilities

Asking a patient to draw a clock can be very helpful in assessing their constructional abilities, as well as executive function (do they have a systematic, planned approach to the task?). Other useful tasks include asking patients to copy intersecting pentagons (as in the MMSE) or a wire cube drawing (as in the ACE-III).

Prosodic components of language (tone, melody/intonation)

These do not require formal testing but should be noted in your conversation with a patient.

Emotional processing

Again, we would rarely perform any formal assessment of emotional processing at the bedside, but inferences can be made from the history (do relatives describe the patient having difficulty reading others' emotions?) or from observations of the patient's behaviour during the consultation.

Gait

Gait and mobility are a particularly useful part of the examination, so they should be assessed wherever possible (and are too often not done in elderly inpatients or those in pain). Look for a good 'get up and go', with regular non-antalgic gait of normal width, stride and symmetry, turning, postural control, and tandem gait walking, without abnormal movements and normal arm swing. Some signs can be missed when walking in an examination room with shoes (e.g. freezing in doorways or dystonic toe in, for example, young Parkinson's disease patients).

Gait and balance are not just neurological in the narrow sense; sensation, orthopaedic abnormalities, pain, balance, vision, and emotions (like fear) play a large role. A poor tandem gait is not a very specific sign of cerebellar disease. If someone struggles to attempt heel–toe walking ('I can't do that doctor') but does not have falls, expectation often plays a large role. The pull test is useful to detect postural instability; however, minimal touch leading to major balance adjustment helpfully illustrates the role of expectation in balance for the patient. Poor postural control can support a PSP diagnosis and is correlated with dementia in Parkinson's disease. Normal pressure hydrocephalus causes a typical 'magnetic gait'. Many movement disorders affect gait, most commonly perhaps drug-induced parkinsonism. Changes in gait also warrant reassessment. We can recommend further reviews (Bronstein and Brandt, 2004; Snijders et al., 2007).

CASE STUDY 2

A psychiatric schizophrenic inpatient with severe retrocollis from tardive dystonia developed a progressive gait disorder but was not examined. Four months later, he was found to have severe leg spasticity as a result of cervical myelopathy requiring surgical intervention. He was left with permanent severe disability.

Cranial nerve examination

(See Box 3.1.)

Box 3.1   The two-minute abbreviated cranial nerve examination

- Observe (for ptosis, facial asymmetry, unequal pupil size)
- Ask, 'Have you noticed any change in your sense of smell?'
- Confrontation visual field testing and visual acuity
- Pupillary light reflexes
- Fundoscopy
- Pursuit eye movements (remember to also look for nystagmus)
- Facial sensation ('Can you feel me touching your face gently on both sides?')
- Facial muscles ('Raise your eyebrows, screw your eyes up tight, puff your cheeks out, show your teeth')
- Tongue: observe for wasting/fasciculation, then test tongue movements

Cranial nerve I

The sense of smell is not routinely examined, but we should ask about it in the history of anyone with personality change, dementia, or parkinsonism. The sense of smell is often impaired in premotor Parkinson's disease. In a patient with constipation, REM sleep behaviour disorder, or new-onset anxiety/depression, impairment of smell would point towards this diagnosis.

CASE STUDY 3

A middle-aged man complained of loss of sense of smell, but this was ignored. Seven years later, after progressive personality changes, including apathy and irritability, he was diagnosed with a 10 × 8 × 7 cm frontal meningioma.

Cranial nerves II, III, IV, and VI

Eye movements can give very useful clues to underlying pathology; they can be abnormal early in, for example, HD and PSP. We recommend testing the range of movement, range, and speed of voluntary saccades and observing whether pursuit is smooth or not. Testing of visual acuity and colour vision is easily done with apps freely available for mobile phones. Fundoscopy remains essential in anyone with a headache (as described earlier). We have now seen several cases of obese patients with comorbid severe functional neurological symptoms and idiopathic intracranial hypertension; again fundoscopy can be crucial in making this diagnosis. Ptosis is important to comment upon, albeit it is rarely present in neuropsychiatric conditions (although depression and myasthenia can go together). Functional 'ptosis' can be identified by overactivity of orbicularis oculi, with a depressed eyebrow (rather than an elevated eyebrow from frontalis overactivity to compensate for levator weakness in true ptosis) and often a raised eyebrow on the opposite side. Pupil size can give a hint towards drug use, and the Argyll-Robertson pupil (and other pupil abnormalities) may point towards syphilis. Convergence paralysis and spasm are quite frequently encountered, and not always associated with clinical symptoms, but seem to be common in other functional movement disorders (Fekete et al., 2012). Functional visual (field) loss often requires ancillary tests, but present pupil reflexes and non-anatomical (e.g. pure tunnel vision) fields on bedside testing support the diagnosis.

CASE STUDY 4

A 60-year-old woman with slowly progressive personality change was admitted to an inpatient psychiatric unit with the diagnosis of (? late-onset) borderline personality disorder. Her inability to reach a target when instructed and move her eyes at request to a target was understood to be part of her personality disorder. These rare signs of optic ataxia and oculomotor apraxia were actually signs of her unusual presentation of Alzheimer's dementia.

Cranial nerve V

In patients with functional neurological symptoms, there can be subjective asymmetry in facial sensation—something not always previously noticed by the patient. If sensation is not delineated in the midline and there are symmetrical corneal reflexes, this sign can be used to support an explanation of functional sensory symptoms to the patient, by describing how it does not match organic sensory loss. Asymmetric perception of a vibration intensity in the forehead also can support a functional sensory diagnosis.

Cranial nerve VII

Facial asymmetry is not infrequently seen in functional disorders. Importantly, facial 'droop' overactivity on the seemingly affected side with variability and platysma activation are diagnostic clues. An excellent recent review describes functional cranial nerve signs in detail (Kaski et al., 2015).

Cranial nerve VIII

Hearing loss is a risk factor for cognitive symptoms in older people, and also a major source of distress and loneliness. It is often undiagnosed and untreated. Rinne's and Weber's tests can be useful to distinguish sensorineural and conductive deafness.

Cranial nerves IX, X, and XI

Cranial nerve IX is not routinely assessed in neuropsychiatry (with the exception of palatal myoclonus which can have a functional origin). Cranial nerve X is essential for many autonomic functions, but also for speech and swallowing. It does not require routine assessment, nor does cranial nerve XI.

Cranial nerve XII

Examination of the tongue for wasting, fasciculation, and speed of movements can be helpful in FTD to consider a motor neurone disease overlap syndrome. Speech is affected by multiple cranial nerves, and they should be examined if speech is abnormal.

Motor systems

(See Box 3.2.)

The motor system comprises multiple elements and is often separated into upper and lower motor neurone disorders—extrapyramidal and cerebellar disorders. Power is best observed

---

Box 3.2 A five-minute abbreviated motor examination

- Observe: wasting, fasciculation, abnormal movements
- Tone: any rigidity or spasticity?
- Power: assess functionally or test muscles systematically
- Bradykinesia: finger-taps
- Reflexes: tendon jerks and the plantar response
- Coordination: finger–nose test
- Gait: get up, walk a few metres, turn and come back, Romberg test, pull test

---

functionally. Good screening assessments include the ability to keep the arms outstretched, to get up from a chair without support (or, even better, up from one knee), and to stand on the heels and toes. Asking patients to show the movement with which they feel they struggle (e.g. writing, drinking with a cup) is essential. Inspection for muscle size asymmetry can be useful.

CASE STUDY 5

A 35-year-old woman with previous complex regional pain syndrome was admitted with rapidly evolving ascending weakness, and complaining of breathing difficulties. She was rapidly intubated on ITU and treated for presumed Guillain–Barré syndrome. On examination, she had profound bilateral hip extension weakness when this was tested directly, but she had normal hip extension whilst extending her trunk against resistance. A diagnosis of functional weakness was made.

Cerebellar disorders can present with isolated gait ataxia, but often eye movement, speech abnormalities, and limb ataxia are present. A brief screening will exclude significant cerebellar disease. Upper motor neurone disorders are generally quite easy to ascertain, with brisk reflexes, spastic tone, typical spastic positioning of the limbs, and a pyramidal pattern of weakness and gait.

The Babinski reflex is one of the few tests that are absolutely essential. In subacute cognitive decline, an abnormal finding should lead to urgent scanning to exclude a subdural haematoma, a recent stroke, or a space-occupying lesion. In patients with chronic cognitive or behavioural symptoms, it might raise the possibility of a diagnosis of multiple sclerosis (Feinstein et al., 2013). Regular practice helps distinguish an extensor plantar from a (normal) withdrawal response, and self-stimulation can also help in this scenario (Sohrab and Gelb, 2016) (see Fig. 3.1). The frequently encountered mute response (and lack of ticklishness) in functional weakness can also be useful. There is a well-established literature on bias and interobserver and intraobserver reliability in the Babinski reflex (Singerman and Lee, 2008; Van Gijn and Bonke, 1977) and whether it should be routine (Miller and Johnston, 2005).

CASE STUDY 6

A 25-year-old woman presented in great distress with right hemisensory disturbance, following a 'military fitness' session. The neurologist initially wondered about a functional disorder, but she had a right extensor plantar (without any other neurological signs).

Investigations showed a left thalamic infarct from a vertebral artery dissection.

Movement disorders

This chapter cannot cover all movement disorders in neuropsychiatry, but some basic principles are outlined (for further reading, see Burn, 2013; Donaldson et al., 2012; Hallett and Cloninger, 2006).

It is useful to separate movement disorders into hyperkinetic and hypokinetic disorders (but they can be mixed). Hyperkinetic movement disorders (or dyskinesias) include chorea, dystonia, tics, myoclonus, and tremor, but also stereotypies and various other abnormal movements. Hypokinetic disorders are the parkinsonian conditions with brady- and/or hypokinesia.

Myoclonus

Myoclonus (brief and mostly non-rhythmic jerking) is frequently seen in neuropsychiatric conditions. This may be part of the disease (e.g. in different types of dementia) or a consequence of treatment (for a review, see Lozsadi, 2012). It can be difficult to distinguish psychogenic jerks from organic myoclonus (especially in axial/propriospinal jerks), and experts frequently do not agree (van der Salm et al., 2013). Specific neurophysiological approaches (e.g. Bereitschaftspotential) can be a useful adjunct to clinical examination in this situation.

Chorea

Quasi-purposeful movements are typical (e.g. adjusting glasses) and sometimes more obvious when walking. Chorea can be subtle, and not always noticed by the patient, so always ask yourself 'could this be chorea?' if you notice someone is fidgety or restless.

Dystonia

Dystonia is sustained or intermittent muscle contractions causing abnormal, often repetitive, postures or movements, or both. Dystonic movements are typically patterned and twisting and may be tremulous. Dystonia is often initiated or worsened

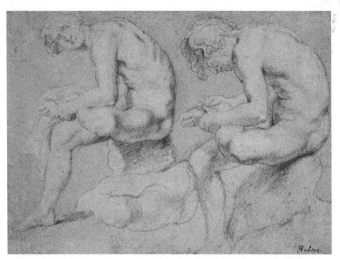

Fig. 3.1 Self-stimulation of the plantar reflex: Spinario—Sir Peter Paul Rubens' 1601 study of the famous Greco-Roman sculpture, showing a person removing a thorn from the sole of his foot.
© The Trustees of British Museum; reproduced with permission.

by voluntary action and associated with overflow muscle activation. It can be classified according to clinical characteristics, including age of onset, temporal features, and body part and associated movement, and according to aetiology (Albanese et al., 2013). Fixed dystonia (defined as immobile dystonic postures that do not return to the neutral position) is best understood as a functional disorder. Typical postures are flexion of the fingers (with digits 4 and 5 more involved than digits 1 and 2, and the thumb often spared) or inversion and plantar flexion of the ankle with curled toes (Schrag et al., 2004).

Tics

Tics are often defined as brief, involuntary (although at times semi-voluntary), stereotyped movements or vocalizations. They are often suppressible, so at times they are not visible during a consultation.

Tremor

Tremors are involuntary, rhythmical oscillations of a body part. It is worth describing the amplitude and body part, and whether at rest or with action (postural, task-specific, or kinetic). Functional tremor is usually distractible, especially with demanding externally paced tasks.

Ask the patient to make finger-tapping movements with one hand (the unaffected hand if the tremor is unilateral) that exactly match the timing of your own (irregular) finger taps. A functional tremor in the contralateral hand will almost always reduce or stop if the task is performed successfully (for video examples, see Thenganatt and Jankovic, 2014). Functional tremors also often entrain (adapt to the variable rhythm presented by the examiner). In our experience, spiral drawing can be very variable between visits, with multiple axes and varying densities within a spiral. At times, with severe functional postural tremor, it can be surprisingly normal.

Hypokinetic movements

Bradykinesia is a very important sign. It is crucial in the diagnosis of parkinsonism but can be over-interpreted if pain or excessive attention makes movements slow and small. True bradykinesia is defined as slowness with progressive reduction in frequency and amplitude (decrement). Assessment therefore requires 15 seconds of unilateral finger tapping (or an alternative like foot tapping). It is not the same as hypokinesia (<50% amplitude of normal controls) which is less specific and seen more often in certain situations such as in PSP (Ling et al., 2012).

Sensory systems

Sensory examination can be particularly subjective and unreliable, so it is unlikely to be useful where there are no sensory symptoms or other abnormal signs on examination.

Where there are symptoms, it is helpful to use a targeted examination to map out the abnormal area. Often pinprick, soft touch, joint position, and vibration can suffice. The absence of anatomical delineation can help explain and support a diagnosis of functional sensory symptoms.

Autonomic systems

There can be disturbance of the autonomic system in neuropsychiatric disorders, including Parkinson's disease, catatonia, and neuroleptic malignant, serotonergic, and cholinergic syndromes. Blood pressure and heart rate are important to measure in both inpatient and outpatient settings, both to detect common comorbidities and side effects of medication. A 30-year-old with new-onset amnesia (and papilloedema on fundoscopy) who proved to have hypertensive encephalopathy recently reminded us of the importance of these routine measures. Autonomic dysregulation is also a feature of NMDA encephalitis, so it may point towards the diagnosis. Bowel, bladder, and sexual function is usually assessed primarily from the history. There is a literature on heart rate variability (and feedback treatment) in dissociation/psychogenic non-epileptic seizures (PNES) (Ponnusamy et al., 2012; van der Kruijs et al., 2014) and postural orthostatic tachycardia syndrome in functional neurological symptoms (Ricciardi et al., 2015), but routine assessment is rarely performed.

Soft neurological signs in mental illness

There is a large literature on soft neurological signs in mental illness, mostly studied with the Neurological Evaluation Scale (NES) (Buchanan and Heinrichs, 1989). These signs range from what is called primary signs (18) to sensory integration (5), motor coordination (4), and sequencing (3) signs on a 0 (normal) to 2 (abnormal) scale. Other scales are available, e.g. the Cambridge Neurological Inventory (Chen et al., 1995). In our opinion, some signs are highly subjective. While they are not infrequently seen in mental illness and as a result of its treatment, their importance is unclear (for a review on schizophrenia, see Chan et al., 2010). Some have many causes (so not always 'neurological'), e.g. gaze impersistence and right/left confusion. Abnormal tone occurs (e.g. in catatonia) for various reasons, and hyperreflexia is not defined (and even if it was, it is highly subjective). Tremor is commonly seen as a result of medication or anxiety. However, soft neurological signs have been found in treatment-naïve patients with schizophrenia (Venkatasubramanian et al., 2003) and their relatives (Neelam et al., 2011), and in cannabis dependence (Dervaux et al., 2013), attention-deficit/hyperactivity disorder (ADHD) (Patankar et al., 2012), social phobia (Hollander et al., 1996), and bipolar disorder (Goswami et al., 2006). They predict poor treatment response in OCD (Hollander et al., 2005) and have structural brain correlates (Dazzan et al., 2004). In our opinion, the scale and the study of the signs would benefit from much more validation, studying test interpretation, and perhaps certification (like the Unified Parkinson's Disease Rating Scale (UPDRS) in Parkinson's disease—see Goetz et al., 2008; or the Unified Huntington's Disease Rating Scale (UHDRS) in HD—see Anon, 1996).

Uses and pitfalls of scales

There are two key clinical areas where rating scales are particularly useful. Firstly, they can provide a standardized approach to brief cognitive assessment with validated norms. Secondly, self-rating scales can be helpful to screen for symptoms that are important but which you might not have time to do justice to in the history.

For a very brief cognitive assessment, the MMSE is frequently used and has the advantage of being widely understood by clinicians. However, as it was designed for the assessment of AD, it is heavily weighted towards orientation and memory. The MoCA assesses frontal function better, so it may be more useful in vascular disease and parkinsonian disorders (Nasreddine and Phillips, 2005). These scales are useful to document longitudinal change in delirium and dementia. For a more standardized cognitive assessment that is still short enough to use in clinic, we would recommend the ACE-III. The limitations of all these standardized instruments also need to be recognized. Age, education, ethnic group, hearing, vision, and first language all influence their interpretation. Low scores frequently arise from non-neurological explanations like pain, medication, effort, or sleep apnoea. In patients with a functional cognitive disorder, we often find it best to avoid doing a scale in the first place, as 'false-positive' low scores are so common and normal scores do not always reassure (see a reply of Coebergh et al., 2016 to Pennington et al.). A patient with functional cognitive symptoms can sometimes be reassured by a good score on the ACE-III, but not by the MMSE as it is often too easy.

We find the FAB a quick and useful bedside test when a more detailed assessment of executive function is required. It has been validated in many neuropsychiatric conditions (Dubois et al., 2000). Scales for the assessment of motor symptoms are probably most useful in the context of trials, rather than everyday clinical practice. However, they can sometimes give structure and support to a diagnosis, especially if disease-specific like in Parkinson's disease, PSP (Golbe et al., 2007), HD, or tic disorders (Leckman et al., 1989). Another useful condition to assess with scales is catatonia (see, for example, Bush et al., 1996; Northoff et al., 1999).

Self-rating scales are particularly useful to detect important symptoms that may not be volunteered by patients in the history. It can be useful to send these out to patients prior to clinic appointments or to ask them to complete them in the waiting room. A good example would be the use of non-motor symptom scales in Parkinson's disease (Rios Romenets et al., 2012). The large impact of apathy on quality of life is frequently not sufficiently appreciated, and the short-form Lille Apathy rating scale (Dujardin et al., 2013) can structure its assessment (for a review, see Stanton and Carson, 2016). A strong argument can be made for using scales to screen for depression and anxiety in a whole range of neurological and neuropsychiatric conditions, e.g. the Hospital and Anxiety Depression Scale (HADS)/Beck Depression Inventory (BDI) (Beck et al., 1993; Zigmond and Snaith, 1983).

The neurological examination as treatment in functional symptoms

In functional disorders, there has been a shift in emphasis from physical examination solely to exclude organic disease towards using positive signs on physical examination as part of making a consultation therapeutic (Stone, 2016). Used well, these physical signs can show patients that there can be reversibility and demonstrate the role of attention, distraction, and expectation (Stone and Edwards, 2012).

Much of the treatment of functional symptoms is in the whole assessment, including the history, examination, and explanation. Some doctors talk little during the examination, but especially with functional symptoms, a joke, reassurance, or a detailed explanation can do a lot (e.g. 'your fundoscopy is normal which tells me the pressure you feel is of no concern to me'). It also is a way to explain complex pathophysiology. For instance, patients can observe that their slowness at finger tapping improves when they tap to a rhythm or that their gait is better when walking backwards. This not only shows that more normal function is possible, but also demonstrates the important role of attention in functional symptoms. In patients with suspected functional hemiparesis, Hoover's sign (see Fig. 3.2) is very useful to make a positive diagnosis. Firstly, demonstrate weakness of hip extension on the affected side. Then re-test hip extension on that side, while the patient flexes the contralateral hip against resistance, to demonstrate that it returns to normal and affirm to the patient they cannot control it voluntarily (Stone and Sharpe, 2001). Patients can appreciate that voluntary movement is much more difficult than automatic movement, particularly using analogies from sport or music (a golfer trying to putt, or a pianist's performance halting if they start to think about what they are doing). We have run through hospital corridors with patients who struggled to walk after showing them a video of a patient with functional symptoms who could do just that (https://open.abc.net. au/explore/114378).

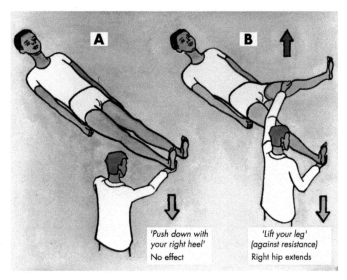

Fig. 3.2 Hoover's sign.
Reproduced with permission from J. Stone. Functional symptoms and signs in neurology: assessment and diagnosis. *Neurology, Neurosurgery & Psychiatry*, 76 (suppl. 1). Copyright © 2005, *British Medical Journal*. http://dx.doi.org/10.1136/ jnnp.2004.061655.

findings (Hallett et al., 2016) (for a brief discussion of functional movement disorders, see Table 3.2).

CASE STUDY 7

An 80-year-old woman presented with a gait disorder since a fall 2 years previously. On examination, her gait normalized when talking about her previous holiday. The neurologist used this finding to explain the important role of attention in her symptoms.

Physical signs may also help explain the concept of dissociation and bodily awareness ('see how your weak foot is not ticklish; that is maybe because it does not feel like it belongs to you'). Demonstrating how you make the diagnosis can give great confidence to patients and those who accompany them, in a way that simply pointing out the absence of organic disease does not. It can also suggest therapeutic strategies ('see how your tremor stops if you tap with your other hand? You might be able to use this to stop it sometimes. There is actually evidence that it works for other people'). The sensitivity and specificity of the various signs of functional disorders are becoming better characterized (Daum et al., 2014).

For functional fixed dystonia, examination under propofol sedation can be helpful to see whether deformity is fixed or not (typically inversion at the feet and flexion at the wrist). With the use of video and ongoing movement activation, often together with physiotherapists, this can kick-start physical recovery, sometimes dramatically after very long periods of abnormal movement (Stone et al., 2014). We highly recommend a recommendation consensus for physiotherapy treatment of functional disorders (parts of which can be attempted by any clinician) (Nielsen et al., 2015) and an extensive review in the *Handbook of Clinical Neurology* of the current state of knowledge, with detailed explanation of examination

Conclusion

The neurological examination in neuropsychiatry is an essential part of the assessment of a patient (see Table 3.3). It supports the role of the brain in psychiatry, but through all the roles of the examination in the doctor–patient ritual, it also supports the role of the mind in neurology. There is no such thing as a 'full neurological examination', but used in a targeted way, it is an extremely powerful tool as part of personalized medicine in neuropsychiatry.

KEY LEARNING POINTS

- This chapter discusses how to approach the neurological examination in neuropsychiatry.
- The neurological examination in neuropsychiatry is as essential as the mental state examination in neurology.
- The neurological examination includes the whole nervous system and is part of the wider physical examination.
- Many neurological signs have limited sensitivity, specificity, and intra- and interobserver reliability, so they need to be interpreted in the context of the assessment as a whole.
- Misinterpretation of the neurological examination can lead to unnecessary investigations and treatment or delay diagnosis and management.
- A focused neurological examination in neuropsychiatry, however, is essential for patient satisfaction and diagnosis and can be part of treatment.

Table 3.2 Clues suggesting a functional/psychogenic cause of a movement disorder

Historic	General examination

Abrupt onset (symptoms often maximal at that time)
Static course
Spontaneous remissions/cures
Paroxysmal symptoms (generally non-kinesigenic)*
Psychiatric comorbidities†
Secondary gain (often not apparent)
Risk factors for conversion disorder (sexual and physical abuse, trauma)
Psychological stressors
Multiple somatizations/undiagnosed conditions
Employed in allied health professions (infrequent)
	Movement inconsistent:
	• Variability over time (frequency, amplitude, direction/distribution of movement)
	• Distractibility reduces or resolves, attention increases movement
	• Entrainment (especially tremor)
	
	Movement incongruous with organic movement disorders:
	• Mixed (often bizarre) movement disorders
	• Paroxysmal attacks (including pseudoseizures)
	• Precipitated paroxysms (often suggestible/startle)
	  Suggestibility
	  Effortful production or deliberate slowness (without fatiguing) of movement
	  Self-inflicted injury (caution: tic disorders)
	  Delayed and excessive startle response to a stimulus
	  Burst of verbal gibberish or stuttering speech
	  False (give-away) weakness
	  Non-anatomic sensory loss or spread of movement
	  Certain types of abnormal movements common in individuals with functional movement disorders‡
	  Functional disability out of proportion to examination findings

* Separation from organic paroxysmal dyskinesias can be challenging, particularly if they occur infrequently with prolonged symptom-free periods.

† Psychiatric diseases can also coincide with organic illness or be present as part of the organic movement disorder.

‡ Such movements include dystonia that begins as a fixed posture (particularly if abrupt-onset, painful, and early contractures are seen); bizarre gait; twisting facial movements that move the mouth to one side or the other (organic dystonia of the facial muscles usually does not pull the mouth side-wise).

Reproduced with permission from M.-P. Stenner and P. Haggard. Voluntary or involuntary? A neurophysiologic approach to functional movement disorders. In *Functional Neurologic Disorders*, 1st Edition, Volume 139. Copyright © 2016 Elsevier B.V. All rights reserved. https://doi.org/10.1016/B978-0-12-801772-2.00011-4. Source data from Gupta, A., and Lang A. E. (2009). Psychogenic movement disorders. *Curr Opin Neurol.*, 22, 4: 53–67.

Table 3.3 Treatable diagnoses not to miss

Diagnosis	Typical clinical context in neuropsychiatry	Key signs to look for on examination	Treatment
Wernicke's encephalopathy	Any recent significant cognitive change or gait disorder, with alcohol history or poor oral intake	Ataxia, ophthalmoplegia	IV Pabrinex®
Hepatic encephalopathy	Any encephalopathic patient, especially with low albumin or impaired coagulation	Asterixis ('liver flap')	Laxatives, reduced protein intake, rifamixin
Neuroleptic malignant syndrome	Patients on antipsychotic medication	Rigidity, autonomic dysfunction, encephalopathy	Stop antipsychotics, supportive care, dantrolene
Serotonin syndrome	Patients on serotonergic medications (especially in combination)	Hyperreflexia, myoclonus, autonomic dysfunction, encephalopathy	Stop serotonergic medication, supportive care
Wilson's disease	Cognitive and behavioural symptoms in younger patients, especially with liver disease	Parkinsonism, dystonia, ataxia, Kayser–Fleischer rings	Dietary change, copper chelation
Anti-NMDA antibody encephalitis	Atypical presentations of psychosis, particularly with seizures	Hyperkinetic movement disorders, autonomic dysfunction	Immunomodulatory therapy
Anti-VGKC complex (LG1/CASP2) encephalitis	Subacute confusion or new-onset seizures (at times resembling brief panic attacks)	Faciobrachial dystonic seizures, memory deficits	Immunomodulatory therapy

NMDA, *N*-methyl-*D*-aspartate; VGKC, voltage-gated potassium channel.

REFERENCES

Albanese, A. et al., 2013. Phenomenology and classification of dystonia: a consensus update. *Movement Disorders*, 28, 863–73.

Allen, C., 2012. Teaching clinical neurology. *Practical Neurology*, 12, 97–102.

Anon, 1996. Unified Huntington's Disease Rating Scale: reliability and consistency. Huntington Study Group. *Movement Disorders*, 11, 136–42.

Beck, A.T., Steer, R.A., and Brown, G.K., 1996. *Manual for the Beck Depression Inventory-II*. San Antonio, TX: Psychological Corporation.

Bronstein, A. and Brandt, M.W., 2004. *Clinical Disorders of Balance, Posture and Gait*, second edition. London: Arnold.

Buchanan, R.W. and Heinrichs, D.W., 1989. The Neurological Evaluation Scale (NES): a structured instrument for the assessment of neurological signs in schizophrenia. *Psychiatry Research*, 27, 335–50.

Burn, D., 2013. *Oxford Textbook of Movement Disorders*. Oxford: Oxford University Press.

Bush, G. et al., 1996. Catatonia. I. Rating scale and standardized examination. *Acta psychiatrica Scandinavica*, 93, 129–36.

Cassidy, A., 2016. The clinical assessment of apraxia. *Practical Neurology*, 16, 317–22.

Chan, R.C.K. et al., 2010. Neurological soft signs in schizophrenia: A meta-analysis. *Schizophrenia Bulletin*, 36, 1089–104.

Chen, E.Y.H. et al., 1995. The Cambridge Neurological Inventory: A clinical instrument for assessment of soft neurological signs in psychiatric patients. *Psychiatry Research*, 56, 183–204.

Coebergh, J.A., Stanton, B.R., and Isaacs, J. 2016. Reply to Functional cognitive disorder: what is it and what to do about it? *Practical Neurology*. Available from: https://pn.bmj.com/content/15/6/436.responses

Coebergh, J.A., Wren, D.R., and Mumford, C.J., 2014. 'Undiagnosing' neurological disease: how to do it, and when not to. *Practical neurology*, 14, 436–9.

Daum, C. et al., 2015. Interobserver agreement and validity of bedside 'positive signs' for functional weakness, sensory and gait disormders in conversion disorder: a pilot study. *Journal of Neurology, Neurosurgery, and Psychiatry*, 86, 425–30.

Dazzan, P. et al., 2004. The structural brain correlates of neurological soft signs in AESOP first-episode psychoses study. *Brain : a journal of neurology*, 127(Pt 1), 143–53.

Dervaux, A. et al., 2013. Neurological soft signs in non-psychotic patients with cannabis dependence. *Addiction Biology*, 18, 214–21.

Donaldson, I. et al., 2012. *Marsden's Book of Movement Disorders*, Oxford: Oxford University Press.

Dubois, B. et al., 2000. The FAB: a Frontal Assessment Battery at bedside. *Neurology*, 55, 1621–6.

Dujardin, K. et al., 2013. Assessing apathy in everyday clinical practice with the short-form Lille Apathy rating scale. *Movement Disorders*, 28, 2014–19.

Feinstein, A. et al., 2013. Cognitive and neuropsychiatric disease manifestations in MS. *Multiple Sclerosis and Related Disorders*, 2, 4–12.

Fekete, R. et al., 2012. Convergence spasm in conversion disorders: prevalence in psychogenic and other movement disorders compared with controls. *Journal of Neurology, Neurosurgery, and Psychiatry*, 83, 202–4.

Folstein, M.F., Folstein, S.E. & McHugh, P.R., 1975. 'Mini-mental state'. A practical method for grading the cognitive state of patients for the clinician. *Journal of Psychiatric Research*, 12, 189–98.

Goetz, C.G. et al., 2008. Movement Disorder Society-Sponsored Revision of the Unified Parkinson's Disease Rating Scale (MDS-UPDRS): Scale presentation and clinimetric testing results. *Movement Disorders*, 23, 2129–70.

Golbe, L.I. et al., 2007. A clinical rating scale for progressive supranuclear palsy. *Brain*, 130(Pt 6), 1552–65.

Goswami, U. et al., 2006. Neuropsychological dysfunction, soft neurological signs and social disability in euthymic patients with bipolar disorder. *British Journal of Psychiatry*, 188, 366–73.

Groopman, J., 2009. Diagnosis: What Doctors Are Missing. *The New York Review of Books*. 56, 26.

Hallett, M. and Cloninger, R., 2006. *Psychogenic Movement Disorders*. Philadelphia, PA: Lippincott Williams & Wilkins.

Hallett, M., Stone, J., and Carson, A., 2016. *Functional Neurologic Disorders*, first edition, Volume 139. Amsterdam: Elsevier.

Hodges, J.R., 2007. *Cognitive Assessment for Clinicians*. Oxford: Oxford University Press.

Hollander, E. et al., 1996. Neurological soft signs in social phobia. *Neuropsychiatry, Neuropsychology, & Behavioral Neurology*, 9, 182–5.

Hollander, E. et al., 2005. Neurological Soft Signs as Predictors of Treatment Response to Selective Serotonin Reuptake Inhibitors in Obsessive-Compulsive Disorder. *Journal of Neuropsychiatry and Clinical Neurosciences*, 17, 472–7.

Hsieh, S. et al., 2013. Validation of the Addenbrooke's Cognitive Examination III in Frontotemporal Dementia and Alzheimer's Disease. *Dementia and Geriatric Cognitive Disorders*, 36, 242–50.

Jaspers, K., Hoenig, J., and Hamilton, M.W., 1997. *General Psychopathology*, Volume II. Berlin Heidelberg: Springer-Verlag.

Kaski, D. et al., 2015. Cranial functional (psychogenic) movement disorders. *The Lancet Neurology*, 14, 1196–205.

Leckman, J.F. et al., 1989. The Yale Global Tic Severity Scale: initial testing of a clinician-rated scale of tic severity. *Journal of the American Academy of Child and Adolescent Psychiatry*, 28, 566–73.

Ling, H. et al., 2012. Hypokinesia without decrement distinguishes progressive supranuclear palsy from Parkinson's disease. *Brain*, 135(Pt 4), 1141–53.

Lozsadi, D., 2012. Myoclonus: a pragmatic approach. *Practical Neurology*, 12, 215–24.

Miller, T.M. and Johnston, S.C., 2005. Should the Babinski sign be part of the routine neurologic examination? *Neurology*, 65, 1165–8.

Moore, F.G.A. and Chalk, C., 2009. The essential neurologic examination: what should medical students be taught? *Neurology*, 72, 2020–3.

Nasreddine, Z. & Phillips, N., 2005. The Montreal Cognitive Assessment, MoCA: a brief screening tool for mild cognitive impairment. *Journal of the American Geriatric Society*, 53, 695–9.

Neelam, K., Garg, D., and Marshall, M., 2011. A systematic review and meta-analysis of neurological soft signs in relatives of people with schizophrenia. *BMC Psychiatry*, 11, 139.

Nielsen, G. et al., 2015. Physiotherapy for functional motor disorders: a consensus recommendation. *Journal of Neurology, Neurosurgery, and Psychiatry*, 86, 1113–19.

Northoff, G. et al., 1999. Catatonia as a psychomotor syndrome: a rating scale and extrapyramidal motor symptoms. *Movement disorders*, 14, 404–16.

Patankar, V.C. et al., 2012. Neurological soft signs in children with attention deficit hyperactivity disorder. *Indian Journal of Psychiatry*, 54, 159–65.

Ponnusamy A, Marques JL, Reuber M., 2012. Comparison of heart rate variability parameters during complex partial seizures and psychogenic nonepileptic seizures. *Epilepsia*, 53, 1314–21.

Ricciardi, L., et al., 2015. *Functional (Psychogenic) Neurological Symptoms In Patients With Postural Tachycardia Syndrome (PoTS)*. MDS 19th International Congress of Parkinson's Disease and Movement Disorders. Volume 30, June 2015 Abstract.

Rios Romenets, S. et al., 2012. Validation of the non-motor symptoms questionnaire (NMS-Quest). *Parkinsonism and Related Disorders*, 18, 54–8.

Schott, J.M., 2003. The grasp and other primitive reflexes. *Journal of Neurology, Neurosurgery, and Psychiatry*, 74, 558–60.

Schrag, A. et al., 2004. The syndrome of fixed dystonia: An evaluation of 103 patients. *Brain*, 127, 2360–72.

Singerman, J. and Lee, L., 2008. Consistency of the Babinski reflex and its variants. *European Journal of Neurology*, 15, 960–4.

Snijders, A.H. et al., 2007. Neurological gait disorders in elderly people: clinical approach and classification. *The Lancet Neurology*, 6, 63–74.

Sohrab, S.A. and Gelb, D., 2016. Value of self-induced plantar reflex in distinguishing Babinski from withdrawal. *Neurology*, 86, 977.

Stanton, B.R. and Carson, A., 2016. Apathy: a practical guide for neurologists. *Practical Neurology*, 16, 42–7.

Stone, J., 2016. Functional neurological disorders: the neurological assessment as treatment. *Practical Neurology*, 16, 7–17.

Stone, J. and Edwards, M., 2012. Trick or treat?: Showing patients with functional (psychogenic) motor symptoms their physical signs. *Neurology*, 79, 282–4.

Stone, J. and Sharpe, M., 2001. Hoover' s sign. *Practical Neurology*, 1, 50–3.

Stone, J., Hoeritzauer, I., Brown, K., and Carson, A., 2014. Therapeutic sedation for functional (psychogenic) neurological symptoms. *Journal of Psychosomatic Research*, 76, 165–8.

Teasdale, G. and Jennett, B., 1974. Assessment Of Coma And Impared Conciousness. *The Lancet*, 304, 81–4.

Thenganatt, M.A. and Jankovic, J., 2014. Psychogenic tremor: a video guide to its distinguishing features. *Tremor and Other Hyperkinetic Movements*, 4, 253.

Van der Kruijs, S.J., et al., 2014. Neurophysiological correlates of dissociative symptoms. *Journal of Neurology, Neurosurgery, and Psychiatry*, 85, 174–9.

Van der Salm, S.M.A. et al., 2013. The eye of the beholder: inter-rater agreement among experts on psychogenic jerky movement disorders. *Journal of Neurology, Neurosurgery, and Psychiatry*, 84, 742–7.

Van Gijn, J. and Bonke, B., 1977. Interpretation of plantar reflexes: biasing effect of other signs and symptoms. *Journal of Neurology, Neurosurgery, and Psychiatry*, 40, 787–9.

Venkatasubramanian, G., et al., 2003. Neurological soft signs in never-treated schizophrenia. *Acta Psychiatrica Scandinavica*, 108, 144–6.

Warlow, C., 2010. Why I have not stopped examining patients. *Practical Neurology*, 10, 126–8.

Wiles, C.M., 2013. Introducing neurological examination for medical undergraduates—how I do it. *Practical Neurology*, 13, 49–50.

Zeman, A., 2014. Neurology is psychiatry—and vice versa. *Practical Neurology*, 14, 136–44.

Zigmond, A.S. and Snaith, R.P., 1983. The hospital anxiety and depression scale (HADS). *Acta Psychiatrica Scandinavica*, 67, 361–70.

4

Philosophy and neuropsychiatry

Norman A. Poole and Derek Bolton

Introduction

A chapter on the philosophy of neuropsychiatry might be expected to comprehensively review the literature on the notoriously thorny mind–body problem, bequeathed to us by Descartes' dictum *cogito ergo sum*. This is not the approach taken here for a variety of reasons. Firstly, that literature is vast and complex, so any review will necessarily be superficial and elide the actual philosophical issues. There are a number of excellent book-length surveys and the interested reader could usefully begin with Robinson's (2016) entry on dualism in the *Stanford Encyclopedia of Philosophy*. Secondly, the mind–body problem is not unique to neuropsychiatry but pervades all of medicine, so its inclusion in a neuropsychiatry textbook is no more or less essential than in any medical textbook. Finally, it is unlikely that neuropsychiatrically inclined neurologists or psychiatrists seriously entertain a philosophy of mind that is not soundly materialist. Clinical phenomena would, on the face of it, seem to refute that mind and body represent distinct ontological realms (dualism) or that reality is a form of thought (idealism). Materialism holds that mind and body are identical, but the precise nature of the identity relation remains obscure and, once again, not of interest to the neuropsychiatrist exclusively. One aspect of this identity relation plays out in a particular manner in the neuropsychiatric domain, however, and it will be the focus of this chapter. If the mind and brain are identical, how do descriptions of normal and abnormal mental phenomena relate to neurobiology? Specifically, while normal-range mental phenomena are described in terms of meanings and reasons, somehow implemented in the living, functional brain, it seems possible that abnormal mental phenomena can be regarded not in those terms, but rather as senseless and reasonless upshots of brain dysfunction.

Identifying the patient

Within the philosophy of psychiatry, doctors have been criticized for a tendency to focus their gaze upon the patient as a person suffering disease, ignoring their own role in a dyadic relationship in which values colour both diagnosis and therapeutics. Foucault is credited with bringing such issues to the fore: 'The asylum of the age of positivism, which it is Pinel's glory to have founded, is not a free realm of observation, diagnosis, and therapeutics; it is a juridical space where one is accused, judged, and condemned' (Foucault, 2006/1967, p. 269).

Psychiatrists do reflect on the nature of this relationship but continue to ignore how the patient came to be regarded as such. Of particular relevance here are judgements made by carers and referrers to neuropsychiatry, typically colleagues in neurology. But what is it about a patient's presentation that suggests neuropsychiatric assessment is warranted? This issue engages the different types of description mentioned above. Neurologists typically invoke causal neurobiological processes, while psychiatric explanation involves mental states and processes.

Nick Haslam has recently proposed a model of 'folk psychiatry' to explain how people come to regard behaviour (including the verbal sort) as abnormal (Haslam, 2005). When carers 'pathologize'[1] behaviour, it is then attributed to one of three potential causes: moral, medical, or psychological. Haslam has argued that judging behaviour to be pathological is a complex process involving at least four elements: (i) infrequently encountered behaviour is, by definition, unfamiliar, hence puzzling; (ii) pathologizing occurs where it is difficult for an observer to provide a coherent explanation for particular acts, and Ahn, Novick, and Kim (2003) have shown that supplying plausible explanations attenuates the perceived abnormality of clinical phenomena;[2] (iii) a behaviour that is deemed unusual or distinctive tends to be attributed internally to the person—such an attribution is reinforced where the behaviour is stable across contexts; and (iv) finally, groups that are considered small (minority), yet held to share common (and threatening) characteristics, are regarded as distinct entities, so are more readily pathologized.

In Haslam's model, while pathologizing opens up an explanatory gap that needs to be filled, it need not necessarily indicate mental disorder. Behaviour that contravenes social norms can be viewed as *morally* reprehensible, remaining the responsibility of the person so behaving. *Medicalizing*, on the other hand, attributes the behaviour to abnormality caused by a disease, hence outside the person's

---

[1] Haslam confusingly uses the term 'pathologize' to refer to all seemingly abnormal or norm-breaking behaviour, whether attributable to disease or not.

[2] Providing brain-based causal explanations, rather than those based on life events, did not make the behaviour any more understandable or normal to the observers.

control. The former explains phenomena in terms of reasons, while the latter looks to brute biological causation. Malle (1999) observes that the majority of philosophers describe reasons as beliefs or desires that both motivate and rationally support action. Haslam describes a third explanatory style—*psychologizing*—that lies between the moralizing and medicalizing poles: 'To psychologize abnormality is to make sense of it using psychological concepts that have causal rather than intentional force' (Haslam, 2003, p. 630). ('Intentional' is here to be understood as reason-type explanations.) To be precise, psychological explanations: (i) invoke mechanistic and functional concepts (e.g. absence of empathy in psychopathic disregard for others); (ii) challenge the principle that actors are aware of their own reasons/motivations *and* that these rationally support the action; (iii) involve causal histories such as the actor's personality traits and psychosocial development; and (iv) appeal to emotions and their relationship to reflex behaviour and somatic processes. This partly causal story of which the actor is only partially aware is unique to psychological explanations and marks it as distinct from fully 'intentional' accounts.

Thus, while the process of pathologizing tells us how carers identify abnormality, there is no clear-cut method pointing to the correct explanatory framework, and this leaves room for conflict between patients, carers, and different professionals, all of whom may adopt different explanations for the seemingly abnormal behaviour (Haslam, 2003). Doctors, one expects, should be inclined towards medicalizing, while carers may, at times, adopt moralizing or psychologizing explanations. The judgements involved in such attributions are, it should be noted, conceptual rather than empirical matters, so empirical studies cannot resolve them. Here is where psychiatry meets philosophy. To see this, consider Horwitz and Wakefield's (2007) arguments in *The Loss of Sadness* about whether a mildly depressed mood is best considered an illness or a psychological reaction to adversity.[3] A carer may account for a loved one's lowered mood in terms of recent losses and a tendency to withdraw from conflict (psychologizing), a lack of resolve (moralizing), or a neurotransmitter deficit (medicalizing). Those authors advise that discerning between these attributions depends on whether one can find an 'appropriate reason' (Horowitz and Wakefield, 2007, p. 6) for the depressed mood. Analogously, the DSM-5 proposes that a pattern of psychological/behavioural phenomena cannot be considered a mental disorder if it is an 'expectable response' to stress or loss. While frequency of response is cited, there is no mention of specific rates, so it seems it is clinicians' intuitions about how people should respond that bear the load. The point here is not to adjudicate on these issues, but to highlight that failure to identify reasons for psychological phenomena is implicated in their attribution as mental disorders. Reason-type explanations are specifically disavowed in empirical science, which seeks to understand statistical correlations and underlying causation; reasons, on the other hand, are concerned with norms, rules, values, and coherence. They are fundamentally different approaches, as discussed at length by Karl Jaspers (1997/1957) in *General Psychopathology* and by other major twentieth-century philosophers such as Donald Davidson (2004), Ludwig Wittgenstein (1953/2001), and Gilbert Ryle (1949/2000).

[3] Note that these arguments can apply either at the pathologizing stage, undermining the initial attribution, or at the second stage where the explanatory gap is resolved.

Attributions in neuropsychiatry

Neuropsychiatry faces these issues in a particularly acute form for a number of inter-related reasons. Neuropsychiatrists are involved in managing conversion/dissociative disorder, but these patients are identified and referred by neurologists. While there are positive physical indicators of some conversion disorders, such as Hoover's sign (Stone and Sharpe, 2000) for the identification of functional leg weakness, these are neither fully reliable nor available for the whole range of functional symptoms. Instead, neurologists utilize psychological and moral concepts, such as deception, trauma, and distress, as part of their diagnostic and explanatory framework for such 'pathologized' phenomena, while admitting this strays outside their professional comfort zone (Kanaan et al., 2009). So, in contrast to the case of depression, here psychological concepts are involved when differentiating functional from 'organic' neurological disorders.

Also, the neuropsychiatric assessment involves 'objective' investigations, such as neuroimaging, blood tests, and neuropsychology, to a greater degree than other psychiatric sub-specialties, but the relationship between the test findings and mental disorder is far from clear. Bortolloti and Broome (2009) make the strong claim that mental disorder can only be identified at the level of norms; hence neuroimaging and other physical investigations are interesting, yet peripheral to psychiatry's main business. But the relationship is more complex in neuropsychiatry. Take a patient with psychological symptoms following traumatic brain injury. While MRI neither conclusively proves nor disproves a neurological aetiology, the results do enter into diagnostic reasoning. But such clinical judgements are based on whether the behaviour correlates with the severity and site of the lesion, the patient's psychosocial context, and premorbid personality and functioning. Lishman (1978, p. 235), for instance, described a 50-year-old man who suffered a mild head injury but developed memory impairment, suggesting 'organic brain damage'. Ultimately it was concluded that he had developed depression following the accident and that 'his wife had colluded and reinforced this aspect of the situation'. In other words, reasons and motivations were invoked which thereby excluded neurological injury as an explanation. The point is not that reason-type explanations take primacy over physical investigations, or vice versa, but rather to show how they are implicit in clinical decision-making while their character and function remain relatively obscure.

To summarize what is at stake, neurologists refer patients to the neuropsychiatric clinic or concerned relatives bring them because some aspect of behaviour has been deemed pathological. Yet part of the discrimination between medicalizing, psychologizing, and moralizing explanations concerns the recognition or otherwise of reasons, a decidedly unmedical and unscientific endeavour. Can philosophy help us understand how these discriminations are made?

Philosophical responses

One strategy within the philosophy of neuroscience, called eliminative materialism, has been to criticize reason-type explanations as hopelessly inadequate. On this view, explanation in terms of reasons (dubbed 'folk psychology') is a theory for why people behave as they do, but a theory so defective it should be abandoned altogether. Folk psychology, Churchland (1989) argues, neither explains nor predicts terribly well, while a whole host of phenomena, such as sleep and mental disorder, remain opaque from its purview.[4] Better, they say, to rid ourselves of the theory entirely and replace it with a neuroscientifically valid psychology, in which mental phenomena can be mapped directly onto neurobiological states. This would abolish the role of reasons when adjudicating between medicalizing, psychologizing, and moralizing explanatory frameworks, because there are no such things as reasons. While it is now some time since Churchland first argued for folk psychology's elimination, the hoped-for replacement language has yet to materialize, yet patients and carers continue to present to clinic, so their largely negative thesis cannot address our current concerns.

Another approach, deriving from the phenomenological[5] tradition in philosophy, is to claim that all morbid psychic phenomena, whether associated with neurological disorder or not, can nevertheless be understood meaningfully, either in and of themselves or as response to disease. It is, such critics argue, the consequence of archaic, yet pervasive, philosophies to think otherwise. Indeed, the phenomenologist Louis Sass observes a tendency 'particularly among organic psychiatrists … to ignore the psychological interpretation or empathic understanding of mental symptoms' (Sass, 1992, p. 376). This tendency is, Sass says, nurtured by the development of neuroimaging and somatic markers of disease, but its roots predate them. Psychiatrists and neurologists, inspired by such icons as J Hughlings Jackson, continue to view mental symptoms as mere defects or deficiency secondary to cerebral disease, in keeping with Haslam's medicalizing attribution. Sass thinks though that psychiatrists have the cart before the horse. Psychopathological phenomena are regarded as meaningless because they are first assumed to be symptoms of underlying disease, as opposed to first finding no reason for the person's experiences and then attributing this finding to disorder. While his argument is primarily addressed to schizophrenia, it can equally well be applied to all neuropsychiatric disorders too as every insult, whether psychological or organic, invokes a personally meaningful response.

Matthew Ratcliffe (2004) offers a phenomenological approach to the Capgras delusion that aims to show it can be understood using everyday psychological concepts. He criticizes folk psychology in its current form as inadequate to the task but recommends enrichment, rather than elimination. Central to his description is the loss of an 'affective familiarity', a taken-for-granted background through which the world is experienced, particularly those objects we value. Following its loss, the sufferer no longer feels at home in the world and 'there is a sense in which an "absence," a "not" is part of the experience' (Ratcliffe, 2004, p. 41). Thus, her altered experience of the world is uncanny. She directly perceives her husband as identical, yet unfamiliar; the *alius* is seen *as* an imposter. According to Ratcliffe, due to its neglect of affect, folk psychology cannot account

for the delusional content, but once incorporated, the delusion becomes understandable. He can be taken as either making the strong claim that phenomenological understanding sufficiently explains the entire Capgras phenomenon or a weaker claim that just the response to a loss of affective familiarity can be so understood. If the strong claim, then he needs to account for this loss of affective familiarity. Even if everyday experiences of unfamiliarity go some way towards understanding its uncanniness, the total absence of familiarity seems to remain unexplained. Also, why such a general experience should produce the relatively circumscribed focus upon intimates and the frequently bizarre accounts of their disappearance (e.g. being beamed into outer space) is unclear. If the weaker claim, then he himself concedes the point that something additional is required to provide a full model of the delusion—common-sense everyday psychological concepts are unequal to the task. Indeed, Sass's (1994) own psychological accounts of schizophrenia, based in Wittgensteinian philosophy, intriguing and ingenious as they are, strike the authors as equally alienating as the reductive biological theories they seek to replace.

The philosopher of neuroscience Daniel Dennett has offered another approach that attempts to reconcile the neurobiology and intentionality of mental states. He does not think mental attitudes involved in reason-giving explanations of behaviour, such as belief and desire, should be eliminated entirely; however, there are occasions when they should be discarded. Folk psychological concepts are visible only from a particular perspective, the 'intentional stance' in Dennett's terminology, while the neurobiology of the brain is seen from either the 'physical' or 'design' stances.

Dennett's stances

Dennett (1981) proposed his highly influential 'intentional stance theory' in part to account for the success of our ability to predict complex systems such as chess-playing computers and human beings. It has been so influential because it is compatible with two contemporary scientific programmes: evolutionary biology and artificial intelligence (AI). He demystified mental content by grounding it in evolution, giving succour to the AI project of creating machines that comprehend and act. Mental disorder, however, is an instance where interpretation and prediction of the afflicted person fail from the intentional stance: 'In cases of even the mildest and most familiar cognitive pathology—where people seem to hold contradictory beliefs, or to be deceiving themselves for instance—the canons of interpretation of the intentional strategy fail to yield clear, stable verdicts about which beliefs and desires to attribute to a person' (Dennett, 1989a, p. 28).

To explain such failures, he recommends a shift to the physical stance, just as Haslam claims happens with medicalizing explanations. So let us consider each of Dennett's three stances in turn. In the physical stance, prediction is based on the application of knowledge of causal processes at the physical and microphysical level. Thus, the location and speed of a comet can be calculated for any time in the past or future, according to Kepler's Laws.[6] Where a system has been designed to perform a particular function, it is

---

[4] Although she ignores precisely this point, that mental disorder may represent a failure in the very neurobiological mechanisms that support folk psychology, hence the latter 'breaks down' prohibiting understanding in its own terms.

[5] Phenomenological approaches to philosophy and psychiatry are, in fact, quite distinct. Chris Walker has argued that Jaspers' phenomenological psychiatry owes little to the philosophical tradition, which is better regarded as descriptive psychopathology. There is, however, a strong tradition of truly phenomenological psychiatry of which Sass and Ratcliffe are successors.

[6] Dennett explicitly disregarded the indeterminacy of subatomic particles.

quicker and easier to adopt the design stance to predict future be-haviour. Basically, one predicts behaviour based upon knowledge of the design and the—somewhat risky—assumption that it is per-forming as designed. In the case of highly complex structures, such as animals and humans, the underlying design is not sufficiently well understood to form the basis of predictions, yet still we do predict future behaviour. One easily predicts the outcome when a cat spots a mouse. Prediction is successful here because it is natural for us to adopt Dennett's so-called intentional stance towards other complex objects and organisms.

> Here is how it works: first you decide to treat the object whose be-haviour is to be predicted as a rational agent; then you figure out what beliefs the agent ought to have, given its place in the world and its purpose. Then you figure out what desires it ought to have, on the same considerations, and finally you predict that this rational agent will act to further its goals in the light of its beliefs. A little practical reasoning from the chosen set of beliefs and desires will in many—but not all—instances yield a decision about what the agent ought to do; that is what you predict the agent will do.
>
> (Dennett, 1989a, p. 17)[7]

One assumes that the cat ought both to believe there is a mouse nearby and to be keen on eating it. Therefore, one predicts the cat will stalk its prey. The intentional stance is, however, a highly abstract and risky stance to adopt—risky because of the various assumptions involved. The first assumption is that an agent holds the beliefs it *ought to*. For Dennett, humans and animals come to believe mostly true and relevant facts about the world they inhabit. Even false be-liefs require a special story to be told that involves predominately true beliefs. Likewise, we hold certain sophisticated beliefs unre-lated to direct experience—the belief that all matter is composed of waves, for instance—that may be true or false or neither. Again, these are grounded in true beliefs related to direct experience of the environment. A related assumption is that the agent desires what it *ought to*—the most basic of which include survival, food, procre-ation, pleasure, comfort, and absence of pain. Belief and desire are interdependent upon each other and come to be known through consideration of the agent's ecological niche. The opportunities and threats in the environment enable the identification and weighting of goals relative to that agent's needs for survival, safety, and nutri-tion. Its beliefs and desires will be evident in behaviour, as beliefs about the environment guide the agent towards the fulfilment of de-sires. Destructive or misevaluated desires require a special story to be told that shows they too derive, in the main, from salutary ones.

What permits these assumptions? Natural selection over pro-longed periods ensures optimal adaptation to the environment, for it is precisely those features that increase the probability of propaga-tion and survival that are selected. Dennett is strongly committed to the view that evolution produces optimal design (Dennett, 1989b) and that biological design can be apprehended only through this assumption of optimality (Dennett, 1990). The third and final assumption—that intentional systems are by and large rational—is the most contentious (see, for example, Kahneman, 2011) and is closely tied to evolutionary optimality. Beliefs and desires can be inferred from behaviour only because the behaviour is rational in terms of those beliefs and desires. If someone wants a glass of milk and believes there to be milk in the fridge, his looking under the bed for milk would appear irrational. Indeed, the belief 'milk is in the fridge' is difficult to ascribe, based upon that behaviour. These failures in rationality indicate the intentional stance is redundant, so a drop to the physical stance level is warranted: 'I hold that such errors, as either malfunctions or the outcomes of misdesign, are un-predictable from the intentional stance […] If there is no saving interpretation—if the person in question is irrational—no inter-pretation at all will be settled on' (Dennett, 1989c, p. 84).

That is, where reason-type explanations falter, physical misdesign and biological dysfunction are implicated, just as Haslam claims, and Dennett points to the ways in which they might fail. Dennett, in other words, may be making explicit what has so far been implicit. It was with this in mind that one of the authors (NP) interviewed patients and their carers for a recent research project.

Dennett in the clinic

The patients Liz and John (not their real names and identifying in-formation has been changed) were participants in that study. Take Liz first.[8] Liz is a pleasant South Londoner in her mid seventies. She is down-to-earth and speaks matter-of-factly, but expressively, about her unusual experiences. Following a severe heart attack and right parietal stroke, she spent time in the intensive care unit (ICU). Thereafter, she began reporting visual hallucinations with occa-sional auditory components. She described a vivid scene involving Victorian buildings and an injured child lying on the street; then a large black door opened to reveal an elderly woman with a large cat in a room filled with red furniture. Since discharge, she has seen her artificial flowers dance, seven-foot 'angels', an octogenarian uni-cyclist in evening attire, and tin soldiers materializing as she ap-proaches sleep. Liz now sleeps with earplugs, avoids her bedroom, checks the house for intruders, and has fled these apparitions, causing her to fall.

On the face of it, she does not believe what she ought to about her environment and so we can safely ignore what she says—dropping instead to the physical level to explain and predict her behaviour. While the intentional stance tolerates some false be-liefs about the environment, provided they are grounded in true belief, hallucination and illusion are not in this camp. Take the vertical–horizontal illusion, for instance (see **Fig. 4.1**). This ef-fect is inexplicable from the intentional stance, and only know-ledge of how visual systems are implemented (design stance) can account for such illusions. Dennett, however, explicitly dis-cussed visual hallucinations in *Consciousness Explained* (1993) and appeared of the view that the hallucinated content reflected the sufferer's individual psychology. Thus, it seems hallucin-ation both does and does not involve reason-type explanations. Can this paradox be resolved or does it demonstrate some inco-herence in Dennett's project? An obvious solution might be to

---

[7] Reproduced from Dennett, D. True believers: the intentional strategy and why it works. In *The Intentional Stance*. Cambridge, MA, US: The MIT Press. Copyright © 1989, MIT Press.

[8] The authors thank Professor Michael Kopleman who recruited Liz to the study from his clinical service at St Thomas' Hospital, London.

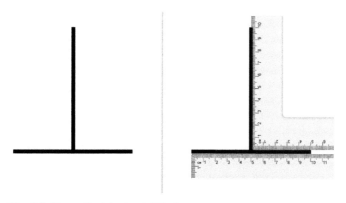

Fig. 4.1 The vertical–horizontal illusion.

reprise the famous form/content dichotomy in psychiatry. Form was said by Jaspers to be universal and biologically determined, while content was filled by culture and individual psychology (Jaspers, 1957/1997, p. 709). Thus, the presence of hallucinations is to be understood as an effect of biological dysfunction, while the hallucinated content reflects more personal factors. While it seems that culture must play some role—dandyish unicyclists are an unlikely universal—visual hallucinations are frequently of animals, children, and gargoyles, moderating the importance of individual factors. In any case, the sharp form/content divide broke down over the twentieth century (Yap, 1974).

A challenging and relevant aspect of Dennett's theory involves the deflated vision of the individual and her own self-reflections. One has no privileged access to mental states or their meaning from the intentional stance perspective, which is avowedly third person-orientated. Just as the novelist has no right to say what her novel definitively means, she has no privileged interpretation of her own behaviour and mental states. One can claim whatever one likes about beliefs and desires etc., but if they are of no use in predicting behaviour, then an observer is licensed to disregard them. There just is no fact of the matter about what the person really means if the claims do not enable one to predict and explain behaviour. This—probably, there have been no empirical studies to date—is exactly how clinicians approach visual hallucinations. They tend not to be overly concerned about the content's meaning beyond its potential assistance diagnosing the underlying cause (ffytche, 2007). Carers and patients, on the other hand, seem more concerned with the meaning of content, and Liz was preoccupied with the symbolism of her hallucinated images, analogous to a need to interpret dreams. Wittgenstein wrote of this in reference to Freud's habit of over-interpreting:

> Freud would ask: 'What made you hallucinate that situation at all?' One might answer that there need not have been *anything* that *made* me hallucinate it.
>
> (Wittgenstein, 1967, p. 49e)

The allure, he explained, of Freudian analysis is twofold: (i) dreams and hallucinations give the impression of being a symbolic language without, in fact, being so; and (ii) the subject feels compelled to accept the wish-fulfilment interpretation in order to prove an initial prejudice thinking has been overcome. But just because one can take a top hat to be a phallic symbol does not make it so in the hallucination. The wish-fulfillment hypothesis precludes alternative interpretations, or none.

There is an inducement to say, 'Yes, of course, it must be like that.' A powerful mythology.

> (Wittgenstein, 1967, p. 52e)

All this seems to suggest that there is a very human proclivity to interpret oneself and others, but while the outcome is interesting, it is far from definitive. So Dennett's intentional stance reading of hallucinations seems to meld this natural tendency with the neuropsychiatrists' drop to the physical stance.

Now let us consider John's extravagant confabulatory claims about his travels. John is a retired 76-year old from Ireland who lived and worked in London for many years. He was abstemious and hard-working until the death of his wife shortly after their fourth child was born. Thereafter, he raised the children alone and continued to work but for a few years he drank heavily. Several years ago, he moved into the same sheltered-housing scheme as his sister, at which point he regained sobriety. All was well until a few months before a recent hospital admission. John began to spend more time away from the flat and would be found at significant locations such as the house where he lived with his wife and old workplaces. He disappeared for 48 hours and was taken to the local emergency department by the police. Neuropsychological testing and neuroimaging were in keeping with the early stages of an Alzheimer's-type dementia, and John was noted to confabulate about his recent past. Coincidentally, confabulation is integral to Dennett's unified theory of mind and meaning. Recall that the agent providing rationales for action is in exactly the same position as her interpreter; she has no direct privileged access to motivations or associated beliefs, so instead she provides what Dennett calls 'approximating confabulations'.

> The agent comes to label its tendencies *as if* they were governed by explicitly represented goals—blueprints for actions—instead of trends of action that emerge from the interplay of the various candidates.
>
> (Dennett, 1996, p. 127)

Thus, for Dennett, confabulation is not restricted to psychopathology but is actually a general state of all our claims to self-knowledge. In Dennett's multiple-drafts vision of consciousness, a multitude of mini-selves constantly produce competing narratives, only one of which enters conscious awareness. The narrative is not selected or composed consciously nor does it arise from an illusory single cohesive self; yet it sustains that illusion.

> Their effect on any audience is to encourage them to (try to) posit a unified agent whose words they are, about whom they are: in short, to posit a *centre of narrative gravity*.
>
> (Dennett, 1996, p. 127)

Pathological confabulation unveils this inherent propensity for self-narration, just as the visual hallucinations exposed the need to self-interpret. Both may be revealing of the utterer's personality and concerns. While recent empirical work has suggested that confabulatory content is affectively weighted towards promoting self-esteem (Fotopoulou, 2010), that is a far cry from it meaning anything in particular. On the other hand, it opposes the frequent description of confabulations as 'purposeless', 'incidental and unmotivated', and 'unintentionally incongruous' noted by Conway and Tacchi (1996). For Dennett, confabulations are epistemically dubious as they are neither justified nor true. That is, they neither cohere with other beliefs nor are grounded in veridical percepts, so they are not the beliefs John ought to hold. When this inconsistency is pointed out,

John does not correct himself but carries on regardless: 'and this is a hospital, it's nearly all hospitals [laughs] wherever you go [laughs], I am telling you, I got the shock of my life'. What is the standard against which the patient's coherence and truth are graded? It consists of shared understandings of what makes sense, which are, to some degree, innate.

> What else, in the end, could one rely on? When considering what we ought to do, our reflections lead us eventually to a consideration of what we in fact do; this is inescapable, for a catalogue of our considered intuitive judgments on what we ought to do is both a compendium of what we do think, and a shining example (by our lights—what else?) of how we ought to think.
>
> (Dennett, 1989c, p. 98)[9]

Uncomfortably perhaps, this reveals the clinician's own sources of values and rationality are deeply involved in evaluating the patient's status.

Conclusion

Dennett's intentional stance theory is appealing to the neuropsychiatrist then for a variety of reasons. He makes hitherto assumed features of our interactions explicit and recognizes that it is erroneous beliefs about the immediate environment and/or the rational inconsistency of actions, beliefs, and desires that point towards psychopathology. But these are obscured from the first-person perspective for there is an inbuilt over-tendency to construct narrative self-reports. Indeed, this tendency is revealed in the psychopathology neuropsychiatrists commonly encounter and is frequently described as impaired insight. As Haslam would say, the professional is medicalizing while the patient is offering a reason-type explanation for his or her current state or even disputing it, should be considered pathological. Of course, as conversion/dissociative disorders show, the divergence need not always be in this direction. Nor is it limited to interactions with patients. Carers (and neurologists) also diverge in their judgements from mental health professionals. And aspects of this disagreement lie in the values of those involved and their ability to empathize and to offer interpretation, as much (or more) than in matters of fact. Similar judgements are involved when evaluating the relevance of physical investigations. Furthermore, the intentional stance theory maintains the conceptual incompatibility of physical-level investigations with intentional-level explanations, while respecting the autonomy of each; one is not prioritized over the other. This is not without cost, however. All of our utterances are seen as provisional only, and meaninglessness becomes a real possibility. But the demarcation between the meaningful and the meaningless cannot be sharply drawn. It is essentially blurred and uncertain, so it has to be negotiated. It is essential because, on the one hand, the mind is inherently meaningful and at least more or less rational, while on the other hand, the mind depends on a well-functioning brain, which can be damaged or otherwise malfunction, with more or less catastrophic effects on mental function. While some cases are clearly of one kind or the other, there are many instances where either or both can occur, and in a fluctuating way.

All parties involved, with their various perspectives and tasks—the patient, the carer, the neurologist, and neuropsychiatrist—have to tolerate uncertainty, disentangle complexities, and find the best ways of managing which they can.

KEY LEARNING POINTS

- This chapter explores the distinction between the mind and the body through the lens of empiricism in neuropsychiatry.
- The argument is made that, although much of our understanding of the relationship between the functioning mind and its abnormalities comes from rationalization, neuropsychiatric practices cannot be based entirely in a materialist idea of the mind and body as identical.
- Although the tests a neuropsychiatrist performs, such as neuroimaging, blood tests, and neuropsychology, appear more objective, the relation between their results and mental disorders is not empirically clear.
- By citing Daniel Dennett's intentional stance theory, the perception that psychopathological phenomena are meaningless is questioned. Dennet's stances are applied to clinical scenarios in order to demonstrate that while physical-level investigations may be conceptually incompatible with those on the intentional level, there is often no way to cleanly separate the two, and both must be considered in the line of a neuropsychiatrist's work.

REFERENCES

Ahn, W., Novick, L.R., and Kim N.S. (2003) Understanding behaviour makes it more normal. *Psychonomic Bulletin and Review*, 746–52.

Bortolotti, L. and Broome M.R. (2009) The future of scientific psychiatry. In: M. Broome and L. Bortolotti (eds.) *Psychiatry as Cognitive Neuroscience: Philosophical Perspectives*. Oxford: Oxford University Press. pp. 365–76.

Churchland, P.S. (1989) *Neurophilosophy: Toward a Unified Science of the Mind/Brain*. Cambridge, MA: MIT Press.

Conway, M. and Tacchi, P.C. (1996) Motivated confabulation. *Neurocase*, 2, 325–39.

Davidson, D. (2004) *Problems of Rationality*. Oxford: Oxford University Press.

Dennett, D.C. (1981) Intentional systems. In: D.C. Dennett. *Brainstorms: Philosophical Essays on Mind and Psychology*. Cambridge, MA: MIT Press. pp. 3–22.

Dennett, D. (1989a) True believers: the intentional strategy and why it works. In: D.C. Dennett. *The Intentional Stance*. Cambridge, MA: MIT Press. pp. 13–42.

Dennett, D. (1989b) Intentional systems in cognitive ethology: the 'Panglossian paradigm' defended. In: D.C. Dennett. *The Intentional Stance*. Cambridge, MA: MIT Press. pp. 236–86.

Dennett, D. (1989c) Making sense of ourselves. In: D.C. Dennett. *The Intentional Stance*. Cambridge, MA: MIT Press. pp. 83–116.

Dennett, D. (1990) The interpretation of texts, people and other artefacts. *Philosophy and Phenomenological Research*, 50, 177–94.

---

[9] Reproduced from Dennett, D. Making Sense of Ourselves. In *The Intentional Stance*. Cambridge, MA, US: The MIT Press. Copyright © 1989, MIT Press.

Dennett, D. (1993) *Consciousness Explained*. London: Penguin Books.

Dennett, D. (1996) *Kinds of Minds: Towards an Understanding of Consciousness*. New York, NY: Basic Books.

ffytche, D.H. (2007) Visual hallucinatory syndromes: past, present, and future. *Dialogues in Clinical Neuroscience*, 9, 173–89.

Fotopoulou, A. (2010) The affective neuropsychology of confabulation and delusion. *Cognitive Neuropsychiatry*, 15, 38–63.

Foucault, M. (2006/1967) *Madness and Civilization: A History of Insanity in the Age of Reason*. New York, NY: Vintage Books. p. 269.

Haslam, N. (2003) Folk psychiatry: lay thinking about mental disorder. *Social Research*, 70, 621–44.

Haslam, N. (2005) Dimensions of Folk Psychiatry. *Review of General Psychology*, 9, 35–47.

Horwitz, A.V. and Wakefield J.C. (2007) *The Loss of Sadness: How Psychiatry Transformed Normal Sorrow into Depressive Disorder*. New York, NY: Oxford University Press.

Jaspers. K. (1997/1957) *General Psychopathology*. Baltimore, MD: John Hopkins University Press.

Kahneman, D. (2011) *Thinking, Fast and Slow*. London: Penguin Books.

Kanaan, R., Armstrong, D., Barnes, P. and Wessely, S. (2009) In the psychiatrist's chair: how neurologists understand conversion disorder. *Brain*, 132, 2889–96.

Lishman, W.A. (1978) *Organic Psychiatry: The Psychological Consequences of Cerebral Disorder*. London: Blackwell Scientific Publications.

Malle, B.F. (1999) How people explain behavior: a new theoretical framework. *Personality and Social Psychology*, 3, 23–48.

Ratcliffe, M. (2004) Interpreting delusions. *Phenomenology and the Cognitive Sciences*, 3, 25–48.

Robinson, H. (2016) Dualism. In: E.N. Zalta (ed.) *Stanford Encyclopedia of Philosophy Archive*. Available at: http://plato.stanford.edu/archives/win2016/entries/dualism/

Ryle, G. (2000/1949) *The Concept of Mind*. London: Penguin Books.

Sass, L.A. (1992) *Madness and Modernisms: Insanity in the Light of Modern Art, Literature, and Thought*. New York, NY: Basic Books.

Sass, L.A. (1994) *The Paradoxes of delusion: Wittgenstein, Schreber and the Schizophrenic Mind*. Ithaca, NY: Cornell University Press.

Stone, J. and Sharpe, M. (2000) Hoover's sign. *Practical Neurology*, 1, 50–3.

Wittgenstein, L. (1953/2001) *Philosophical Investigations*, second edition, London: Blackwell.

Wittgenstein, L. (1967) Conversations on Freud. In: C. Barrett (ed.) *Lectures and Conversations on Aesthetics, Psychology, and Religion*. Compiled from notes taken by Y. Smythies, R. Rhees, and J. Taylor. Berkeley, CA: University of California Press.

Yap, P.M. (1974) *Comparative Psychiatry: A Theoretical Framework*. Toronto, ON: University of Toronto Press.

5

Phenomenology: a neuropsychiatric perspective

Michael Trimble

'Our life is spent filling voids.'

Bergson H, 1911, (p. 298)

Introduction

In order to follow the development of phenomenology, as it later became of importance for neuropsychiatry, it is relevant to understand that the pre-nineteenth-century continental philosophy was an idealistic one, and one of the pillars of establishment was Immanuel Kant (1724–1804). From his time, German philosophy has been concerned with the structure of the mind, forms of thinking, and knowing. Kant distinguished between the noumenon and the phenomenon, in other words things in themselves (*Ding an sich*), in contrast to our experience of them. This led to the conundrum of how the two are united.

His assertion that 'Our intellect does not draw its laws from nature, but imposes its laws upon nature' might be a starting point (Popper, 1963, p. 244). This served as a counterpoint to the embedded empiricist approach to our understanding of the world around us (that what we know must be derived only from the senses) and to the Cartesian assertion that mind and body are quite distinct. Descartes' cleavage of *res cogitans* from *res extensa* provided the logocentric perspective, which became embraced in the split between psychiatry and neurology. The view that the mind can be hived off from the body, and that *logos*, reason, logical sequential thinking was unassailable and, for some (including Descartes), was assured by God, was received dogma.

This rift between the mind and the world has preoccupied neurothinkers exploring the mind–brain problem, and also philosophy, referred to as dualism. An alternative stream of ideas, monism, has insisted not only that there is a world out there, but also that we are a part of that world. Further frames of reference for an understanding of ourselves might begin not with reasoning, but with feeling, and acknowledge our place as one of the millions of species in the world as *Homo sapiens*. The small, but so important, deictic words 'I', 'here', and 'now' place each of us firmly in a time–space context, and with time, things change, meanings change, that which is, including ourselves, always 'becoming' never static.

Of the several philosophical approaches which preoccupied the early twentieth century was logical positivism, which would only accept scientific or verifiable statements as meaningful. But the theoretical role of the natural sciences was diminished by a hermeneutical approach, seeking via interpretation, not so much knowledge but understanding, and psychoanalysis. Another was phenomenology.

Phenomenology: understanding and explanation

Like so many words used in philosophy and science, phenomenology has no secure meaning and has been used quite liberally, especially in clinical practice. To study the science of phenomena begs the question as to what exactly a phenomenon is, and then to ask how one might gain knowledge of it and how one might experience it. The first question is perhaps more of a philosophical issue; the latter two immediately bring us to the subjective actualization of mental states, and their exploration in psychopathology.

Derived from the Greek *phainómenon*—'that which appears'—and *logos*—discourse or study, this chapter will begin with the work of Edmund Husserl (1859–1938). This is not to ignore that others contributed greatly to the philosophies underlying phenomenology, including Max Scheler (1874–1928) and Martin Heidegger (1889–1986), but from a neuropsychiatric perspective, Husserl is an appropriate stepping-off stone.

He states, 'I am conscious of a world endlessly spread out in space, endlessly becoming and having become in time. I am conscious of it: that signifies, above all, that intuitively I find it immediately, that I experience it' (Cerbone, 2006, p. 9). Husserl's philosophical intention was to 'bracket' out all questions of whether things actually exist and other extraneous factors and assumptions, and to isolate mental experiences in order to get to the essence of conscious experiences without prior theoretical judgements. This technique is referred to as *epochē* or 'reduction'.

Another theoretical concept which requires discussion is that of 'intentionality'. Initially linked to medieval scholastic philosophy, it is now associated with Franz Brentano (1838–1917), who used the term to mean that every mental phenomenon has a content (intentional in-existence), which is directed towards an object (but not necessarily a thing), the intentional object. The intentional in-existence is exclusively psychical, and mentation is always about something and directed. Brentano wanted to bring a scientific approach to psychology (*Psychology from an Empirical Standpoint*, 1874) and distinguished between genetic (*genetische Psychologie*) and subjectively descriptive psychology (*beschreibende Psychologie*). The former is the study of psychological phenomena from a third-person perspective, essentially a 'scientific' approach setting up empirical investigations, and the latter is exclusively devoted to the study of consciousness from the first-person perspective.

There was also an important background to these ideas which related to the German language distinctions between two different ways of interpreting history. The empirical view, preferred by the Anglo-Saxon tradition, would try to base history firmly on facts, as if there were natural 'laws' of history which are discoverable. The alternative sought not so much knowledge, but 'understanding', derived from European schools of hermeneutics or text interpretation. 'Meaning' in this latter approach precedes knowledge, with the historian taking what scattered pieces of documentation or artefacts are available and working them into a woven tapestry of identifiable ideas, however incomplete the picture. The historian–psychologist Wilhelm Dilthey (1833–1911) realized that there were no natural 'laws' for history, as there are in the physical sciences. His introduction of the distinction between genetic and descriptive psychology (above) led onto a differential between the study of the sciences of nature (*Naturwissenschaften*) and the human sciences (*Geisteswissenschaften*). Dilthey saw interpretative 'understanding' (to understand—*Verstehen*) as the key for the latter, in contrast to the natural sciences which seek to explain explanation (*Erklären*) by way of cause and effect. The humanities need to 'understand' humans in their *Umwelt*, the perceived world in which we all live. Thrown into the ollapodria is the work of psychologists such as Wilhelm Wundt (1832–1920), the so-called father of experimental psychology and the developing Gestalt school of cognitive operations.

Changing times

The latter half of the nineteenth and first half of the twentieth centuries saw quite radical changes in Western cultures, which went *pari passu* with the various strands of philosophical thought discussed earlier. As summed up by George Lakoff and Mark Johnson (1999), the main stream of Western philosophy which had for so long clung to a view that held that rational thought is conscious, logical, transcendent, and dispassionate, had to evolve, along with changing perspectives in the arts, literature, and music. Impressionism, Symbolism, Dadaism, Cubism,

Surrealism, Suprematism, and other -isms proliferated. Kasimir Malevich (1879–1935) and the antirationalist Russian Futurists called for a dissolution of language, wanting a language of sounds without meaning. If words had no meanings, then pictorial representations could be abandoned, leading to the paintings of Malevich, in which colours and forms had no links to things in the physical world, no perspective, and no logic. From the Renaissance, we have looked at the world knowing where to look; suddenly there was no focus.

In music, the great romantic sounds of Giuseppe Verdi (1813–1901) and Giacomo Puccini (1858–1924) were confronted by the style of sustained chromaticism and 'endless melody', developed by Richard Wagner (1813–1883), whose operas matured from the dramas of action, such as his *Rienzi*, to *Tristan and Isolde* and his *The Ring of the Nibelung* in which the music depicts the lived emotional strata of the protagonists. Musical phrases and *leitmotifs* constantly intermingle and undergo transformations through which the present is entwined with recollections of the past and presentiments of the future, a *déjà acuté* presenting narrative ideas as yet to be fully developed. Music then lost its tonal gravity, with the advent first of the free atonality and then of the serially structured 12-tone atonality of Arnold Schoenberg (1874–1951), in which all 12 pitches of the octave were treated as equal.

As the twentieth century moved on, interest in narrated time, instead of actual time, and in interior monologues, as opposed to description and depiction of external things and events, dominated the intellectual and cultural *Zeitgeist*. James Joyce (1882–1941) gave us *Ulysses*, a book with no overall plot, but with much interior monologue and verbal artefact exploring the psyche of its protagonist Leopold Bloom over the course of one day in Dublin. Likewise, Virginia Woolf (1882–1941), Thomas Mann (1875–1955), and William Faulkner (1897–1962) developed new ways of exploring the mind and emotions in literature.

Two other great influences were William James (1842–1910) and Sigmund Freud (1856–1939). James, in his *Principles of Psychology* (1890), emphasized the goal-directed nature of our activities. He was after a physiological psychology, without a Cartesian homunculus or the hidden mental processes of Kantian categories. Our inner life, our consciousness, is a stream of thought; there is no linking together of disconnected ideas. Thoughts have a 'feeling' of belonging together with other thoughts—we have a sense of continuity through time and experience being unified, not discontinuous. His developed philosophy was one of functionalism, which implied that mental life was organic, active, and pragmatic, but he made us aware of the fourth dimension that permeated thoughts.

Freud studied with Brentano and took from him ideas which included intentionality. This was re-worked as an object–relations theory in the form in which, in the development of the individual mental life, someone else is always involved. Further elaboration of these ideas included cathexis and libidinal investment.

While Freud was by no means the first to bring attention to the unconscious mind, his attempt to bring a scientific framework to the role of unconscious forces in human behaviour, from the simplest twist of the tongue to the development of the world's religions, had a profound influence on psychology and the developing discipline of a psychological psychiatry.

Phenomenology and psychiatry: early intuitions

Brentano considered that science should underlie philosophy, while for Husserl it was the other way round—philosophy should underlie science. Husserl rejected psychologism, the application of the techniques of a scientific psychology to philosophy, emphasizing that the laws of logic are not those of psychological processes. Arguing for 'antinaturalism' and seeking to grasp the 'essence' of experience, Husserl wanted to give phenomenology ('pure phenomenology'—a 'science of essences') an apparent independence from other natural sciences.

Although Husserl had a brief 'realistic' phase and later embraced notions of a 'life world', his overall philosophy was what can be referred to as a 'transcendental idealism'. The word transcendental may sound both allusive and illusive, and its origins take us back to earlier religious doctrines associated with concepts that lie outside Aristotelian categories. It was reintroduced to philosophy by Kant as ' … all knowledge which is occupied not so much with objects as with the mode of our knowledge of objects in so far as this mode of knowledge is to be possible a priori'[1] (Kant, 1929, B,25). This refers to the conditions of possibility, conditions that allow something to exist for us. For the romantic philosopher Friedrich Schelling (1775–1854), a basic task of philosophy was to develop a 'transcendental' philosophy which did not try to make intelligence out of nature, but nature out of intelligence. For Levinas (1906–1995), the transcendental is 'that which cannot be encompassed' (Levinas, 1969, p. 293).

Husserl's 'transcendental subjectivity', explored with his *epochē* or 'transcendental reduction', was disconnected from the natural world and independent of the realm of direct experience. But such an attempt to try to discern underlying psychic phenomena places his ideas within the framework of the disembodied Cartesian ego and is unhelpful for neuropsychiatry.

A problem with Brentano's approach was his deriding of the unconscious (a major difference from Freud's); likewise Husserl (also a student of Brentano), along with many philosophers, has looked askance at the role of the unconscious in the conscious. Husserl's legacy lives on in the egocentric and logocentric perspectives which are retained today by many theoreticians. In part, this emphasizes the split between Continental and Analytic approaches to philosophy. The former is firmly linked to phenomenology. The philosophies of interest in this chapter are those lamenting the failure of much philosophy and science to integrate different realms of human life and to explore how *Naturwissenschaften* and *Geisteswissenschaften* are related. The distinctions between to 'understand' (*Verstehen*) and to 'explain' (*Erklären*) are especially relevant to neuropsychiatry (Trimble, 2016).

Psychopathology and phenomenology

In the mid- to late nineteenth century, alienists and forerunners of today's neuropsychiatrists were brilliant at collecting descriptions of patients' mental states and were often also neuropathologists.

Psychiatry, as it developed in the twentieth century, more and more divorced from neurology and had little truck with neuroscience, and even attempts to retain finesse with psychopathology has, in various settings, been either downgraded or obliterated. The use of rating scales and computerized profiling of responses to committee-determined questions in the search for a spurious diagnostic purity has sacrificed validity for reliability, the latter having a fragile subsoil, quite dependent on the agreement of like-minded people to agree. The interest in memory which preoccupied earlier theorists, such as Théodule-Armand Ribot (1839–1916), William James, and Henri Bergson (1859–1941), and which was central to Marcel Proust (1871–1922) became addled and degraded by standardized neuropsychological tests and scales. The 'involuntary' unconscious remembrances written about by Proust, along with the 'affective' memories of Ribot, embodied and embedded, have been forgotten since no rating scale has been able to capture them. But for Proust's protagonist in *À la Recherche du Temps Perdu* (also called Marcel), these were the bases for his theory of art, with time as the artist. They were also Proust's own justification for becoming a writer. Notions of the 'self' as a coherent identity were brushed aside by a number of philosophies. Behaviouralist psychologies even eschewed the patients' inner world.

A re-turn of the mind

An interest in phenomenology for psychiatry, especially for neuropsychiatry, re-emerged in the last part of the last century (Trimble, 2016). The revival has been more pronounced in European, as opposed to American, psychiatry and includes a shift of perspective away from 'knowledge' about the external world to internal experiences and 'meaning' (*Bedeutung*), a shift away from earlier obsessions with 'truth'. In this framework, it is acknowledged that the perceived object is not the same as the object of experience. A further consequence of the 'stream of consciousness', an expression also used by Husserl, is that our minds are always moving forwards, with the past embedded within. Finally there has been an attempt to heal the subject–object split, so reinforced by Descartes. The sensorimotor underpinning of intentionality, that is mentally going into something, and not just intending to do something, and a re-evaluation of the association between consciousness and perception, in which perception follows consciousness (i.e. the perceptual object and the physical object are not the same), and not vice versa have reversed much of the empirically bound earlier thinking.

The psychiatrist Ludwig Binswanger (1881–1966), heavily influenced by both Husserl and Martin Heidegger (1889–1976), set out a method to explore the human being as present in the world and interacting with that world. There was an *Umwelt* ('around-world'), the *Mitwelt* ('with-world'), and the *Eigenwelt* ('own world'). He set this in an anthropological context. All sentient animals have an *Umwelt*, and the *Mitwelt* is our shared world, while the *Eigenwelt* is our own subjective experience. As a member of the species *Homo sapiens*, the individual as a historical being dwells in the world unfolding over time. 'In this context the term "anthropological" means elucidating the dimensions and dimensionality of the unfolding of human *Dasein* (being or existence), and quite especially of human "space". Spatial standards (in a metaphorical sense) must serve for the categorical understanding and articulating of human Da-sein in

---

[1] Reproduced from Kant I. *Critique of Pure Reason*. Trans: Kemp Smith N. McMillan and co, London 1929.

general.' (*Dasein*: literally 'being here' (Blankenburg, 1982, p. 39)). Several philosophers, all with some interest in medical science, contribute to the next part of the story. They are Bergson, Scheler, Maurice Merleau-Ponty (1908–1961), and Karl Jaspers (1883–1969).

Creativity, evolution, the active embodied mind

Henri Ellenberger (1905–1993), in his magnificent book *The Discovery of the Unconscious* (1970), devotes no less than 277 pages to the emergence of what he refers to as Dynamic Psychiatry. The history begins in the late eighteenth century. The first phase, lasting from 1775 to 1900, covers Romanticism, the philosophies of *Naturphilosophie* (Nature philosophy), the development of Darwinism, the philosophies of Karl Marx, and the potential eclipse of the Enlightenment, all of which he linked with various political and cultural crises in Europe. This brings us up to the time discussed earlier and the development of phenomenology. While Ellenberger was much concerned with the evolution of psychodynamic ideas, Russell Meares in a discussion of a 'new philosophy of psychiatry' used the term Dynamic Psychiatry to mean something that is involved with 'the notion of personal existence' and considered that 'In philosophy the dominant voice was that of Henri Bergson' (Meares, 2003, p. 43).

Henri Bergson, related to Proust through marriage, was familiar with the ideas of Charles Darwin and Herbert Spencer (1820–1903) (who adopted some of Darwin's ideas towards contemporary society), was a friend of William James, and brought the biological sciences into his theories. *Matter and Memory* was published in 1903, and his concept of an *élan vital* first appeared in his book *Creative Evolution* published in 1907.

Some quotes giving a flavour of Bergson's unique ideas include:

> 'Our intellect ... is intended to secure the perfect fitting of our body to its environment' (Bergson, 1911, p. ix).

> 'Memories, messengers from the unconscious, remind us of what we are dragging behind us unawares ... our past then as a whole ... is felt in the form of a tendency ...' (Bergson, 1911, p. 5).

> 'The present contains nothing more than the past, and what is found in the effect was already in the cause (Bergson, 1911, p. 14)'.

> 'We maintain that the brain is an instrument of action, and not of representation' (Bergson, 1912, p. 83).[2]

Bergson thought that modern science had become divorced from our ordinary experiences and emotions, in which time is the central vessel of reality—time, not space, being the important feature of life. In complete contrast to Husserl, he rejected any bracketing of conscious experience (*epochē*), accepted a biological approach to life, and, *pace* Darwin, expressed the view that adaptation was more than merely the adoption of the unadapted, but was due to an inner directing principle, which 'springs from the very effort of the living being to adapt itself to the circumstances of its existence' (Bergson, 1911, p. 76).

Bergson further proposed that 'Action in the world ... implies anticipation of several possible actions, these being marked out before

action itself' (Bergson, 1911, p. 96). Moving beyond the moment of existence is the link to the future. Our actions in this philosophy are the outcome of a preceding series of anticipatory potentials, and action itself is involved with what he refers to as the body image of our conscious states.

Bergson refers frequently to the brain in his writings, 'as an instrument of action'. He considered that 'to know how to use a thing ... is to take a certain attitude, to have a tendency to do so through what the Germans call motor impulses (*Bewegungsantriebe*)'. Motor tendencies give us feelings of recognition, such that perception is no photographic reproduction (Bergson, 1912, pp. 83, 111). Bergson quotes clinical cases, for example of Charcot and Heinrich Lissauer (1861–1891), bringing in apraxia, aphasia, word blindness, echolalia, and loss of topographical orientation to his understanding. He was highly critical of the ever more complicated wire diagrams that were produced to explain simply the complicated to the simple, and refuted the idea of 'centres' in the brain.

Maurice Merleau-Ponty (1908–1961) in 1949 became Professor of Child Psychology at the Sorbonne where he collaborated with Jean Piaget (1896–1980) who influenced his understanding of early infant cognitive development. He took a scientific approach to philosophy, and his most celebrated work is *The Phenomenology of Perception* (1945, English translation 1962). Taking a theme raised by Bergson that 'there is no perception which is not full of memories' (Bergson, 1912, p. 24), Merleau-Ponty's philosophy emphasized the body and its engagement with the world—he was after the nature of the body–world dialogue. The body was, for him, the intermediary between mind and matter, the 'body subject' being anchored in a pre-cognitive, pre-objective, pre-reflexive disposition. He followed Bergson's maxim that 'The essential process of recognition is not centripetal, but centrifugal' (Bergson, 1912, p. 168).

Merleau-Ponty rejected the Cartesian perspective inherent in Husserl's philosophy and considered the *Lebenswelt*, the lived world in which our bodies move around, as most relevant to his developing philosophy, a further break from Husserl's pure phenomenological reduction. From Heidegger, he took the idea that humans were not worldless subjects but were everyday *in-der-Welt-sein*—a state or structure of being in the world. Merleau-Ponty wanted 'to return to that world which precedes knowledge, of which knowledge always speaks ...' (Merleau-Ponty, 2002, p. x). Phenomenology for him was a transcendental philosophy for which the world is always 'already there' for us before reflection begins. Our efforts are concentrated upon achieving a direct and positive contact with the world and endowing that contact with a philosophical status. Perception for him was not just passive, but also an active process of exploration of the environment—the 'body subject' had a 'grip' on objects, which was nevertheless ambiguous and time-bound. Things in our perception 'speak', so to speak, for themselves, 'The object which presents itself to the gaze or touch arouses a certain motor intention ... (there is) a coition ... of our body with things' (Merleau-Ponty, 2002, pp. 370, 372).

Merleau-Ponty was influenced by the infant development theories of Piaget, the anthropology of Claude Lévi-Strauss (1908–2009), and the philosophies of Kant, Husserl, Heidegger, and Jean-Paul Sartre (1905–1980). While so much philosophical and neuroscience discussion, especially of the empiricist schools, was concerned with vision, Merleau-Ponty was concerned with other senses, especially the tactile—that of touching and being touched. The empiricists,

---

[2] Reproduced from Bergson H. (1988). *Creative Evolution*. Trans Mitchell A. New York, US: Dover Publications.

who would conceive of each of the senses as being separate, lacked a framework for what is referred to as a 'binding problem'—that is, how do we experience the combined sensations of say viewing a rose as an object, complete and fragrant as is a rose? The whole is more than the sum of the parts.

For Merleau-Ponty, the importance of perception was not to be found in the perceived object, but in our experience of it. He was concerned with the phenomenal field, that which is presented to the perceiver, which is ontological, referring to the structure and the very meaning of *being*. Merleau-Ponty considered that sensations are intentional—one sees blue things, not just bluenesss. Further, phenomena have figure/background constructions. Since our perceptual horizons are always moving, sense experience is not to be confused with sensation, a fundamental philosophical mistake.

One of the key ideas in *The Phenomenology of Perception* is motor intentionality, the way in which the body directs itself towards, and 'grasps' objects in a pre-cognitive manner. We explore the world, and gain knowledge of it from our very first stirrings with our phenomenal body, as we move towards objects to be grasped (*greifen* to grasp, *begreifen* to understand). In doing, so we feel our way in the world. Even a baby infant has 'embodied intentionality' prior to the invasion of language, the latter enhancing the development of subjectivity. Included in sensory perceptions are proprioceptive ones, which give us information about our own bodies, coming from our limbs and interior organs. Further, perceptual experience gives us access to things which have value for us; we have meaningful interactions with them.

Perceiving is a *motor skill* based on a (pre-cognitive) 'motor intentionality'. This is a fundamental change of perspective for philosophy, psychology, and neurology. It is not that perception leads to action, with stimulus leading to response, but rather that there is a palimpsest to perception, based on motor possibilities. The environment draws the subject to action, whereby the body's 'being-in-the-world' is offered the world: ' … motility as basic intentionality. Consciousness is in the first place not a matter of 'I think', but of "I can"'. (Merleau-Ponty, 2002, pp. 159, 164, 169). Such an approach is extremely relevant for an understanding of aesthetics and our appreciation of the arts,. As expressed by the philosopher John Dewey (1859–1952), 'There must be indirect and collateral channels of response prepared in advance in the case of one who really sees a picture or hears music. This motor preparation is a large part of esthetic education in any particular line. To know what to look for and see how to see it is an affair of readiness on the part of the motor equipment'[3] (Dewey, 1934, p. 102).

Karl Jaspers

Karl Jaspers studied medicine and worked with Franz Nissl (1860–1919) (of Nissl tissue staining fame) at Heidelberg; the latter was a student of Kraepelin (1856–1926). Jaspers was well grounded in scientific method, as it was at that time, and the link with medical practice. He became recognized as an outstanding philosopher of the twentieth century, but his importance for neuropsychiatry came with his book *Allgemeine Psychopathogie* (General Psychopathology). It was written when he was recuperating from

illness and was first published in German in 1913 and ran to nine editions. The seventh edition was translated into English in 1963. It is not a philosophical treatise but contains descriptions and definitions of various mental states. He refers to his approach as phenomenological, seeking authentic experiences and describing psychopathological states with no bias to any particular theory. However, it is not the phenomenology of Husserl, Heidegger, or others, such as Scheler, which reflects on the different approaches that various philosophers have adopted under the term phenomenology. His dual approach was much influenced by Dilthey and the sociologist Max Weber (1864–1920) (Ghaemi, 2010).

With regard to the psychology of meaning, Jaspers wrote, 'When the contents of thoughts emerge one from another in accordance with the rules of logic, we understand the connections rationally. But if we understand the contents of thoughts as they have arisen out of moods, wishes and fears of the person who thought them, we understand the connections psychologically or empathetically. Only the latter can be called psychological understanding … Whereas rational understanding is only an aid to psychology, empathic understanding *is* psychology itself' (Jaspers, 1913/1997, p. 83)[4].

The philosophies of Kant, Dilthey, and, to some extent, Husserl were influential for him in his attempt to capture the essences of mental states and give an 'objective' descriptive psychology of patients' inner experiences. He was very critical of Freudian theories and wanted to describe individual components of mental states in the way he might have learnt from Nissl: 'Whoever has no eyes to see cannot practice histology: whoever is unwilling or incapable of actualising psychic events and representing them vividly cannot acquire an understanding of phenomenology' (Jaspers, 1912/2012, p. 94).

Jaspers brought to neuropsychiatry the necessity of distinguishing *Verstehen*—to understand—which is about the meaning of existence (*verstehende* psychopathology), from *Erklären* (to explain) which has to do with causal connections (explanatory psychopathology). The latter is concerned with establishing general laws, while *Understanding* seeks literally an understanding of the individual. This breaks not only with Cartesian logic, but also with Kantian categories of understanding.

Understanding requires empathy with which to immerse oneself in the patient's mental life, along with the therapist's own experience, and through both a realization that there are some whose experiences are beyond such understanding, essentially the psychotic. Meaningful connections—how one psychic event merges with and emerges from another, what he called *genetic* understanding, the longitudinal dissection of the psyche—were central to this process. Causal explanations are different. Psychic processes alter psychic life without destroying it, while organic processes despoil it.

Jaspers' scientific background did not lead him to reject objectivity, but he tried to rescue psychiatry from both the progressive reductionism of materialism and psychological speculation (e.g. Freud). His ideas influenced diagnostic manuals such as the later International Classification of Diseases (ICD) and DSM publications, although his contributions are hardly ever acknowledged.

[3] Reproduced from Dewey J. (1934). *Art as Experience*. New York, US: Penguin Group.

[4] Reproduced from Jaspers K. (1997). *General Psychopathology*. Trans Hoenig J, Hamilton WW. Baltimore, US: Johns Hopkins Press.

For the practising neuropsychiatrist, Jaspers is the most important phenomenological theorist. Accepting that psychic events were caused by cerebral events and eschewing the humbug of Wernicke's neuromythology and Freudian psychomythology, he tried to put psychopathology and issues of causality of mental disorders 'in order'. A brave attempt at the time, yet even more pertinent today. Straddling the line between psyche and soma, *Verstehen* and *Erklären* are both a part of the diagnostic and therapeutic endeavours, and the identification of any contributing somatic basis to a patient's signs and symptoms is key for neuropsychiatry. At the other end of the spectrum, and no less important in neuropsychiatry, is the identification of personality features and problems of living, which require a different clinical approach entirely.

Jaspers outlined a psychotherapeutic method, which is not so different for patients with or without an organic substrate for their problems, but very much based in the doctor–patient relationship.

Nassir Ghaemi (2010), in his coruscating criticism of the 'Biopsychosocial Model' of current lubricity, asks how Jaspers would practise psychiatry today.

> 'Avoid overpathologising, overdiagnosis, social construction and abuse of medical power. The corrective to these risks is to remember that diseases, though real objective entities in the natural world, happen to individual human beings, free men and women, with *feelings* about having or not having a disease. And sometimes there is no disease at all, but only problems of individual free human beings … in which case the disease model does not apply.'
>
> (Ghaemi, 2010, p. 208)[5]

Conclusion

Kant's separation of phenomena and noumena, the latter for him being unattainable, left out our living world, which was also lost with Husserl's phenomenological reduction. While Husserl emphasized the great importance of consciousness and meaning for philosophy, his method separated essence (outside time and place) from existence. Bergson and Merleau-Ponty placed human experience firmly back into the temporal flux, along with the human mind's necessity of seizing the meaning of the lived-in world. This 'transcendental' subjectivity was also an inter-subjectivity. The true 'cogito' is 'being in the world' (Merleau-Ponty, 2002, p. xvi). Intentionality is related to the body–world dialogue, through premotor dispositions, perceptions which allow direction for action, the organism in its environment capturing the temporal flow of existence. This is an incarnate intentionality, the body subject having a 'grip' on objects and the surrounding world, a process which is never complete, only ambiguous, and always becoming. Such views are at odds with a scientific perspective in which the subjective is simply made objective, and with a traditional philosophy in which consciousness is not usually viewed as embodied.

A task of twentieth-century Continental philosophy has been to seek how meaning emerges for us in and from the world, an exercise not available via empirical philosophy. Phenomenology takes us beyond the limited realm of empirical psychology to consider transcendental phenomena. It is a generative, not a reflexive, psychology and rejects the core tenets of Descartes. The phenomenologist places consciousness and experience at the heart of mental life. The upshot of all this is that the role of emotion and the fundamental principle of embodiment are now respectable subjects of study in neuroscience. There is much interest in 'the social brain', Theory of Mind (that other people have minds like one's own), empathy, mirror neurones, and mental time travel (how we see the possibility of future events based on past experiences) (Trimble, 2012). Merleau-Ponty opined that 'Sensations, 'sensible qualities', are then far away from being reducible to a certain indescribable state or *quale*; they present themselves with a motor physiognomy and are enveloped in a living significance' (Merleau-Ponty, 2002, p. 243).

Such ideas place the body's physiological processes and anatomical structures as fundamental, not only for the rise of consciousness, but also for knowledge, reasoning, and creativity. To quote John Cutting (2016) in a summary of the achievements of the phenomenologists discussed in this chapter: 'In one stroke they solved the centuries old dispute between idealists—who thought that the mind of the knower one-sidedly created the experience that the human being deemed real, albeit out of some undifferentiated "soup" out there—and realists—who thought that the knower was merely a passive recipient of some already established order out there.'[6] 'The incontestable truth of (the everyday realist) becomes invalid when empirical reality is presumed to be wholly and conclusively known and when it claims to determine alone what is at issue. Against this must be maintained that the real world by no means is so simply present' (Jaspers, 1947/1959, pp. 25/26).

Neuropsychiatry should claim the phenomenological approach of Jaspers as a philosophy which distinguishes it from an empirically based neurology or a Cartesian freely floating ego of conventional psychiatry. Jaspers would, I am sure, have been delighted to have available all of the somatic treatments we have today at his disposal and investigations such as EEG and brain imaging. While he acknowledged that the psychic life is only partially cognizable, he favoured a precise description of a patient's experience and would have been in favour of identification of syndromes, rather than diseases, in a descriptive psychopathology and horrified by the reductive use of diagnostic manuals such as the DSM series of diversions (largely invalidated) and rating scales. He quoted Kraepelin favourably, even if remaining somewhat ambivalent about the construction and constriction of the latter's diagnostic entities. Earlier enthusiasm for Jasper's ideas, especially in British psychiatry, faded with DSM-III and, with successors, was later lost in translation. Many neuropsychiatric presentations do not fit neatly into such blind alleys, and neuropsychiatrists should be wary of affixing such categories to all the clinical syndromes they assess.

Jaspers would have rejected ideas of localization of function, suggesting an interplay of anatomical parts, stimulating and inhibiting one another, ideas now in favour. He would have also rejected newer psychologies and exclusive implications that social factors explain all mental events, any understanding that justified reductionist behaviour therapies, and too ready an assumption that we understand 'causes'.

[5] Reproduced from Ghaemi N. (2010). *The Rise and Fall of the Biopsychosocial Model. Reconciling Art and Science in Psychiatry*. Baltimore, US: Johns Hopkins University Press.

[6] Cutting J. *Phenomenology and Phenomenological Psychiatry*. 2016.

Ghaemi refers to the Jasperian approach as 'method-based psychiatry'. It takes 'the biologically reductionist model of disease and applies it where appropriate, but always with a humanistic awareness of the importance of the person, the individual who has the disease … This is best understood through an understanding of literature, to the uniqueness of humanity and of each individual human being, which is best approached, though never completely captured in poetry and fiction' (Ghaemi, 2010, p. 209).[7]

KEY LEARNING POINTS

- To understand the development of phenomenology, one must also understand the Kantian influence on pre-nineteenth-century continental philosophy, namely his distinction between the noumenon (the thing itself) and the phenomenon (the thing as it appears to us). This chapter explores the effects of phenomenology's evolution on the field of psychiatry and then neuropsychiatry, following the pari passu shifts in Western culture and its prevailing philosophies.
- By examining the intellectual trajectories of philosophers such as Edmund Husserl and Karl Jaspers, it traces the development of our understanding of consciousness, arguing Jasper's 'method-based psychiatry', heavily reliant on the patient's description of their experience, to be the best fit for neuropsychiatry, neither tied entirely to empirical neurology or the 'Cartesian freely floating ego' of conventional psychiatry.

ACKNOWLEDGEMENTS

I am very grateful to John Cutting, Nassir Ghaemi, and Michael Graubart who have all contributed to my thoughts in this chapter, and with whom I have enjoyed discussions and diversions over many years on these and other topics.

REFERENCES

Bergson H. *Creative Evolution*. Trans. Mitchell A. Dover Publications, New York, NY. 1988 (1911).

Bergson H. *Matter and Memory*. Dover Philosophical Classics, New York, NY. 2004 (1912).

Blankenburg W. A dialectical conception of anthropological proportions. In: De Kooning AJJ, Jenner FA, eds. *Phenomenology and Psychiatry*. Academic Press, London, 1982.

Cerbone DR. *Understanding Phenomenology*. Acumen, Chesham, 2006.

Cutting J. *Phenomenology and Phenomenological Psychiatry*. 2016.

Dewey J. *Art as Experience*. Penguin Group, New York, NY. 1934.

Ellenberger H. *The Discovery of the Unconscious: The History and Evolution of Dynamic Psychiatry*. Basic Books, New York, NY. 1970.

Ghaemi N. *The Rise and Fall of the Biopsychosocial Model. Reconciling Art and Science in Psychiatry*. Johns Hopkins University Press, Baltimore, MD. 2010.

Jaspers K. The phenomenological approach in psychopathology. Trans. Curran JN. Reproduced in: *The Maudsley Reader in Phenomenological Psychiatry*. Broome MR, Harland R, Owen GS, Stringaris A, eds. Cambridge University Press, Cambridge, 1912/2012.

Jaspers K. *General Psychopathology*. Trans. Hoenig J, Hamilton WW. Johns Hopkins Press, Baltimore, MD. 1913/1997.

Jaspers K. *Truth and Symbol*. Trans. Wilde JT, Kluback W, Kimmel W. College and University Press, New Haven CT. 1947/1959.

Kant I. *Critique of Pure Reason*. Trans. Kemp Smith N. McMillan and Co, London. 1929.

Lakoff G, Johnson M. *Philosophy in the Flesh*. Basic Books, New York, NY. 1999.

Levinas E. *Totality and Infinity*. Trans. Lingis A. Duquesne University Press, Pittsburg, PA. 1969.

Meares R. Towards a psyche for psychiatry. In: Fulford B, Morris K, Sadler J, Stanghellini G, eds. *Nature and Narrative: An Introduction to the New Philosophy of Psychiatry*. Oxford University Press, Oxford. 2003, pp 43–56.

Merleau Ponty M. *The Phenomenology of Perception*. Trans. Smith C. Routledge, London. 2002.

Popper K. *Conjectures and Refutations: The Growth of Scientific Knowledge*. Routledge, London. 1963.

Trimble M. *Why Humans Like to Cry. Tragedy, Evolution and the Brain*. Oxford University Press, Oxford. 2012.

Trimble M. *Intentional Brain: Motion, Emotion, and the Development of Modern Neuropsychiatry*. Johns Hopkins University Press, Baltimore, MD. 2016.

---

[7] Reproduced from Ghaemi N. (2010). *The Rise and Fall of the Biopsychosocial Model. Reconciling Art and Science in Psychiatry*. Baltimore, US: Johns Hopkins University Press.

6

Basic neuroanatomy review

John Hart Jr

Introduction

The following is a review of the neuroanatomy that is considered to be the most relevant to cognition.[1] Neuroanatomy is not easily learnt by reading a text because it is a three-dimensional (3-D) set of relationships. This text assumes some background in neuroanatomy and is not a substitute as an initial comprehensive presentation of neuroanatomy. If one is unfamiliar with neuroanatomy, there will be a reasonable amount of memorization required or at least use of this chapter as a reference to locate regions when anatomic references are made in later chapters.

Although knowledge of the locations of anatomic regions is essential to understanding neuroanatomy, understanding the connections between regions and how regions interact with each other provides the optimal grasp of neuroanatomy. This 3-D grasp of how regions are related in space to each other and interconnect will allow for the optimal understanding of how cognitive–anatomic units (CAUs) connect and inter-relate to perform a task. Having a 3-D model in hand, while going through this chapter, may greatly aid in both grasping the localization of regions and understanding their connections.

The key neuroanatomic structures that are most commonly associated with cognitive processing and behaviour are the cerebral cortex, white matter, and subcortical nuclei. One approach of a 3-D conceptualization of the brain is to start with the most deep and midline structures and build layers on top of them. That starting point is the subcortical nuclei. Overlaying these structures are the white matter connections, and then the most external layer are the cortices of the frontal, parietal, temporal, and occipital lobes. If you keep this layering model in mind, it provides both a structural organization on how to envision the neuroanatomic regions and a clearer understanding of how regions are connected and communicate with each other. The layers chosen anatomically also segregate three general functional divisions (cortex—cognitive processing and representation, white matter—connections, and subcortical nuclei—relay and control circuits). We will revisit and elaborate on

this layering of brain regions as a guide to organizing and learning neuroanatomy.

Before describing these anatomic structures, some basic principles describing directions and orientation of brain structures are established. Many of the anatomic figures used in this text are from radiological images, and thus brain orientation and directionality are explained as applied in that framework.

Fig. 6.1 demonstrates the lateral view of the human brain with the directional terms used to orient one in relative terms to a particular brain region. Regions located more at the front of the brain are referred to as anterior (or rostral) in location (direction of the forehead), with the back of the brain referred to as the posterior (or caudal) direction. The top of the brain is referred to as the superior (or dorsal) direction (towards the crown of the head), with the bottom of the brain being the inferior (or ventral) direction. Regions that are more towards the midline of the brain are referred to as more medial, and those towards the outside (nearest cortex) of the brain are said to be more lateral.

Most of the images of the brain presented in this book are from MRI or computed tomography (CT) scans. The presentation of the MRI images varies, depending on the orientation in which the brain is 'sliced' when the image was acquired or 're-sliced' to assess structures from a different perspective. The typical view in which most MRI/CT images are acquired and presented is the axial view, in which the images are oriented through the brain from anterior to posterior that is parallel to the ground if a person is standing upright (see Fig. 6.2).

Sagittal images are vertically oriented from superior to inferior, with the plane of the slices dividing the brain into right and left halves (see Fig. 6.3). Another common orientation is referred to as the coronal plane, which is oriented vertically from superior to inferior but, compared to the sagittal plane, is oriented to slice the brain from front to back (see Fig. 6.4).

There is one additional point to consider when viewing MRI images in this text and elsewhere. If the MRI images are in 'radiological' convention, then the right side of the images is actually depicting the left side of the brain. Standard or conventional orientation has the left side of the brain represented on the left side of the image. When a figure is in radiological orientation, it is noted in the figure legend. If there is no notation, then the image is in conventional orientation.

---

[1] This chapter is reproduced from a previously published book *The Neurobiology of Cognition and Behavior*, by John Hart, Jr, (January 2016), pp. 23–41, Copyright © 2016 Oxford University Press USA.

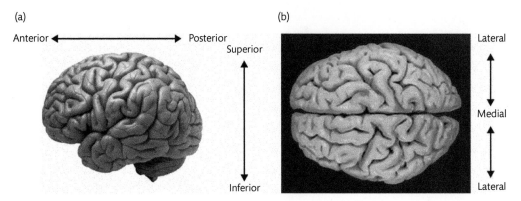

Fig. 6.1 Labels for directional orientation used in referring to brain structures. Anterior (rostral) refers to being more towards the front (forehead) aspect of the brain, with posterior (caudal) towards the back of the brain and head. Superior (dorsal) refers to the topward direction of the brain (crown of the head), and inferior (ventral) towards the bottom of the brain. When referring to more midline brain structures, the term medial is used. The term lateral is used to refer to the outside aspects of the brain, towards the cortical areas.

Reproduced with permission from John Hart Jr. Basic Neuroanatomy Review. In *The Neurobiology of Cognition and Behavior*. Oxford, UK: Oxford University Press. Copyright © 2015, Oxford University Press. DOI: 10.1093/med/9780190219031.001.0001. Reproduced with permission of the Licensor through PLSclear.

Brain lobes

The basic organization used in this text for cognition is the cortex, the white matter, and the subcortical structures. The organization of the cortex is discussed first, beginning with a description of the general organization of the brain into two halves, or hemispheres, split down the middle of the brain from the anterior to posterior aspects, dividing it into two relatively equal halves—the right and left hemispheres. Each hemisphere is divided into four lobes: frontal, parietal, temporal, and occipital lobes (see Fig. 6.5). Each of these lobes consists of gyri, which are outfoldings of the cerebral cortex consisting of grey matter and its adjacent underlying white matter. When two gyri meet, the contour that forms between them is referred to as a sulcus (see Fig. 6.6). Each lobe and its gyral/sulcal organization are discussed in the following sections.

Frontal lobe

The frontal lobes (one in the right hemisphere and the other in the left) are in the most anterior aspect of the brain, the largest brain lobes, and typically support higher-order cognitive functions controlling numerous cognitive control operations. The frontal lobe is bordered on the posterior aspect by the central sulcus, which separates it from the parietal lobe, and inferiorly by the Sylvian fissure, which is its border separating it from the temporal lobe (see Fig. 6.5).

In the posterior aspect of the frontal lobe, there are two prominent vertically oriented gyri, one in front of the other—the motor cortex, referred to as the precentral gyrus because it is just in front of the central sulcus, and the premotor cortex, which lies just anterior to the precentral gyrus (see Fig. 6.7).

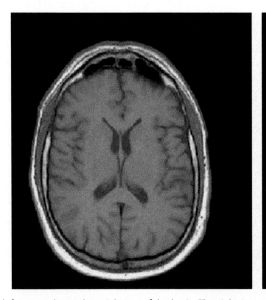
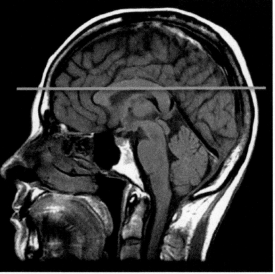

Fig. 6.2 The left image shows the axial view of the brain. The right image shows a side view of the brain; the blue line designates the plane through the brain in which the axial slice is oriented.

Reproduced with permission from John Hart Jr. Basic Neuroanatomy Review. In *The Neurobiology of Cognition and Behavior*. Oxford, UK: Oxford University Press. Copyright © 2015, Oxford University Press. DOI: 10.1093/med/9780190219031.001.0001. Reproduced with permission of the Licensor through PLSclear.

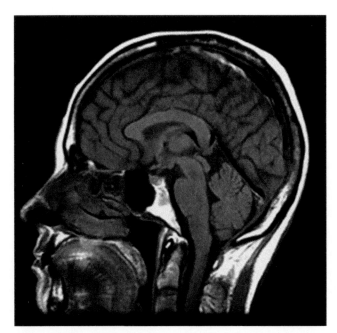

Fig. 6.3 This orientation is the sagittal axis view of the brain.

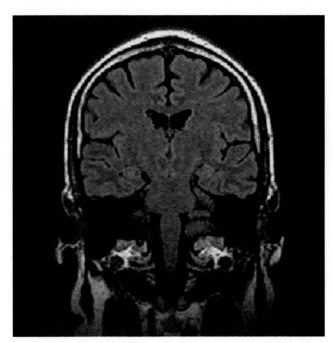

Fig. 6.4 Coronal orientation view of the brain.

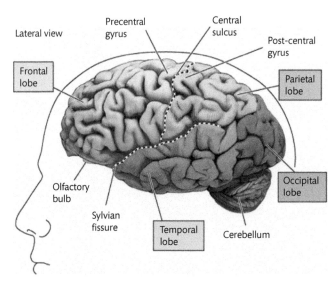

Fig. 6.5 Lateral view of the brain separated into lobes. The frontal lobe is separated from the parietal lobe by the north–south-oriented central sulcus. The central sulcus extends from the superior aspect of the brain inferiorly to the Sylvian fissure. The horizontally oriented Sylvian fissure separates the temporal lobe from both the frontal and parietal lobes. The parietal lobe is separated from the occipital lobe by the horizontally oriented parieto-occipital sulcus.

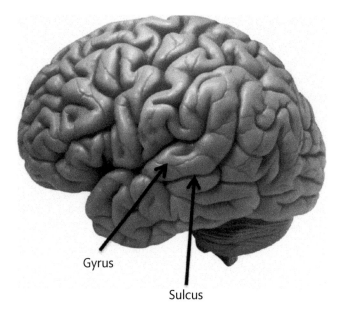

Fig. 6.6 A gyrus, depicted in the photo of a brain, is the rounded, elevated convolutions on the surfaces of the cerebral hemispheres of the brain. A sulcus is the crevice between two gyri.

The motor cortex encodes the motor functions for the opposite side of the body and is organized by body region, referred to as the homunculus (see Fig. 6.8). The homunculus demonstrates what part of the body is represented for its motor control by a specific region of the motor cortex. In general, the face and mouth region is located at the most inferior aspect of the gyrus, the hand in the middle, and the leg at the most superior aspect. The largest part of the motor cortex is dedicated to the part of the body that requires

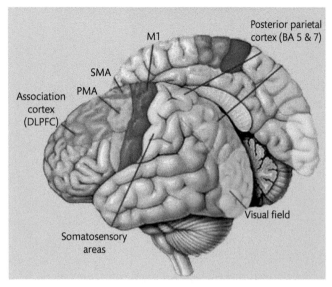

Fig. 6.7 The red gyrus labelled M1 (to designate the primary motor cortex) is the precentral gyrus that encodes for primary motor system control. The light blue gyrus labelled PMA is the premotor gyrus. The purple region at the top of the premotor gyrus is the supplementary motor area (SMA). The green area designates the dorsolateral prefrontal cortex (DLPFC).

Reproduced with permission from *The Brain from Top to Bottom. The Motor Cortex.* www.thebrain.mcgill.ca.

the most motor control. Thus, the largest regions of the motor cortex are dedicated to the tongue, face, and hand, as would be expected, considering the degree of complexity required to control the motor aspects of these regions. From a spatial perspective, starting at the most inferior aspect of the motor gyrus, the order of representation extending up superiorly is the tongue, face, hand, arm, hip, leg, and foot.

The premotor cortex, anterior to the motor cortex, aids in the planning and preparation of motor movements. It follows the same general orientation as the motor cortex, and the functions of planning for motor movement for each body region align in the same general location where that body region is located in the motor cortex.

Anterior to the premotor gyrus are three horizontally oriented gyri that extend up to the most anterior aspects of the frontal lobe—the superior, middle, and inferior frontal gyri (see Fig. 6.9). A key region in cognition is the most posterior aspect of the inferior frontal gyrus in the left hemisphere, referred to as Broca's area (see Fig. 6.10). This is the region described by Paul Broca in the 1890s as being associated with speech production, and it represents one of the first instances of a brain–behaviour correlation.

Another region of the frontal lobe that is involved in cognitive operations is the dorsolateral prefrontal cortex (DLPFC). The DLPFC is not strictly defined anatomically by gyral/sulcal borders but, rather, has been delineated based on the functional activities associated with

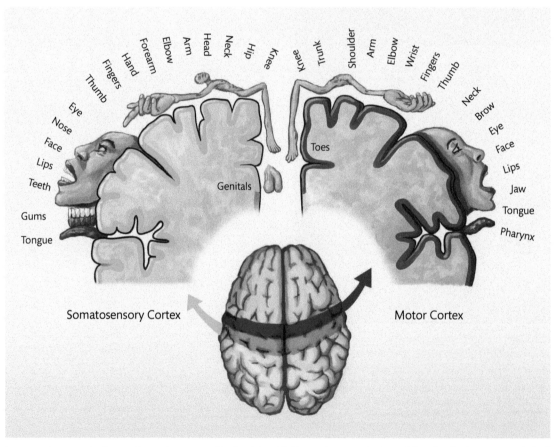

Fig. 6.8 The homunculus organization to the motor cortex. On the right-side figure, the organization of function in the motor strip is shown, with the tongue and face region at the most inferior aspect of the gyrus. Proceeding superiorly up the motor strip, the hand, arm, shoulder, trunk, and leg are represented in that order.

Science History Images/Alamy Stock Photo.

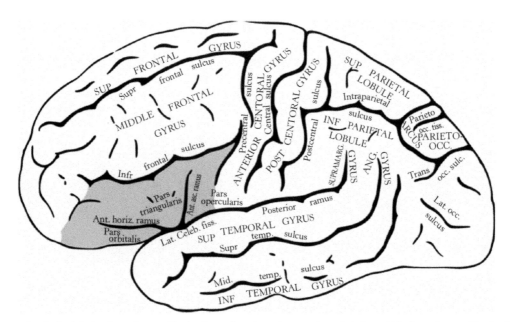

Fig. 6.9 The yellow region is the inferior frontal gyrus. The horizontally oriented gyrus above it is the middle frontal gyrus. The horizontally oriented gyrus above the middle frontal gyrus is the superior frontal gyrus.

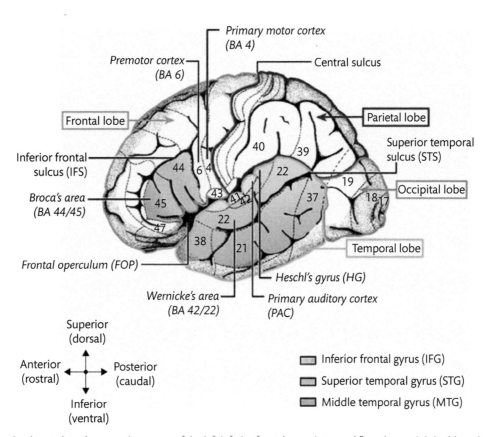

Fig. 6.10 The pink region located on the posterior aspect of the left inferior frontal gyrus is termed Broca's area. It is in this region where the inferior frontal gyrus undulates upwards and downwards. The area marked 44, Brodmann area 44, which is the posterior 'curve' to the inferior frontal gyrus, is called the pars opercularis. Brodmann area 45, at the bottom of the next to the last curve of the inferior frontal gyrus, is called the pars triangularis. These two regions together constitute the majority of Broca's area.

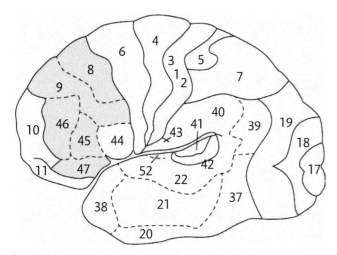

Fig. 6.11 Regions that have been purported to be the DLPFC. It is a generally held belief that BA 9 and 46 constitute the DLPFC, but some have suggested that BA 8, 9, and 10 better represent the DLPFC.

Reproduced with permission from John Hart Jr. Basic Neuroanatomy Review. In *The Neurobiology of Cognition and Behavior*. Oxford, UK: Oxford University Press. Copyright © 2015, Oxford University Press. DOI: 10.1093/med/9780190219031.001.0001. Reproduced with permission of the Licensor through PLSclear.

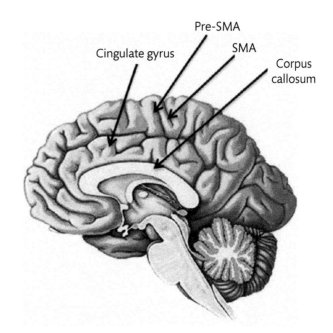

Fig. 6.12 Medial aspects of the frontal lobe. The corpus callosum is the dominant white matter tract connecting the two hemispheres. Just superior to the corpus callosum is the horizontally oriented cingulate gyrus. The supplementary motor area (SMA) is a superior region just anterior to the motor cortex and is engaged in movement control. Anterior to the SMA is the pre-SMA, which is involved in planning motor acts and cognition.

Reproduced with permission from John Hart Jr. Basic Neuroanatomy Review. In *The Neurobiology of Cognition and Behavior*. Oxford, UK: Oxford University Press. Copyright © 2015, Oxford University Press. DOI: 10.1093/med/9780190219031.001.0001. Reproduced with permission of the Licensor through PLSclear.

the region. Although there is not a clear definition for the boundaries of the DLPFC, it is generally postulated to include the middle frontal gyrus, including the lateral part of Brodmann area (BA) 9 and BA 46 (see the introduction to the Brodmann system later in this chapter) (see Fig. 6.11). Other investigators have defined the borders of the DLPFC to include regions of BA 8, 9, and 10 (Cieslik et al., 2013). The DLPFC has been associated with a variety of cognitive control and other operations, including working memory, decision-making, planning, abstract reasoning, and inhibition.

The medial aspect of the frontal lobe consists of a prominent gyrus on its most inferior aspect—the cingulate gyrus (see Fig. 6.12). This gyrus lies directly on top of the largest white matter tract connecting the two hemispheres—the corpus callosum. The white matter fibres of the corpus callosum carry tracts that communicate between the cortices of the two hemispheres for mediating cognitive processes that require cross-hemispheric coordination. In addition, there are two superior medial cortical regions that are engaged directly or indirectly with cognitive functions—the supplementary motor area (SMA) and the pre-SMA. The SMA lies just in front of the primary motor cortex and is engaged in the control of movement. The pre-SMA lies anterior to the SMA and is involved with planning of motor acts, as well as several cognitive operations to be addressed later in this text.

The inferior aspects of the frontal lobes consist of four gyri—anterior, lateral, posterior, and medial orbitofrontal gyri (see Fig. 6.13). As a group, these gyri are also referred to as the ventromedial frontal lobe and play a key role in decision-making that is discussed in further detail later. Posterior to the orbitofrontal cortices lies the insular cortex, a region that when viewed from a lateral perspective lies underneath (medial to) the temporal and frontal lobes. The insular cortex has been imputed to be engaged in a variety of functions, most notably language- and speech-related functions, as well as body awareness.

Parietal lobe

The parietal lobe is delineated by three borders. It is separated from the frontal lobe on its anterior aspect by the central sulcus.

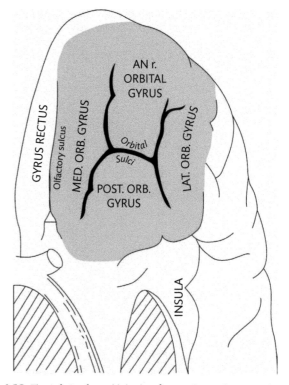

Fig. 6.13 The inferior frontal lobe has four gyri: anterior, posterior, medial, and lateral orbitofrontal gyri. Posterior to the orbitofrontal gyri is the insula. If the Sylvian fissure is separated, the insula can be seen underlying the superior temporal and inferior frontal gyri.

Source: http://www.wikipedia.org.

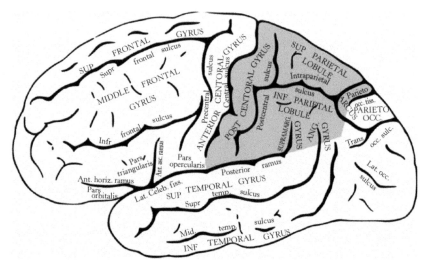

Fig. 6.14 Gyri of the parietal lobe. The post-central gyrus is a vertically oriented region that encodes for somatosensory (touch) representations for the opposite side of the body. The inferior parietal lobule consists of the supramarginal gyrus, which wraps around the end of the Sylvian fissure, and the angular gyrus, which is at the end of the superior temporal sulcus and extends up superiorly. The superior parietal lobule is situated above the intraparietal sulcus and is posteriorly bounded by the parieto-occipital sulcus.
Source: https://commons.wikimedia.org/.

Its inferior border dividing the parietal from the temporal lobe is the Sylvian fissure. The posterior border separating the parietal from the occipital lobe is the parieto-occipital sulcus (see Fig. 6.14).

The gyral pattern of the parietal lobe consists of the post-central gyrus, which is at the anterior aspect of the parietal lobe and is oriented vertically. This region is also referred to as the primary somatosensory cortex because it encodes the sensory representations for touch for the opposite side of the body. Posterior to the somatosensory cortex is a region described collectively as the posterior parietal cortex. This general region is subdivided into the superior parietal lobule and the inferior parietal lobule, which are separated by the intraparietal sulcus. The inferior parietal lobule consists of two gyri of great significance in cognition—the supramarginal and angular gyri. The supramarginal gyrus wraps around the end of the Sylvian fissure connecting the temporal to the parietal lobe. The angular gyrus is situated posterior to the supramarginal gyrus as it starts at the end of the superior temporal sulcus, extending superiorly into the parietal region (see Fig. 6.14).

Another key structure for cognition that is medially located in the parietal lobe and just superior to the parieto-occipital sulcus is the region referred to as the precuneus (see Fig. 6.15B). This region borders superiorly on the cuneus area of the occipital lobe and is considered part of the superior parietal lobule. It has been imputed to contribute to episodic and working memory functions, but it has received recent interest in studies of functional connectivity networks in the brain. It is one of the least well cognitively mapped areas in the cortex, mostly attributable to its deep location, leaving it rarely damaged by either trauma or stroke.

Occipital lobe

The occipital lobe is the smallest lobe and is primarily responsible for visual processing. Although the gyral organization to the occipital

(a)

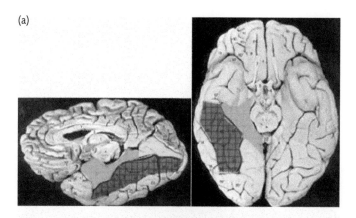

(b)

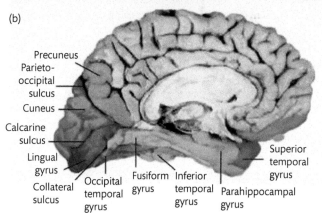

Fig. 6.15 (a) Gyri of the medial and inferior occipital lobe. The yellow region is the lingual gyrus; the purple region is the fusiform gyrus, and the green region is the parahippocampal gyrus (part of the temporal lobe). (b) Medial view of the occipital lobe. The cuneus is coloured orange and located on the posterior aspect of the occipital lobe, and includes the primary visual cortex. Anterior to the cuneus on the most medial aspect is the lingual gyrus, with the fusiform gyrus immediately lateral and the occipito-temporal gyrus the most lateral.

lobe is covered here, it is typically and most effectively described using BA distinctions that are explained further later in this chapter.

The most posterior aspect of the occipital lobe is the primary visual cortex, also referred to as the striate cortex due to the striations in the cortices. This region encodes for the low-level (colour, orientation, etc.) visual characteristics received directly from the optic radiations that transmit information derived originally from the peripheral visual system. Another name applied to the wedge-shaped region that encompasses the primary visual cortex (BA 17) is the cuneus, which is the region that extends from the parieto-occipital sulcus superiorly to the calcarine sulcus inferiorly (see Fig. 6.15B).

The visual information processed in the primary visual cortex extends out to the visual association cortices neighbouring the striate cortices, which are named the lateral occipital gyri. Information then proceeds inferiorly to the base of the occipital lobe. The gyri located in this region include the lingual gyrus, which is medial and anterior to the lateral occipital gyri. The fusiform gyrus is lateral to the lingual gyrus, and the occipitotemporal gyrus is lateral to the fusiform gyrus (see Fig. 6.15A). The fusiform gyrus extends anteriorly to become part of the temporal lobe. At its most anterior aspect, the fusiform gyrus lies between the inferior temporal (laterally) and the parahippocampal (medially) gyri.

These regions (lingual, fusiform, and occipitotemporal gyri) perform higher-order visual processing from the previous analyses performed in the early visual cortices and have been referred to as the 'what' system. The 'what' system is the region where visual information is integrated to form whole object representations and where the visual memories for these objects are stored. There are further subdivisions of these regions that will be specified throughout the text.

The other method by which the visual system is segregated and described, as opposed to gyri, is via BAs. The BA numbers cross gyral boundaries but best describe the functional role each region plays in visual processing. The primary visual cortex is referred to as BA 17, with the regions proceeding more anteriorly being areas BA 18 and BA 19 (see Fig. 6.11). As the BA numbers increase, the regions designated by them perform more complex visual processing.

Temporal lobe

The temporal lobes from the lateral view have three horizontally oriented gyri—the superior, middle, and inferior temporal gyri. These regions, particularly in the left hemisphere, have been associated with language-related cognitive operations, with several key areas being associated with specific cognitive operations. The superior temporal region is where the primary auditory cortex resides. This region encodes sounds that are delivered in raw form from the peripheral auditory system and processes the information in units that are organized by the frequency of the sound. It is referred to as the transverse temporal gyrus of Heschl and is located in the superior aspect of the superior temporal gyrus and tucked into the Sylvian fissure (BA 42). Another part of the superior temporal gyrus, the posterior and superior aspects, forms a region referred to as the planum temporale, which also plays a role in language-related auditory processing and is larger on the left than right side in most individuals (see Fig. 6.16). The surrounding cortices, referred to as secondary auditory association cortices, are where these basic frequencies are integrated into meaningful sounds.

Also localized at the most posterior aspect of the superior temporal gyrus is Wernicke's area. This region, described by Wernicke

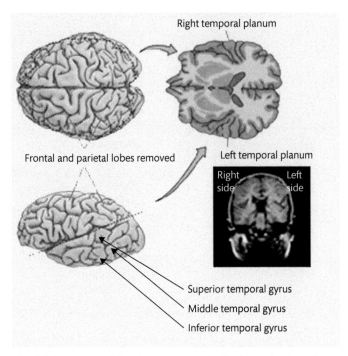

Fig. 6.16 Location of the planum temporale. The brain drawings show the location and relative size of the planum temporale region of the superior aspect of the superior temporal gyri that has been implicated in language processing. The left planum temporale is typically larger than the right side.

Reproduced with permission from *The Brain from Top to Bottom. Broca's Area, Wernicke's Area, And Other Language-Processing Areas In The Brain.* www.thebrain.mcgill.ca.

in the 1800s, has been associated with language comprehension and converting sounds to meaning (see Fig. 6.10). More details of its role in cognitive operations are discussed in later chapters.

The basal surface of the temporal lobes consists of the hippocampus at its most medial aspect, with the amygdala just anterior to it, but still on the most medial aspect of the temporal lobe. The next gyrus lateral and inferior to the hippocampus is the parahippocampal gyrus, which extends from the temporal pole posteriorly back to the posterior aspect of the corpus callosum (see Fig. 6.17). The anterior aspect of the parahippocampal gyrus has a protrusion that projects medially and is called the uncus. Lateral to the parahippocampal gyrus is the inferior temporal gyrus, with the border between these two gyri forming the junction of the lateral and basal temporal lobes.

The hippocampus is divided into three parts—head, body, and tail. The head is referred to as the pes hippocampus. The body of the hippocampus extends medially, narrowing into the tail that disappears as a ventricular structure (see Fig. 6.18). The hippocampus, the parahippocampal gyrus, and other related structures form the hippocampal formation. These regions are essential to episodic memory functions and are disrupted in patients with amnesia and Alzheimer's disease.

Another key structure located in the temporal lobe that has a substantial impact on cognition and behaviour is the amygdala. This almond-shaped structure, located immediately anterior to the pes hippocampus in the medial temporal lobe, is involved in memory and emotional responses such as arousal and fear.

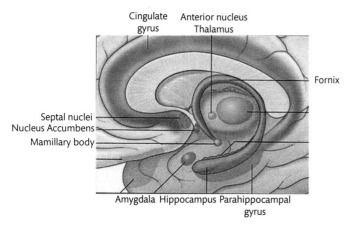

Fig. 6.17 Caricature of the relative locations of the parahippocampal and hippocampal gyri. The parahippocampal gyrus lies adjacent to (inferior and lateral to) the hippocampus. The hippocampus lies on the medial aspect of the temporal lobe.

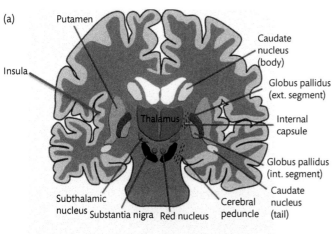

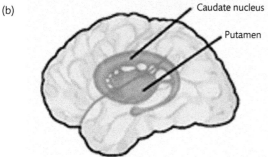

Fig. 6.18 (a) Basal ganglia structures. The heads of the caudate nuclei are located next to the ventricles and extend around in a curved manner to terminate at the amygdala. The middle set of nuclei are on the most medial aspect of the internal segment of the globus pallidus, with the external segment of the globus pallidus being just lateral to that and the most lateral of the group being the putamen. The subthalamic nucleus lies just inferior to the thalamus, and the substantia nigra is located in the midbrain. (Note that the thalamus, red nucleus, and cerebral peduncle are not part of the basal ganglia.) (b) Caricature of the caudate nucleus. The caudate consists of the head, body, and tail. The head starts on the superior and anterior aspects of the caudate, with the body encompassing the extent of the curved aspect of the caudate and the tail terminating at the amygdala.

Subcortical nuclei

The basal ganglia and thalamus are grey matter nuclei located deep in the brain and are supportive of numerous cognitive and behavioural operations. The following discussion does not detail all of the regions of these subcortical areas but, rather, highlights those that are most central to cognition and behaviour.

Basal ganglia

The basal ganglia consists of the striatum (caudate and putamen), globus pallidus (internal and external), substantia nigra, subthalamic nucleus, nucleus accumbens, and ventral tegmental area (see Fig. 6.18). The caudate nucleus has a head and tail component, with the tail extending through the frontal gyrus and curving into the temporal lobe terminating next to the amygdala. The next most medial nucleus of the basal ganglia group is the globus pallidus. The globus pallidus is separated into two segments—an internal and an external segment. The putamen is the most lateral of the basal ganglia nuclei, lateral to the external segment of the globus pallidus. These three sets of nuclei have been shown to be engaged in cognitive control functions, procedural memory, and action selection.

Inferiorly (situated near the brainstem) and midline in location is another set of basal ganglia nuclei—the substantia nigra. The substantia nigra is located in the brainstem and midbrain region, and neighbouring the cerebral peduncles, with its major function to provide dopamine via its projections to the basal ganglia (see Fig. 6.18). This is the brain area that shows significant loss of dopamine neurones in patients with Parkinson's disease, resulting in motor dysfunction due to this lack of dopamine. Another deep basal ganglia nucleus is the subthalamic nucleus, which is located more inferiorly to the striatum and globus pallidus, inferiorly to the thalamus, and superiorly to the substantia nigra. It functions in mediating movements via its inputs to other basal ganglia structures. If unilaterally damaged, the patient develops a movement disorder termed hemiballismus. Degenerative changes in the subthalamic nucleus are associated with progressive supranuclear palsy, a progressive movement and cognitive disorder.

The substantia nigra's role is to provide dopamine input to the basal ganglia structures. The caudate and putamen receive input from the cortices, with outputs to other basal ganglia structures only. The role of the globus pallidus is to provide inhibitory motor control. The subthalamic nucleus projects to the globus pallidus, while receiving input mainly from the cerebral cortex. With this rich set of interactions with other cortical and subcortical structures related to motor movements, it is important to note that these structures are also engaged in a vast array of cognitive operations and behaviours, including, but not limited to, cognitive control/executive functions, processing speed, coordination of cognitive and motor operations, procedural memory, motivation, and emotion processing.

Thalamus

The thalamus, known as the brain's relay station, is a set of nuclei located centrally in the brain between the cerebral cortex and the midbrain. The thalamus maintains an extensive set of connections between its numerous nuclei and the cerebral cortices, providing a rich set of bidirectional circuits. One set of major functions of the thalamus is to relay sensory and/or motor signals to cortical structures. Other functions subsumed by the thalamus and its cortical connections are to relay synchronizing rhythms from the brainstem to mediate sleep/wake states, level of alertness, and aspects of cognition.

Some of the major nuclei of the thalamus act purely as relays of sensory perceptual information to their cortical end-target region. For example, the lateral geniculate nucleus acts as a relay nucleus between the retina and the primary visual cortex. The medial geniculate nucleus functions as an auditory relay between midbrain structures and the primary auditory cortex. The ventral posterior nucleus is a relay to the somatosensory cortex.

Several of the nuclei of the thalamus play essential roles in behaviour and cognition (see Fig. 6.19). The dorsomedial nucleus is associated with episodic memory via its connections to medial

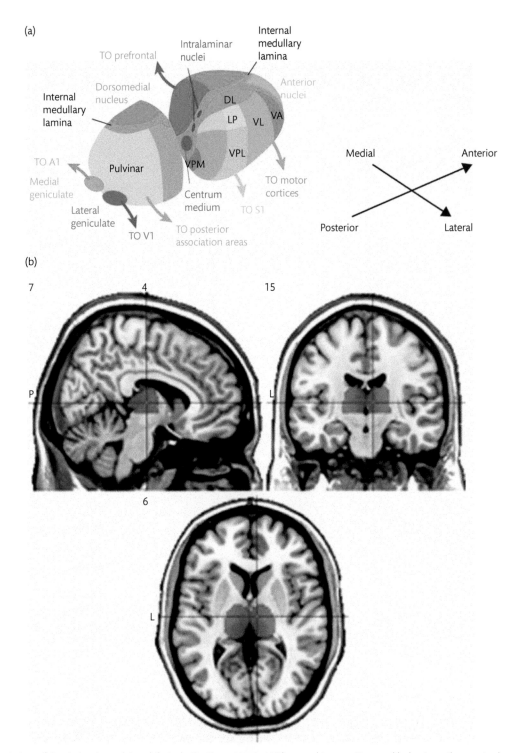

Fig. 6.19 (a) Depiction of the thalamic nuclei and their destination outputs. With regard to cognition and behaviour, the most relevant nuclei are the dorsomedial (blue; connecting to the prefrontal and medial temporal areas), pulvinar (pink; connecting to the posterior association cortices and cingulate and prefrontal cortices), anterior (green; connecting to the mammillary bodies and cingulate), and dorsal lateral nuclei (aqua; connecting to the visual and parietal cortices). (b) Magnetic resonance images in sagittal, coronal, and axial orientations, depicting in red the location of the thalamus.

Reproduced with permission from John Hart Jr. Basic Neuroanatomy Review. In *The Neurobiology of Cognition and Behavior*. Oxford, UK: Oxford University Press. Copyright © 2015, Oxford University Press. DOI: 10.1093/med/9780190219031.001.0001. Reproduced with permission of the Licensor through PLSclear.

temporal lobe and frontal lobe structures. The pulvinar nucleus has widespread connections to the visual, posterior parietal, cingulate, and prefrontal cortices and is associated with a variety of cognitive functions, including attention, memory, and higher-order visual processing. The anterior nuclei play a key role in learning and memory due to their connections with the mammillary bodies and cingulate gyrus. The dorsal lateral nucleus receives input from the visual cortex and has output to the parietal cortices that are engaged in emotion and behavioural functions.

Overall, thalamic involvement in cognition, other than its role as a relay station of information derived from the senses, is evolving with improved experimental designs and advanced neuroimaging techniques. The area where the thalamus appears to have a continually evolving role in cognition and behaviour is in mediating and modulating synchronized electrical oscillations (e.g. EEG power spectra and time–frequency oscillations—Başar et al., 2013). It is becoming evident from a variety of electrophysiological (e.g. EEG and magnetoencephalography) and from a different aspect of neuroimaging studies (e.g. functional connectivity MRI—Buckner et al., 2013) that synchronized firing of groups of neurones in a rhythmic pattern communicates signals between cortical regions for cognitive operations and may, in fact, be a method of encoding object representations (e.g. integrated object concept) (Hart et al., 2007, 2013; see also Griessenberger et al., 2012).

White matter

White matter tract integrity is essential to effective cognition and behaviour. Whereas grey matter has demonstrated notable adaptability and plasticity after injury, white matter does not demonstrate significant reorganization and plasticity. Even if neighbouring grey matter cortices develop adaptive, plastic changes, if there are inadequate white matter connections to connect the adapted regions to the proper targets, then functions such as cognition and behaviour do not recover.

In addition to the increasingly evident importance of the white matter's role in cognition, it is clear that there are specializations as to the types of white matter tracts present in the brain. Currently, three major different types of white matter tracts can be specified: (1) projection tracts that extend vertically between cortical regions and lower brain/spinal cord centres (e.g. spinocerebellar tracts); (2) commissural tracts crossing from one cerebral hemisphere to the other; and (3) association tracts connecting different gyri within the same hemisphere of the brain.

There are several long association tracts that convey key cognitive information between cortical regions. The inferior longitudinal fasciculus (ILF) is a long white matter tract that extends from the visual cortices anteriorly to the temporal lobe (see Fig. 6.20). This connection transfers visual information to both language and memory centres. There is an analogue superior version of the ILF— the superior longitudinal fasciculus (SLF)—which bidirectionally connects visual and temporal cortices to prefrontal regions (see Fig. 6.21). This tract has been further subdivided into four different bundles (SLF I, II, and III, and arcuate fasciculus) that are engaged in a range of cognitive functions, including regulating motor behaviour, spatial attention, language functions, working memory, and auditory processing.

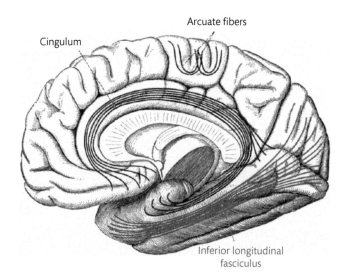

Fig. 6.20 Diagram of the inferior longitudinal fasciculus (red)—the white matter tract connecting the visual system to the temporal lobe. Source: http://www.wikipedia.org.

The uncinate fasciculus connects the hippocampus and the amygdala with the orbitofrontal cortex (see Fig. 6.21). This foreshortened pathway obviates having to go around the Sylvian fissure to access the frontal lobe from the temporal lobe and has been implicated in memory functions and behaviour (see Fig. 6.21). The arcuate fasciculus is a much studied cortico-cortical connection in cognition because it is the primary white matter pathway involved in language as the connection between Wernicke's and Broca's areas (see Fig. 6.22). A lesion of the arcuate fasciculus leads to a disconnection of Wernicke's area from Broca's area and results in the aphasic syndrome of conduction aphasia, a condition known for a prominent deficit in the ability to repeat words.

The largest and most significant white matter bundle in the brain is the corpus callosum—a commissural tract connecting the two hemispheres (see Fig. 6.23). This tract provides extensive cross-hemispheric cortico-cortical communication that leads to

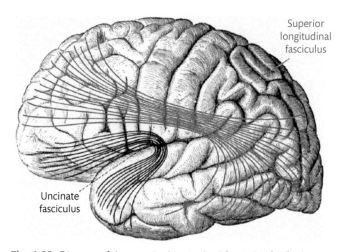

Fig. 6.21 Diagram of the superior longitudinal fasciculus (red)—the white matter tract connecting the occipital and temporal lobes to the frontal lobe. The uncinate fasciculus (black) connects the hippocampus and amygdala to the orbitofrontal cortex. Source: http://www.wikipedia.org.

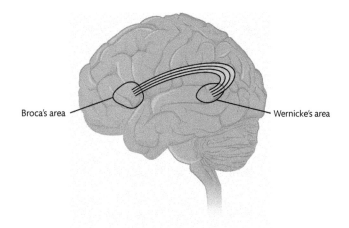

Fig. 6.22 Diagram of the arcuate fasciculus white matter pathway that connects Wernicke's area to Broca's area.

synergistic communication and/or inhibition between hemispheres. Lesioning of the corpus callosum has occurred previously by transection of the anterior two-thirds as a treatment for intractable epilepsy. These patients developed multiple cognitive and behavioural

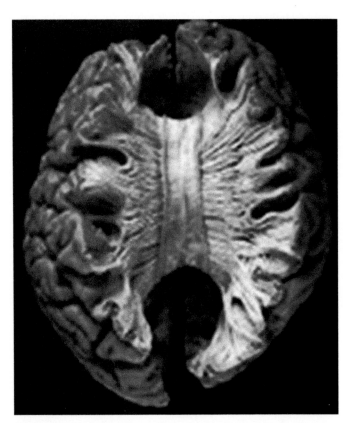

Fig. 6.23 The corpus callosum white matter tract in a dissected brain specimen.

dysfunctions, demonstrating how disconnection between the two hemispheres can disrupt coordination of cognitive operations.

Limbic system

The limbic system is a collection of deep brain structures, referred to as the paleomammalian brain, that lies beneath the cerebral cortex. The structures include the olfactory bulb, hippocampus, amygdala, anterior thalamus, fornix, mammillary body, septum pellucidum, cingulate gyrus, parahippocampal gyrus, and upper midbrain (see Figs 6.17 and 6.24). These structures, present in many species of animals, are engaged in a variety of functions, including smell, emotion, and motivation. These regions are also involved in the formation of episodic and long-term memories.

Many of these regions have been described as part of the lobe or brain region where they reside (parahippocampal gyrus and hippocampus with the temporal lobe) or will be explained in detail in Chapter 6 as part of the Papez circuit. Their existence is raised at this point to demonstrate the organization of these structures in one system and the evolutionary significance of this group of structures across species.

Brodmann areas

In addition to the gyral/sulcal localization schema used traditionally for functional–anatomic assignment, there exist other organizational schema to classify brain locations, with the most popular being the use of Brodmann areas. Brodmann initially described this organization in 1909, based on characterization of different patterns of layers of neurones in the cerebral cortex. He numbered these areas by regions that had similar neuronal organization in the cortical layers. These areas crossed over boundaries of the traditional gyral/sulcal patterns (see Fig. 6.25). The effectiveness of this organization extends from the number of significant correlations of these BAs with specific cognitive and other brain functions.

Sensory cortices map effectively to BA organization. BA 1–3 correspond to primary somatosensory cortices, BA 17 to the primary visual cortex, BA 4 to the primary motor cortex, and BA 41 and 42 are the primary auditory cortices. Related association cortices include the visual association cortex in BA 18 and 19 and the somatosensory association cortices in BA 7.

The following are other key BAs that are relevant to cognitive and behavioural functions:

- Frontal lobe:
  - Premotor cortex and SMA are BA 6.
  - Frontal eye fields are BA 8.
  - DLPFC is BA 9 and 46.
  - Broca's area is BA 44 and 45.
  - Orbitofrontal cortex is BA 11 and 12.
  - Insular cortex is BA 13, 14, and 16.
  - Cingulate cortex is BA 24, 32, and 33 (anterior) and BA 23, 26, and 29–31 (posterior).
- Temporal lobe:
  - Anterior temporal lobe is BA 15.

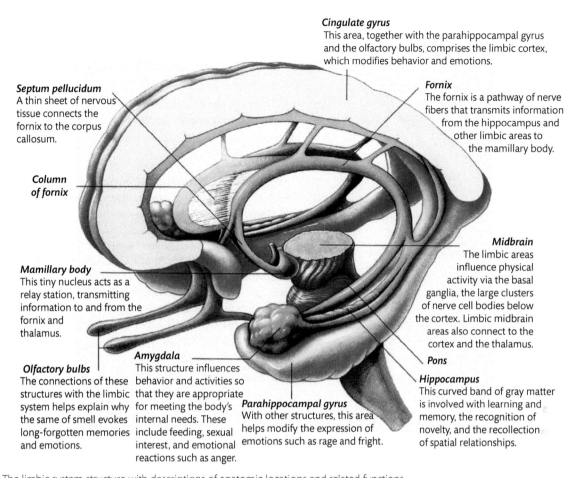

Cingulate gyrus
This area, together with the parahippocampal gyrus and the olfactory bulbs, comprises the limbic cortex, which modifies behavior and emotions.

Septum pellucidum
A thin sheet of nervous tissue connects the fornix to the corpus callosum.

Fornix
The fornix is a pathway of nerve fibers that transmits information from the hippocampus and other limbic areas to the mamillary body.

Column of fornix

Midbrain
The limbic areas influence physical activity via the basal ganglia, the large clusters of nerve cell bodies below the cortex. Limbic midbrain areas also connect to the cortex and the thalamus.

Mamillary body
This tiny nucleus acts as a relay station, transmitting information to and from the fornix and thalamus.

Pons

Amygdala
This structure influences behavior and activities so that they are appropriate for meeting the body's internal needs. These include feeding, sexual interest, and emotional reactions such as anger.

Olfactory bulbs
The connections of these structures with the limbic system helps explain why the same of smell evokes long-forgotten memories and emotions.

Parahippocampal gyrus
With other structures, this area helps modify the expression of emotions such as rage and fright.

Hippocampus
This curved band of gray matter is involved with learning and memory, the recognition of novelty, and the recollection of spatial relationships.

Fig. 6.24 The limbic system structure with descriptions of anatomic locations and related functions.

Reproduced with permission from John Hart Jr. Basic Neuroanatomy Review. In *The Neurobiology of Cognition and Behavior*. Oxford, UK: Oxford University Press. Copyright © 2015, Oxford University Press. DOI: 10.1093/med/9780190219031.001.0001. Reproduced with permission of the Licensor through PLSclear.

- Superior temporal gyrus is BA 22 (Wernicke's area is part of BA 22).
- Middle temporal gyrus is BA 21.
- Inferior temporal gyrus is BA 20.
- Anterior temporal pole is BA 38.
- Parietal lobe:

- Angular gyrus is BA 39 (part of which is Wernicke's area).
- Supramarginal gyrus is BA 40 (also part of Wernicke's area).
- Occipital lobe:
  - Fusiform gyrus is BA 37.

All of the frameworks presented provide different perspectives on how to view the brain's anatomical divisions. Throughout

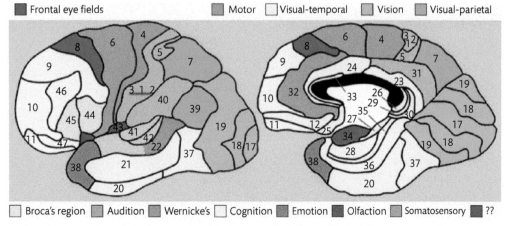

Fig. 6.25 Schematic of Brodmann areas, with the lateral view of the brain on the left and the medial view on the right.
Courtesy of Professor Mark Dubin.

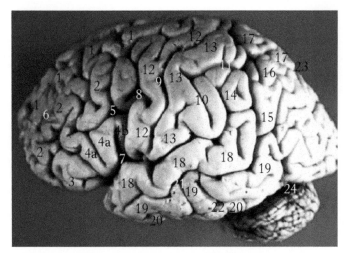

Fig. 6.26 Numbers designating the cortical regions on the lateral view of the brain: 1, superior frontal gyrus; 2, middle frontal gyrus; 3, orbital gyrus; 4, inferior frontal gyrus—(a) pars triangularis and (b) pars opercularis; 5, inferior frontal sulcus; 6, superior frontal sulcus; 7, lateral sulcus; 8, precentral sulcus; 9, central sulcus; 10, post-central sulcus; 11, intraparietal sulcus; 12, precentral gyrus; 13, post-central gyrus; 14, supramarginal gyrus; 15, angular gyrus; 16, inferior parietal lobule; 17, superior parietal lobule; 18, superior temporal gyrus; 19, middle temporal gyrus; 20, inferior temporal gyrus; 21, superior temporal sulcus; 22, middle temporal sulcus; 23, parieto-occipital sulcus; 24, preoccipital incisures.

investigations in neuroscience, studies are reported using the anatomic localization system that best fits reporting of the data. This chapter is not meant to be an exhaustive review of all of neuroanatomy or organizational frameworks, but rather as a reference and roadmap to use to frame the findings of behavioural and cognitive correlates described in the ensuing chapters. As an additional summary figure of anatomic locations from the lateral view of one hemisphere of the brain, Fig. 6.26 is included as a convenient reference for finding anatomical locations for the correlations reported in the ensuing chapters.

Conclusion

For those learning neuroanatomy, as one adopts a conceptual framework of anatomical structures and their inter-relationships in the brain, it is again recommended to have a 3-D model of the brain available, particularly one that allows for opening to see deep structures. One approach of a 3-D conceptualization of the brain is to start with the most deep and midline structures and build layers on top of them. That starting point is the thalamus, midline and deep in location. It is neurally efficient because the 'relay station' connecting all cortical and subcortical brain regions (thalamus) would be located centrally in the brain (see Figs. 6.18 and 6.19).

The next layer placed on top of the thalamus is the limbic system. Evolutionarily speaking, the limbic system is a primitive set of structures like the thalamus. It supports functions such as learning and memory, smell, and fear/threat. One can take the amygdala,

hippocampus, fornix, and mammillary body and sit them on top of the thalamus. These can then be wrapped in the parahippocampal gyrus inferiorly and the cingulate gyrus posteriorly and superiorly (see Figs. 6.17 and 6.24).

The basal ganglia are the next layer to overlay on the model. Because these structures modulate cortical to brainstem and, in some cases, cortical to thalamic communications, this is an ideal location for these structures. The globus pallidus and then the putamen are laid laterally around our building brain, with the caudate head placed superiorly and anteriorly by the lateral ventricle, and the body and tail extending posteriorly and curving inferiorly to complete the basal ganglia structure overlay (see Fig. 16.18).

The last layer are the cortices of the frontal, parietal, temporal, and occipital lobes. The area that can be confusing among the cortical regions is the area underneath the temporal lobe that is the inferior part of the frontal lobe containing the insula. With regard to how this follows the surface of the frontal lobe, this is best conceptualized by following the inferior frontal gyrus cortical surface inferiorly. This cortical surface then tucks in medially over the top of the superior temporal gyrus at the Sylvian fissure and then continues inferiorly downward (see Figs. 6.4 and 6.18). This latter aspect of the inferior extension of the frontal lobe is the insula, the part of the frontal lobe you see when you pull apart the frontal lobe and temporal lobe at the Sylvian fissure. The posterior aspect of the insular region then joins with the medial extension of the superior temporal gyrus in the most posterior aspect of the frontal and temporal lobes. This is best seen in the coronal view of the brain in Fig. 6.18.

Again, this is one formulation to conceptualize the brain structure and inter-relationships. It is left to each individual to best develop a framework that is most effective for his or her use.

KEY LEARNING POINTS

- Knowledge of basic neuroanatomic organization is essential to understanding cognitive anatomic correlations.
- This chapter provides a descriptive overview of the basic neuroanatomic structures in the human brain, with a particular emphasis on the structures that are associated with cognitive and behavioural functions.
- These structures include the lobes of the brain (frontal, parietal, occipital, and temporal), the subcortical nuclei (basal ganglia and thalamus), the white matter, and the limbic system.
- A conceptual framework is presented that can be utilized to organize the anatomical locations, as well as the interconnections between regions.

REFERENCES

Başar E, Başar-Eroğlu C, Güntekin B, Yener G. Brain's alpha, beta, gamma, delta, and theta oscillations in neuropsychiatric diseases: Proposal for biomarker strategies. *Supplements to Clinical Neurophysiology* 2013;62:19–54.

Buckner R, Krienen F, Yeo B. Opportunities and limitations of intrinsic functional connectivity MRI. *Nature Neuroscience* 2013;16:832–7.

Cieslik E, Zilles K, Caspers S, et al. Is there 'one' DLPFC in cognitive action control? Evidence for heterogeneity from co-activation-based parcellation. *Cerebral Cortex* 2013;23:2677–89.

Griessenberger H, Hoedlmoser K, Heib D, Lechinger J, Klimesch W, Schabus M. Consolidation of temporal order in episodic memories. *Biological Psychology* 2012;91:150–5.

Hart J, Anand R, Zoccoli S, et al. Neural substrates of semantic memory. *Journal of the International Neuropsychological Society* 2007;13:865–80.

Hart J, Maguire M, Motes M, et al. Semantic memory retrieval circuit: Role of BA6 and thalamus. *Brain and Language* 2013;126:89–98.

7

Neurophysiology in neuropsychiatry

Elisaveta Sokolov and Nandini Mullatti

Introduction

Electroencephalography (EEG) is a widely available, non-invasive, and relatively inexpensive test that can help identify or exclude functional or structural factors that may be contributing to psychiatric syndromes. This chapter defines the clinical usefulness of EEG in evaluating neuropsychiatric disorders and also highlights the use of other techniques, including transcranial magnetic stimulation in such conditions.

The clinical specialties of neurology and neuropsychiatry are overlapping more, as we progress in our understanding of the close links between structural and functional brain disorders. The pathophysiology of many psychiatric illnesses, such as depression and bipolar disorder, are now being described in terms of their anatomy, physiology, genetics, proteomics, and metabolomics. There is increasing overlap in these two specialties, for example, in the management of dementia or traumatic head injury. EEG analysis often can support our understanding of the physiologic or pathologic changes associated with such disorders.

Commonly used terminology in electroencephalography

In this section, we explain the terms typically used in EEG and the methods for communicating EEG results to others. A clear and precise interpretation of an EEG tracing is central to the use of EEG in clinical practice. Careful use and understanding of EEG terminology is key to non-ambiguous communication of EEG findings to others. Standard EEG terms were published initially in 1974 and updated in 1999. In addition, by using a standard nomenclature, EEG findings can be associated clearly with clinical syndromes ('A glossary of terms most commonly used by clinical electroencephalographers', 1974; Noachtar et al., 1999]. EEG waves should be described in terms of their location corresponding to the cortical region, voltage (amplitude), rhythmicity, frequency, morphology, and continuity. For example, a right parietal theta wave could be described as follows: 'Occasional intermittent high-voltage sinusoidal 6-Hz waves are evident in the right parietal region during drowsiness.' The frequency of waves on the EEG includes delta, theta, alpha, and beta, which are rhythms in specific frequency bands and are described

in Table 7.1. EEG recording at the scalp rarely exceeds frequencies of 30–40 Hz (high-frequency filters are applied to filter frequencies higher than this when presumed to be artefactual or noise). Frequency can be described using two interchangeable terms—hertz (Hz) or cycles per second (cps). EEG is a complex summation of frequencies. Different frequencies sometimes add or cancel each other out. A harmonic results when two waves are combined, and one has a frequency that is a multiple of the other. For example, there may be a 5-Hz base frequency and a superimposed 10-Hz frequency due to mixing of these waves.

The locations of EEG electrodes are typically best described in terms of which electrodes are involved. Either the 10–20 system of electrode placement or the Modified Maudsley system can be used. Fig. 7.1 demonstrates the 10–20 electrode placement system. In addition, the EEG can employ terms such as 'generalized', 'focal', 'lateralized', or 'multifocal' to better categorize results. A focal discharge or wave is one isolated to a specific (single) brain area. A generalized seizure involves all or almost all brain areas at once. A lateralized event is specific to a single hemisphere, and a multifocal event should involve three or more brain areas.

EEG acquisition

EEG acquisition and set-up are typically performed by clinical neurophysiologists. Experienced technicians take about 10 minutes to correctly place scalp electrodes. This requires scrubbing the scalp and carefully positioning the electrodes in the correct place. Scrubbing helps to reduce impedance which may interfere with accurate EEG acquisition. Impedance can be measured and should be maintained as low as possible. Impedance can be defined as the effective resistance of an electric circuit or component within an electric circuit to an alternating current. This typically arises from the combined effects of resistance and reactance.

Electrodes and montages

Montages define the topographic display of EEG channels. It is the electrical map that is developed from the spatial array of recording electrodes. EEG standards require at least three

Table 7.1 EEG wave frequencies

Wave	Frequency
Beta	>13 Hz
Alpha	8–13 Hz
Theta	4–8 Hz
Delta	0–4 Hz

montages—referential, transverse bipolar, and longitudinal bipolar. Thus, several montages are used throughout a 20-minute EEG recording. Bipolar and referential montages are the two most commonly used EEG montages. A longitudinal bipolar montage runs in the sagittal orientation. A transverse bipolar montage runs in the coronal orientation. In referential montages, all electrodes are referred back to one reference electrode and a resultant average is produced. Generalized activity is usually displayed accurately in a referential montage. In the referential montage, all activity is compared to a common average—the 'average electrode'. A referential montage uses an active electrode site as the initial input and then at least one neutral electrode to depict the absolute voltage through amplitude measurement that represents the area of maximum electropositivity or negativity.

To lateralize temporal recordings, a midline electrode may be useful. In some cases, it may be useful to use two reference electrodes for more generalized discharges. This is any chosen electrode, typically in the midline. Bipolar montages may be arranged in many different spatial formats, including longitudinal, transverse, or circumferential. Bipolar montages compare active electrodes next to each other and indicate sites of maximum negativity by way of phase reversals. A bipolar montage is thus particularly useful for localizing focal discharges. If the voltage difference between electrode 1 is more negative than electrode 2, the waveform deflection is 'up'. This is purely by convention. Recordings are usually performed at the following settings: amplifier sensitivities 7 µV/mm, visual display 30 mm/s, and filter settings as discussed below.

Filters

EEG filters are required to remove unnecessary potentials. A low-frequency filter blocks low-frequency artefact such as potentials generated from slight temperature changes, skin conductance, or patient movement. The standard setting for a low-frequency filter is 1 Hz. A high-frequency filter removes high-frequency artefact such as muscle noise. The standard setting for a high-frequency filter is 70 Hz. The third type of filter is a notch filter. This can remove

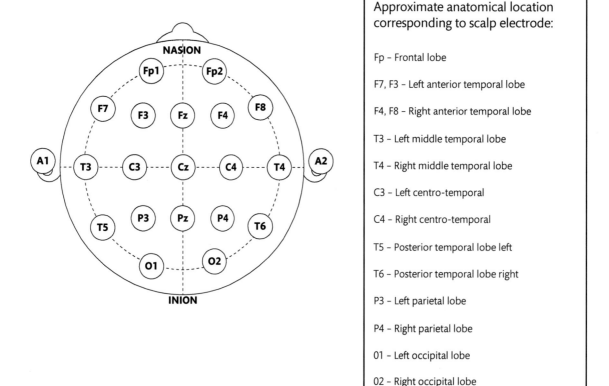

Approximate anatomical location corresponding to scalp electrode:

Fp – Frontal lobe

F7, F3 – Left anterior temporal lobe

F4, F8 – Right anterior temporal lobe

T3 – Left middle temporal lobe

T4 – Right middle temporal lobe

C3 – Left centro-temporal

C4 – Right centro-temporal

T5 – Posterior temporal lobe left

T6 – Posterior temporal lobe right

P3 – Left parietal lobe

P4 – Right parietal lobe

01 – Left occipital lobe

02 – Right occipital lobe

Fig. 7.1 The electrode nomenclature for the 10–20 EEG electrode system. Odd-numbered electrodes represent the left cerebral cortex and even-numbered electrodes represent the right cerebral cortex. FP, F, P, T, and O correspond to frontal polar, frontal, parietal, temporal, and occipital electrodes.

specific frequencies from a signal, for example, 60 Hz. This is mediated through the ground electrode.

Electroencephalographic artefacts

The purpose of an EEG is to record intracerebral physiologic processes. However, it also records electrical activities that occur from extra-cerebral sites. This is artefact. There are physiological and extra-physiological artefacts. Physiological artefacts arise from body parts other than the brain. Extra-physiological artefacts arise from environmental objects such as pieces of equipment. Muscle artefact (see Fig. 7.2) is common and may pertain to movement of the frontalis and temporalis muscles. Myogenic potentials commonly have a shorter latency and an increased frequency, compared to cortical potentials. Some movement disorders can give rise to particular myogenic artefacts on EEG; for example, essential tremor and Parkinson's disease can create rhythmic 4- to 6-Hz sinusoidal artefacts. The eyeball has a dipole, with a positive pole (cornea) and a negative pole (retina). When the eyeball moves, it produces a current which is detected by electrodes in proximity, giving an 'eye movement artefact' on the EEG. A blink results in the positive pole (cornea) moving towards the frontopolar electrodes (Fp1–Fp2) and producing symmetric positive deflections on the EEG. The opposite occurs during downward movement of the eye. The positive pole of the eyeball moves away from the frontal electrodes, producing a negative deflection on the EEG. Lateral eye movements typically affect F7 and F8. When the eyes make a lateral movement to the right,

the positive pole of the eyeball moves towards F8 and away from F7. With left lateral eye movement, the opposite occurs.

Electroencephalography: wakefulness and sleep

Assessment of the background rhythm on the EEG is the first step in its interpretation. The background or posterior rhythm is analysed. The main finding in the awake patient in a normal tracing is a posteriorly dominant alpha rhythm. This is maximally noted in the occipital regions. This typically has a frequency of 8–13 Hz. This is seen in 'quiet wakefulness', as opposed to those who are concentrating or are agitated, in which case there is an attenuation of this alpha rhythm. The voltage of the alpha rhythm may be slightly higher in the right-sided channels, compared to the left; however, amplitude differences of >50% are considered pathological. The waking posterior rhythm is present in most infants by the age of 3 years. Prior to this, slower rhythms are present typically. Wakefulness is most reliably determined by observation for spontaneous eye opening. Agitation and restlessness are other evidence of wakefulness.

Sleep can be catagorized into stages 1–4 (Table 7.2).

Stages 1–4 are frequently categorized as non-REM sleep. Most adults will spend 75% of their time in non-REM sleep and 25% in REM sleep. It is necessary to distinguish the sleep state from pathological states on the EEG. EEG features of sleep are depicted in Table 7.2. There is a slowing or attenuation of the background

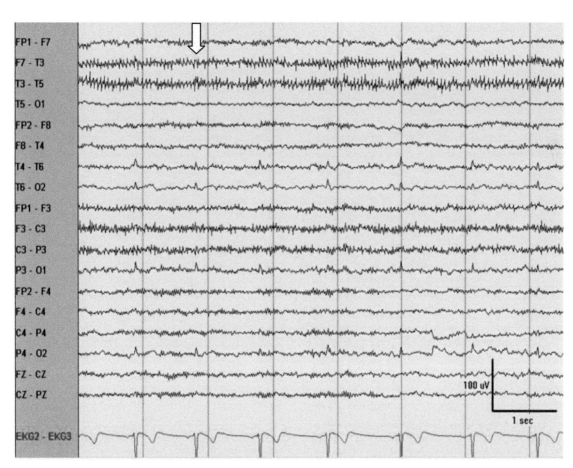

Fig. 7.2 EEG demonstrating muscle and ECG artefact. Muscle artefact is mainly evident in the left temporal region (see arrow).

Table 7.2 Sleep stages

Stage	Name	EEG frequency	Electromyography	Eye movement
Stage W	Wakefulness	Alpha	++	++
1	Drowsiness	Theta	+	+ (slow rolling)
2	Light sleep	Theta	–	+
3 and 4	Deep sleep	Delta	–	+
REM	REM sleep	Alpha/theta	++	–

rhythm in drowsiness, with emergence of diffuse generalized theta activity. It is common to see lateral 'rolling' eye movements in the anterior channels at the beginning of sleep. Stage 2 sleep is defined by sleep spindles. These are centrally predominant 10- to 12-Hz rhythms and mainly seen fronto-centrally. K-complexes appear during light sleep as polyphasic or biphasic midline slow-wave bursts with high amplitude. Vertex sharp waves can appear near or linked to K-complexes. In addition, it is possible to see positive occipital sharp transients of sleep (POSTS) during stage 1 or 2 sleep. These are sharp transients which are varied in amplitude and synchronous in the occipital region with a positive potential (these are described in more detail in Normal variants in EEG below).

Normal variants in EEG

Here we discuss a few of the normal variants that can be identified on the EEG. The literature is extensive, so only a pertinent few are discussed. On eye closure, squeak phenomenon can occur. This is a transient increase in alpha activity. This is named after the short squeaking noise made by historical EEG systems after eye closure and rapid onset of activity. Fast alpha variant with a frequency of approximately 25 Hz can arise when this faster harmonic activity predominates over the slower alpha activity. Similarly to alpha rhythm, fast alpha variant is present during wakefulness and attenuates with eye closure. Mu rhythm with a frequency within the alpha range (10–11 Hz) is scallop-shaped activity seen in parasagittal regions. It may often be unilateral only and attenuates with contralateral limb movement. Mu rhythm is a reflection of activity within the awake sensorimotor cortex. It is evident in 10–15% of tracings. Beta activity (>13 Hz) can often be seen on EEG tracings, with varying significance. Posteriorly, on the EEG, in the occipital electrodes, it is important not to confuse lambda waves with POSTS. Lambda waves occur in the occipital regions bilaterally as positive (upgoing) waves. They are triangular-shaped and usually symmetrical. These occur in the awake patient and are said to be most evident when the subject stares at a blank surface. Lambda waves can arise when reading, for example. Morphologically, they are similar to POSTS and both are seen in an occipital distribution. POSTS are also triangular waveforms that are evident in bilateral occipital regions as positive waves. They can be multiple and usually are also symmetric, as with lambda waves. POSTS, however, arise in the asleep patient (notably stage 2 sleep). Benign epileptic transients of sleep (BETS) are sharp waves occurring on one or both hemispheres (typically asynchronously), often in the temporal and frontal brain regions. BETS are more frequently seen in adults, compared to children. BETS often are seen in individuals without epilepsy and can be regarded as a probable normal variant, although they can occur in epileptic patients (see Fig. 7.3).

Interictal epileptiform discharges

These are EEG events which arise during a tracing, while a clinical seizure is not occurring, which are indicative of epilepsy (see Table 7.3). We also outline EEG events which may provide some evidence of a tendency to seizures but are not definitively diagnostic for epilepsy.

EEG in neuropsychiatry

In this section, we cover EEG features of common conditions that may be seen in the neuropsychiatric setting.

Temporal lobe epilepsy

This is the commonest focal epilepsy (localization-related). Complex partial seizures are the commonest seizure type seen with temporal lobe epilepsy (TLE), but TLE is not the only cause of complex partial seizures. If a cause for the seizures is identified, for example, a hamartoma or cortical dysplasia, then the TLE is considered a symptomatic epilepsy. One of the commonest causes for TLE is hippocampal sclerosis (see Fig. 7.4). If no cause is identified, then the TLE is considered cryptogenic (Pataraia et al., 1998).

The typical temporal lobe seizure may start with an aura. These auras can be any of the following types: somatosensory, visual, auditory, gustatory, olfactory, autonomic, abdominal, and psychic. Automatisms of the hands typically occur ipsilateral to the seizure focus. Dystonic posturing of a hand, if present, is typically contralateral to the seizure focus. TLE may secondarily generalize, leading to tonic–clonic convulsions of all four limbs. The typical EEG correlate of TLE is a spike or sharp wave over the anterior temporal lobe (see Fig. 7.5). These focal discharges may generalize with varying amounts of interhemispheric discharges. Sleep may activate focal temporal discharges. Temporal intermittent rhythmic delta activity (TIRDA), a form of slow-wave activity in the temporal lobe, may be present. Focal slowing and spikes correlate clearly with the ictal onset zone, with focal delta waves occurring in 82% of cases analysed and spikes occurring in 90% (Blume et al., 1993).

Ictal recordings are often required, as patients can have non-epileptic attacks such as psychogenic non-epileptic seizures (PNES), in addition to TLE.

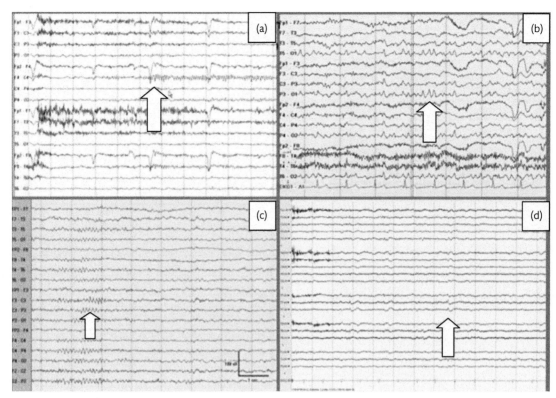

Fig. 7.3 (a) Mu rhythm. (b) Lambda waves. (c) Positive occipital sharp transients of sleep (POSTS). (d) Benign epileptiform transients of sleep (BETS) (see arrows).

Non-convulsive status epilepticus

Non-convulsive status epilepticus (NCSE) can be described as a change in behaviour from baseline, accompanied by continuous epileptiform discharges in the EEG. However, there is ongoing debate regarding the diagnosis of NCSE. It is generally classified as generalized or focal. Generalized NCSE consists of absence, *de novo* late-onset absence, and atypical absence. Some authors include myoclonic status epilepticus under this category (Power et al., 2015). Absence status is characterized by confusion or decreased responsiveness, with infrequent blinking, lasting hours to days, with an EEG showing generalized spike and slow-wave discharges. Focal NCSE includes simple and complex focal status epilepticus. Complex partial status comprises repetitive or prolonged complex partial seizures and produces confusion or a labile level of consciousness. Other confused or comatose patients with rhythmic, rapid epileptiform discharges on the EEG may have so-called 'electrographic' status epilepticus and can be regarded within the same diagnostic category. In terms of EEG findings, when differentiating NCSE from encephalopathies, the overall picture of the EEG discharge should be taken into account, including its evolution in space and time. NCSE is indicated by an incremental evolution of regional or generalized rhythmic discharges and decremental features with flat periods associated with clinical seizure activity (Hirsch et al., 2005). Coma patients can have periodic and rhythmic EEG changes that are not usually pathognomonic, and the diagnosis of NCSE generally therefore should not be based on EEG changes alone. The diagnosis of NCSE usually involves an abnormal mental status examination, with decreased responsiveness, a supportive

Table 7.3 Interictal epileptiform discharges

EEG event	Clinical significance
Sharp wave	Any sharp transient that interrupts and stands out from ongoing background activity has a sharp component and a duration measured at its base of between 70 and 200 ms. This can often be followed by a slow wave potential. If these criteria are met, this is termed a sharp wave, a finding that carries a significant association with epileptic seizures. Typically, the sharp component and after-coming slow wave have a surface negative potential. Many surface-positive discharges indicate a benign origin
Spike	A sharp transient that meets the criteria for sharp waves, except the duration is briefer (between 20 and 70 ms). Spikes and sharp waves are both referred to as interictal epileptiform discharges (IEDs) and both are associated with susceptibility to recurrent seizures
Transient	General term for any brief potential encountered in a tracing
Sharp transient	Any transient potential with an epileptiform (sharp) morphology. Note that epileptiform is synonymous with sharp and is a morphologic descriptor, rather than a clinical predictor. A sharp transient may or may not have a clinical significance, and not all are necessarily associated with epilepsy

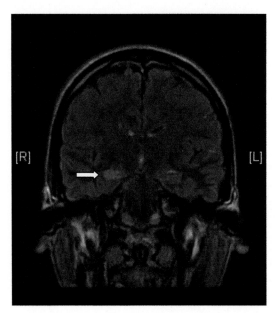

Fig. 7.4 Right mesial temporal sclerosis in a patient with temporal lobe epilepsy.

EEG, and usually a good response to antiepileptic treatment. Although a positive electroclinical response to acute anticonvulsant therapy can be helpful in the diagnosis, a poor response does not rule out the diagnosis. NCSE is not associated with extensive morbidity; rather it is the underlying disease which is. However, in cases of prolonged NCSE or those with focal lesions, systemic illness, or very fast epileptiform discharges, more permanent damage may ensue. Although clinical studies show little evidence of permanent neurologic injury, there is evidence to support prolonged memory dysfunction, and in some cases, NCSE can be fatal and lead to severe sequelae, suggesting that NCSE should be treated expeditiously (Drislane et al., 1999).

Epilepsy partialis continua

Epilepsia partialis continua (EPC) can be regarded as status epilepticus equivalent of simple focal motor seizures. There is focal motor clonic activity. Clonic activity in EPC can involve any muscle group and is more common in the upper limb. The frequency of the clonic activity is typically 0.1–6 Hz. The seizures remain in the part of the body in which they originally started in the majority of cases. However, in some cases, there can be a Jacksonian spread of the seizure, which can lead to a secondary generalized seizure. The focal clonic activity can continue for many hours or even weeks, and awareness is not typically impaired. Post-ictal weakness is frequently present in these patients.

EPC typically originates in the cortex; however, subcortical mechanisms have been hypothesized. EPC can constitute part or all of the clinical phenotype of a pre-existing cortical lesion or a progressive disease such as Rasmussen syndrome (Bancaud et al., 1970).

It is now defined as a form of partial status epilepticus with simple motor manifestations, continuing for longer than 1 hour, with clonic activity restricted to one body part, and recurring at fairly regular intervals. It should also be noted that the motor activity often is modified by sensory stimulation. About 60% of patients have other types of seizures besides EPC. EPC can be sub-classified, as described in Table 7.4. In terms of neurophysiology, in Rasmussen encephalitis, frequently, lateralized, asymmetrical background slowing is noted. The EEG may also provide evidence of other seizure types or projected abnormalities suggestive of widespread, but lateralized, pathology. Evoked-potential techniques, particularly somatosensory evoked potentials (SSEPs), have been used to understand the physiology and anatomical origins of EPC. Giant SSEPs are often present and may indicate cortical hyperexcitability, which is hypothesized as an essential mechanism of EPC.

Psychogenic non-epileptic seizures

PNES, also known as non-epileptiform attack disorders (NEADs), consist of events presenting clinically in a similar way to an epileptic seizure, however, without the concomitant EEG correlate. Nevertheless, between 5% and 20% of patients with PNES also have epilepsy. The terminology on the topic has been variable. Differing terms are used, including non-epileptic seizures, pseudoseizures, dissociative seizures, non-epileptic attacks, and psychogenic seizures. PNES is the preferred term in the literature. PNES is a

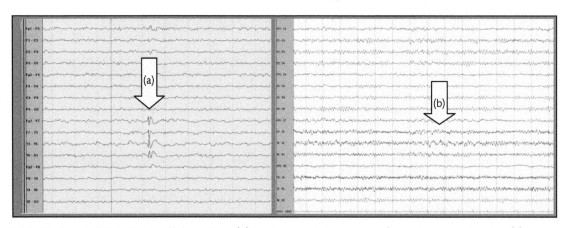

Fig. 7.5 Interictal EEG abnormalities in temporal lobe epilepsy. (A) Spike-wave activity over the left anterior temporal region. (B) Slow waves over the left anterior temporal region.

Table 7.4 Sub-classification of epilepsy partialis continua

Type 1 (classic)	Type 2 (Rasmussen)
Rolandic isolated lesion	Normal development and history until seizure onset
Neurological deficit preceding partial motor seizures	Partial motor seizures
Myoclonic jerks	Myoclonic jerks
EEG: focal abnormalities	EEG: abnormal background with focal and diffuse intermittent abnormalities
Non-progressive course. Surgery usually effective	Progressive course. Intractable epilepsy

neuropsychiatric disorder, specifically a functional disorder, classified under the diagnostic category of somatic symptom disorders in the DSM-5 (American Psychiatric Association, 2013). In the general population, PNES is common, with an estimated prevalence of 2–33 cases per 100,000 population. PNES are common at epilepsy centres where they are seen in 20–30% of patients referred for refractory seizures. Often certain features of the phenotype can point towards PNES, rather than true seizures. Resistance to antiepileptic drugs (AEDs) is common. A psychogenic aetiology can be considered when the reported frequency of seizures is not improved by AEDs. Other presenting clinical features can point towards PNES, for example, emotional triggers such as stress. Pain may be a feature, but this is not exclusive to PNES, although it is unusual in epilepsies. In addition, if particular lights are said to always trigger an episode, this may also indicate PNES. PNES do not result from any aberrant electrical discharges from the cortex. Therefore, the EEG is typically within normal limits. PNES can provide a specific clinical phenotype as a manifestation of the psychological disturbance. In terms of prognosis, PNES markedly affects the quality of life, and outcomes in adults are poor. At 10 years post-PNES onset, 50% of patients may still have seizures (Meierkord et al., 1991).

EEG in dementia

Dementia is defined as memory loss, confusion, and poor judgement. Pathologically, there is degeneration of cortical neurones. This is usually generalized throughout all lobes of the brain. The EEG recorded in Alzheimer's disease is not static but is dependent upon the degree of progression of the disease (see Fig. 7.6). Initially the EEG may be within normal limits. As neurodegeneration progresses, the alpha activity is diminished and the overall amplitude drops. There can be theta activity seen, with intermittent delta activity, i.e. progressive slowing of background rhythms occur. It is also possible to see sharpened theta waves or indeed sharp waves, especially in Alzheimer's disease; however, clear epileptic foci are unusual. The typical sleep architecture can be disrupted with sparse K-complexes.

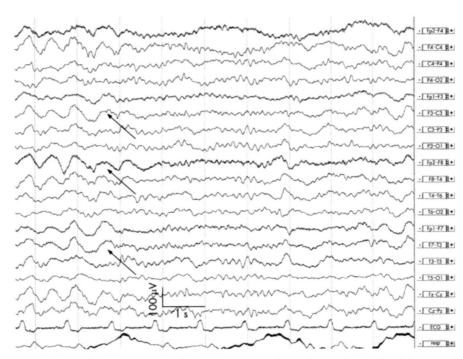

Fig. 7.6 An EEG in a patient with dementia with Lewy bodies. The EEG has a posterior background within the alpha range. Frequent generalized bursts and runs of slow waves are seen.

Metabolic encephalopathies

A metabolic encephalopathy is generalized dysfunction of cerebral neurones, associated with changes in the brain's normal environment caused by metabolic or toxic factors. This pathology is potentially reversible if it has not been ongoing for long enough to cause permanent brain damage. The primary clinical change in a patient suffering from metabolic encephalopathy is an alteration in conscious level. This can range from deep coma to mild confusion. The EEG characteristics are typically non-focal (see Fig. 7.7). Typically there is slowing of the alpha rhythm into the theta range. This can further develop into polymorphic delta or frontal intermittent rhythmic delta activity (FIRDA). The EEG may become lower in voltage and lose reactivity. Periodic discharges may develop, changing to burst suppression activity, and ultimately may not recover, resulting in electro-cerebral inactivity. There may be focal features which can be varied.

Hepatic encephalopathy

This is typically associated with cirrhosis of the liver due to either hepatitis or high alcohol intake. It can present as a type of metabolic encephalopathy, with fluctuating consciousness from confusion to deep coma. Blood ammonia levels are often elevated in these patients. The precise cause of intracerebral dysfunction remains to be determined. In the earlier phases of hepatic encephalopathy, patients may have an EEG which is within normal limits or with some generalized slowing of background rhythms. As encephalopathy progresses, triphasic waveforms appear. These typically have a voltage of 150–300 µV and the frequency is 1.5–3 Hz, repeating periodically

(see Fig. 7.8). They are positive sharp transients that are preceded and followed by negative waves of relatively lower amplitude. The triphasic waves are bilaterally symmetrical and are predominantly frontal but can be seen in a generalized distribution (Janti et al., 2015). Triphasic waves are not specific for hepatic encephalopathy, and their presence has been described in uraemia, anoxia, and hypercalcaemia, amongst others. These changes are usually present in stage 3 coma. Patients with level 1 and 2 coma with hepatic encephalopathy may have an EEG which is within normal limits or with some generalized slowing. Cortical irritation can be seen in triphasic wave encephalopathy. There may be aberrant function of the thalamocortical relay neurones due to structural or metabolic disturbance. These are hypothesized to be responsible for the EEG and clinical findings associated with triphasic wave encephalopathy.

Creutzfeldt–Jakob disease

This is a subacutely progressive brain disorder which can lead to severe brain damage. Prion proteins deposit within the cerebral cortex and precipitate the clinical presentation. The patient may present with rapid cognitive decline and memory impairment, change in personality, loss of balance and coordination, slurred speech, visual disturbance, abnormal jerking movements, and progressive loss of brain function and mobility. Diagnosing Creutzfeldt–Jakob disease (CJD) may be difficult due to the huge variation in presentation. There are four broad types of CJD: sporadic, variant, iatrogenic, and familial. Recently, a CSF protein 14-3-3 has been found to be highly sensitive and specific to CJD and greatly aids diagnosis. Radiology can also play a significant role in the diagnosis of CJD, and together with EEG and CSF results for 14-3-3, the diagnosis can be made

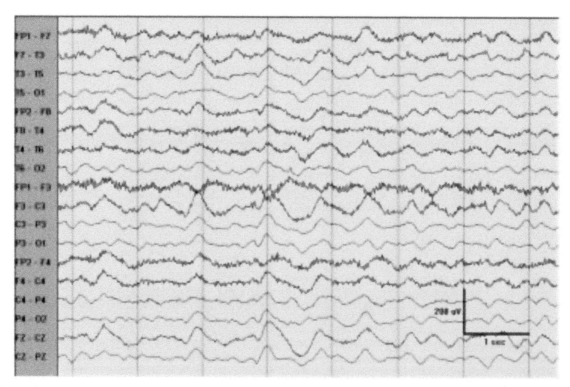

Fig. 7.7 The EEG has a posterior background which is diffusely slowed (3 Hz). This may be in keeping with a moderate to severe encephalopathy.

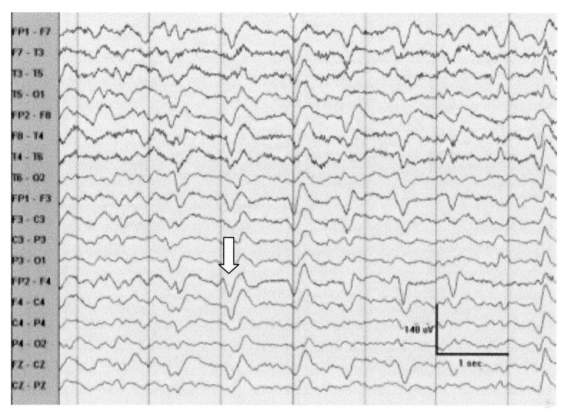

Fig. 7.8 EEG demonstrating triphasic waves (see arrow).
Reproduced with permission from S. R. Benbadis. Introduction to Sleep Electroencephalography. In *Sleep: A Comprehensive Handbook*. T. Lee-Chiong (ed.). Oxford, UK: Wiley. Copyright © 2006 John Wiley & Sons, Inc. https://doi.org/10.1002/0471751723.ch130.

more readily. EEG is part of the World Health Organization's diagnostic classification criteria for CJD. FIRDA can be seen in sporadic CJD, especially in the early stages. Typical classical EEG features of CJD include periodic sharp wave complexes (PSWCs); however, these are only present in approximately 60% of cases. PSWCs may disappear during sleep and can be attenuated by external stimulation and sedative medication. Seizures are not a common finding but are seen in approximately 12% of patients with sporadic CJD. In cases of iatrogenic CJD, PSWCs usually present with more regional EEG findings corresponding to the site of inoculation of the transmissible agent. In genetic CJD, PSWCs in their typical form are uncommon, occurring in about 10%. No PSWCs occur in EEG recordings of patients with variant CJD.

Autoimmune encephalitis

This most commonly occurs in young females. As with encephalopathies in general, all areas of cognition tend to be impaired. Occasionally, rarer focal features, such as those of FTD, occur. Neuropsychiatric features can be present in >50% of cases. Other manifestations can include hallucinations, headache, hypersomnolence, language difficulties, and stroke-like episodes. Seizures are more frequent in paraneoplastic limbic encephalitis, and some cases of status epilepticus are reported which are refractory to antiepileptic medications. EEG is useful to exclude subclinical seizures or NCSE as the primary cause of encephalopathy (Duffey et al., 2003). Diffuse slowing or epileptiform abnormalities

in the temporal lobes are the commonest findings. Rapidly progressive dementia can arise from autoimmune encephalopathy that can be mistaken for CJD (see Fig. 7.9) (Coral et al., 2005). The MRI and EEG features typical of CJD have been described in patients with autoimmune encephalopathy. Despite EEG, CSF, and serological findings, a brain biopsy is occasionally needed to verify the diagnosis. With autoantibodies to voltage-gated potassium channels, limbic encephalitis predominates. Patients with leucine-rich glioma inactivated 1 (LGI1), antibody-associated limbic encephalitis present with symptoms of memory loss, seizures, myoclonus, and a syndrome of limbic encephalitis. Laboratory serology testing commonly reveals hyponatraemia. On EEG, there may be epileptiform discharges in the temporal regions. MRI can demonstrate hyperintensity in the mesial temporal lobes. Many patients improve with immunosuppressive treatment, but this may be only a partial response (see Fig. 7.10).

CASE STUDY 1

Patient RP presents with a 'feeling in her stomach which stays there'. This is a strange 'crawling' and 'nauseating' sensation which spreads from her stomach to her mouth. After this, she is unable to remember what happens next. It takes her several minutes to come back around. She has no post-event speech problems or tongue bites and no weakness. On rare occasions, she has been incontinent. After the event, she is often very tired for several hours.

She feels she has 'memory gaps' for these events. These events have improved over the last few years in terms of frequency.

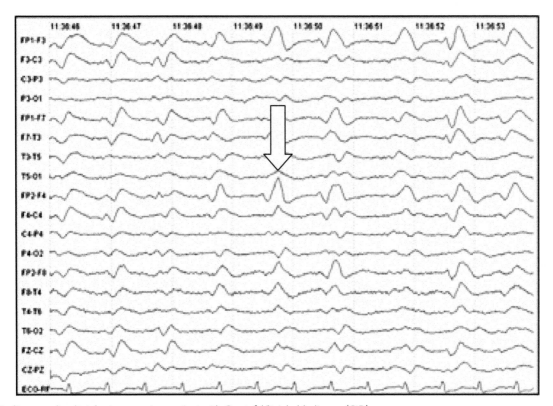

Fig. 7.9 Periodic generalized triphasic waves in a patient with Creutzfeldt–Jakob's disease (CJD).

Reproduced from Coral, P. *et al*. Creutzfeldt-Jakobs disease – case report with emphasis on the electroencephalographic features. *J. Epilepsy Clin. Neurophysiol*. vol.11 no.4. Copyright © 2005, Scielo. http://dx.doi.org/10.1590/S1676-26492005000400007.

Currently she has one event per week, with an interval of 1–2 weeks. They can occur at any time of day and also from sleep. Triggers for these events include stress and lack of sleep. Patient RP has a further medical history, including glaucoma and eczema. She had otherwise normal developmental milestones and no childhood illnesses.

Patient RP underwent an EEG to assess for an organic cause for her presentation which showed spike and slow-wave discharges over the right temporal region (see Fig. 7.11). MRI brain demonstrated right hippocampal sclerosis. The patient was diagnosed with temporal lobe epilepsy and commenced on levetiracetam. Her symptoms have now completely resolved. This history is classical for TLE. In a patient with abdominal sensations, TLE should remain within the differential diagnosis.

CASE STUDY 2

Patient EG underwent an extensive right-sided stereotactic EEG exploration. Single pulse electrical stimulation (SPES) and functional stimulation were also carried out. This was with the aim to consider neurosurgical removal of the main epileptic focus.

EG suffers from tuberous sclerosis with epilepsy from the age of 2. This was diagnosed when she presented with seizures and was found to have a shagreen patch. In 2009, she underwent transcallosal resection of a mass lesion at the right foramen of Monro for a subependymal giant cell astrocytoma (SEGA). There may have been some slight delay in her speech development and she required some input at school.

She has multiple tubers in both cerebral hemispheres, but telemetry has consistently shown right-sided changes, more often over the anterior quadrant.

The current commonest seizure type consists of a feeling of déjà vu and feeling sick. She feels as if she is being enclosed in. She remains conscious and knows where she is. These last about 5 minutes. She finds them very disturbing.

In the second type of seizure, objects or people or things around her change shape and distort. They can become bigger or smaller. Colours remain the same.

The third type of event seems to be some form of auditory illusion. She hears a word and goes over and over it in her head and then sees an object relating to the word. These three seizure types had clear ictal correlates on the EEG and were considered epileptic in origin.

She was also describing a number of hallucinatory experiences which included seeing many death-related and blood-related scenes which were frightening to her. We captured several of these hallucinations, while carrying out the EEG recording, and no clear ictal EEG correlate was seen. These hallucinations were deemed non-epileptic and, in fact, were thought possibly due to a side effect of topiramate and have gone away since reducing this.

This case nicely illustrates the use of EEG in differentiating epileptic from non-epileptic events and the need for further considerations in the event that a symptom is non-epileptic.

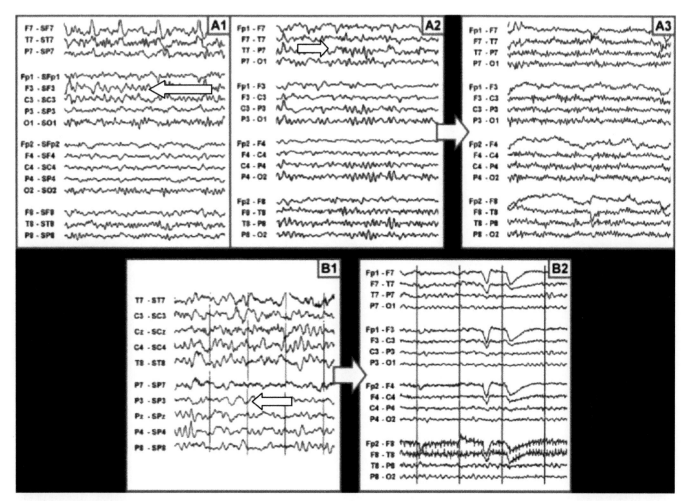

Fig. 7.10 EEG of patients with autoimmune encephalopathy pre- and post-immunotherapy. A1: EEG in a 60-year-old man pre-treatment, demonstrating a left anterior temporal lobe seizure. A2: intermittent rhythmic delta and sharp wave activity over the left temporal region. A3: resolution after phenytoin loading and intravenous methylprednisolone. B1: EEG in a 71-year-old man, demonstrating diffuse theta and delta waves, particularly over the left hemisphere. B2: post-treatment with intravenous methylprednisolone.

CASE STUDY 3

Patient AD was brought by ambulance to the emergency department in status epilepticus involving convulsions of all four limbs. He was intubated and ventilated and sedated in order to try to stop the seizures. He has known idiopathic generalized epilepsy but is often non-compliant with his medications. His EEG after treatment with propofol, Keppra®, and lorazepam demonstrated the pattern seen in Fig. 7.12. This patient fully recovered within 2 days. This is a medically induced burst suppression pattern which is used to prevent ongoing electrical seizure activity in the brain. Often when a patient has been 'burst-suppressed' for some hours, they make a good recovery from status epilepticus. The EEG is key to monitoring such cases, for the initial diagnostic clarification, and then to monitor the burst suppression pattern.

Conclusion

Overall it is clear that the scalp or surface EEG is a useful tool to aid in the diagnosis of numerous brain pathologies. To reiterate a few, it can aid in the diagnosis of neurodegenerative disorders, such as dementia, as well as neuroinflammatory disorders, including autoimmune encephalitis. In addition, the EEG has a key supportive role in the diagnosis of epilepsy.

The advent of depth electrode mapping for epilepsy surgery is revolutionizing this branch of medicine. We are beginning to slowly understand, with the aid of EEG technology, the importance of seizure spread and white matter tracts, especially in the context of focal refractory epilepsies.

There is a large degree of overlap between psychiatry and neurology and the neurosciences, probably to a greater degree than we currently fully appreciate. Thus, it is perhaps not surprising that the EEG can also be a useful tool for the psychiatrist. It is often

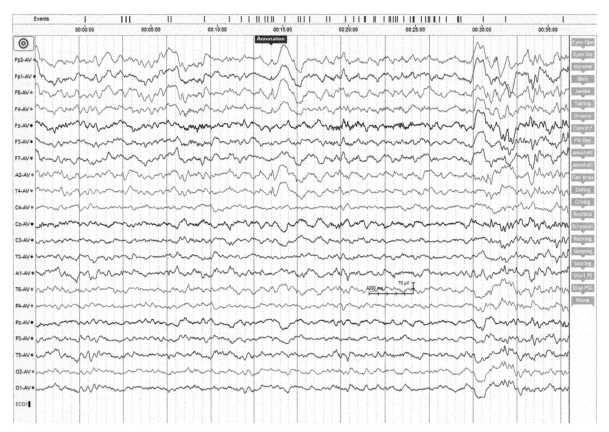

Fig. 7.11 Spike and slow wave discharges over the right temporal region in a patient with temporal lobe epilepsy.

important to distinguish organic versus non-organic pathology, and the EEG may aid with this. For example, it can provide clarity in the diagnosis of non-epileptic attack disorder or patients presenting with features which may constitute TLE. It is important to note that certain antipsychotic medications such as olanzapine can mimic epileptiform discharges on the EEG. This needs to be closely considered when referring your patient for an EEG. The use of EEG technology is ever expanding and we are excited for its future. For further reading, a comprehensive review of EEG can be found in the comprehensive handbook by Bendabis (2006).

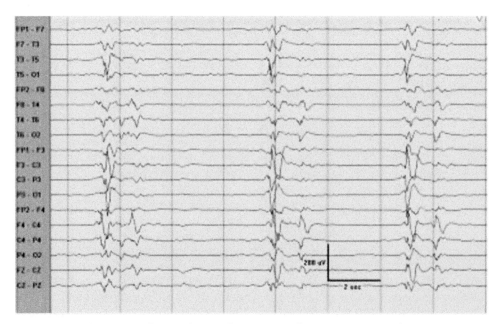

Fig. 7.12 Burst suppression pattern. This consists of bursts of activity (combination of sharp and slow waves) periodically interrupted by periods of suppression (activity <10 μV). Usually the periods of suppression are longer (5–10 s) than the bursts of activity (1–3 s).

KEY LEARNING POINTS

- EEG is a widely available, non-invasive, and relatively inexpensive test that can determine or rule out which functional or structural factors may be contributing to psychiatric syndromes.
- In this chapter, the clinical usefulness of EEG in evaluating neuropsychiatric disorders is defined, while the application of other techniques such as transcranial magnetic stimulation is highlighted.
- The chapter presents different diseases, such as Alzheimer's disease, epilepsy, and various forms of encephalitis, and describes how each would present itself on an EEG. Case studies are presented to demonstrate the role EEG plays in determining neuropsychiatric disorders and monitoring their treatment.

REFERENCES

American Psychiatric Association. *Diagnostic and Statistical Manual of Mental Disorders*, fifth edition. American Psychiatric Association, Arlington, VA, 2013.

Bancaud J, Bonis A, Talairach J, Bordas-Ferrer M. Kojewnikow syndrome and somato-motor attacks (clinical EEG, EMG and SEEG study). *Encephale* 1970;59950:391–438.

Bendabis SR. Introduction to EEG. In: Lee-Chiong T, ed. *Sleep: A Comprehensive Handbook*. Wiley & Sons, Hoboken, NJ, 2006. pp. 989–1024.

Blume WT, Borghesis JL, Lemieux JF. Interictal indices of temporal seizure origin. *Annals of Neurology* 1993;34:703–9.

Coral P, Germiniani FMB, Silvado CE. Creutzfeldt–Jakobs disease—case report with emphasis on the electroencephalographic features. *Journal of Epilepsy and Clinical Neurophysiology* Porto Allegre Dec 2005;11(no.4).

Drislane FW. Evidence against permanent neurologic damage from non-convulsive status epilepticus. *Journal of Clinical Neurophysiology* 1999;16:323–31.

Duffey P, Yee S, Reid IN, et al. Hashimoto's encephalopathy: postmortem findings after fatal status epilepticus. *Neurology* 2003;61:1124–6.

Hirsch LJ, Brenner RP, Drislane FW, et al. The ACNS subcommittee on research terminology for continuous EEG monitoring: proposed standardized terminology for rhythmic and periodic EEG patterns encountered in critically ill patients. *Journal of Clinical Neurophysiology* 2005;22:128–35.

Janti AB, Alghasab N, Umair M. Focal triphasic sharp waves and spikes in the electroencephalogram. *Neurological Sciences* 2015;36:221–6.

Meierkord H, Will B, Fish D, Shorvon S. The clinical features and prognosis of pseudoseizures diagnosed using video-EEG telemetry. *Neurology* 1991;41:1643–6.

Noachtar S, Binnie C, Ebersole J, et al. A glossary of terms most commonly used by clinical electroencephalographers and proposal for the report form for the EEG finding. *Electroencephalography and Clinical Neurophysiology Suppl* 1999;52:21–41.

[No authors listed] A glossary of terms most commonly used by clinical electroencephalographers. *Electroencephalography and Clinical Neurophysiology* 1974;37:538–48.

Pataraia E, Lurger S, Series W, et al. Ictal scalp EEG in unilateral mesial temporal lobe epilepsy. *Epilepsia* 1998;39:608–14.

Power KN, Gramstad A, Gilhus NE, et al. Adult non-convulsive status epilepticus in a clinical setting: Semiology, aetiology, treatment and outcome. *Seizure* 2015;24:102–6.

8

Structural imaging in neuropsychiatry

Naga Kandasamy and Dana Niry

Introduction

Medicine is ever changing and progressing. In the last few decades, imaging is perhaps one of the specialties in medicine which has made remarkable progress. To put things into perspective, it is known that the first medical use of X-ray was in 1895 when Roentgen obtained a radiograph of his wife's left hand. While X-rays have been in medicine since then, it was not until the early 1970s that computed tomography (CT) scanning, which also utilizes X-rays, although with differing principles, was invented. Since then, within a few decades, CT scanning has rapidly progressed in terms of capability and dose reduction, with the most modern CT scanners being capable of acquiring an image, i.e. a 'slice', in around 200 ms, down from 300 s in 1972 and 1–2 s in 1989. This has been accompanied by a reduction in 'slice' thickness, from 13 mm in 1972 to sub-millimetres currently, to increase spatial resolution.

The provision to obtain near-isotropic images with multidetector CT has made it possible to reconstruct images in several planes, with no loss of image resolution. Dose reduction and significant reduction in scanning times have enabled increasing application of CT scanning, particularly in patients who cannot 'tolerate scans'. (See Fig. 8.1.)

In contrast to CT, magnetic resonance imaging (MRI) uses the principle of nuclear magnetic resonance to obtain images. The physics of MRI is beyond the remit of this chapter; however, fundamentally, this does not involve ionizing radiation.

Magnetic resonance imaging

The differences between CT and MR and the advantages of one modality over the other are mentioned in numerous articles and book chapters, but it should be noted that both of these modalities complement, rather than compete with, each other.

In our own practice, we have seen increased application of CT, given its availability and, as previously mentioned, the reduction in radiation dose, although it is important to note that there is no 'safe' radiation dose. Multiplanar reconstructions with the more recent CT scanners offers a major advantage in that multiplanar capability was initially only possible with MRI. While CT has no 'absolute' contraindications, for patients who cannot have an MRI

examination (e.g. MR-incompatible aneurysm clips, pacemakers, metallic implants—be it medical or non-medical, or prosthesis), CT may be the only available imaging option.

In routine clinical practice, CT and MRI are most commonly used for structural imaging purposes. Table 8.1 summarizes the considerations for choice of imaging modality.

Applications using CT and MRI to assess brain function, i.e. measuring changes related to brain metabolism or changes in blood flow, constitute functional imaging. Functional imaging aims at measuring neuronal activity, either by assessing regional metabolic changes, e.g. positron emission tomography (PET), or by assessing changes to regional blood flow, e.g. functional MRI (fMRI). fMRI utilizes the paramagnetic properties of deoxyhaemoglobin to assess regional variations in blood flow.

Broadly speaking, imaging for neuropsychiatric purposes may be indicated in (Cooper et al., 2013; Ikram et al., 2010):

- New-onset psychosis.
- New-onset mood/memory symptoms.
- Occurrence of new or atypical symptoms.
- New-onset personality changes.
- Anorexia without body dysmorphic symptoms.

Equally, situations in which neuroimaging for neuropsychiatric issues may or may not be required include:

- Recurrence of previously controlled psychiatric symptoms, and
- Patients who are refractory to treatment.

Imaging features

First-episode psychosis

The diagnostic yield and the need for structural imaging in patients presenting with first-episode psychosis has been found to be minimal in the young and adolescent age groups (Williams et al., 2014). In patients presenting with first-episode psychosis, neuroimaging, ideally with MRI examination, should be considered when the presentation is with atypical features (e.g. visual hallucinations, disorientation, memory loss, and decreased consciousness); in the presence of neurological signs; in older age groups; in epilepsy, inflammatory (vasculitis)/demyelinating conditions; or when

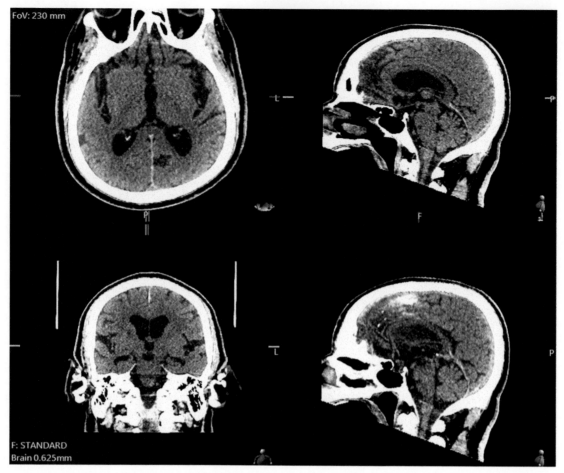

Fig. 8.1 The image shows multiplanar reformatting of a CT examination acquired in the axial plane in an 81-year-old patient. Note that there is only minimal peri-Sylvian volume loss (white arrow), better assessed on the coronal image. This CT examination should be sufficient enough to exclude large tumours and extra-axial collections/haemorrhage and also to assess for selective/regional volume loss. Note that the slice thickness in the acquisition is 0.625 mm.

neoplastic conditions are being considered (Madhusoodanan et al., 2015; Silva-Dos-Santos and Salina, 2016).

Neurodegenerative conditions

In the setting of dementia and other neurodegenerative conditions (Royal College of Radiologists, 2017), MRI (preferably) or CT can be used to:

1. Exclude other cerebral pathology.
2. Establish a subtype for diagnosis.

It should be noted that the DSM-5 does not include imaging findings as criteria/requirements for diagnosis.

In a small proportion of patients with suspected dementia, imaging may identify potentially reversible or alternative causes, e.g. hydrocephalus, tumour, and subdural haemorrhage.

Diagnostic sensitivity may increase if imaging is restricted to patients with an atypical presentation, e.g. presentation with focal neurological signs, gait ataxia, or a history of trauma. MRI may also help with diagnosis in acute/rapidly progressive conditions such as limbic encephalitis and CJD (Royal College of Radiologists, 2017).

Alzheimer's dementia

Alzheimer's dementia is the commonest neurodegenerative disorder. Given the later age of presentation, this is usually associated with other brain pathology, notably small-vessel ischaemic change.

The prominent imaging feature of Alzheimer's dementia is atrophy of the entorhinal cortex and hippocampi, features which are considered to be biomarkers of the disease (Jack et al., 2002).

Hippocampal atrophy is shown to be a risk factor in normally ageing people for cognitive decline and dementia, but also for progressing from amnesic MCI to Alzheimer's dementia (Ikram et al., 2010).

In routine clinical practice, hippocampal volume loss is diagnosed by visual assessment, although manual volumetry and automated voxel-based methods (using dedicated software) are available, but limited in use, particularly manual volumetry, in view of the tedious process and potential lack of reproducibility. (See Fig. 8.2.)

Fronto-temporal dementia

FTD is the third commonest dementia for individuals aged 65 years and older, and the second commonest form for individuals aged 65 years and younger (Brunnstorm et al., 2009). FTD defines a

Table 8.1 Factors to consider when choosing an imaging modality

	CT	MRI
Availability	Mostly universally available, both in terms of location and time. Cheaper option	Available in majority of centres, although may have limited access in many centres 'out of hours'
Radiation	Ionizing radiation and hence may be a relative contraindication in certain conditions, e.g. in pregnancy	Non-ionizing and hence more universal application
Use of contrast (Royal College of Radiologists, 2015)	While contrast is not routinely used in CT examinations, the contrast agent being iodinated will have implications in patients with documented iodine allergy and deranged renal function (eGFR <40 mL/min)	While contrast-enhanced scans are less commonly used, contrast agents are relatively contraindicated in pregnancy/breastfeeding and deranged renal function (eGFR <30 mL/min)
Time	Approximately 3–4 minutes and hence more relevant in uncooperative/unstable patients	Approximately 30 minutes, depending on sequences required. Challenging in patients who cannot keep still for a long period of time
Contraindications	No absolute contraindication for a non-contrast CT examination. Contraindications to the use of ionizing radiation and iodinated contrast agents apply	MRI-incompatible implants (e.g. pacemakers, aneurysm clips, ferromagnetic foreign bodies) are absolute contraindications. Recent use of MR-conditional pacemakers and MRI-compatible surgical implants (e.g. cerebral aneurysm clips and surgical prosthesis) is on the rise. Claustrophobia is a relative contraindication as these patients can have an MRI examination under anaesthesia, if required, or open/wide-bore MRI scanners may be considered in this situation. Pregnancy is not a contraindication, on the basis that MRI on the fetus has not been shown to cause harmful effects, although the long-term effects continue to be studied (Bulas et al., 2013)
Indications (within the remit of neuropsychiatry)	1. To exclude acute abnormality, e.g. haemorrhage/infarction/extra-axial collections 2. To exclude large space-occupying lesions 3. To monitor ventricular dimension 4. To identify regional/lobar atrophy, given that multiplanar reconstruction is possible with multislice CT scanners	Given better contrast resolution, MRI is ideal when: 1. Looking for smaller space-occupying lesions, e.g. temporal lobe/cortical lesions in epilepsy, and better localization of lesions shown on CT 2. Looking for small infarction (stroke) and when no imaging correlate is shown on CT examination 3. Quantifying the extent of small vessel ischaemic change, especially looking for microhaemorrhage 4. Considering conditions affecting white matter (e.g. demyelination, toxic encephalopathy) 5. Investigating infective processes (encephalitis/meningitis)

heterogenous group of clinical syndromes marked by progressive focal neurodegeneration of the frontal and anterior temporal lobes (Pasquier et al., 1997).

A psychiatric prodrome, neuropsychiatric symptoms, and language difficulties are common in FTD (Bott et al., 2014).

FTD affects brain regions implicated in motivation, reward processing, personality, social cognition, attention, executive functioning, and language. Currently, FTD incorporates three clinical subtypes. Behavioural variant FTD (BvFTD) accounts for about half of all FTD cases (Johnson et al., 2005) and involves initial and progressive decline in social functioning and changes in personality. BvFTD is characterized by focal and prominent bilateral frontal atrophy, although some reports suggest more right hemispheric involvement than left (Perry et al., 2006). The remaining subtypes are classified as variants of primary progressive aphasia (PPA) and are marked by initial and prominent disturbance and decline of language functioning. Loss of semantic knowledge is associated with the semantic variant of PPA, while agrammatism and motor–speech difficulties are associated with the non-fluent variant of PPA (Gorno-Tempini et al., 2011). The semantic variant is characterized by bilateral anterior temporal lobe atrophy, associated with language dysfunction and impairment in emotional processing. Most patients present initially with greater left hemisphere atrophy. However, approximately a quarter of cases present with initial right anterior temporal lobe atrophy and is associated with a more behavioural presentation of symptoms,

including social awkwardness, loss of insight, and difficulty with face recognition (Thompson et al., 2003). The non-fluent variant of PPA is accompanied by left inferior frontal and insular atrophy. Expressive speech and syntax difficulties are characteristic of the disease early in its course.

Neuroimaging findings consistent with FTD include frontal or anterior temporal lobe atrophy, or both, on CT or MRI, depending on the subtype, with sparing of the parietal and occipital lobes. There is a knife blade appearance of the atrophied gyri and prominent enlargement (ballooning) of the frontal horns and inferior horns of the ventricles. There is variable degree of gliosis in the atrophic lobes. (See Fig. 8.3a and b.)

Parkinson's disease

A hallmark of Parkinson's disease (PD) is progressive neurodegeneration of dopaminergic neurones in the substantia nigra pars compacta (SNc).

The disease features motor parkinsonism (rigidity, tremor, bradykinesia, and postural imbalance), visual hallucinations, and potentially changes in cognition. Seventy to 80% of patients with PD develop cognitive impairment and/or dementia over the course of the disease (Watson et al., 2009).

CT shows non-specific cerebral atrophy.

On MRI, the SNc is narrowed and difficult to differentiate from the adjacent pars reticulata of the substantia nigra and red nucleus. The volume of the putamen is decreased, and there are T2

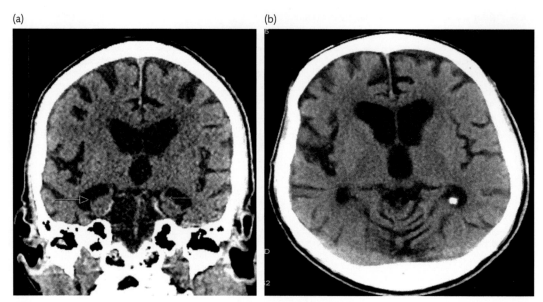

Fig. 8.2 (a) Coronal (reconstructed) and (b) axial CT image in a 78-year-old male who presented with slowly declining memory and cognitive impairment with a Mini-Mental State Examination (MMSE) score of 20/30. The images show no significant white matter low attenuation to suggest small vessel ischaemic change. Note that there is excessive hippocampal volume loss (white arrow) bilaterally. The high-density focus on the left lateral ventricle is choroid plexus calcification, which is physiological. (Compare with **Fig. 8.1** which is a CT examination of a normal 81-year old.)

hyperintense foci in the putamen and globus pallidus in some PD patients.

Imaging may differentiate 'idiopathic' Parkinson's disease from secondary, mostly vascular, forms of the disease and from other disorders with extrapyramidal signs, PSP, multiple system atrophy (MSA), DLB, and late-stage AD (Brundin et al., 2000).

Huntington's disease

Huntington's disease (HD) is an inherited neurodegenerative disorder characterized by progressive impairment of motor and cognitive function and progressive neuropsychiatric disturbance.

It is autosomal dominant with complete penetrance (Dormont et al., 2008).

CT and MRI demonstrate progressive reductions in striatal volume. Atrophy of the putamen is greater than that in the caudate early in the disease, and later atrophy expands to the globus pallidus and nucleus accumbens. The most striking and best known feature is that of caudate head atrophy, resulting in enlargement of the frontal horns, often giving them a 'box'-like configuration (Dormont et al., 2008).

Atrophy is also seen in other grey matter and white matter regions, including cerebral thinning throughout the cortex, atrophy

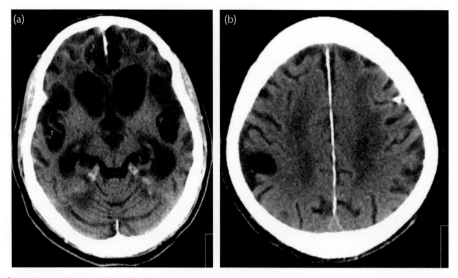

Fig. 8.3a and b CT performed in a 75-year-old male who was noted to be increasingly withdrawn and unable to speak. Minor left-sided weakness suggested stroke or transient ischaemic attack. (a) Axial CT images show marked frontal (F) and temporal/peri-Sylvian (T) cortical and white matter volume loss. Note relative preservation of the cortex in the superior frontal and parietal convexities (panel (b), same patient).

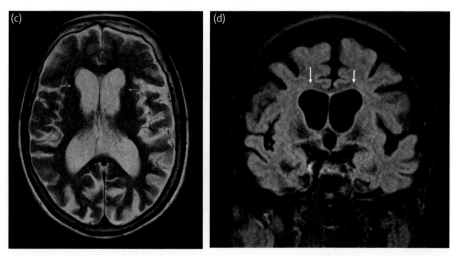

Fig. 8.3c and d Axial T2-weighted and Cor FLAIR images showing marked caudate head atrophy (arrow in panel (c)), with 'squaring' of the frontal horns of both lateral ventricles (white arrows in panel (d)). This was a 52-year-old female who had presented with choreiform movements over a period of 2 months. She also had a family history of Huntington's disease.

in the cingulate gyrus and thalamus, and atrophy of the white matter tracts near the striatum, as well as the corpus callosum, posterior white matter tract, and frontal lobe white matter (Georgiou-Karistianis et al., 2013). (See Fig. 8.3c and d.)

Creutzfeldt–Jakob disease

CJD is a fatal neurodegenerative disease caused by the accumulation of a pathogenic isoform of a prion protein in neurones that is responsible for subacute dementia (Clarençon et al., 2008).

The accumulation of abnormal prion proteins can occur sporadically (sporadic CJD), due to exposure to food (variant CJD) or tissues (iatrogenic CJD) containing the abnormal prion protein, or due to a genetic variation in the prion protein gene (PRNP) (genetic CJD) (Risacher et al., 2013).

Serial CT imaging demonstrates progressive atrophy and ventricular dilatation.

The commonest MRI abnormality in sporadic CJD is hyperintense signal intensity on T2-weighted imaging in the basal ganglia, thalami, and less often in the cortex. On DWI, there is restricted diffusion in the caudate, putamen, cerebellum, globus pallidus, and regions of the cerebral grey matter and white matter (Macfarlane et al., 2007). There are gyriform hyperintense areas in the cerebral cortex—the 'cortical ribbon sign'. Changes in the basal ganglia are associated with faster disease progression. However, these signal alterations may disappear as the disease progresses in the presence of more severe atrophy (Shiga et al., 2004).

DWI and T2-weighted imaging studies in variant CJD show abnormalities in the pulvinar of the thalamus and sometimes in the dorsomedial thalamic nuclei. Other alterations are seen in the periaqueductal grey, caudate, and parieto-occipital white matter (Macfarlane et al., 2007). Similar to sporadic CJD, these alterations may disappear as the disease progresses and atrophic changes expand (Risacher et al., 2013). (See Fig. 8.4.)

Vascular dementia

Vascular dementia (VaD) is a leading form of dementia, after AD, affecting the elderly population (Venkat et al., 2015).

VaD/vascular cognitive impairment is a heterogenous group of disorders with variable clinical and morphological findings and variable pathophysiology, but substantially it means 'disease with a cognitive impairment resulting from cerebrovascular disease and ischaemic or haemorrhagic brain injury' (Iemolo et al., 2009).

Pathogenesis is multifactorial, and cognitive decline is commonly associated with small ischaemic/vascular lesions, often involving subcortical and strategically important brain areas (thalamus, frontobasal, limbic system) (Jellinger, 2008).

Vascular mechanisms are many but chiefly include large artery disease, cardiac embolic events, small vessel disease, ischaemic white matter lesions, lacunar infarcts, and haemodynamic mechanisms.

On cranial CT, there is typically generalized atrophy, with focal cortical infarction.

Neuroimaging findings include hypodensity in the periventricular white matter (leukoaraiosis), which may be discrete to confluent, as well as in cortical grey matter, subcortical white matter, basal ganglia, and pontine infarcts.

MRI is more sensitive, especially to small vessel ischaemic change in the white matter, as well as microhaemorrhages seen in cerebral amyloid angiopathy and chronic hypertensive encephalopathy.

On fluid-attenuated inversion recovery (FLAIR), T2-weighted, and proton density sequences, there are punctate or confluent white matter hyperintensities and hyperintense foci (lacunes = old infarcts) within the basal ganglia and central pons.

On T1-weighted sequences, there is generalized atrophy, with enlargement of the ventricles and widened sulci.

T2*-weighted gradient-recalled echo (GRE)/susceptibility weighted imaging (SWI) sequences demonstrate multiple 'blooming' hypointensities in the cortex and along the pial surface.

In chronic hypertensive encephalopathy, subcortical arteriosclerotic encephalopathy, or Binswanger's disease, there is evidence of confluent white matter disease and lacunes in the basal ganglia, thalami, and brainstem, with a typical feature of hypertensive encephalopathy being microhaemorrhages (best seen on T2*-GRE/SWI sequences), with a predilection for the basal ganglia, thalami, brainstem, and cerebellum.

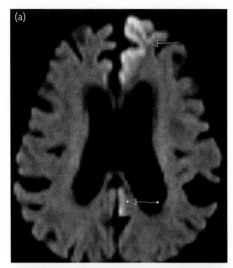

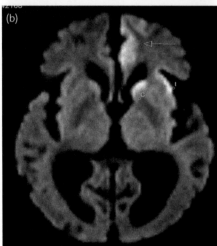

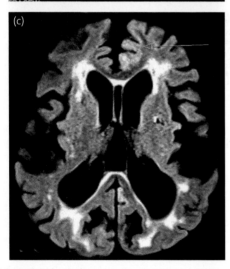

Fig. 8.4 (a) and (b) are DWI sequences on MRI which show cortical restricted diffusion (cortical ribbon sign—arrows) in the left superior frontal and left posterior cingulate gyri. Further restricted diffusion is also shown involving the left insula (I) and the head of left caudate nucleus (c). Panel (c) shows FLAIR sequence with cortical hyperintensity in the left superior frontal gyrus (arrow). The marked periventricular and deep white matter signal change is most likely to represent moderate to severe small vessel ischaemic change. This was an 85-year old with new-onset seizure/myoclonus. The appearances were thought to represent CJD.

A genetically transmitted form is known as familial arteriopathic leukoencephalopathy or CADASIL (cerebral autosomal dominant arteriopathy with subcortical infarcts and leukoencephalopathy). It is seen in young adults and is a non-arteriosclerotic, amyloid-negative hereditary angiopathy, primarily affecting leptomeningeal and long perforating arteries of the brain (Auer et al., 2001).

In CADASIL, the white matter lesions have a predilection for the anterior temporal regions and the external capsule. (See Fig. 8.5.)

Cerebral amyloid angiopathy

Cerebral amyloid angiopathy (CAA) occurs in approximately half of elderly individuals (Yamada et al.,1987). It results from focal to widespread amyloid-β protein (Aβ) deposition within leptomeningeal and cerebral cortical vessels.

These, in turn, lead to the development of haemorrhagic lesions (lobar intracerebral macrohaemorrhage, cortical microhaemorrhage, and cortical superficial siderosis/focal convexity subarachnoid haemorrhage), ischaemic lesions (cortical infarction and ischaemic changes of the white matter), and encephalopathies that include subacute leukoencephalopathy caused by CAA-associated inflammation/angiitis (Yamada et al., 2015).

CAA thus causes vascular lesions that potentially lead to (vascular) dementia and may further contribute to dementia by impeding the clearance of solutes out of the brain and transport of nutrients across the blood–brain barrier. Severe CAA is an independent risk factor for cognitive decline (Attems et al., 2011).

The clinical diagnosis of CAA is based on the assessment of associated cerebrovascular lesions which are now possible to establish, based on imaging findings.

Cranial CT demonstrates macrohaemorrhages. However, sensitive MRI methods, such as T2(*) GRE imaging and SWI, are useful for detecting cortical microhaemorrhages and cortical superficial siderosis (Nandigam et al., 2009).

Encephalitis

Encephalitis refers to an acute, usually diffuse, inflammatory process affecting the brain. An infection by a virus is the commonest and important cause of encephalitis, although other organisms may sometimes cause encephalitis (Kennedy, 2004).

In individuals who survive this condition, post-encephalitic impairments of elemental neurologic, cognitive, emotional, and behavioural function are common (Arciniegas et al., 2004).

Herpes simplex encephalitis

Herpes simplex encephalitis (HSE) is one of the most commonly recognized forms of viral encephalitis (Kapur et al., 1994).

In adults, herpes simplex virus type 1 (HSV-1) is the causative agent. It is a human neurotropic virus that establishes latent infection in dorsal root ganglia (DRG) for the entire life of the host and can reactivate from there to cause morbidity and mortality (Steiner et al., 2013).

MRI is the imaging modality of choice in acute encephalitis, although it may be simpler to obtain a CT scan quickly and easily in restless patients (Chaudhuri et al., 2002).

On imaging, there is a predilection for the limbic system: temporal lobes, insula, subfrontal areas, and cingulate gyri. The changes are typically bilateral and often asymmetric.

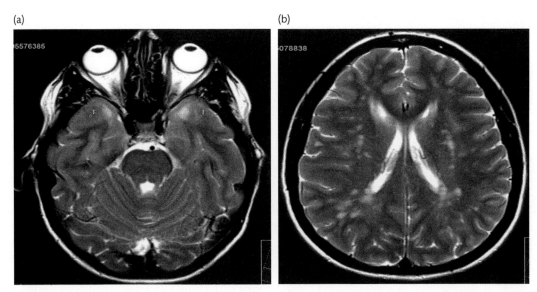

Fig. 8.5 Axial T2-weighted MRI images showing numerous scattered T2 hyperintense foci in the white matter, in excess for that expected for the patient's age. Panel (a) shows subcortical white matter T2 hyperintensity in the anterior temporal pole bilaterally (T), typical of CADASIL. This was a 39-year-old male with a history of migraine and a strong family history of CADASIL.

CT may be normal in HSE, especially early in the illness, with the earliest CT findings 3 days after symptom onset. CT characteristically shows reduced attenuation in one or both medial temporal lobes and insula, with mass effect. On contrast-enhanced CT, in the late acute/subacute stage, there is patchy or gyriform enhancement in the temporal lobes. Haemorrhage may be seen in the late stages.

MRI is sensitive in the early stages of HSE, although rarely it may be normal in this condition. The typical MRI features in HSE are areas of focal oedema in the temporal lobes and on the orbital surface of the frontal lobes, as well as the insular cortex and angular gyrus (Kennedy, 2004).

The initial changes may be seen only on DWI, with restricted diffusion in the limbic system. There is cortical swelling and mass effect, with cortical and subcortical signal abnormality. On post-gadolinium T1 imaging, early there is only mild, patchy enhancement affecting the limbic system. Gyriform enhancement is usually seen around 1 week after initial symptoms and occasionally there is meningeal enhancement.

In the subacute/chronic stage, there is atrophy, as well as encephalomalacia, in the affected areas. T2* imaging will show hypointensity in haemorrhagic areas (Osborn, 2004). (See Fig. 8.6.)

HIV encephalopathy

Neurological involvement in human immunodeficiency virus (HIV) infection is commonly associated with cognitive impairment. While severe and progressive neurocognitive impairment has become rare in HIV in the era of potent antiretroviral therapy, moderate cognitive impairment is common despite good virologic response to therapy. A majority of HIV patients worldwide perform below expectations on formal neurocognitive tests (Clifford et al., 2013). Independent of opportunistic conditions, advanced HIV is associated with cognitive impairment—the consequence of HIV infection within the nervous system. Acquired immune deficiency syndrome (AIDS) dementia complex (ADC), a subcortical dementia, was characterized as a progressive, disabling condition

that manifested with increasing loss of attention and concentration, marked motor slowing, and variable behavioural components, generally leading to death in less than a year (Clifford et al., 2013; Navia et al., 1986).

On CT imaging, there is atrophy, with bilateral periventricular/diffuse white matter hypodensity. Basal ganglia, cerebellum, and brainstem hypodensity can also be seen.

MRI demonstrates diffuse 'hazy' white matter on T2/FLAIR sequences.

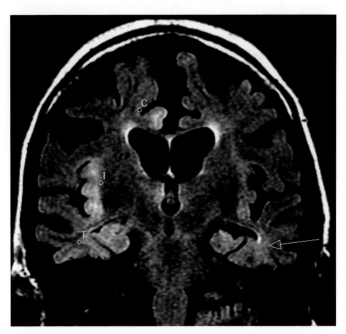

Fig. 8.6 Coronal FLAIR sequence of an MRI examination showing signal change involving the right temporal lobe (T), the insula (I), and the cingulate gyrus (C). The temporal lobe signal change is asymmetrical, with less conspicuous signal change also present in the left temporal lobe. This was a 58-year old who presented with seizure and confusion.

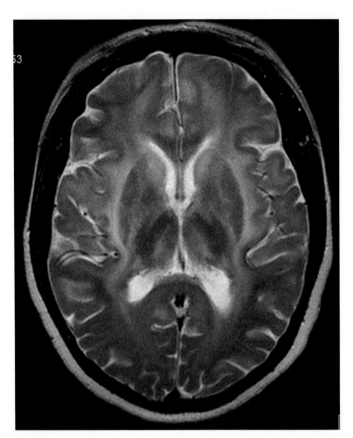

Fig. 8.7 Axial T2-weighted sequence of an MRI examination showing confluent bihemispheric white matter signal change. No abnormal enhancement was shown (no images provided). In the given context, the appearances are most in keeping with HIV encephalopathy. This was a 44-year-old known HIV patient with persistent viraemia and a CD4 count of 190 cells/mm³ who was admitted with confusion.

The white matter lesions are non-enhancing, and if enhancement is present, opportunistic infections and immune reconstitution inflammatory syndrome (IRIS) should be considered (Osborn, 2004). (See Fig. 8.7.)

Progressive multifocal leukoencephalopathy

Progressive multifocal leukoencephalopathy (PML) is a demyelinating disease caused by reactivation of the DNA virus JC polyomavirus in immunocompromised patients. It is seen in patients with AIDS and those with chronic diseases associated with compromised immune response, such as cancer, organ transplantation, chemotherapy, myeloproliferative disease, and in patients undergoing immunosuppressive therapy, including steroids for treatment in multiple sclerosis and rheumatic diseases. It most commonly presents with altered mental status/cognitive deficits, progressive neurological symptoms, headache, and lethargy (Shah et al., 2010).

On CT imaging, there are low attenuation changes in the subcortical and periventricular white matter, without mass effect. The white matter lesions may be unilateral but more often are bilateral and asymmetric. Frontal and parieto-occipital locations are the commonest.

The characteristic MRI appearance of PML is single or multifocal white matter lesion(s) that are round to oval at first and become confluent and large with progressive disease. The involvement of arcuate fibres (U fibres) creates a sharp border with the cortex. The lesions are hypointense on T1-weighted and hyperintense on T2-weighted imaging, compared to normal white matter. The involvement is most often asymmetric, with relative sparing of the periventricular white matter. Usually there is no mass effect or enhancement. Involvement of the parieto-occipital white matter and corpus callosum is commonly seen. Posterior fossa involvement, especially in the middle cerebellar peduncles, is also frequently seen. Occasionally, lesions may be limited to the cerebellum and/or brainstem or demonstrate selective pyramidal tract involvement (Boster et al., 2009).

Although PML lesions typically involve the white matter, grey matter involvement can be seen in up to 50% of patients.

Marked mass effect and robust contrast enhancement are rare in PML and should suggest an alternative diagnosis. However, minimal mass effect and faint peripheral enhancement can also be seen.

In PML, newer lesions and the advancing edge of large lesions have high signal on DWI and normal-to-low ADC values, signifying restricted diffusion. Older lesions and the centre of large lesions have increased ADC values (da Pozzo et al., 2006). (See Fig. 8.8a–c.)

Acute disseminated encephalomyelitis

Acute disseminated encephalomyelitis (ADEM) is an immune-mediated disorder of the CNS. It is a monophasic demyelinating disease, typically affecting the grey and white matter of the brain and spinal cord in multiple locations. Disease typically starts with an abrupt onset of neurologic symptoms and signs within days to weeks after a viral infection or immunization (Noorbakhsh et al., 2008).

Common psychiatric symptoms include lethargy, irritability, and confusion. Ataxia, seizures, and other signs representing involvement of various areas of the brain and spinal cord are common neurologic presentations (Patel et al., 1997).

CT imaging is generally normal at onset and usually becomes abnormal 5–14 days later. The typical CT appearance is that of low attenuation, with multifocal lesions in the subcortical white matter (Lukes et al., 1983).

Demyelinating lesions of ADEM are better visualized by MRI. These demyelinating lesions of ADEM usually exhibit no mass effect and can be seen scattered throughout the white matter of the posterior fossa and cerebral hemispheres. Involvement of the cerebellum and brainstem is more common in children. Characteristic lesions seen on MRI appear as bilateral, asymmetric patchy areas of increased signal intensity on conventional T2-weighted images and on FLAIR. Lesions may be multifocal punctate to large flocculent, tumour-like hyperintensities. Though white matter involvement predominates, grey matter can also be affected, with frequent involvement of the thalami and basal ganglia, which is typically asymmetric. Unlike multiple sclerosis, there is usually no involvement of the calloso-septal interface in ADEM. MRI lesions may demonstrate punctate, ring, incomplete ring, or peripheral enhancement after gadolinium administration. In order to qualify as ADEM, lesions on MRI should be of the same age and no new lesion should appear on CNS imaging studies after the initial clinical attack (Garg, 2003). (See Fig. 8.8d–f.)

Paraneoplastic autoimmune encephalitis

Paraneoplastic autoimmune encephalitis is considered one of the classic paraneoplastic neurological syndromes which are defined as

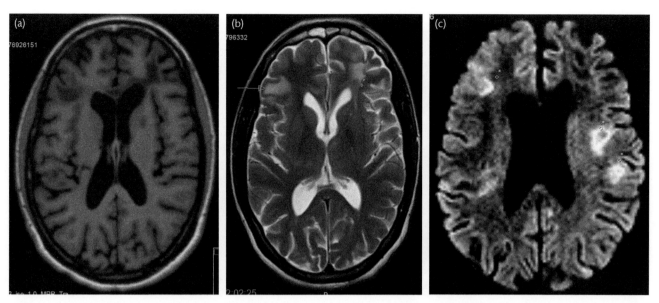

Fig. 8.8a–c. Panels (a), (b) and (c) are axial T1-weighted, axial T2-weighted, and diffusion-weighted MRI sequences, respectively. There is bihemispheric subcortical white matter signal change (T1 hypointense and T2 hyperintense), extending to involve the subcortical 'U' fibres (arrow and *), with no associated mass effect (swelling)—appearances typical of progressive multifocal leukoencephalopathy. The DWI sequence shows restricted diffusion (*) in the 'advancing edge' of these lesions. This was in a 41-year-old newly diagnosed HIV patient presenting with left-sided upper and lower limb weakness and blurring of vision.

neurological symptoms not associated with local or metastatic activity due to malignancy and sometimes supported by the presence of specific onconeural antibodies (Graus et al., 2004).

Limbic encephalitis is the commonest clinical paraneoplastic syndrome. It is a disorder characterized by personality changes, irritability, confusion, depression, seizures, memory loss, and sometimes dementia (Gultekin et al., 2000).

It is clinically suggested by the subacute onset, in days or up to 12 weeks, and psychiatric symptoms suggesting involvement of the limbic system (Sarria-Estrada et al., 2014).

The imaging appearances simulate those of HSE.

CT is initially normal. Rarely, a low density is seen within the mesial temporal lobes.

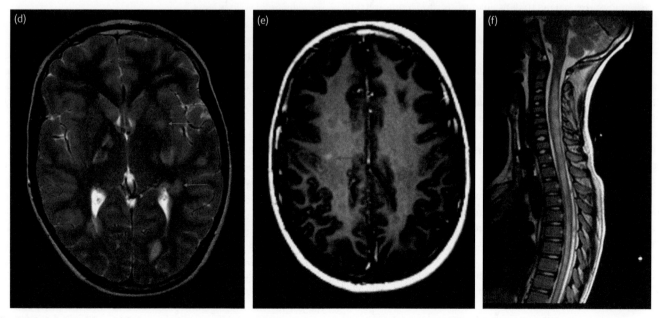

Fig. 8.8d–f Panels (d) and (e) show axial T2-weighted and post-contrast axial T1-weighted images of the brain, respectively, with asymmetric multiple T2 hyperintense lesions involving the white matter and also the lentiform nucleus (blue arrow). The contrast-enhanced sequence shows a white matter lesion with nodular enhancement, with the further lesion sited anteriorly, demonstrating subtle incomplete peripheral enhancement (red arrows). Panel (f) shows a sagittal T2-weighted sequence through the spine with extensive signal change involving the cervical and thoracic segments of the spinal cord and with patchy brainstem signal changes also present. This was a 15-year-old male who presented with limb weakness and decreased consciousness following a recent upper respiratory tract infection.

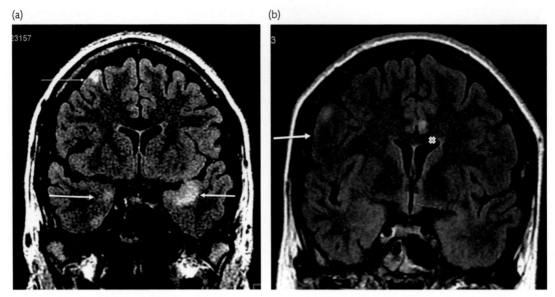

Fig. 8.9 Panels (a) and (b) are coronal FLAIR images showing asymmetric signal change involving the left mesial temporal lobe (arrow) and left cingulate gyrus (x), with further signal change in the right frontal lobe (white arrows). This was a 39-year old who presented with seizures, with extensive evaluation revealing the patient was positive for voltage-gated potassium channel (VGKC) antibody.

On MRI, there is usually bilateral (though it may be unilateral in 40%) and extensive disease in the mesial temporal lobes (hippocampus and amygdala), insula, cingulate gyrus, subfrontal cortex, and inferior frontal white matter, which is hypointense on T1-weighted imaging and hyperintense on T2-weighted imaging and FLAIR. There may be minimal mass effect.

Atrophy of the temporal lobes may be seen in chronic cases.

Patchy enhancement is common, but haemorrhage is exceedingly uncommon (if blood products are seen, herpes encephalitis should be considered).

Abnormal signal intensity in the brainstem or hypothalamus may be seen in approximately 10–20% of cases of limbic encephalitis (Yousem et al., 2010). (See Fig. 8.9.)

Toxic encephalopathy

The term 'toxic encephalopathy' is used to indicate brain dysfunction caused by toxic exposure (Kim et al., 2012).

Few neurotoxins cause patients to present with a pathognomonic neurological syndrome. The symptoms and signs of neurotoxin exposure may be mimicked by various psychiatric, metabolic, inflammatory, neoplastic, and degenerative diseases of the nervous system (Spencer et al., 2000).

Alcohol encephalopathy

Ethanol causes diverse neurologic conditions caused by acute and chronic brain damage. Chronic alcohol dependence causes cognitive problems and impaired memory.

In patients with alcohol dependence, CT and MRI reveal generalized atrophy, with symmetric enlargement of the lateral ventricles and cerebral sulci. There is disproportionate superior vermian atrophy.

Wernicke's encephalopathy (WE) is an uncommon, but severe, neurological syndrome, caused by thiamine (vitamin B1) deficiency. It is characterized by sudden onset of altered consciousness, ophthalmoplegia, and ataxia (Thomson et al., 2008).

On MRI, there are bilateral and symmetrical T2-weighted and FLAIR hyperintensities in the thalami, mammillary bodies, tectal plate, and periaqueductal area. Signal intensity alterations in the dorsal medulla and the pons, cerebellar dentate nuclei, red nuclei, the substantia nigra of the midbrain, cranial nerve nuclei, the vermis and the paravermian regions of the cerebellum, the corpus callosum, the fornices, the head of the caudate nucleus, and the frontal–parietal cortex represent atypical MRI findings; they are almost always found in association with the typical findings.

The atypical findings, moreover, are found more frequently in non-alcoholic WE patients.

Patients with alcoholic WE typically have chronic atrophic mammillary bodies and third ventricular enlargement.

Contrast enhancement is seen in the mammillary bodies, periaqueductal grey, and medial thalamus in 50% of cases. Restricted diffusion is seen in or around the third ventricle, periaqueductal region, bilateral dorsomedial thalami, and brainstem (Manzo et al., 2014).

Marchiafava–Bignami disease (MBD) is a rare disease associated with alcoholism, though rarely also seen in patients without alcoholism. It is characterized by demyelination and necrosis of the corpus callosum. Clinical symptoms can vary from cognitive impairment, gait disturbance, and hemiparesis to stupor, coma, and death.

CT of MBD patients shows diffuse periventricular low density and focal areas of low density in the genu and splenium of the corpus callosum (Ihn et al., 2007). On MRI, patients with MBD show areas of low signal intensity on T1-weighted images. There is high signal intensity on T2 and FLAIR images in the body of the corpus callosum, genu, splenium, and adjacent white matter. During the acute phase, the lesions may show peripheral contrast enhancement. As the disease progresses, signal alterations become less evident, but residual atrophy of the involved structure is usually observed (Zuccoli et al., 2010).

Drug abuse

Illicit drug use often causes cerebrovascular disease. The illicit drugs more commonly associated with stroke are psychomotor stimulants such as amphetamines and cocaine. Less commonly implicated are opioids and psychotomimetic drugs, including cannabis (Fonseca et al., 2013).

Cocaine is the hallmark drug well known for producing both ischaemic stroke and intracranial haemorrhage (Toossi et al., 2010). The drug blocks the reuptake carrier of monoamines, ultimately resulting in vasoconstriction of blood vessels, elevation of blood pressure, tachycardia, and increased cardiac output (Fessler et al., 1997). These well-known effects can lead to detrimental acute neurologic complications, including stroke and subarachnoid and intraparenchymal haemorrhage, as well as other complications secondary to chronic abuse (Tamrazi et al., 2012).

Acute haemorrhage is demonstrated on CT imaging.

Acute infarcts secondary to the vasoconstrictor effects of cocaine are also easily detected with imaging, which demonstrates changes in the calibre of the involved vessels, as well as restricted diffusion on diffusion-weighted MRI. In addition to depicting focal calibre changes of the involved vessels, MR angiography with contrast material can also aid in potentially differentiating isolated vasospasm from vasculitis, demonstrating vessel wall enhancement in the latter case (Geibprasert et al., 2010).

Tumours

While the clinical presentation of brain tumours can be varied, psychiatric symptoms like mood changes, psychosis (particularly in the older age group), memory problems, personality changes, anxiety, or anorexia may be a less common presentation, which may complicate the clinical picture.

Given that early diagnosis of a brain tumour is more likely to improve patient outcome, neuroimaging would need to be considered in patients presenting with the above.

Keschner et al. (1938) noted that while 78% of the 530 brain tumour patients in their cohort had psychiatric symptoms, only 18% in the same cohort presented with psychiatric symptoms as the first clinical manifestation of the brain tumour. Treatment of these symptoms would primarily be with use of antidepressants, antipsychotics, mood stabilizers, and anxiolytics (Madhusoodanan et al., 2007).

The clinical presentation of tumours is mainly related to the location of the tumour. There has been some, albeit weak, correlation shown with various psychiatric presentations and tumour location (Madhusoodanan et al., 2010). Depression is one of the commonest accompanying psychiatric symptoms and may occur at presentation or following tumour diagnosis. Associations with changes in personality with frontal lobe tumours and appetite disturbances with hypothalamic lesions are well-known conditions.

Given that psychiatric symptoms are the clinical presentation in only a small proportion of patients with brain tumour, neuroimaging, ideally with MRI examination, would need to be considered appropriately. Management of these patients is multidisciplinary, with treatment of the tumour either standalone or involving a combination of surgery, radiotherapy and chemotherapy, and appropriate management of the neurological symptoms (e.g. seizures) or psychiatric symptoms. (See Fig. 8.10.)

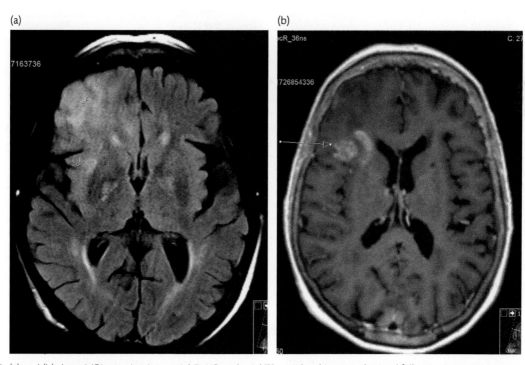

(a)   (b)

Fig. 8.10 Panels (a) and (b) show MRI examination—axial FLAIR and axial T1-weighted images obtained following intravenous contrast showing extensive signal change involving the right frontal lobe (F) and insula (I). There are patchy areas of enhancement (arrow). Note that there is swelling and mass effect. This was a 75-year-old patient presenting with progressive memory decline and possible seizure. The patchy area of enhancement represents disruption in the blood–brain barrier and is usually indicative of a higher-grade tumour, with new enhancement most likely to represent tumour upgrade.

Conclusion

Imaging plays a key role in the diagnosis and management of neurological and neuropsychiatric disorders. Given that there is some overlap of imaging findings between various clinical conditions, it is vital that the imaging findings are interpreted in conjunction with clinical findings and other parameters (e.g. CSF analysis).

The main imaging modalities (CT and MRI) have their distinct strengths and weaknesses, and optimal use of techniques may improve patient outcome.

KEY LEARNING POINTS

- CT and MRI are key imaging modalities for structural neuroimaging.
- The wider availability of CT and quicker scanning time, with multiplanar capabilities of newer CT scanners, should be remembered as CT may provide an answer to most clinical questions, particularly in the acute setting.
- CT and MRI have their own advantages and pitfalls. Both of these imaging modalities complement, rather that compete, with each other.
- Various clinical conditions have characteristic imaging appearances. However, images need to be interpreted in the appropriate clinical setting in the light of clinical information and supplementary results.
- Imaging is a useful tool to monitor disease progression/regression and effects of treatment.

REFERENCES

Arciniegas DB, Anderson CA. 2004. Viral Encephalitis: Neuropsychiatric And Neurobehavioral Aspects. *Current Psychiatry Reports* 6:372–9.

Attems J. et al. 2011. Review: Sporadic Cerebral Amyloid Angiopathy. *Neuropathology and Applied Neurobiology* 37:75–93.

Auer DP, et al. 2001. Differential Lesion Patterns In CADASIL And Sporadic Subcortical Arteriosclerotic Encephalopathy: MR Imaging Study With Statistical Parametric Group Comparison. *Radiology* 218:443–51.

Boster A, et al. 2009. Progressive Multifocal Leukoencephalopathy And Relapsing-Remitting Multiple Sclerosis. *Archives of Neurology* 66:593–9.

Bott NT, et al. 2014. Frontotemporal Dementia: Diagnosis, Deficits And Management. *Neurodegenerative Disease Management* 4:439–54.

Brundin P. 2000. Bilateral Caudate And Putamen Grafts Of Embryonic Mesencephalic Tissue Treated With Lazaroids In Parkinson's Disease. *Brain* 123:1380–90.

Brunnström H, et al. 2009. Prevalence Of Dementia Subtypes: A 30-Year Retrospective Survey Of Neuropathological Reports. *Archives of Gerontology and Geriatrics* 49:146–9.

Bulas D, Egloff A. 2013. Benefits and risks of MRI in pregnancy. *Seminars in Perinatology* 37:301–4.

Chaudhuri A. 2002. Diagnosis And Treatment Of Viral Encephalitis. *Postgraduate Medical Journal* 78:575–83.

Clarençon, F. et al. 2008. MRI And FDG PET/CT Findings In A Case Of Probable Heidenhain Variant Creutzfeldt-Jakob Disease. *Journal of Neuroradiology* 35:240–3.

Clifford DB, Ances BM. 2013. HIV-Associated Neurocognitive Disorder. *The Lancet Infectious Diseases* 13:976–86.

Cooper D, Limet N, McClung I, Lawrie SM. 2013. Towards clinically useful neuroimaging in psychiatric practice. *British Journal of Psychiatry* 203:242–4.

da Pozzo S, et al. 2006. Conventional And Diffusion-Weighted MRI In Progressive Multifocal Leukoencephalopathy: New Elements For Identification And Follow-Up. *La Radiologia Medica* 111:971–7.

Dormont D, Seidenwurm DJ. 2008. Dementia And Movement Disorders. *American Journal of Neuroradiology* 29: 204–6.

Fessler RD, et al. 1997. The Neurovascular Complications Of Cocaine. *Surgical Neurology* 47:339–45.

Fonseca AC, Ferro JM. 2013. Drug Abuse And Stroke. *Current Neurology and Neuroscience Reports* 13:325.

Garg RK. 2003. Acute Disseminated Encephalomyelitis. *Postgraduate Medical Journal* 79:11–17.

Geibprasert S, Gallucci M, Krings T. 2010. Addictive Illegal Drugs: Structural Neuroimaging. *American Journal of Neuroradiology* 31:803–8.

Georgiou-Karistianis N, et al. 2013. Structural MRI In Huntington's Disease And Recommendations For Its Potential Use In Clinical Trials. *Neuroscience and Biobehavioral Reviews* 37:480–90.

Gorno-Tempini ML, et al. 2011. Classification Of Primary Progressive Aphasia And Its Variants. *Neurology* 76:1006–14.

Graus F. 2004. Recommended Diagnostic Criteria For Paraneoplastic Neurological Syndromes. *Journal of Neurology, Neurosurgery and Psychiatry* 75:1135–40.

Gultekin SH. 2000. Paraneoplastic Limbic Encephalitis: Neurological Symptoms, Immunological Findings And Tumour Association In 50 Patients. *Brain* 123:1481–94.

Iemolo F, et al. 2009. Pathophysiology Of Vascular Dementia. *Immunity and Ageing* 6:13.

Ihn YK, Hwang SS, Park YH. 2007. Acute Marchiafava-Bignami Disease: Diffusion-Weighted MRI In Cortical And Callosal Involvement. *Yonsei Medical Journal* 48:321.

Ikram MA, et al. 2010. Brain tissue volumes in relation to cognitive function and risk of dementia. *Neurobiology of Aging* 31:378–86.

Jack CR Jr, et al. 2002. Antemortem MRI findings correlate with hippocampal neuropathology in typical aging and dementia. *Neurology* 58:750–7.

Jellinger KA. 2008. Morphologic Diagnosis Of 'Vascular Dementia'—A Critical Update. *Journal of the Neurological Sciences* 270:1–12.

Johnson JK, et al. 2005. Frontotemporal Lobar Degeneration. *Archives of Neurology* 62:925–30.

Kapur N, et al. 1994. Herpes Simplex Encephalitis: Long Term Magnetic Resonance Imaging And Neuropsychological Profile. *Journal of Neurology, Neurosurgery and Psychiatry* 57:1334–42.

Kennedy PGE. 2004. Viral encephalitis: causes, differential diagnosis, and management. *Journal of Neurology, Neurosurgery and Psychiatry* 75:10i–15.

Keschner M, Bender MB, Strauss I. 1938. Mental symptoms associated with brain tumor: a study of 530 verified cases. *JAMA* 110:714–18.

Kim Y, Kim JW. 2012. Toxic Encephalopathy. *Safety and Health at Work* 3:243–56.

Lukes SA, Norman D. 1983. Computed Tomography In Acute Disseminated Encephalomyelitis. *Annals of Neurology* 13:567–72.

Macfarlane RG, et al. 2007. Neuroimaging Findings In Human Prion Disease. *Journal of Neurology, Neurosurgery and Psychiatry* 78:664–70.

Madhusoodanan S, Danan D, Moise D. 2007. Psychiatric manifestations of brain tumors: diagnostic implications. *Expert Review of Neurotherapeutics* 7:343–9.

Madhusoodanan S, et al. 2010. Brain tumor location and psychiatric symptoms: is there any association? A meta-analysis of published case studies. *Expert Review of Neurotherapeutics* 10:1529–36.

Madhusoodanan S, et al. 2015. Psychiatric aspects of brain tumors: A review. *World Journal of Psychiatry* 5:273–85.

Manzo G, et al. 2014. MR Imaging Findings In Alcoholic And Nonalcoholic Acute Wernicke'S Encephalopathy: A Review. *BioMed Research International* 2014:1–12.

Nandigam RNK, et al. 2009. MR Imaging Detection Of Cerebral Microbleeds: Effect Of Susceptibility-Weighted Imaging, Section Thickness, And Field Strength. *American Journal of Neuroradiology* 30:338–43.

Navia BA, Jordan BD, Price RW. 1986. The AIDS Dementia Complex: I. Clinical Features. *Annals of Neurology* 19:517–24.

Noorbakhsh F, et al. 2008. Acute Disseminated Encephalomyelitis: Clinical And Pathogenesis Features. *Neurologic Clinics* 26:759–80.

Osborn AG. *Diagnostic Imaging: Brain.* Amirsys, Salt Lake City, UT, 2004.

Pasquier F, Henri P. 1997. Frontotemporal Dementia: Its Rediscovery. *European Neurology* 38:1–6.

Patel SP, Friedman RS. 1997. Neuropsychiatric Features Of Acute Disseminated Encephalomyelitis: A Review. *Journal of Neuropsychiatry* 9:534–40.

Perry RJ, et al. 2006. Patterns Of Frontal Lobe Atrophy In Frontotemporal Dementia: A Volumetric MRI Study. *Dementia and Geriatric Cognitive Disorders* 22:278–87.

Risacher S, Saykin A. 2013. Neuroimaging Biomarkers Of Neurodegenerative Diseases And Dementia. *Seminars in Neurology* 33:386–416.

Robert WS, Yukio Koyanagi C, Shigemi Hishinuma E. 2014. On the usefulness of structural brain imaging for young first episode inpatients with psychosis. *Psychiatry Research* 224:104–6.

Royal College of Radiologists. 2015. *Standards for intravascular contrast agent administration to adult patients*, third edition. Royal College of Radiologists, London.

Royal College of Radiologists. 2017. *iRefer: Making the Best Use of Clinical Radiology*, eighth edition. Royal College of Radiologists, London.

Sarria-Estrada S. et al. 2014. Neuroimaging In Status Epilepticus Secondary To Paraneoplastic Autoimmune Encephalitis. *Clinical Radiology* 69:795–803.

Shah R, et al. 2010. Imaging Manifestations Of Progressive Multifocal Leukoencephalopathy. *Clinical Radiology* 65:431–9.

Shiga Y, et al. 2004. Diffusion-Weighted MRI Abnormalities As An Early Diagnostic Marker For Creutzfeldt-Jakob Disease. *Neurology* 63:443–9.

Silva-Dos-Santos A, Talina MC. 2016. Retrospective study on structural neuroimaging in first-episode psychosis. *Peer-Reviewed Journal* 4:e2069.

Spencer PS, Schaumburg HH, Ludolph AC. 2000. *Experimental and Clinical Neurotoxicology*. Oxford University Press, New York, NY.

Steiner I, Benninger F. 2013. Update On Herpes Virus Infections Of The Nervous System. *Current Neurology and Neuroscience Reports* 13:414.

Tamrazi B, Almast J. 2012. Your Brain On Drugs: Imaging Of Drug-Related Changes In The Central Nervous System. *RadioGraphics* 32:701–19.

Thomson AD, et al. 2008. Wernicke's Encephalopathy Revisited. Translation Of The Case History Section Of The Original Manuscript By Carl Wernicke 'Lehrbuch Der Gehirnkrankheiten Fur Aerzte And Studirende' (1881) With A Commentary. *Alcohol and Alcoholism* 43:174–9.

Thompson SA, Patterson K, Hodges JR. 2003. Left/Right Asymmetry Of Atrophy In Semantic Dementia: Behavioral-Cognitive Implications. *Neurology* 61:1196–203.

Toossi Shahed, et al. 2010. Neurovascular Complications Of Cocaine Use At A Tertiary Stroke Center. *Journal of Stroke and Cerebrovascular Diseases* 19:273–8.

Venkat P, Chopp M, Chen J. 2015. Models And Mechanisms Of Vascular Dementia. *Experimental Neurology* 272:97–108.

Watson R, Blamire AM, O'Brien JT. 2009. Magnetic Resonance Imaging In Lewy Body Dementias. *Dementia and Geriatric Cognitive Disorders* 28:493–506.

Yamada M. 2015. Cerebral Amyloid Angiopathy: Emerging Concepts. *Journal of Stroke* 17:17.

Yamada M, et al. 1987. Cerebral Amyloid Angiopathy In The Aged. *Journal of Neurology* 234:371–6.

Yousem DM, Grossman RI. 2010. *Neuroradiology*. Mosby/Elsevier, Philadelphia, PA.

Zuccoli G, et al. 2010. Neuroimaging Findings In Alcohol-Related Encephalopathies. *American Journal of Roentgenology* 195:1378–84.

9

Functional neuroimaging in neuropsychiatry

Robin A. Hurley, Shane C. Masters, and Katherine H. Taber

Introduction

Functional neuroimaging techniques (e.g. single-photon emission computed tomography [SPECT], positron emission tomography [PET], functional magentic resonance imaging [fMRI], electroencephalography [EEG], magnetoencephalograpy [MEG]) provide measures that are directly (MEG, EEG) or indirectly (SPECT, PET, fMRI) related to brain activity. The functional neuroimaging techniques presently applicable to clinical practice in neuropsychiatry are SPECT and PET, which provide indirect measures [e.g. cerebral blood flow (CBF), cerebral metabolic rate (CMR)] of brain activity. Additional newer SPECT and PET techniques are transitioning from research into highly advanced clinical arenas. Those include amyloid and tau imaging, amino acid scanning, and targeted neurotransmitter imaging.

Guiding principles

Neuroimaging is making increasing contributions to multiple aspects of clinical neuropsychiatry, including differential diagnosis, prognosis, clinical management, and development of new interventions (Filippi et al., 2012; Osuch and Williamson, 2006). A study of patients with dementia admitted to a medical psychiatry unit in a general university hospital found that more than one-third of structural imaging examinations (CT, MRI) and almost three-quarters of functional imaging examinations (SPECT, PET) resulted in a change in diagnosis (Tanev et al., 2012). The commonest reasons for ordering neuroimaging were to rule out stroke or tumour or for dementia differentiation. A study in a small rural hospital of psychiatric patients (inpatients and outpatients) referred for SPECT imaging due to clinical indicators (e.g. history of TBI, stroke or seizures, atypical presentation) reported that 81% of scans were abnormal (Sheehan and Thurber, 2008). A change in treatment and/or diagnosis resulted in 79% of cases, including 13% in which the new diagnosis was a previously unrecognized TBI syndrome. A case series presented three elderly individuals with recent resurgence of idiopathic OCD that had resolved decades earlier, all with structural and/or functional neuroimaging abnormalities in the frontal lobes and basal ganglia (Salinas et al., 2009).

Unlike structural neuroimaging, functional neuroimaging is dynamic and state-dependent. Many factors can influence scan results of a particular individual on a particular day. Thus, it has had less penetrance into the clinical arena. Functional neuroimaging is particularly useful for areas that are dysfunctional yet look normal on structural neuroimaging (e.g. the 'hidden' lesions). Evaluation of the resting state also has shown potential for prediction of treatment response in some conditions. In general, patients whose clinical symptoms do not fit the classic historical picture for the working diagnosis should be considered for some form of functional neuroimaging (Defense Centers of Excellence, 2013).

Current clinical techniques

SPECT and PET are the most widely available methods. Both PET and SPECT involve intravenous injection of a radioactive compound (tracer or ligand) that distributes in the brain and emits radiation that is detected and used to form an image. The chemical properties of the compound determine its distribution. As noted earlier, both can provide indirect measures of brain activity, either regional CBF (rCBF) or regional CMR (rCMR). For clinical studies, both SPECT and PET are usually acquired under resting conditions, providing a way to assess the baseline functional state of brain areas. In some cases, pharmacological challenges are also used. Tracers are also available to measure various aspects of neurotransmitter systems. The only contraindication to a SPECT or PET scan is pregnancy, and even this is only a relative contraindication. Although very rarely necessary, the study could be performed in uncommon situations in which the scan result is critical. In addition, breastfeeding should be discontinued for a variable length of time (depending on the radiotracer, most often 1 day or less) after tracer injection. It is important to recognize that the tracers used in all diagnostic nuclear medicine examinations are 1000 to 1 million times too low a concentration to have any pharmacological effects (other than placebo); thus, renal and hepatic functions are less critical. The radiation dose to the patient as a result of a nuclear brain scan is comparable to that of a CT scan.

Clinician considerations

Clear and complete clinical information on the imaging request should be provided (not just 'rule out pathology' or 'new-onset mental status changes'). Examples of the types of information that are of most value to the nuclear medicine physician include: a lesion is suspected in a particular location; a specific disease process might be present; dominant symptoms prompting the examination; and comorbid conditions that may complicate interpretation. The imaging physician and technical staff also need to be fully informed on any aspect of the patient's current condition that might alter tracer uptake or create difficulties during the scan. Sending a current problem list and medication list or a recent clinic note with the order can be helpful in some cases. Examples of conditions that can alter tracer uptake include: the patient's emotional state, some psychoactive medications, and diabetes. Examples of conditions that would require special management include: delirium, psychosis, paranoia, agitation, significant tremor, and high BMI.

It is important to explain the procedure to the patient beforehand. Although each imaging centre has specific detailed protocols, the following describes the basics. A common requirement is that the patient fast for 4–6 hours prior to the tracer injection when FDG-PET is to be performed. In preparation for resting state scanning, the patient waits in a quiet and darkened room with an intravenous line in place. A technologist enters the room quietly and injects the radioactive tracer. The patient typically remains in the room for 30–60 minutes, although the darkness and quiet are essential only during the tracer uptake period (12 minutes for clinical SPECT; 20–30 minutes for clinical PET). Although the patient could be imaged immediately following the uptake period, image quality is improved by waiting until the tracer washes out from adjacent facial and scalp areas. Nuclear cameras are not confining and rarely cause claustrophobic reactions. The scanning table is quite hard and can be uncomfortable for patients with back pain. All types of neuroimaging require absolute head immobility. Often the head is held still with support from a head-holder attachment on the imaging table, sometimes with additional support from light taping. SPECT and PET scans take approximately 30 minutes. If the patient is unable to remain still for the length of the examination, an anti-anxiety medication or other sedative medication can be given immediately prior to imaging, after the tracer distribution in the brain has become fixed.

Clinical neuroimages are most often presented as a series of two-dimensional sections through the brain, in which the patient's right is on the viewer's left and the patient's left is on the viewer's right (radiographic perspective). Regional CBF and rCMR are high in grey matter areas and lower in white matter. Consequently, SPECT and PET using standard radiotracers are not good techniques for evaluating white matter diseases. In addition to visual interpretation of scan results, many centres also utilize computer-based analytics that provide semi-quantitative measures or allow the patient's results to be compared to a database of results from healthy individuals (Eisenmenger et al., 2016 ; Salmon et al., 2015; Scholl et al., 2014).

If the scan is read as abnormal, it would be of value to review the scan and radiology report with the nuclear medicine physician. Ask the nuclear medicine physician to point out normal anatomical markers and any pathology observed on the images. This information can be of great value when explaining the abnormal findings to the patient and family. Note that PET and SPECT scans are always interpreted as digital images. Reasonable copies can be printed on photographic paper. However, paper reproductions are often quite suboptimal for image interpretation. Images printed on X-ray film are rarely diagnostically useful and should be avoided. Three-dimensional renderings are sometimes available. Note that if the patient has provided you with the neuroimaging examination (e.g. on CD or a flash-drive), it is important to verify that the name and other identifiers match.

PET: technical details, advantages, and limitations

Radioactive compounds used in PET contain positron-emitting radionuclides.

Virtually all current clinical PET tracers use fluorine-18 (^{18}F). The positrons released as the radiotracer decays travel a few millimetres in tissue before encountering an electron. The mass of the two colliding particles is converted into two high-energy photons travelling in opposite directions. The PET scanner recognizes when two photons have struck the ring of detectors simultaneously (annihilation coincidence detection). By combining the results of millions of such coincidence detection events, the scanner's computer can generate a high-resolution image of the distribution of radiotracer. Most centres prefer 3-D acquisition for brain PET scanning. It allows a high-quality brain PET scan to be acquired in as little as 6–8 minutes. A comparable two-dimensional brain scan would take approximately 15–20 minutes. The theoretical limit for spatial resolution is about 2.5 mm (Turner and Jones, 2003), whereas the resolution of clinical PET is in the order of 4–5 mm (Slough et al., 2016).

Both photons from an annihilation must be detected to register an event, making PET very sensitive to attenuation artefact and necessitating attenuation correction. This was formerly done using transmission scans from rod sources. It now is typically performed using a CT scan obtained immediately before or after PET in a hybrid PET-CT scanner (Salmon et al., 2015; Werner et al., 2015). For the attenuation correction to be accurate, it is necessary to minimize patient motion, as the correction requires the PET and CT data sets to be co-registered. Misregistration will produce artefact due to incorrect attenuation correction. This often presents as regionally decreased counts in the cortex of one of the anterior frontal lobes but can have other appearances, depending on the degree and type of motion. If recognized, registration can be adjusted prior to attenuation correction. It is often more efficient to reacquire the images, particularly if the misregistration is severe. MR images can also be used for attenuation correction, and recently PET-MRI scanners have been developed.

There is considerable value in combining (co-registering) PET with structural imaging (CT, MRI) to improve anatomical localization, especially for small structures (Salmon et al., 2015; Werner et al., 2015). It is important to realize that, in an effort to reduce radiation dose, many PET-CT protocols use very low-dose CT. While the CT scan obtained with these protocols will be completely adequate for attenuation correction, it will not be diagnostic and likely of little benefit in co-registration. A diagnostic CT scan can be ordered for the time of the PET, if desired, or a recent prior CT scan can be co-registered. Although there is certainly better anatomic detail from a PET-CT scan than a PET scan alone, fusion of PET and

MRI is even more advantageous (Werner et al., 2015). MRI provides much better structural anatomic detail (e.g. higher contrast between grey matter and white matter, superior resolution of posterior fossa and subcortical structures), as well as the ability to add additional sequences to view other aspects of the brain (e.g. tractography, iron deposition from haemorrhage, water diffusion properties, angiography). The MRI can be obtained at the time of the PET in a hybrid PET-MRI scanner (Werner et al., 2015). However, very few of these instruments are available for clinical use. Co-registration of scans obtained on separate instruments is more common at this time. The disadvantages include the standard contraindications for MRI (e.g. implanted medical devices, metal fragments), eliminating the availability of hybrid PET-MRI scanning for these patients.

Overall, PET uses in neuropsychiatry include examination of rCBF, rCMR, receptor density, amino acid activity, and/or protein accumulation. The different PET tracers each have specific clinical applications. The most commonly used of the PET tracers approved for clinical use in the United States is ^{18}F-fluorodeoxyglucose (^{18}F-FDG). FDG is taken up into cells and undergoes metabolism to a form that is trapped (FDG-6-phosphate), providing a measure of rCMR. This imaging tracer was first synthesized in 1976 (Scholl et al., 2014). Since that time, uses in the brain sciences, both clinical and research, have become widespread. FDG is taken up by the neuronal cell bodies; thus, these examinations are for conditions that largely involve the grey matter (see Figs. 9.1 and 9.2a, b, and e), rather than those largely involving the white matter (Salmon

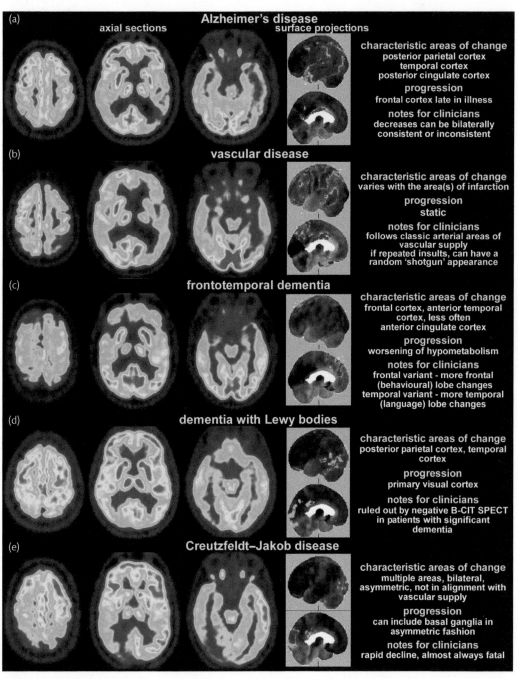

Fig. 9.1 Classic FDG-PET hypometabolic patterns in common dementias.

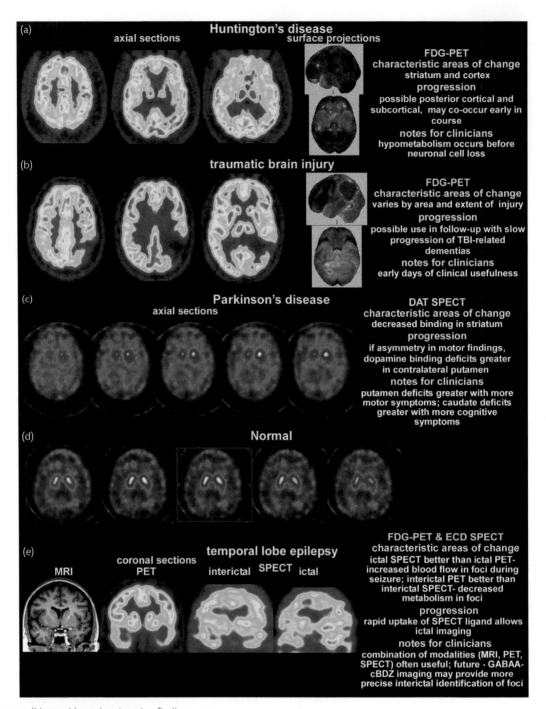

Fig. 9.2 Other conditions with nuclear imaging findings

et al., 2015; Scholl et al., 2014; Werner et al., 2015). In many clinical centres, the major current clinical use is in neuro-oncology. Amyloid imaging allows identification of β-amyloid accumulation in the brain (Eisenmenger et al., 2016; Narayanan and Murray, 2016; Slough et al., 2016; Villemagne, 2016). The first compound to achieve widespread study for its application to differential diagnosis in dementia was Pittsburg Compound B (¹¹C-PiB). This compound has a short half-life of 20 minutes, requiring an on-site cyclotron; thus, it had limited clinical utility. The development of 'second-generation' ¹⁸F-labelled compounds improved clinical utility, and three (florbetaben, NeuraCeq˝; florbetapir, Amyvid˝;

flutemetamol, Vizamyl˝) are approved for clinical use in Europe and the United States. Florbetapir was the first to be approved and is still the most widely used (see Fig. 9.3), A negative scan excludes a diagnosis of AD in patients with dementia (Salmon et al., 2015; Werner et al., 2015). Many additional radiotracers have been extensively studied and may soon be useful, although they are not yet approved for clinical use in the United States. The fluorinated PET tracer dihydroxyphenylalanine (¹⁸F-DOPA) provides a measure of dopamine presynaptic synthetic capacity, and therefore nigrostriatal dopaminergic integrity (Lu and Yuan, 2015; Salmon et al., 2015). This can also be assessed using the fluorinated PET tracer FP-CIT

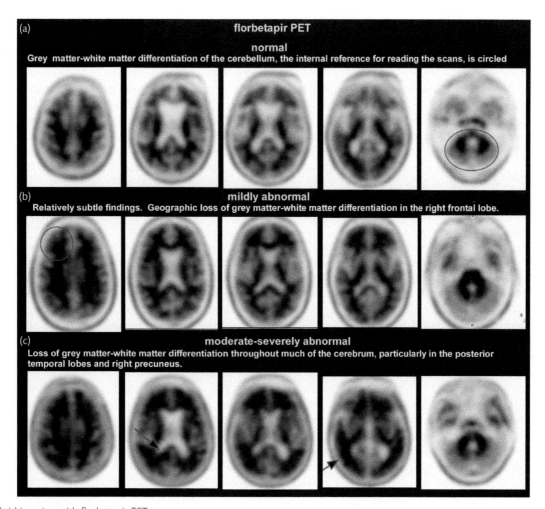

Fig. 9.3 Amyloid imaging with florbetapir PET.

(^{18}F-FP-CIT) which binds to the presynaptic dopamine transporter (DAT) (Lizarraga et al., 2016). Several radiolabelled amino acids that have been developed as PET tracers (e.g. ^{11}C-methionine, MET; ^{18}F-fluoroethyltyrosine, FET) may be useful for primary brain tumour diagnosis and differentiating tumour recurrence from radiation-induced changes (Lu and Yuan, 2015; Salmon et al., 2015; Werner et al., 2015). As is always the case, all should only be utilized as part of a full clinical work-up, and never in isolation.

SPECT: technical details, advantages, and limitations

As the radiotracers utilized in SPECT decay, they emit photons that are detected by a gamma camera and used to reconstruct a tomographic image, similar to the procedure for standard CT (Warwick, 2004). Resolution is heavily dependent on the age and sophistication of the equipment. Most modern SPECT cameras have a theoretical resolution of about 6–7 mm. In practice, the shoulders physically prevent the camera heads from being positioned close enough to the patient's head, reducing clinical resolution to about 1–1.3 cm (Van Heertum et al., 2004).

The major SPECT tracers approved for clinical use in the United States provide measures of rCBF (^{99m}Tc-HMPAO, Ceretec˜; ^{99m}Tc-ECD, Neurolite˜). Tracer uptake, which occurs during the first 1–2 minutes after injection, is roughly proportional to blood flow. After that, the tracer is 'fixed' in the brain. These are lipophilic compounds that quickly diffuse across the blood–brain barrier and into cells (neurones and/or glia). There they are converted into hydrophilic compounds that cannot diffuse back out. Abnormalities in intracellular esterase or glutathione metabolism might lead to SPECT abnormalities, independent of rCBF changes. Iodoamphetamine (^{123}I-IMP), a previously used perfusion tracer, is no longer commercially available in the United States and is infrequently used elsewhere. SPECT tracers for imaging presynaptic DAT (see Fig. 9.2d) are commonly available in Europe and Asia (Warwick, 2004). In 2011, a DAT tracer (^{123}I-FP-CIT, ioflupane, DaTscan) was approved for clinical SPECT in the United States to distinguish parkinsonian syndromes (see Fig. 9.2c) from essential tremor (Bajaj et al., 2013).

Clinical conditions

Dementia

Dementia is most commonly the result of either a primary neurodegenerative disorder (e.g. AD) or a vascular disease (including large and small vessel; cortical and subcortical) (Eisenmenger et al., 2016; Narayanan and Murray, 2016; Scholl et al., 2014). The changes in regional perfusion/metabolism considered characteristic for these conditions are summarized in Fig. 9.1. As noted previously and as is standard of practice, all imaging techniques are considered tool(s) within the evaluation, and reports from these should not be considered conclusive evidence for a particular dementing illness in the absence of a full clinical evaluation, appropriate laboratory testing, and clinical history.

Vascular diseases (see Fig. 9.1b), which remain the second commonest cause of cognitive decline after AD (see Fig. 9.1a), can usually be differentiated by the abrupt (rather than gradual) onset of symptoms, 'step-wise' (as opposed to 'progressive') decline, and structural imaging findings that support a vascular aetiology (e.g. characteristic lesion pattern, atrophy that does not match AD) (Eisenmenger et al., 2016; Narayanan and Murray, 2016). However, nuclear imaging (e.g. rCBF, rCMR) may be a secondary addition to the clinical evaluation; identified deficits follow the pattern of vascular supply to the affected areas.

Although widespread reductions in cortical rCBF or rCMR often indicate the presence of a neurodegenerative process, this appearance is sometimes misleading, as illustrated by two recent case reports (Hassamal et al., 2016; Lajoie et al., 2013). In both cases, a degenerative dementia was suspected, based on FDG-PET and the patients received ECT to address neuropsychiatric symptoms unresponsive to medications. Of particular note, at 2 months post-treatment, both showed sustained improvements in cortical metabolism and remission of neuropsychiatric symptoms, highlighting the false-positive findings of suspected dementia in patients with psychotic depression. As noted in one paper, such cases do not provide insight into ECT's mechanism(s) of action (Hassamal et al., 2016). Although nuclear imaging has been used in multiple investigations of ECT, results have been quite mixed, with both increases and decreases in perfusion/metabolism reported post-treatment (Bolwig, 2014). This may be due to differences in patient population, study design, and/or time of imaging after treatment.

The decision to choose between PET and SPECT for imaging in dementia remains a function of both availability and limitations of technique. A recent small study comparing FDG-PET (rCMR) to IMP SPECT (rCBF) found that both were equally good in differentiating between AD and dementia with Lewy bodies disease (DLBD) in patients with dementia (Chiba et al., 2016). However, FDG-PET was more useful than IMP SPECT for differentiating between AD (see Fig. 9.1a) and DLBD (see Fig. 9.1d) in patients with MCI. Additional studies have reaffirmed the greater specificity and sensitivity of PET over SPECT for dementia differentiation (Eisenmenger et al., 2016). However, a 2015 Cochrane review determined that routine use of FDG-PET in the clinical setting to identify those patients with MCI who will develop AD is not supported by the evidence to date, due to the wide range in sensitivity and specificity across studies (Smailagic et al., 2015). A later editorial noted that the wide variance in PET imaging techniques, interpretation of the imaging results, and what clinically constitutes 'MCI' may account for such differences in specificity and sensitivity in diagnostic accuracy within the cited studies (Morbelli et al., 2015). Of note, the authors advocated for more standardized technique and for software-assisted interpretation that may reduce the variance and lead to stronger evidence for routine use.

Amyloid imaging (see Fig. 9.3) is extremely useful, as a negative scan (see Fig. 9.3a) excludes a diagnosis of AD in patients with dementia (Salmon et al., 2015, Werner et al., 2015). However, the presence of amyloid (see Fig. 9.3b and c) does not necessarily indicate the presence of AD, as many cognitively healthy individuals and patients with MCI also have β-amyloid accumulations identified on autopsy and/or amyloid imaging (Slough et al., 2016). Of note, recent summaries indicate that MCI patients with positive amyloid scans do develop AD at a higher rate than MCI patients with negative amyloid scans (Narayanan and Murray, 2016). The presence of amyloid on imaging in non-clinically demented patients potentially indicates a population in the pre-clinical stage, for which any future plaque-reducing agents might be helpful, if developed. β-amyloid can also be found in DLBD, Parkinson's disease (PD) with dementia (PDD), and other dementias, so clinical correlation is critical if the examination is positive (Eisenmenger et al., 2016).

Early studies are ongoing with both FDG-PET and amyloid imaging in cognitively normal subjects who might be at risk for AD and those individuals with high 'cognitive reserve'(Kato et al., 2016). In both cases, nuclear imaging is contributing to the understanding of the pathophysiology of AD. Many at-risk individuals have lower FDG uptake before conversion to AD. Cognitively impaired patients who are highly educated have significantly lower FDG uptake than patients with similar cognitive impairments, but lower levels of education—indicating the protective nature of education before clinically disabling symptoms overcome the patient (higher cognitive reserve) (Kato et al., 2016). To date, there are no currently standardized recommendations on when to re-image a patient with PET for progressive dementia (Eisenmenger et al., 2016).

As noted in a recent Cochrane review, if the clinical presentation of cognitive decline does not clearly match the criteria for DLBD versus AD, DAT SPECT imaging can be of assistance (McCleery et al., 2015). Although only one study was found that used autopsy confirmation for the validity of DAT SPECT for the diagnosis of DLBD, the authors concluded that it was valuable in this population (moderate to severe dementia, clinical criteria met for probable DLBD). Thus, the evidence supports elimination of DLBD from consideration as the cause of dementia if the scan results in a normal uptake pattern. The authors also noted the need for studies that address the value of DAT imaging in the diagnosis of DLBD in earlier stages of disease (McCleery et al., 2015). Criteria for formal diagnosis of DLBD now includes decreased DAT binding on either PET or SPECT (Narayanan and Murray, 2016).

Tau is an abundant protein in the brain that stabilizes microtubules (Eisenmenger et al., 2016; Slough et al., 2016). There is neocortical accumulation of tau in several progressive dementias, including frontotemporal dementia (FTD) and AD. It is often used as an adjunct to amyloid imaging. Very early investigations are also occurring for the use of tau imaging in suspected cases of chronic traumatic encephalopathy (CTE) and other severe traumatic injury-related dementias.

Movement disorders

Although useful in the diagnosis of DLBD, DAT imaging was largely researched for its utility is distinguishing PD (see Fig. 9.2c) from familiar/essential tremors and other dementias with movement components such as AD and DLBD (Eisenmenger et al., 2016; Lizarraga et al., 2016). Dopamine imaging that reflects integrity of the nigrostriatal dopamine system can be very clinically beneficial in treatment planning, with reference to the different clinical trajectories and 'usual' symptom course. In PD, binding of presynaptic tracers (DAT, DOPA) in the putamen is decreased more contralateral to the side with greater motor deficits (Lizarraga et al., 2016). If there is a cognitive component, the caudate may demonstrate binding deficits. Although Huntington's disease (HD), a degenerative movement disorder with dementia, is diagnosed by chromosomal analysis (autosomal dominant inheritance with repeats of the CAG sequence on chromosome 4), studies indicate that nuclear imaging (see Fig. 9.2a) may demonstrate decreased function before any structural degeneration is evident on MRI (Lizarraga et al., 2016; Pagano et al., 2016). FDG-PET (and secondarily dopamine imaging) can be used clinically for informing/monitoring progression of the disease (Pagano et al., 2016).

Temporal lobe epilepsy

Both PET and SPECT are widely used in the clinical investigations of epilepsy (see Fig. 9.2e), particularly with the differential diagnosis of non-epileptic (pseudoseizures) and epileptic seizures and for defining the boundaries of a seizure focus for pre-surgical planning (Sarikaya, 2015). The rapid uptake with SPECT allows for fixation of the ligand during a seizure (ictal), even if brief. The longer uptake time for FDG-PET makes it more useful when a seizure is not present (interictal). Ictal SPECT commonly demonstrates increased rCBF in the epileptic area (see Fig. 9.2e). Interictal FDG-PET commonly demonstrates a decreased rCMR (see Fig. 9.2e). FDG-PET, particularly when combined with structural imaging (MRI or CT), can give much greater neuroanatomical detail for pre-surgical planning of intractable epileptogenic foci. PET imaging utilizing ligands for various receptors is showing increasing clinical promise. For example, recent studies suggest that PET imaging utilizing ^{11}C-flumazenil [binds to gamma aminobutyric acid (GABA) A—a central benzodiazepine receptor] may provide more precise delineation of epileptic foci than FDG-PET. There are also early indications that it may assist in informing whether or not patients with temporal lobe epilepsy can achieve a 'seizure-free' state after surgery, as those with high periventricular binding have poor outcome (Sarikaya, 2015).

Brain tumours

Although FDG-PET has been utilized historically to identify areas of tumour-associated increased metabolism, the high metabolic rate of healthy brain limits sensitivity (Galldiks et al., 2015). The more recently developed PET amino acid tracers methionine (^{11}C-MET) and tyrosine (^{18}F-FET) combine high uptake by tumours with relatively low uptake by healthy brain, and so provide better tumour-to-background contrast. The difference is particularly noticeable with gliomas both for detection and for detailing of glioma boundaries. These amino acid tracers are now utilized in initial diagnostic work-ups of brain tumours, for identifying post-radiation necrosis, in ascertainment of treatment response, and in assessing for recurrence following treatment (Galldiks et al., 2015; Salmon et al., 2015). As with other PET tracers, ^{11}C-MET requires an on-site cyclotron, so ^{18}F-FET scans are more widely available. Neither is yet approved for clinical use in the United States.

Promising future applications

The wide range of PET and SPECT ligands under development for eventual clinical use in neuropsychiatry include imaging the multiple aspects of the cholinergic system; translocator proteins (TSPO), a marker for microglia; serotonin transporter and receptors; noradrenaline transporter; and histaminergic receptors (Eisenmenger et al., 2016; Roy et al., 2016). Impaired functioning of the cholinergic system, which plays a critical role in cognition and memory, is highly implicated in the pathophysiology of dementia. There are now tracers for the cholinergic system targeting post-synaptic receptors (muscarinic and nicotinic), the enzyme that degrades acetylcholine (acetylcholinesterase, AChE), and the presynaptic vesicular acetylcholine transporter (VAChT) (Eisenmenger et al., 2016; Roy et al., 2016). An intriguing early finding in AD is that the anatomic patterns of decreases on AChE PET and VAChT SPECT do not match the areas of reduced metabolism identified by FDG-PET. Preliminary studies indicate that AChE PET imaging may have potential to improve the differential diagnosis, as some conditions are associated with reductions in cortical areas (e.g. PD, PDD, AD), whereas others are associated with reductions in subcortical areas (e.g. PSP). Alterations in the serotonergic system, which have been implicated in the development of mood and anxiety symptoms, can now be studied with tracers that bind to presynaptic (serotonin transporter) and post-synaptic (serotonin receptors) targets (Chi et al., 2015; Eisenmenger et al., 2016). A few investigative groups have used serotonin transporter PET to compare patients with major depressive disorder (MDD) prior to treatment in an effort to identify biomarkers that predict responders versus non-responders (Chi et al., 2015). The results have been very mixed, indicating that it is very, very early days for using PET as a possible tool to predict medication response in MDD.

Additional uses of nuclear imaging (PET and SPECT) include both investigations of the pathophysiology and limited patient diagnostic evaluation before ECT. Across studies, results have been quite mixed, with both increases and decreases in perfusion/metabolism reported after ECT (Bolwig, 2014). This may be due to differences in study design and time of imaging after treatment.

Conclusion

Functional neuroimaging is coming into increasing use for the clinical evaluation and case formulation of neuropsychiatric patients. These techniques can contribute to differential diagnosis, assist treatment planning, and provide information for prognostic decisions. Although PET has the advantage of higher spatial resolution and often the disadvantage of higher cost than SPECT, the modality is ultimately dictated by the radiotracer required to evaluate the suspected pathology. There are many advancements happening within the field of nuclear imaging, with rapidly improving contributions to the field of neuropsychiatry. As the newer neurotransmitter ligands receive approval for clinical use, the potential for functional neuroimaging to contribute to the diagnosis, treatment planning, and prognostic decisions in neuropsychiatry is innumerable.

KEY LEARNING POINTS

- Functional imaging includes measures that are directly (MEG, EEG) or indirectly (SPECT, PET, fMRI) related to brain activity.
- Patients whose clinical symptoms do not fit the classic historical picture for the working diagnosis should be considered for some form of functional neuroimaging.

- Providing clear and complete clinical information on the imaging request (not just 'rule out pathology' or 'new-onset mental status changes') is critical for obtaining the most meaningful information from functional imaging.
- SPECT and PET using standard radiotracers are best for grey matter processes and of less value for evaluation of white matter diseases.
- Amyloid imaging allows identification of β-amyloid accumulation in the brain. A negative scan excludes a diagnosis of AD in patients with dementia. A positive scan does not necessarily indicate AD, as many cognitively healthy individuals have amyloid accumulations. Clinical correlation is indicated for a positive scan.
- Dopamine imaging can be used to distinguish parkinsonian syndromes from essential tremor.
- The decision to choose between PET and SPECT for imaging in dementia remains a function of both availability and limitations of technique—although PET has the advantage of higher spatial resolution and often the disadvantage of higher cost than SPECT.

REFERENCES

Bajaj, N., R. A. Hauser, and I. D. Grachev. 2013. Clinical utility of dopamine transporter single photon emission CT (DaT-SPECT) with (123I) ioflupane in diagnosis of parkinsonian syndromes. *J Neurol Neurosurg Psychiatry* 84:1288–95.

Bolwig, T. G. 2014. Neuroimaging and electroconvulsive therapy: a review. *J ECT* 30:138–42.

Chi, K. F., M. Korgaonkar, and S. M. Grieve. 2015. Imaging predictors of remission to anti-depressant medications in major depressive disorder. *J Affect Disord* 186:134–44.

Chiba, Y., E. Iseki, H. Fujishiro, et al. 2016. Early differential diagnosis between Alzheimer's disease and dementia with Lewy bodies: Comparison between (18)F-FDG PET and (123)I-IMP SPECT. *Psychiatry Res* 249:105–12.

Defense Centers of Excellence. 2013. *Neuroimaging following mild traumatic brain injury in the non-deployed setting*. Washington, DC: Defense and Veterans Brain Injury Center.

Eisenmenger, L. B., E. J. Huo, J. M. Hoffman, et al. 2016. Advances in PET Imaging of Degenerative, Cerebrovascular, and Traumatic Causes of Dementia. *Semin Nucl Med* 46:57–87.

Filippi, M., F. Agosta, F. Barkhof, *et al.* 2012. EFNS task force: the use of neuroimaging in the diagnosis of dementia. *Eur J Neurol* 19:e131–40, 1487–501.

Galldiks, N., K. J. Langen, and W. B. Pope. 2015. From the clinician's point of view—What is the status quo of positron emission tomography in patients with brain tumors? *Neuro Oncol* 17:1434–44.

Hassamal, S., P. Jolles, and A. Pandurangi. 2016. Reversal of cerebral glucose hypometabolism on positron emission tomography with electroconvulsive therapy in an elderly patient with a psychotic episode. *Psychogeriatrics* 16:376–81.

Kato, T., Y. Inui, A. Nakamura, and K. Ito. 2016. Brain fluorodeoxyglucose (FDG) PET in dementia. *Ageing Res Rev* 30:73–84.

Lajoie, C., M. A. Levasseur, and N. Paquet. 2013. Complete normalization of severe brain 18F-FDG hypometabolism following electroconvulsive therapy in a major depressive episode. *Clin Nucl Med* 38:735–6.

Lizarraga, K. J., A. Gorgulho, W. Chen, and A. A. De Salles. 2016. Molecular imaging of movement disorders. *World J Radiol* 8:226–39.

Lu, F. M., and Z. Yuan. 2015. PET/SPECT molecular imaging in clinical neuroscience: recent advances in the investigation of CNS diseases. *Quant Imaging Med Surg* 5:433–47.

McCleery, J., S. Morgan, K. M. Bradley, A. H. Noel-Storr, O. Ansorge, and C. Hyde. 2015. Dopamine transporter imaging for the diagnosis of dementia with Lewy bodies. *Cochrane Database Syst Rev* 1:CD010633.

Morbelli, S., V. Garibotto, E. Van De Giessen, et al. 2015. A Cochrane review on brain [(1)(8)F]FDG PET in dementia: limitations and future perspectives. *Eur J Nucl Med Mol Imaging* 42:1487–91.

Narayanan, L., and A. D. Murray. 2016. What can imaging tell us about cognitive impairment and dementia? *World J Radiol* 8:240–54.

Osuch, E., and P. Williamson. 2006. Brain imaging in psychiatry: from a technique of exclusion to a technique for diagnosis. *Acta Psychiatr Scand* 114:73–4.

Pagano, G., F. Niccolini, and M. Politis. 2016. Current status of PET imaging in Huntington's disease. *Eur J Nucl Med Mol Imaging* 43:1171–82.

Roy, R., F. Niccolini, G. Pagano, and M. Politis. 2016. Cholinergic imaging in dementia spectrum disorders. *Eur J Nucl Med Mol Imaging* 43:1376–86.

Salinas, C., G. Davila, M. L. Berthier, C. Green, and J. P. Lara. 2009. Late-life reactivation of obsessive-compulsive disorder associated with lesions in prefrontal-subcortical circuits. *J Neuropsychiatry Clin Neurosci* 21:332–4.

Salmon, E., C. Bernard Ir, and R. Hustinx. 2015. Pitfalls and Limitations of PET/CT in Brain Imaging. *Semin Nucl Med* 45:541–51.

Sarikaya, I. 2015. PET studies in epilepsy. *Am J Nucl Med Mol Imaging* 5:416–30.

Scholl, M., A. Damian, and H. Engler. 2014. Fluorodeoxyglucose PET in Neurology and Psychiatry. *PET Clin* 9:371–90.

Sheehan, W., and S. Thurber. 2008. Review of two years of experiences with SPECT among psychiatric patients in a rural hospital setting. *J Psychiatr Prac* 14:318–23.

Slough, C., S. C. Masters, R. A. Hurley, and K. H. Taber. 2016. Clinical Positron Emission Tomography (PET) Neuroimaging: Advantages and Limitations as a Diagnostic Tool. *J Neuropsychiatry Clin Neurosci* 28:A4, 67–71.

Smailagic, N., M. Vacante, C. Hyde, S. Martin, O. Ukoumunne, and C. Sachpekidis. 2015. (1)(8)F-FDG PET for the early diagnosis of Alzheimer's disease dementia and other dementias in people with mild cognitive impairment (MCI). *Cochrane Database Syst Rev* 1:CD010632.

Tanev, K., M. Sablosky, J. Vento, and D. O'Hanlon. 2012. Structural and functional neuroimaging methods in the diagnosis of dementias: a retrospective chart and brain imaging review. *Neurocase* 18:224–34.

Turner, R., and T. Jones. 2003. Techniques for imaging neuroscience. *Br Med Bull* 65:3–20.

Van Heertum, R.L., E.A. Greenstein, and R.S. Tikofsky. 2004. 2-Deoxy-fluroglucose-positron emission tomography imaging of the brain: Current clinical applications with emphasis on the dementias. *Semin Nucl Med* 34:300–12.

Villemagne, V. L. 2016. Amyloid imaging: Past, present and future perspectives. *Ageing Res Rev* 30:95–106.

Warwick, J.M. 2004. Imaging of brain function using SPECT. *Metab Brain Dis* 19:113–23.

Werner, P., H. Barthel, A. Drzezga, and O. Sabri. 2015. Current status and future role of brain PET/MRI in clinical and research settings. *Eur J Nucl Med Mol Imaging* 42: 512–26.

10

Proteomics and metabolomics in neuropsychiatry

Suman Ray

Introduction: what are metabolomics and proteomics?

The term 'metabolome' was first used in 1998. It is defined as the level of the metabolite pool in a cell, tissue, or organism, analogous to that of the term 'genome' for the level of the genetic pool. This definition, initially limited to the 'quantitative complement of all the low molecular weight molecules present in a cell in a particular physiological or developmental state', has widened so that 'metabolomics' is a comprehensive analysis of all metabolites in a biological system that can be identified and quantified (Fiehn et al., 2000). Metabolomics is therefore a tool to measure disturbance in metabolic pathways and networks in human diseases or disorders on the basis of a global assessment of the metabolites present in any given biological system. Metabolomics is made possible by detecting early biochemical changes in the diagnosis and identification of key metabolic features which describe certain pathological and physiological states of a disease (Mamas et al., 2011). Metabolomics has the potential to play a significant role in the investigation of neurological pathologies which lack reliable diagnostic markers, for example, AD (Ibanez et al., 2015).

The term 'proteome' is defined as the set of all expressed proteins in a cell, tissue, or organism, including any post-translational modifications (PTMs) occurring at a particular time that play an important role in several signalling cascades (Jungblut et al., 2008). Proteomic technology includes two-dimensional (2-D) gel electrophoresis, image analysis, mass spectrometry (MS), amino acid sequencing, and bioinformatics to comprehensively resolve, quantify, and characterize proteins. It is possible to estimate which proteins or groups of proteins are responsible for a specific function or phenotype of disease using proteomic tools. An illustrative proteomic method from sample collection to protein identification and analysis by MS is described in Fig. 10.1. The various biomarker sources used for biomarker discovery research in neuropsychiatry include blood, urine, amniotic fluid, saliva, CSF, nipple aspirate fluid, and synovial fluid.

Metabolomics and proteomics approaches

1. Disease diagnosis and treatment: the metabolomic approach offers promise for the identification of potential diagnostic and treatment response biomarkers in the context of neuropsychiatric disorders. It involves analysis of metabolites in biological samples from patients suffering from the disease under investigation. Information generated from metabolite profiling has potential for individualized therapies, which may be more effective in disease treatment.

2. Biomarker discovery and disease understanding: biomarker development is the preferred twenty-first-century approach for neuropsychiatric disease diagnosis, treatment, and management. A metabolomic approach may make it more possible to develop effective diagnostic biomarkers. This involves quantitative and qualitative metabolite assessment within biological systems (Arakaki et al., 2008; Zhang et al., 2012). Metabolic profiling may also help increase insight into the pathogenesis of disease states. The method has potential to be simple, sensitive, accurate, and specific.

3. Drug discovery and development: metabolomics provides a means to drug discovery and development due to its diverse applicability in pre-clinical and clinical research. The approach provides better ways of drug screening, drug toxicity profiling, and monitoring of adverse drug reactions. This reduces the failure rate and other risks associated with drug discovery and development which is highly expensive (Kumar et al., 2014).

4. Pharmacometabolomics and personalized medicine: metabolomics is a rapidly developing new discipline that has important potential implications for pharmacologic science. Metabolomic studies may enhance understanding of disease mechanisms and add to new diagnostic markers. It may also inform pharmacometabolomics, which is the capacity to predict individual variation in drug response phenotypes (Kaddurah-Daouk et al., 2008).

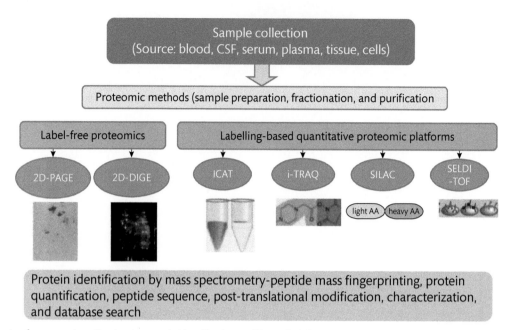

Fig. 10.1 Proteomics: from sample collection to protein identification and its analysis by mass spectrometry.
Reproduced with permission from Patel S. Role of proteomics in biomarker discovery and psychiatric disorders: current status, potentials, limitations and future challenges. *Expert Rev Proteomics*, 9(3):249–65. Copyright © 2012, Rights managed by Taylor & Francis. https://doi.org/10.1586/epr.12.25. www.tandfonline.com.

5. Metabolic engineering/biotechnology: the production of primary and secondary metabolites is called 'metabolic engineering' and requires a quantitative understanding of microbial metabolism.

The areas of various proteomic approaches include:

1. Expression proteomics: it involves quantitative and qualitative proteome analysis.
2. Functional proteomics: it is the study of functional properties of individual proteins and their organization into substructures, complexes, and networks.
3. Clinical proteomics: it focuses on the identification of biomarkers and disease mechanisms.

Strength of proteomics over genomics

Proteomics is considered a step progression beyond genomics in several ways:

1. Unlike proteomics, genome-wide analysis cannot be used successfully in biological fluids due to the difficulty in isolating good-quality messenger ribonucleic acid (mRNA).
2. Genomic-based studies do not give a very good representation of the various protein modifications, but proteomic studies can overcome this.
3. Proteomic approaches are able to identify mRNA splices, but this is not possible by current mRNA analysis methods.
4. Proteomic technologies have the advantage over genomics when it comes to a deeper understanding of disease mechanisms and conditions, as more proteins than genes exist because of modifications made to gene products by alternative splicing.

5. Proteomics over genomics is preferred due to its potential to identify even smaller amounts of protein from increasingly complex mixtures and because proteins are directly involved in performing most biological functions.

Metabolomic technologies

Metabolic technologies that are used to identify metabolites in various neuropsychiatric disorders are summarized in Table 10.1. Metabolic changes in various disease states can be captured using metabonomics based on comprehensive analysis of low-molecular weight endogenous metabolites in a biological sample.

Non-targeted metabolomic mapping is possible by using analytical techniques such as nuclear magnetic resonance (NMR) spectroscopy, gas chromatography–mass spectroscopy (GC-MS), liquid chromatography electrochemical array detection (LCECA), and liquid chromatography–mass spectroscopy (LC-MS) (Kristal, 2007; Money and Bousman, 2013; Villas-Boas, 2007; Weckwerth, 2007). These techniques are useful in the identification of diagnostic biomarkers for neuropsychiatric disorders, including stroke, multiple sclerosis, schizophrenia, and autism (Jungblut et al., 2008; Nicholson and Lindon, 2008; Noga et al., 2012). For example, several potential metabolite biomarkers in the plasma and urine of patients with MDD have been demonstrated using NMR and GC-MS (Zheng et al., 2012; Zheng et al., 2013).

Metabolomics-based technologies provide an opportunity to develop predictive biomarkers that serve as indicators of pathological abnormalities prior to the development of clinical symptoms in neuropsychiatric disorders (Sethi and Brietzke, 2015). The metabolomic approach has been used to identify disease-specific metabolic profiles and biomarkers in CNS disorders, including MDD (Kaddurah-Daouk and Krishnan, 2009; Quinones and

Table 10.1 Metabolic technologies used to identify metabolites of various neuropsychiatric disorders

Neuropsychiatric disorders	Model/ subject	Tissue, blood, cells (sample)	Method	Status of metabolites identified	Pathways involved/ functions	References
Bipolar disorder	Human	Urine	NMR spectroscopy and GC-MS	Increased α-hydroxybutyrate, decreased 2,4-dihydroxypyrimidine	Increased oxidative stress, disturbance of glutamine	Chen et al., 2014
	Human	Plasma	High-performance liquid chromatography	Increased 3-methoxy-4-hydroxyphenylglycol (MHPG)	Regulation of noradrenaline levels	Kurita et al., 2015
Schizophrenia	Human	Plasma	Matrix-assisted laser desorption/ionization time-of-flight mass spectrometry(MALDI-TOF/TOF) and peptide mass fingerprinting	Decreased level of apolipoprotein A-I (APOA-I)	Lipid transportation and metabolism	Song et al., 2014
	Human	Serum, CSF	LC-MS, ^{1}H-NMR spectroscopy	Fatty acid amide (pFAA) abnormalities, increased glucose, decreased acetate and lactate	Endocannabinoid system, glucoregulatory process	Holmes et al., 2006; Schwarz et al., 2011
	Human	Plasma	Multiplex immunoassays, mass spectrometry	Alterations in level of diacylglycerides (DG), triacylglycerides (TG), cholestenone, α-ketoglutarate, and malate	Energy metabolism pathways—TCA cycle	Paredes et al., 2014
Alzheimer's disease	Human	Serum	Gas chromatography coupled with mass spectrometry	Increased lactic acid, α-ketoglutarate, isocitric acid, glucose, oleic acid, adenosine, and cholesterol, as well as decreased urea, valine, aspartic acid, pyroglutamate, glutamine, phenylalanine, asparagine, ornithine, pipecolic acid, histidine, tyrosine, palmitic and uric acid, tryptophan, stearic acid, and cystine	Energy deficiencies, oxidative stress	González-Domínguez et al., 2015c
Stress and anxiety	Wistar rats	Bilateral amygdala	Proton magnetic resonance spectroscopy (^{1}H-MRS)	Increase in N-acetylaspartate (NAA)/creatine (Cr), choline moieties (Cho)/Cr	Divergent mitochondrial pathways	Filiou et al., 2011
Depression	Rodent model	Rat cerebellum	GC-MS	Increased glycolytic and TCA cycle enzyme levels, perturbation of ATP biosynthesis	Cerebellar energy metabolism	Shao et al., 2015

Kaddurah-Daouk, 2009; Schwarz and Bahn, 2008). This approach captures the overall health status of an individual, based on the metabolic state of organisms at the global or '-omics' level. It provides information about what has been encoded by the genome and modified by environmental factors (Quinones and Kaddurah-Daouk, 2009). Psychiatric disorders can be investigated by using metabolic signatures in CSF, plasma/serum, erythrocytes, urine, or post-mortem brain tissue (Money and Bousman, 2013). Pharmacometabolomics is gaining importance in medical practice by identifying metabolic signatures (biomarkers) that embody global biochemical changes in disease states. In this way, precise prediction of responses to treatment or medication side effects (Quinones and Kaddurah-Daouk, 2009) is possible. It is anticipated that metabolomics will become a powerful tool in psychiatric research to investigate disease susceptibility, clinical course, and treatment response.

^{1}H (proton)-NMR tracks the behaviour of protons when introduced into strong magnetic fields. This approach is useful for metabolomic and small molecule analyses (Guest et al., 2016). Although less sensitive, compared to MS, ^{1}H-NMR has several potential advantages:

1. It does not require separation or pre-fractionation of the molecules in some cases.
2. It has the analytical reproducibility and sheer simplicity of the sample preparation step.
3. It gives information on the structural properties of molecules and is therefore suited for identification purposes.

Since the frequency of rotation is related to the chemical and physical environment of the atom within the molecule, using different combinations of radio-pulses, it is possible to determine how each atom interacts with other atoms in the same molecule. This yields the structure, and therefore the identification of the molecule (Guest et al., 2016).

Proteomic technologies

Proteomic technologies have been used to identify protein biomarkers in various neuropsychiatric disorders. These are summarized in Table 10.2.

Table 10.2 Proteomic technologies used to identify protein biomarkers in various neuropsychiatric disorders

Neuropsychiatric disorders	Model/ subject	Tissue, blood, cells	Method	Status of proteins identified	Pathways involved/ functions	References
Bipolar disorder	Human	Brain (pituitary)	Chromatography–mass spectrometry (liquid chromatography–mass spectrometry (E)) analysis	Increased levels of the major pituitary hormones POMC and galanin	Stress response, lipid metabolism, and growth signalling	Stelzhammer et al., 2015
	Human	PBMCs and serum	LC-MS(E) and multi-analyte profiling (human Map®) platforms	Cytoskeletal and stress response-associated proteins	Cell death/survival pathways	Herberth et al., 2011
Schizophrenia	Human	Serum	Affinity capture protein chips (IMAC30), surface-enhanced laser desorption-ionization time-of-flight mass spectrometry, matrix-assisted laser desorption/ ionization mass spectrometry	Decreased level of N-terminal fragments of fibrinogen	N-terminal fragments of fibrinogen are a useful biomarker for molecular diagnosis of schizophrenia	Ding et al., 2015
	Human	Brain (DLPFC)	2-D gel electrophoresis and mass spectrometry	Increased level of synaptic proteins, septin isoforms	Synaptic-associated-presynaptic machinery and NMDA receptor activity	Pennington et al., 2008
Alzheimer's disease	Human	CSF	Antibody-based detection method	Decreased level of eight proteins (A2GL, APOM, C1QB, C1QC, C1S, FBLN3, PTPRZ, and SEZ6)	Cell adhesion and migration, synapse, and the immune system	Khoonsari et al., 2016
Anxiety	Mouse	Brain (cingulate cortex)	^{15}N metabolic labelling and mass spectrometry	Differential expression of about 300 proteins and metabolites found	Energy metabolism, mitochondrial import and transport, oxidative stress, and neurotransmission	Filiou et al., 2011
	Zebrafish	Brain	Sodium dodecyl sulfate–polyacrylamide gel electrophoresis (SDS-PAGE) and immunoblotting	Increased level of corticotropin-releasing factor (CRF) and calcineurin, and decreased level of phospho CREB (cyclic AMP response element binding protein)	Mitochondrial dysfunction	Chakravarty et al., 2013
Depression	Human	Brain (pituitary)	LC-MS profiling	Decreased levels of the prohormone-converting enzyme carboxypeptidase E, decreased activity of prolyl-oligopeptidase convertase	Intracellular transport and cytoskeletal signalling	Stelzhammer et al., 2015
	Rat	Cerebellum	iTRAQ, GC/MS	Increased glycolytic and TCA cycle enzyme levels	Energy metabolism	Shao et al., 2015
	Human	Serum	Liquid chromatography-tandem mass spectrometry for protein profiling	Increased level of caeruloplasmin, inter-alpha-trypsin inhibitor heavy chain H4 and complement component 1qC	Inflammation	Lee et al., 2015

Multiplex immunoassay

This is a highly sensitive method for detecting important bioactive or regulatory molecules (such as hormones, growth factors, and cytokines) present in blood plasma and serum. The steps involved in multiplex immunoassay are shown in Fig. 10.2. Simple Plex is a microfluidic multiplex immunoassay device that offers miniaturized and automated analysis of protein biomarkers (Cao et al., 2015). Multiplex immunoassay is a widely used approach for quantitative multiplexing of proteins. It represents a promising platform for use in translational research to measure protein biomarkers in clinical samples.

Two-dimensional gel electrophoresis

In this method, the sample containing proteins is first separated, according to their isoelectric points (the point at which there is no net charge on the protein), using isoelectrofocusing. In the second step, separation of the proteins is achieved according to their molecular weight. The subsequent protein spots in the gels are visualized with any number of stains (such as Coomassie blue or Sypro Ruby) and then quantitated using imaging software. This method, however, has a number of drawbacks. For example, very abundant proteins, such as albumin, and less abundant proteins, such as the cytokines, are difficult to separate.

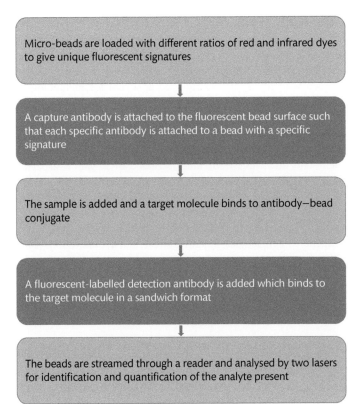

Micro-beads are loaded with different ratios of red and infrared dyes to give unique fluorescent signatures

↓

A capture antibody is attached to the fluorescent bead surface such that each specific antibody is attached to a bead with a specific signature

↓

The sample is added and a target molecule binds to antibody–bead conjugate

↓

A fluorescent-labelled detection antibody is added which binds to the target molecule in a sandwich format

↓

The beads are streamed through a reader and analysed by two lasers for identification and quantification of the analyte present

Fig. 10.2 Steps involved in multiplex immunoassay.

Mass spectrometry

This comprises an ion source, a mass analyser, and a detection unit. There are two broad types based on the difference of ion source specifically in the field of proteomics:

1. electrospray ionization (ESI), and
2. matrix-assisted laser desorption/ionization (MALDI) instruments.

Various mass analysers, such as ion trap, triple quadrupole, time-of-flight (TOF), and Fourier-transform ion cyclotron (that differ in their mechanisms of ion separation, mass accuracy, resolution, and complementary protein identification), are used in MS-based approaches for protein identification (Chandramouli et al., 2009).

Metabolomic signatures in psychiatric disorders

Bipolar affective disorder

The hypothalamic–pituitary–adrenal (HPA) axis has been implicated in the pathophysiology of bipolar affective disorder (BPAD). BPAD cannot be diagnosed by objective laboratory-based modalities. This is due to the complex and diverse nature of clinical symptoms in the disease, often resulting in underdiagnosis and misdiagnosis. However, this can be overcome by using the combined approach of NMR-based and GC-MS-based metabonomic methods to characterize the urinary metabolic profiles of bipolar disorder subjects and healthy controls (Chen et al., 2014). It has been shown that the urinary biomarker panel (using the complementary nature of NMR spectroscopy and GC-MS for metabonomic analysis) is an effective diagnostic tool in BPAD (Chen et al., 2014). Investigations have identified increased levels of glutamate, creatine, and

myo-inositol in post-mortem brain tissue of bipolar disorder (BD) patients (Lan et al., 2009). However, long-term treatment with valproate and lithium decreased the ratio of glutamate/glutamine and increased the level of GABA (Lan et al., 2009). It has been suggested that plasma level of MHPG (3-methoxy-4-hydroxyphenylglycol) could be used as a biomarker of mood states in BD I (Kurita et al., 2015).

Schizophrenia

The importance of metabolomics in psychiatric disorders is illustrated by metabolic dysregulation in schizophrenia patients which renders them at increased risk of metabolic syndrome (MetS), compared to controls. Second-generation antipsychotics (SGAs) used to treat schizophrenia may result in metabolic disturbances, and hence MetS, in a subset of patients. Paredes et al. (2014) analysed the comprehensive metabolomic profiling of 60 schizophrenia patients. When compared to a cohort of 20 healthy controls, patients undergoing treatment with SGAs were designated at high (clozapine, olanzapine), medium (quetiapine, risperidone), or low (ziprasidone, aripiprazole) risk of developing MetS (Paredes et al., 2014). Earlier studies have shown a significant increase in serum fatty acids, and CSF metabolic profile with increased glucose and decreased acetate and lactate (Holmes et al., 2006; Schwarz et al., 2011). It was observed that treatment with atypical antipsychotics for 9 days normalized the CSF metabolic profile of 50% of patients with schizophrenia (Holmes et al., 2006; Schwarz et al., 2011). Findings based on a general population-based study of the metabolome suggest that specific metabolic abnormalities, related to glucoregulatory processes and proline metabolism, are specifically associated with schizophrenia and reflect two different disease-related pathways (Orešič et al., 2011). It was found that schizophrenia had significantly higher metabolite levels in six lipid clusters containing mainly saturated triglycerides, and in two small-molecule clusters containing, among other metabolites, branched-chain amino acids, phenylalanine, and tyrosine, and proline, glutamic, lactic, and pyruvic acids (Orešič et al., 2011). Plasma protein analysis using 2-D gel electrophoresis (2-DE), matrix-assisted laser desorption/ionization time-of-flight mass spectrometry (MALDI-TOF/TOF), and peptide mass fingerprinting suggested that apolipoprotein A-I might be a novel biomarker (related to metabolic side effects) in first-episode schizophrenia treated with risperidone (Song et al., 2014).

Depression

Combined proteomic and metabolomic approaches have been used to understand the aetiology of MDD. A recent study based on the analysis of differentially expressed proteins and metabolites using isobaric tags for relative and absolute quantitation (iTRAQ) in a rodent model of MDD revealed significant alterations associated with cerebellar energy metabolism (Shao et al., 2015). This investigation showed significant alterations associated with cerebellar energy metabolism such as: (1) abnormal amino acid metabolism, accompanied by corresponding metabolic enzymatic alterations and disturbed protein turnover; (2) increased glycolytic and tricarboxylic acid (TCA) cycle enzyme levels paralleled by changes in the concentrations of associated metabolites; and (3) perturbation of adenosine triphosphate (ATP) biosynthesis through adenosine, accompanied by perturbation of the mitochondrial respiratory chain (Shao et al., 2015). Another study involving a rat model of depression showed that amino acid metabolism, in particular glutamate metabolism, cysteine and methionine metabolism, and arginine and proline metabolism, are significantly perturbed in the prefrontal cortex (Zhou et al., 2017). Although a comprehensive understanding of the underlying molecular mechanism in major depression remain unclear, proteomic and metabolomic analyses have proven to be useful in understanding the pathophysiological mechanism(s) underlying MDD.

Stress and anxiety

A non-targeted metabolomic approach based on GC-MS of the prefrontal cortex in chronic restraint stress (CRS)-treated rats revealed metabolic disturbances in the prefrontal cortex of the CRS rat model of depression (Liu et al., 2016). Other findings suggest that metabolic abnormalities in the amygdala and hippocampus are involved in male Wistar rats exposed to a single prolonged stress (SPS) in an animal model of post-traumatic stress disorder (PTSD) (Han et al., 2015). Proton magnetic resonance spectroscopy (¹H-MRS) analysis revealed that N-acetylaspartate (NAA)/creatine (Cr) and choline moieties (Cho)/Cr ratios increased in bilateral amygdala, whereas this ratio was decreased in the left hippocampus (Han et al., 2015). Metabolic analysis of a trait anxiety mouse model revealed divergent mitochondrial pathways pointing towards a molecular network of anxiety pathophysiology, with a focus on mitochondrial contribution to anxiety-related behaviour (Filiou et al., 2011). Overall, these findings indicate the importance of the metabolomic approach in understanding the mechanisms underlying stress and anxiety.

Alzheimer's disease

AD is a progressive neurodegenerative disorder characterized by amyloid plaque accumulation, loss of synapses and neurones, extracellular senile plaques, and intracellular neurofibrillary tangles (NFTs). AD pathology involves perturbed polyamine metabolism in both brain and blood plasma, based on a study using APPswe/PS1deltaE9 double transgenic and wild-type mice. Brain and blood metabolome analysis showed disturbances in essential amino acids, branched-chain amino acids, and neurotransmitter serotonin, in addition to pronounced imbalances in phospholipid and acylcarnitine homeostasis (Pan et al., 2016). Delineation of metabolic alterations in transgenic CRND8 mice, urinary metabolomics based on high-resolution MS revealed alterations of aromatic amino acid metabolism. This included upregulation of serotonin pathways and downregulation of the kynurenine pathway and aromatic L-amino acid decarboxylase deficiency (Tang et al., 2016). The application of a metabolomic approach based on direct MS analysis for the elucidation of altered metabolic pathways in serum from the APP/PS1 transgenic model of AD revealed increased levels of di- and tri-acylglycerols, eicosanoids, inosine, choline, and glycerophosphoethanolamine; reduced content of cholesteryl esters, free fatty acids, lysophosphocholines, amino acids, energy-related metabolites, phosphoethanolamine, urea; and also abnormal distribution of phosphocholines, depending on the fatty acid linked to the molecular moiety (González-Domínguez *et al.*, 2015a). Serum metabolome analysis based on the combination of GC-MS and ultra-high-performance LC-MS revealed the involvement of multiple metabolic networks

in the underlying pathology such as deficiencies in energy metabolism, altered amino acid homeostasis, abnormal membrane lipid metabolism, and other impairments related to the integrity of the CNS (González-Domínguez et al., 2015b). Gas chromatography coupled with MS is also being used as a tool for metabolomic profiling of low-molecular weight metabolites. Exploitation of this tool in serum comparing AD patients and healthy controls showed altered levels of 23 metabolites that included increased lactic acid, α-ketoglutarate, isocitric acid, glucose, oleic acid, adenosine, and cholesterol, and decreased urea, valine, aspartic acid, pyroglutamate, glutamine, phenylalanine, asparagine, ornithine, pipecolic acid, histidine, tyrosine, palmitic and uric acid, tryptophan, stearic acid, and cystine. Metabolic pathway analysis revealed involvement of multiply affected pathways associated with energy deficiencies, oxidative stress, and hyperammonaemia (González-Domínguez et al., 2015c).

Proteomic signatures in psychiatric disorders

Bipolar disorder

BD patients showed changes in proteins associated with gene transcription, stress response, lipid metabolism, and growth signalling, based on the proteomic profiling of post-mortem pituitaries from 13 BD and 14 MDD patients, in comparison to 15 controls using liquid chromatography–mass spectrometry (LC-MS(E)) analysis (Stelzhammer et al., 2015). The study demonstrated that BD patients had significantly increased levels of the major pituitary hormones pro-opiomelanocortin (POMC) and galanin (Stelzhammer et al., 2015). Comparative analysis of 17 patients diagnosed with BD and 31 healthy subjects revealed an increase in α-defensins 1–4, S100A12, cystatin A, and S-derivatives of cystatin B levels (Iavarone et al., 2014). Data from comprehensive 2-D difference-in-gel electrophoresis (DIGE) investigations of post-mortem human hippocampus of people with BD have shown involvement of 14-3-3 signalling, aryl hydrocarbon receptor signalling, and glucose metabolism (Schubert et al., 2015).

Analysis of peripheral biomarkers in patients affected by acutely psychotic BD using a proteomic approach showed upregulation of LIM and SH3 domain protein 1 and short-chain specific acyl-CoA dehydrogenase mitochondrial protein (Giusti et al., 2014). Another study involving multiplex immunoassay analysis of plasma revealed prominent upregulation of growth factor activity pathways linked to GSK3β signalling in BD patients (Haenisch et al., 2014). Surface-enhanced laser desorption/ionization time-of-flight mass spectrometry (SELDI-TOF-MS) protein profiling of post-mortem prefrontal cortex tissue from BD and psychiatric-free controls ($n = 35$ in each group) showed 13 protein peaks distinguishing BD versus control (Lakhan et al., 2012). Other studies have shown apolipoprotein A-I as a candidate serum marker for the response to lithium treatment in BD (Sussulini et al., 2011). Approximately 60 differentially expressed molecules involved predominantly in cell death/survival pathways were identified through proteome profiling of peripheral blood mononuclear cells (PBMCs) and serum from BD patients who were not experiencing mania or major depression (euthymia), compared to matched healthy controls, using LC-MS(E) and multi-analyte profiling (Herberth et al., 2011).

Schizophrenia

Characterization of salivary proteins from 32 schizophrenic patients, compared with 31 healthy subjects, using top-down proteomics has confirmed schizophrenia-associated dysregulation of the immune pathway of peripheral white blood cells (Iavarone et al., 2014). Involvement of 14-3-3 signalling, aryl hydrocarbon receptor signalling, and glucose metabolism has been shown, based on data obtained from comprehensive 2-D DIGE investigations of post-mortem human hippocampus of individuals diagnosed with schizophrenia (Schubert et al., 2015). Proteomics-based biomarker discovery in investigation of psychiatric disorders has many advantages— incorporation of multiplex biomarker approaches into clinical assessment may lead to better patient characterization and delivery of novel treatment approaches (Steiner et al., 2017). In addition, the development of such approaches using lab-on-a-chip and smartphone platforms may help to shift diagnosis and treatment of schizophrenia patients into a point-of-care setting for improved patient outcomes (Steiner et al., 2017).

Proteomics-based approaches have shown that within postsynaptic density (PSD)-associated proteins, NMDA-interacting and endocytosis-related proteins contribute to disease pathophysiology (Föcking et al., 2015). Similar studies involving proteomic analysis of the DLPFC in schizophrenia revealed prominent synaptic and metabolic abnormalities (Pennington et al., 2008). Protein biomarker candidates such as myelin basic protein and myelin oligodendrocyte protein contributing to disease pathogenesis were identified in schizophrenia patients (Martins-de-Souza et al., 2010). Prefrontal cortex shotgun proteome analysis has shown altered calcium homeostasis and immune system imbalance in schizophrenia (Martins-de-Souza et al., 2009). Alterations in limbic system-associated membrane protein (LAMP), synaptic function [syntaxin-binding protein 1 (STXBP1)], and brain abundant membrane-attached signal protein 1 (BASP1) have been shown in a study involving proteomic analysis of membrane microdomain-associated proteins in the DLPFC in schizophrenia (Behan et al., 2009). Other investigations have shown that apolipoprotein A-1 is consistently downregulated in the CNS, as well as peripheral tissues, of schizophrenia in patients (Huang et al., 2008).

Depression

Proteomic profiling of post-mortem pituitaries from 13 BD and 14 MDD patients, in comparison to 15 controls, using LC-MS(E) analysis showed that BD patients had significantly increased levels of the major pituitary hormones POMC and galanin (Stelzhammer et al., 2015). Combination (iTRAQ)-based proteomic and GC-MS metabolomic techniques, using major depression in an animal model, revealed perturbed energy metabolism in the chronic mild-stressed rat cerebellum (Shao et al., 2015). This included abnormal amino acid metabolism accompanied by corresponding metabolic enzymatic alterations and disturbed protein turnover, increased glycolytic and TCA cycle enzyme levels, paralleled by changes in the concentrations of associated metabolites, and perturbation of ATP biosynthesis through adenosine, accompanied by perturbation of the mitochondrial respiratory chain (Shao et al., 2015). Proteomics-based approaches have also been used to compare depressive and remission-state patients with MDD (Lee et al., 2015). Proteomic analysis showed that three proteins— caeruloplasmin, inter-alpha-trypsin inhibitor heavy chain H4, and complement component 1qC—to be upregulated during depressed states (Lee et al., 2015).

Stress and anxiety

Divergent mitochondrial pathways have been shown in a study based on proteomic and metabolomic analysis using a trait anxiety mouse model (Filiou et al., 2011). The study revealed altered levels of up to 300 proteins and metabolites, differentiating high anxiety-related behaviour (HAB) and low anxiety-related behaviour (LAB) mice (Filiou et al., 2011). Altered protein networks in the brain proteome in a mouse model of anxiety have also been demonstrated by other investigators (Szego et al., 2010). The identified proteins were linked to different cellular functions such as synaptic transmission, metabolism, proteolysis, protein biosynthesis and folding, cytoskeletal proteins, brain development and neurogenesis, oxidative stress, and signal transduction. Alterations in serotonin receptor-associated proteins, carbohydrate metabolism, the cellular redox system, and synaptic docking are associated with anxiety (Szego et al., 2010). Similarly, other studies, based on brain proteomic analysis, have implicated mitochondrial dysfunction in chronic unpredictable stress (CUS)-induced anxiety and related mood disorders in a zebrafish model (Chakravarty et al., 2013).

Alzheimer's disease

Analysis of the CSF proteome in a recent study showed lower levels ($p < 0.05$) of eight proteins (A2GL, APOM, C1QB, C1QC, C1S, FBLN3, PTPRZ, and SEZ6) in AD patients, compared to controls, using an antibody-based detection method (Khoonsari et al., 2016). These identified proteins play various biological roles such as cell adhesion and migration, regulation of synapse, and in the immune system. Unwanted platelet activation, as revealed by clinical proteomics, is known to be involved in the pathophysiology of AD (García, 2016). Proteomics is considered an ideal analytical tool for platelet research, based on the identification of platelet biomarkers and drug targets (García, 2016). Clinical proteomics is a relevant tool in early diagnosis of AD, as it allows the detection of various proteins in fluids such as urine, plasma, and CSF for the diagnosis of AD (Martins, 2016). Other research findings based on the proteomic differences in amyloid plaques in rapidly progressive and sporadic AD have been useful for diagnosis, as they provide an important insight into the factors that contribute to plaque development (Drummond et al., 2017).

Conclusion

Proteomics-based technologies have great potential for biomarker discovery. This is because alterations in protein expression, presence in abundance, structure, or function may be used as indicators of pathological abnormalities prior to the development of clinical symptoms in neuropsychiatric disorders. Metabolomics also has great potential for improving diagnosis, therapeutic treatment, and management of disease. Metabolomic analysis of biofluids can be used to detect early biological changes to the host due to perturbations in disease.

KEY LEARNING POINTS

- Metabolomics is a tool for measuring perturbations in metabolic pathways and networks in human disease or disorders on the basis of global assessment of the metabolites present in a biological system.
- Proteomics is a powerful tool to predict the development, course, and outcome of a disease towards personalized ailments. Proteomics has advanced in psychiatric disorders.
- The metabolic changes in various disease states can be captured using metabonomics which is based on the comprehensive analysis of low-molecular weight endogenous metabolites in a biological sample.
- Proteomics-based techniques have great potential for biomarker discovery.
- Further research on the applicability of proteomics and metabolomics as routine diagnostic tools for investigating neuropsychiatric disorders in the clinical laboratory is a necessity.
- An array of reliable and sensitive biomarkers for tracking psychiatric disorders and developing personalized medicine, which is patient-specific, remains an aspiration in the future of psychiatric diagnosis, care, and treatments in the twenty-first century.

REFERENCES

Arakaki AK, Skolnick J and McDonald JF. Marker metabolites can be therapeutic targets as well. *Nature*. 2008;456:443.

Behan AT, Byrne C, Dunn MJ, Cagney G, Cotter DR. Proteomic analysis of membrane microdomain-associated proteins in the dorsolateral prefrontal cortex in schizophrenia and bipolar disorder reveals alterations in LAMP, STXBP1 and BASP1 protein expression. *Mol Psychiatry*. 2009;14:601–13.

Cao J, Seegmiller J, Hanson NQ, Zaun C, Li D. A microfluidic multiplex proteomic immunoassay device for translational research. *Clin Proteomics*. 2015;12:28.

Chakravarty S, Reddy BR, Sudhakar SR, et al. Chronic unpredictable stress (CUS)-induced anxiety and related mood disorders in a zebrafish model: altered brain proteome profile implicates mitochondrial dysfunction. *PLoS One*. 2013;8:e63302.

Chandramouli K, Qian PY. Proteomics: Challenges, techniques and possibilities to overcome biological sample complexity. *Hum Genomics Proteomics*. 2009;2009:239204.

Chen JJ, Liu Z, Fan SH, et al. Combined application of NMR- and GC-MS-based metabonomics yields a superior urinary biomarker panel for bipolar disorder. *Sci Rep*. 2014;28:5855.

Ding YH, Guo JH, Hu QY, Jiang W, Wang KZ. Protein Biomarkers in Serum of Patients with Schizophrenia. *Cell Biochem Biophys*. 2015;72:799–805.

Drummond E, Nayak S, Faustin A, et al. Proteomic differences in amyloid plaques in rapidly progressive and sporadic Alzheimer's disease. *Acta Neuropathol*. 2017;133:933–54.

Fiehn O, Kopka J, Dörmann P, Altmann T, Trethewey RN, Willmitzer L. Metabolite profiling for plant functional genomics. *Nat Biotechnol*. 2000;18:1157–61.

Filiou MD, Zhang Y, Teplytska L, et al. Proteomics and metabolomics analysis of a trait anxiety mouse model reveals divergent mitochondrial pathways. *Biol Psychiatry*. 2011;70:1074–82.

Föcking M, Lopez LM, English JA, et al. Proteomic and genomic evidence implicates the postsynaptic density in schizophrenia. *Mol Psychiatry*. 2015;20:424–32.

García Á. Platelet clinical proteomics: Facts, challenges, and future perspectives. *Proteomics Clin Appl*. 2016;10:767–73.

García Á. 2016. Platelet Clinical Proteomics: Facts, challenges and future perspectives. *Proteomics Clin Appl*. 2016;10:767–73.

Giusti L, Mantua V, Da Valle Y, et al. Search for peripheral biomarkers in patients affected by acutely psychotic bipolar disorder: a proteomic approach. *Mol Biosyst*. 2014;10:1246–54.

González-Domínguez R, García-Barrera T, Vitorica J, Gómez-Ariza JL. Application of metabolomics based on direct mass spectrometry analysis for the elucidation of altered metabolic pathways in serum from the APP/PS1 transgenic model of Alzheimer's disease. *J Pharm Biomed Anal*. 2015a;107:378–85.

González-Domínguez R, García-Barrera T, Vitorica J, Gómez-Ariza JL. Deciphering metabolic abnormalities associated with Alzheimer's disease in the APP/PS1 mouse model using integrated metabolomic approaches. *Biochimie*. 2015b;110:119–28.

González-Domínguez R, García-Barrera T, Gómez-Ariza JL. Metabolite profiling for the identification of altered metabolic pathways in Alzheimer's disease. *J Pharm Biomed Anal*. 2015c;107:75–81.

Guest PC, Guest FL, Martins-de Souza D. Making Sense of Blood-Based Proteomics and Metabolomics in Psychiatric Research. *Int J Neuropsychopharmacol*. 2016;19.pii:pyv138.

Haenisch F, Alsaif M, Guest PC, et al. Multiplex immunoassay analysis of plasma shows prominent upregulation of growth factor activity pathways linked to GSK3β signaling in bipolar patients. *J Affect Disord*. 2014;156:139–43.

Han F, Xiao B, Wen L, Shi Y. Effects of fluoxetine on the amygdala and the hippocampus after administration of a single prolonged stress to male Wistar rates: In vivo proton magnetic resonance spectroscopy findings. *Psychiatry Res*. 2015;232:154–61.

Herberth M, Koethe D, Levin Y, et al. Peripheral profiling analysis for bipolar disorder reveals markers associated with reduced cell survival. *Proteomics*. 2011;11:94–105.

Holmes E, Tsang TM, Huang JT, et al. Metabolic profiling of CSF: evidence that early intervention may impact on disease progression and outcome in schizophrenia. *PLoS Med* 2006;3:e327.

Huang JT, Wang L, Prabakaran S, et al S. Independent protein-profiling studies show a decrease in apolipoprotein A1 levels in schizophrenia CSF, brain and peripheral tissues. *Mol Psychiatry*. 2008;13:1118–28.

Iavarone F, Melis M, Platania G, et al. Characterization of salivary proteins of schizophrenic and bipolar disorder patients by top-down proteomics. *J Proteomics*. 2014;103:15–22.

Ibáñez C, Simó C, Valdés A, et al. Metabolomics of adherent mammalian cells by capillary electrophoresis-mass spectrometry: HT-29 cells as case study. *J Pharm Biomed Anal*. 2015;110:83–92.

Jungblut PR, Holzhütter HG, Apweiler R, Schlüter H. The speciation of the proteome. *Chem Cent J*. 2008;2:16.

Kaddurah-Daouk R, Krishnan K. Metabolomics: a global biochemical approach to the study of central nervous system diseases. *Neuropsychopharmacology* 2009;34:173–86.

Kaddurah-Daouk R, Kristal BS, Weinshilboum RM. Metabolomics: a global biochemical approach to drug response and disease. *Annu Rev Pharmacol Toxicol* 2008;48:653–83.

Khoonsari PE, Häggmark A, Lönnberg M, et al. Analysis of the Cerebrospinal Fluid Proteome in Alzheimer's Disease. *PLoS One.* 2016;11:e0150672.

Kristal BS. Metabolomics: concept and potential neuroscience application. In: Lajtha A, Gibson GE, Dienel GA, eds. *Handbook of Neurochemistry and Molecular Neurobiology: Brain Energetics. Integration of Molecular and Cellular Processes.* Springer, New York, NY; 2007.

Kumar B, Prakash A, Ruhela RK, Medhi B. Potential of metabolomics in preclinical and clinical drug development. *Pharmacol Rep.* 2014;66:956–63.

Kurita M, Nishino S, Numata Y, Okubo Y, Sato T. The noradrenaline metabolite MHPG is a candidate biomarker between the depressive, remission, and manic states in bipolar disorder I: two long-term naturalistic case reports. *Neuropsychiatr Dis Treat.* 2015;11:353–8.

Lakhan SE. Mass spectrometric analysis of prefrontal cortex proteins in schizophrenia and bipolar disorder. *Springerplus.* 2012;1:3.

Lan MJ, McLoughlin GA, Griffin JL, et al. Metabonomic analysis identifies molecular changes associated with the pathophysiology and drug treatment of bipolar disorder. *Mol Psychiatry.* 2009;14:269–79.

Lee J, Joo EJ, Lim HJ, et al. Proteomic analysis of serum from patients with major depressive disorder to compare their depressive and remission statuses. *Psychiatry Investig.* 2015;12:249–59.

Liu L, Zhou X, Zhang Y, et al. The identification of metabolic disturbances in the prefrontal cortex of the chronic restraint stress rat model of depression. *Behav Brain Res.* 2016;305:148–56.

Mamas M, Dunn WB, Neyses L, Goodacre R. The role of metabolites and metabolomics in clinically applicable biomarkers of disease. *Arch Toxicol.* 2011;85:5–17.

Martins-de-Souza D, Gattaz WF, Schmitt A, et al. Prefrontal cortex shotgun proteome analysis reveals altered calcium homeostasis and immune system imbalance in schizophrenia. *Eur Arch Psychiatry Clin Neurosci.* 2009;259:151–63.

Martins-de-Souza D, Maccarrone G, Wobrock T, et al. Proteome analysis of the thalamus and cerebrospinal fluid reveals glycolysis dysfunction and potential biomarkers candidates for schizophrenia. *J Psychiatr Res* 2010;44:1176–89.

Martins IJ. The Role of Clinical Proteomics, Lipidomics, and Genomics in the Diagnosis of Alzheimer's Disease. *Proteomes.* 2016;4.pii:E14.

Money TT, Bousman CA. Metabolomics of Psychotic Disorders. *Metabolomics* 2013;3:117.

Nicholson JK, Lindon JC. Systems biology: metabonomics. *Nature.* 2008;455:1054–6.

Noga MJ, et al. Metabolomics of cerebrospinal fluid reveals changes in the central nervous system metabolism in a rat model of multiple sclerosis. *Metabolomics* 2012;8:253–63.

Orešič M, Tang J, Seppänen-Laakso T, et al. Metabolome in schizophrenia and other psychotic disorders: a general population-based study. *Genome Med.* 2011;3:19.

Pan X, Nasaruddin MB, Elliott CT, et al. Alzheimer's disease-like pathology has transient effects on the brain and blood metabolome. *Neurobiol Aging.* 2016;38:151–63.

Paredes RM, Quinones M, Marballi K, et al. Metabolomic profiling of schizophrenia patients at risk for metabolic syndrome. *Int J Neuropsychopharmacol.* 2014;17:1139–48.

Pennington K, Beasley CL, Dicker P, et al. Prominent synaptic and metabolic abnormalities revealed by proteomic analysis of the dorsolateral prefrontal cortex in schizophrenia and bipolar disorder. *Mol Psychiatry.* 2008;13:1102–17.

Quinones MP, Kaddurah-Daouk R. Metabolomics tools for identifying biomarkers for neuropsychiatric diseases. *Neurobiol Dis.* 2009;35:165–76.

Schubert KO, Föcking M, Cotter DR. Proteomic pathway analysis of the hippocampus in schizophrenia and bipolar affective disorder implicates 14-3-3 signaling, aryl hydrocarbon receptor signaling, and glucose metabolism: potential roles in GABAergic interneuron pathology. *Schizophr Res.* 2015;167(1–3):64–72.

Schwarz E, Bahn S. The utility of biomarker discovery approaches for the detection of disease mechanisms in psychiatric disorders. *Br J Pharmacol.* 2008;153:S133–6.

Schwarz E, Whitfield P, Nahnsen S, et al. Alterations of primary fatty acid amides in serum of patients with severe mental illness. *Front Biosci (Elite Ed).* 2011;3:308–14.

Sethi S, Brietzke E. Omics-based biomarkers: application of metabolomics in neuropsychiatric disorders. *Int J Neuropsychopharmacol.* 2015;19:pyv096.

Shao WH, Chen JJ, Fan SH, et al.. Combined Metabolomics and Proteomics Analysis of Major Depression in an Animal Model: Perturbed Energy Metabolism in the Chronic Mild Stressed Rat Cerebellum. *OMICS.* 2015;19:383–92.

Song X, Li X, Gao J, et al. APOA-I: a possible novel biomarker for metabolic side effects in first episode schizophrenia. *PLoS One.* 2014;9:e93902.

Steiner J, Guest PC, Rahmoune H, Martins-de-Souza D. The Application of Multiplex Biomarker Techniques for Improved Stratification and Treatment of Schizophrenia Patients. *Methods Mol Biol.* 2017;1546:19–35.

Stelzhammer V, Alsaif M, Chan MK, et al. Distinct proteomic profiles in post-mortem pituitary glands from bipolar disorder and major depressive disorder patients. *J Psychiatr Res.* 2015;60:40–8.

Sussulini A, Dihazi H, Banzato CE, et al. Apolipoprotein A-I as a candidate serum marker for the response to lithium treatment in bipolar disorder. *Proteomics.* 2011;11:261–9.

Szego EM, Janáky T, Szabó Z, et al. A mouse model of anxiety molecularly characterized by altered protein networks in the brain proteome. *Eur Neuropsychopharmacol.* 2010;20:96–111.

Tang Z, Liu L, Li Y, et al. Urinary Metabolomics Reveals Alterations of Aromatic Amino Acid Metabolism of Alzheimer's Disease in the Transgenic CRND8 Mice. *Curr Alzheimer Res.* 2016;13:764–76.

Villas-Boas SG. *Metabolome Analysis: An Introduction.* Wiley, Hoboken, NJ; 2007.

Weckwerth W. *Metabolomics: Methods and Protocols.* Humana Press, Totowa, NJ; 2007.

Zhang A, Sun H, Wu X, Wang X. Urine metabolomics. *Clinica Chimica Acta.* 2012;414:65–9.

Zheng P, Gao HC, Li Q, et al. Plasma metabonomics as a novel diagnostic approach for major depressive disorder. *J Proteome Res.* 2012;11:1741–8.

Zheng P, Wang Y, Chen L, et al. Identification and validation of urinary metabolite biomarkers for major depressive disorder. *Mol Cell Proteomics.* 2013;12:207–14.

Zhou X, Liu L, Zhang Y, et al. Metabolomics identifies perturbations in amino acid metabolism in the prefrontal cortex of the learned helplessness rat model of depression. *Neuroscience.* 2017;343:1–9.

11

Neuropsychological assessment of dementia

James R. Burrell, John R. Hodges, and Olivier Piguet

Introduction

Dementia is an umbrella term encompassing a range of progressive neurodegenerative brain conditions, characterized by variable changes in cognition, behaviour, and movement. Overall, age is the commonest risk factor for dementia. Specifically, the incidence of dementia rises from 3.9 per 1000 person-years at age 60–64 to 104.8 per 1000 person-years at age >90 (Prince et al., 2015). In high-income countries, it is expected that the number of individuals diagnosed with dementia will increase threefold in the next 30 years, due to ageing of the population and medical advances in treating other age-related diseases.

Clinically, dementia presents in many different guises. Most common is Alzheimer's disease (AD), which accounts for 60–70% of all dementia cases. Vascular dementia (VaD) (i.e. dementia associated with vascular pathology) and dementia with Lewy bodies (DLB) are also common. Rarer forms include frontotemporal dementia (FTD) and a range of dementia syndromes associated with motor disorders such as progressive supranuclear palsy (PSP) or corticobasal syndrome. Importantly, FTD is much more common in younger-onset dementia (before age 65 years), being almost as common as AD in this age group.

Dementia is also pathologically variable. The location and pathological features of the dementia syndromes are relatively well known and include abnormal protein accumulations, inflammatory processes, and neuronal loss. Reliable *in vivo* clinical biomarkers of dementia do not currently exist, despite significant advances in neuroimaging, pathology, and genetics. As such, the diagnosis of dementia is made primarily on clinical grounds. History, examination, neuroimaging, and performance on neuropsychological assessment all contribute towards a diagnosis. Careful consideration of a diagnosis of dementia has important implications with regard to management and interventions (and potential treatments). This is particularly important in younger-onset dementia patients where the risk of misdiagnosis (e.g. in favour of psychiatric conditions) is greater, delaying appropriate interventions.

Diagnosis of dementia and patterns of deficits

Numerous clinical diagnostic criteria for dementia exist. These include broad indices, such as the DSM-5, as well as those focusing on specific entities, including AD (McKhann et al., 2011), FTD (Rascovsky et al., 2011), and primary progressive aphasias (PPAs) (Gorno-Tempini et al., 2011). Increasingly, these criteria emphasize the need for supporting evidence from biomarkers, such as imaging, blood, or CSF, which may improve diagnostic accuracy in early or even prodromal cases (Dubois et al., 2014; McKhann et al., 2011).

Clinical diagnostic criteria for the main dementia syndromes are important tools but may be difficult to implement in individual cases because of the variability in clinical features at presentation and their overlap across dementia syndromes. Rather than discussing their merits and limitations, we provide a précis of the common neuropsychological profiles associated with the major dementia syndromes. While this discussion is not intended to be exhaustive, it will provide the foundations for neurologists, psychiatrists, and other clinicians interested in these conditions (see Table 11.1).

Alzheimer's disease

The typical, or amnestic, presentation of AD is characterized by marked deficits in episodic memory (verbal and visual), as well as variable changes in concentration/attention and visuospatial abilities. A subset of patients will present with marked early executive deficits. In contrast, language skills, behaviour, and social cognition are relatively intact, at least in the initial stages (Miller, 2012). This pattern of cognitive deficits predicts an underlying AD pathology with >85% accuracy. In a small proportion of cases, AD may present in an atypical fashion with predominant deficits in language (i.e. logopenic progressive aphasia), executive function, motor function (i.e. corticobasal syndrome), or vision (i.e. posterior cortical atrophy) (McKhann et al., 2011; Stopford et al., 2008). The role of specific memory testing in patients with MCI, often considered a prodromal form of AD, remains controversial.

Table 11.1 Profiles of cognitive deficits in the common dementia syndromes

Cognitive domain	AD			FTD			Atypical parkinsonian diseases		
	Amnestic AD	LPA	VaD	bvFTD	SD	PNFA	DLB	PSP	CBS
Attention and concentration	++ – +++	+ – ++	+ – ++	–	–	–	+ – ++	–	–
Memory									
Encoding	+++	Variable	+	Variable	–	–	+ – ++	–	Variable
Retrieval	+++	Variable	+++	Variable	–	–	+ – ++	–	Variable
Recognition	+++	Variable	+	Variable	–	–	+ – ++	–	Variable
Language									
Speech	Fluent	Non-fluent	Fluent	Fluent	Fluent	Non-fluent	Fluent	Sparse and adynamic	Sometimes non-fluent
Motor speech errors	+	+ – ++	–	–	–	++ – +++	–	–	Variable
Object naming	+	+ – ++	–	–	+++	–	–	–	Variable
Word knowledge	+	–	–	–	++ – +++	–	–	–	Variable
Single word repetition	–	+	–	–	–	+ – ++	–	–	Variable
Sentence repetition	–	++ – +++	–	–	–	–	–	–	Variable
Word production	Preserved	Impaired	Preserved	Preserved	Preserved	Impaired	Preserved	Preserved	Variable
Visuospatial									
Visuoperception deficits	Variable	–	–	–	–	–	++ – +++	–	+++
Visuoconstruction deficits	++	+ – ++	+	–	–	–	+ – ++	–	+++
Executive	+ – ++	–	+ – +++	++ – +++	–	–	+	+	Variable
Social cognition									
Behavioural disturbances	+ – ++	–	+ – ++	++ – +++	++	–	+ – ++	–	–
Emotion	+	–	–	++ – +++	+ – +++	–	–	–	+
Motor symptoms/ signs	–	–	+ – ++	Variable	–	–	++ – +++	++ – +++	++ – +++
Impaired performance on MMSE	++	++	+ – ++	–	–	–	++	–	Variable

Note: + mild deficit; ++ moderate deficit; +++ severe deficit.

MMSE, Mini-Mental State Examination; AD, Alzheimer's disease; LPA, logopenic progressive aphasia; VaD, vascular dementia; bvFTD, behavioural variant frontotemporal dementia; SD, semantic dementia; PNFA, progressive non-fluent aphasia; DLB, dementia with Lewy bodies; PSP, progressive supranuclear palsy; CBS, corticobasal syndrome.

Concerns about declining memory, sometimes accompanied by subtle memory deficits on cognitive screening, become increasingly common with ageing. Importantly, only a proportion of the individuals experiencing these changes will develop AD or another dementia, and it remains difficult to predict with certainty the outcome in any individual patient. The pattern of deficits on memory tasks may help, whereby impaired encoding of information, together with impaired recall and recognition, appears to associate with the early hippocampal pathology seen in AD. In contrast, impaired recall, but relatively preserved recognition, is suggestive of an alternative diagnosis (Dion et al., 2014; Pike and Savage, 2008; Sarazin et al., 2007). Unfortunately, such memory deficit profiles may not be as specific as initially thought for the early diagnosis of AD (Pike et al., 2008).

Vascular dementia

At a clinical level, VaD can be difficult to distinguish from AD; the two conditions often coexist pathologically, particularly in very old individuals. A history of multiple strokes and focal neurological signs on examination are suggestive of VaD, as is marked white matter signal change on MRI (Miller, 2012). On cognitive examination, VaD patients demonstrate variable memory and executive impairment, like patients with AD, although subtle differences may be detectable (Miller, 2012). For example, unlike AD patients who demonstrate impairment in *encoding* and *retrieval* of new information, patients with VaD may show a relatively spared ability to encode novel information, but impaired retrieval of information. In addition, reduced cognitive processing speed is also common in VaD, thought to reflect the subcortical burden of pathology (Miller, 2012; Schoenberg and Scott, 2011).

Dementia with Lewy bodies and with other movement disorders

DLB is another important dementia syndrome, which exists clinically in a disease continuum with idiopathic Parkinson's disease; true DLB presents with a combination of cognitive deficits and motor impairment, although patients with long-standing Parkinson's disease can develop dementia late in the disease course (often referred to as Parkinson's disease dementia) (Lippa et al., 2007). DLB is often associated with mixed brain pathology, with features of both AD (i.e. amyloid plaques and tau tangles) and Parkinson's disease (i.e. α-synuclein) pathologies. Clinically, DLB is characterized by impaired, but fluctuant, concentration throughout the day and visual hallucinations (Miller, 2012), although fluctuation may be difficult to assess neuropsychologically. Memory deficits, similar to those seen in AD, are also common. Importantly, cognitive dysfunction in DLB often responds to treatment with anticholinesterase inhibitors (Mayo and Bordelon, 2014).

Atypical parkinsonian disorders are associated with variable cognitive deficits (Burrell et al., 2014a; Miller, 2012). PSP is associated with poverty of verbal output, as well as subtle executive dysfunction (Burrell et al., 2014a). Corticobasal syndrome, on the other hand, is associated with a wide range of cognitive deficits, including memory, language, and visuospatial impairments (Burrell et al., 2014a). Perhaps the most consistent abnormality identified in corticobasal syndrome is visuospatial impairment, which is often closely related to limb apraxia (Burrell et al., 2014b). In addition, patients with corticobasal syndrome may develop a non-fluent speech disorder, which can be difficult to distinguish from progressive non-fluent aphasia (PNFA) in the early stages (see Frontotemporal dementia).

Frontotemporal dementia

FTD is the commonest cause of dementia in younger patients after AD and presents with a range of behavioural and cognitive deficits (Burrell et al., 2016; Snowden et al., 2011). About half of FTD patients present with the behavioural variant of FTD (bvFTD), which is characterized by marked changes in personality, behaviour (e.g. disinhibition or apathy), and interpersonal conduct. Performance on cognitive testing may appear intact initially, although detailed testing usually demonstrates evidence of executive dysfunction and disinhibition (Hornberger et al., 2008). Deficits in language and memory may become increasingly prominent as the disease progresses (Hornberger et al., 2010).

A diagnosis of bvFTD is relatively straightforward in the presence of marked and progressive behavioural disturbance, accompanied by atrophy or hypometabolism in the frontotemporal regions on brain imaging. Importantly, however, patients with atypical AD (e.g. the frontal variant) can present with apathy and executive deficits, despite relatively preserved memory. Alternatively, some patients with a clinical presentation identical to bvFTD may have no cortical atrophy on MRI or perform normally on neuropsychological testing. Whether such patients have FTD, or a neuropsychiatric mimic of FTD, remains to be resolved. Finally, an atypical or slowly progressive bvFTD phenotype has been described in carriers of the *C9ORF72* repeat expansion, now recognized as an important cause of familial and apparently sporadic FTD (DeJesus-Hernandez et al., 2011; Renton et al., 2011).

Almost half of FTD patients will present with striking, but differing, patterns of language impairment which can be fluent or non-fluent (Miller, 2012; Savage et al., 2013). The semantic dementia (SD) phenotype is characterized by severe deficits in word and object knowledge, surface dyslexia (i.e. difficulty reading irregular words), and behavioural disturbances, with preserved single word and sentence repetition (Hodges et al., 1992). On neuroimaging, the typical presentation is that of asymmetric anterior temporal lobe atrophy (generally left > right). Once encountered, SD is easily recognized but may be missed by the uninitiated. Pathologically, SD is tightly associated with underlying TDP-43-positive intraneuronal inclusions (Davies et al., 2005), so recognition of the syndrome is very helpful diagnostically. In contrast, non-fluent speech characterized by motor speech errors (called apraxia of speech) and grammatical errors, or agrammatism, is typical of PNFA, which is more commonly associated with underlying tau positive pathology (Caso et al., 2014). On MRI, these patients tend to exhibit focal atrophy involving the left inferior frontal and anterior insula regions of the left hemisphere. PNFA is difficult to differentiate from another atypical language form of AD called logopenic progressive aphasia (LPA) (Gorno-Tempini et al., 2011). LPA is characterized by marked word-finding difficulties and impaired sentence repetition, despite relatively preserved single word repetition, and only minor phonological or grammatical errors in spontaneous speech (Leyton et al., 2012). Unlike PNFA, LPA is almost always associated with underlying AD pathology (Leyton et al., 2011), with brain atrophy involving more posterior (parietal) left hemispheric regions.

The distinction between the different aphasia syndromes can be difficult, even for experienced clinicians, especially in non-fluent cases. Reliance on clinical neuropsychological features alone may not be sufficient. For example, syntactic or grammatical errors may occur in both PNFA and LPA, as can disturbances of word and sentence repetition. Similarly, impaired naming and word-finding difficulties occur in both LPA and SD, even though the two disorders are quite distinct clinically and neuroradiologically. Despite the publication of diagnostic criteria based on clinical features (Gorno-Tempini et al., 2011), specific markers of underlying pathology are required to improve clinicopathological correlations.

Neuropsychological assessment in the context of suspected dementia

Used in the right context and with the right tools, neuropsychological testing provides invaluable and reliable information on cognitive function. It helps establish an individual's cognitive profile, strengths, and weaknesses, will inform about their functional capacity, and will document progression and/or evolution of cognitive deficits over time. The pattern of cognitive deficits provides insights into normal brain function and underlying pathological processes. Nonetheless, the interfaces between neuropsychology and related disciplines, such as neurology and psychiatry, in the assessment of dementia are complex. An understanding of the general framework underpinning a neuropsychological assessment is important, as it will guide the investigations of cognitive functions and improve diagnostic accuracy.

What is neuropsychological testing?

A neuropsychological assessment encompasses a series of different tasks designed to probe specific aspects of cognition. Six independent, but overlapping, domains are outlined in the fifth edition of the *Diagnostic and Statistical Manual of Mental Disorders* (DSM-V): complex attention, learning and memory, perceptual/visuospatial/visuoconstructive, language, executive function, and social cognition (Sachdev et al., 2014). Each domain can be further subdivided into specific sub-domains. These cognitive domains have relatively well-defined biological substrates, although evidence from lesion and neuroimaging studies has demonstrated that most involve distributed neural networks and multiple brain regions. Readers interested in the neuroanatomy of cognition and associated networks are referred to Chapters 5, 7, and 8 of this volume, which cover these aspects in detail.

Although cognitive dysfunction may be suspected following a careful clinical assessment, neuropsychological testing quantifies the extent and severity of change. Furthermore, the pattern of cognitive deficits may evolve over time, prompting revision of the syndromic diagnosis in individual patients. The next sections will review the types of tests most commonly used to examine each cognitive domain. It is not meant to be an exhaustive list of recommended tests or instruments but rather is meant to provide a heuristic regarding the types of processes clinicians interested in the cognitive assessment of dementia patients may need to consider during their evaluation.

General cognitive screening tests

A vast array of neuropsychological tasks is available to probe *specific* cognitive abilities, many of which are time-consuming and labour-intensive (see Table 11.2). Clearly, a comprehensive neuropsychological examination for every individual is not always possible or necessary. Nonetheless, even busy clinicians can administer a brief cognitive screening task, which provides an estimate of overall cognitive function and helps identify patients who require a detailed cognitive evaluation.

Mini-Mental State Examination

The MMSE, which was originally designed to distinguish cognitive deficit due to dementia from apparent cognitive impairment in psychiatric illnesses (Folstein et al., 1975) is probably the most recognized cognitive screening test. Its administration usually takes <10 minutes, even in patients with dementia, and it provides a broad index of cognitive function where a score of 25 or below, out of a possible total of 30 points, is indicative of cognitive deficits.

The MMSE is widely used by clinicians from all levels (e.g. junior hospital doctors, registrars, specialists) and specialties (e.g. general practitioners, neurologists, psychiatrists, geriatricians). Importantly, the MMSE was not designed to distinguish different forms of dementia. It is heavily weighted towards the orientation/attention and memory domains (70% of the available points). Assessments of language and visuospatial function are very brief, and executive function is essentially ignored. As such, the MMSE is insensitive to cognitive deficits encountered in some dementias like FTD. Despite these potential inadequacies, the MMSE has been the de facto clinical gold standard to determine cognitive function in the clinic and in many drug trials for the last four decades. Unfortunately, it is now subject to copyright, making it an expensive option for routine clinical practice. Alternatives to the MMSE are provided below.

Montreal Cognitive Assessment

The MoCA is a recent instrument first published in 2005 (Nasreddine et al., 2005). Similar to the MMSE, the MoCA samples a range of cognitive functions and is scored out of 30. Its administration time is comparable to that of the MMSE. Unlike the MMSE, however, attention and memory make up only half of the available points. Tests of language, executive function, and visuospatial abilities are also included. The MoCA offers a number of advantages over the MMSE. Firstly, the assessment of a broader range of cognitive deficits results in a higher sensitivity of the MoCA in detecting MCI; a cut-off of 26/30 detects MCI with a sensitivity of ~90% and a specificity of 87% (Nasreddine et al., 2005). It has been validated in many different languages.

Addenbrooke's Cognitive Examination-III

The ACE-III is the most detailed cognitive screening test in common usage (Hsieh et al., 2013). Similar to the MoCA, the ACE-III covers a range of cognitive domains, including attention/concentration, memory, verbal fluency (executive function), language, and visuospatial ability. It is scored out of 100 points, and a cut-off of <88/100 detects dementia with high sensitivity and specificity (Hsieh et al., 2013). Subscores for each of the cognitive domains can also be obtained. Rather than providing a single index of the severity of any cognitive deficits, the ACE-III has the ability to distinguish across different dementia syndromes by considering the *pattern* of cognitive deficits. In particular, the ACE-III reliably distinguishes FTD and AD, primarily because of the detailed language and executive assessments. These benefits are achieved with only a modest increase in the administration time (12–20 minutes) (Lonie et al., 2009), compared to other screening tools. In addition, its broad range of scores makes the ACE-III useful for tracking the progression of cognitive deficits over time.

Overall, it is important to remember that cognitive screening instruments are just that—they may not be sensitive to subtle cognitive deficits, especially in very intelligent or highly educated individuals. This emphasizes the need for specific and cognitively demanding tasks in such individuals, in the very early stages of a dementing illness.

Domain-specific neuropsychological testing

A neuropsychological assessment aims to specifically probe each of the main cognitive domains. In practice, however, most cognitive tasks are not 'pure' measures of a single cognitive domain and optimal performance usually relies on a combination of cognitive processes. An understanding of the domains tested by each task is required to interpret the results. Comprehensive neuropsychological testing may take between 2 and 7 hours, depending on the presenting symptoms and severity of deficits.

Estimating general premorbid cognitive ability

An estimate of premorbid general cognitive function is an internal benchmark against which performance on cognitive testing is interpreted. Individuals of high cognitive aptitude are expected to perform better on neuropsychological tasks than others with low cognitive capacity, even in the context of early dementia. The

Table 11.2 Common neuropsychological tests

Test	Domain(s) tested	Clinical utility
Screening tools		Useful in the clinic for brief screening
Mini-Mental State Examination (MMSE)	Attention, memory, language (brief), visuospatial ability	Brief administration time, but especially weighted towards attention and memory, with limited testing of language
Montreal Cognitive Assessment (MoCA)	Attention, memory, executive abilities, language, visuospatial ability	Brief administration time, with more balanced assessment across range of cognitive domains
Addenbrooke's Cognitive Examination (ACE-III)	Attention, memory, executive abilities, language, visuospatial ability	Slightly longer administration time, compared to MMSE or MoCA, but more comprehensive assessment of language. Helpful breakdown of tasks into subtasks of specific cognitive domains
Specific neuropsychological tests		Used by clinical neuropsychologists to characterize cognitive deficits in depth
Oddball tasks (i.e. response to infrequent and irregular stimuli)	Sustained attention and concentration	Impaired in delirium; also impaired in AD
Reciting numbers, days of week, months of year (forward and backward)	Attention and concentration; working memory	Impaired in delirium; also impaired in AD
Digit span forwards	Attention and concentration	Impaired in delirium; also impaired in AD
Digit span backwards	Working memory	Impaired in delirium; also impaired in AD
Paired Associate Learning	Verbal learning and memory (cued recall)	Impaired in amnestic AD
Free and Cued Selective Reminding Test	Verbal learning and memory	Impaired in amnestic AD
Rey Adult Verbal Memory Learning Test (RAVLT)	Verbal learning and memory (immediate and delayed recall; recognition)	Impaired in amnestic AD; also impaired in other dementias, including bvFTD
Doors and People Test	Visual learning and memory (immediate recognition)	Impaired in amnestic AD
Rivermead Behavioural Memory Test	Ecological measures of everyday memory	More 'ecological' measure in everyday life; impaired in amnestic AD; infrequently administered in clinical practice
Boston Naming Test	Language (naming); semantic knowledge	Profoundly impaired in SD; may be mildly impaired in amnestic AD, or LPA, and other dementias
'Pyramid and Palm Trees' and 'Camel and Cactus'	Language (semantic association); semantic knowledge	Profoundly impaired in SD; may be mildly impaired in amnestic AD, or LPA, and other dementias
SYDBAT	Language (single word repetition, naming, word association, and semantic knowledge)	Useful in assessing PPA; single word repetition impaired in PNFA, whereas naming, word association, and semantic knowledge are impaired in SD. LPA shows milder impairment across the subtasks
TROG	Language (syntactic comprehension)	Impaired in PNFA; LPA may show mild impairment
Copy tasks (wire cube, interlocking pentagons, clock face)	Visuospatial and constructional abilities, executive (planning), motor function	Highly sensitive to deficits, but may show poor specificity
Rey Complex Figure	Visuospatial and constructional abilities, executive (planning), motor function, visual memory	May show poor specificity, but recall component useful in testing visual memory
Visual Object Space Perception (VOSP)	Visuospatial abilities	May show poor sensitivity for visuospatial impairment, but highly specific
Trail Making Test	Speed of information processing (Part A); executive abilities (set-shifting; Part B)	Common test of executive impairment
Verbal fluency tasks (phonemic, semantic)	Executive abilities (phonemic fluency); semantic knowledge (semantic fluency)	Frequently used in clinical practice
Behavioural Assessment of the Dysexecutive Syndrome (BADS)	Executive abilities (multiple facets assessed)	Comprehensive tool; administration time may limit ability to complete the task in its entirety
Iowa Gambling Test and Wisconsin Card Sorting Test	Executive abilities (set-shifting; mental flexibility)	Complex tests with lengthy administration time; may be helpful when assessing mild deficits in patients with high premorbid abilities
The Awareness of Social Inference Test (TASIT)	Social cognition	Useful in assessing the social cognition deficits characteristic of FTD
Neuropsychiatric Inventory (NPI), Cambridge Behavioural Inventory (CBI), Frontal Behavioral Inventory (FBI)	Behavioural disturbance and functional capacity	Useful in screening for, quantitating, and characterizing behavioural deficits; especially useful in FTD

AD, Alzheimer's disease; FTD, frontotemporal dementia; bvFTD, behavioural variant frontotemporal dementia; SD, semantic dementia; PNFA, progressive non-fluent aphasia; LPA, logopenic progressive aphasia; PPA, primary progressive aphasia.

simplest method to estimate premorbid ability is to use educational and vocational attainment. Another common approach is to assess word-reading ability, which reflects lifelong learning/knowledge capacity and is relatively resistant to the effects of cognitive decline and ageing (Schoenberg and Scott, 2011). In English, one such task is the National Adult Reading Task (NART) (Strauss et al., 2006), which is composed of 50 irregular words of decreasing frequency. Knowledge and pronunciation of irregular words (e.g. 'cello'), which cannot be read correctly with the application of common phonetic rules, can only be acquired through exposure and correlate with general intelligence.

Attention and concentration

Cognition may be considered hierarchical, with attention and concentration representing the building blocks that are necessary for other cognitive abilities. Indeed, in the clinic, patients must be able to concentrate on the cognitive tasks at hand during the examination or testing will, at best, be uninterpretable and, at worst, impossible to perform. As such, concentration is often investigated first, either by assessing the ability to respond to simple questions or commands (provided language is intact) or by observing distractibility, lethargy, and drowsiness during interactions and testing.

Formal tests of attention are varied but include span tasks. Digit span forwards, for example, examines the ability to sustain attention. A series of digits is repeated in order, with the number of digits increasing as the test proceeds. English-speaking adults are generally able to repeat 6–8 digits in the correct order. Separately, the ability to divide attention can be assessed by so-called 'Oddball' tasks, which require a response to an infrequent (and irregular) target stimulus presented among a series of standard stimuli (Huettel and McCarthy, 2004). Other simple tasks include counting from 1 to 20, reciting the days of the week or months of the year, followed by the same tasks in reverse order.

Working memory represents the capacity to manipulate information 'online' in real time, such as remembering a phone number while you get your phone and start dialling. Because of its limited capacity, information in working memory is rapidly discarded or 'pushed out' when other information comes in. Working memory is sometimes conceptualized as a domain that is aligned with, but distinct from, executive function. Clinically, however, it is often examined with attention/concentration abilities with such tasks as digit span backwards. This task requires a sequence of digits to be repeated in reverse order (Hodges, 2007; Lezak et al., 2012; Strauss et al., 2006). Most adults can repeat at least four digits in reverse, but patients with significantly impaired working memory may be unable to repeat >2 digits.

Learning and memory

Given its prominent role in everyday functioning and its breakdown in many neurological and psychiatric conditions, memory has attracted a great deal of interest. Memory is conceptualized in different ways such as 'declarative' or 'explicit' when referring to conscious recollection of facts, or 'non-declarative' or 'implicit' when referring to memory for skills and procedures. Declarative memory is further subdivided into episodic memory (e.g. where you went to dinner on your last birthday) or semantic memory (e.g. knowledge of the Australian states or English counties). In the

clinic, only declarative memory, particularly episodic memory, is routinely tested, with verbal and visuospatial (non-verbal) aspects tested separately.

Most memory tests assess various components necessary for adequate memory performance and can be summarized as follows: (i) encoding (i.e. capacity to take in novel information); (ii) retention (i.e. capacity to hold this information over time); and (iii) retrieval (i.e. capacity to bring back this information after a delay). Retrieval can be examined further using free recall (no external assistance), cued recall (in response to a general or specific cue), or recognition. In general, free recall is more difficult than cued recall, which is, in turn, more difficult than recognition.

In clinical practice, verbal memory is tested using verbal information that varies in grammatical and semantic structure (see Lezak et al., 2012 for a comprehensive review of existing tests). In addition to prose passages (e.g. Wechsler Memory Scale Logical Memory subtest), common tasks include pairs, arrays, or lists of words with variable semantic relations (e.g. Paired-Associate Learning, Free and Cued Selective Reminding Test (FCSRT), Rey Auditory Verbal Learning Test) (Lezak et al., 2012; Strauss et al., 2006). Most of these tasks include immediate and delayed (i.e. after 30 minutes) recall (free and/or cued) components, as well as recognition. The FCSRT appears to be particularly sensitive in differentiating episodic memory deficits due to MCI from those due to early AD (Lemos et al., 2015; Sarazin et al., 2007) and in the distinction of AD and FTD (Lemos et al., 2014). The FCSRT has been incorporated into trials of anti-amyloid therapies.

Memory for visual (non-verbal) information is assessed by recognition of visual stimuli or by recollection and reproduction of line drawings from memory. For example, in one of the four components of the Doors and People test (Strauss et al., 2006), patients are presented with 12 pictures of different types of doors to memorize. Responses with correct recognition of doors from an array of four similar doors is scored. Reproduction from memory of a complex line drawing, e.g. the Rey Complex Figure (Lezak et al., 2012; Schoenberg and Scott, 2011; Strauss et al., 2006) (see Visuospatial and constructional ability) is another common test of visuospatial memory.

Semantic memory is generally examined using tests of word knowledge, knowledge of famous faces, or less commonly world events. Aspects of autobiographical and procedural memory are seldom tested in routine clinical practice.

One criticism of many memory tasks is that they bear little relevance to functional day-to-day memory ability. The Rivermead Behavioural Memory Test was developed as an ecological measure of memory in order to address this confound. It comprises tasks such as memory for faces and objects, appointments, messages, and location of a hidden object (Strauss et al., 2006).

Language

Although predominantly the realm of speech and language pathologists, examination of the integrity of verbal and written language skills is also part of a comprehensive neuropsychological assessment. Aspects to consider include speech fluency, prosody (i.e. the intonation of verbal output), rate of speech, errors in grammar, and motor speech problems (e.g. effortful, distorted speech). This is often accomplished by engaging the patient in unstructured conversation, or perhaps by asking them to describe a complex visual scene such as the 'Cookie theft' (Strauss et al., 2006) or 'Beach' scenes from the Western Aphasia Battery (Kertesz, 1982).

Formal language instruments may include tasks of naming, picture–word matching, single word repetition, and sentence repetition. A common naming task is the Boston Naming Test, which consists of 60 line-drawn objects of increasing difficulty (Lezak et al., 2012; Strauss et al., 2006). Common word–picture matching tasks include the 'Pyramid and Palm Trees' (Howard and Patterson, 1992) or 'Camel and Cactus' (Bozeat et al., 2000) tasks. The Sydney Language Battery (SYDBAT) is a recent test that combines a number of these aspects into a single task (Savage et al., 2013). The advantage of the SYDBAT is that it consists of four subtests, including confrontation naming, word comprehension, semantic association, and single word repetition using the same stimulus set. The profile of impairment across SYDBAT subtests is useful in distinguishing subtypes of PPA such as SD, PNFA, and LPA (Savage et al., 2013).

Other aspects of language, such as production and interpretation of grammar, are less frequently assessed. The Test of Reception of Grammar (TROG) is used to probe grammatical understanding (Lezak et al., 2012; Strauss et al., 2006). The TROG requires patients to interpret a number of short sentences, which become increasingly complex grammatically as the test proceeds. Ability to follow 1-, 2-, or 3-step commands is another simple way to test grammatical understanding, especially if complex sentence structures are used (e.g. 'Hand me the pen after touching the paper').

Visuospatial and constructional ability

Visuospatial and constructive function is assessed by measuring the ability to interpret various types of visual information. Simple copy or drawing tasks, such as interlocking pentagons, wire cube, interlocking figure of eights, or the reproduction of a clock face (see Fig. 11.1), are widely used to assess constructional ability (Strauss et al., 2006). These tasks are easily administered, even with very impaired individuals. The clock face test requires the individual to draw a clock face from memory, with the numbers and hands set at a specific time. Distortions or inability to draw the numbers within the clock face have been found to be sensitive, but non-specific, indicators of cognitive deficits (Strauss et al., 2006). Another common, and more difficult, measure of visuoconstructive ability is the Rey–Osterrieth Complex Figure task (Lezak et al., 2012; Strauss et al., 2006) where the person is asked to copy a complex line drawing (see Fig. 11.2). The accuracy of the copy (scored out of 36 points), the time taken to copy the figure, and the approach to the task are recorded. Obviously, pronounced motor dysfunction (e.g. limb weakness, dystonia, parkinsonism, or apraxia) may confound performance.

Basic visual processing can be assessed using line bisection or object cancellation tasks (Schoenberg and Scott, 2011; Strauss et al., 2006). Another common test—the Visual Object and Space Perception Battery (VOSP) (Strauss et al., 2006)—involves the interpretation of information that varies in visual complexity (e.g. dot counting, position discrimination, and cube analysis). Cognitively intact individuals are expected to obtain perfect, or near-perfect, scores on VOSP subtests (>90% correct). As such, even a small decline in performance is suggestive of cognitive impairment.

Higher-order visual processing deficits are also easily investigated. For example, a verbal description of a complex visual scene (e.g. the 'Cookie theft' picture) can be used to assess for simultanagnosia (the inability to interpret a complex visual scene). Similarly, visual agnosia—the impaired ability to recognize objects despite intact basic visual perception—may be suspected by observing how a patient approaches naming common objects. For example, the patient may have difficulty naming an object by sight but produce the correct name when other sensory modalities (e.g. touch) are employed. Prosopagnosia is a special case of visual agnosia and refers to the difficulty or inability to recognize faces. This can be assessed using facial recognition tasks which require the matching of a target face with an array of similar-looking faces presented from different angles (Strauss et al., 2006).

Executive function

Executive function comprises different cognitive skills, including the ability to abstract, set-shift, plan, organize, and adapt behaviour to current circumstances (Schoenberg and Scott, 2011), and is tested using a combination of approaches. For example, abstraction can be tested by concept formation or similarities tasks (e.g. 'what do "bicycle" and "train" have in common?'). The type of responses will inform the examiner as to the capacity of the patient to reason in abstract terms (e.g. 'They are both modes of transport') or in concrete terms (e.g. 'They both have wheels').

Set-shifting can be tested using the Trail Making Test (Hodges, 2007; Strauss et al., 2006). Part A of the Trail Making Test requires the participant to draw lines between circles labelled with consecutive numbers (i.e. '1', '2', '3', etc.). In Part B, the task is made more difficult by alternating consecutive numbers with consecutive letters (i.e. '1', 'A', '2', 'B', '3', 'C', etc.). Individuals with executive impairment may take longer to complete these tasks, or make errors, or both.

Fluency tasks, such as letter (e.g. F, A, and S) or category (e.g. animals, vegetables) fluency, also assess the capacity to follow specific rules and to modify behaviour flexibly (i.e. set-shifting). Fluency tasks require the generation of as many words as possible in

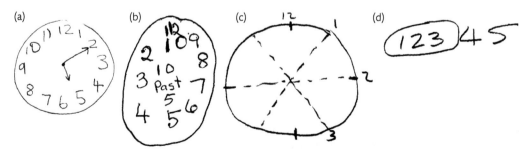

Fig. 11.1 The clock face. Patients are instructed to draw a clock face, including all the numbers, and to set the time from memory. (a) Control subject; (b) to (d) Three examples of impaired clock faces from different individual patients with dementia.

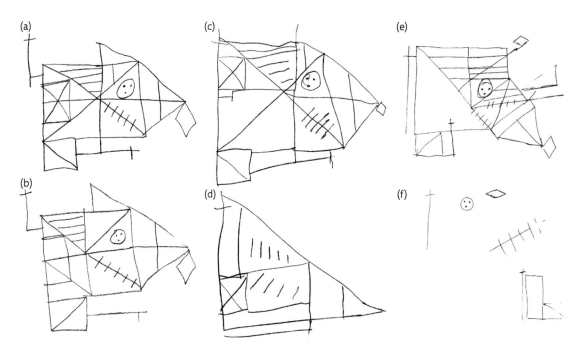

Fig. 11.2 The Rey Complex Figure. The Rey Complex Figure copy (a, c, e) and reproduction from memory (b, d, f) after a 3-minute delay. Time taken to produce the copy is recorded and accuracy is scored. Examples of Rey Complex Figure task performance in a control subject (Copy a, Recall b). Performance in patients with dementia is shown in (c) to (f) (Copy c and e, corresponding Recall d and f).

1 minute, according to the rule set. Patients with executive dysfunction produce fewer correct responses on verbal fluency tasks than normal controls, although language proficiency and/or deficits need to be considered. Other non-verbal equivalents (e.g. design fluency) also exist but are less commonly used.

Planning and organization deficits might become apparent by observing the approach taken to complete a task. For example, a slow and disorganized approach to a copy task might suggest executive impairment. Disinhibition, and behaviour modulation more generally, is infrequently tested in clinical practice. One option is the Hayling Sentence Completion test, which requires suppression of a prepotent responses by completion of sentences with nonsensical endings (Hodges, 2007; Strauss et al., 2006).

A number of different aspects of executive functioning, including temporal judgement, set-shifting, planning, and strategy, can be tested formally using such tasks as the Behavioural Assessment of the Dysexecutive Syndrome (BADS) (Hodges, 2007). Complex tasks, such as the Iowa Gambling Test or the Wisconsin Card Sorting Test, which were designed primarily for research, are sometimes used clinically to detect subtle executive dysfunction (Hodges, 2007), although they tend to be lengthy (e.g. 150 trials for the Iowa Gambling Test and 128 for the Wisconsin Card Sorting Test).

Social cognition

Social cognition is a complex construct that encompass skills, such as emotion processing and recognition and knowledge of social rules and social norms, as well as empathy. These skills are necessary to navigate interpersonal interactions and social structures successfully. Disturbances of social cognition in dementia, and their interactions with other cognitive domains, have been increasingly recognized over the last 20 years. Although still not widely used in clinical practice, tests of social cognition are gaining ground in the assessment of dementia syndromes.

Tests of social cognition investigate emotion recognition, disinhibition, or theory of mind. One of the most commonly used tests to measure facial emotion recognition is the Ekman 60 where participants are required to match photographs to one of six basic facial emotions (anger, disgust, fear, sadness, surprise, and happiness) (Kumfor et al., 2014). This test has been variously criticized, in part because of its use of static stimuli (black and white photographs). The Awareness of Social Inference Test (TASIT) was designed to address these shortcomings and provide more naturalistic situations. The TASIT uses videotaped vignettes to assess the evaluation of basic emotions, as well as complex situations that require intact knowledge of social interference (e.g. sarcasm detection) (Kumfor et al., 2014). Other tasks have been developed to test recognition of social faux pas (Baron-Cohen et al., 1999) and theory of mind, which reflects the ability of an individual to imagine the inner thoughts of another person, an ability normally acquired throughout childhood and adolescence (Gregory et al., 2002). This field is fast-evolving, with particular interest in the interactions between social cognition, neuroeconomics, and complex decision-making in individuals with dementia.

Behaviour and functional assessment

Behavioural disturbances and functional capacity are often measured together, through the use of carer-based questionnaires. For example, the occurrence and severity of behavioural disturbances are probed with instruments like the Neuropsychiatric Inventory (NPI) or the Cambridge Behavioural Inventory (CBI) (Bozeat et al., 2000; Wedderburn et al., 2008). The NPI is a structured carer interview that uses screening questions, as well as detailed sub-questions, to probe neuropsychiatric symptoms like delusions, hallucinations, dysphoria, anxiety, agitation, euphoria, apathy, irritability, disinhibition, aberrant motor behaviour, night-time behaviour disturbances, and changes in appetite and eating (Cummings, 1997). Partly based on the NPI, the CBI examines a wider range of symptoms (Wedderburn et al., 2008) and may be administered in written form, either before or during the clinical assessment. Responses to the NPI and CBI are graded in terms of frequency and severity and can be converted into scores to indicate the level of behavioural disturbance. In addition, the CBI includes several items designed to measure functional abilities (e.g. use of electrical appliances, handling money, self-grooming, etc.).

A number of tools have been developed to probe different aspects of behavioural disturbance more specifically. For example, the Geriatric Depression Scale, composed of 30 'yes'/'no' questions, was developed to explore affective symptoms in older adults, both healthy and demented (Yesavage et al., 1982). Other measures examine apathy (Starkstein et al., 1992), stereotypical behaviours (Shigenobu et al., 2002), and changes in eating and appetite (Ikeda et al., 2002) through the use of structured questions, posed to carers or patients themselves. The BADS is a test battery, which includes six components designed to probe rule set-shifting, problem-solving, planning, and judgement. It was developed to assess executive dysfunction in a range of everyday activities, and thereby provide an objective measure of functional performance (Strauss et al., 2006). Its usefulness is mitigated by its length of administration and is therefore rarely administered in its entirety to dementia patients.

Several instruments have been developed to specifically assess functional impairment in patients with FTD. For example, the Frontal Behavioral Inventory (FBI) is a 24-item face-to-face caregiver interview designed to document the types of behavioural disturbances commonly seen in bvFTD (Kertesz et al., 1997). The Functional Rating Scale (FRS) is another commonly used assessment that includes a functional assessment. The FRS examines performance in: behaviour, outings and shopping, household chores and telephone use, finances, medications, meal preparation and eating, and self-care/mobility (Mioshi et al., 2010). Importantly, measures of functional impairment, such as the FBI or FRS, may detect behavioural changes in patients with FTD who perform well on cognitive testing initially.

The progression of functional impairment in dementia can be measured using tools such as the Clinical Dementia Rating Scale (CDR), which was specifically developed for use in AD (Morris, 1997). The CDR incorporates patient- and informant-derived information to grade performance in: memory, orientation, judgement, problem-solving, community affairs, home and hobbies, and personal care. Each section is rated individually and then combined to produce a global CDR score. A CDR score rates dementia as 0 (no dementia), 0.5 (questionable), 1 (mild), 2 (moderate), and 3 (severe) (Morris, 1997). The CDR has now been modified for use in FTD (CDR-FTD) to include behavioural and language sections (Knopman et al., 2008). By comparing current with previous patient ability, the CDR may be less influenced by education, language, and culture than traditional neuropsychological testing (Morris, 1997).

What are the pitfalls in neuropsychological testing?

It is important to emphasize that results from a neuropsychological assessment needs to be interpreted within the broad context of the person's medical and personal history (obtained from both the patient and the family), psychiatric history, neurological examination, neuroimaging, and, where available, other investigations (e.g. blood tests, genetic testing).

A number of medical and non-medical variables may influence cognitive performance on testing. Firstly, reduced or variable effort, which may be inherent to the underlying disease prompting the referral, will affect the person's capacity to sustain concentration for long periods of time. Comorbid physical and psychological illnesses (e.g. respiratory, renal, or hepatic failure, drug intoxication, depression, anxiety) can also affect performance.

Secondly, most neuropsychological tests are administered using verbal instructions—and often require a verbal or written response. As such, ensuring that patient and examiner can communicate with each other appropriately is important. The use of medical interpreters only partly accounts for this potential confound. Culturally biased tests and level of education are other potential confounds. Additionally, it is important to bear in mind that language deficits are inherent to a number of dementia syndromes. Such deficits are likely to interfere with the assessment of non-language cognitive domains, regardless of the language used to perform testing.

Finally, performance on cognitive testing is not meaningful in itself and scores need to be compared to a relevant benchmark (i.e. comparative or normative scores). Normative scores are usually derived from testing of healthy individuals, generally controlling for such variables as age and/or education. Norms, however, may not be able to control for all relevant variables, e.g. premorbid cognitive ability. It is worth emphasizing that, while people perform better on some tests than others, healthy individuals tend to obtain a fairly homogenous test performance across cognitive domains (e.g. memory, language, executive function). A disproportionate impairment in one or more cognitive domains, while not pathognomonic in itself, may reflect a disorder of cognition. It is also the pattern of deficits that is the most informative diagnostically.

Conclusion

Like many other clinical tools, a detailed neuropsychological assessment can play a central role in the diagnosis and grading of cognitive deficits in dementia syndromes, provided the benefits and limitations are clearly understood by referring clinicians. An understanding of cognitive (e.g. attention and orientation, memory, language, visuospatial function, and executive function) and behavioural domains is central to the interpretation of neuropsychological reports (see Box 11.1). It is important to understand how 'normal' performance on cognitive tests is defined, whether this is relative to an estimate of premorbid function or to a set of population norms. Finally, the pattern of deficits can be helpful in defining clinical phenotypes, which can sometimes accurately predict the underlying molecular pathology. Such clinicopathological correlation will become invaluable, as disease-modifying treatments for dementia are developed and implemented.

This chapter describes the main types of dementia and their characteristic cognitive profiles and outlines the importance of a comprehensive neuropsychological assessment to help with the diagnosis and monitor progression. General cognitive screening tools, appropriate for use by (neuro)psychiatrists and related clinicians, as well

Box 11.1 What to look for in a neuropsychology report

1 Premorbid cognitive ability (how was it estimated?)
2 History
3 Test conditions
   a Effort
   b Medical/medication confounds
   c Comorbid depression/anxiety
   d Linguistic/cultural background
4 Cognitive screening task
   a MMSE
   b MoCA, or
   c ACE-III
5 Domain-based cognitive testing (with reference to 'normal' performance)
   a Attention/orientation/working memory
   b Memory
   c Language
   d Executive function
   e Visuospatial ability
   f Social cognition
6 Summary of findings
7 Neuropsychological diagnosis

as specific cognitive tests examining the main cognitive domains (attention and orientation, memory, visuospatial function, language, and executive function) in dementia patients are considered. Finally, we discuss how to interpret the results when assessing individuals with suspected dementia.

KEY LEARNING POINTS

• Neuropsychological testing is helpful for the diagnosis and management of dementia.

• Patients need to be able to perform at their best for the testing to be meaningful; medical illnesses, medications, anxiety/depression, and testing in the patient's second language can all confound the results.

• Testing may not be reliable in patients with severe deficits—especially language deficits.

• All main cognitive domains should be considered.

• Cognitive screening tasks (e.g. MoCA or ACE-III) are helpful in flagging the need for further investigations of cognitive functions.

• The assessment of behaviour and social cognition is an important part of the neuropsychological assessment.

REFERENCES

Baron-Cohen, S., O'Riordan, M., Stone, V., Jones, R., Plaisted, K. 1999. Recognition of faux pas by normally developing children and children with Asperger syndrome or high-functioning autism. *J Autism Dev Disord* 29, 407–18.

Bozeat, S., Gregory, C.A., Ralph, M.A., Hodges, J.R. 2000. Which neuropsychiatric and behavioural features distinguish frontal and temporal variants of frontotemporal dementia from Alzheimer's disease? *J Neurol Neurosurg Psychiatr* 69, 178–86.

Burrell, J.R., Halliday, G.M., Kril, J.J., et al. 2016. The frontotemporal dementia-motor neuron disease continuum. *Lancet* 388, 919–31.

Burrell, J.R., Hodges, J.R., Rowe, J.B. 2014a. Cognition in corticobasal syndrome and progressive supranuclear palsy: a review. *Mov Disord* 29, 684–93.

Burrell, J.R., Hornberger, M., Vucic, S., Kiernan, M.C., Hodges, J.R. 2014b. Apraxia and motor dysfunction in corticobasal syndrome. *PLoS One* 9, e92944.

Caso, F., Mandelli, M.L., Henry, M., et al. 2014. *In vivo* signatures of nonfluent/agrammatic primary progressive aphasia caused by FTLD pathology. *Neurology* 82, 239–47.

Cummings, J.L. 1997. The Neuropsychiatric Inventory Assessing psychopathology in dementia patients. *Neurology* 48, 10S–16S.

Davies, R.R., Hodges, J.R., Kril, J.J., Patterson, K., Halliday, G.M., Xuereb, J.H. 2005. The pathological basis of semantic dementia. *Brain* 128, 1984–95.

DeJesus-Hernandez, M., Mackenzie, I.R., Boeve, B.F., et al. 2011. Expanded GGGGCC hexanucleotide repeat in noncoding region of C9ORF72 causes chromosome 9p-linked FTD and ALS. *Neuron* 72, 245–56.

Dion, M., Potvin, O., Belleville, S., et al. 2014. Normative Data for the Rappel libre/Rappel indicé à 16 items (16-item Free and Cued Recall) in the Elderly Quebec-French Population. *Clin Neuropsychol* 28 Suppl 1, S1–19.

Dubois, B., Feldman, H.H., Jacova, C., et al. 2014. Advancing research diagnostic criteria for Alzheimer's disease: the IWG-2 criteria. *Lancet Neurol* 13, 614–29.

Folstein, M.F., Folstein, S.E., McHugh, P.R. 1975. 'Mini-mental state'. A practical method for grading the cognitive state of patients for the clinician. *J Psychiatr Res* 12, 189–98.

Gorno-Tempini, M.L., Hillis, A.E., Weintraub, S., et al. 2011. Classification of primary progressive aphasia and its variants. *Neurology* 76, 1006–14.

Gregory, C., Lough, S., Stone, V., et al. 2002. Theory of mind in patients with frontal variant frontotemporal dementia and Alzheimer's disease: theoretical and practical implications. *Brain* 125, 752–64.

Hodges, J.R. 2007. *Cognitive Assessment for Clinicians*, second edition. Oxford University Press, New York, NY.

Hodges, J.R., Patterson, K., Oxbury, S., Funnell, E. 1992. Semantic dementia. Progressive fluent aphasia with temporal lobe atrophy. *Brain* 115 (Pt 6), 1783–806.

Hornberger, M., Piguet, O., Graham, A.J., Nestor, P.J., Hodges, J.R. 2010. How preserved is episodic memory in behavioral variant frontotemporal dementia? *Neurology* 74, 472–9.

Hornberger, M., Piguet, O., Kipps, C., Hodges, J.R. 2008. Executive function in progressive and nonprogressive behavioral variant frontotemporal dementia. *Neurology* 71, 1481–8.

Howard, D., Patterson, K. 1992. *Pyramids and Palm Trees Test: A Test of Semantic Access from Words and Pictures*. Harcourt Assessment, London.

Hsieh, S., Schubert, S., Hoon, C., Mioshi, E., Hodges, J.R. 2013. Validation of the Addenbrooke's Cognitive Examination III in Frontotemporal Dementia and Alzheimer's Disease. *Dementia and Geriatric Cognitive Disorders* 36, 242–50.

Huettel, S.A., McCarthy, G. 2004. What is odd in the oddball task? Prefrontal cortex is activated by dynamic changes in response strategy. *Neuropsychologia* 42, 379–86.

Ikeda, M., Brown, J., Holland, A.J., Fukuhara, R., Hodges, J.R. 2002. Changes in appetite, food preference, and eating habits in frontotemporal dementia and Alzheimer's disease. *J Neurol Neurosurg Psychiatr* 73, 371–6.

Kertesz, A. 1982. *Western Aphasia Battery*. The Psychological Corporation, San Antonio, TX.

Kertesz, A., Davidson, W., Fox, H. 1997. Frontal behavioral inventory: diagnostic criteria for frontal lobe dementia. *Can J Neurol Sci* 24, 29–36.

Knopman, D.S., Kramer, J.H., Boeve, B.F., et al. 2008. Development of methodology for conducting clinical trials in frontotemporal lobar degeneration. *Brain* 131, 2957–68.

Kumfor, F., Irish, M., Leyton, C., et al. 2014. Tracking the progression of social cognition in neurodegenerative disorders. *J Neurol Neurosurg Psychiatry* 85, 1076–83.

Lemos, R., Cunha, C., Marôco, J., Afonso, A., Simões, M.R., Santana, I. 2015. Free and Cued Selective Reminding Test is superior to the Wechsler Memory Scale in discriminating mild cognitive impairment from Alzheimer's disease. *Geriatr Gerontol Int* 15, 961–8.

Lemos, R., Duro, D., Simões, M.R., Santana, I. 2014. The free and cued selective reminding test distinguishes frontotemporal dementia from Alzheimer's disease. *Arch Clin Neuropsychol* 29, 670–9.

Leyton, C.E., Piguet, O., Savage, S., Burrell, J., Hodges, J.R. 2012. The neural basis of logopenic progressive aphasia. *J Alzheimers Dis* 32, 1051–9.

Leyton, C.E., Villemagne, V.L., Savage, S., et al. 2011. Subtypes of progressive aphasia: application of the International Consensus Criteria and validation using β-amyloid imaging. *Brain* 134, 3030–43.

Lezak, M.D., Howieson, D.B., Bigler, E.D., Tranel, D. 2012. *Neuropsychological Assessment*, fifth edition. Oxford University Press, Oxford and New York, NY.

Lippa, C.F., Duda, J.E., Grossman, M., et al.; DLB/PDD Working Group. 2007. DLB and PDD boundary issues: diagnosis, treatment, molecular pathology, and biomarkers. *Neurology* 68, 812–19.

Lonie, J.A., Tierney, K.M., Ebmeier, K.P. 2009. Screening for mild cognitive impairment: a systematic review. *Int J Geriatr Psychiatry* 24, 902–15.

Mayo, M.C., Bordelon, Y. 2014. Dementia with Lewy bodies. *Semin Neurol* 34, 182–8.

McKhann, G.M., Knopman, D.S., Chertkow, H., et al. 2011. The diagnosis of dementia due to Alzheimer's disease: recommendations from the National Institute on Aging-Alzheimer's Association workgroups on diagnostic guidelines for Alzheimer's disease. *Alzheimers Dement* 7, 263–9.

Miller, B.L. 2012. *The Behavioral Neurology of Dementia*. Cambridge University Press, Cambridge.

Mioshi, E., Hsieh, S., Savage, S., Hornberger, M., Hodges, J.R. 2010. Clinical staging and disease progression in frontotemporal dementia. *Neurology* 74, 1591–7.

Morris, J.C. 1997. Clinical dementia rating: a reliable and valid diagnostic and staging measure for dementia of the Alzheimer type. *Int Psychogeriatr* 9 Suppl 1, 173–6; discussion 177–8.

Nasreddine, Z.S., Phillips, N.A., Bédirian, V., et al. 2005. The Montreal Cognitive Assessment, MoCA: a brief screening tool for mild cognitive impairment. *J Am Geriatr Soc* 53, 695–9.

Pike, K.E., Rowe, C.C., Moss, S.A., Savage, G. 2008. Memory profiling with paired associate learning in Alzheimer's disease, mild cognitive impairment, and healthy aging. *Neuropsychology* 22, 718–28.

Pike, K.E., Savage, G. 2008. Memory profiling in mild cognitive impairment: can we determine risk for Alzheimer's disease? *J Neuropsychol* 2, 361–72.

Prince, M., Wimo, A., Guerchet, M., Ali, G., Wu, Y.T., Prina, M. 2015. *World Alzheimer report 2015—the global impact of dementia: an analysis of prevalence, incidence, cost and trends*. Alzheimer's Disease International, London.

Rascovsky, K., Hodges, J.R., Knopman, D., et al. 2011. Sensitivity of revised diagnostic criteria for the behavioural variant of frontotemporal dementia. *Brain* 134, 2456–77.

Renton, A.E., Majounie, E., Waite, A., et al. 2011. A hexanucleotide repeat expansion in C9ORF72 is the cause of chromosome 9p21-linked ALS-FTD. *Neuron* 72, 257–68.

Sachdev, P.S., Blacker, D., Blazer, D.G., et al. 2014. Classifying neurocognitive disorders: the DSM-5 approach. *Nat Rev Neurol* 10, 634–42.

Sarazin, M., Berr, C., De Rotrou, J., et al. 2007. Amnestic syndrome of the medial temporal type identifies prodromal AD: a longitudinal study. *Neurology* 69, 1859–67.

Savage, S., Hsieh, S., Leslie, F., Foxe, D., Piguet, O., Hodges, J.R. 2013. Distinguishing subtypes in primary progressive aphasia: application of the Sydney language battery. *Dement Geriatr Cogn Disord* 35, 208–18.

Schoenberg, M.R., Scott, J.G. 2011. *The Little Black Book of Neuropsychology: A Syndrome-Based Approach*. Springer, New York, NY.

Shigenobu, K., Ikeda, M., Fukuhara, R., et al. 2002. The Stereotypy Rating Inventory for frontotemporal lobar degeneration. *Psychiatry Res* 110, 175–87.

Snowden, J.S., Thompson, J.C., Stopford, C.L., et al. 2011. The clinical diagnosis of early-onset dementias: diagnostic accuracy and clinicopathological relationships. *Brain* 134, 2478–92.

Starkstein, S.E., Mayberg, H.S., Preziosi, T.J., Andrezejewski, P., Leiguarda, R., Robinson, R.G. 1992. Reliability, validity, and clinical correlates of apathy in Parkinson's disease. *J Neuropsychiatry Clin Neurosci* 4, 134–9.

Stopford, C.L., Snowden, J.S., Thompson, J.C., Neary, D. 2008. Variability in cognitive presentation of Alzheimer's disease. *Cortex* 44, 185–95.

Strauss, E., Sherman, E.M.S., Spreen, O. 2006. *A Compendium of Neuropsychological Tests: Administration, Norms, and Commentary*, third edition. Oxford University Press, New York, NY.

Wedderburn, C., Wear, H., Brown, J., et al. 2008. The utility of the Cambridge Behavioural Inventory in neurodegenerative disease. *J Neurol Neurosurg Psychiatr* 79, 500–3.

Yesavage, J.A., Brink, T.L., Rose, T.L., et al. 1982. Development and validation of a geriatric depression screening scale: a preliminary report. *J Psychiatr Res* 17, 37–49.

12

Genetics of neuropsychiatric disease

Stefania Bruno and Nayana Lahiri

Introduction

In the practice of modern medicine, an understanding of the genetic basis of disease, genomic technologies, and the interpretation of increasingly complicated genomic data is essential for all clinicians. This is particularly true for neurologists and neuropsychiatrists who are confronted with conditions, such as developmental disorders, epilepsy, movement disorders, and dementia, for which the genetic basis is becoming both clearer and more complex in equal measure.

All disease is the result of a combination of genetic and environmental factors. Clearly some conditions, such as meningitis or traumatic brain injury, are primarily environmental. Only very few, for example, Huntington's disease (HD), are related to a single gene. The majority of disorders encountered by neuropsychiatrists are related to a number of different genetic factors or arise from an interaction between environmental factors and a complex interplay of multiple genetic influences. Even in a single-gene disorder like HD, features such as the age of onset and individual clinical characteristics can be extremely variable due to a combination of modifier genes and environmental factors.

To better understand the complexity of genetic influences in neuropsychiatric disease, it is necessary first to have a basic understanding of the models of human inheritance, as well as an understanding of current diagnostic techniques. An appreciation of the principles of genetic counselling is also important, as with genetic diagnoses comes the complication that results of genetic testing might not only affect the individual concerned, but potentially their siblings, their children, and their, as yet, unborn children.

The aims of this chapter are to revise basic genetic principles and outline current applications and emerging uses of genomic technologies in the field of neurogenetics and their implications for neuropsychiatry, with some clinical examples of genetically determined conditions.

Chromosomal disorders

The human genome contains approximately 3 billion base pairs, which are packaged in 23 pairs of chromosomes within the nucleus of human cells. Each chromosome contains hundreds to thousands of genes which carry the instructions for making proteins. Each of the estimated 25,000 genes in the human genome makes an average of three proteins (Pertea, 2010).

There are 22 pairs of autosomal chromosomes, one of each pair being inherited from each parent. The twenty-third pair are the sex chromosomes—an X chromosome is inherited from the mother. For males, a Y chromosome is inherited from the father, and in females a second X chromosome is inherited from the father.

Structural chromosomal abnormalities and copy number variation

Errors of chromosomal replication or recombination can result in structural defects that are microscopically visible during karyotyping. These include inversions, translocations, deletions, duplications, or insertions (see Fig. 12.1). These structural defects involve relatively large gene segments and may cause impairment of many genes, resulting in severe clinical manifestations, often with neurological problems. Trisomy 21, or Down's syndrome, is a common cause of mental retardation, in which the prevalence of epilepsy is in the order of 5%. Alzheimer's disease frequently develops after the age of 40 years in affected individuals (Menéndez, 2005).

Small 'submicroscopic' chromosome deletions or duplications, which can still produce defects in several adjacent genes (contiguous gene deletion syndromes), are not visible on karyotype. Targeted molecular cytogenetic techniques, such as fluorescence *in situ* hybridization (FISH) (see Fig. 12.2), can be used to identify such conditions, e.g. the 22q11.2 deletion associated with DiGeorge syndrome (see Box 12.1).

Microarray-based comparative genomic hybridization (array CGH) allows for high-resolution evaluation of submicroscopic chromosome abnormalities without having to select a specific target chromosomal region, as required for FISH. It is a method for identifying gains or losses in the chromosomal material by comparison of patient DNA with a reference DNA (see Fig. 12.3). When a chromosome imbalance is detectable by array CGH, this is referred to as a copy number variation (CNV). CNV is common—at least 4% of the human genome varies in copy number, much of which is benign. However, CNVs that are recurrent in multiply affected individuals have been identified as a major risk factor in neuropsychiatric disorders, such as autism, intellectual disability, and schizophrenia, and are known as 'neurosusceptibility loci'. For example, both deletions

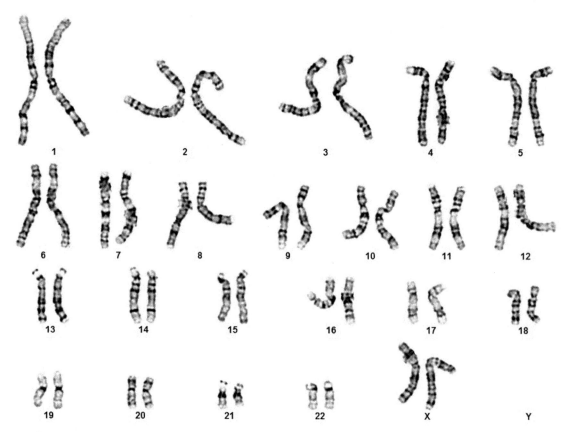

Fig. 12.1 Normal karyotype. Conventional cytogenetic G-banded karyotype showing a normal female 46, XX.

and duplications of the 16p11.2 chromosomal regions confer a risk for autistic spectrum disorder, intellectual disability, and schizophrenia but can equally be carried by normal unaffected parents, thereby showing 'reduced penetrance' (Kirov, 2014).

Most chromosomal aberrations are sporadic, with very small recurrence risks for future children of unaffected parents (typically in the order of 1% or less). Occasionally, a chromosomal syndrome can be inherited through normal carriers of a balanced *chromosomal translocation* who are at risk for an unbalanced rearrangement in the fetus. Balanced chromosomal translocations are not detectable by array CGH, only by karyotype. Balanced chromosomal translocation carriers are at risk of infertility, recurrent miscarriage, or having a child with an unbalanced chromosome rearrangement. The risk is dependent on the nature of the translocation, but empirically it is approximately 15% (Barišic, 1996). Once present, chromosomal microdeletions and CNVs are inherited in a dominant pattern but often exhibit variable penetrance and expression.

Single-gene disorders

Depending on the gene involved, single-gene disorders can be inherited in one of several Mendelian patterns—autosomal dominant,

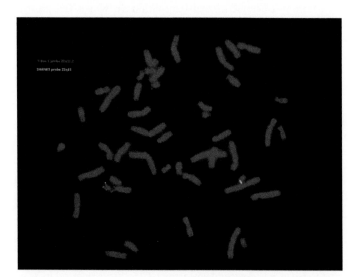

Fig. 12.2 Fluorescence *in situ* hybridization. FISH is based on DNA probes annealing to specific target sequences of sample DNA. Attached to the probes are fluorescent reporter molecules, which confirm the presence or absence of a particular submicroscopic chromosome aberration when viewed under fluorescence microscopy. This figure shows both copies of chromosome 22q showing the presence of the SHANK3 probe, but only one copy of the T-Box probe specific to the 22q11.2 region, deletions of which are associated with di George syndrome.

Box 12.1 DiGeorge syndrome

DiGeorge syndrome is the most common micro-deletion syndrome in humans, with a prevalence of 1:2000. It is also known as velo-cardio-facial syndrome, to describe the frequent occurrence of cleft palate, facial dysmorphisms and congenital cardiac abnormalities. Neuropsychiatric features are very common, with mild learning disability, and a strong association with schizophrenia; twenty times more likely than in the general population (Murphy et al., 1999).

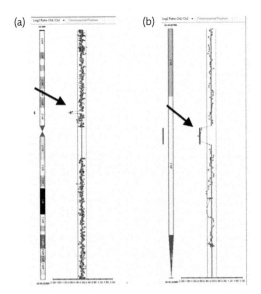

Fig. 12.3 Array CGH. A deletion in chromosome 16p11.2, detected by an array CGH test. Each black dot represents an oligonucleotide probe; there are several probes in the deleted region (shown in red) in panel A, and enlarged in panel B. The microarray comprises tens of thousands of oligonucleotide probes arranged on a glass chip. Digested DNA from the patient is labelled with a coloured fluorescent dye (green). Digested reference DNA is labelled with a different coloured fluorescent dye (red). Samples are mixed together and hybridized to the chip which is scanned in a microarray scanner, which measures the amount of red and green fluorescence on each probe. Too much patient DNA (due to a chromosome duplication) would show as an excess of green fluorescence. Too little patient DNA (due to a chromosome deletion) would be shown as an excess of red fluorescence.

autosomal recessive, or X-linked (see Fig. 12.4)—or non-Mendelian patterns in the case of mitochondrial and imprinting disorders.

Autosomal dominant disorders

In autosomal dominant conditions, a mutation in one copy of the gene (*heterozygote*) is sufficient for a person to be affected. Each child of a person affected with an autosomal dominant disease has a 50% risk of inheriting the mutation and potentially developing the disease. Males and females are equally at risk of being affected, and usually the disease appears over multiple generations. It is not unusual for dominant disorders to display variable penetrance and expression where the features of a condition vary between family members. Examples of autosomal dominant neuropsychiatric disorders include HD (see Box 12.2), tuberous sclerosis, CADASIL, and some forms of familial Alzheimer's disease.

Autosomal recessive disorders

In autosomal recessive inheritance, an individual will only be affected with the condition if both copies of the gene have a mutation—'homozygous'. The parents of an individual with an autosomal recessive condition each carry one copy of the mutated gene; they do not typically show signs and symptoms of the condition and are 'unaffected carriers'. Autosomal recessive disorders are typically not seen in every generation of a family. Both males and females can be affected. In small families, autosomal recessive disorders may appear as isolated or sporadic cases. In isolated populations or in consanguineous families, autosomal recessive disorders can occur in multiple generations. In couples where both individuals are a carrier for an autosomal recessive condition, there is a 25% risk for

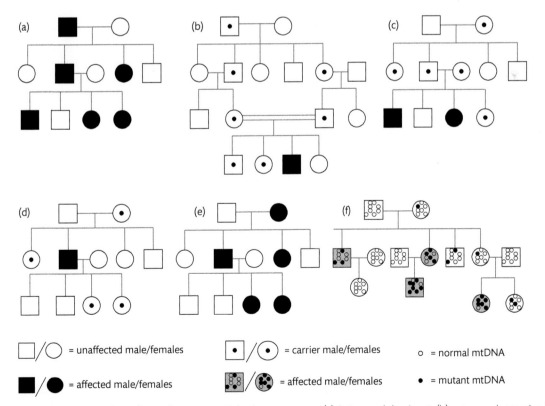

□/○ = unaffected male/females

■/● = affected male/females

⊡/⊙ = carrier male/females

▨/◍ = affected male/females

○ = normal mtDNA

● = mutant mtDNA

Fig. 12.4 Inheritance patterns: example pedigrees for common inheritance patterns. (a) Autosomal dominant; (b) autosomal recessive (double line shows consanguinity); (c) autosomal recessive; (d) X-linked recessive; (e) X-linked dominant; (f) mitochondrial inheritance.

Huntington's disease (HD) is an autosomal dominant neurodegenerative disorder caused by abnormal expansion of a cytosine-adenine-guanine (CAG) repeat in the Huntingtin (*HTT*) gene, located on the short arm of chromosome 4. HD was first described by George Huntington (1872), who captured the characteristic triad of motor, cognitive and psychiatric symptoms. The motor symptoms are often preceded by cognitive and psychiatric disorder by several years (for a full clinical description see Chapter 18). Huntingtin is a ubiquitous protein and, as well as nervous system involvement, metabolic and systemic abnormalities, including severe weight loss, are now recognized as an integral part of the condition. The pathogenic effect of the mutation is generally attributed to a toxic gain of function, but it has been suggested that loss of function may also be relevant, as *HTT* has a role in vesicular transport and membrane scaffolding in several cellular pathways, including, amongst others, pathways relevant for mood regulation and hippocampal neurogenesis (Pla et al., 2014). The average normal number of CAG repeats on the HTT gene is 17-20 (Kremer et al., 1994). The age of onset of the disease, determined by the appearance of motor symptoms, is inversely correlated with the number of repeats, so that an expansion of more than 60 repeats leads to the rare juvenile form, with onset before the age of 20 (5% of HD cases), while most commonly the illness starts in midlife (mean age of onset = 40) (Ross and Tabrizi, 2011). Forty repeats are inevitably associated with full penetrance, while 36-39 repeats have incomplete penetrance, with milder phenotype or absence of manifestation. 27-35 repeats represent an intermediate genotype where individuals will not develop the disease but there may be an increased risk for the offspring. It is thought that DNA replication instability in spermatogenesis is the reason for which larger expansions are more likely to be inherited paternally, and may explain 'new mutations' in individuals without a family history (8% of cases), due to expansion of an intermediate allele into the pathogenic range, and 'anticipation', an earlier age of onset from one generation to the next (Walker, 2007).

Fragile X syndrome and fragile X-associated tremor/ataxia syndrome (FXTAS) are X-linked conditions which are an example of how the same gene mutation can cause two different diseases. The full expansion (>200 repeats) of the CGG trinucleotide repeat on the *FMR1* gene causes loss of function. Affected individuals develop fragile X syndrome in childhood, with mental retardation, autism, and hyperactivity, as well as characteristic dysmorphic features. The 'pre-mutation' of the gene (55–100 repeats) results instead in the production of an abnormal protein with gain-of-function toxicity. Adults carrying the pre-mutation may develop premature ovarian failure or FXTAS, characterized by ataxia, parkinsonism, and cognitive decline.

the X chromosome are usually recessive, meaning that only males, who do not have a normal working copy of the gene, are affected. Female carriers tend to remain unaffected, though they may have some mild features due to X-inactivation of the normal copy of the gene. The commonest neurogenetic conditions caused by X-linked recessive genes are Duchenne muscular dystrophy and fragile X syndrome (see Box 12.4).

X-linked dominant conditions, e.g. Rett syndrome, which causes physical and intellectual disability, are rare. Females tend to show a higher prevalence of X-linked dominant disorders because they have more chance of inheriting a mutated X chromosome. Some X-linked dominant disorders are fatal to males, and therefore, only females with these conditions survive.

Y-linked disorders

Y-linked disorders are caused by mutations on the Y chromosome. These conditions may only be transmitted by males to their male offspring and they cannot affect females. They are very rare, given that there are only approximately 200 genes located on the Y chromosome; the commonest involve mutations of the *SRY* gene, which cause gonadal dysgenesis and sex reversal (Mohnach, 2008).

Mitochondrial disorders

Mitochondria are essential double-membrane subcellular organelles, present in all nucleated mammalian cells. Their primary function is to support aerobic respiration and produce cellular ATP by oxidative phosphorylation. Mitochondria contain a compact, double-stranded circular genome, with several hundreds or thousands of copies of the mitochondrial genome present in a single cell (mitochondrial DNA—mtDNA). Human mtDNA contains only 37 genes, which encode 13 polypeptides, all core subunits of respiratory chain complexes I, III, IV, and V, and the RNA necessary for mtDNA translation. Nuclear genes (located on chromosomes) encode the remaining components of oxidative phosphorylation and all the other proteins required for mitochondrial metabolism and maintenance. When all mtDNA molecules within a cell are identical, this is called homoplasmy. When two or more mitochondrial genomes are present within an organism, this is called heteroplasmy (Tuppen, 2010).

Mitochondrial diseases are a clinically heterogenous group of disorders that arise as a result of dysfunction of the mitochondrial respiratory chain. While some mitochondrial disorders only affect a single organ (i.e. the eye in Leber hereditary optic neuropathy), others may involve multiple organs and often present with prominent neurologic and myopathic features. There are some mtDNA mutations that are associated with particular mitochondrial

each child of being affected. For unaffected siblings of an affected individual, there is a 2/3 probability of being a carrier. Examples of autosomal recessive neuropsychiatric disorders include Wilson's disease and phenylketonuria (see Box 12.3).

X-linked disorders

An X-linked gene is located on the X chromosome. Males will have one copy only of each X-linked gene, whereas women will have two. X-linked conditions can never be inherited from father to son.

In women, each cell expresses only one copy of the X chromosome and the other is randomly inactivated. Mutations of genes on

Wilson's disease is an autosomal recessive disorder caused by a mutation in the *ATP7B* gene, encoding a copper-transporting ATPase (Bull et al., 1993). This results in impaired formation of the copper-transporting protein *caeruloplasmin*, with failure of the mechanisms of removal of excess copper by hepatocytes, abnormal transit of copper through the blood-brain barrier, and accumulation in the liver, brain, kidney, and cornea. Major mutations, causing absent or malfunctioning caeruloplasmin, lead to a rare, severe hepatic form of the disease with childhood onset (Merle et al., 2010), while for the more common adult-onset form, there are over 500 possible mutations with poor genotype–phenotype correlations (Bandmann et al., 2015). The clinical picture is characterized by an extrapyramidal disorder, with tremor, parkinsonism, and dystonia, frequent psychiatric features (Zimbrian and Schilsky, 2014), and cognitive decline, mainly affecting executive functions. The diagnosis is generally based on serum and 24-hour urine copper, serum caeruloplasmin, and slit-lamp eye examination looking for Kayser–Fleischer rings (dark staining of the outer margins of the cornea due to copper deposition). Genetic testing for the *ATP7B* gene to identify homozygous mutations confirms the diagnosis.

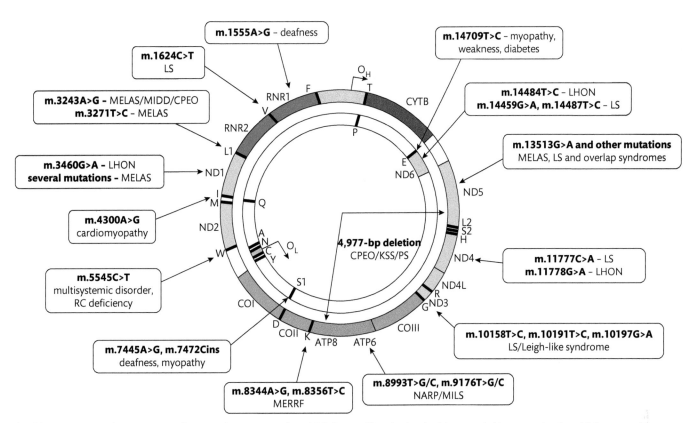

Fig. 12.5 Genotype:phenotype correlations in human mitochondrial disease. The circular double-stranded human mitochondrial genome is depicted with sites of common mtDNA mutations highlighted. Associated clinical presentations are also highlighted. CPEO, chronic progressive external ophthalmoplegia; LHON, Leber's hereditary optic neuropathy; LS, Leigh syndrome; MELAS, mitochondrial myopathy, encephalopathy, lactic acidosis, and stroke-like episodes; MERRF, myoclonic epilepsy and ragged red fibres; MILS, maternally inherited Leigh syndrome; NARP, neurogenic weakness, ataxia, and retinitis pigmentosa; PS, Pearson syndrome.

disorders, but there is considerable clinical variability with an overlapping spectrum of disease phenotypes (see Fig. 12.5).

As mitochondria are under the dual genetic control of both the mitochondrial and nuclear genomes, mutations within either may result in mitochondrial disease. Mitochondrial mutations in genes encoded by nuclear DNA are inherited in an autosomal recessive or autosomal dominant manner. However, mtDNA is almost exclusively maternally inherited in mammals. This means that men with mtDNA disease cannot pass the disorder on to their offspring, but women who carry an mtDNA mutation can transmit mutated mtDNA to their children (see Box 12.5).

Many pathogenic mtDNA mutations are *heteroplasmic*, which means that only a proportion of the mitochondria carry the mutation. The ratio of wild-type to mutant mtDNA determines the onset of clinical symptoms. The percentage of heteroplasmy may be estimated by determining the ratio of mitochondrial mutations in different tissues (e.g. blood lymphocytes, muscle, urine) but may not reflect the level of the mutation in the brain or ovary. During mitosis, mitochondria are randomly segregated, with variation in mtDNA heteroplasmy also occurring during oogenesis and early embryonic development (Tuppen, 2010). These features of mitochondria contribute to the variability in phenotype and clinical symptoms within families.

Box 12.5 Epilepsy in mitochondrial disorders

Mitochondrial disorders should be suspected in patients presenting with multi-organ involvement, as well as neurological abnormalities, and a suggestion of maternal inheritance. The neurological symptoms are very variable, ranging from epilepsy to headaches, stroke-like episodes, and ataxia; cognitive impairment and psychiatric features are very common (Finsterer, 2012). Epilepsy is a frequent feature because defects of the mitochondrial respiratory chain result in decreased intracellular ATP levels, deficits of the sodium–potassium ATPase activity, and increased neuronal excitability with epileptogenic effect (Kunz, 2002). Myoclonic epilepsy with ragged red fibres (MERRF) and mitochondrial myopathy encephalopathy, lactic acidosis, and stroke-like episodes (MELAS) are two of the clinical syndromes that are relatively more frequent in clinical practice. MERRF is characterized by progressive myoclonic epilepsy, deafness, ataxia, myopathy, and cognitive decline. 'Ragged red fibres' are the histological hallmark, visible on microscopy of tissue from muscle biopsy, using a modified **Gömöri** trichrome stain, and represent muscle fibres with an intracellular accumulation of damaged mitochondria. Patients with MELAS often present with seizures, headaches, and stroke-like episodes, with slowly evolving MRI changes, more often involving the temporal and occipital lobes (Iizuka et al., 2003); diabetes, deafness, and myopathy can also be present.

Box 12.6 Imprinting disorders: Prader–Willi and Angelman syndrome

Angelman syndrome (AS) is characterized by seizures, severe intellectual disability, ataxia, and microcephaly. It is caused by loss of the maternally expressed *UBE3A* gene. Analysis of parent-specific DNA methylation imprints in the 15q11.2-q13 chromosome region detects approximately 80% of individuals with AS, including those with a deletion of the maternal allele, paternal uniparental disomy (two paternally inherited copies of chromosome 15), or an imprinting defect, with 11% having a pathogenic variant in the *UBE3A* gene (Dagli et al., 1998). This is in contrast to Prader–Willi syndrome (PWS), a condition characterized by infantile hypotonia, early childhood obesity, short stature, intellectual disability, and behavioural problems, which is caused by abnormalities of the same 15q11.2-q13.3 chromosome region, but in PWS, it is a deletion of the paternal allele or maternal uniparental disomy or, rarely, an imprinting defect that causes the disease (Driscoll et al., 1998).

Disorders of imprinting

As described earlier, an individual inherits two complete sets of chromosomes, one from their father and one from their mother. Most autosomal genes are expressed from both maternal and paternal alleles. However, approximately 1% of all mammalian genes are imprinted and only show expression from one allele. Expression is determined by the parent of origin, with the second copy being epigenetically silenced. Some genes are exclusively maternally expressed, and others exclusively paternally expressed. Genomic imprints are erased in the germline and reset during egg and sperm formation. Imprinted genes may affect growth, development, and viability and are known to impact on behaviour, language development, vulnerability to alcohol dependency, schizophrenia, and bipolar affective disorder, as well as predisposition to cancer (Butler, 2009). Several imprinting disorders are well characterized (see Box 12.6); however, it is thought that epigenetic regulation and dysfunction of imprinted genes may be associated with vulnerability to several common psychiatric disorders, though the mechanisms underlying this are, as yet, incompletely understood.

Sporadic cases of genetic disease

A single case of an apparently genetic disease may occur sporadically in a family. There are several possible explanations for this, which complicates genetic counselling. Autosomal recessive disorders may often appear as isolated cases in small, unrelated families, but the risk for subsequent children is 25%. The risk to the children of an individual with an autosomal recessive disease is very small, unless that individual has children with a carrier of the same disease. The population carrier frequency for most recessive conditions is low, unless there is a history of consanguinity.

Sporadic instances of dominant disease may represent *de novo* (new) mutations at the time of conception or arise due to germline mosaicism (where only a proportion of the gametes of one parent carry the mutation) and occur in people with no history of the disorder in the family. Sporadic instances of dominant disease may also appear as the first case in a family due to expansion from an intermediate allele into the disease causing an expanded range in triplet repeat disorders. This genetic phenomenon of *anticipation* with lengthening size of triplet repeats from generation to generation

also provides the explanation for juvenile cases of HD and cases of congenital muscular dystrophy. Sporadic instances of a genetic condition in a family may also be explained by non-paternity.

Genomic technologies in single-gene disorders

Karyotyping, FISH, and array CGH techniques are used to identify large-scale genomic variation, usually loss or gain of more than one gene. The resolution of array CGH is occasionally sensitive enough to identify single-gene disorders, such a neurofibromatosis type 1 or Duchenne muscular dystrophy, which can sometimes be due to large intragenic deletions. However, most single-gene disorders are caused by small-scale disease-causing sequence alterations or repeat expansions, which are beyond the resolution of array CGH.

DNA sequencing is the process of determining the order of the nucleotide bases—adenine (A), guanine (G), cytosine (C), and thymine (T)—in a molecule of DNA. Though the structure of DNA was identified in 1953, due to an inability to separate and fragment DNA molecules in a controlled fashion, it was not until 1977 that DNA sequencing became a staple of molecular biology (Sanger et al., 1977).

The Human Genome Project generated a reference sequence of the human genome in 2003. It took 4 years and hundreds of millions of dollars to complete the project. Using next-generation sequencing (NGS), the cost per genome has fallen by the end of 2015, for the first time, to less than $1000, and it now takes only a few days (https://www.genome.gov/27565109/the-cost-of-sequencing-a-human-genome/).

Sanger sequencing

Sanger sequencing (Sanger et al., 1977) utilizes polymerase chain reaction (PCR) technology to denature DNA and attach primers complementary to a known DNA sequence that flanks the regions of interest. DNA polymerase then binds to the primers and starts to incorporate new nucleotides complementary to the template (patient) DNA. In current Sanger sequencing techniques, a proportion of nucleotides (nucleotide triphosphates—NTPs) in the mix are fluorescently labelled (dideoxynucleotide triphosphates, ddNTPs). Each ddNTP is labelled with an adherent fluorescent tag, so that A, G, T, and C can be distinguished from each other. The DNA polymerase randomly incorporates either an NTP or a ddNTP to the growing strand. Incorporation of an NTP will allow the DNA polymerase to add further nucleotides, but when a ddNTP is incorporated, this terminates the DNA strand, resulting in a set of fragments differing in length from each other by a single fluorescent base. The fragments are then separated by size using capillary electrophoresis in a sequencing machine, and the fluorescent bases at the end of each fragment are detected as a coloured peak and can be aligned and compared to a reference sequence (see Fig. 12.6). Current methods can directly sequence only relatively short (300–1000 nucleotides long) DNA fragments in a single reaction and are expensive and time-consuming (Metzker, 2005). However, Sanger sequencing remains the gold standard for identifying mutations and, in most cases, the results from NGS tests are confirmed using Sanger sequencing (Box 12.7).

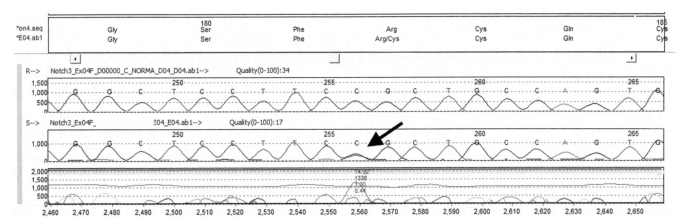

Fig. 12.6 Sanger sequencing. A Sanger sequence chromatograph showing (with arrow) a common heterozygous missense *NOTCH3* mutation c.544C>T, which results in a substitution of arginine to cysteine at amino acid position 182 in exon 4, resulting in CADASIL phenotype (cerebral autosomal dominant arteriopathy with subcortical infarcts and leukoencephalopathy).

Multiplex ligation-dependent probe amplification (MLPA)

Although for most genetic conditions, partial-gene deletions or duplications account for <10% of all disease-causing mutations, for some disorders, it is much higher than this. Sanger sequencing would not detect these, and array CGH may lack the resolution to detect smaller CNVs. MLPA is a low-cost technique for detecting CNV that is often used alongside Sanger sequencing for identifying single-gene disorders (Schouten, 2002). Essentially, MLPA probes, which consist of two oligonucleotide sequences that bridge a target DNA region, are hybridized and ligated to target DNA. Ligation will only occur when both probes are hybridized to their adjacent targets. The ligated probes are then amplified using PCR, and the relative amount of patient probes are compared to a reference to allow identification of CNV.

A variation of the technique—methylation-specific MLPA (MS-MLPA)—is used for both copy number quantification and methylation profiling, and it is a very useful method for the detection of imprinting diseases (Nygren, 2005).

Next-generation sequencing

NGS enables faster, less expensive genomic sequence data, compared to Sanger sequencing. There are a number of different techniques, but the final outcome is that the DNA sequence is generated from thousands of fragmented DNA templates, which are aligned to a reference genome in order to identify differences in the sequenced DNA from the reference (Metzker, 2010) (see Fig. 12.7). There are a number of different NGS platforms, but essentially the steps are: template preparation, sequence, and imaging, followed by data analysis (Bahassi, 2014). Template preparation involves fragmenting DNA to form fragments of 300–500 base pairs. 'Libraries' are then created by attaching oligonucleotides of a known sequence to the ends of the DNA fragments, and these are then amplified in preparation for sequencing. The nucleic acid sequence is obtained by sequencing and imaging from the amplified libraries of short fragments.

Data analysis involves several steps. Initially, sequence data for each of the short reads are aligned to a known reference sequence. Then, sequence analysis of the compiled sequence occurs, using a variety of bioinformatics and data analysis tools.

Whole genome/whole exome sequencing

When an entire genome is being sequenced, the process is called 'whole genome sequencing'. An alternative to whole genome sequencing is the targeted sequencing of part of a genome. Most often, this involves just sequencing the protein-coding regions of a genome—the exons—which correspond to approximately 1.5% of

---

Box 12.7 Examples of mutation types

- *Missense mutation*: a change in one DNA base (A, C, T, or G) that results in the substitution of one amino acid for another in the protein made by a gene.
- *Nonsense mutation*: this is also a change in one DNA base. However, the altered DNA sequence leads to a premature STOP codon (TAG, TAA, TGA). This type of mutation results in a shortened protein that may function improperly or not at all.
- *Insertion*: this changes the number of DNA bases in a gene by adding a piece of DNA. As a result, the protein made by the gene may not function properly.
- *Deletion*: a deletion changes the number of DNA bases by removing a piece of DNA. Small deletions may remove one or a few base pairs within a gene, while larger deletions can remove an entire gene or several genes. The deleted DNA may alter the function of the resulting protein.
- *Indel*: a mutation which involves both removing and inserting a piece of DNA.
- *Duplication*: this consists of a piece of DNA that is abnormally copied one or more times. This type of mutation may alter the function of the resulting protein.
- *Frameshift mutation*: this type of mutation occurs when the addition or loss of DNA bases changes a gene's reading frame. A reading frame consists of groups of three bases that each code for one amino acid. A frameshift mutation shifts the grouping of these bases and changes the code for amino acids. The resulting protein is usually non-functional. Insertions, deletions, and duplications can all be frameshift mutations.
- *Repeat expansion*: nucleotide repeats are short DNA sequences that are repeated a number of times in a row. For example, a trinucleotide repeat is made up of 3-base pair sequences, and a tetranucleotide repeat is made up of 4-base pair sequences. A repeat expansion is a mutation that increases the number of times that the short DNA sequence is repeated. This type of mutation can cause the resulting protein to function improperly.

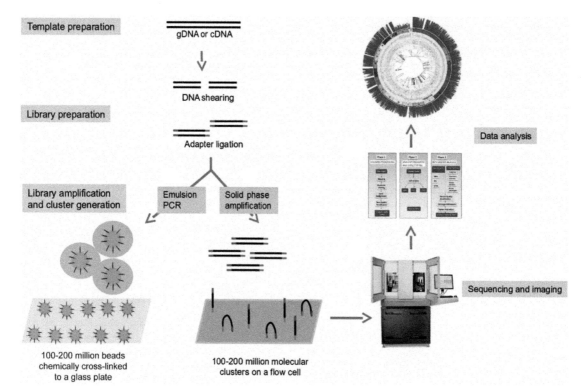

Fig. 12.7 NGS technologies: template preparation, sequencing and imaging, and data analysis. For whole genome sequencing, genomic DNA is sheared by sonication or nebulization to form fragments of 300–500 base pairs. Library amplification can be done by either emulsion PCR (emPCR) or solid-phase amplification. In emPCR (A), a reaction mixture consisting of an oil–aqueous emulsion is created to encapsulate bead–DNA complexes into single aqueous droplets. PCR amplification is performed within these droplets to create beads containing several thousand copies of the same template sequence. emPCR beads can be chemically attached to a glass slide or deposited into PicoTiterPlate wells. Solid-phase amplification (B) is composed of two basic steps: initial priming and extending of the single-stranded, single-molecule template, and bridge amplification of the immobilized template with immediately adjacent primers to form clusters. (C) Sequencing and imaging using one of several platforms. (D) Data analysis using the available software or an integrated workflow.

Reproduced with permission from Bahassi *et al*. Next-Generation sequencing technologies: breaking the sound barrier of human genetics. *Mutagenesis*, 29(5): 303–310. Copyright © 2014, with permission from Oxford University Press on behalf of the UK Enironmental Mutagen Society. https://doi.org/10.1093/mutage/geu031.

the whole genome. At present, this is the best understood part of the human genome, creates less data, and is currently cheaper than whole genome sequencing.

Panel testing

Traditional Sanger sequencing methods screen single or only small groups of genes that are selected, based on a patient's phenotype. Where a patient has a clear phenotype, but multiple genes are implicated in that phenotype, an NGS panel of genes may be more efficient and cost-effective than whole genome or whole exome sequencing, while still allowing effective simultaneous screening of multiple genes in less time than required for several serial Sanger sequencing analyses. In the diagnostic setting, challenges remain as not all areas of each gene on a panel are necessarily covered well using NGS methodology. In addition, deletions or duplications are not always detected, and therefore MLPA or array CGH should be considered, alongside NGS, for genes with high rates of partial deletions or duplications.

Genetic testing for repeat disorders

Repeat disorders can involve expansions of the various repeats in coding and non-coding regions of a gene. Fragile X is caused by a CGG trinucleotide repeat expansion in the 5′ untranslated

region (UTR) of the *FMR1* gene. Friedreich's ataxia is caused by an expansion of an intronic GAA trinucleotide in the *FXN* gene, and HD is caused by a CAG trinucleotide in the first coding exon of the *HTT* gene. Expanded GGGGCC hexanucleotide repeats in the *C9orf72* gene are associated with a number of different neurogenetic phenotypes (see Box 12.8). It is important to appreciate that neither Sanger sequencing nor current NGS technologies are accurate methods for detecting repeat sequence expansions and that specific techniques, such as triplet repeat primed PCR, Southern blotting, methylation status, or immunoassays, may be required.

Applications of genomic technology in clinical neuropsychiatry

Management of the patient

Utility of diagnostic testing

Psychiatric diagnoses are generally based on operational criteria, i.e. on the recognition of a group of symptoms that identify a syndrome, rather than on biological tests. This presents a challenge in the field of neuropsychiatry where cases are often complex and may have come to the attention of the neuropsychiatrist, having posed a

Box 12.8 *C9orf72*—one gene, many diseases

The discovery that a hexanucleotide expansion (GGGGCC) in the first intron of chromosome 9 open reading frame 72 (C9orf72) is the commonest cause of frontotemporal dementia (FTD), familial amyotrophic lateral sclerosis (ALS), and 5–20% of cases of sporadic ALSL (Dejesus-Hernandez et al., 2011; Renton et al., 2011) has had a major impact on the understanding of these two devastating diseases, with immediate repercussions on clinical practice. The neurotoxic effects of the mutation are thought to be related to three different mechanisms: loss of function of C9orf72, a protein with a putative role in cellular trafficking, gain of function due to toxic RNA, and accumulation of dipeptide repeat proteins encoded by the nucleotide repeat expansion (Haeusler et al., 2016). Genetic testing for the mutation is now commonly adopted in the diagnostic work-up of FTD, and there is awareness of increased cognitive and behavioural problems in ALS patients carrying the mutation (Rohrer et al., 2015), in a condition traditionally seen as an essentially motor disease. C9orf72 expansions are also the commonest cause of HD phenocopies (Hensman et al., 2013), and screening for this mutation has been incorporated in the clinical algorithm for the diagnostic assessment of 'HD look-alike' patients.

diagnostic conundrum to others. Genetic testing can, at times, resolve a diagnostic impasse and may be requested by neuropsychiatrists or neurologists as part of a range of investigations addressing a differential diagnosis. Clarifying the diagnosis may have immediate consequences on pharmacological treatment choices, avoiding unnecessary medications and unwanted side effects. In addition, the clinician may be able to give a more accurate prognosis and likely course of illness. This enables patients to make informed decisions on their care, including life and career choices, and arranging advance directives or lasting power of attorney. Generally, patients and their carers value a definitive diagnosis, as this often ends periods of uncertainty and fear, allowing them to move on to the next phase of adjustment and, very importantly, providing the possibility of meeting others who are experiencing the same condition and may be able to offer peer support.

There are several conditions in which identification of the disease through genetic testing is crucial, as the timely introduction of treatment can alter significantly the clinical course or even be lifesaving. For example, episodic ataxia type 2, caused by mutations in *CACNA1A*, is associated with episodic vertigo and ataxic symptoms lasting up to several hours, which are often elicited by stress, physical activity, or alcohol. Acetazolamide and the potassium channel blocker 4-aminopyridine are known to be beneficial in reducing the number and duration of attacks (Kalla et al., 2016). In Wilson's disease, early introduction of a low-copper diet and treatment with copper chelators and zinc salts (the former facilitating copper excretion, and the latter reducing copper accumulation in tissues) can prevent irreversible liver and brain damage and ultimately have lifesaving effects (Bandmann et al., 2015).

Choosing the right test

In terms of clinical decision-making, it is important to balance the costs of genomic testing with the likelihood and utility of obtaining a diagnosis. When the clinical presentation is strongly suggestive of a specific disease, single-gene or panel testing may be appropriate.

As discussed previously, if the presenting phenotype is less clear, gene panels are available for some genetically heterogenous conditions such as Parkinson's disease (see Box 12.9). Whole exome sequencing is currently available in clinical practice where a genetic disorder is suspected, but the phenotype may not be clear or testing for known disease genes for a particular phenotype may not be routinely available. A National Genomic Test Directory now specifies which genomic tests are commissioned by the NHS in England, the technology by which they are available, and the patients who will be eligible to access a test (https://www.england.nhs.uk/publication/national-genomic-test-directories/).

Box 12.9 Several genes, one disease?

Parkinson's disease (PD) is a very common neurodegenerative disorder, clinically defined by the presence of tremor, rigidity, bradykinesia, and postural instability. Cognitive and psychiatric problems almost inevitably occur during the course of the illness, with up to 80% of patients developing dementia. The pathological hallmarks of the disease are loss of dopaminergic neurones in the substantia nigra and the midbrain, and accumulation of intracellular inclusions of α-synuclein, called Lewy bodies. Despite being first described by James Parkinson in 1817 (Goetz, 2011), the aetiology of PD is yet to be fully understood. While the majority of cases are sporadic, i.e. likely to be caused by a combination of predisposing genes and environmental factors, 5–10% of cases are hereditary. Several genes have been identified, causing disease with autosomal dominant or recessive inheritance, or representing risk factors without being directly causative (Kalinderi et al., 2016). In general, early-onset PD (i.e. before the age of 40) is likely to be caused by autosomal recessive mutations, while autosomal dominant mutations tend to cause later-onset disease. The first autosomal dominant mutation to be discovered was in the gene encoding α-synuclein (*SNCA*, *PARK1*). Patients with α-synuclein mutations tend to have a more aggressive clinical course, but these mutations, perhaps surprisingly, are not common. The commonest cause of autosomal dominant PD are instead mutations in the *LRRK2* (leucine-rich repeat kinase 2) gene, resulting in a phenotype resembling the classic late-onset disease, but with less cognitive impairment. All mutations linked to PD phenotypes have been named PARK in numerical succession (*PARK1*, *PARK2*, etc.). The great majority of early-onset cases are caused by mutations in the *Parkin* gene (*PARK2*). The phenotype is generally benign, with slow progression and without dementia, but with psychiatric/behavioural symptoms in over 50% of cases (Kahn et al., 2003). Other genes associated with early-onset PD are *PINK1* and *DJ-1*, both producing similar clinical features to the Parkin phenotype, but with a higher incidence of psychiatric symptoms and dementia. Among the susceptibility genes increasing the risk of developing the sporadic disease, an interesting example is the mutation in the glucocerebrosidase gene (*GBA*), which, in homozygous individuals, causes Gaucher's disease, a recessive lysosomal storage disorder, while heterozygous carriers have a significantly higher risk of developing a form of PD (Lesage et al., 2011), with a higher incidence of dementia (Seto-Salvia et al., 2012).

A pressing question is: do these different phenotypes really represent the same illness? For example, the *Parkin* mutation causes a disease with absence of Lewy bodies, which are a classic pathological hallmark of PD. It is important, in particular for future treatments, to identify the final common pathway by which different gene mutations can lead to similar clinical phenotypes. This is a work in progress. Current theories under exploration involve faults in the autophagy–lysosomal system and inadequate removal of dysfunctional mitochondria, very important for dopaminergic neurones that are cells with high energy expenditure (Kalinderi et al., 2016).

Interpreting the results of genetic testing

The results from diagnostic genetic testing may be 'yes—pathogenic genetic mutation identified' or 'no—genetic mutation not identified'. However, interpretation of results is often not quite as straightforward as this, in particular in the interpretation of less targeted genetic testing (i.e. whole genome or whole exome sequencing). Interpretation of the results often requires close collaboration between clinician and geneticists but can yield precious information, at times revealing new mutations and opening up previously unexplored therapeutic possibilities.

If a mutation is identified, it is important for the clinicians to consider if it is in keeping with the features seen in their patient. In addition, is there any doubt about the pathogenicity of the mutation? Is this an 'intermediate allele' or a 'variant of unknown significance', and are any further family studies or other investigations warranted to investigate causality? If a mutation has not been identified, particularly for genetically heterogenous disorders, it is important to consider which genes have been tested and how comprehensively. Does a negative result, given the testing that has been carried out, exclude a genetic cause or perhaps simply reduce the possibility, given that all known disease-associated genes may not have been tested?

Counselling prior to diagnostic genetic testing

Genetic diagnosis has consequences not only for the individual patient, but also for other family members, and once the implications have been fully absorbed, it may cause distress for both the immediate and extended family. Careful attention to timing and the needs of the family can maximize the potential therapeutic value of the diagnostic testing process, and guidelines for diagnostic genetic testing in HD are relevant to other genetic disorders with neuropsychiatric features (Craufurd et al., 2015). In cases where diagnostic genetic testing is being considered, it is best practice to inform both the patient and immediate relatives about the hereditary nature of the disease before carrying out the test. If the diagnosis is confirmed, the clinician must recognize the needs of the entire family, as well as the individual patient, and ensure that family members can access appropriate genetic counselling services.

Management of the family

Presymptomatic genetic testing

Predictive testing is available to 'at-risk' family members for a number of conditions where diagnostic testing in a relative has revealed a genetic cause for their symptoms. The decision regarding presymptomatic testing for incurable, adult-onset neurodegenerative disease is a complex and personal one and best considered following specialist genetic counselling. Historically, up to 85% of individuals in the UK have chosen not to have predictive testing for HD (Harper et al., 2000), and this proportion is likely to be similar, if not greater, for other adult-onset neurodegenerative disorders. Recommendations for genetic counselling prior to predictive testing for HD have been developed, which also apply to other late-onset neurodegenerative diseases such as familial frontotemporal dementia and spinocerebellar ataxia (International Huntington Association, World Federation of Neurology, 1994; MacLeod et al., 2013).

Family planning

Once a genetic diagnosis has been confirmed in an individual or family, this presents opportunities for family planning, which should be discussed in the context of genetic counselling. If a couple wishes to have children, genetic family planning options are available. These include prenatal testing (via chorionic villus sampling) and pre-implantation genetic diagnosis (PGD). These techniques are not without risk and are not always effective, and emotional impact should not be underestimated. In practice, many couples choose not to intervene.

Research opportunities

Where a diagnosis is not made through routine genetic investigations, research studies, such as The 100,000 Genomes Project (http://www.genomicsengland.co.uk/the-100000-genomes-project/), may provide an additional avenue for pursuing a genetic diagnosis.

Where a genetic diagnosis of a rare disorder has been made, opportunities to participate in observational or clinical research can be helpful for patients and their families, especially for those for have had predictive testing but remain asymptomatic. These studies advance scientific knowledge of the natural history of these rare monogenic conditions and increase the likelihood of potential therapeutic interventions. Since the discovery of the genetic basis for HD, for example, it is hoped that reducing the levels of the mutant huntingtin protein will slow or halt disease progression. Animal studies of antisense oligonucleotide and small RNAs have been promising, and human studies are in progress (Aronin and DiFiglia, 2014).

Emerging applications of genomic technology

Pharmacogenomics

On 30 January 2015, the President of the United States Barack Obama launched the *Precision Medicine Initiative*, calling experts from all fields of science to unite their efforts towards the achievement of treatments tailored to individual patients, as opposed to the current 'one-size-fits-all approach' (http://www.whitehouse.gov/precision-medicine) (for more on precision medicine, see Jameson and Longo, 2015). Pharmacogenomics aims to identify the genetic factors behind inter-individual variations in drug efficacy and tolerability, taking into account biological complexity and clinical heterogeneity. Precision medicine is based on the concepts of 'deep phenotyping' and 'genetic stratification' of clinical populations for the study of treatment response.

Neurology and psychiatry are among the areas of major development, together with oncology and cardiovascular medicine. In the United States, the FDA issues pharmacogenomic information on several antidepressants, antipsychotics, and anticonvulsants. Dose adjustments are suggested for patients identified as 'poor metabolizers', based on polymorphisms of the genes that encode the enzyme cytochrome CYP2D6 and CYP2C19. Other genetic markers (HLA-B* 1502, CPS1, and OTC) indicate vulnerability to adverse effects for carbamazepine, phenytoin, and valproic acid (Drodza et al., 2014).

Complex disease genomics

The emergence of NGS technologies providing the ability to measure genetic variation at hundreds of thousands of markers across the genome in a large number of individuals, in the form of genome-wide association studies (GWAS), has begun to transform our understanding of the genomic variants associated with disease. Most genetic variants associated with inherited susceptibility to late-onset neurodegenerative diseases, such as Alzheimer's and Parkinson's disease, are likely to interact with each other (and with non-genetic factors) to modulate susceptibility to disease and disease phenotype. This is probably reflected in the clinical and biological heterogeneity of these disorders. Large post-mortem studies of ageing brains of demented and non-demented subjects have shown that the majority of individuals, including those cognitively intact, presented with a combination of Alzheimer's disease and Lewy body pathology, and vascular disease (Huntington, 1872; Kremer et al., 1994; Pla et al., 2014; Ross and Tabrizi, 2011; Sonnen et al., 2011; Walker, 2007) (see Box 12.10). Thus, precision medicine aims to target the pathological processes behind the individual clinical presentation, rather than artificially constructed nosological entities (Chorleton et al. 2016).

This complexity of interaction between genetic and non-genetic factors is mirrored in the more common psychiatric disorders such as schizophrenia, mood disorders, or autistic spectrum disorders.

Box 12.10 Genetics of a very common disease

Alzheimer's disease (AD) affects 40 million individuals in the world (Alzheimer's Disease International, 2015). Its neuropathology is characterized by the extracellular accumulation of amyloid-β (Aβ) plaques and the intracellular accumulation of tau neurofibrillary tangles in the brain (Braak and Braak, 1991). Onset before the age of 65 defines 'early-onset' AD. Although the object of ongoing debate, the dominant theory to explain the neurodegeneration in AD has been the 'amyloid cascade hypothesis', according to which it would be the accumulation of amyloid oligomers in the brain that triggers the neurodegenerative cascade leading to neuronal death and loss of volume (atrophy) (Hardy and Higgins, 1992; Hyman, 2012). This hypothesis seems supported by the observation that, to this day, there are only three autosomal dominant genes known to cause familial AD, all involved in the production of amyloid: presenilin1 (PSEN1), presenilin 2 (PSEN2), and amyloid precursor protein (APP). Nevertheless, APP, PSEN1, and PSEN2 only account for about 5–10% of cases of autosomal dominant AD, while the majority of cases remain unexplained (Cacace, 2016).

For the vast majority of people with AD, inheritance is complex. More than 20 risk variants have been identified through GWAS. This has revealed several other genes that have variants linked to increased or decreased risk of AD. These genes include CLU, CR1, PICALM, BIN1, ABCA7, MS4A, CD33, EPHA1, and CD2AP. These are thought to have roles in inflammation and immunity, fat metabolism, or transport within cells (Schu, 2012). The variants of these genes affect a person's risk of developing AD much less than APOE. Researchers suspect that there are many more risk genes that have not yet been discovered.

The gene with the greatest contribution is APOE. APOE has three alleles: APOE ε2, APOE ε3, and APOE ε4. APOE ε4 is associated with a higher risk of AD. Approximately 25% of the population carries one copy of the APOE ε4 allele, and the presence of this allele could as much as double the lifetime risk of AD. Approximately 2% of the population has two copies of the APOE ε4 allele, and this could increase the lifetime risk of AD by up to five times. There is some suggestion that the APOE ε2 allele may lower the risk of AD (Van Giau, 2015).

Genetic testing for risk alleles is not currently widely available or recommended by health professionals, due to the complexity of interpreting multiple risk variants in conjunction with environmental risk factors. However, the identification of genetic factors associated with increased or decreased risk of developing common disease has helped to elucidate pathways important in the neurodegenerative process.

These are all highly aetiologically complex disorders. In schizophrenia, for example, studies have found large numbers of variants that each have a small effect on disease risk—a recent primary GWAS of 34,241 individuals with schizophrenia and 45,604 controls revealed 108 associations (Schizophrenia Working Group of the Psychiatric Genomics Consortium, 2014), but these loci collectively explain only 3% of the variance of schizophrenia. On the positive side, even variants with small effect sizes may provide clues to the underlying biological processes that lead to disease and potentially provide novel therapeutic targets, although this is limited by technological developments and understanding of gene regulation. Recent technological advances, such as the CRISPR–Cas9 genome editing system, are already improving our ability to unravel the biology of GWAS associations.

Another feature common to many psychiatric disorders is the marked pleiotropy, which means that the same genetic risk variants are shared by several diseases. For example, the genetic risk factors for schizophrenia, bipolar disorder, major depressive disorder, ADHD, and autistic spectrum disorders overlap in various degrees (Cross-Disorder Group of the Psychiatric Genomics, 2013). This, again, raises the issue of the validity of psychiatric categorical diagnoses that have proven, over the years, of solid descriptive reliability but have been perhaps less useful as therapeutic targets.

Conclusion

Advances in genomic technology have already heralded the identification of a number of highly penetrant genes for rare inherited forms of neuropsychiatric disorders. These rare disease genes have also provided important insights into the mechanisms of more common psychiatric diseases such as schizophrenia or primary mood disorders.

Despite recent technological advances and an increase in knowledge of the underlying genetic mechanisms, routine genetic testing in common psychiatric diseases is unlikely to be useful in day-to-day clinical practice for risk determination and family studies for several years to come. However, the increased knowledge of the underlying biological mechanisms is likely to yield in the near future new therapeutic targets and a more personalized and successful approach to the treatment of psychiatric disease.

KEY LEARNING POINTS

- It is important for clinicians to have a basic understanding of the main patterns of genetic inheritance and genomic technologies in neuropsychiatric disease to aid clinical practice and assist diagnosis.
- The lower cost and rapid execution times of NGS make it a tool that can be now used routinely for diagnosis, but the interpretation of findings can prove challenging.
- Early discussion with clinical genetics colleagues for cases with a likely genetic component can be helpful to direct diagnostic investigations and interpretation of results.
- Genetic counselling should be offered to all families at risk of genetic disease.

REFERENCES

Alzheimer's Disease International. (2015). *World Alzheimer Report 2015. The Global Impact of Dementia: An Analysis of Prevalence, Incidence, Cost and Trends*. Alzheimer's Disease International, London.

Aronin, N., DiFiglia, M. (2014). Huntingtin-lowering strategies in Huntington's disease: antisense oligonucleotides, small RNAs and gene editing. *Movement Disorders*, **29**, 1455–61.

Bahassi, el M., Stambrook, P.J. (2014). Next-generation sequencing technologies: breaking the sound barrier of human genetics. *Mutagenesis*, **29**, 303–10.

Bandmann, O., Weiss, K.W., Kaler S.G. (2015). Wilson's disease and other neurological copper disorders. *The Lancet Neurology*, **14**, 103–13.

Barišic, I., Zergollern, L., Mužinic, D., Hitrec, V. (1996). Risk estimates for balanced reciprocal translocation carriers—prenatal diagnosis experience. *Clinical Genetics*, **46**, 145–51.

Braak, H., Braak, E. (1991). Demonstration of amyloid deposits and neurofibrillary changes in whole brain sections. *Brain Pathology*, **1**, 213–16.

Bull, P.C., Thomas, G.R., Rommens, J.M., Forber, J.R., Cox, D.W. (1993). The Wilson's disease gene is a putative copper transporting P-type ATPase similar to the Menkes gene. *Nature Genetics*, **5**, 327–37.

Butler, M.G. (2009). Genomic imprinting disorders in humans: a mini-review. *Journal of Assisted Reproduction and Genetics*, **26**, 477–86.

Cacace, R., Sleegers, K., Van Broeckhoven C. (2016). Molecular genetics of early onset Alzheimers' Disease revisited. *Alzheimer's and Dementia*, **12**, 733–48.

Chorleton, B., Larson, E.B., Quinn, J.F., et al. (2016). Precision medicine: clarity for the complexity of dementia. *American Journal of Pathology*, **186**, 500–6.

Craufurd, D., Macleod, R., Frontali, M., et al.; on behalf of the Working Group on Genetic Counselling and Testing of the European Huntington's Disease Network (EHDN). (2015). Diagnostic genetic testing for Huntington's disease. *Practical Neurology*, **15**, 80–4.

Cross-Disorder Group of the Psychiatric Genomics. (2013). Genetic relationship between five psychiatric disorders estimated from genome-wide SNPs. *Nature Genetics*, **45**, 984–94.

Dagli, A.I., Mueller, J., Williams, C.A. (1998, updated 14 May 2015). Angelman syndrome. In: Pagon RA, Adam MP, Ardinger HH, et al., editors. GeneReviews® [Internet]. Seattle, WA: University of Washington; pp. 1993–2016.

Dejesus-Hernandez, M., et al. (2011). Expanded GGGGCC hexanucleotide repeat in non-coding region of C9orf72 causes chromosome 9p-linked FTD and ALS. *Neuron*, **72**, 245–56.

Driscoll, D.J., Miller, J.L., Schwartz, S., et al. (1998, updated 4 February 2016). Prader-Willi Syndrome. In: Pagon RA, Adam MP, Ardinger HH, et al., editors. GeneReviews® [Internet]. Seattle, WA: University of Washington; pp. 1993–2016.

Drozda, K., Müller, D.J., and Bishop, J.R. (2014). Pharmacogenomic Testing for Neuropsychiatric Drugs: Current Status of Drug Labeling, Guidelines for Using Genetic Information, and Test Options. *Pharmacotherapy*, **34**, 166–84.

Finsterer, J. (2012). Cognitive Dysfunction in mitochondrial disorders. *Acta Neurologica Scandinava*, **126**, 1–11.

Goetz, C.G. (2011). The history of Parkinson's Disease: early clinical descriptions and neurological therapies. *Cold Spring Harbor Perspectives in Medicine*, **1**, a008862.

Haeusler, A.R., Donnelly, C.J., Rothstien, J.D. (2016). The expanding biology of the C9orf72 nucleotide repeat expansion in neurodegenerative disease. *Nature Reviews Neuroscience*, **12**, 383–95.

Hardy, J.A., Higgins, G.A. (1992). Alzheimers' disease: the amyloid cascade hypothesis. *Science*, **256**, 184–5.

Harper, P., Lim C., Craufurd, D.; on behalf of the UK Huntington's Disease Prediction Consortium. (2000). Ten years of presymptomatic testing for Huntington's Disease: the experience of UK Huntington's disease Prediction Consortium. *Journal of Medical Genetics*, **37**, 567–1.

Hensman, D., Poulter, M., Beck, J., Tabrizi, S.J. (2013). C9orf72 expansion are the most common genetic cause of Huntington's disease phenocopies. *Neurology*, **82**, 292–9.

Huntington, G. (1872). 'On Chorea'. *Medical and Surgical Reporter of Philadelphia*, **26**, 317–21.

Hyman, B.T., Phelps, C.H., Beach, T.G., et al. (2012). National Institute on Aging-Alzheimer's Association guidelines for the neuropathologic assessment of Alzheimer's disease. *Alzheimer's and Dementia*, **8**, 1–13.

Iizuka, T., Sakai, F., Kan, S., Suzuki, N. (2003). Slowly progressive spread of the stroke-like lesions in MELAS. *Neurology*, **61**, 1238–44.

International Huntington Association, World Federation of Neurology. (1994). Guidelines for the molecular genetics predictive testing in Huntington's disease. *Journal of Medical Genetics*, **44**, 1533–6.

Jameson, J.L., Longo, D.L. (2015). Precision Medicine—Personalized, Problematic, and Promising, *New England Journal of Medicine*, **372**, 2229–34.

Kahn, N.L., Graham, E., Critchley, P., et al. (2003). Parkin disease: a phenotypic study of a large case series. *Brain*, **126**, 1279–92.

Kalinderi, K., Bostantjopoulou, S., Fidani, L. (2016). The genetic background of Parkinson's disease: current progress and future prospects. *Acta Neurologica Scandinavica*, **134**, 314–26.

Kalla, R., Teufel, J., Fiiel, K., Muth, C., Strupp, M. (2016). Update on the pharmacotherapy of cerebellar and central vestibular disorders. *Journal of Neurology*, **263**, 24–9.

Kirov, G., Rees E., Walters, J.T.R., et al. (2014). The penetrance of copy number variations for schizophrenia and developmental delay. *Biological Psychiatry*, **75**, 378–85.

Kremer, B., Goldberg, P., Andrew, S.E., et al. (1994). A worldwide study of the Huntington's disease mutation. The sensitivity and specificity of measuring CAG repeats. *New England Journal of Medicine*, **330**, 1401–6.

Kunz, W.F. (2002). The role of mitochondria in epileptogenesis. *Current Opinion in Neurology*, **15**, 179–84.

Lesage, S., Anheim, M., Condroyer, C., et al. (2011). Large-scale screening of the Gaucher's disease related glucocerebrosidase gene in Europeans with Parkinsons's disease. *Human Molecular Genetics*, **20**, 202–10.

Macleod, R., Tibben, A., Frontali, M., et al.; and Editorial Committee and Working Group 'Genetic Testing Counselling' of the European Huntington Disease Network (EHDN). (2013). Recommendations for the predictive genetic test in Huntington's disease. *Clinical Genetics*, **83**, 221–31.

Menéndez, M. (2005). Down syndrome, Alzheimer's disease and seizures. *Brain Development*, **27**, 246–52.

Merle, U., Weiss, K.H., Eisenbach, C., Tuma, S., Ferenci, P., Stremmel, W. (2010). Truncating mutations in the Wilson disease gene *ATP7B* are associated with very low serum ceruloplasmin oxidase activity and an early onset of Wilson disease. *BMC Gastroenterology*, **10**, 8.

Metzker, M.L. (2005). Emerging technologies in DNA sequencing. *Genome Research*, **205**, 1767–76.

Metzker, M.L. (2010). Sequencing technologies—the next generation. *Nature Reviews Genetics*, **11**, 31–6.

Mohnach, L., Fechner, P.Y., Keegan, C.E. (2008, updated 2 June 2016). Nonsyndromic disorders of testicular development. In: Pagon RA, Adam MP, Ardinger HH, et al., editors. GeneReviews˚ [Internet]. Seattle, WA: University of Washington; pp. 1993–2016.

Murphy, K.C., Jones, L.A., Owen, M.J. (1999). High rates of schizophrenia in adults with cello-cardio-facial syndrome. *Archives of General Psychiatry*, **56**, 940–5.

Nygren A.O., et al. (2005). Methylation-specific MLPA (MS-MLPA): simultaneous detection of CpG methylation and copy number changes of up to 40 sequences. *Nucleic Acids Research*, **33**, e128.

Pertea, M., Salzberg, S.L. (2010). Between a chicken and a grape: estimating the number of human genes. *Genome Biology*, **11**, 206.

Pla, P., Orvoen, S., Saudou, F., David, D.J., Humbert, S. (2014). Mood disorders in Huntington's disease. *Frontiers of Behavioural Neurosciences*, **8**, 135.

Renton, A.E., et al. (2011). A hexanucleotide repeat expansion in C9orf72 is the cause of chromosome 9p21-linked ALS-FTD. *Neuron*, **72**, 257–68.

Rohrer, J.D., Isaacs, A.M., Mizielinska, S., et al. (2015). C9orf72 expansions in frontotemporal dementia and amyotrophic lateral sclerosis. *The Lancet Neurology*, **14**, 291–301.

Ross, C.A., Tabrizi, S. (2011). Huntington's disease: from molecular pathogenesis to clinical treatment. *The Lancet Neurology*, **10**, 83–98.

Sanger, F., Nicklen, S., Coulson, A.R. (1977). DNA sequencing with chain-terminating inhibitors. *Proceedings of the National Academy of Sciences of the United States of America*, **74**, 15463–7.

Schizophrenia Working Group of the Psychiatric Genomics Consortium. (2014). Biological insights from 108 schizophrenia-associated genetic loci. *Nature*, **511**, 421–7.

Schu, M.C., et al. (2012). The genetics of Alzheimer's disease. Modernizing Concept, Biological Diagnosis and Therapy. *Adv Biol Psychiatry*, **28**, 15–29.

Schouten, J.P. et al. (2002). Relative quantification of 40 nucleic acid sequences by multiplex ligation-dependant probe amplification. *Nucleic Acids Research*, **30**, E57.

Seto-Salvia, N., Pagonabarraga, J., Houlden, H., et al., (2012). Glucocerebrosidase mutations confer a greater risk of dementia during Parkinson's disease course. *Movement Disorders*, **27**, 393–9.

Sonnen, J.A., Santa Cruz, K., Hemmy, L.S., et al. (2011). Ecology of the aging human brain. *Archives of Neurology*, **68**, 1049–56.

Tuppen, H.A.L., Blakely, E.L., Turnbull D.M., Taylor, R.W. (2010). Mitochondrial DNA mutations and human disease. *Biochimica and Biophysica Acta*, **1797**, 113–28.

Van Giau, V., Bagyinszky, E., An, S.S.A., Kim, S.Y. (2015). Role of apolipoprotein E in neurodegenerative diseases. *Neuropsychiatric Disease and Treatment*, **11**, 1723–37.

Walker, F.O. (2007). Huntington's disease. *The Lancet*, **369**, 218–28.

Zimbrian, P.C., Schilsky M.L. (2014). Psychiatric aspects of Wilson's disease: a review, *General Hospital Psychiatry*, **36**, 53–62.

13

Neuropsychiatry curriculum and key clinical competencies

Perminder S. Sachdev and Adith Mohan

Introduction

Inexorable and welcome advances in neuroscience in the last three decades are resulting in the greater underpinnings of psychiatry by neuroscience and its closer rapprochement with neurology. Since neuropsychiatry (NP), in its broader conceptualization, entails the application of the principles of neuroscience to the understanding and treatment of emotional, behavioural, and cognitive disorders, one could question the need for a subdiscipline of NP. Indeed, all of psychiatry, and much of neurology, could be regarded as NP. In practice, however, the future of the disciplines of psychiatry and neurology as distinct disciplines appears secure and they are unlikely to be subsumed under one super-discipline of NP. This is not simply the consequence of historical tradition, but the fact that psychiatry and neurology require distinct skill sets and have vastly different demands placed upon them (Sachdev, 2005).

The strengths of psychiatry are manifold and range from the rich description of its mental phenomena (phenomenology), well-developed interviewing skills, understanding of multiple causations (behavioural, biological, and psychological), accounting for individual variation, dealing with ambiguity, the interpersonal context, and the skill to combine biological with psychological and behavioural treatments. Equally, neurology excels in its rigorous clinical examination skills, empiricism, and objectivity. The training experiences necessary for both disciplines are distinct, and an amalgamation of the two runs the risk of diluting both.

In practice, there is a set of conditions and disorders that traverse the two traditional disciplines and require a combined set of skills and experiences. These have come to define the territory of NP as a broader discipline with its own history and prevailing zeitgeist (Price et al., 2000). Here, one can distinguish between neuropsychiatric 'territory' and the neuropsychiatric 'approach', although the need for the latter influences the former. As an example, the management of Tourette syndrome requires an understanding of movement disorders, as well as obsessive–compulsive disorder, attention-deficit disorder, conduct disorder, mood disorders, specific developmental disabilities, and sleep disorder, as well as skills in pharmacotherapy, behaviour therapy, family therapy, genetic counselling, and rehabilitation. A skilled neuropsychiatrist is capable of managing such a case arguably far better than a combination of clinicians from different disciplines. The neuropsychiatrist brings individual skills of psychiatry and neurology, combined with expertise in neuroimaging, neuropsychology, and neurophysiology, to bear upon the condition in question, thereby demonstrating the neuropsychiatric approach (Sachdev, 2002).

The discipline of NP needs consideration in relation to behavioural neurology (BN). In many respects, NP and BN are two slightly different approaches to the same set of disorders and conditions—the former is biased towards a traditional psychiatric approach, and the latter has its route through neurology (Marsel Mesulam, 2000). The core competencies are similar, with perhaps differences in emphasis. The United Council for Neurologic Subspecialties (UCNS) of the United States has a common core curriculum for BN and NP (https://www.ucns.org/Online/Accreditation/Program_Requirements.aspx), a position that we support. This chapter concerns a curriculum for NP; an effort will, however, be made to identify specific areas that are particularly important to BN, so that the curriculum can be readily adapted to BN.

Currently, there are few training programmes worldwide that are exclusive to NP and lead to a specific NP specialist accreditation. In most countries, trainees who gain experience in NP do so within general adult psychiatry, old age psychiatry, child psychiatry, or forensic psychiatry. This is true even for countries in which a number of NP specialist positions exist. Some countries, in particular the United States, have provision for dual training in neurology and psychiatry, with certification in both disciplines. While this approach meets some of the requirements of training in NP, it is important to appreciate that this may not be enough for competence in NP, as training separately in the two disciplines could skirt the core business of NP, and a period of training in NP per se is essential. This period of NP training is often set at a minimum of 1 year, but a 2-year period should be recommended, considering the wide range of experiences necessary to produce a well-rounded neuropsychiatrist (see Fig. 13.1).

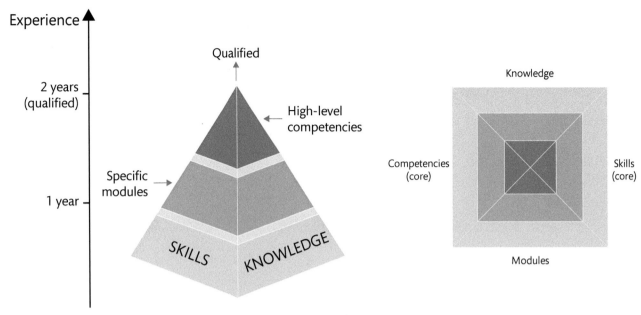

Fig. 13.1 The neuropsychiatry training pyramid shows how to produce a qualified, well-rounded neuropsychiatrist.

Goals of an NP training programme

The purpose of a training programme in NP is to produce specialists who are competent in the diagnosis and management of neuropsychiatric disorders. For this, they will need a sound knowledge in neuroscience, in particular neuroanatomy, neurophysiology, neurochemistry, and neuropharmacology. They will have expertise in the use of specialized neuropsychiatric investigations (such as neuroimaging—both structural and functional; neurophysiology, in particular EEG; and neuropsychology). They will need to be competent in the recognition and management of common psychiatric and neurologic disorders, with further exposure to disorders that are regarded as neuropsychiatric (see later). They will have developed specialized skills in physical treatments in NP, without ignoring the principles of psychotherapeutic and rehabilitative approaches. As a result, they will be able to provide secondary- and tertiary-level consultations to general physicians, psychiatrists, and neurologists. A neuropsychiatrist will also combine academic pursuit with clinical work and therefore will be able to critically evaluate research evidence and be actively involved in the advancement of empirical knowledge in this field. Due to their specialized role, neuropsychiatrists must also train to be good teachers and mentors to advance the discipline into the future.

Structure of an NP training programme

With these goals in mind, there is no one model that suits all training programmes in NP. However, it is important to recognize and incorporate the basic tenets of an ideal programme that will train specialists who will be able to provide secondary and tertiary level of care (service) and education. In most instances, NP training will begin with basic training in psychiatry for a period of about 3 years and in neurology for about a year. This could be reversed, with primary training being in neurology and BN specialization in

perspective. What is important is that the first 4 years of training include substantive periods in both psychiatry and neurology, with the longer period being in the specialty of primary affiliation, as would be required by training Colleges or Boards or by regulatory agencies.

This would be followed by a period of training, generally for 2 years, in NP, as an advanced trainee or a Fellow. Such training should only occur in a tertiary training centre, staffed by at least two or more neuropsychiatrists and one or more clinical neuropsychologists, with close working relationships with general psychiatric, clinical neurology, and neurosurgical services. Many NP training centres also have a behavioural neurologist as a staff member. The NP training centre would, in consequence, usually be part of a general teaching hospital and have easy access to a neurophysiology service and up-to-date neuroimaging to include structural MRI and functional imaging. It should also have a research programme and the facilities necessary for an educational institution such as a modern library and research infrastructure (Sachdev, 2010).

The training programme should have, as its primary focus, assessment, diagnosis, and treatment of neuropsychiatric disorders from a broad perspective. The training is usually in an apprenticeship style, with some didactic work. There is generally a continuous evaluation process, based on several formal assessments and/or a series of informal assessments by the supervisors. A project, based on original research or systematic reviews, should form part of this training to prepare the trainee for a lifelong period of education and professional enhancement. In a rapidly advancing field, this lifelong commitment is critical, and preparation for this should begin in the early years of training. It is important that all of this occurs in a setting of the highest ethical standards of conduct in clinical practice and scholarly work.

Different models for training are found internationally. In the United Kingdom and Australia, training in NP follows the apprenticeship model, adopting key elements of the neuropsychiatric curriculum such as that proposed by the International

Neuropsychiatric Association (INA) (Sachdev, 2010). In this model, trainees seek to obtain clinical experience in a range of settings that include memory clinics, movement disorder clinics, and tertiary (liaison) consultation in the general hospital and epilepsy services, among others, through clinical placements within each of these services. Research projects and academic writing are undertaken contemporaneously, with peer-reviewed publication being encouraged. A typical period of training in this model would span 24 months (and possibly more), with a large proportion of this being spent in a specialist NP centre that offers supervision and service access, as set out earlier. In the United States, on the other hand, 32 accredited Fellowship Programs across the country offer a structured 2-year clinical and research experience, following a prescribed curriculum, with a certification examination at the end prior to the Fellowship being awarded. Individual programmes require accreditation by the UCNS, ensuring standardized delivery of clinical teaching and supervision.

Specific aims

A training programme is designed to develop high-level skills on a sound knowledge base. The training should also foster an attitude of care and advocacy for neuropsychiatric patients.

Understanding disability (attitudinal)

Neuropsychiatric disorders produce great disability in sufferers and can be a burden on carers and supporters (Global Burden of Disease Study 2013 Collaborators, 2015). This is compounded by the relative lack of appropriately targeted services in most places and the social stigma still prevalent in many societies. It is incumbent on the trainee in NP to be aware of this and to become an advocate for the needs of neuropsychiatric patients and their carers. The attitudinal objectives therefore relate to interactions with the patient, their supporters, the health system, and society in general, with the needs of the patient being paramount in all the determinations (Benjamin et al., 2014).

Foundations of knowledge

NP is based on a rapidly expanding corpus of empirical neuroscience, keeping up with which poses major challenges. There is, however, a basic body of neuroscientific knowledge that the trainee needs to master to enable competent clinical practice.

Basic neuroscience

This begins with knowledge of the brain structure and organization at the macroscopic and microscopic levels, in particular an understanding of neuronal networks, the limbic system, the neuroanatomical substrates of cognition, and the brain's structure–function relationships. It is important to have a sound understanding of neurotransmitter and receptor function, which provide the biochemical basis of neuropsychopharmacology. Knowledge of brain development and the drivers of neuronal migration and organization provide a lifespan context for the later development of neuropsychiatric disorders. The basic principles of neurophysiology should be studied as they apply to the diagnosis and assessment of neuropsychiatric disorders. The same applies to the principles of neuroimaging, both structural and functional, with an emphasis on

MRI and PET. With rapid advances in neurogenetics, a good understanding of the basic principles of genetics is important. Trainees may anchor their study to a basic textbook of neuroscience (Kandel et al., 2012; Squire et al., 2012).

Applied neuroscience

The neuroscientific basis of investigations and treatments in NP deserves particular attention. A basic understanding of EEG and event-related potentials (ERPs) is necessary for their appropriate application in assessment. A neuropsychiatrist must understand how the principles of neuroimaging apply to structural imaging using CT and MRI, and functional imaging using fMRI, PET, SPECT, quantitative EEG, and MEG. The principles of ECT and the emerging brain stimulation technologies—transcranial magnetic stimulation (TMS), transcranial direct current stimulation (tDCS), vagus nerve stimulation (VNS), and deep brain simulation (DBS), among others—must be understood (Reti, 2015). Other developments in relation to neurofeedback, brain–computer interface, and virtual reality may be of interest. Since NP is at the forefront of other physical treatments, keeping abreast of the scientific basis of new drug treatments and novel approaches to treating mental disorders is important. Notable examples include the use of ketamine in depression (Katalinic et al., 2013) and the focus on targeting inflammatory and neuroimmune pathways in psychosis and mood disorders (Miller et al., 2016).

Neuropsychology and cognitive neuroscience

Neuropsychology is a distinct discipline within NP, and a thorough knowledge of the principles of neuropsychology are critical for neuropsychiatric practice. Neuropsychology examines the brain basis of mental phenomena, in particular cognition (Lezak et al., 2012). Recent years have seen the emergence of the related discipline of cognitive neuroscience, which studies the biological principles underlying cognition and includes cognitive psychology, computational modelling, and behavioural genetics (Gazzaniga et al., 2002). Neuropsychiatrists collaborate closely with neuropsychologists in diagnosis and treatment, requiring that a basic training in neuropsychology should be embedded in any neuropsychiatric curriculum.

The brain–mind relationship

A basic grasp of issues related to the mind–brain debate, the biology of consciousness, and other neurophilosophical issues is important for helping the neuropsychiatrist bridge the gulf between psychiatry and neurology (Bickle, 2013). It falls to the neuropsychiatrist, for instance, to provide a balanced view on contemporary neuroethical debates surrounding brain stimulation and the augmented self, authenticity, and alienation of self-experience (Kraemer, 2013).

Neuropsychiatric disorders

By completion of training, neuropsychiatry trainees should be knowledgeable about the epidemiology, aetiology, psychopathology, clinical features (including complications), and the natural history of a range of neuropsychiatric disorders, including concepts of impairment, disability, and handicap. A sound knowledge of the assessment and care of these conditions is also required. Particular attention is to be paid to atypical presentations of illness such as psychosis, 'pseudodementia', 'masked' depression, 'conversion' disorders, and behavioural disorders.

While it is difficult to fully delineate the territory of neuropsychiatric disorders, the following disorders are likely to be assessed and managed by neuropsychiatrists: neurocognitive disorders, including the dementias and pre-dementia syndromes; delirium and related syndromes; disorders of arousal (coma, persistent vegetative state, catatonia), seizure disorders, especially in relation to their psychiatric and behavioural aspects, and non-epileptic seizures; movement disorders, especially drug-induced movement disorders (tardive dyskinesia, akathisia, parkinsonian side effects, and neuroleptic malignant syndrome); psychiatric aspects of movement disorders such as Parkinson's disease, Huntington's disease, and dystonia; psychogenic movement disorders; psychiatric aspects of traumatic brain injury; secondary psychiatric disorders, i.e. psychosis, depression, mania, and anxiety disorders secondary to 'organic' brain disease; substance-related psychiatric disorders—alcohol, drugs of abuse, etc.; attentional disorders (adult ADHD and related syndromes); tic disorders, including Tourette syndrome; neurodevelopmental disorders; and psychiatric aspects of sleep disorders (David et al., 2012; Yudofsky et al., 2007).

Appropriate management plans for neuropsychiatric disorders include the interpretation of medical, psychological, and neurodiagnostic investigations and assessments; expert use of psychopharmacology (Stahl, 2013), ECT, and other physical treatments (in particular, novel brain stimulation therapies such as repetitive TMS, tDCS, VNS, DBS), including the frequency and management of side effects (Hamani et al., 2016); application of psychotherapies, including supportive, cognitive behavioural, and group and family therapies as they relate to neuropsychiatric patients; use of behaviour modification, environmental adaptation, and preventive measures; situations in which referral to, or consultation with, colleagues in psychiatry and other disciplines is appropriate; programmes involving changes in lifestyle; rehabilitation programmes; management in forensic settings; and strategies that meet the needs of carers, including the role of self-help groups such as Alzheimer's Association, Tourette Syndrome Association, and other consumer organizations.

The neuropsychiatrist should understand the influence of specific factors on diagnosis, treatment, and care of neuropsychiatric disorders, including age, intellectual capacity (including intellectual disability), medical illness and disability, gender, culture, spiritual beliefs, socio-economic status, psychiatric comorbidity, polypharmacy, and support factors. In their practice, neuropsychiatrists would be expected to give due importance to the evidence base and evaluate the relative cost-effectiveness of any proposed intervention.

Medicine in relation to neuropsychiatry

By completion of training, neuropsychiatry trainees should be knowledgeable about medical and surgical conditions in general. Higher levels of knowledge are expected in those areas of medicine that particularly relate to psychiatric practice such as neurology, neurosurgery, geriatrics, and rehabilitation medicine. The neuropsychiatrist should be familiar with the principles of liaison consultation with medical specialties, in particular the clinical neurosciences. Due to the common occurrence of neuropsychiatric disorders in geriatric patients, issues of ageing, in particular brain ageing, should be part of the curriculum.

Medicolegal context

The medicolegal aspects relevant to the practice of NP, with particular emphasis on mental health and guardianship legislation, including its local application, testamentary capacity, lasting powers of attorney, informed consent, assessment of older offenders, and fitness to plead and stand trial, should form part of the core curricular requirements in NP training (Appelbaum et al., 2006).

Prevention and health promotion in neuropsychiatry

Issues specific to mental health promotion in relation to NP should be addressed. There is increasing evidence that risk factors for neuropsychiatric disorders begin early in life, and the focus of prevention should move to mid life for many of the late-life neuropsychiatric disorders.

Research methods

By completion of training, NP trainees should be knowledgeable about the principles of scientific method in their practice and the use of this knowledge to evaluate developments in neuropsychiatric research. This can be achieved through seminars, journal clubs, targeted courses, personal study, and participation in research. Knowledge of commonly used techniques in biostatistics and data management is crucial.

Service issues

By completion of training, NP trainees should be knowledgeable about the organization and delivery of mental healthcare to neuropsychiatric patients, including the ethical, economic, geographical, and political constraints within which these services operate.

Professional responsibility

By completion of training, NP trainees should be knowledgeable about the principles of medical ethics, the development of professional attitudes, and processes for the development and maintenance of clinical competence, acknowledging the need for professional and public accountability.

Skills required

Assessment of neuropsychiatric patients

By completion of training, trainees should possess the skills necessary for performing a comprehensive neuropsychiatric assessment. They will demonstrate interviewing skills adapted to the needs of neuropsychiatric patients; appropriately use and interpret cognitive tests and document these accurately; perform a competent neurological assessment (Kaufman et al., 2013); appropriately refer people for neuropsychological assessment, interpret the neuropsychological report with expertise, interact with the clinical neuropsychologist in relation to the findings, if necessary, and effectively utilize the results; be adept at using neuroimaging and neurophysiological investigations as part of the assessment; be competent in liaising with expert neuroradiologists, nuclear physicians, and neurophysiologists when appropriate; conduct assessments in a range of hospital and community settings, including assessment of the environmental context of the illness and the socio-cultural determinants of behaviour; perform a functional assessment, including activities of daily living, and apply it to the determination of the most appropriate form of living arrangements for the individual; and recognize and assess relevant features of the family context, including the family's role as carers, carer stress, and elder abuse.

Competent management of neuropsychiatric patients

By completion of training, trainees should have experience in the management of common neuropsychiatric conditions, as listed in Neuropsychiatric disorders (p. 143), in various hospital, outpatient, and community settings. This involves the use of both physical and psychological therapies (Klonoff, 2010), although the expertise should be particularly manifest in the use of physical treatments. The neuropsychiatrist will use a comprehensive treatment approach and involve the family and significant others, where necessary, including liaison with other medical disciplines, as indicated.

Medicolegal assessments

Perform medicolegal assessments, with particular emphasis on testamentary capacity, guardianship, enduring power of attorney, competency, and informed consent. In addition, assessments for brain injury in relation to trauma may be necessary, and the neuropsychiatrist should be familiar with the requirements for providing medicolegal opinions (Rosner, 2003).

Prevention and health promotion

By completion of training, the NP trainee should be able to apply specific knowledge of the principles and processes of health promotion and illness prevention. This may include lifestyle factors, physical exercise, cognitive training, nutrition, control of vascular risk factors, prevention of brain trauma, and control of substance use. They will recognize and address risk factors for common neuropsychiatric problems in the community, hospitals, and long-term care such as falls, confusion, and depression. They will be able to recognize and address the needs of carers of neuropsychiatric patients.

Neurorehabilitation

While neurorehabilitation is a growing specialty in its own right, the neuropsychiatrist should be familiar with its principles and be able to guide the patient towards the best practice and strategies. A number of new techniques are being applied to engage the plastic properties of the brain, and the neuropsychiatrist should attempt to exploit these for the patient (Dietz et al., 2015).

Research project

There is no better way to develop research skills than to engage in an original research project. It is recommended that this should involve the development of a research plan, an ethics approval process, data collection, analysis, and preparation of a dissertation or paper for publication. An alternative is to perform a systematic review. A trainee should aim for a first author publication in a peer-reviewed journal by the end of their training.

Competency

The aims of an NP training programme are to deliver/develop competencies throughout the period of training. Competency is measured at specific points and continuously.

To be certified, the trainee must be assessed throughout the period of the training. The methods of assessment should comprise a combination of validated self-assessment, observed interviews by a supervisor, case presentations, maintenance of a clinical log book, and some formal review of progress. A continuous assessment process, rather than exclusive reliance on an exit examination, is recommended, but this will only be possible if appropriate procedures for evaluation and redress are in place. In Australia, in line with the current competency-based training system in place for trainees in other subdisciplines of psychiatry, a series of formative assessments to evaluate the acquisition of key competencies in NP has been proposed.

Key competencies in neuropsychiatry

The curriculum (with examples as illustrated below) identifies some core competencies in the skill base and specific modules of specialist knowledge base acquired over 2 years. The competencies are described as 'modules', but they are not necessarily independent of each other. The importance of the Core Skills Modules is highlighted. The aims and objectives of this module will normally be covered within the specific clinical modules undertaken but should represent an additional and specific focus of study within the individual clinical modules. The level of expertise in each of the specific modules will vary, depending upon the facilities available, but a basic level of competence in each module is expected in a 2-year training programme. Limitations on space allow only the Core Skills Modules and two Specific Modules to be described (see Appendix 1 for detailed descriptions) as exemplars for other modules.

Example: Core Skills Modules

- Knowledge base in clinical neuroscience.
- Clinical skills in NP:
  - Neuropsychiatric diagnosis, including history and examination, neurophysiological investigations, neuroimaging, neuropsychology, and other investigations.
  - Treatment, including pharmacology and other physical treatments (ECT, repetitive TMS, other brain stimulation techniques, surgical interventions), without neglecting psychotherapeutic and rehabilitative interventions.
- Critical thinking in neuropsychiatry—research and scholarship.

Example: Specific Modules

- Neurocognitive disorders—dementia in the elderly (AD, VaD, DLB, FTD, PDD, HD, CJD, mixed, other), early-onset dementia, mild neurocognitive disorders (including neurodegenerative disorders, infectious disorders, e.g. HIV, TBI, substance-related); focal cognitive disorders (amnesia, aphasia, apraxia, abulia, disinhibition, impulse control disorders, Kluver Bucy syndrome, etc.) (see Appendix 2 for a detailed description).
- General hospital liaison NP (see Appendix 3 for a detailed decription).
- Disorders of arousal (e.g. coma, persistent vegetative state, MCS, etc.).
- Disorders of attention (e.g. delirium, confusion, neglect/visuospatial disturbances).
- Cerebrovascular disease and neuropsychiatric disorders (neurocognitive disorders, depression, other).
- Seizure disorders, epileptic and non-epileptic (psychiatric aspects).

- Movement disorders—drug-induced (tardive dyskinesia, akathisia, parkinsonism, neuroleptic malignant syndrome), psychiatric aspects of other movement disorders (PD, idiopathic dystonia, etc.), tic disorders.
- TBI and its psychiatric consequences.
- Secondary psychiatric disorders, i.e. psychosis, depression, mania, anxiety disorders, and obsessive–compulsive symptoms, and disorders secondary to 'organic' brain disease.
- Substance-related psychiatric disorders—alcohol, drugs of abuse, etc.
- Psychiatric aspects of immunological disorders, including autoimmune encephalitides and chronic fatigue syndrome.
- ADHD and behavioural disorders.
- Sleep disorders, neuropsychiatric aspects.
- Developmental NP (learning disorders, developmental disability, including intellectual handicap, pervasive developmental disorders, and related syndromes).
- Neuropsychiatric rehabilitation.
- Forensic NP.

Conclusion

While the brain basis of mental illness has always been of interest to physicians, the importance of neuroscience in contemporary psychiatry cannot be over-emphasized. There has been a recent push to reconfigure psychiatric disorders on the basis of underlying neuroscientific principles (Insel et al., 2005). Basic neuroscience and the principles of NP should therefore be part of any psychiatric training programme (Benjamin, 2013). The knowledge base upon which to rely is no different from that discussed earlier, except that the depth and breadth will necessarily be limited in a general psychiatry context. It is important that all psychiatry training programmes aim to achieve this training goal and the teachers and training facilities are adequately equipped to do so. Neuropsychiatrists have a central role to play in imparting this knowledge and training and, as such, will be required to develop skills in the teaching, supervision, and assessment of postgraduate trainees. The role of the neuropsychiatrist as an academic and scholar is thus emphasized.

Much progress has been made in the last two decades in uncovering the structural, genetic, and biochemical underpinnings of mental disorders, and the long-enshrined Cartesian mind-body duality is increasingly being rejected in favour of integrated models of formulating mental illness. The opportunities for clinical interactions between general adult psychiatrists and neuropsychiatrists are growing, as is the need for collaboration in the care of patients with epilepsy and psychiatric comorbidities offering a ready example. The general psychiatrist is often called upon by colleagues in neurological specialties to assist in the care if such patients, reflective, in part, of the relative inaccessibility of tertiary NP services and their concentration in centres of excellence within metropolitan settings. Formalized pathways for referral between general psychiatry and NP services need further development, so collaborative care models can be readily implemented (Jethwa et al., 2016).

Taken together, there is a growing recognition of the need for NP services to restructure themselves so as to provide pathways for clinical consultation, as well as contribute to the upskilling of the general psychiatric workforce through joint working and dissemination of research findings with translational potential. The 'hub and spoke' model proposed in the UK, with a tertiary NP service embedded at the centre offering outreach services that combine direct clinical contact with service-level consultation, is an example of the way forward (Agrawal et al., 2008). Indeed, the continuing momentum of neuroscientific discovery with direct relevance to core mental disorders requires such innovation in the development and delivery of NP services, and the neuropsychiatrist is tasked with developing an appreciation of the principles of service development, all the while incorporating the skills and attributes set out in the curriculum described earlier.

KEY LEARNING POINTS

- In many respects, neuropsychiatry (NP) and behavioural neurology (BN) can be seen as two different approaches to the same set of disorders and conditions. The treatment of many conditions, such as Tourette syndrome, requires an understanding of both.
- As such, while this chapter is focused on a curriculum for NP, it also identifies areas of relevance to BN to allow for the curriculum to be adapted to both.
- The goals and structure of an NP training programme are laid out, followed by a more comprehensive discussion of the course's aims and the skills required to complete it, from the assessment and management of neuropsychiatric patients to neurorehabilitation.
- Finally, the key competencies are outlined, with examples drawn from the Core Skills Modules and then modules specific to subspecialties and certain types of disorders which bridge the fields of NP and BN such as neurocognitive disorders, movement disorders, and substance-related psychiatric disorders.

REFERENCES

Agrawal N, Fleminger S, Ring H, Deb S. Neuropsychiatry in the UK: planning the service provision for the 21st century. *Psychiatr Bull* 2008;32:303–6.

Appelbaum PS, Gutheil TG. *Clinical Handbook of Psychiatry and the Law*, fourth edition. Philadelphia, PA: Lippincott Williams & Wilkins; 2006.

Benjamin S. Educating psychiatry residents in neuropsychiatry and neuroscience. *Int Rev Psychiatry* 2013;25:265–75.

Benjamin S, Travis MJ, Cooper JJ, Dickey CC, Reardon CL. Neuropsychiatry and neuroscience education of psychiatry trainees: attitudes and barriers. *Acad Psychiatry* 2014;38:135–40.

Bickle J (ed) *Oxford Handbook of Philosophy and Neuroscience*. New York, NY: Oxford University Press; 2013.

David A, Fleminger S. *Lishman's Organic Psychiatry: A textbook of neuropsychiatry*, fourth edition. Oxford: Blackwell Scientific; 2012.

Dietz V, Ward N (eds). *Oxford Textbook of Neurorehabilitation*. Oxford: Oxford University Press; 2015.

Gazzaniga MS, Ivry RB, Mangun GR. *Cognitive Neuroscience: The Biology of the Mind*, second edition. New York, NY: W.W. Norton; 2002.

Global Burden of Disease Study 2013 Collaborators. Global, regional, and national incidence, prevalence, and years lived with disability for 301 acute and chronic diseases and injuries in 188 countries, 1990–2013: a systematic analysis for the Global Burden of Disease Study 2013. *Lancet* 2015;386:743–800.

Hamani C, Holtzheimer P, Lozano AM, Mayberg H (eds.). *Neuromodulation in Psychiatry*. West Sussex: Wiley-Blackwell; 2016.

Insel TR, Quirion R. Psychiatry as a clinical neuroscience discipline. *JAMA* 2005;294:2221–4.

Jethwa KD, Joseph V, Khosla, Cavanna AE. The interface between general adult psychiatry and behavioural neurology/neuropsychiatry. *BJPsych Advances* 2016;22:127–31.

Kandel ER, Schwartz JH, Jessell TM, Siegelbaum SA, Hudspeth AJ (eds.). *Principles of Neuroscience*, fifth edition. New York, NY: McGraw-Hill; 2012.

Katalinic N, Lai R, Somogyi A, Mitchell PB, Glue P, Loo CK. Ketamine as a new treatment for depression: a review of its efficacy and adverse effects. *Aust N Z J Psychiatry* 2013;47:710–27.

Kaufman DM, Milstein MJ. *Kaufman's Clinical Neurology for Psychiatrists*, seventh edition. New York, NY: Elsevier Saunders; 2013.

Klonoff PS. *Psychotherapy after Brain Injury: Principles and Techniques*. New York, NY: Guilford Press; 2010.

Kraemer F. Me, Myself and My Brain Implant: Deep Brain Stimulation Raises Questions of Personal Authenticity and Alienation. *Neuroethics* 2013;6:483–97.

Lezak MD, Howieson DB, Bigler ED, Tranel D. *Neuropsychological Assessment*, fifth edition. New York, NY: Oxford University Press; 2012.

Marsel Mesulam M (ed) *Principles of Behavioral and Cognitive Neurology*, second edition. New York, NY: Oxford University Press; 2000.

Miller AH, Raison CL. The role of inflammation in depression: from evolutionary imperative to modern treatment target. *Nat Rev Immunol* 2016;16:22–34.

Price BH, Adams RD, Coyle JT. Neurology and psychiatry: closing the great divide. *Neurology* 2000;54:8–14.

Reti I (ed) *Brain Stimulation: Methodologies and Interventions*. New Jersey: Wiley-Blackwell; 2015.

Rosner R (ed) *Principles and Practice of Forensic Psychiatry*. Boca Raton, FL: CRC Press; 2003.

Sachdev P. Neuropsychiatry—a discipline for the future. *J Psychosom Res* 2002;53:625–7.

Sachdev P. Core curriculum in neuropsychiatry of the International Neuropsychiatric Association. In: Miyoshi K, Morimura Y, Maeda K (eds). *Neuropsychiatric Disorders*. Tokyo: Springer Japan; 2010. pp. 317–46.

Sachdev PS. Whither neuropsychiatry? *J Neuropsychiatry Clin Neurosci* 2005;17:140–4.

Squire L, Berg D, Bloom FE, Lac SD, Ghosh A, Spitzer NC (eds). *Fundamental Neuroscience*, fourth edition. Oxford: Academic Press; 2012.

Stahl SM (ed) *Stahl's Essential Psychopharmacology: Neuroscientific Basis and Practical Applications*, fourth edition. New York, NY: Cambridge University Press; 2013.

Yudofsky SC, Hales RE (eds). *Textbook of Neuropsychiatry and Clinical Neurosciences*, fifth edition. Washington DC: American Psychiatric Publishing; 2007.

APPENDIX 13.1
Core skills module

Knowledge base in neuroscience

- Knowledge of the brain structure at the macroscopic and microscopic levels, in particular knowledge of neuronal networks, the limbic system, the neuroanatomical substrates of memory, and the frontal executive system.
- A knowledge of CNS structure–function correlations.
- Knowledge of neurochemistry, especially neurotransmitter and receptor function.
- The biochemical basis of neuropsychopharmacology.
- The basic principles of neurophysiology.
- The basic principles of neuroimaging—structural and functional.
- The basic principles of genetics and immunology, as they apply to the CNS.
- The basic principles of neuropsychology and cognitive neuroscience.
- A basic grasp of issues related to the mind–brain debate, the biology of consciousness, and other neurophilosophical issues.
- Research methods and biostatistics.

Clinical skills in neuropsychiatry

1. Undertake clinical assessment of patients with apparent or possible neuropsychiatric problems

Take a neuropsychiatric history

This includes all of the information routinely gathered as part of a psychiatric and medical history, but with special emphasis on gathering information about possible illnesses or injury to the CNS and about sudden or gradual changes in intellectual functioning, level of consciousness, personality, and judgement, as well as changes in motor and sensory functions, which might indicate neurological disease.

Perform a neuropsychiatric assessment

This will again involve and encompass all of the routine skills required to carry out a psychiatric examination but, in addition, will include demonstration of the ability to elicit information relevant to possible neuropsychiatric disorders and neurological conditions, e.g. the ability to list the history of stepwise cognitive decline or psychomotor seizure activity.

Perform a cognitive examination (simple and extended)

The trainee will develop the ability to carry out simple tests 'at the bedside' to determine a patient's level of orientation, attention, concentration, memory, etc. and to do so in the context of a psychiatric examination. A neuropsychiatrist would be competent in assessing deficits in language, praxis, gnosis, visuospatial function, and other cognitive syndromes. This would not require the ability to administer formal neuropsychological tests, as carried out by a neuropsychologist, but may involve carrying out paper and pencil tests and the use of simple material such as word lists or pictures.

A neuropsychiatrist should have competency in interpreting the results of such an examination in order to determine whether the patient is suffering from a dementing illness, a confusional state, or a specific cognitive deficit, as well as competency in diagnosing the range of adult psychiatric conditions. Part of the skill would involve placing the results of the examination in the context of the patient's educational and social background and premorbid level of functioning.

Perform a neurological examination

The trainee should be able to carry out a full and detailed neurological examination, with particular emphasis on higher cortical functioning. The trainee should be able to demonstrate the ability to interpret any abnormal signs elicited and place them in the context of the patient's presentation and a differential diagnosis. This may include eliciting signs, which require further specialist investigation, either within the realm of neuropsychiatry or neurology or electrophysiology.

Construct a neuropsychiatric differential diagnosis

The trainee neuropsychiatrist should be able to demonstrate familiarity with multi-axial forms of classification. S/he should be able to arrange multiple diagnoses into a rational hierarchy and be able to summarize the key elements of the history and examination, which support that differential diagnosis. S/he should be able to evaluate the extent to which patterns of psychiatric symptomatology and presentation may be due to underlying organic brain disease and be familiar with the range of organic disorders that may account for particular presentations. S/he should be able to communicate this in a clear and concise way to other health professionals, as well as to patients and their carers.

2. Undertake and plan investigation of a patient with apparent or possible neuropsychiatric problems

Trainees should be familiar with the relevant haematological, metabolic, bacteriological, virological, immunological, and toxicological investigations of relevance to NP. This will include demonstrating knowledge and judgement that the relevant parameter is of central importance to the neuropsychiatric presentation and knowing which investigations need to be pursued with further tests and which may be incidental or within normal limits; interpretation of examination of CSF, nerve, muscle, and brain biopsies will also be required, although detailed knowledge is not necessary; unlike many other specialties within psychiatry, NP requires familiarity with EEG and other neurophysiological investigations and their interpretation. The trainee should be able to discuss the advantages and limitations of routine EEG, sleep EEG, and longer-term EEG telemetry in patients with possible neuropsychiatric problems. While the trainee is not expected to be competent in reading EEGs independently, s/he should have working knowledge of the profiles of normal and abnormal EEGs. In addition, s/he should understand the use and application of sensory evoked potentials and nerve conduction studies and electromyography (EMG), as they occur in neurological disorders with neuropsychiatric complications and also as a tool to exclude neurological causes of abnormal function, which may, in fact, have a psychological basis. The trainee should be familiar with the settings in which these investigations are carried out and should be able to query the interpretation with a consultant or an experienced technician in the area and to convey this information to members of the multidisciplinary team, carers, and patients alike.

NP requires a sound understanding of the indications for, and interpretations of, the various forms of brain imaging, both structural and functional, including MRI, CT, SPECT, and PET. The trainee should have sufficient familiarity with these techniques to be able to describe them to a patient and their family/carer and to interpret the results. The trainee should know when such investigations are likely to alter management or treatment decisions and should have some understanding of their theoretical importance. The trainee should have sufficient first-hand knowledge of CT and MRI brain scans to be able to detect salient abnormalities and critically assess an expert neuroradiological report.

3. Manage patients with neuropsychiatric disorders, including those with psychiatric and behavioural symptoms and coexisting neurological disorder

The trainee should have sufficient skills to explain the mode of action, benefits, and side effects of these treatments to fellow health professionals, patients, and their families and be familiar with the principles of treatment of major neurological disorders and with neuropsychiatric complications of such treatment. The neuropsychiatrist should also be aware of the neurological manifestations and complications of psychiatric treatment, and advise patients and professionals on evaluating the importance of these and in minimizing their occurrence and severity. S/he must be familiar with potential drug interactions between psychiatric and neurological medications and other treatments. This will include the awareness of the risks associated with prescribing psychotropic drugs to patients with neurological and neurosurgical diseases and have a working knowledge of non-pharmacological treatments in neurological and neuropsychiatric disorders. The trainee will have competence in the assessment for, and the administration of, ECT in its current form. The trainee should have some understanding of the newer physical treatments such as TMS, VNS, DBS, and other physical treatments. S/he should also acquire knowledge of the principles of neurorehabilitation and familiarity with the concepts of disability and handicap. Overall, the trainee should be familiar with social, psychological, and biological interventions for neuropsychiatric disorders.

4. Diagnose and treat patients with medically unexplained symptoms presenting as neurological and neuropsychiatric problems

NP training should include competence in understanding the possible social, cultural, and family influences on unexplained neurological symptoms. The trainee should be able to grasp the principles behind cognitive behavioural treatments for such patients and be able to plan and oversee such treatments carried out by another professional such as a trained nurse or a clinical psychologist. The trainee should be aware of the relationship between NP and allied psychiatric subspecialties, such as old age, child, and learning disability psychiatry, and by which sub-discipline patients might most appropriately be served. The neuropsychiatry trainee must become adept at working with colleagues in other disciplines to determine which further tests and investigations are necessary and prudent, and which might further hinder the patient's treatment and care.

5. Critical thinking in neuropsychiatry—research and scholarship

A specialist training in NP will equip the trainee to think critically in the field. The trainee should be able to critically assess the empirical evidence in support of any clinical practice, including the ability to evaluate published material. This skill can be developed by means of journal clubs, attendance at research meetings, research presentations, short-term courses, etc. It is expected that the trainee will undertake a research project. This should ideally involve all the steps in an empirical project (background review, design of study, applying for ethics clearance, data gathering and analysis, and report preparation). However, it may take the form of a critical review of a current topic or a case series. The trainee will produce a report of a publishable standard, as judged by the supervisors, and will be encouraged to publish in a peer-reviewed journal. The research report is a mandatory component of the training.

APPENDIX 2
Examples of specific modules

Module: Neurocognitive disorders

Specific competencies

Dementias and pre-dementia syndromes

- Be competent in the diagnosis and investigation of dementias resulting from:
  - AD.
  - Vascular cognitive disorder (VCD).
  - DLB.
  - FTD, including behavioural variant FTD, semantic dementia, primary progressive aphasia, etc.
  - Dementias related to Parkinsonism plus syndromes (progressive supranuclear palsy, corticobasal degeneration, multiple system atrophy).
  - Prion diseases, especially CJD and variant CJD.
  - HD.
  - Dementia resulting from head injury, alcohol use, medical conditions including HIV, brain tumours, encephalitis, etc.
  - Combination of pathologies.

Domain-specific cognitive disorders

- Be familiar with the diagnosis and investigation of *specific memory disorders* (amnesic syndromes), in particular Wernicke–Korsakoff's syndrome due to alcohol abuse and other causes of thiamine deficiency, brain infection such as herpes encephalitis or other encephalopathies, brain dysfunction resulting from cerebral hypoxia, e.g. carbon monoxide poisoning, and vascular disorders such as thalamic infarction or subarachnoid haemorrhage.
- Be familiar with the diagnosis and investigation of other 'specific' cognitive disorders, including language disorders (anomias and disorders of comprehension or expression), reading disorders (surface and deep dyslexia), mental calculation (whether or not part of Gerstmann's syndrome), disorders of visuospatial awareness, perception (hallucinations, illusions, derealization), and construction, the agnosias, and disorders of social cognition. The Kluver Bucy syndrome is one example of a historical syndrome.
- Be familiar with the diagnosis and investigation of psychologically based cognitive impairments:
  - Dissociative disorder and other causes of psychogenic amnesias.
  - Pseudodementias, as in depression, factitious disorder, and other.
  - Cognitive impairment as part of somatization, factitious, or malingering syndromes.
- Be familiar with the status and controversies regarding MCI or mild neurocognitive disorder.

Diagnostic techniques

- Clinical assessment, including neurological and clinical cognitive examination.
- Be familiar with the role, importance, and principles of neuropsychological testing.
- Be familiar with the interpretation of occupational therapy and speech and language therapy assessments and reports.
- Be familiar with the relevant investigations in a clinical blood screen.
- Be familiar with routine and urgent requirements of an EEG.
- Be familiar with the purpose and interpretation of CT and MRI brain scans.
- Be familiar with the putative roles of other forms of neuroimaging, including SPECT, PET, diffusion tensor imaging (DTI), and fMRI.

Be familiar with the main principles involved in the management and treatment of cognitive disorders, including dementias

- The work of a multidisciplinary team.
- The contribution of cognitive behaviour therapy and psychological counselling in specific conditions.
- The use of cognitive-enhancing drugs, including cholinesterase inhibitors and memantine.
- The use of other medications in NP, including antiepileptics and antidepressants.
- The management of behavioural and psychiatric disturbances in dementia.
- The use of outreach and community support services.

Learning and assessment methods

Suggested learning methods	Suggested assessment methods
Observation/modelling	Clinical supervision
Working as a team member	Direct observation
Supervise clinical practice	Clinical log book
Review of suitable texts and papers in scientific publications, including review articles	Clinical audit
	Case presentations

APPENDIX 3

Example module–General hospital liaison neuropsychiatry

Specific competencies

Undertake assessment of patients with unexplained neurological symptoms

- Take an appropriate neuropsychiatric history.
- Interpret previously performed investigations.
- Perform examination of mental and physical status.
- Assess the patient's function in the context of their disability.
- Understand the concepts of conversion, somatization, and dissociation in a neurological context.
- Formulate appropriate management plans.
- Communicate information to the neurology team.

Learning and assessment methods

- Take an appropriate neuropsychiatric history (see other sections).
- Interpret previously performed investigations.

Suggested learning methods	Suggested assessment methods
Observation/modelling	Validated self-assessment
Supervised clinical practice	Clinical supervision
Specific teaching from relevant health professionals (e.g. radiologist)	Case presentation

- Perform examination of physical and mental status (see other sections).
- Assess the patient's function in the context of their disability.

Suggested learning methods	Suggested assessment methods
Observation/modelling	Validated self-assessment
Supervised clinical practice	Clinical supervision
Specific teaching from relevant health professionals (e.g. occupational therapist)	Clinical log book
	Case presentation

- Understand the concepts of conversion, somatization, and dissociation

Suggested learning methods	Suggested assessment methods
Supervised clinical practice	Clinical supervision
Reading relevant texts	Clinical log book
Peer group discussion	Case presentation

- Formulate appropriate management plans (see other sections).
- Communicate information to the neurology team.

Suggested learning methods	Suggested assessment methods
Observation/modelling	Clinical supervision
Supervised clinical practice	Direct observation

Undertake assessment of patients with delirium

- Take a relevant clinical history from the patient and informants.
- Gather information from clinical staff.
- Perform examination of physical and mental status.
- Construct an appropriate differential diagnosis (delirium versus depression versus dementia).
- Perform investigation to ascertain the aetiology.
- Initiate and monitor treatment where appropriate.

Learning and assessment methods

- Take a relevant clinical history from the patient and informants (see other sections).
- Gather information from clinical staff.

Suggested learning methods	Suggested assessment methods
Observation/modelling	Clinical supervision
Supervised clinical practice	Direct observation
Working as a team member	

- Perform examination of physical and mental status (see other sections).
- Construct an appropriate differential diagnosis (e.g. delirium versus depression versus dementia).

Suggested learning methods	Suggested assessment methods
Supervised clinical practice	Clinical supervision
Appropriate reading	Case presentation
	Clinical log book
	Validated self-assessment

- Perform investigation to ascertain the aetiology.

Suggested learning methods	Suggested assessment methods
Supervised clinical practice	Clinical supervision
Appropriate reading	Case presentation
Specific teaching from other health professionals	Clinical log book
	Validated self-assessment

- Initiate and monitor treatment where appropriate (see other sections).

14

Immunology relevant to neuropsychiatry

Rachel Patel and Neil A. Harrison

Introduction

From long sitting at the fringes of psychiatric research, psycho-neuroimmunology, the study of bidirectional immune–brain interactions, has rapidly emerged to become a major psychiatric research priority. A particular focus has been the role of innate immune activation in the aetiology of major depressive disorder (MDD). This has been fuelled by recognition that acute immune activation rapidly impairs mood (Harrison et al., 2009a). When inflammation is prolonged, pro-inflammatory cytokines, such as interferon-alpha (IFN-α) can also precipitate major depressive episodes, even in previously euthymic individuals (Capuron et al., 2002). Conversely, raised pro-inflammatory cytokines, particularly interleukin (IL)-6 and acute phase proteins such as C-reactive protein (CRP), are consistently reported in MDD patients (Dowlati et al., 2010). Initial attempts to block inflammation using anti-cytokine therapies like anti-tumour necrosis factor (TNF) have been shown to improve mood in patients with psoriasis (Tyring et al., 2006), as well as some patients with treatment-resistant depression (Raison et al., 2013). This potential to repurpose immune-active compounds has generated considerable excitement within the psychiatric research community and stimulated the first industry-funded trial of an anti-IL-6 therapy in MDD.

Aside from MDD, the immune system is implicated in the aetiology and progression of a number of other common neuropsychiatric illnesses. For example, infective episodes are linked to accelerated decline in AD (Holmes et al., 2009), relapse in multiple sclerosis (Correale et al., 2006), and severe, even persistent, cognitive impairment in previously healthy older individuals (Iwashyna et al., 2010). Infections/inflammation have long been recognized to precipitate delirium. Recent advances in neuroimmunology are beginning to identify the importance of age-related priming of microglial cells (dedicated brain immune cells) in this common neuropsychiatric disorder (Cunningham, 2011). Indeed, immunotherapeutics targeting microglia are being actively developed, offering the potential for new therapies directly targeting a key mediator of this common, and often devastating, condition. Immune mechanisms are also strongly linked to the aetiology of schizophrenia. For example, polymorphisms within the major histocompatibility complex (MHC), the key mechanism used to differentiate self from non-self, are among the strongest associations in GWAS (Corvin et al., 2014).

In this fast-evolving field, there is a pressing need for psychiatrists to refresh their knowledge of the workings of the immune system to facilitate assimilation of new knowledge and lay the foundation for safe and efficacious use of emerging immunotherapies. In this chapter, we provide an overview of the structure of the immune system, with a particular emphasis on components implicated in psychiatric illness. We provide an accessible primer on how the immune system acts on, and within, the brain and an update on increasingly obsolete concepts of the CNS as an immune-privileged site.

Overview of the immune system

The key function of the immune system is to identify, memorize, and ultimately eliminate threats to bodily integrity. These threats are frequently exogenous, e.g. viruses and bacteria, but can also include endogenous threats such as tissue damage from trauma or malignancy. At the most fundamental level, the immune system can be divided into three effector mechanisms: natural barriers, e.g. the skin and blood–brain barrier (BBB) that prevent tissue infection; innate immunity, e.g. macrophages, neutrophils, and natural killer (NK) cells that provide an immediate response to infection; and adaptive immunity, e.g. B- and T-lymphocytes that provide a highly specific response leading to long-term immunological memory. These three arms of the immune system use a range of cellular and molecular mechanisms to carefully coordinate and integrate responses to threat and preserve bodily integrity.

Historically, the CNS has been conceptualized as an immune-privileged site, reflecting the notion that it lacked the sophisticated immune mechanisms seen in the periphery. However, as will be illustrated in the following sections, this view has been challenged and revised to incorporate evidence of a highly complex and active CNS immune system (Louveau et al., 2015a). This CNS immune system includes each of the three fundamental effector mechanisms—it has a highly dynamic BBB that facilitates bidirectional communication between the peripheral and central immune systems (Banks, 2016) and contains specialized parenchymal macrophages (microglia) that, in addition to providing immune surveillance, regulate pruning of neuronal dendrites (Schafer et al., 2012). The meninges host a broader range of innate immune cells, including eosinophils and dendritic cells, as well as numerous types of B- and particularly T-lymphocytes that provide an adaptive immune response.

Overturning decades of neuroscience dogma, the CNS has recently been shown to contain a dedicated lymphatic system (Louveau et al., 2015b) and a 'glymphatic' system that allows the CSF to enter, and interstitial solutes to exit, the brain parenchyma along the perivascular (Virchow–Robin) spaces (Nedergaard et al., 2013). Aside from their immunological roles, parenchymal microglia and meningeal lymphocytes appear to play important functions in normal cognition and have been implicated in the pathophysiology of a range of neuropsychiatric disorders, including depression, AD, and autism (Kipnis et al., 2012; Schafer et al., 2012).

Finally, the immune system does not act in isolation. In the face of an infective threat to the body, it rapidly reorients our behaviour, prioritizing resources to fighting the infection. These changes in behaviour are known collectively as 'sickness behaviour' and are discussed in the final section. Together, these developments in our understanding of the CNS immune system suggest that should we continue to use the term 'immune privilege', and we should perhaps do so to more correctly indicate a dynamic system that is adapted for the special environment of the brain and spinal cord.

Barriers

Natural barriers, such as the epithelial cells of the skin, act as dynamic physical shields against pathogens in the environment that can be modulated by behavioural actions, e.g. wearing gloves or handwashing in humans and grooming in animals. Within the CNS, the BBB provides a similar function, preventing access of harmful systemic pathogens. However, it is important to recognize that the BBB is a highly interactive barrier that continually adapts to dynamically serve the needs of the CNS, leading some researchers to suggest renaming it the blood–brain interface (BBI) (Banks, 2016). This adaptive nature facilitates brain–body communication, enables resident brain macrophages (microglia) to respond to immune challenges within the body, and regulates access of innate immune cells to the brain.

Blood–brain barrier

The BBB is a semi-permeable membrane, which, together with its partner the blood–CSF barrier in the choroid plexus, plays a key role in controlling the CNS environment and defending it against insult. Tight junctions between brain endothelial cells form the basis of the physical barrier. However, close communication between endothelial cells and neighbouring astrocytes, microglia, neurones, mast cells, and pericytes within the brain, as well as circulating immune cells, plays a critical role in refining and maintaining barrier characteristics. Neuroimmune modulators, such as cytokines and other immune-active substances released from astrocytes, microglia, leucocytes, and even endothelial cells themselves, modify a host of BBB functions, altering BBB integrity, BBB transporters, and the permeability of the BBB to pathogens and circulating immune cells (Banks et al., 2015).

A few regions of the brain, such as the circumventricular organs, express a specialized BBB comprising loops of fenestrated capillaries that increase permeability and enhance sensing of circulating molecules (Gross, 1991). Others, such as large vessels

in the subarachnoid space, the sensory ganglia of spinal/cranial nerves, and the nucleus tractus solitarius, contain 'functional leaks' that allow small amounts of circulating substances to pass through extracellular pathways to reach the Virchow–Robin spaces and the glymphatic system (Banks, 2016). The importance of this latter pathway is that it is the likely route through which antibodies (including therapeutic anti-Aβ antibodies being trialled in AD) gain access to the brain.

Innate immune system

The innate immune system consists of both cellular and non-cellular components that together provide rapid detection and response to infecting agents or tissue damage. Unlike cells of the adaptive immune system, innate immune cells recognize pathogens and tissue damage through expression of a set of invariant pattern recognition receptors (PRRs) that recognize highly conserved pathogen-associated molecular patterns (PAMPs) broadly shared by pathogens or damage-associated molecular patterns (DAMPs) associated with cell components released during cell damage or death (Chen and Nuñez, 2010). In the periphery, the innate immune system includes a range of different cell types with varying immunological functions. These include phagocytic cells such as tissue-resident macrophages, monocytes, and neutrophils that engulf, or 'phagocytose', pathogens, antigen-presenting cells such as reticular cells, and mast cells, and granulocytes such as basophils and eosinophils. The innate immune system also includes specific types of lymphocytes, most notably NK cells that play a critical role in the identification and removal of virally infected cells.

Within the CNS, the range of innate immune cells is more limited. The most prevalent innate immune cells in the brain parenchyma are microglia, dedicated brain macrophages that make up 10–15% of all brain cells (Ransohoff and Cardona 2010). The brain parenchyma also contains mast cells, particularly within the thalamus, hypothalamus, and the median eminence. Mast cells are granulocytes. However, unlike other granulocytes, their functional phenotype matures following tissue entry (Stone et al., 2010). They secrete a broad range of mediators, including histamine, serotonin, corticotropin-releasing hormone (CRH), prostaglandins, leukotrienes, and a variety of chemokines and cytokines (da Silva et al., 2014). Within the body, histamine released from mast cells plays an important role in dilating post-capillary venules and increasing blood vessel permeability, leading to oedema, warmth, and redness associated with classical inflammation. Within the CNS, mast cells also play a critical role in regulating BBB permeability and have been implicated in increases in BBB permeability associated with stress (Esposito et al., 2001).

Innate immune system: cells

Though the innate immune system includes a diversity of innate immune cells, there are two main classes of cells: macrophages/microglia and NK cells that have particular relevance for neuropsychiatry. These are discussed in more detail below.

Macrophages and microglia

Macrophages (from the Greek meaning 'big eater') are professional phagocytes that engulf and digest dead and dying cells, microbes, cancer cells, and even aged neutrophils, the commonest phagocytic cell type in the periphery. They are found in all tissue types, including the brain, and display substantial anatomical and functional diversity. This diversity is partly reflected in tissue-specific naming, e.g. Kupffer cells in the liver, osteoclasts in bone, and microglia in the brain (Wynn et al., 2013). Classically, macrophages were defined as deriving from circulating monocytes originating in the bone marrow. However, this position has recently undergone a significant revision. It is now acknowledged that most tissue-resident macrophages (including brain microglia) do not derive from the bone marrow but instead originate from the primitive ectoderm of the embryonic yolk sac (Schultz et al., 2012) (see Fig. 14.1). This revision has important implications for neuropsychiatric disorders linked to central inflammation, as it means that microglia are a self-sustaining cell population that are highly adapted to their environment, with little, if any, contribution from circulating monocytes.

Macrophages, including microglia, are highly plastic cells and undergo a variety of structural and functional changes, according to changes in their local environment. Within the healthy brain, so-called 'resting' microglia exist in a highly dynamic state, expanding and retracting multiple branched ramifications to continuously sample the extracellular space and neighbouring cells (Nimmerjahn et al., 2005). In this state, microglia can secrete a range of neurotrophic factors, including brain-derived neurotrophic factor (BDNF), transforming growth factor-beta (TGF-β), and insulin-like growth factor 1 (IGF-1) (Kreutzberg, 1996). Upon detection of homeostatic disruption, including infection, trauma, or marked alteration in neuronal activity, resting microglia rapidly activate, changing their morphometry, motility, cell number, and function (Ransohoff and Perry, 2009). Specifically, they adopt an increasingly amoeboid shape, with the loss of ramifications, and migrate to the location of the insult where they proliferate, enhance their phagocytic activity, and produce a number of cytokines and other molecular mediators of inflammation. Importantly, this shift from a resting to an 'activated' state is associated with increased expression of translocator protein (TSPO), which can be detected clinically using a number of PET tracers such as PK11195, FEPPA, and PBR28 (Setiawan et al., 2015).

Microglial activation typically serves to maintain homeostasis and resolve CNS insult. However, in some circumstances, activated microglia can have detrimental neurotoxic effects. Increased microglial activation has also been reported in a number of neuropsychiatric and neurodegenerative diseases, including motor neurone disease, AD, PD, depression, and schizophrenia (Block et al., 2007; Bloomfield et al., 2016; Lucin and Wyss-Coray, 2009; Perry and Holmes, 2014; Saijo and Glass, 2011; Setiawan et al., 2015).

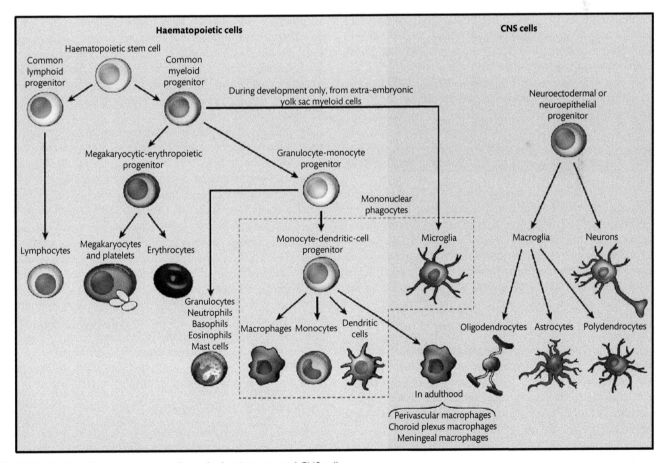

Fig. 14.1 Relationship between microglia and other immune and CNS cells.

Reproduced with permission from R. M. Ransohoff and A. E. Cardona. The myeloid cells of the central nervous system parenchyma. *Nature*, 468: 253–262. Copyright © 2010, Springer Nature. https://doi.org/10.1038/nature09615.

In addition to these immunological roles, macrophages are also critical to tissue modelling during development and throughout adult life. For example, macrophage-deficient mice are unable to develop haemopoietic cavities within bones and, during pregnancy, do not show the typical changes in ductal expansion and breast tissue architecture. This remodelling function also extends to the CNS. Within the brain, microglia are critically dependent on colony-stimulating factor-1 (CSF-1) for their survival. Congenital absence of CSF-1 in mice disrupts normal brain circuitry, resulting in enlarged ventricles, increased cortical neuronal density, and reduced oligodendrocytes. In humans, a mutation in the CSF-1 receptor causes 'hereditary diffuse leukoencephalopathy with spheroids', a syndrome associated with loss of myelin sheaths and axonal destruction (Wynn et al., 2013). Recently, microglia have also been shown to play important roles in activity-dependent synaptic plasticity and pruning of excess or redundant synapses (Schafer et al., 2012). This process is dependent on complement, a key molecular component of the innate immune system. Remarkably, this mechanism appears to be central to the early loss of synapses observed in mouse models of AD where inhibition of complement factors C1q or C3 is sufficient to reverse this process (Hong et al., 2016).

NK cells

NK cells are another type of innate immune cells that has been implicated in the aetiology of depression. Briefly, NK cells detect the loss of MHC class I on 'stressed' host cells infected with a virus or undergoing malignant change. Their name 'natural killer' reflects their ability to initiate cytotoxicity without the need for activation by CD4$^+$ T-cells of the adaptive immune system. Studies have repeatedly shown reduced NK cell number in patients with MDD, and some have also shown reduced NK cell activity (Park et al., 2015). It has been proposed that this reduction in NK cell number and function may underlie the increased rates of cancer and viral infection in MDD patients.

Innate immune system: molecules

The innate immune system uses a plethora of different molecules to recognize, respond, and ultimately destroy invading pathogens and infected dead or dying host cells. Illustrating the thriftiness of biology, many of these molecules are being found to play additional roles in diverse aspects of normal mental function and some are even implicated in the pathophysiology of psychiatric disease. The most important from the perspective of a neuropsychiatrist are detailed below.

(Primitive) pattern recognition receptors

As highlighted previously, the innate immune system uses a number of different PRRs to rapidly identify PAMPs and DAMPs. These can be broadly classified into membrane-bound and cytoplasmic receptors, though secreted forms, such as CRP, also exist. The best well-known PRRs are a group of 11 transmembrane proteins known as Toll-like receptors (TLRs). TLRs are expressed on surface or endosomal membranes of a range of innate immune cells, including macrophages, NK cells, and dendritic cells, as well as some adaptive immune (B- and T-lymphocytes) and non-immune cells, e.g. endothelial cells. TLRs have also been identified on glia, neurones, and

neural progenitor cells within the brain where they modulate axonal growth, hippocampal neurogenesis, and structural plasticity (Okun et al., 2011).

Individual TLRs recognize specific molecular signatures that are shared across classes of pathogens. For example, TLR4 recognizes lipopolysaccharide found in the outer membrane of Gram-negative bacteria, as well as heat shock proteins and other polysaccharides. Interestingly, TLR4 has also been shown to bind opioids, an action implicated in maintaining established neuropathic pain (Hutchinson et al., 2008). In contrast, TLR3 recognizes double-stranded RNA. With the exception of TLR3, all TLRs signal via the MyD88-dependent pathway to induce NF-κB signalling. This leads to secretion of pro-inflammatory cytokines and the subsequent activation of immune cells. TLRs play an important role in linking innate and adaptive immune responses. TLR3 and TLR4 also activate the TRIF-dependent signalling pathway, leading to production of type-I interferons that stimulate macrophages and NK cells to trigger potent antiviral responses. Of importance to psychiatry, heightened activation of both NF-κB and type-I interferon pathways have been implicated in the aetiology of MDD (Jansen et al., 2016).

The innate immune system also utilizes a number of other PRRs beyond TLRs. These include cytoplasmic PRRs, such as nucleotide-binding oligomerization domain (NOD)-like receptors, which have been implicated in Crohn's disease, and a subgroup of NOD-like receptor proteins, known as NLRPs, that are involved in forming the inflammasome. The inflammasome plays an important role in triggering inflammatory cascades; it promotes the maturation of IL-1β (which also promotes fever through actions at the organum vasculosum, one of the circumventricular organs) and cleavage of the IL-18 precursor to induce IFN-gamma (γ) secretion and NK cell activation. Though playing a critical role in inflammatory processes, contributions of inflammasome activation to common mental illnesses are currently poorly understood (Krishnadas and Harrison, 2016).

The final group of PRRs of importance to neuropsychiatry are the secreted forms. These include mannose-binding lectin (MBL), which recognize carbohydrate patterns found on the surface of many pathogens, including bacteria, viruses, protozoa, and fungi, leading to activation of the complement system, the complement proteins themselves, and CRP. CRP was the first PRR to be discovered (Tillett and Francis, 1930). It is an acute phase protein, produced by the liver in response to IL-6 released by macrophages and other cells, including adipocytes. It binds to the surface of dead or dying cells, leading to activation of the complement system. CRP is a commonly measured marker of inflammation that has consistently been shown to be elevated in depression (Dowlati et al., 2010). In addition to indexing cardiovascular risk (Koenig et al., 1999), CRP is beginning to show promise as a potential marker for guiding between serotonergic or noradrenergic antidepressants (Uher et al., 2014) and is finding utility in stratifying patients for trials of novel immunotherapeutics (Raison et al., 2013).

Cytokines and chemokines

Cytokines are small proteins that are important in cell signalling and coordinating innate and adaptive immune responses. Chemokines are a subset of cytokines that act as chemoattractants to guide cell migration. Though discussed here under the innate immune system, cytokines are a broad collection of proteins that are released by both innate and adaptive immune cells, as well as endothelial cells, fibroblasts, and stromal (connective tissue) cells. They include ILs, IFNs (involved in antiviral responses), TNF, CSFs, and chemokines, e.g. CCL and CXCL nomenclatures. Cytokines typically circulate in very low concentrations, e.g. picomolar (10^{-12} M), though the concentration can increase up to 1000-fold during infection or trauma. Their immunomodulatory functions are achieved through a combination of autocrine, paracrine, and endocrine signalling. Examples of the latter include the fever response triggered by IL-1 and TNF acting on the organum vasculosum and the induction of sickness behaviours. Cytokines typically display a high degree of redundancy and pleiotropy and often enhance or inhibit the action of other cytokines in complex ways. This has impeded simple functional classification. Nevertheless, one clinically useful division is between pro-inflammatory cytokines, including IL-1, TNF, and IL-6, and chemokines that up-regulate inflammatory reactions and anti-inflammatory cytokines such as the IL-1 receptor antagonist (IL-1ra) and IL-10 that promote healing and reduce inflammation.

Within the CNS, microglia, particularly in their activated state, can release the pro-inflammatory cytokines IL-1, IL-6, and TNF, as well as a number of chemokines, including CCL2. Some cytokines can also gain access to the CNS through expression of dedicated transporters in the BBB (Banks, 2016). In addition to their immunological roles, a number of cytokines, including IL-1, IL-6, and TNF, have been shown to regulate a range of complex cognitive processes, including hippocampus-dependent learning (Pugh et al., 2001) and sleep (Krueger et al., 2008). Increased CNS CCL2 has also been linked to the pathology of a number of neuropsychiatric disorders, including multiple sclerosis, stroke, AD, epilepsy, and head injury (Conductier et al., 2010).

Elevated circulating pro-inflammatory cytokines, particularly IL-6 and TNF, have been linked in meta-analyses to MDD (Dowlati et al., 2010) and schizophrenia (Miller et al., 2011). Higher plasma IL-6 in childhood has also been associated with an increased prevalence of depression in adult life (Khandaker et al., 2015). Childhood adversity is an important risk factor for the later development of a number of common mental illnesses, particularly depression. It is therefore noteworthy that childhood neglect and maltreatment result in elevated IL-6 responses to stress, suggesting a putative role for IL-6 as a molecular mediator linking early life adversity to depression (Carpenter et al., 2010).

Another group of cytokines important to neuropsychiatry are the IFNs. IFNs are powerful signallers of viral infection and are used therapeutically for the treatment of chronic viral infections such as hepatitis C. However, sustained therapeutic use precipitates major depressive episodes in up to a third of patients (Musselman et al., 2001). This finding has provided powerful evidence for an aetiological role for pro-inflammatory cytokines in depression.

Adaptive immune system

The adaptive immune system consists of specialized cells (B- and T-lymphocytes) and molecular systems (e.g. antibodies) that produce highly specific responses to pathogens and induce long-term immunological memory. It is the basis of vaccination. Unlike the primitive PRRs of the innate immune system, adaptive immune cells express hugely variable surface receptors and 'acquire' specificity

to pathogens through clonal selection of pathogen specific cells. This allows the adaptive immune system to mount a highly targeted immune response to almost any plausible antigen, including self-antigens. Its ability to differentiate self- from non-self antigens (immune tolerance) relies upon a number of factors. Firstly, all nucleated self-cells express MHC class I on their cell surface, while professional antigen-presenting cells, e.g. reticular cells, B-cells, and monocytes/macrophages, express MHC class II. T-cells can only recognize antigen bound to MHC. During T- and B-lymphocyte development in the thymus and bone marrow, respectively, self-reactive clones are deleted. Any remaining self-reactive lymphocytes are regulated by the action of regulatory T-cells (T_{reg}) in the peripheral tissues and lymph nodes.

Lymphocytes are generally absent from the healthy brain parenchyma, though T- and, to a lesser extent, B-lymphocytes, together with dendritic cells (professional antigen-presenting cells), are present in the meningeal space (Kipnis, 2016). This reflects strategic positioning at sites that are first exposed to blood-borne pathogens. The route of entry of lymphocytes into the CSF is currently uncertain though likely occurs via meningeal blood vessels. Lymphocytes then circulate through the meningeal space, exiting via the recently discovered CNS lymphatics adjacent to the large cerebral veins, before draining into the deep cervical lymph nodes (Louveau et al., 2015b). Many of these T-cells have a memory (RO45[+]) phenotype and play a protective immune surveillant role. However, recent evidence suggests that they may also play a role in cognition, as absence of meningeal T-cells is associated with impaired hippocampus-dependent memory. Furthermore, IL-4 released from T-cells increases astrocyte release of BDNF and enhances hippocampus-dependent learning in mice (Kipnis et al., 2012). Interestingly, meningeal T-cell release of IFN-γ also appears to play a critical role in rodent social behaviour and, though actions on GABAergic interneurons, fronto-cortical brain connectivity (Filiano et al., 2016).

Outside of autoimmune psychosis (reviewed in Chapter 22), the role of the adaptive immune system in neuropsychiatry is currently an under-investigated area. However, the recent discovery of cognitive actions of lymphocytes and T-cell-related cytokines is likely to change this over coming years.

Adaptive immune system: cells

Lymphocytes

There are three main types of lymphocytes: T-cells, B-cells, and NK cells. NK cells are classified as innate immune cells and are discussed earlier. Most of the body's lymphocytes circulate through the body tissues and lymphatic system, with perhaps only 2% present in the blood. They move to their target tissue through expression of homing receptors that bind to tissue-selective addressins. Together, lymphocytes have a total mass equivalent to a large organ such as the brain. T-cells (which mature in the thymus) are involved in cell-mediated immunity, while B-cells (which mature in the bone marrow) are responsible for humoral immunity and secretion of antibodies.

Following maturation in the thymus, T-cells circulate throughout the body as naïve CD4[+] helper (T_H) or regulatory (T_{reg}) T-cells that recognize antigen expressed with MHC class II, and CD8[+] cytotoxic

T-cells (T_C) that recognize antigen expression on MHC class I. T_H cells assist in a broad range of immunological actions. Upon antigen recognition, naïve T_H rapidly proliferate and further differentiate into a range of subtypes that are associated with discrete patterns of cytokine release and immunological actions. This includes T_{H1} cells that, following IL-12 and IL-2 stimulation, secrete IFN-γ to activate macrophage and cytotoxic T-cell phagocytosis of intracellular bacteria. In contrast, T_{H2} cells are triggered by IL-4 to secrete IL-4, IL-5, IL-9, IL-10, and IL-13, leading to activation of eosinophils, basophils, B-cells, and mast cells, which attack extracellular pathogens, including helminths (parasitic worms). T_{reg} cells are crucial for the maintenance of immune tolerance. They down-regulate the activation of cytotoxic T-cells, following resolution of infection, and suppress autoreactive T-cells that survive clonal deletion in the thymus. T_H cells also regulate the maturation of B-cells into plasma cells (that secrete large volumes of antibodies) and long-lived memory B-cells. In contrast to CD4+ T_H cells, CD8+ T_C cells recognize antigen presented with MHC class I, which is expressed on all nucleated self-cells. Once activated, T_C release cytotoxins like perforin that play a central role in killing virus-infected, malignant, and damaged cells. Following resolution of an infection, a subset of both CD4+ and CD8+ cells persist as memory cells (indicated by the marker RO45) that can rapidly proliferate in response to antigen re-exposure. It is these RO45+ memory cells that are typically found in the CSF space.

Following maturation, B-cells migrate to the secondary lymphoid tissue, such as the spleen and lymph nodes, where they sample the circulating lymph, which is rich in antigens. Some antigens, such as foreign polysaccharides, can directly activate B-cells without the need for T-cell help. B-cell responses to these antigens are generally rapid, though the antibodies produced typically show weak affinity. Most antigens, however, e.g. foreign proteins, require T_H cell support and presentation of the antigen on MHC class II. B-cell responses to these antigens are slower (typically several days), though they produce antibodies of greater affinity and allow for antibody class switching (e.g. immunoglobulin M (IgM) to immunoglobulin G (IgG)) and formation of long-lived plasma and memory cells.

Adaptive immune system: major histocompatibility complex

MHC is critical to self/non-self differentiation and presentation of antigens to adaptive immune cells. It contains >200 genes, many of which are among the most polymorphic in the genome. In humans, these are called *human leucocyte antigen* (*HLA*) genes. Given their crucial role in immunity, it is perhaps unsurprising that many different HLA haplotypes have been linked to disease, particularly diseases with an autoimmune aetiology such as type 1 diabetes mellitus, rheumatoid arthritis, and systemic lupus erythematosus. This includes neuropsychiatric disease. Indeed, one of the strongest links with HLA is narcolepsy where the HLA-DQB1*0602 haplotype is found in up to 98% of patients (Dauvilliers et al., 2007). This finding in an HLA class II region strongly implicates a T-cell aetiology. Further support for this comes from epidemiological studies that have shown spikes in narcolepsy incidence following H1N1 influenza outbreaks and/or vaccination against H1N1 (Partinen et al., 2014). Though yet to be proven, it is hypothesized that the

characteristic loss of hypothalamic orexin neurones in narcolepsy results from autoimmune destruction of these cells.

Another example of HLA associations in psychiatry stemmed from early work in rheumatoid arthritis which showed higher-than-expected expression of HLA-DRB1*04, but lower-than-expected comorbidity with schizophrenia. Rates of the HLA-DRB1*04 allele have since been shown to be lower than expected in schizophrenia (Torrey and Yolken, 2001). Furthermore, there is preferential non-transmission of HLA-DRB1*04 alleles from heterozygous parents to offspring with schizophrenia, suggesting a protective role for HLA-DRB1*04. More recently, GWAS have repeatedly confirmed the association between the MHC locus and schizophrenia (Shi et al., 2009).

MHC class I was once considered to be absent in neurones. However, pioneering work by Carla Shatz and colleagues has revealed that not only is MHC class I expressed in neurones, but it also plays a critical role in neuronal development (Shatz, 2009). This is another example of biology 'recycling' molecules for different purposes. These studies have shown that neuronal MHC class I genes are dynamically regulated during critical periods of brain development and continue to be expressed in specific areas of the adult brain, including the hippocampus. MHC class I signalling appears to be essential for hippocampal function, as when it is blocked (by removing the receptor CD3z), it results in aberrant long-term potential (LTP), a process considered critical to learning and memory and the remodelling of neural connections (Shatz, 2009). Together, these important studies are beginning to provide clues about how infections during critical developmental periods may contribute to the aetiology of neurodevelopmental disorders such as autism and schizophrenia.

Glymphatics and the meningeal lymphatic pathway

Our understanding of how cells and solutes circulate around the CNS has undergone a major revision in recent years. Firstly, Nedergaard and colleagues have demonstrated the presence of an intraparenchymal clearance pathway (named the glymphatic system) that is central to the clearance of solutes, including β-amyloid from the brain parenchyma (Nedergaard, 2013). Secondly, Kipnis's group have shown that the CNS contains a dedicated lymphatic system that drains CNS immune cells from the meninges into the deep cervical lymph nodes (Louveau et al., 2015b).

In the periphery, toxic metabolites and cell debris are removed from tissue by drainage of interstitial fluid into local lymphatics, lymph nodes, and ultimately blood. However, the CNS parenchyma lacks a classical lymphatic system for draining interstitial fluid. The first hint at how this may be achieved in the brain came in the 1980s when tracers injected into the ventricles were shown to accumulate in the 'Virchow–Robin' spaces surrounding small penetrating blood vessels (Rennels et al., 1985). Subsequent work by Nedergaard has shown that tracers injected into mouse CSF appear in the para-arterial spaces within 10 minutes, and then the paravenous spaces 30 minutes later (Nedergaard, 2013). This suggests that CSF diffuses from the periarterial to the perivenous spaces through the brain parenchyma (Nedergaard, 2013). Tracers injected directly into the brain parenchyma accumulate only in the paravenous spaces, confirming this as a likely exit path for brain solutes. Flow through this 'glymphatic' system is driven by pulsatile arterial contractions and, interestingly, increases dramatically during sleep. Of importance to neuropsychiatry, glymphatic flow appears to be the major route for clearing Aβ from the brain parenchyma (Iliff et al., 2012). Furthermore, glymphatic flow reduces markedly with age (the most important risk factor for AD) and paravenous drainage of Aβ is impeded by APOE4, the most important genetic risk factor for late-onset AD (see Fig. 14.2).

In the second major conceptual advance, Kipnis and colleagues have shown that, contrary to popular belief, the CNS does indeed contain a rudimentary lymphatic system that facilitates the flow of macromolecules and cells out of the CSF and into the deep cervical lymph nodes (Louveau et al., 2015b). As illustrated in Fig. 14.3,

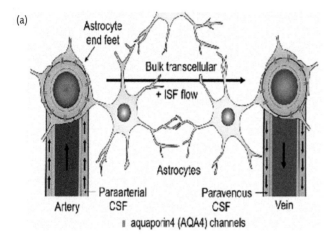

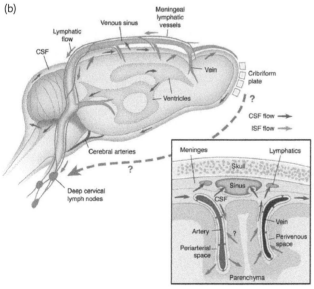

Fig. 14.2 CNS lymphatic and glymphatic pathways. (a) Schematic of the glymphatic system. The CSF enters the brain parenchyma through the Virchow–Robin spaces surrounding penetrating arterioles, then leaves via the perivenous spaces. Dense expression of aquaporin4 (AQA4) channels on astrocytes that surround blood vessels facilitate water and solute flow. (b) Schematic of the CNS lymphatic system. The CSF and meningeal immune cells leave the meningeal space via lymphatic vessels travelling adjacent to the venous sinuses terminating in the deep cervical lymph nodes.

these meningeal lymphatic vessels lie adjacent to the large venous sinuses. Though still in its infancy, research is actively exploring the role of this system in diseases such as AD and multiple sclerosis and the potential of modulating this system as a potential novel therapeutic target.

Communication between peripheral and central immune systems

A number of parallel humoral and neural pathways link the peripheral and central immune systems (Critchley and Harrison, 2013; Dantzer et al., 2008). Autonomic afferents travelling with the vagus and possibly sympathetic nerves can rapidly sense changes in circulating pro-inflammatory cytokines signalling to the brainstem solitary nucleus (Goehler et al., 2000). Subsequent projections to subcortical and cortical (e.g. insula) components of the interoceptive pathway coordinate behavioural responses to infection known as 'sickness behaviours' (Harrison et al., 2009b). In addition, peripheral inflammation activates a number of humoral pathways. For example, microglia residing in the circumventricular organs rapidly activate, following peripheral inflammation. This may occur in response to direct sensing of circulating cytokines (Laflamme and Rivest, 2001) or prostaglandin E2 (Saper et al., 2012) produced by perivascular and endothelial cells. These activated microglia then produce TNF, which acts on adjacent cells, leading to a cascade of microglial activation that propagates across the brain parenchyma. Additionally, the BBB has been shown to express specific cytokine transporters, which further facilitate the entry of some cytokines into the brain (Banks, 2015).

Sickness behaviours

In addition to immune system activation, infections anywhere in the body rapidly induce a cluster of mood, motivational, and cognitive changes, collectively known as 'sickness behaviours' (Hart, 1988). These include changes in mood, experienced as mild depression, anxiety, and fatigue (Harrison et al., 2009a), heightened sensitivity to punishments, compared to rewards (Harrison et al., 2016), cognitive changes such as subtle impairments in memory (Harrison et al., 2014), social withdrawal and neurovegetative symptoms such as sleep disturbance, anorexia, fatigue, and psychomotor slowing (Brydon et al., 2008; Yirmiya and Goshen, 2011). Sickness behaviours are typically short-lasting and rapidly resolve, following resolution of the infection. Though once considered to be non-specific actions of the infecting organism, demonstration that they are readily induced by pro-inflammatory cytokines, such as IL-1, TNF, and IL-6, has identified them as an integral part of the host response. Running concurrent with activation of the innate immune system, pro-inflammatory cytokines act on the brain to reorient motivation and prioritize whole organism responses to fighting the infection and preserving bodily integrity (Dantzer et al., 2008).

The relevance of sickness behaviours to psychiatry stems from their remarkable similarity to symptoms of depression. Furthermore, when inflammation is severe or prolonged, true major depressive episodes frequently emerge (Raison et al., 2006). Elevated pro-inflammatory cytokines are also consistently reported

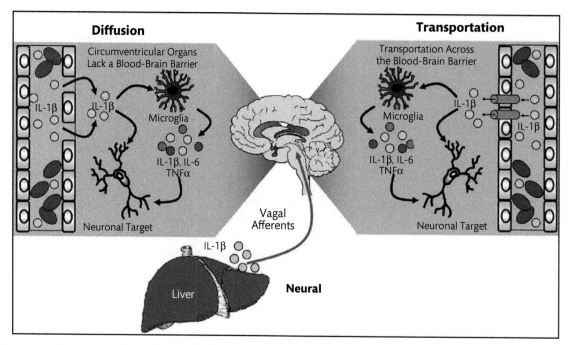

Fig. 14.3 Immune–brain communicating pathways. The figure illustrates the three main immune–brain communicating pathways, including cytokine activation of visceral afferents, cytokine diffusion at regions expressing a fenestrated BBB and active cytokine transport. Pro-inflammatory cytokines can also signal across the BBB by triggering the endothelial release of prostaglandin E2. Innate immune cells, such as monocytes/macrophages, may also cross the BBB in small numbers.

in patients with MDD (Dowlati et al., 2010). One of the most important recent developments in psychiatry was the discovery that prolonged administration of pro-inflammatory cytokines, notably IFN-α, can precipitate major depressive episodes, even in previously euthymic individuals (Musselman et al., 2001). Subsequently, studies of patients with IFN-α -induced depression have shown marked similar patterns of brain dysfunction to those observed in idiopathic MDD (Harrison, 2017). They have also demonstrated that pro-inflammatory cytokines modulate a number of enzymes involved in monoamine synthesis, including indoleamine 2,3-deoxygenase (IDO), a key enzyme in the synthesis of serotonin (Dantzer et al., 2008). Recently, immunotherapeutics, such as etanercept that blocks TNF signalling, have also been shown to improve depressive symptoms (Tyring et al., 2006), even in some patients with treatment-resistant depression (Raison et al., 2013). These trials offer a potentially bright future for immunotherapies in psychiatry.

Conclusion

This chapter serves to introduce the clinician to a number of important immunological concepts that are fundamental to understanding the immune system's role in healthy brain development and function and its contribution to neuropsychiatric disorders. It is by no means a complete overview of the immune system but instead focuses on processes and pathways that are of particular relevance to psychiatry. As we hope we have illustrated in this chapter, recent conceptual advances have identified a multitude of different mechanisms through which the immune system may (or does) contribute to mental illness. This ranges from the role of MHC in neural development and possibly schizophrenia aetiology to the ability of pro-inflammatory cytokines to induce MDD. As we learn more about the mechanisms through which the immune system interacts with our brain to alter behaviour, we step closer to untangling the complex aetiological processes behind many neuropsychiatric diseases. Excitingly, the nascent field of immunopsychiatry offers a range of new therapeutic options for tackling what are currently some of the most common and disabling human illnesses.

KEY LEARNING POINTS

* Neuroimmunology is a rapidly developing field, challenging the age-old notion of the CNS as an immune-privileged site with limited immune function.
* Within the last two decades, new technologies have demonstrated that immune processes play a critical role in normal CNS development, are integral to fundamental neurological processes such as long-term potentiation and synaptic plasticity, and are implicated in pathologies ranging from narcolepsy to depression, schizophrenia, and AD.

- They indicate that immunology and mental illness are fundamentally intertwined, opening exciting new avenues for future immunotherapies tackling psychiatric disease. Here we review basic immune mechanisms, specifically highlighting processes that are of particular relevance to neuropsychiatry.

REFERENCES

Banks, W.A. (2015) The blood-brain barrier in neuroimmunology: Tales of separation and assimilation *Brain, Behavior, and Immunity* 44, 1–8.

Banks, W.A. (2016) From blood-brain barrier to blood-brain interface: new opportunities for CNS drug delivery. *Nature Reviews Drug Discovery* 15, 275–92.

Banks, W.A., Gray, A.M., Erickson, M.A., et al. (2015) Lipopolysaccharide-induced blood-brain barrier disruption: roles of cyclooxygenase, oxidative stress, neuroinflammation, and elements of the neurovascular unit. *Journal of Neuroinflammation* 2, 223.

Block, M.L., Zecca, L., Hong, J.S. (2007) Microglia-mediated neurotoxicity: uncovering the molecular mechanisms. *Nature Reviews Neuroscience* 8, 57–69.

Bloomfield, P.S., Selvaraj, S., Veronese, M., et al. (2016) Microglial Activity in People at Ultra High Risk of Psychosis and in Schizophrenia: An [(11)C]PBR28 PET Brain Imaging Study. *American Journal of Psychiatry* 173, 44–52.

Brydon, L., Harrison, N.A., Walker, C., Steptoe, A., Critchley, H.D. (2008) Peripheral Inflammation is Associated with Altered Substantia Nigra Activity and Psychomotor Slowing in Humans. *Biological Psychiatry* 63, 1022–9.

Capuron, L., Gumnick J.F., Musselman D.L., et al. (2002) Neurobehavioral Effects of Interferon-alpha in Cancer Patients: Phenomenology and Paroxetine Responsiveness of Symptom Dimensions *Neuropsychopharmacology* 12, 643–52.

Carpenter, L.L., Gawuga, C.E., Tyrka, A.R., Lee, J.K., Anderson, G.M., Price, L.H. (2010) Association between Plasma IL-6 Response to Acute Stress and Early-Life Adversity in Healthy Adults. *Neuropsychopharmacology* 35, 2617–23.

Chen, G.Y., Nuñez, G. (2010) Sterile inflammation: sensing and reacting to damage. *Nature Reviews Immunology* 10, 826–37.

Conductier, G., Blondeau, N., Guyon, A., Nahon, J.L., Rovere, C. (2010) The role of monocyte chemoattractant protein MCP1/CCL2 in neuroinflammatory diseases. *Journal of Neuroimmunology* 224, 93–100.

Correale, J., Fiol, M., Gilmore, W. (2006) The risk of relapses in multiple sclerosis during systemic infections. *Neurology* 67, 652–9.

Corvin, A., Morris, D.W. (2014) Genome-wide association studies: Findings at the major histocompatibility complex locus in psychosis. *Biological Psychiatry* 75, 276–83.

Critchley, H.D., Harrison, N.A. (2013) Visceral influences on brain and behavior. *Neuron* 77, 624–38.

Cunningham, C. (2011) Systemic inflammation and delirium—important co-factors in the progression of dementia. *Biochemical Society Transactions* 39, 945–53.

Dantzer, R., O'Connor, J.C., Freund, G.G., Johnson, R.W., Kelley, K.W. (2008) From inflammation to sickness and depression: when the immune system subjugates the brain. *Nature Reviews Neuroscience* 9, 46–56.

da Silva, E.Z., Jamur, M.C., Oliver, C. (2014) Mast cell function: a new vision of an old cell. *Journal of Histochemistry and Cytochemistry* 62, 698–738.

Dauvilliers, Y., Arnulf, I., Mignot, E. (2007) Narcolepsy with cataplexy. *Lancet* 369, 499–511.

Dowlati, Y., Herrmann, N., Swardfager, W., et al. (2010) A Meta-Analysis of Cytokines in Major Depression. *Biological Psychiatry* 67, 446–7.

Esposito, P., Gheorghe, D., Kandere, K., et al. (2001) Acute stress increases permeability of the blood-brain-barrier through activation of brain mast cells. *Brain Research* 888, 117–27.

Filiano, A.J., Xu, Y., Tustison, N.J., et al. (2016) Unexpected role of interferon-γ in regulating neuronal connectivity and social behaviour. *Nature* 535, 425–9.

Goehler, L.E., Gaykema, R.P.A., Hansen, M.K., Anderson, K., Maier, S.F., Watkins, L.R. (2000) Vagal immune-to-brain communication: A visceral chemosensory pathway. *Autonomic Neuroscience: Basic and Clinical* 85, 49–59.

Gross, P.M. (1991) Morphology and physiology of capillary systems in subregions of the subfornical organ and area postrema. *Canadian Journal of Physiology and Pharmacology* 69, 1010–25.

Harrison, N.A. (2017) Brain Structures Implicated in Inflammation-Associated Depression. *Current Topics in Behavioral Neurosciences* 31, 221–48.

Harrison, N.A., Brydon, L., Walker, C., Gray, M.A., Steptoe, A., Critchley, H.D. (2009a) Inflammation Causes Mood Changes Through Alterations in Subgenual Cingulate Activity and Mesolimbic Connectivity. *Biological Psychiatry* 66, 407–14.

Harrison, N.A., Brydon, L., Walker, C., et al. (2009b) Neural Origins of Human Sickness in Interoceptive Responses to Inflammation. *Biological Psychiatry* 66, 415–22.

Harrison, N.A., Doeller, C.F., Voon, V., Burgess, N., Critchley, H.D. (2014) Peripheral Inflammation Acutely Impairs Human Spatial Memory via Actions on Medial Temporal Lobe Glucose Metabolism. *Biological Psychiatry* 76, 585–93.

Harrison, N.A., Voon, V., Cercignani, M., Cooper, E.A., Pessiglione, M., Critchley, H.D. (2016) A Neurocomputational Account of How Inflammation Enhances Sensitivity to Punishments Versus Rewards. *Biological Psychiatry* 80, 73–81.

Hart, B.L. (1988) Biological basis of the behavior of sick animals. *Neuroscience and Biobehavioral Reviews* 12, 123–37.

Holmes, C., Cunningham, C., Zotova, E., et al. (2009) Systemic inflammation and disease progression in Alzheimer disease. *Neurology* 73, 768–74.

Hong, S., Beja-Glasser, V.F., Nfonoyim, B.M., et al. (2016) Complement and microglia mediate early synapse loss in Alzheimer mouse models. *Science* 352, 712–16.

Hutchinson, M.R., Zhang, Y., Brown, K., et al. (2008) Non-stereoselective reversal of neuropathic pain by naloxone and naltrexone: involvement of toll-like receptor 4 (TLR4). *European Journal of Neuroscience* 28, 20–9.

Iliff, J.J., Wang, M., Liao, Y., et al. (2012) A Paravascular Pathway Facilitates CSF Flow Through the Brain Parenchyma and the Clearance of Interstitial Solutes, Including Amyloid β. *Science Translational Medicine* 4, 147ra111.

Iwashyna, T.J., Ely, E.W., Smith, D.M., Langa, K.M. (2010) Long-term cognitive impairment and functional disability among survivors of severe sepsis. *JAMA* 304, 1787–94.

Jansen, R., Penninx, B.W.J.H., Madar, V., et al. (2016) Gene expression in major depressive disorder. *Molecular Psychiatry* 21, 339–47.

Khandaker, G.M., Pearson, R.M., Zammit, S., Lewis, G., Jones, P.B. (2015) Association of serum interleukin 6 and C-reactive protein in childhood with depression and psychosis in young adult life: a population-based longitudinal study. *JAMA Psychiatry* 71, 1121–8.

Kipnis, J. (2016) Multifaceted interactions between adaptive immunity and the central nervous system. *Science* 353, 766–71.

Kipnis, J., Gadani, S., and Derecki, N.C. (2012) Pro-cognitive properties of T cells. *Nature Reviews Immunology* 12, 663–9.

Koenig, W., Sund, M., Frohlich, M., et al. (1999) C-Reactive protein, a sensitive marker of inflammation, predicts future risk of coronary heart disease in initially healthy middle-aged men: results from the MONICA (Monitoring Trends and Determinants in Cardiovascular Disease) Augsburg Cohort Study, 1984 to 1992. *Circulation* 99, 237–42.

Kreutzberg, G.W. (1996) Microglia: a sensor for pathological events in the CNS. *Trends in Neurosciences* 19, 312–18.

Krishnadas, R., Harrison, N.A. (2016) Depression Phenotype, Inflammation, and the Brain: Implications for Future Research. *Psychosomatic Medicine* 78, 384–8.

Krueger, J.M., Rector, D.M., Roy, S., Van Dongen, H.P., Belenky, G., Panksepp, J. (2008) Sleep as a fundamental property of neuronal assemblies. *Nature Reviews Neuroscience* 9, 910–19.

Laflamme, N., Rivest, S. (2001) Toll-like receptor 4: the missing link of the cerebral innate immune response triggered by circulating gram-negative bacterial cell wall components. *FASEB* 15, 155–63.

Louveau, A., Harris, T.H., Kipnis, J. (2015a) Revisiting the Mechanisms of CNS Immune Privilege. *Trends in Immunology* 36, 569–77.

Louveau, A., Smirnov, I., Keyes, T.J., et al. (2015b) Structural and functional features of central nervous system lymphatic vessels. *Nature* 523, 337–41.

Lucin, K.M., Wyss-Coray, T. (2009) Immune Activation in Brain Aging and Neurodegeneration: Too Much or Too Little? *Neuron* 64, 110–22.

Miller, B.J., Buckley, P., Seabolt, W., Mellor, A., Kirkpatrick, B. (2011) Meta-analysis of cytokine alterations in schizophrenia: clinical status and antipsychotic effects. *Biological Psychiatry* 70, 663–71.

Musselman, D.L., Lawson, D.H., Gumnick, J.F., et al. (2001) Paroxetine for the Prevention of Depression Induced by High-Dose Interferon Alfa. *New England Journal of Medicine* 344, 961–6.

Nedergaard, M. (2013) Garbage truck of the brain. *Science* 340, 1529–30.

Nimmerjahn, A., Kirchhoff, F., Helmchen, F. (2005) Resting microglial cells are highly dynamic surveillants of brain parenchyma *in vivo*. *Science* 308, 1314–18.

Okun, E., Griffioen, K.J., Mattson, M.P. (2011) Toll-like receptor signaling in neural plasticity and disease. *Trends in Neurosciences* 34, 269–81.

Park, E.J., Lee, J.-H., Jeong, D.-C., Han, S.-I., Jeon, Y.-W. (2015) Natural killer cell activity in patients with major depressive disorder treated with escitalopram. *International Immunopharmacology* 28, 409–13.

Partinen, M., Kornum, B.R., Plazzi, G., Jennum, P., Julkunen, I., Vaarala, O. (2014) Narcolepsy as an autoimmune disease: the role of H1N1 infection and vaccination. *The Lancet Neurology* 13, 600–13.

Perry, V.H., Holmes, C. (2014) Microglial priming in neurodegenerative disease. *Nature Reviews Neurology* 10, 217–24.

Pugh, C.R., Fleshner, M., Watkins, L.R., Maier, S.F., Rudy, J.W. (2001) The immune system and memory consolidation: a role for the cytokine IL-1β. *Neuroscience and Biobehavioral Reviews* 25, 29–41.

Raison, C.L., Capuron, L., Miller, A.H. (2006) Cytokines sing the blues: inflammation and the pathogenesis of depression. *Trends Immunology* 27, 24–31.

Raison, C.L., Rutherford, R.E., Woolwine, B.J., et al. (2013) A randomized controlled trial of the tumor necrosis factor antagonist infliximab for treatment-resistant depression: the role of baseline inflammatory biomarkers. *JAMA Psychiatry* 70, 31–41.

Ransohoff, R.M., Cardona, A.E. (2010) The myeloid cells of the central nervous system parenchyma. *Nature* 468, 253–62.

Ransohoff, R.M., Perry, V.H. (2009) Microglial physiology: Unique stimuli, specialized responses. *Annual Review of Immunology*, 119–45.

Rennels, M.L., Gregory, T.F., Blaumanis, O.R., Fujimoto, K., Grady, P.A. (1985) Evidence for a 'Paravascular' fluid circulation in the mammalian central nervous system, provided by the rapid distribution of tracer protein throughout the brain from the subarachnoid space. *Brain Research* 326, 47–63.

Saijo, K., Glass, C.K. (2011) Microglial cell origin and phenotypes in health and disease. *Nature Reviews Immunology* 11, 775–87.

Saper, C.B., Romanovsky, A.A., Scammell, T.E. (2012) Neural circuitry engaged by prostaglandins during the sickness syndrome. *Nature Neuroscience* 15, 1088–95.

Schafer, D.P., Lehrman, E.K., Kautzman, A.G., et al. (2012) Microglia Sculpt Postnatal Neural Circuits in an Activity and Complement-Dependent Manner. *Neuron* 74, 691–705.

Schulz, C., Gomez Perdiguero, E., Chorro, L., et al. (2012) A lineage of myeloid cells independent of Myb and hematopoietic stem cells. *Science* 336, 86–90.

Setiawan, E., Wilson, A.A., Mizrahi, R., et al. (2015) Role of translocator protein density, a marker of neuroinflammation, in the brain during major depressive episodes. *JAMA Psychiatry* 72, 268–75.

Shatz, C.J. (2009) MHC Class I: An Unexpected Role in Neuronal Plasticity. *Neuron* 64, 40–5.

Shi, J., Levinson, D.F., Duan, J., et al. (2009) Common variants on chromosome 6p22.1 are associated with schizophrenia. *Nature* 460, 753–7.

Stone, K.D., Prussin, C., Metcalfe, D.D. (2010) IgE, mast cells, basophils, and eosinophils. *Journal of Allergy and Clinical Immunology* 125 Supplement 2, S73–80.

Tillett, W.S., Francis, T. (1930) Serological reactions in pneumonia with a non-protein somatic fraction of pneumococcus. *Journal of Experimental Medicine*, 52, 561–71.

Torrey, E.F., Yolken, R.H. (2001) The schizophrenia-rheumatoid arthritis connection: Infectious, immune, or both? *Brain, Behavior, and Immunity* 15, 401–10.

Tyring, S., Gottlieb, A., Papp, K., et al. (2006) Etanercept and clinical outcomes, fatigue, and depression in psoriasis: Double-blind placebo-controlled randomised phase III trial. *The Lancet* 367, 29–35.

Uher, R., Tansey, K.E., Dew, T., et al. (2014) An inflammatory biomarker as a differential predictor of outcome of depression treatment with escitalopram and nortriptyline. *American Journal of Psychiatry* 171, 1278–86.

Wynn, T.A., Chawla, A., Pollard, J.W. (2013) Macrophage biology in development, homeostasis and disease. *Nature* 496, 445–55.

Yirmiya, R., Goshen, I. (2011) Immune modulation of learning, memory, neural plasticity and neurogenesis. *Brain, Behavior, and Immunity* 25, 181–213.

15

Neuropsychiatry of consciousness

David Linden

Introduction

The definition and understanding of consciousness is a matter of ongoing philosophical enquiry (Cavanna and Nani, 2012 and 2014; Linden, 2015). For clinical purposes, a working definition might be that consciousness denotes a combination of wakefulness and awareness that enables people to process and respond to sensory stimuli. This capacity can be diminished through disturbances of wakefulness, awareness, or both. The impairment of wakefulness and awareness is captured by the hierarchy of levels of consciousness that range from the normal vigilant state to deep coma. Isolated impairments of awareness with a preserved sleep–wake cycle can be ordered along a hierarchy of minimally conscious states/unresponsive wakefulness (Laureys, 2005). Transient states of reduced awareness with preserved wakefulness occur during epileptic attacks. There are also states in which wakefulness is reduced, but participants have very active mental processing, Dreaming is a classical example, but we would generally not equate the sensory experiences of a dream with awareness, except perhaps in the rare cases of lucid dreaming.

In addition to these impairments of consciousness, also termed 'quantitative disorders of consciousness', psychopathologists, especially in the German tradition, have also classified 'qualitative disorders of consciousness', which include dissociative states, psychotic experiences, and states of disorientation and delirium.

This chapter provides an overview of clinical presentations that include quantitative and/or qualitative disturbances of consciousness (see Box 15.1) and discusses the associated pathologies and underlying neurophysiological mechanisms. It finally sets out a number of challenging clinical scenarios that involve—or may appear to involve—disturbed consciousness and in which neuropsychiatric expertise is particularly needed in order to arrive at the correct diagnosis and management plan.

Clinical syndromes with impaired or altered consciousness

Impaired consciousness

In standard clinical terminology, the gradual reduction of consciousness during pathological states follows the steps of 'somnolence', 'stupor' ('sopor' is also used to describe a broadly similar state

and is a more specific term because 'stupor' is used differently in psychiatry), and 'coma' (ICD-10: R40). The level of reduced consciousness can be measured with several observational scales, the best known of which is the Glasgow Coma Scale (GCS). The GCS evaluates a patient's eye movements and motor and verbal responses. Whereas a patient in sopor can be aroused from the state of unresponsiveness by vigorous and repeated stimuli, patients in deep coma will not even respond to intensely painful stimuli. A similar state can be induced pharmacologically (general anaesthesia).

Delirium, in the definition of the DSM-5 (American Psychiatric Association and American Psychiatric Association. DSM-5 Task Force, 2013), is characterized by a 'disturbance in attention (i.e. reduced ability to direct, focus, sustain, and shift attention) and awareness' (see also Chapter 36). Although this disturbance is largely quantitative (a reduction in awareness of the environment and one's own relationship to it, as also described by the term 'clouding of consciousness'), delirium is commonly subsumed under qualitative, rather than quantitative, disorders of consciousness (in traditions where such a distinction is made—this applies more to Continental Europe than to Anglo-American psychiatry). A reason may be that motor and perceptual symptoms that often form part of delirium resemble the altered mental states (e.g. hallucinations, twilight states) discussed later.

Transient states of unresponsiveness occur during epileptic and non-epileptic seizures and syncope and pseudosyncope (Blumenfeld and Meador, 2014; Mostacci et al., 2011; Raj et al., 2014) These are generally self-limiting and can be accompanied by purposeless movements ('automatisms') or tonic–clonic movements in different types of seizures (see Chapter 17). Unresponsiveness is also a feature of the motionless form of catatonia (see Chapter 37), which is characterized by stupor, mutism, and negativism. Because, in many cases, no meaningful communication is possible, it will be very difficult to assess the patient's level of alertness and awareness.

At the other end of the spectrum, states of hypervigilance that are characterized by abnormally increased arousal and constant scanning of the environment for potential threats have been associated with anxiety disorders, particularly post-traumatic stress disorder (PTSD). Another type of heightened awareness or 'expanded consciousness' can accompany acute episodes of psychotic disorder or be induced by psychedelic drugs. Patients often report particularly intensive sensations, e.g. extraordinary brightness of

Box 15.1 A classification of disorders of consciousness

Impairments of awareness and wakefulness
- Somnolence
- Sopor (stupor)
- Syncope/pseudosyncope
- Generalized seizures
- Concussion
- Coma

Globally impaired awareness with preserved wakefulness
- Persistent:
  - UWS
  - MCS
  - Akinetic mutism
- Transient:
  - Complex partial seizures
  - Some dissociative states
  - Some catatonic states

Partially impaired awareness with preserved wakefulness
- Neglect/extinction
- Anosognosia
- Alien limb syndromes

Qualitative disturbances of consciousness
- Delirium
- Derealization/ depersonalization
- Fugue
- Twilight states
- Hallucinations

This list is not exhaustive, and overlap and transitions between the different types of disturbed consciousness are possible.

light and trance-like or ecstatic experiences. Because of the alteration of perceptual experiences and their particular affect, these psychedelic states are also classified among the qualitative disorders of consciousness.

Dissociations between wakefulness and awareness

Persistent vegetative state (PVS)—also called apallic syndrome or unresponsive wakefulness syndrome (UWS) (Laureys et al., 2010)—and minimally conscious state (MCS) are disorders of consciousness with partly preserved wakefulness, but absent (UWS) or diminished (MCS) awareness (Bernat, 2009). Patients in UWS breathe independently, can have their eyes open, and move spontaneously, but not purposefully. Moreover, they do not communicate and do not follow any commands. However, they have an intact sleep–wake cycle. Patients with MCS respond variably and show some directed movements, but their communication is limited to simple gestures or verbal responses. Both UWS and MCS patients are bed-bound and totally dependent on 24-hour care. Patients can stay in UWS or MCS for many years, and some can fully recover awareness, even after years or decades (Gosseries et al., 2011). Another disorder of communication (but not of consciousness) arises when the higher brain areas are separated from their output pathways by a stroke or other lesion of the upper brainstem. In this 'locked-in syndrome', patients are fully alert and aware but may only be able to give 'yes' and 'no' signals through vertical eye or lid movements. In the very rare cases where even these movements are no longer possible, e.g. as a consequence of late-stage motor neurone disease, communication

can be attempted through brain–computer interfaces (BCIs). BCIs use brain signals, picked up by EEG or fMRI, for the control of an output device, e.g. a computer mouse. If a patient is capable of controlling the relevant brain signal, he/she would also be able to give answers through the BCI (Linden, 2014).

Several studies of patients with UWS who apparently followed commands to engage in a specific mental activity during fMRI attracted widespread attention. In one such study, a patient was asked to imagine playing tennis, and higher motor areas showed activity during these instructions. Such findings suggest that purely clinical measures of responsiveness may underestimate the level of cortical activity (Bernat, 2009). In a study that examined the ability of 54 patients with a long-standing disorder of consciousness to modulate their brain activity with fMRI, five patients showed signs of awareness and cognitive activity (Monti et al., 2010). Because patients can survive in UWS or MCS for many years—generally life expectancy is between 2 and 5 years—and the average survival time in the locked-in state is about 6 years (Gosseries et al., 2011), such improved diagnostic and prognostic assessments are of great clinical importance.

Akinetic mutism describes a syndrome of immobility and lack of communication, although occasional reactions to strong stimuli can occur and patients may pursue an object with their gaze. Unlike patients with locked-in syndrome, patients do not show any interest in communication. By the nature of the syndrome, it is often impossible to distinguish whether it is produced by impaired consciousness or severely reduced motivation and drive, although it is hard to see how full awareness could be preserved in the absence of communicative intentionality. It has also been suggested that akinetic mutism is a subtype of MCS (Formisano et al., 2011).

Altered mental states

Most of the disorders described earlier (with the exception of the hypervigilant states and the transient loss of consciousness during seizures, syncopes, and similar attacks) were characterized by a pervasive and often long-lasting disturbance of consciousness that entailed severe restrictions in basic functions and dependency on care. However, consciousness can also be impaired in a more circumscribed and/or transient fashion. These largely qualitative disorders of consciousness or altered mental states can be associated with a variety of psychiatric or neurological conditions. They include depersonalization, derealization, fugue, twilight states, and hallucinations.

Depersonalization and derealization denote changes in the awareness of oneself or the environment, respectively. In depersonalization, people find it difficult to experience their body and their own emotions and often describe a feeling of being detached from their own body. Derealization describes the feeling that other people or other aspects of the outside world are somehow not real. Patients with derealization also find it difficult to engage emotionally with the environment. Depersonalization and derealization, which often occur in combination, are classified as dissociative symptoms and have to be distinguished from delusional beliefs of unreality. Fugue, another classical dissociative state, describes periods of hours or days (rarely of longer duration) during which patients engage in seemingly purposeful activities (e.g. boarding a train), for which, however, they later have no memory and cannot give an explanation. Although classified as a subtype of dissociative amnesia in the DSM-5, dissociative fugue can also be regarded as a disorder of consciousness because it is often accompanied by changes in self-awareness (adopting a new identity) and confusion. Episodes of fugue can also occur as part of post-ictal states in patients with epilepsy and, rarely, as the sole manifestation of non-convulsive status epilepticus (Khwaja et al., 2013). Fugues have overlapping symptoms with 'twilight states', which are also characterized by automatic movements, confusion, and reduced responsiveness, but generally have a more dream-like character and do not generally include the travelling of the classical fugue.

Hallucinations are perceptual experiences in the absence of adequate sensory stimuli. They can occur in any sensory modality. People experiencing hallucinations might be aware of the particular nature of their experience (that, albeit vivid, their sensations are not produced by outside stimuli). Hallucinations with preserved awareness of the source are sometimes called 'pseudohallucinations', although the intensity of the altered sensory experience may be equal to that of other types of hallucinations. Patients who develop hallucinations as part of a psychotic syndrome are often not aware of the self-generated nature of the sensory experience and may assign delusional meanings to their content, e.g. thinking that they have to obey the instructions provided through so-called command hallucinations.

Acute psychosis, severe affective disorders, and dissociative disorders can also lead to unresponsive states that are sometimes difficult to distinguish from disorders of consciousness. Depressive stupor generally develops as part of a melancholic or psychotic depression and is characterized by lack of verbal and non-verbal communication and general immobility and much reduced intake of food and drink. However, patients are awake and may have a very active inner thought process (such as guilty ruminations), register external stimuli, and/or engage in vivid mental imagery. Thus, unlike the 'stupor' (better termed 'sopor') that marks the transition from somnolence to coma in the hierarchy of quantitative disturbances of consciousness, this 'psychiatric' stupor may occur in a patient who is very much aware of themselves and their environment. Catatonic stupor can arise during different psychotic states or as a component of neuroleptic malignant syndrome (NMS) (White and Robins, 2000) and other medical and neurological conditions (Ahuja, 2000). Because of the absent or severely diminished interaction with the patient, it is difficult to determine whether patients are aware of their surroundings. Patients who develop stupor as part of schizophrenia or an isolated catatonic syndrome may still have active mental processing, whereas NMS generally entails a state of obtundation. Dissociative stupor is another of the rare 'psychiatric' causes of unresponsiveness.

It is impossible to define clear boundaries between (qualitative) disorders of consciousness and other related, and often co-occurring, psychopathological and neuropsychological symptoms and deficits such as thought disorder and amnesia. Clearly, many of the altered mental states described in this section involve impairments of memory and clarity of thought. Conversely, autobiographical amnesia might be described as loss of awareness of past events, and Schneiderian first-rank symptoms of schizophrenia involve altered self-awareness. However, thought disorder and amnesia are considered elsewhere in textbooks of psychopathology and neuropsychology (and indeed, disorders of memory are discussed in detail in Chapter 25). Confining the discussion to the classical disorders of consciousness hence seems to be appropriate for the purposes of this introduction into the neuropsychiatry of consciousness.

Neuroanatomy and neurophysiology of disturbances of consciousness

The dissociation of preserved wakefulness and impaired awareness in UWS and MCS is thought to be caused by the different neural representation of these functions. Wakefulness is supported by the ascending reticular activating system (ARAS), which can be unaffected in patients with cortical lesions, whereas awareness relies on cortico-thalamic systems. The reticular formation in the brainstem is the core of the ARAS. The reticular formation is composed of groups of neurones that are chemically and functionally heterogenous and spread throughout the medulla oblongata, pons, and midbrain. Its median strand—the raphe nuclei—contains serotonergic nuclei. Other main neurotransmitters of the reticular formation are acetylcholine, histamine, and noradrenaline, and orexin (hypocretin) also seems to play a role. The ARAS projects to the cortex via thalamic and intralaminar nuclei, and to the basal forebrain and limbic system through the hypothalamus. Cholinergic nuclei linked to the ARAS include the nucleus basalis of Meynert and the mesopontine and pedunculopontine nuclei. The main noradrenergic nucleus is the locus caeruleus of the pons, which has multiple cortical projections. It is thought that, whereas a functioning ARAS is required for basic arousal and wakefulness, its cortical projections are needed to enable sensory perception and awareness (Jellinger, 2009).

Both a sufficient level of arousal and intact cortical processing are likely required for awareness of externally or internally generated stimuli and sensory experiences. A sufficient level of arousal generally amounts to wakefulness, although a special case of awareness—dreaming—occurs during sleep, but only if some level of arousal is provided, which is the case during REM sleep. During wakefulness, which requires intact function of the ARAS, coordinated activity between primary sensory areas, association areas in the occipital, parietal, temporal, and lateral frontal cortices, and medial frontal areas (including the cingulate cortex) for monitoring of the environment is required for full awareness of external sensory stimuli (Rees, 2013).

Coma can be caused by a primary disturbance of parts of the ARAS in the brainstem or thalamus or by primary cerebral or cerebellar lesions that disrupt its function. Direct lesions of the ARAS can arise from thalamic and brainstem strokes and TBI. Mass lesions in parts of the cortex and white matter can cause compression of subthalamic and mesencephalic parts of the ARAS, e.g. through transtentorial herniation of the temporal lobe, and cerebellar lesions can compress adjacent parts of the brainstem. Coma can also result from diffuse and widespread damage to the thalamus and cortex, e.g. caused by TBI with contusions and diffuse axonal injury, hypoxia, or inflammatory processes. Widespread thalamocortical damage resulting in coma is not always accompanied by discernible pathological signs on brain imaging. If the underlying process is metabolic or toxic or a generalized seizure, current structural imaging techniques may not be sensitive enough to detect the correlates of nerve damage. However, in these cases, functional techniques, such as EEG, or perfusion imaging with SPECT or PET will often show marked abnormalities (Haupt et al., 2015).

Disturbances of consciousness arise if the general metabolic activity of the brain and its blood supply system drop below a certain level. The normal rate of cerebral blood flow is approximately 55 mL/min/100 g of brain tissue, and an acute drop of 50% generally causes impaired consciousness, accompanied by slowing of the EEG, and a drop below 12–15 mL/min/100 g leads to loss of consciousness. To maintain alertness, it is also necessary that the brain extracts sufficient amounts of oxygen from blood, and a cerebral metabolic rate of oxygen below 2 mg/min/100 g generally leads to disturbed consciousness (Ropper et al., 2014). These metabolic changes can be caused by global ischaemia, anoxia, or a wide range of other homeostatic and toxic disturbances, leading to generalized encephalopathies, as discussed in standard textbooks of neurology, e.g. see Chapter 40, 'The acquired metabolic disorders of the nervous system' in Adams and Victor's *Principles of Neurology* (Ropper et al., 2014). Of course, coma can also be induced in medical settings by inhalation or intravenous anaesthetics, most of which depress neural activity through direct action on inotropic neurotransmitter (GABA or glutamate) receptors or other ion channels (Khan et al., 2014a and b).

Loss of consciousness resulting from brain damage can be transient, lasting from only minutes to several days, particularly in acute, reversible conditions such as epilepsy, drug overdose, treatable brain haemorrhage, or encephalitis. Prolonged loss of consciousness is called coma. In many cases, particularly those caused by anoxia, ischaemia, and widespread traumatic damage, prognosis is poor and the patient may never wake up again, although basic vital functions may remain intact for some time. In patients who do not fully recover from their coma, the possible outcomes are brain death, locked-in syndrome, and UWS, defined as a state of wakefulness without awareness that persists over a month after the initial brain injury. Although brainstem functions are intact in UWS, brain metabolism remains low at about 40–50% of its normal level. Patients may progress to MCS, which is characterized by a less severe reduction in brain metabolism (20–40%) and signs of some recovered cortical function such as occasional responses to verbal commands (Gosseries et al., 2011).

Akinetic mutism, which describes a clinical syndrome similar to MCS, has been associated with lesions of the paramedian strands of the reticular formation in the diencephalon or midbrain or of the bilateral frontal lobes, particularly bilateral lesions of the anterior cingulate cortex after anterior cerebral artery strokes (Devinsky et al., 1995).

Locked-in syndrome can occur after lesions of the upper brainstem. The main cause of sudden locked-in syndrome is basilar artery stroke, whereas it develops surreptitiously in motor neurone disease. If cortical functions are spared, patients may be completely alert and cognitively able, although cognitive deficits can occur if cortical areas are affected as well.

Reduced cerebral perfusion associated with loss of consciousness also occurs as part of the normal sleep–wake cycle (deep or 'slow-wave' sleep) and transiently in patients with autonomic dysregulation syndromes (syncope). However, there are also instances in which consciousness is transiently impaired with normal (psychogenic pseudosyncope), or even increased (epileptic seizures), perfusion and EEG activity, the pathophysiological mechanisms of which

are poorly understood. The transient unresponsive states with automatisms that are subsumed under the syndrome of complex partial seizures are most commonly associated with foci in the medial temporal lobes.

Delirium, twilight states, and dissociative alterations of consciousness are not associated with any characteristic focal lesions. In post-ictal twilight states, cerebral perfusion may be reduced and EEG activity suppressed, but the metabolic changes associated with dissociative states have not been clarified and delirium can be associated with a wide range of primary intra- and extracranial pathologies.

Focal brain lesions can lead to loss of, or altered, awareness that is confined to particular objects or locations. The classical example of reduced spatial awareness is hemineglect, which occurs after unilateral (commonly right-sided) lesions to cortical (superior temporal and inferior parietal lobes) and subcortical (pulvinar, putamen, caudate nucleus) structures (Karnath et al., 2001 and 2002; Karnath and Rorden, 2012). Hemineglect is characterized by inability to report stimuli presented on the contralesional side (often affecting multiple sensory domains) and a reduced orienting response, although active exploration of the affected side may still be possible (Karnath, 2015). In some cases, loss of awareness for the stimulus on the affected side of egocentric space is only induced if another stimulus is presented simultaneously on the unaffected side. This 'extinction' phenomenon is generally explained through competition for limited attentional resources (de Haan et al., 2012) and highlights the close link between the concepts of 'attention' and 'awareness'.

Disturbed awareness can also affect individual limbs, most famously in the (rare) 'alien hand syndrome' (AHS). It is characterized by involuntary and apparently purposeful movements, of which the patient is often not aware. In fact, the patient may be convinced that the affected hand does not belong to them. AHS has been observed after a contralateral stroke or other lesions affecting the frontal or parietal lobes or the corticospinal tract, but also after callosal lesions (Kikkert et al., 2006). Another rare syndrome of deficient awareness of a limb can occur in patients who develop hemiparesis or paralysis after a stroke or other lesions affecting the corticospinal tract. This phenomenon, called anosognosia, may be associated with additional lesions to the insula (Karnath and Baier, 2010). Anosognosia in its broader definition describes a lack of awareness for the wider range of consequences of brain damage, e.g. the ensuing cognitive and sensory deficits. It has been associated with (mainly right-sided) lesions of cortical (frontal, parietal, and temporal lobes) structures or the thalamus.

Experimental psychologists have developed techniques to assess the level of processing of stimuli or aspects of stimuli of which patients do not demonstrate any awareness. For example, words presented in the affected hemifield of neglect patients can induce priming, even if they are not consciously perceived (Schweinberger and Stief, 2001). Some patients with hemianopia resulting from unilateral damage of the primary visual cortex in the occipital lobe nevertheless answer forced-choice questions about visual stimuli presented in the 'blind' field, e.g. about their shape or direction of motion. This phenomenon, called 'blindsight' (Stoerig, 2006), points to a crucial role of primary sensory cortices for perceptual awareness, while association areas may be able to support some level of object recognition, even in the absence of a functioning primary cortex.

Physiological techniques can also be useful in showing preserved processing of some aspects of stimuli that are not consciously perceived. For example, skin conductance responses revealed emotional processing of affective stimuli—the emotional content of which was not reported by the patient—in Balint syndrome (Denburg et al., 2009). Balint syndrome is a triad of failure to scan the whole visual scene, failure to coordinate gaze and hand movements, and inability to perceive simultaneously all aspects of a complex visual scene (simultanagnosia). It is generally associated with bilateral damage to the parietal and/or occipital lobes, excluding the primary visual areas. The partial deficits in conscious perception resulting from lesions of association cortices (as discussed here using the examples of Balint syndrome and neglect) reveal that both primary and higher sensory areas need to be intact to enable full awareness of the environment.

The neurophysiological correlates of hallucinations can also provide insight into the mechanisms of perceptual awareness and how it can be uncoupled from sensory processing of external stimuli. We know from the research programme led by the Canadian neurosurgeon Wilder Penfield that direct cortical stimulation in the temporal lobe can induce sensory experiences. Musical hallucinations were most commonly reported by Penfield's patients, followed by other auditory and visual experiences and gustatory and olfactory hallucinations (Linden, 2014; Penfield and Perot, 1963). Functional imaging studies in patients with schizophrenia have shown activity in primary sensory areas during auditory (Dierks et al., 1999) and visual hallucinations (Oertel et al., 2007). A wider network of frontotemporal areas involved in speech production and perception has also been implicated in auditory verbal hallucinations (Jardri et al., 2011). Patients with Charles Bonnet syndrome who develop visual (pseudo-)hallucinations after a decline in their visual function (e.g. with progressing diabetic retinopathy) had increased activity in higher visual areas (Ffytche et al., 1998). These findings again point to the interplay between higher and primary sensory areas in generating fully formed perceptual experiences, which, interestingly, do not necessarily require external sensory input.

Little is known about the neurochemical mechanisms underlying hallucinations occurring as part of neuropsychological or psychopathological syndromes, but the hallucinogenic properties of certain prescription and illicit drugs indicate that stimulation of dopamine and serotonin receptors can lead to hallucinations, particularly in the visual domain (Geyer and Vollenweider, 2008; Hill and Thomas, 2011; Lees, 2016). For neuropsychiatrists, one particular challenge is to balance the beneficial effects of dopaminergic drugs on the motor symptoms of PD against their tendency to induce hallucinations after long-term use in some patients.

Clinical scenarios for the neuropsychiatrist

The specific multidisciplinary expertise of neuropsychiatrists should equip them to evaluate clinically challenging scenarios posed by altered states of consciousness that allow for multiple underlying diagnostic possibilities. In addition, three clinical scenarios

are highlighted that show how the syndromes introduced earlier may be differentiated in clinical practice.

Unresponsiveness

A patient who is awake, but unresponsive, can suffer from an enduring disturbance of awareness (UWS, MCS, akinetic mutism) or from a transient disturbance of awareness and/or communication. In the former case, there will be generally a clear indication as to the long-standing and persistent nature of the problem from the clinical history and evidence for an underlying major brain injury. Transient states of impaired awareness or lack of communication can occur in the context of delirium, epileptic seizures, post-ictal twilight states, dissociative, depressive, or catatonic stupor, and also during intoxications, although in those cases, wakefulness generally would be impaired as well. A thorough investigation of possible general medical, neurological, or psychiatric causes is therefore needed to establish the diagnosis and initiate appropriate treatment. The expertise of the neuropsychiatrist will be helpful in delineating the exact clinical syndrome and prioritizing the necessary investigations, as well as advising on psychotropic medication and, where needed, psychological and behavioural interventions.

Depersonalization and derealization

An altered sense of awareness of one's own body (or a particular part of it) and/or one's environment can occur as part of dissociative syndromes, but also in the context of a wide range of other mental disorders, including depression, generalized anxiety disorder, borderline personality disorder, and psychotic disorders. It can also accompany complex partial seizures or arise as a consequence of a focal brain lesion, as in the case of the 'alien hand syndrome' discussed in the previous section. Intoxication, especially with hallucinogenic substances such as lysergic acid diethylamide (LSD) (Schmid et al., 2015) or cannabis (Johns, 2001), and drug withdrawal can also lead to depersonalization and derealization. A clinical history and neurological and mental state examination will generally reveal the underlying syndrome and its comorbid features, but additional assessments, such as drug testing, EEG, or neuroimaging, may be needed to achieve diagnostic certainty.

Hallucinations

Hallucinations and pseudohallucinations can occur as part of a number of psychiatric/neuropsychiatric syndromes and as a consequence of intoxication or drug withdrawal or as a side effect of prescription drugs. Among the mental disorders, hallucinations are most frequently encountered in schizophrenia and acute and transient psychoses, but they can also occur during episodes of mania or psychotic depression. Pseudohallucinations can be part of the spectrum of dissociative symptoms and perceptual abnormalities reported in borderline personality disorder. Hallucinations can also accompany all types of dementia, most characteristically in the form of visual hallucinations in Lewy body dementia (Linden, 2019). Pseudohallucinations, particularly in the visual domain, are also a common feature of PD (Fénelon et al., 2000), although long-term treatment with dopaminergic drugs may also contribute to their causation. Inflammatory (e.g. in systemic lupus erythematosus) and metabolic encephalopathies also sometimes lead to hallucinations, as do focal lesions caused by brain tumours or strokes. Hallucinations in all sensory domains can also be caused by complex partial seizures. Many drugs of abuse can induce hallucinations during states of both intoxication and withdrawal (Linden, 2019), and hallucinations can occur as side effects of prescription drugs, e.g. visual hallucinations during antidepressant treatment (Cancelli et al., 2004).

Acute visual hallucinations are also a hallmark of delirium and can occur more chronically as part of deafferentation syndromes (Manford and Andermann, 1998; Teeple et al., 2009), e.g. in Charles Bonnet syndrome. Complex visual pseudohallucinations are also part of the auras experienced by many migraine patients (Sacks, 1999), and hypnagogic and hypnopompic hallucinations are classically associated with narcolepsy. This non-exhaustive list of diagnostic possibilities underlines the complexity of the neuropsychiatric assessment of patients presenting with altered mental states and the need for detailed documentation of both the clinical history and the exact nature of the altered perceptual experience.

Conclusion

Consciousness requires wakefulness and awareness, and disturbances of these functions play a central role in many neuropsychiatric syndromes. Neuropsychiatric assessment therefore crucially involves the evaluation of a patient's wakefulness and sleep–wake cycle and of any quantitative or qualitative disturbances of awareness. Beyond global deficits and alterations of awareness, it is also important to explore changes of awareness that are specific to particular situations (e.g. dissociative states), parts of the body (e.g. alien limb syndrome), the environment (e.g, hemineglect) or sensory domains (e.g. hallucinations).

KEY LEARNING POINTS

- Consciousness requires wakefulness and awareness.
- Both are disrupted in deep sleep, general anaesthesia. and coma.
- Dissociation between preserved wakefulness and lack of awareness can persist for many years after coma (UWS).
- Transient disruptions of awareness occur in many neuropsychiatric syndromes, e.g. during complex partial seizures.
- The ARAS of the brainstem is a key driver of arousal and wakefulness.
- Both direct and indirect lesions of the ARAS and its thalamo-cortical projections can lead to coma.
- Specific disorders of awareness, e.g. for aspects of one's own body or certain locations in space, can occur after a variety of focal lesions.
- Neuropsychiatric assessment of consciousness takes account of the medical history and the overall context of the mental state, in order to define the clinical syndrome, and utilizes the appropriate diagnostic tests to identify the underlying disease process.

REFERENCES

Ahuja, N. (2000) Organic catatonia: a review. *Indian J Psychiatry,* 42, 327–46.

American Psychiatric Association DSM-5 Task Force. (2013) *Diagnostic and Statistical Manual of Mental Disorders (DSM-5),* fifth edition. Washington, DC: American Psychiatric Association.

Bernat, J. (2009) Chronic consciousness disorders. *Annu Rev Med,* 60, 381–92.

Blumenfeld, H. and Meador, K.J. (2014) Consciousness as a useful concept in epilepsy classification. *Epilepsia,* 55, 1145–50.

Cancelli, I., Marcon, G., and Balestrieri, M. (2004) Factors associated with complex visual hallucinations during antidepressant treatment. *Hum Psychopharmacol,* 19,577–84.

Cavanna, A.E. and Nani, A. (2012) *Consciousness: States, Mechanisms and Disorders.* Hauppauge, NY: Nova Science.

Cavanna, A.E. and Nani, A. (2014) *Consciousness: Theories in Neuroscience and Philosophy of Mind.* New York, NY: Springer.

de Haan, B., Karnath, H.O., and Driver, J. (2012) Mechanisms and anatomy of unilateral extinction after brain injury. *Neuropsychologia,* 50, 1045–53.

Denburg, N.L., Jones, R.D., and Tranel, D. (2009) Recognition without awareness in a patient with simultanagnosia. *Int J Psychophysiol,* 72, 5–12.

Devinsky, O., Morrell, M.J., and Vogt, B.A. (1995) Contributions of anterior cingulate cortex to behaviour. *Brain,* 118 (Pt 1), 279–306.

Dierks, T., Linden, D.E.J., Jandl, M., et al. (1999) Activation of Heschl's Gyrus during auditory hallucinations. *Neuron,* 22, 615–21.

Ffytche, D., Howard, R., Brammer, M., David, A., Woodruff, P. and Williams, S. (1998) The anatomy of conscious vision: an fMRI study of visual hallucinations. *Nature Neurosci,* 1, 738–42.

Fénelon, G., Mahieux, F., Huon, R., and Ziégler, M. (2000) Hallucinations in Parkinson's disease: prevalence, phenomenology and risk factors. *Brain,* 123 (Pt 4), 733–45.

Formisano, R., D'Ippolito, M., Risetti, M., et al. (2011) Vegetative state, minimally conscious state, akinetic mutism and Parkinsonism as a continuum of recovery from disorders of consciousness: an exploratory and preliminary study, *Funct Neurol,* 26,15–24.

Geyer, M. and Vollenweider, F. (2008) Serotonin research: contributions to understanding psychoses. *Trends Pharmacol Sci,* 29, 445–53.

Gosseries, O., Vanhaudenhuyse, A., Bruno, M.-A., et al. (2011) Disorders of consciousness: coma, vegetative and minimally conscious states. In: Cvetkovic, D. and Cosic, I. (eds.) *States of Consciousness: Experimental Insights into Meditation, Waking, Sleep and Dreams.* Berlin, Heidelberg: Springer, pp. 29–55.

Haupt, W.F., Hansen, H.C., Janzen, R.W., Firsching, R., and Galldiks, N. (2015) Coma and cerebral imaging. *Springerplus,* 4, 180.

Hill, S.L. and Thomas, S.H. (2011) Clinical toxicology of newer recreational drugs. *Clin Toxicol (Phila),* 49,705–19.

Jardri, R., Pouchet, A., Pins, D., and Thomas, P. (2011) Cortical activations during auditory verbal hallucinations in schizophrenia: a coordinate-based meta-analysis. *Am J Psychiatry,* 168, 73–81.

Jellinger, K.A. (2009) [Functional pathophysiology of consciousness]. *Neuropsychiatr,* 23, 115–33.

Johns, A. (2001) Psychiatric effects of cannabis, *Br J Psychiatry,* 178, 116–22.

Karnath, H.O. (2015) Spatial attention systems in spatial neglect, *Neuropsychologia*, 75, 61–73.

Karnath, H.O. and Baier, B. (2010) Right insula for our sense of limb ownership and self-awareness of actions. *Brain Struct Funct*, 214(5–6), 411–17.

Karnath, H.O., Ferber, S., and Himmelbach, M. (2001) Spatial awareness is a function of the temporal not the posterior parietal lobe. *Nature*, 411, 950–3.

Karnath, H.O., Himmelbach, M., and Rorden, C. (2002) The subcortical anatomy of human spatial neglect: putamen, caudate nucleus and pulvinar. *Brain*, 125(Pt 2), 350–60.

Karnath, H.O. and Rorden, C. (2012) The anatomy of spatial neglect. *Neuropsychologia*, 50, 1010–17.

Khan, K.S., Hayes, I. and Buggy, D.J. (2014a) Pharmacology of anaesthetic agents I: intravenous anaesthetic agents. *Continuing Education in Anaesthesia, Critical Care & Pain*, 14, 100–5.

Khan, K.S., Hayes, I., and Buggy, D.J. (2014b) Pharmacology of anaesthetic agents II: inhalation anaesthetic agents. *Continuing Education in Anaesthesia, Critical Care & Pain*, 14, 106–11.

Khwaja, G.A., Duggal, A., Kulkarni, A., et al. (2013) Recurrent prolonged fugue states as the sole manifestation of epileptic seizures. *Ann Indian Acad Neurol*, 16, 561–4.

Kikkert, M.A., Ribbers, G.M., and Koudstaal, P.J. (2006) Alien hand syndrome in stroke: a report of 2 cases and review of the literature. *Arch Phys Med Rehabil*, 87, 728–32.

Laureys, S. (2005) The neural correlate of (un)awareness: lessons from the vegetative state. *Trends Cogn Sci*, 9, 556–9.

Laureys, S., Celesia, G.G., Cohadon, F., et al. (2010) Unresponsive wakefulness syndrome: a new name for the vegetative state or apallic syndrome. *BMC Med*, 8, 68.

Lees, A. (2016) *Mentored by a Madman*. Notting Hill Editions.

Linden, D. (2014) *Brain Control*. Basingstoke: Palgrave.

Linden, D.E. (2015) Consciousness: theories in neuroscience and philosophy of mind, *Cogn Neuropsychiatry*, 1–3.

Linden, D. (2019) *The Biology of Psychological Disorders*. Red Globe Press.

Manford, M. and Andermann, F. (1998) Complex visual hallucinations. Clinical and neurobiological insights. *Brain*, 121 (Pt 10), 1819–40.

Monti, M., Vanhaudenhuyse, A., Coleman, M., et al. (2010) Willful modulation of brain activity in disorders of consciousness. *N Engl J Med*, 362, 579–89.

Mostacci, B., Bisulli, F., Alvisi, L., Licchetta, L., Baruzzi, A., and Tinuper, P. (2011) Ictal characteristics of psychogenic nonepileptic seizures: what we have learned from video/EEG recordings—a literature review. *Epilepsy Behav*, 22, 144–53.

Oertel, V., Rotarska-Jagiela, A., van de Ven, V.G., Haenschel, C., Maurer, K. and Linden, D.E. (2007) Visual hallucinations in schizophrenia investigated with functional magnetic resonance imaging. *Psychiatry Res*, 156, 269–73.

Penfield, W. and Perot, P. (1963) The brain's record of auditory and visual experience. A final summary and discussion. *Brain*, 86, 595–696.

Raj, V., Rowe, A.A., Fleisch, S.B., et al. (2014) Psychogenic pseudosyncope: diagnosis and management. *Auton Neurosci*, 184, 66–72.

Rees, G. (2013) Neural correlates of consciousness. *Ann N Y Acad Sci*, 1296, 4–10.

Ropper, A., Samuels, M. and Klein, J. (2014) *Adams and Victors Principles of Neurology*, tenth edition. McGraw-Hill Education.

Sacks, O. (1999) *Migraine*. New York, NY: Vintage Books.

Schmid, Y., Enzler, F., Gasser, P., et al. (2015) Acute Effects of Lysergic Acid Diethylamide in Healthy Subjects. *Biol Psychiatry*, 78, 544–53.

Schweinberger, S.R. and Stief, V. (2001) Implicit perception in patients with visual neglect: lexical specificity in repetition priming. *Neuropsychologia*, 39, 420–9.

Stoerig, P. (2006) Blindsight, conscious vision, and the role of primary visual cortex. *Prog Brain Res*, 155, 217–34.

Teeple, R.C., Caplan, J.P., and Stern, T.A. (2009) Visual hallucinations: differential diagnosis and treatment. *Prim Care Companion J Clin Psychiatry*, 11, 26–32.

White, D.A. and Robins, A.H. (2000) An analysis of 17 catatonic patients diagnosed with neuroleptic malignant syndrome. *CNS Spectr*, 5, 58–65.

GLOSSARY

Absence seizure: Epileptic attack, generally of brief (15–20 s) duration, with loss of consciousness with or without other symptoms.

Akinetic mutism: Syndrome of immobility and lack of communication generally attributed to focal brain lesions or neurodegenerative disorders. Patients may show some spontaneous motor activity and response to salient stimuli. This syndrome has also been classified as a subtype of minimally conscious state.

Catatonia: Motor syndrome with reduced or increased psychomotor activity (or a combination of both) and characteristic symptoms such as stereotypic movements, echolalia and echopraxia, and waxy flexibility, which is associated with a range of psychiatric and medical conditions and can arise from toxic effects of psychotropic drugs.

Coma: Prolonged loss of consciousness. Patients cannot be aroused and, depending on the level of brain damage, reflexes may be impaired.

Complex partial seizure: Epileptic attack with lack of awareness and responsiveness and loss of memory for the episode, often involving purposeless movements (automatisms).

Depersonalization: Sense of detachment from one's own person/body.

Derealization: Sense of detachment from the outside world.

Dissociation: Generic term for states and symptoms thought to involve some detachment from reality and often expressed through somatic or psychological symptoms.

Fugue: Transient loss of sense of identity, often coupled with aimless wandering or travelling.

Hallucination: Sensory experience in the absence of adequate external stimulus.

Locked-in syndrome: Inability to communicate because of loss of motor control with preserved consciousness. Causes include ischaemic or neurodegenerative lesions of the midbrain. In incomplete locked-in syndrome, vertical eye movements are still preserved, allowing for some level of communication. Brain computer interfaces may enable communication, even for completely 'locked-in' patients.

Lucid dreaming: A somewhat controversial concept that describes awareness of dreams.

Minimally conscious state (MCS): Severely reduced awareness and communication with preserved sleep–wake cycle.

Non-epileptic attack disorder (NEAD): Dissociative disorder characterized by recurrent attacks that resemble epileptic seizures but are not accompanied by paroxysmal neural activity.

Pseudohallucination: A term sometimes used to describe hallucinations in patients who are aware that their experiences are not evoked by external stimuli.

Pseudosyncope: Transient loss of consciousness without an observable neurological cause and without accompanying reduction in cerebral blood flow or electroencephalographic activity.

Somnolence: A state of drowsiness without spontaneous speech production, but patients can still be aroused and reflexes are preserved.

Sopor: A state resembling sleep that entails reduced consciousness, but patients can be aroused with painful or other strong stimuli, and reflexes are preserved.

Stupor: Lack of responsiveness, as observed in psychotic, affective, catatonic, and dissociative syndromes. This term is sometimes also used to describe sopor, although it is important to remember that these are different concepts, and stupor, as defined by a lack of responsiveness, can be accompanied by preserved awareness.

Syncope: Transient loss of consciousness, caused by a sudden drop in blood perfusion, with a variety of medical causes.

Tonic–clonic seizure: Generalized epileptic seizure with loss of consciousness and involuntary movements and muscle contractions.

Unresponsive wakefulness syndrome (UWS): Also called apallic syndrome or persistent vegetative state. Loss of awareness with preserved sleep–wake cycle and some spontaneous, but not purposeful, movements.

SECTION 2
Core neuropsychiatric conditions

16

Brain injury

Niruj Agrawal

Introduction

Brain injury is a major cause of disability and mortality all around the world, particularly in younger men. Advances in the early management of brain injury, with improvements in imaging techniques, development of brain injury pathways, and better neurosurgical and intensive care management, have improved survival following brain injury. Long-term sequelae with persistent neurocognitive, emotional, and behavioural problems, often collectively referred to as neuropsychiatric, have become increasingly recognized. These problems often determine the functional outcomes, quality of life, and burden on carers, family, and society in general.

Various terms, such as brain injury, head injury, and acquired brain injury (ABI), are often used loosely and interchangeably in clinical settings, creating unnecessary confusion. Clinicians in the past used to differentiate between head injury and brain injury by looking at imaging evidence of structural damage to the brain. Such a differentiation is now considered obsolete, as it is recognized that not all traumatic brain injuries (TBIs) are structurally visible on currently available brain scans, including MRI brain scans with routine sequences. Head injury now often refers to injury to the scalp or skull only without injury to the brain.

Injuries to the brain could be described under the overarching umbrella term 'acquired brain injury' (see Fig. 16.1). This includes the categories of TBIs and non-TBIs. TBIs can be sub-classified into open/penetrating TBIs where there is a fracture of the skull and a breach of the dura mater, or closed TBIs where there is no breach of the skull and dura mater. Closed TBIs are often caused by blunt trauma (assault), fall, accidents at home or work, road traffic collisions, and blast injuries. Blast injuries are commonly encountered in war veterans returning from battlefields. These could result in brain injury, in addition to other injuries, including limb injuries. Non-traumatic ABIs include a range of 'injuries' to the brain, including hypoxic–ischaemic injury, cerebrovascular events (stroke), or other mechanisms, including infections and metabolic or chemical/toxic factors affecting brain functions. This chapter will focus mainly on TBIs and briefly touch upon anoxic brain injury, as some of the other non-TBIs, including stroke, infections, and metabolic and toxic injuries are covered in other chapters. Blast injuries are outside the scope of this chapter.

There can be various mechanisms involved in causing a TBI. These include direct impact on the skull/brain, acceleration–deceleration injuries, and rotational injuries. Blast injuries are also a common cause in battlegrounds. Secondary causes of brain injury include increased intracranial pressure, infection, lack of blood supply, or bleeding inside the skull. Shearing of blood vessels could cause additional injury to the brain, in addition to the mechanism of the initial injury. Generally, the inferior surface of the frontal lobes and the frontal and temporal poles are the most commonly affected areas of visible structural damage to the brain following a TBI.

Extent of the problem

European data from a systematic review involving studies from a number of countries indicate an aggregated hospitalized plus fatal TBI incidence rate of about 235 per 100,000 population per year (Tagliaferri et al., 2006). A mortality rate of about 15 per 100,000 per year was reported. It is widely estimated that 4–8 times this number sustain a brain injury, most of whom either do not attend hospital or may not be recognized to have had a brain injury in accident and emergency departments. In the United States, population-based studies suggest that the incidence of TBI is between 180 and 250 per 100,000 population per year (Bruns and Hauser, 2003). More recently, a study from New Zealand reported a higher incidence of 790 per 100,000 person-years of TBI, but it is argued that this higher incidence is partly due to a wider definition and inclusion of people not admitted to hospital (Andelic, 2013).

Males are about twice as likely as females to sustain a TBI. Children aged 0–4 years and adolescents aged 15–19 years are more likely to sustain a TBI than persons in other age groups (Langlois et al., 2006), For hospitalizations only, adults aged 75 years or older have the highest incidence of TBI. Mortality varies by severity of TBI and is high in those with severe injury and in the elderly.

Commonly, the severity of TBI is defined by a combination of indices, including the Glasgow Coma Scale (GCS) score, the duration of loss of consciousness (LOC), and the duration of post-traumatic amnesia (PTA). In addition, neuroradiological evidence of the extent of damage to the brain can be a useful criterion. The duration of PTA is considered to be the most useful measure in terms of functional outcomes of injury (Ponsford et al., 2016).

Over three-quarters of TBIs are classed as mild and only approximately 6–8% of injuries are classified as severe (see Table 16.1). In

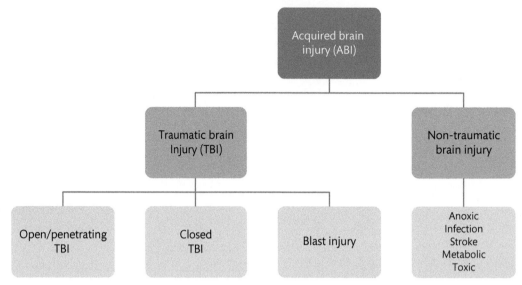

Fig. 16.1 Types of brain injury.

European populations (Tagliaferri et al., 2006), the TBI severity ratio of hospitalized patients was about 22:1.5:1 for mild versus moderate versus severe TBI, respectively.

In recent years, the Mayo Classification System for Traumatic Brain Injury Severity (Malec et al., 2007) has become popular with clinicians and is widely used. This classification system not only takes into account the GCS score and PTA and LOC duration, but also includes other available indicators that include death due to TBI, trauma-related neuroimaging abnormalities, and specified post-concussive symptoms. This system classifies TBI severity into the following three categories: (A) moderate–severe (definite) TBI; (B) mild (probable) TBI; and (C) symptomatic (possible) TBI. For the diagnostic criteria, see Malec et al. (2007).

Aetiology

There are a number of factors, which can determine the occurrence of neuropsychiatric conditions following a TBI (Fig. 16.2). Traditionally, the location of injury-related lesions, its severity, and the extent of structural damage were considered the most important. However, a number of factors not related to the injury can be important determinants of various emotional and behavioural problems. These include pre-injury vulnerability factors, including genetic predisposition for psychiatric problems, premorbid personality, and past or pre-existing psychiatric problems. Environmental factors, such as circumstances of injury, availability of subsequent psychosocial support, the patient's belief about the nature and severity of the injury, and litigation factors could

determine the neuropsychiatric outcome. Some of the post-injury biological processes, such as subclinical epileptiform discharges, endocrinal abnormalities such as hypopituitarism, and various prescribed medications can lead to various emotional and behavioural problems and should be carefully considered, as part of a detailed assessment.

Mild TBI and post-concussion syndrome

Over three-quarters of TBIs are mild in severity. Mild TBI (mTBI) commonly presents with a combination of somatic symptoms, such as headache, dizziness, blurred vision, and neurocognitive

Table 16.1 Severity of TBI

Severity	GCS	PTA	LOC
Mild	13–15	<1 hour	<15 minutes
Moderate	9–12	1–24 hours	15 minutes to 6 hours
Severe	<9	>24 hours	>6 hours

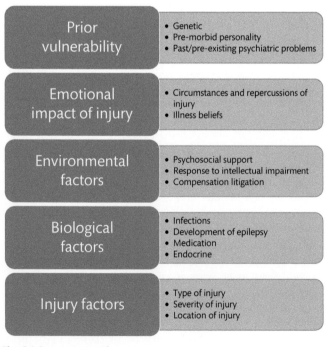

Fig. 16.2 Aetiological factors.

difficulties with attention, concentration, and memory, along with neuropsychiatric symptoms of irritability, anxiety, low mood, fatigue, and sleep disturbance. These features are collectively described as post-concussion syndrome (PCS). This condition, despite being included in the ICD-10, remains a controversial entity because of the non-specific nature of symptoms, which have a huge overlap with various other psychiatric conditions such as anxiety disorders and PTSD. More recently, there have been calls for removing the term PCS completely (Sharpe and Jenkins, 2015) from routine clinical use and diagnostic manuals such as the ICD-10, though others (Marshall et al., 2015) have recommended the development of clear guidelines for clinical use to provide an up-to-date framework for healthcare professionals treating patients with concussion/mTBI. The American classification system in the DSM-5 does not have a specific diagnostic category for this condition.

Generally, the majority of people who have mTBI and develop PCS would show full recovery from PCS in days or weeks after the mTBI, with over 60% improving by 3 months post-injury. However, up to 15% of individuals with mTBI are recognized to continue to experience persisting symptoms, even after 1 year (Marshall et al., 2012). Factors that predispose to a more severe or longer-lasting PCS include: being over the age of 40, female gender, past mTBI, pre- or post-mTBI psychopathology or substance misuse, and pursuing a compensation claim (King and Kirwilliam, 2013). Conditions that frequently occur concurrently with PCS, such as pain, anxiety, depression, and PTSD, are likely to be associated with persistent PCS symptoms. Illness perceptions about the consequences of mTBI on physical, social, and psychological well-being, including the belief that an mTBI will have a serious negative consequence, predicted the development and persistence of PCS (Whittaker et al., 2007).

Various pharmacological and psychological treatments have been proposed for PCS. None of the pharmacological treatments are specifically approved or licensed by the regulatory bodies for this condition. Medications often target the comorbid condition or predominant symptoms such as anxiety and low mood. The commonest medications prescribed are antidepressants, particularly selective serotonin reuptake inhibitors (SSRIs), which are thought to be efficacious in several small, non-randomized, uncontrolled studies and case reports (Hadanny and Efrati, 2016). Non-pharmacological treatment approaches include education and reassurance, cognitive rehabilitation, cognitive behavioural therapy (CBT), and mindfulness-based intervention. Potter, Brown, and Fleminger (2016) carried out a randomized controlled trial (RCT) and reported that outpatient-based CBT can improve quality of life for adults with persistent PCS and potentially reduce symptoms. Future treatments may include exercise-based rehabilitation, repetitive transcranial magnetic stimulation (rTMS), and hyperbaric oxygen therapy, but further studies are needed to prove their clinical effectiveness (Hadanny and Efrati, 2016).

Acute post-traumatic amnesia/post-traumatic agitation

PTA is very common immediately after TBI. It is characterized by confusion, disorientation, and agitation, along with an inability to learn new information (Marshman et al., 2013). It could be of variable duration and its duration correlates with the severity of injury and functional outcomes. PTA can be associated with focal lesions and decreased cerebral perfusion in the frontal and temporal lobes (Metting et al., 2010). However, PTA and associated agitation post-TBI can be seen in patients without any visible structural lesions on brain scans. De Simoni et al. (2016) suggest that the symptoms of PTA are caused by functional disconnection within the default mode network.

A significant clinical manifestation of PTA is associated abnormal behavioural state, often loosely termed as agitation. This is characterized by psychomotor restlessness, emotional lability, disturbed diurnal rhythm, impaired insight, impulsiveness, automatisms, and verbal and physical aggression. There may be autonomic changes associated in the form of tachycardia, transient pyrexia, and clamminess (Marshman et al., 2013).

Post-TBI agitation can also be associated with epilepsy, particularly non-convulsive status, depression, frontal lobe and paralimbic pathology, and a history of alcohol and substance misuse. There is no clear association reported with gender or age. Post-TBI agitation can also be associated with higher chances of subsequent neuropsychiatric problems. Worse outcomes for agitation are associated with a longer duration of agitation, the severity of agitation behaviour, and structural abnormalities on the brain scan (Singh et al., 2014).

Prospective objective assessment of PTA in people after TBI is recommended. Such an assessment not only contributes to the determination of the severity of TBI, but also helps with the diagnosis and in determining the cause of agitation post-brain injury. Scales such as the Westmead PTA Scale (Shores et al., 1986) are now increasingly used prospectively in specialist brain injury services. Detailed clinical assessment of an agitated patient after brain injury will not only involve assessment of PTA but also require a detailed neuropsychiatric assessment to establish past and family history of psychiatric problems, including any personality issues and alcohol and substance misuse, and performing a detailed mental state examination.

Management of agitated behaviour during PTA requires careful management of the environment, with minimization of excessive stimulation, reorientation, and avoidance of restraints while maintaining safety. A wide range of pharmacological agents have been used in agitation following TBI. The evidence base for any pharmacological agents or even classes of medication is poor. Currently, no medication is approved for treatment of agitation after TBI by the FDA in the United States or in any European countries. However, various medications such as atypical neuroleptics and antiepileptic agents, such as carbamazepine, are widely used in the management of patients with acute agitation or aggression.

A Cochrane review found β-blockers, e.g. propranolol and pindolol, in relatively high doses to be effective in controlling post-head injury agitation (Fleminger et al., 2006). However, two RCTs included in this review were of small size and this finding has not been replicated. This review did not find enough evidence for efficacy of other agents such as valproate or carbamazepine. Use of β-blockers need to be carefully monitored due to effect on blood pressure and chances of inducing falls due to postural hypotension.

For acute severe agitation, atypical antipsychotic agents, such as risperidone, olanzapine, and quetiapine, remain in common use, though the evidence base remains poor. Atypical antipsychotic medications are preferred over typical neuroleptic agents, such as haloperidol, which are not commonly used now due to concerns about extrapyramidal side effects. Concerns have been raised about the use of neuroleptics in patients with TBI with an increased risk of worsening of motor and cognitive functions. A recent French guideline (Plantier and Luauté, 2016) noted that there are no standards or consensus regarding the use of neuroleptics. A greater sensitivity to their adverse effects post-TBI was noted.

The antiepileptic agents carbamazepine and valproate are commonly used as mood stabilizers to treat agitation after TBI. The North American Neurobehavioral Guidelines Working Group noted that carbamazepine seems to be effective in some patients experiencing aggression after TBI, though the published literature did not support a recommendation for use of carbamazepine at that time (Warden et al., 2006). They concluded that there is insufficient evidence to support the development of any standards for the treatment of aggression following TBI. More recently, French guidelines noted that carbamazepine and valproate seem effective for the treatment of agitation and aggression and are recommended as first-line treatment (Plantier and Luauté, 2016). Other antiepileptic agents such as oxcarbazepine, lamotrigine, or gabapentin do not have any evidence to support their use. Levetiracetam has no positive effect on aggressiveness post-TBI and can make agitation and aggressiveness worse, as well as carries risks of behavioural and mood disorders; hence it should be avoided.

Benzodiazepines can sometimes be used in an acute emergency for sedation, but generally its regular use should be avoided as it can have a negative effect on neurocognition and brain plasticity and can make aggression paradoxically worse. Other pharmacological agents which have been tried for agitation and aggression following TBI include amantadine, buspirone, modafinil, and methylphenidate. Of these agents, methylphenidate seems to be the most promising, though further evidence is required before routine clinical use can be recommended.

Long-term consequences of severe brain injury

Neuropsychiatric consequences of severe TBI include various neurocognitive and neurobehavioural problems such as mood swings, impulsivity, apathy, irritability and agitation, aggression, and impaired attention, concentration and memory. Deb et al. (1999) used the Schedules for Clinical Assessment in Neuropsychiatry Interview to reach a formal ICD-10 diagnosis and found that, in comparison with the general population, a higher proportion of adult patients had developed psychiatric illnesses 1 year after a TBI (21.7%), though the rates of neurobehavioural symptoms which do not fulfil diagnostic criteria for a psychiatric disorder were much higher.

Using DSM-IV criteria in a 30-year follow-up study, Koponen et al. (2002) found that 48.3% had an axis I disorder that began after TBI and 61.7% had an axis I disorder during their lifetime. In addition, 23.3% had an axis II personality disorder and 15% had a DSM-IIIR organic personality syndrome. The commonest psychiatric disorders following TBI were major depression (26.7%), alcohol abuse or dependence (11.7%), panic disorder (8.3%), specific phobia (8.3%), and psychotic disorders (6.7%). They suggested that TBI may cause decade-lasting vulnerability to psychiatric illness, as many individuals develop psychiatric problems for the first time many years after a TBI.

More recently, Alway et al. (2016) in a prospective examination of axis I psychiatric disorders in the first 5 years following moderate to severe TBI using DSM-IV found that 75.2% received a psychiatric diagnosis, commonly emerging within the first year in 77.7% of cases. Anxiety, mood, and substance use disorders were the commonest diagnostic classes, often presenting comorbidly. Over half of patients experienced a completely new post-TBI psychiatric condition not present prior to injury. The strongest predictors of post-TBI psychiatric disorders were a pre-injury disorder and accident-related limb injury. Their findings suggest the first year post-injury is a critical period for the emergence of psychiatric disorders. Disorder frequency declines thereafter, with anxiety disorders showing greater resolution than mood and substance use disorders.

Mood disorders

Depression is the most commonly reported psychiatric problem following TBI, with reports suggesting that up to 60% of patients with TBI develop depression in the first year after injury (Fann et al., 2009). The prevalence of depression reported in the literature varies from 17% to 60% and this variation is mostly due to the use of different screening tools, different study populations, differences in the study design, and the diagnostic criteria/threshold used. The cumulative 1-year prevalence of MDD (DSM-IV) has been reported to be 53.1% among a cohort of patients hospitalized for TBI. MDD was associated with a past history of MDD (Bombardier et al., 2010). The prevalence of depressive symptoms remains stable over time, if untreated, emphasizing the importance of recognizing and treating depression early after the injury (Sigurdardottir et al., 2013).

Complex interaction of neurological, psychological, and social factors is generally accepted to contribute to the development of post-TBI depression (Williams and Evans, 2003). Psychosocial stressors and employment status were also noted to contribute to depressive symptoms and psychological distress, whereas injury severity did not have any predictive value (Sigurdardottir et al., 2013). However, injury severity is reported to be important in other studies, with a higher prevalence reported in severe TBI, as compared to mTBI. In contrast, using self-report measures of depression, the prevalence of depression is higher following mTBI (64%), compared with severe TBI (39%). A number of factors may contribute to this finding, including higher rates of memory problems and reduced self-awareness associated with severe TBI (Osborn et al., 2014).

It is suggested that MDD may be the most disabling psychiatric condition in individuals with TBI. Poorer cognitive functioning, aggression and anxiety, greater functional disability, poorer recovery, and greater healthcare costs are thought to be associated with MDD after TBI (Bombardier et al., 2010). Depression is noted to be an independent predictor of poorer health-related quality of life in people after TBI. Risk of suicide is significantly increased following TBI (Teasdale and Engberg, 2001). TBI with a structural lesion has a higher risk than TBI with no structural lesions, with standardized mortality ratios increased by up to four times, compared to the general population.

A number of symptoms of depression could overlap with the core features of brain injury, including tiredness, poor concentration, and sleep and appetite changes. This makes assessment of depression more difficult. Depression should ideally be routinely screened through the use of standardized depression screening instruments, followed by a full neuropsychiatric assessment. Attempts should be made to rule out possibilities such hypopituitarism and apathy–amotivation which could mimic depression after TBI. Affective dysregulation due to frontal lobe damage may also be confused with depression.

Evidence suggests that antidepressants are effective in treating depression in neurological settings (Agrawal and Rickards, 2011). Hence, clinicians should have a low threshold for diagnosing and treating depression, given the costs for not doing so in terms of outcomes and quality of life. A systematic review looking at treatment for depression after TBI included 27 studies but noted that there is a paucity of RCTs for depression following TBI. It noted that serotonergic antidepressants and cognitive behavioural interventions appear to have the best preliminary evidence for treating depression following TBI (Fann et al., 2009). SSRIs, particularly sertraline and citalopram, were found to be well tolerated. Clinically, as routine, these are recommended as first-line treatment. Tricyclic antidepressants do not have good evidence for efficacy and have a higher risk of side effects, so are generally avoided. Monoamine oxidase inhibitors (MAOIs) are not recommended due to a lack of efficacy data and potentially serious side effects, specifically with difficulties in adhering to dietary restrictions due to cognitive difficulties. Psychological treatments, such as CBT, have comparable efficacy to antidepressants. Other psychological treatments often used include goal setting, behavioural activation, and problem-solving therapy (Cuijpers et al., 2007) in multidisciplinary neurorehabilitative settings.

Anxiety disorders

Anxiety disorders are commonly seen after a TBI. These include acute stress reaction, generalized anxiety, panic disorder, specific phobic disorder, PTSD, and obsessive–compulsive symptoms.

Preliminary data from a large prospective cohort study on post-TBI anxiety showed a high proportion of participants suffered from significant levels of anxiety during the first year post-TBI, regardless of TBI severity and gender. At 4, 8, and 12 months, respectively, 29.9%, 29.2%, and 30.8% of participants presented with clinically significant anxious symptoms (Laviolette et al., 2014). They noted participants with a positive premorbid history of anxiety disorders had greater anxiety on the HADS, compared to those with a negative premorbid anxiety history. Koponen et al. (2002) reported post-TBI prevalence of panic disorder of 8.3%, specific phobia 8.3%, and generalized anxiety disorder 1.7%. A much higher lifetime rate of these anxiety disorders was noted.

Commonly, patients who are involved in TBI also experience other physical and psychological trauma, including fear of death or fear of subsequent treatment, including subsequent intensive medical care (Hiott and Labbate, 2002). These traumatic experiences may result in, or contribute to, the development of PTSD. The diagnosis of PTSD may be difficult following TBI because of overlap with symptoms of TBI, particularly with PCS. Various post-TBI neurobehavioural symptoms, such as increased alcohol consumption, depression, impulsivity, or irritability, may alter PTSD presentation, making it harder to diagnose.

An accurate diagnosis of these anxiety disorders requires awareness of these overlaps between anxiety disorders, depression, and other neurobehavioural problems due to TBI. Management is often best delivered as part of neurorehabilitative care, with a combination of anxiety management techniques, CBT, and pharmacological treatment with SSRI.

Apathy

Apathy or amotivation is commonly seen following TBI and can be confused with depression. Apathy is associated with reduced goal-directed behaviour, lack of motivation, impaired initiative, diminished activity, and lack of concern. These symptoms of apathy are commonly divided into three dimensions: behavioural, cognitive, and emotional. Apathy can be associated with poor outcomes due to lack of engagement in neurorehabilitation and may impact on family, social, and occupational functioning and can cause increased caregiver distress.

Various terms have been used to describe apathy, including amotivation and abulia, and it is generally described by lay people as 'reduced get up and go'. Assessment consists of a good history and an account of symptoms from carers and a wider multidisciplinary team. Distinction should be made between apathy as a symptom of mood disorder, altered level of consciousness, or cognitive impairment and apathy as a syndrome of acquired changes in mood, behaviour, and cognition not due to mood disorder, altered level of consciousness, or cognitive impairment (van Reekum, 2005). Use of measures such as the Apathy Evaluation Scale (Marin, 1991) can help with diagnosis, but other causes such as depression should be excluded.

Treatment in the initial instance can be only non-pharmacological, particularly in milder cases. In more severe cases, a combination of pharmacological and non-pharmacological approaches is recommended. Cognitive interventions are the most commonly used strategy, but other interventions such as music therapy and cognitive rehabilitation have been used (Lane-Brown and Tate, 2009). Practical behavioural approaches, such as activity scheduling, are also used clinically. Various pharmacological treatments, including dopaminergic drugs such as selegiline, stimulants such as methylphenidate, cholinesterase inhibitors such as donepezil, and others such as SSRIs and modafinil, have been tried. For more details on apathy and its management, see Chapter 37.

Psychosis

Growing evidence from a number of studies points towards a higher prevalence of psychosis following TBI. Rates of psychosis in TBI are estimated to be up to 10%, with a range of 1.35–9.2% (Batty et al., 2013). Various risk factors such as male gender, alcohol and substance use, such as cannabis, and pre-existing psychiatric conditions, such as mood disorders, are noted. Increased vulnerability in people with frontal, temporal, or hippocampal lesions has been reported, though the evidence is still emerging. Neuropsychological impairment of memory and executive functions are the commonest correlates.

Psychosis following TBI most commonly presents as delusional disorders or schizophrenia-like psychoses. Delusional disorders may present with Capgras syndrome, reduplicative paramnesia, delusional jealousy, Cotard syndrome, or somatic delusions (11%). Schizophrenia-like psychosis commonly presents with auditory hallucinations and persecutory delusions, and negative symptoms are not common. Onset of psychosis after TBI could be delayed by years, with a mean latency between TBI and onset of psychosis reported as 3–5 years (Fujii and Ahmed, 2014). Delusional disorders tend to develop earlier, generally in the first year after TBI.

Clinical assessment should focus on establishing the phenomenology of psychotic symptoms and ruling out other causes of psychosis, including substance-induced psychosis, psychosis related to epilepsy, and a primary psychotic disorder. Initial post-TBI presentation with agitation and behavioural problems associated with PTA can be commonly confused with psychosis. Diagnosis of psychosis when a patient is still in PTA should be avoided. Treatment of psychosis after TBI is similar to treatment of psychosis in general. Consideration should be given to interactions with other medications, sensitivity to side effects, and impact on neurocognitive functions.

Organic personality and behavioural change

Persistent changes in behaviours and emotions after TBI are commonly reported by patients, carers, and relatives, often collectively referred to as personality change. These are often reported as the most distressing consequence of injury. General presentation of changes in personality and behaviour includes irritability, anger, aggression, frustration, impulsivity, emotional lability, social or sexual disinhibition, impairment of judgement, and poor insight. People are described as child-like and self-centred, with difficulties in social behaviours and appropriate expression of affection. Symptoms of personality change can have some overlap with mood problems such as depression or impact of cognitive impairment but cannot be fully explained by either.

Approximately a quarter of patient with TBI have a pre-existing personality disorder; particularly common is antisocial personality disorder. However, the prevalence of such pre-existing personality disorder is similar to the community prevalence and is not particularly over-represented in TBI patients. Using the Structured Clinical Interview for DSM-IV Personality Disorders, Hibbard et al. (2000) reported 66% of people post-TBI met criteria for at least one personality disorder. No specific correlation was reported with TBI severity, age at injury, and time since injury. In a 30-year follow-up study, Koponen et al. (2002) reported the prevalence of at least one personality disorder as 23.3% and 15% the rates of 'organic personality syndrome'. Others have suggested the severity of brain injury as measured by the duration of LOC and the degree of cognitive impairment as an important predictor of personality dysfunction following TBI (Golden and Golden, 2003).

Organic personality change is associated with poor psychosocial adjustment, poor emotional functioning, increased caregiver distress, poor engagement with rehabilitative treatment, and poor occupational functioning. Frontal lobe lesions (particularly the orbitofrontal area), anterior temporal lesions, disruption to the limbic system, and impairment of frontal lobe functions on neurocognitive assessment are commonly associated with organic personality change. Widespread damage caused by shearing stress, such as diffuse axonal injury, can commonly result in organic personality change. However, personality change can occur in the absence of any discernible cognitive impairment or without any identifiable structural brain lesions. Individuals with pre-existing psychiatric conditions or personality disorders can be at a greater risk of developing organic personality change. In the absence of structural lesions, patients may present with a combination of exacerbation of pre-existing personality traits, organic orderliness and obsessionality, and adjustment to post-injury life, along with persistent irritability and morbid anxiety, impacting on personality and behaviour.

A good clinical assessment would usually include assessment of current and past axis I psychiatric conditions, assessment of neurocognitive functions, and collateral history from family and carers. Detailed neurocognitive assessment helps in establishing the nature and severity of neurocognitive difficulties which may have an impact on behaviour. Specific measures, such as the Frontal Systems Behaviour Scale (FrSBe), the Behaviour Rating Inventory of Executive Functions (BRIEF), and the Dysexecutive Questionnaire (DEX) can be used to help with diagnosis. Management of organic personality change is best delivered in the context of brain injury rehabilitative services, with a combination of behavioural programme and pharmacological management. Currently, the evidence base to support pharmacological treatment remains poor, but agents such as SSRIs, mood stabilizers (such as carbamazepine), and atypical antipsychotic agents (such as risperidone) are commonly used in clinical practice. Other agents tried include stimulants, such as methylphenidate, or dopaminergic drugs such as bromocriptine. These are more likely to be used when there is an overlap with apathy symptoms.

Alcohol and drugs

Alcohol is a major risk factor for injury, and 30–50% of all patients hospitalized with trauma are intoxicated at the time of injury. Even so, the effect of alcohol on TBI outcomes is still controversial (Tien et al., 2006). There is evidence that alcohol use does not result in a clinically significant reduction in GCS scores in trauma patients (Stuke et al., 2007) and hence may not influence the assessment of severity in the aftermath of injury. Alcohol consumption on the day of injury is well recognized to increase the risk of sustaining a TBI, but evidence so far suggests that alcohol consumption on the day of injury does not appear to be associated with substantially poorer outcomes after a TBI, except for poorer cognitions in individuals with high day-of-injury blood alcohol levels (Mathias and Osborn, 2016). It is suggested that alcohol may be neuroprotective in small amounts, as it has been shown that low levels of blood alcohol are associated with lower mortality, as compared to no alcohol, but high levels of blood alcohol are associated with higher mortality (Tien et al., 2006).

However, alcohol use after TBI carries several risks. These include an increased risk of recurrent TBI, more atrophy of the cerebral cortex, development of post-traumatic seizures, and deterioration of behavioural functioning (Opreanu et al., 2010). In addition, people may have worsening of neurocognitive difficulties, increased emotional difficulties, and aggression. Generally, people after a TBI stop alcohol consumption for a while, but those with a past history of alcohol misuse and high levels of use are more likely to restart. Hence there is a need for intervention at an early stage after a TBI to educate people about the impact of alcohol, with motivational interviewing, particularly in individuals with heavy use prior to their TBI.

Substance abuse, similarly to alcohol misuse, is a risk factor for TBI due to its impact on cognitive function, behaviour, and judgement. Substance misuse pre- and post-TBI is commonly associated with alcohol misuse. Evidence suggests approximately 50–60% of persons with TBI have significant issues with alcohol and/or drugs. Substance misuse may increase after the TBI, with odds of 4.5 within the first year post-injury and 1.4 at 3 years post-injury (Allen, 2016). However, others suggest that there may be a decline in substance misuse for a while after a TBI, similarly to what is reported in relation to alcohol misuse. A history of substance abuse predicts increased disability, poorer prognosis, and delayed recovery. Even in people with mTBI, subtle impairments in neurocognitive functions, when combined with difficulties in psychosocial adjustment and coping skills that the substance user had pre-injury, may increase the risk of chronic substance abuse (Allen, 2016). Substance misuse post-injury could lead to problems with emotions, behaviour, motivation, neurocognitive functions, and overall outcome from TBI.

Risk of dementia after TBI

Traditionally, TBI is considered to be a static condition, which is not progressive in its course and rather tends to show gradual improvement, especially in the first few years after the injury. Neurocognitive impairments post TBI generally show some improvement in the initial recovery phase. There is now growing evidence that the risk of dementia is increased in people with moderate to severe TBI. One of the mechanisms often postulated is that of a diminished cognitive reserve, which increases the impact of neurodegenerative changes in later life (Vincent et al., 2014). Another mechanism suggested is acceleration of brain atrophy caused by TBI, thus increasing the susceptibility for dementia. Radiological studies of the brains of TBI patients estimated these to be older than their chronological age (Cole et al., 2015). These studies indicate this discrepancy increases with time since injury, suggesting that TBI accelerates the rate of brain atrophy.

While the increased risk associated with moderate to severe TBI is increasingly accepted, emerging evidence suggests that mTBI, particularly repeated mild injuries, may also increase the risk of dementia. However, this remains a controversial issue. Repeated sports-related concussion is reported to produce chronic neurocognitive and behavioural problems associated with neuropathological changes previously called dementia pugilistica and more recently termed chronic traumatic encephalopathy (McKee et al., 2013). This is thought to be associated with a reduced cognitive reserve and increased chances of a neurodegenerative process becoming clinically apparent. However, Cole et al. (2015) in their neuroradiological study noted that the degree of apparent ageing was only associated with moderate and severe TBI, with mTBI showing no brain atrophy.

TBI is postulated to be the best established environmental risk factor for dementia. It is noted that individuals who had a TBI of sufficient severity to result in LOC were at approximately 50% increased risk of dementia, while the estimated odds ratios are reported to be 4.0 for TBI with LOC and 2.0 for TBI without LOC (Shiveley, 2012). The risk of dementia is reported to be higher with increased severity of injury, multiple TBIs, and increased age at injury.

Childhood brain injuries

Childhood is a common time to have a TBI. Boys are more likely to have TBIs than girls. TBIs could be commonly related to abuse, falls, or pedestrian or bicycle injuries in children and are more likely to be bicycle injuries and road traffic accidents in older adolescents. As in adults, over three-quarters of injuries are mild and only <10% of injuries are severe. Children who have a TBI are more likely to have pre-injury behavioural problems and psychiatric disorders. Rates of a pre-injury psychiatric disorder are reported to be between one-third and half of children (Max et al., 2012). Following TBI, the rates of neuropsychiatric problems in children 2 years after a severe TBI have been reported to be 54–63%, and following mild/moderate TBI to be 10–21% (Max et al., 2012). The range of neuropsychiatric problems following a TBI in children includes PCS after mTBI, personality change, secondary ADHD, oppositional defiant or conduct disorder, depression, PTSD, and anxiety disorders.

Childhood TBI can significantly affect schooling and alter educational achievements and subsequent occupational outcomes. Outcomes were reported to be poorer for children with moderate to severe TBI than for children with orthopaedic injuries only. Children with TBI had more behaviour problems and lower competence by parent report, lower teacher ratings of academic performance, poorer adaptive functioning, and weaker maths and writing skills (Taylor et al., 2002). Environmental factors, particularly family support, can influence the long-term outcome.

Management of neuropsychiatric problems post-TBI involves additional school-based intervention for extra educational support and family interventions, along with general post-TBI neurorehabilitation and psychological and pharmacological management. Behavioural intervention, traditional contingency management procedures, and positive behaviour support procedures are recommended as a treatment guideline based on positive evidence (Ylvisaker et al., 2007).

Anoxic brain injuries

Anoxic brain injury is also known as hypoxic brain injury and can be used synonymously with the term hypoxic–ischaemic brain injury, though the mechanisms and pathophysiology are generally different. While hypoxic brain injury is primarily due to reduced oxygen supply to the brain, hypoxic–ischaemic injuries are due to reduced cerebral blood flow, reduced oxygen supply, or both. Hypoxic–ischaemic brain injury is commonly seen after a cardiac arrest, due to severe hypotension, or after a prolonged seizure in hospital settings. Hypoxic brain injuries are seen after suffocation, strangulation, respiratory obstruction, or carbon monoxide poisoning. In psychiatric settings, anoxic brain injuries occur after deliberate self-harm such as hanging or by exhaust fume inhalation resulting in carbon monoxide poisoning.

The clinical presentation of anoxic brain injury includes a range of motor, neurocognitive, and neuropsychiatric problems. Motor symptoms include gait abnormality and involuntary movements. Cognitive impairment is a prominent part of the presentation, including impairments in memory, executive function, attention, and visuospatial functions. Changes in personality and behaviour are commonly seen (Caine and Watson, 2000), including emotional lability, impulsivity, irritability, disinhibition, or lack of insight and emotional reactivity.

Commonly affected structures of the brain include damage to the hippocampus, watershed areas of the cerebral cortex, basal ganglia, thalamus, and cerebellum. Early CT scan may show diffuse swelling, attenuation of grey–white matter differentiation, hypodensity of the cortical grey matter and basal ganglia, and hypodensity of the white matter. MRI brain scan would show widespread hyperintensity in the basal ganglia, hippocampus, thalamus, cerebral cortex, and subcortical white matter. These abnormalities on MRI scan are more likely to be seen in FLAIR and DWI sequences. Generally, T1 and T2 sequences can be reported as normal. EEG would show increased low-voltage generalized slow waves.

Treatment for brain anoxia needs urgent attention, and generally initial treatment may be with general medics, in intensive care settings, or with neurologists. Acute interventions include therapeutic hypothermia and ventilator support, which may improve global outcomes. Treatments for cognitive impairments are generally akin to treatment for TBI in similar neurorehabilitative settings. Neuropsychiatric consequences require a comprehensive assessment, and management is generally along similar lines to management of various neuropsychiatric consequences of TBI.

Patients with anoxic brain injury generally have similar lengths of stay in hospital, as compared to TBI patients, but may make slower progress, with poorer outcomes, and may be more likely to be transferred to residential care. These patients have more severe impairments on cognitive assessment, relative to those with TBI, being particularly susceptible to memory impairments, especially visual or short-term memory (Fitzgerald et al., 2010). A slower rate of recovery for patients with anoxic brain injury, compared with those with TBI, was also noted in another study (Cullen et al., 2009), with physical recovery being slower than cognitive recovery during inpatient rehabilitation. In terms of psychosocial outcomes, cardiac arrest survivors experiencing anoxic brain injury experience more psychosocial difficulties, as compared to those without anoxia. This is postulated to be due to a combination of neuropsychological, social, and psychological factors (Wilson et al., 2014). There were more anxiety, depression, and post-traumatic stress symptoms, but there was no difference in self-reported quality of life.

Principles of management

Patients with TBI are generally managed within multidisciplinary trauma pathways, with involvement of various therapists, including neuropsychologists, physiotherapists, occupational therapists, and speech and language therapists. Neuropsychiatrists would be an integral part of such teams. Treatments are individualized following detailed assessment of the patient's problems and their strengths and weaknesses using a goal-planning approach. Neuropsychiatric conditions following a TBI are treated by such neurorehabilitative

teams, with a combination of pharmacological, psychological, behavioural, and social approaches.

Pharmacological approaches require attention to issues specific to TBIs, including sensitivity to side effects, impact on energy levels and cognitive functions, interactions with other medications, and risk of post-traumatic epilepsy. The general rule is to start low and go slow and to remove medications which are not helpful in regular, planned reviews. Many patients will, however, require a full therapeutic trial symptomatically, as in non-TBI populations. There is a dearth of evidence-based pharmacological treatments post-TBI, supported by strong RCT evidence. Almost any psychotropic medication which is used for any psychiatric disorder has been used in patients following a TBI. This is a growing field with a gradual accumulation of evidence. Currently, no medications are specifically approved to be used post-TBI by the FDA or European or UK regulators. Hence, currently, treatment is often based on available evidence from often open-label studies and clinical experience. Various expert consensus guidelines (Plantier and Luaute, 2016; Warden et al., 2006) and pragmatic reviews (Bhatnagar et al., 2016; Chew and Zafonte, 2009; Deb and Crownshaw, 2004) are available, which can guide management of neuropsychiatric problems post-TBI.

Conclusion

Brain injury is a common condition, and while the vast majority of brain injuries are mild, these are commonly associated with a wide range of neuropsychiatric consequences. These neuropsychiatric comorbidities and consequences include depression, anxiety, affective dysregulation, apathy–amotivation, agitation/aggression, and personality changes. These have a significant impact on initial neurorehabilitative treatment, quality of life, and overall functioning. Early recognition and management of these neuropsychiatric problems is likely to result in improved outcomes.

KEY LEARNING POINTS

- Acquired brain injuries (ABIs) can be categorized as traumatic or non-traumatic brain injuries.
- Traumatic brain injuries (TBIs), sub-classified as either open or closed TBIs, depending on whether there is a fracture of the skull or a breach in the dura mater, are typically caused by a physical impact such as blunt trauma or a fall.
- Severity of TBI is commonly determined based on a combination of GCS score, duration of LOC and PTA along with any structural abnormalities on brain scans.
- mTBI are the most common form of TBI and present with a range of somatic, neurocognitive and neuropsychiatric symptoms traditionally referred to as PCS.
- Moderate to severe TBI lead on to a wide range of neuropsychiatric conditions such as depression, anxiety, apathy, personality change etc.
- Anoxic brain injury commonly results in neurocognitive impairments and can be associated with neuropsychiatric symptoms including personality change.

REFERENCES

Agrawal, N. and Rickards, H., 2011. Detection and treatment of depression in neurological disorders. *Journal of Neurology, Neurosurgery & Psychiatry* 82, 828–29.

Allen, S., Stewart, S. H., Cusimano, M., and Asbridge, M., 2016. Examining the Relationship Between Traumatic Brain Injury and Substance Use Outcomes in the Canadian Population. *Substance Use & Misuse*, 51, 1577–86.

Alway, Y., Gould, K.R., Johnston, L., McKenzie, D., and Ponsford, J., 2016. A prospective examination of Axis I psychiatric disorders in the first 5 years following moderate to severe traumatic brain injury. *Psychological Medicine*, 46, 1331–41.

Andelic, N., 2013. The epidemiology of traumatic brain injury. *The Lancet Neurology*, 12, 28–9.

Batty, R.A., Rossell, S.L., Francis, A.J., and Ponsford, J., 2013. Psychosis following traumatic brain injury. *Brain Impairment*, 14, 21–41.

Bhatnagar, S., Iaccarino, M.A., and Zafonte, R., 2016. Pharmacotherapy in rehabilitation of post-acute traumatic brain injury. *Brain Research*, 1640, 164–79.

Bombardier, C.H., Fann, J.R., Temkin, N.R., Esselman, P.C., Barber, J., and Dikmen, S.S., 2010. Rates of major depressive disorder and clinical outcomes following traumatic brain injury. *JAMA*, 303, 1938–45.

Bruns, J. and Hauser, W.A., 2003. The epidemiology of traumatic brain injury: a review. *Epilepsia*, 44, 2–10.

Caine, D. and Watson, J.D., 2000. Neuropsychological and neuropathological sequelae of cerebral anoxia: a critical review. *Journal of the International Neuropsychological Society*, 6, 86–99.

Chew, E. and Zafonte, R.D., 2009. Pharmacological management of neurobehavioral disorders following traumatic brain injury–a state-of-the-art review. *Journal of Rehabilitation Research and Development*, 46, 851.

Cole, J.H., Leech, R., and Sharp, D.J., 2015. Prediction of brain age suggests accelerated atrophy after traumatic brain injury. *Annals of Neurology*, 77, 571–81.

Cuijpers, P., van Straten, A., and Wamerdam, L. (2007). Problem solving therapies for depression: A meta-analysis. *European Psychiatry*, 22, 9–15.

Cullen, N.K., Crescini, C., and Bayley, M.T., 2009. Rehabilitation outcomes after anoxic brain injury: a case-controlled comparison with traumatic brain injury. *PM&R*, 1, 1069–76.

Deb, S. and Crownshaw, T., 2004. Review of subject The role of pharmacotherapy in the management of behaviour disorders in traumatic brain injury patients. *Brain Injury*, 18, 1–31.

Deb, S., Lyons, I., Koutzoukis, C., Ali, I., and McCarthy, G., 1999. Rate of psychiatric illness 1 year after traumatic brain injury. *American Journal of Psychiatry*, 156, 374–8.

De Simoni, S., Grover, P.J., Jenkins, P.O., et al., 2016. Disconnection between the default mode network and medial temporal lobes in post-traumatic amnesia. *Brain*, 139, 3137–50.

Fann, J.R., Hart, T., and Schomer, K.G., 2009. Treatment for depression after traumatic brain injury: a systematic review. *Journal of Neurotrauma*, 26, 2383–402.

Fitzgerald, A., Aditya, H., Prior, A., McNeill, E., and Pentland, B., 2010. Anoxic brain injury: Clinical patterns and functional outcomes. A study of 93 cases. *Brain Injury*, 24, 1311–23.

Fleminger, S., Greenwood, R.R.J., and Oliver, D.L., 2006. Cochrane Injuries Group. Pharmacological management for agitation and aggression in people with acquired brain injury. *Cochrane Database of Systematic Reviews*, 73, CD003299.

Fujii, D.E. and Ahmed, I., 2014. Psychotic disorder caused by traumatic brain injury. *Psychiatric Clinics of North America*, 37, 113–24.

Golden, Z. and Golden, C.J., 2003. Impact of brain injury severity on personality dysfunction. *International Journal of Neuroscience*, 113, 733–45.

Hadanny, A. and Efrati, S., 2016. Treatment of persistent post-concussion syndrome due to mild traumatic brain injury: current status and future directions. *Expert Review of Neurotherapeutics*, 16, 875–87.

Hibbard, M.R., Bogdany, J., Uysal, S., et al., 2000. Axis II psychopathology in individuals with traumatic brain injury. *Brain Injury*, 14, 45–61.

Hiott, D.W. and Labbate, L., 2002. Anxiety disorders associated with traumatic brain injuries. *NeuroRehabilitation*, 17, 345–55.

King, N.S. and Kirwilliam, S., 2013. The nature of permanent post-concussion symptoms after mild traumatic brain injury. *Brain Impairment*, 14, 235–42.

Koponen, S., Taiminen, T., Portin, R., et al., 2002. Axis I and II psychiatric disorders after traumatic brain injury: a 30-year follow-up study. *American Journal of Psychiatry*, 159, 1315–21.

Lane-Brown, A.T. and Tate, R.L., 2009. Apathy after acquired brain impairment: a systematic review of non-pharmacological interventions. *Neuropsychological Rehabilitation*, 19, 481–516.

Langlois, J.A., Rutland-Brown, W., and Wald, M.M., 2006. The Epidemiology and Impact of Traumatic Brain Injury: A Brief Overview. *Journal of Head Trauma Rehabilitation*, 21, 375–8.

Laviolette, V., Ouellet, M.C., Beaulieu-Bonneau, S., and Giguere, M., 2014. Anxiety in the first year after traumatic brain injury: Evolution and risk factors. *Brain Injury*, 28, 705–6.

Malec, J.F., Brown, A.W., Leibson, C.L., et al., 2007. The Mayo Classification System for Traumatic Brain Injury Severity. *Journal of Neurotrauma*, 24, 1417–24.

Marin, R.S., Biedrzycki, R.C., and Firinciogullar, S., 1991. Reliability and validity of the Apathy Evaluation Scale. *Psychiatry Research*, 38, 143–62.

Marshall S, Bayley M, McCullagh S, et al., (2015) Updated clinical practice guidelines for concussion/mild traumatic brain injury and persistent symptoms. *Brain Injury*, 29, 688–700.

Marshall, S., Bayley, M., McCullagh, S., Velikonja, D., and Berrigan, L., 2012. Clinical practice guidelines for mild traumatic brain injury and persistent symptoms. *Canadian Family Physician*, 58, 257–67.

Marshman, L.A., Jakabek, D., Hennessy, M., Quirk, F., and Guazzo, E.P., 2013. Post-traumatic amnesia. *Journal of Clinical Neuroscience*, 20, 1475–81.

Mathias, J.L. and Osborn, A.J., 2016. Impact of day-of-injury alcohol consumption on outcomes after traumatic brain injury: A meta-analysis. *Neuropsychological Rehabilitation*, 1, 1–22.

Max, J.E., et al., 2012. Psychiatric disorders after pediatric traumatic brain injury: a prospective, longitudinal, controlled study. *Journal of Neuropsychiatry and Clinical Neuroscience*, 24, 427–36.

McKee, A.C., Stein, T.D., Nowinski, C.J., et al. 2013. The spectrum of disease in chronic traumatic encephalopathy. *Brain*, 136, 43–64.

Metting, Z., Rödiger, L.A., de Jong, B.M., Stewart, R.E., Kremer, B.P., and van der Naalt, J., 2010. Acute cerebral perfusion CT abnormalities associated with posttraumatic amnesia in mild head injury. *Journal of Neurotrauma*, 27, 2183–9.

Opreanu, R.C., Kuhn, D., and Basson, M.D., 2010. The Influence of Alcohol on Mortality in Traumatic Brain Injury. *Journal*

of the American College of Surgeons, 210, doi: 10.1016/
j.jamcollsurg.2010.01.036.

Osborn, A.J., Mathias, J.L., and Fairweather-Schmidt, A.K., 2014. Depression following adult, non-penetrating traumatic brain injury: A meta-analysis examining methodological variables and sample characteristics. *Neuroscience & Biobehavioral Reviews*, 47, 1–15.

Plantier, D. and Luauté, J., 2016. Drugs for behavior disorders after traumatic brain injury: Systematic review and expert consensus leading to French recommendations for good practice. *Annals of Physical and Rehabilitation Medicine*, 59, 42–57.

Ponsford, J.L., Spitz, G., and McKenzie, D., 2016. Using Post-Traumatic Amnesia To Predict Outcome after Traumatic Brain Injury. *Journal of Neurotrauma*, 33, 997–1004.

Potter, S.D.S., Brown, R.G., and Fleminger, S., 2016. Randomised, waiting list controlled trial of cognitive–behavioural therapy for persistent postconcussional symptoms after predominantly mild–moderate traumatic brain injury. *Journal of Neurology, Neurosurgery, and Psychiatry*, 87, 1075–83.

Sharp, D.J. and Jenkins, P.O., 2015. Concussion is confusing us all. *Practical Neurology*, 15, 172–86.

Shively, S., Scher, A.I., Perl, D.P., and Diaz-Arrastia, R., 2012. Dementia resulting from traumatic brain injury: what is the pathology? *Archives of Neurology*, 69, 1245–51.

Shores, E.A., Marosszeky, J.E., Sandanam, J., and Batchelor, J., 1986. Preliminary validation of a scale for measuring the duration of post-traumatic amnesia. *Medical Journal of Australia*, 144, 569–72.

Sigurdardottir, S., Andelic, N., Røe, C., and Schanke, A.K., 2013. Depressive symptoms and psychological distress during the first five years after traumatic brain injury: Relationship with psychosocial stressors, fatigue and pain. *Journal of Rehabilitation Medicine*, 45, 808–14.

Singh, R., Venkateshwara, G., Nair, K.P., Khan, M., and Saad, R., 2014. Agitation after traumatic brain injury and predictors of outcome. *Brain Injury*, 28, 336–40.

Stuke, L., Diaz-Arrastia, R., Gentilello, L.M., and Shafi, S., 2007. Effect of alcohol on Glasgow Coma Scale in head-injured patients. *Annals of Surgery*, 245, 651–5.

Tagliaferri, F., Compagnone, C., Korsic, M., Servadei, F., and Kraus, J., 2006. A systematic review of brain injury epidemiology in Europe. *Acta Neurochirurgica*, 148, 255–68.

Taylor, H.G., Yeates, K.O., Wade, S.L., Drotar, D., Stancin, T. and Minich, N., 2002. A prospective study of short-and long-term outcomes after traumatic brain injury in children: behavior and achievement. *Neuropsychology*, 16, 15.

Teasdale, T.W. and Engberg, A.W., 2001. Suicide after traumatic brain injury: a population study. *Journal of Neurology, Neurosurgery & Psychiatry*, 71, 436–40.

Tien, H.C., Tremblay, L.N., Rizoli, S.B., et al., 2006. Association between alcohol and mortality in patients with severe traumatic head injury. *Archives of Surgery*, 141, 1185–91.

van Reekum, R., Stuss, D.T., and Ostrander, L., 2005. Apathy: why care? *Journal of Neuropsychiatry and Clinical Neurosciences*, 17, 7–19.

Vincent, A.S., Roebuck-Spencer, T.M., and Cernich, A., 2014. Cognitive changes and dementia risk after traumatic brain injury: implications for aging military personnel. *Alzheimer's & Dementia*, 10, S174–87.

Warden, D.L., Gordon, B., McAllister, T.W., et al., 2006. Guidelines for the pharmacologic treatment of neurobehavioral sequelae of traumatic brain injury. *Journal of Neurotrauma*, 23, 1468–501.

Whittaker, R., Kemp, S., and House, S., 2007. Illness perceptions and outcome in mild head injury: a longitudinal study. *Journal of Neurology, Neurosurgery, and Psychiatry*, 78, 644–6.

Williams, W.H. and Evans, J.J., 2003. Brain injury and emotion: An overview to a special issue on biopsychosocial approaches in neurorehabilitation. *Neuropsychological Rehabilitation*, 13(1–2), 1–11.

Wilson, M., Staniforth, A., Till, R., Das Nair, R., and Vesey, P., 2014. The psychosocial outcomes of anoxic brain injury following cardiac arrest. *Resuscitation*, 85, 795–800.

Ylvisaker, M., Turkstra, L., Coehlo, C., et al., 2007. Behavioural interventions for children and adults with behaviour disorders after TBI: A systematic review of the evidence. *Brain Injury*, 21, 769–805.

17

Neuropsychiatric aspects of epilepsy

Marco Mula and Mahinda Yogarajah

Introduction

Epilepsy is among the commonest serious neurological conditions, with incidence rates in high-income countries ranging between 40 and 70/100,000 persons/year and generally higher in young children and the elderly (Duncan et al., 2006). In resource-poor countries, the incidence is usually much higher, often above 120/100,000 persons/year, and in high-income countries, poorer people also seem to have a higher incidence (Ngugi et al., 2011). Prevalence studies have reported lifetime rates of between 4 and 10/1000 in developed countries, but data from resource-poor countries clearly suggest higher lifetime prevalence rates in the region of 23.2–32.1/1000 up to 57/1000 in some selected cases in rural areas (Sander and Shorvon, 1996).

As captured by the new International League Against Epilepsy (ILAE) definition (Fisher et al., 2014), epilepsy is now recognized as a disorder of the brain, characterized not only by recurrent seizures, but also by its neurobiological, cognitive, psychological, and social consequences. For a long time, the mutual relationships among epilepsy, seizures, and behaviour have fascinated generations of clinicians and neuroscientists. In his famous quote, Hippocrates reported that '*melancholics ordinarily become epileptics, and epileptics, melancholics: what determines the preference is the direction the malady takes; if it bears upon the body, epilepsy, if upon the intelligence, melancholy*' (Temkin, 2010). In more modern times, a number of epileptologists have extensively contributed to the expansion of neuropsychiatry of epilepsy. Wilder Penfield (Penfield, 1946) and subsequently Gloor (Gloor et al., 1982) described the neurophysiological basis of experiential phenomena. Landolt described the electroclinical correlates of epileptic psychoses (Landolt, 1962). Normand Geschwind and his fellows described a number of personality traits typical of patients with temporal lobe epilepsy (Geschwind, 1997), while Michael Trimble and his fellows pointed out to the role of antiepileptic drug (AED) treatment and epilepsy surgery in psychiatric problems of epilepsy (Trimble and Schmitz, 2011).

In general, psychiatric disorders show a uniformly increased prevalence in epilepsy, as compared to the general population (see Table 17.1). The first step in the management of any neuropsychiatric problem in epilepsy is to identify the various elements that may contribute to the final clinical picture such as psychosocial issues, treatment-emergent adverse effects of AEDs, or neurobiological factors directly related to the seizures or the epileptic disorder (Mula, 2016). In fact, patients with epilepsy may experience a number of psychiatric manifestations around the ictus that have to be clearly distinguished from true psychiatric comorbidities. The practicality of classifying such symptoms according to their temporal relation to seizure occurrence (peri-ictal/para-ictal symptoms versus interictal symptoms) is well established (see Table 17.2). Peri-ictal phenomena have been well described by Gowers (Gowers, 2015) and Jackson (Jackson, 1958), but also by Kraepelin (Kraepelin and Johnstone, 2015) and Bleuler (Bleuler, 2013), and the differentiation between peri-ictal and interictal psychiatric symptoms has relevant implications in terms of prognosis and treatment.

The present chapter will cover major axis I disorders that are epidemiologically relevant, such as mood and anxiety disorders, or clinically relevant, such as psychoses, in adults with epilepsy. However, it is important to emphasize that a number of other topics, such as behavioural problems in intellectually disabled patients, autism, and ADHD, may be of relevance to child psychiatrists reviewing children with epilepsy. Patients with multiple neurological problems such as post-traumatic epilepsy may develop psychiatric complications that are linked to both the epilepsy and the TBI.

Mood and anxiety disorders

Epidemiology

Data from community-based studies in epilepsy report prevalence rates for mood disorders in the region of 20–22% (Tellez-Zenteno et al., 2007). Data on anxiety disorders are limited mainly because they are commonly comorbid with mood disorders, but they seem to have prevalence rates comparable to those of depression (Brandt and Mula, 2016). In selected populations, such as tertiary referral centres or surgery programmes, the prevalence rate is even higher and ranging between 30% and 50% (Ring et al., 1998). Such differences partially reflect the severity of the seizure disorder; in fact, depression seems to occur in only 4% of seizure-free patients (Baker et al., 1996). However, the relationship between mood disorders and epilepsy seems to be more complex than that. In fact, a number of epidemiologic studies have suggested that the association between epilepsy and depression is not necessarily unilateral,

Table 17.1 Prevalence of psychiatric disorders in unselected samples

Psychiatric disorder	General population, % (95% CI)	Epilepsy, % (95% CI)
Any mental health disorder (lifetime)	20.7 (19.5–20.7)	35.5 (25.9–44.0)
Any mental health disorder (12 month)	10.9 (10.4–11.3)	23.5 (15.8–31.2)
Mood disorder (lifetime)	13.2 (12.7–13.7)	24.4 (16.0–32.8)
Mood disorder (12 months)	5.2 (4.9–5.5)	14.1 (7.0–21.1)
Anxiety disorder (lifetime)	11.2 (10.8–11.7)	22.8 (14.8–30.9)
Anxiety disorder (12 months)	4.6 (4.3–4.9)	12.8 (6.0–19.7)
Mood and anxiety disorders (12 months)	8.0 (7.6–8.5)	19.9 (12.3–27.4)
Suicidal ideation (lifetime)	13.3 (12.8–13.8)	25.0 (17.4–32.5)
Autism spectrum disorder	1.4 (0.5–2.2)	8.1 (2.2–25.9)
Attention-deficit/hyperactivity disorder	3.4 (2.6–4.5)	15.9 (9.2–24.7)

CI, confidence interval.

but rather bidirectional, and some patients may present with a psychiatric disorder before the emergence of seizures (Hesdorffer et al., 2012). Such a bidirectional relationship is described in a number of other chronic conditions such as PD, stroke, dementia, diabetes, and cardiovascular disease, suggesting that depression is a systemic disorder probably interlinked with a number of chronic medical conditions. In the case of epilepsy, a number of variables, both neurobiological and psychosocial, have to be taken into account. In fact, the burdens of stigma, social limitations, and discrimination can potentially lead to demoralization and poor self-esteem (de Boer et al., 2008), but the pathophysiology of epilepsy per se seems to be interlinked with mood problems. In fact, the involvement of the temporal lobes (Quiske et al., 2000) and the psychotropic effects of AEDs (Perucca and Mula, 2013) seem to be relevant contributors to the increased rates of mood problems in epilepsy.

Clinical features

Peri-ictal mood and anxiety symptoms

Premonitory symptoms preceding seizures are reported by one-third of patients with localization-related epilepsies and they usually occur before secondarily generalized tonic–clonic seizures (Scaramelli et al., 2009). Patients can report depressed mood or irritability lasting hours to days that are typically relieved by the convulsion (Blanchet and Frommer, 1986).

Ictal fear or ictal panic is the most frequently reported ictal psychiatric manifestation and has a strong localizing value (Mula,

2014). In fact, ictal fear has been associated with the right mesial temporal lobe structures (Guimond et al., 2008). It is more common in women than men (Chiesa et al., 2007) and seems to have a poor prognostic value for surgery (Feichtinger et al., 2001). Ictal depression is the second most frequently reported ictal psychiatric manifestation and is characterized by intense anhedonia, feelings of guilt, and/or suicidal ideation, and it is reported by around 1% of patients with temporal lobe epilepsy (TLE) (Gaitatzis et al., 2004).

Post-ictal mood changes are still not easily recognized in clinical practice, but they seem to be frequently reported by patients and relatives. A case series in a monitoring unit reported 18% of patients having at least five symptoms of depression lasting more than 24 hours (Kanner et al., 2004). Manic/hypomanic symptoms are reported post-ictally in 22% of patients, often with associated psychotic symptoms (Kanner et al., 2004). It seems that post-ictal mania has a distinct position among psychiatric manifestations observed in the post-ictal period. In fact, such manic episodes last for a longer period and have a higher frequency of recurrence than post-ictal psychoses, being associated with older age at onset, EEG frontal discharges, and non-dominant hemisphere involvement (Nishida et al., 2006).

Post-ictal anxiety is reported by 45% of patients (Kanner et al., 2004). The median duration of symptoms ranges from 6 to 24 hours. In one-third of cases, post-ictal anxiety may last 24 hours or longer. In about 33% of cases, post-ictal anxiety is reported by patients with a previous history of an anxiety disorder.

Table 17.2 Classification of psychiatric symptoms according to their temporal relationship with epileptic seizures

Relationship with seizures		Duration	Description
Peri-ictal	Pre-ictal	Hours (max 24–48 hours)	Preceding seizures (from hours to days) should be distinguished from the 'aura' which is already a seizure
	Ictal	Minutes	It is a seizure with psychic symptoms (i.e. ictal fear, etc.)
	Post-ictal	Hours to days (maximum 7 days)	Usually following generalized tonic–clonic seizures, very rarely after focal seizures. Mostly stereotyped. These symptoms can be evident immediately after the post-ictal confusional state or after a lucid interval, as in the case of post-ictal psychoses
Para-ictal		Hours to days	Also known as the forced normalization phenomenon
Interictal		Days to years	Mostly chronic disorders

All these symptoms are usually seen in patients with a pre-existing psychiatric disorder and often represent a post-ictal exacerbation.

Interictal mood and anxiety disorders

For many years, the phenomenology of depression in patients with epilepsy has represented a matter of debate. From a clinical perspective, this is a crucial point. In fact, the existence of specific clinical endophenotypes of mood disorders in epilepsy implies the need for specific clinical instruments for the diagnosis, specific guidelines of treatment, and ultimately a different prognosis. Although it is established that patients with epilepsy can develop mood disorders that are identical to those of patients without epilepsy (Jones et al., 2005), an increasing number of authors have pointed out that mood disorders in epilepsy are characterized by atypical features that are poorly reflected by conventional classificatory systems such as the DSM and ICD (Kanner et al., 2000; Mula, 2016b). Pre-modern psychiatrists, such as Kraepelin and Bleuler, observed that patients with epilepsy might develop a pleomorphic pattern of depressive symptoms intermixed with euphoric moods, irritability, fear, and anxiety, as well as anergia, pain, and insomnia (Bleuler, 2013; Kraepelin and Johnstone, 2015). This concept has been revitalized during the twentieth century by Blumer who coined the term interictal dysphoric disorder to refer to this type of somatoform depressive disorder claimed as typical of patients with epilepsy (Blumer, 2000). Modern studies pointed out that such a condition is a mood disorder probably not specific to epilepsy, being diagnosed also in patients with other neurological problems, burdened by a significant component of comorbid anxiety (social phobia and/or generalized anxiety disorder) and quite evident mood instability (Mula et al., 2008b). What seems to be typical of patients with epilepsy is the presence of a specific pattern of mood symptoms (i.e. dysphoria and mood swings) occurring around the seizure and probably responsible for the pleomorphic features of the so-called interictal dysphoric disorder (Mula et al., 2010). The psychopathological spectrum of mood disorders in epilepsy is likely to be large, and it is clear that the underlying brain pathology can influence the expression of mood disorder symptoms, making less evident some aspects or emphasizing others. In the case of epilepsy, a number of variables may account for the atypical phenomenology of mood symptoms like peri-ictal symptoms, the high rates of comorbidity between mood and anxiety disorders (up to 73%), the presence of cognitive problems due to the underlying neurologic condition, and the psychotropic effect of AEDs (Mula, 2013). These issues have relevant implications in terms of prognosis and treatment. On one hand, it emphasizes the need to dissect out peri-ictal manifestations from interictal ones, the former being related to the prognosis and treatment of the epileptic syndrome. On the other hand, the presence of mood instability as an essential element of mood disorders in epilepsy suggests the need to prescribe mood-stabilizing AEDs as the preferred treatment and the utility of antipsychotic drugs in selective cases (Mula, 2013).

Epileptologists are now increasingly recognizing the importance of routine screening for depression in epilepsy clinics. Screening instruments specifically developed for patients with epilepsy are now available and are widely used internationally (Gilliam et al., 2006).

Suicide

In the general population, suicide represents the eleventh cause of death and the second in the group aged 25–34 years. It seems to be more common in men than in women, particularly in developed countries (Wasserman and Wasserman, 2009). In patients with epilepsy, the overall risk of committing suicide is about three times higher than that of the general population (Bell et al., 2009; Christensen et al., 2007). Several studies have attempted to identify reasons for such an increased risk. Although epilepsy is frequently associated with psychiatric comorbidities, this does not seem to explain the reported increased risk. A Danish study pointed out that the rate ratio of suicide in people with epilepsy is still double, even after excluding people with psychiatric comorbidity and adjusting for various factors (Christensen et al., 2007). Some authors have suggested a link with TLE (Park et al., 2015), but others found no association with epilepsy-related variables (Hecimovic et al., 2012). As per mood disorders in general, the relationship between suicide and epilepsy seems to be bidirectional (Hesdorffer et al., 2016). During the last 10 years, the issue of suicide in epilepsy has been linked with AEDs as potentially responsible for such an increased risk (Mula and Sander, 2015). It seems evident now that there are no robust data supporting a causal role, although clinicians (Mula et al. 2013) should always consider treatment-emergent psychiatric adverse events of AEDs. Suicide prevention strategies are increasingly recognized in tertiary epilepsy clinics, and possible screening instruments have been suggested (Mula et al., 2016).

Treatment of mood and anxiety disorders

Data on treatment of depression in epilepsy are still limited and relies heavily on clinical experience. The only double-blind trial on antidepressants in epilepsy was published 30 years ago and compared nomifensine, amitriptyline, and placebo (Robertson and Trimble, 1985). Since then, a number of open studies in small samples of unselected patients with different epilepsy types have been published (i.e. sertraline, citalopram, reboxetine, mirtazapine, and fluoxetine) (Mula, 2016c). One study is of particular interest because it is the only published study in children and adolescents with epilepsy and depression (Thomé-Souza et al., 2007). All these antidepressants were shown to be effective and well tolerated, but due to a lack of controlled data, the Epilepsy Foundation (Barry et al., 2008) and the ILAE (Kerr et al., 2011; Mula and Kanner, 2013) published a number of recommendations to guide clinicians. In general terms, it is reasonable to follow internationally accepted guidelines for the treatment of mood disorders outside epilepsy, applying individual adjustments, in the individual patient, according to the epilepsy type and the concomitant AEDs (Mula and Kanner, 2013). Data on treatment response are limited. It is still unknown whether patients with epilepsy and depression have similar remission and recovery rates as patients with depression but without epilepsy, although it is reasonable to hypothesize so.

Seizure worsening has represented for a long time a major barrier to the use of antidepressants in epilepsy. However, this was based on a priori assumption, rather than on clinical evidence. In reality, the issue of drug-related seizures is quite complex and it is not only confined to psychotropic medications. In general terms, multiple factors have to be taken into account (see Box 17.1) and, on the contrary, studies in animal models suggest that serotonin potentiation is anticonvulsant (Leander, 1992). Among all antidepressants, a clear association with seizures has been established only for maprotiline, high doses of clomipramine and amitriptyline (>200 mg), and high doses of bupropion in the immediate-release formulation (>450 mg). For all other antidepressant drugs, there is no clear evidence of an increased risk of seizures. In this regard, it is important to bear in mind that current knowledge on seizure prevalence during antidepressant drug treatment is based on psychiatric populations and it is still unknown whether these data can be transferred to patients with epilepsy and whether some epileptic syndromes are more at risk than others. If we take into account the increased risk of seizures given by the bidirectional relationship, the reported prevalence of epileptic seizures during treatment with antidepressants in patients with mood disorders (Alper et al., 2007) is even lower than the expected one (Mula, 2016c), suggesting, in conclusion, that antidepressant drugs reduce the risk of seizures.

Psychoses

Epidemiology

Psychoses and thought disorders are relatively rare in patients with epilepsy but represent serious complications affecting prognosis, morbidity, and mortality. Epidemiological evidence pointed out that the incidence of non-organic, non-affective psychoses, including schizophrenia and related disorders, is generally increased (around 4–5%) in epilepsy, as compared to the general population or other chronic medical conditions (Adelow et al., 2012; Qin, 2005). Higher prevalence rates are found in selected samples such as hospital case series (Mendez et al., 1993). Interestingly, both a family history of psychoses and a family history of epilepsy are associated with

psychotic disorders in epilepsy, suggesting strong neurobiological underpinnings between the two disorders (Qin, 2005).

Clinical features

Peri-ictal psychotic symptoms

As per mood and anxiety symptoms, psychotic symptoms of epilepsy are classified according to their relationship with seizures. Among peri-ictal psychoses, the so-called 'ictal psychosis' is, in reality, a non-convulsive status epilepticus, mostly of temporal lobe origin, rarely extra-temporal (i.e. the frontal lobe) (Trimble, 1991). The presence of automatisms and other typical epileptic phenomena can help the clinician in distinguishing a non-convulsive status with psychic symptoms from a brief psychotic episode, and the final diagnosis is based on the EEG (Mula, 2014). Post-ictal psychoses represent the most commonly encountered peri-ictal psychoses, accounting for approximately 25% of all psychoses of epilepsy (see Table 17.3). They are usually precipitated by a cluster of secondarily generalized tonic–clonic seizures and are characterized by peculiar clinical and phenomenological features (Kanemoto at al., 1994; Logsdail and Toone, 1988). Post-ictal psychoses seem to occur in patients with a later age of onset of the epilepsy and with TLE with temporal and extra-temporal structural lesions. Post-ictal psychoses are very rarely reported in subjects with a generalized epilepsy type. The lucid interval (i.e. a period of normal mental state preceding the onset of the psychotic episode) is another typical feature described in almost all patients, lasting from 1 to 6 days (Adachi et al., 2007; Logsdail and Toone, 1988). The psychopathology of post-ictal psychoses is polymorphic, but most patients present with an abnormal mood (either depressed or manic and a paranoid delusion). Some patients are confused throughout the episode, but others present with fluctuating consciousness and disorientation. Delusions of grandiosity and religiosity, often associated with an elevated mood, are also reported, as well as suicidal attempts (Kanemoto et al., 2010). Psychotic symptoms usually remit spontaneously within days or weeks, without the need for psychotropic drug treatment, which is mainly prescribed to reduce mortality and morbidity. In one out of four cases, post-ictal psychosis may progress into chronic psychosis (Adachi et al., 2007).

Interictal psychoses

Psychoses without a clear temporal relationship with epileptic seizures are less frequent than peri-ictal psychoses. However, they are clinically more significant in terms of severity and duration than peri-ictal ones, being chronic disorders. Interictal psychoses develop after several years of active TLE (Adachi et al., 2000). Clinical (Mula et al., 2008a) and neuroimaging findings (Tebartz Van Elst et al., 2002) support a link between mesial temporal structures and psychosis. Neuropathology studies of resected temporal lobes

Table 17.3 Psychoses in relation to seizure activity

	Proportion among all psychotic episodes of epilepsy	Consciousness	EEG	Duration
Interictal	20%	Normal	Unchanged	Months/years
Ictal	10%	Impaired	Non-convulsive status epilepticus	Hours
Post-ictal	60%	Normal/impaired	Slowing	Hours/days
Forced normalization	10%	Normal	Normal	Days

from patients with interictal psychoses have suggested a link with hamartomas and gangliogliomas, rather than mesial temporal sclerosis (Taylor, 1971), but gross abnormalities, such as enlarged ventricles or periventricular gliosis, have also been noted (Bruton et al., 1994). The association with the dominant hemisphere was initially suggested by early studies on interictal psychoses (Flor-Henry, 1983), but subsequent authors showed a complex network reflecting the interplay of psychosis-related genetic factors and the cumulative effects of seizure activity on the brain, rather than a simple laterality effect (Gutierrez-Galve et al., 2012).

Clinical studies have pointed out that the phenomenology of interictal psychoses of epilepsy differs from that of schizophrenia. Some authors described the typical presence of religious mystical experiences and the preservation of affect (Trimble, 1991), while other authors stressed the rarity of negative symptoms and catatonic states (Getz et al., 2003). In addition, the long-term prognosis of interictal psychosis seems to be better than that of schizophrenia, with less reported long-term institutionalization (Ashidate, 2006; Fiseković and Burnazović, 2007), and this is probably due to the tendency of psychotic symptoms to attenuate over time and the rarity of personality deterioration.

Treatment of psychotic disorders

Data on treatment of psychoses of epilepsy are more than scant. As already discussed for mood and anxiety disorders, the Commission on Neuropsychiatry of the International League Against Epilepsy published a collection of papers about treatment strategies in adults with epilepsy and psychiatric disorders and one paper was dedicated to the treatment of psychoses (Adachi et al., 2013). Psychotic symptoms in interictal psychoses can be difficult to manage for a variety of reasons that commonly include poor response to treatment, individual differences in tolerability to antipsychotic drugs, potential interactions with AEDs, and effect on seizure threshold (Mula, 2016c). In addition, it has to be considered that approximately 15% of psychotic episodes may remit with no antipsychotic treatment (Adachi et al., 2013). While the supposed proconvulsant effect of antidepressants is still a matter of debate, this seems to be established for antipsychotics. However, it has to be acknowledged that this is an issue mainly for clozapine, while all other antipsychotics seem to have a low proconvulsant propensity (Alper et al., 2007). For clozapine, the risk is both titration- and dose-dependent. A case series in the United States documented a mean prevalence of seizures during clozapine treatment of 2.9%, with prevalence rates of 1%, 2.7%, and 4.4% for dosages of <300 mg, 300–600 mg, and >600 mg, respectively (Devinsky et al., 1991). Prevalence rates are much lower in patients without a previous history of seizures (Pacia and Devinsky, 1994), confirming that clozapine can deteriorate seizures in predisposed individuals. Up to 5% of patients treated with clozapine can have EEG abnormalities (Varma et al., 2011), but whether this is a predictive factor for clozapine-induced seizures is still unknown. In general, clozapine seems to deteriorate mainly myoclonic jerks, but generalized tonic–clonic seizures or even focal seizures have been reported in predisposed individuals (Varma et al., 2011).

The concept that patients with epilepsy may have abnormal personality profiles is not new but remains controversial for a number of reasons. The main issue relates to whether personality changes are related to the biology of the underlying epilepsy, or a consequence of the epilepsy such as recurrent head injuries, social stigmatization, and use of AEDs. In addition, there are clearly also sociological contributions to personality development in patients. Moreover, the instruments used to detect personality changes, such as the Minnesota Multiphasic Personality Inventory (MMPI), are themselves far from robust and may not be particularly sensitive in patients with epilepsy. The two subtypes of epilepsy for which there is the most robust evidence of specific personality types in some patients are TLE and juvenile myoclonic epilepsy (JME). To overcome the shortcomings of conventional instruments like the MMPI, many groups have developed their own instruments to permit the identification of epilepsy-specific features of behavioural and personality disorders. Bear and Fedio (Bear and Fedio, 1977) developed a rating scale consisting of 18 behavioural features thought to be associated with TLE. They reported that patients with TLE scored significantly higher on subscales, including dependency, obsessionality, humourless sobriety, and religious and philosophical concerns, when compared to healthy or neurological controls. This interictal behavioural syndrome in patients with TLE, emphasizing alterations in sexual behaviour (typically hyposexuality), hyper-religiosity, emotional viscosity, and a tendency towards extensive and compulsive writing (hypergraphia), was actually originally described in the nineteenth century, but better publicized with the work of Gastaut in France and Geschwind in America (Waxman and Geshwind, 1975). The viscosity of the syndrome refers to a bradyphrenia, or slowness of thought processes, and increased social adhesion, such that patients tend to prolong social encounters beyond that indicated by social cues (Trimble, 2013). Although these findings are not present in all patients with TLE, they may be present in a proportion, particularly those with medial sites or limbic temporal lobe lesions who are more susceptible to psychiatric disturbances, including personality disorders.

Although most of the literature has focused on interictal personality changes in TLE, distinctive personality types have also been described in association with generalized epilepsy syndromes. The best known is that described by Janz in patients with JME (Janz, 2002). He described a personality profile in these patients characterized by 'unsteadiness, lack of discipline, hedonism, and indifference towards their illness'. These patient characteristics could often lead to poor compliance with medications and difficulties in managing their epilepsy. Intriguingly, recent studies highlight that patients with JME appear to have subtle frontal lobe neuropsychological deficits, and advanced neuroimaging techniques demonstrate functional and structural abnormalities in the frontal cortex and thalamus that are otherwise not seen in conventional MRI scans (Wandschneider, 2012). These findings are in keeping with the behavioural and personality problems reported in patients with JME and may, in part, explain them.

Recognition of personality subtypes in patients with epilepsy has two main uses. Firstly, it may aid the classification of epilepsy syndromes, though other information such as EEG and seizure semiology play a greater role in this process. Perhaps more importantly, recognition of personality subtypes may aid the management of these patients. A patient's personality may be linked to their compliance with treatment and any breakdown of their relationship with family, friends, and colleagues and may help in adapting consultation's styles and prevent further psychiatric problems.

Psychiatric complications of epilepsy treatment

Post-surgery psychiatric problems

Temporal lobectomy is an established treatment for patients with intractable epilepsy. Ever since the early series, the possibility that surgery may be associated with the development of psychiatric disorders, in particular psychoses, has been discussed. Most centres have stopped operating floridly psychotic patients, based on the observation that psychoses generally do not improve with the operation. Only a few centres, however, regularly include psychiatric screening as part of their preoperative assessment and even fewer centres consider post-operative psychiatric follow-up, in contrast to the often scrupulous recording of neuropsychological deficits.

A number of post-surgical psychiatric complications have been reported, including exacerbation of pre-existing conditions and *de novo* depressive and/or anxiety or psychotic disorders, as well as PNES. The early post-operative phase is dominated by physical problems that may initiate early psychiatric disturbances, especially in patients with preoperative psychiatric comorbidities. The second phase after discharge from hospital is the typical time in which various psychiatric disorders may develop (either *de novo* or exacerbations of known disorders). During that period, it is mandatory to keep in contact with patients, to start psychiatric treatments, if necessary, and to screen for suicidal risk (Koch-Stoecker et al., 2013). The majority of post-surgical complications start within 1 year from epilepsy surgery, and it is important to inform patients and relatives that up to one-third of subjects may experience mood or anxiety symptoms requiring treatment during the first trimester after surgery. Psychoses can start later on during the first year and may complicate the outcome. Further studies are needed in order to identify patients at increased risk of post-surgical complications.

AED-related psychiatric problems

AEDs have a number of mechanisms of action that are likely to be responsible for their anti-seizure activity, but also for their effect on mood and behaviour. It is now established that some AEDs, especially GABAergic compounds, can be associated with the development of depressive symptoms in patients with epilepsy (Mula and Sander, 2007). Patients with a previous history of a mood disorder seem to be more vulnerable to negative psychotropic effects of AEDs, sometimes with unpredictable outcomes, even for compounds with well-known mood-stabilizing properties like valproate or lamotrigine (Perucca and Mula, 2013). In these patients, it is recommended to adopt slow titration rates whenever a new AED is started.

AED-related psychotic symptoms tend to occur in the context of toxic encephalopathies or, more rarely, the so-called forced normalization phenomenon. This concept refers to the publications of Heinrich Landolt who reported a group of patients who had florid psychotic episodes with 'forced normalization' of the EEG (Landolt, 1962). Subsequently, Tellenbach (Tellenbach, 1965) introduced the term 'alternative psychosis' for the clinical phenomenon of the reciprocal relationship between abnormal mental states and seizures, which did not, as Landolt's term did, rely on EEG findings (Trimble and Schmitz, 1998). Since the early observations of Landolt, a number of patients with alternative psychoses have been documented to put their existence beyond doubt and an association with the prescription of all AEDs was noted, suggesting that this is not a drug-specific phenomenon but rather is linked to the neurobiological mechanisms underlying seizure control. In fact, a case of an alternative psychosis secondary to vagus nerve stimulation has been documented (Gatzonis et al., 2000), and it is likely that the forced normalization phenomenon plays a role in patients who develop *de novo* psychosis following successful epilepsy surgery. For many years, there has been a strong debate on whether there is an epilepsy syndrome most commonly associated with the forced normalization phenomenon. Initially, drug-refractory TLE was claimed to be the prototype, but subsequent literature on alternative psychoses favoured generalized epilepsies (Trimble and Schmitz, 1998). Nowadays, there is general agreement that the forced normalization phenomenon occurs with both generalized and focal epilepsies, but it is rare in patients with mainly generalized tonic–clonic seizures (e.g. idiopathic generalized epilepsy of awakening) and in extratemporal lobe epilepsy (Mula, 2010).

Psychogenic non-epileptic seizures

PNES are paroxysmal, time-limited alterations in motor, sensory, autonomic, and/or cognitive signs and symptoms. Superficially, they resemble epileptic seizures, but they are not caused by ictal epileptiform activity (LaFrance et al., 2013a). They are typically reported as being beyond voluntary control, and most fulfil the diagnostic criteria of dissociative (conversion) disorder (ICD-10) or conversion (functional neurological symptom) disorder (DSM-5). Controversy exists over the most appropriate term for these episodes (Stone et al., 2002). Terms such as hysterical seizures or pseudoseizures are both pejorative and oversimplified, and fail to capture the broad range of underlying causes. The term PNES is popular, because it is more specific than 'non-epileptic attack disorder (NEAD)', which encompasses multiple causes for paroxysmal events that resemble epileptic seizures (Smith, 2012). However, the term PNES is also problematic because it makes unsubstantiated presumptions about the aetiology of these paroxysmal episodes and maintains an unhelpful dichotomy between mental and physiological processes (Stone et al., 2002). Nevertheless, given its current widespread use, we have elected to use it here.

Epidemiology

The incidence of PNES is between 1.4 and 4.9/100,000/year, and its prevalence between 2 and 33 per 100,000 (Asadi-Pooya and Sperling, 2015). Onset is commonest between the second and fourth decades of life and is commonest in women at a ratio of 3:1 in this age range. However, in the pre-adolescent and elderly age ranges, there is an equal distribution between both sexes (Asadi-Pooya and Sperling, 2015). As many as 25% of patients referred to epilepsy centres for refractory seizures are diagnosed with PNES, and up to 50% of patients with refractory 'status epilepticus' have PNES, rather than epilepsy (Reuber, 2008). Patients receive a correct diagnosis, on average, 7.6 years after seizure onset and therefore receive inappropriate treatment with anticonvulsants (Reuber et al., 2002a). One-third of patients with PNES are admitted to an intensive care unit during the course of their illness (Dickinson and Looper, 2012). The cost of undiagnosed PNES can therefore be equivalent to the cost of treating epilepsy over the lifetime of the patient (Dickinson and Looper, 2012). Moreover, there are significant, but unquantifiable, socio-economic costs for patients that result from lost work days, unemployment, and quality of life constraints (Reuber, 2008).

Clinical features of PNES

A systematic approach to the semiology of the episodes helps discriminate between PNES and epileptic seizures.

Setting and triggers

Most episodes of PNES occur in front of witnesses, and not during sleep (Avbersek and Sisodiya, 2010), in contrast to epileptic seizures. Patients with PNES may report that seizures occur during sleep and may appear to be asleep, but the EEG in these cases demonstrates wakefulness (Avbersek and Sisodiya, 2010). While stress may trigger PNES, it is also a well-documented seizure precipitant in patients with epilepsy (Galtrey et al., 2016). Furthermore, witness responders are more likely than patients to associate emotional stress as a trigger for events (Reuber et al., 2011).

Frequency, duration, ictal, and post-ictal features

PNES are often frequent, and fewer than one event a week is uncommon (Reuber et al., 2003). The lack of even small improvements in seizure control despite multiple therapeutic trials suggests a diagnosis of PNES (Reuber, 2008). During an event, unresponsive behaviour with motor manifestations mimicking a generalized convulsion or a complex partial seizure is the commonest manifestation, while events that mimic atonic, absence, or simple partial seizures are less common (Hubsch et al., 2011). Features of the clinical event may be useful in distinguishing PNES from epileptic seizures (see

Table 17.4). One systematic review found that long duration, fluctuating course, asynchronous movements, pelvic thrusting, side-to-side head or body movements, forced ictal eye closing, ictal crying, and memory recall reliably favoured PNES. Post-ictal confusion, seizures arising from sleep, and stertorous breathing favoured epileptic seizures (Avbersek and Sisodiya, 2010). However, no single feature is diagnostic for PNES, and the psychiatric, neurological, and psychological background of a patient must be considered.

Diagnosis and investigations

The commonest differential for PNES is epileptic seizures, caused by abnormal, synchronous neuronal activity in the brain. In contrast, the EEG during PNES reveals preserved background rhythms and normal reactivity. However, some epileptic seizures arising from mesial or basal areas of the brain show no ictal EEG changes, because these areas are insensitive to scalp EEG. Frontal lobe seizures may therefore present a particular diagnostic challenge because of their unusual semiology (see Table 17.4). Less commonly, other non-epileptic paroxysmal disorders may sometimes be mistaken for PNES or epileptic seizures, including sleep and movement disorders, and syncope (Smith, 2012).

Though semiological features are diagnostically useful, eyewitness descriptions are unreliable (Syed et al., 2011). The ILAE has determined that video-electroencephalography (video-EEG) is the gold standard investigation for the diagnosis of PNES (LaFrance et al., 2013b). Without video-EEG, the level of diagnostic certainty varies according to the combination of patient history, witness observations, and ictal/interictal EEG data available (see Table 17.5).

Table 17.4 Ictal and post-ictal features distinguishing between epileptic seizures and PNES

Feature	Epileptic	PNES
Duration	Often brief, <1–2 minutes	Often long, >2 minutes
Eyes	Usually open during event	Usually closed during event Forced eye closure may be present
Consciousness during seizure	Complete LOC during convulsive seizure	Often incomplete LOC during convulsive seizure
Motor activity	Stereotyped	Variable (though PNES can be stereotyped, multiple seizure types may be present in one episode)
	Synchronized	Asynchronous*, forward pelvic thrusting*, rolling side to side, opisthotonus
	Gradually builds up	Waxes and wanes
Vocalization	Uncommon during convulsion (can occur at onset)	May occur during convulsion
Prolonged ictal atonia	Rare	May occur
Incontinence and tongue biting	Common in convulsive seizures	Uncommon**
Autonomic signs	Cyanosis, tachycardia with major convulsion	Uncommon
Post-ictal symptoms	Confused, drowsy, amnestic for seizure	Quickly awakens and reorientated, may recall events during seizure*
	Deep and prolonged inspiratory and expiratory breathing after convulsive seizure	Shallow, rapid respiration after convulsive seizure*
	Headache common	Headache rare

* Frontal lobe seizures may present a particular diagnostic challenge. Seizures arising from the dorsolateral aspect of the frontal lobe may have manifestations of activation of primary motor cortices such as forced eye version, clonic or tonic movements, head version, or aphasia. Seizures arising from the prefrontal cortex manifest as 'hypermotor seizures', with variable clinical manifestations, including bizarre gestures, laughing, shouting, and alternating limb movements such as peddling and thrashing of the extremities. Seizures originating from the cingulate gyrus can display complex stereotypic movements, such as kicking, grasping, or running, with or without vocalizations. Seizures arising from the supplementary sensorimotor area in the mesial frontal region are characterized by sudden, brief, and asymmetric tonic posturing of one or more extremities, with repetitive vocalizations, and may cluster. Patients may rapidly reorientate after frontal lobe seizures and may have a post-ictal breathing pattern similar to that seen in PNES.

** Tongue biting, incontinence, and self-injury, though more common in epileptic seizures, can occur in up to 30% of PNES patients. A tongue bitten on the side is more specific for an epileptic seizure than when bitten on the tip.

Adapted with permission from Avbersek, A., & Sisodiya, S. Does the primary literature provide support for clinical signs used to distinguish psychogenic nonepileptic seizures from epileptic seizures? *Journal of Neurology, Neurosurgery, and Psychiatry*, 81(7): 719–725. Copyright © 2010, *British Medical Journal*. http://dx.doi.org/10.1136/jnnp.2009.197996.

Table 17.5 ILAE diagnostic criteria for PNES

Diagnostic classification	History	Witnessed event	EEG
Possible	+	By witness or self-report/description	No epileptiform activity in routine or sleep-deprived interictal EEG
Probable	+	By clinician who reviewed video recording or in person, showing semiology typical of PNES	No epileptiform activity in routine or sleep-deprived interictal EEG
Clinically established	+	By clinician experienced in diagnosis of seizure disorders (on video or in person), showing semiology typical of PNES, while not on EEG	No epileptiform activity in routine or ambulatory ictal EEG during a typical ictus/event in which the semiology would make ictal epileptiform EEG activity expectable during equivalent epileptic seizures
Documented	+	By clinician experienced in diagnosis of seizure disorders, showing semiology typical of PNES, while on video EEG	No epileptiform activity immediately before, during, or after ictus captured on ictal video-EEG with typical PNES semiology

+, history characteristics consistent with PNES.
EEG, electroencephalography.
Source data from LaFrance, W. C., Reuber, M., & Goldstein, L. H. (2013). Management of psychogenic nonepileptic seizures. *Epilepsia*, 54, 53–67.

Other investigations can provide support for the diagnosis or evaluate comorbidities that affect management.

Electroencephalography

Routine EEG records activity for a short period and is unlikely to capture an event. A normal interictal EEG does not exclude the possibility of epilepsy or confirm PNES. Similarly, interictal epileptiform abnormalities do not exclude PNES and can be seen in up to 18% of patients with PNES alone, or more, if there is a past/concurrent history of epilepsy or other underlying neurologic injury or disease (Reuber et al., 2002b). Video-EEG monitoring combines extended EEG with time-locked video acquisition. Up to 96% of patients will have typical PNES within the first 48 hours (Woollacott et al., 2010). However, only 15–30% of simple partial seizures or seizure auras, which involve a limited and deep brain area, are associated with surface EEG changes. Consequently, a normal ictal EEG does not always exclude epilepsy.

Serum prolactin and other biomarkers

Prolactin testing may be useful because levels can rise after epileptic seizures. However, this increment is limited to 60% of generalized tonic–clonic seizures and 46% of complex partial seizures, and is even lower for simple partial seizures (Chen et al., 2005). The same limitations apply to other serum biomarkers such as creatine phosphokinase, lactate dehydrogenase, or pCO_2 (Petramfar et al., 2009).

Neuroimaging

When a structural abnormality is seen on brain MRI, it suggests a neuroanatomical cause for epileptic seizures and provides support for a diagnosis of epilepsy. However, abnormal brain MRI can be present in 10% of patients with PNES (Reuber et al., 2002c), and many patients with epilepsy have normal brain MRI.

Neuropsychological testing

Deficits in attention and memory are present in both PNES and epilepsy patients, and limit the utility of neuropsychological testing for distinguishing between these diagnoses (Willment et al., 2015). Personality testing with the MMPI during neuropsychological evaluation may be helpful in both highlighting comorbid psychiatric disturbances and differentiating patients with PNES and those with epilepsy (see later).

Psychiatric evaluation

Psychiatric evaluation does not have a diagnostic role in PNES but is important for identifying comorbid or underlying psychiatric conditions. These include depression, anxiety, somatoform, dissociative, and other disorders (Reuber et al., 2003).

Aetiology and comorbidities

Patients with PNES typically present to neurologists who define PNES by what they are not (epileptic seizures), instead of by their underlying pathophysiology and psychopathology. PNES is therefore typically attributed to 'psychological causes' and is, at best, described within a framework of predisposing, precipitating, and perpetuating comorbid factors (Reuber, 2009). Recently, efforts have been made to describe mechanistic models of PNES and the relevance of these comorbid factors (Brown and Reuber, 2016a and b). This is the framework we adopt here (see Table 17.6).

PNES as dissociative phenomena

In this model, PNES result from the activation of memory fragments dissociated from awareness as a result of some traumatic experience (Brown and Reuber, 2016a). Patients with PNES have a history of increased exposure to head injuries and traumatic and stressful life events, including abuse, compared to patients with epilepsy or healthy controls (Brown and Reuber, 2016a). Up to 39% of patients with PNES may meet the diagnostic criteria for PTSD, compared to 21% in epilepsy patients (Fiszman et al., 2004). Amnesia for ictal events may represent evidence of actual dissociation during PNES (Kuyk et al., 1999). Alternatively, PNES may represent 'a paroxysmal dissociative response to heightened arousal' with a lack of accompanying fear, reflecting the dissociation of distress during an attack ('panic without panic') (Goldstein et al., 2010). The evidence that patients with PNES report more comorbid dissociative symptoms, compared to patients with epilepsy, is more mixed (Lawton et al., 2008). However, there is evidence to suggest PNES have a deficit in their ability to integrate mental states. Patients with PNES have higher hypnotic suggestibility (Kuyk et al., 1999) and attentional dysfunction (Willment et al., 2015). They have heightened vigilance

Table 17.6 Models of PNES and relevant comorbid factors

Model	Comorbid factors
PNES as dissociative phenomena	• Trauma and PTSD • Stressful life events • Dissociation during PNES • Presence of other dissociative symptoms • Suggestibility • Attentional and executive dysfunction
PNES as a psychological function	• Dysfunctional family relationships • Insecure attachment styles • Anxiety and arousal symptoms • Somatization/conversion disorders • Emotional dysregulation • Alexithymia
PNES as a learnt behaviour	• Exposure to seizure models, e.g. family history of epilepsy or concurrent epilepsy • Reinforcement with primary and secondary gain

It should be noted that PNES occur in a heterogenous patient population and no single mechanism or factor can explain its occurrence in all patients. Thus, multiple mechanisms and comorbid factors may be present in an individual patient.

Adapted from Brown, R. J., & Reuber, M. (2016a). Psychological and psychiatric aspects of psychogenic non-epileptic seizures (PNES): A systematic review. *Clinical Psychology Review*, 45, 157–182. © 2016 Elsevier Ltd. All rights reserved.

and a reduced ability to ignore irrelevant sensory stimuli, compared to epilepsy patients (Willment et al., 2015). This may manifest in attentional and executive dysfunction, including in verbal memory and fluency, and aberrant cognitive–emotion integration. That is, the attentional bias to perceived social threat may result in reduced cognitive flexibility under emotive or stressful conditions (Willment et al., 2015).

PNES as a psychological function

In this model, PNES represent a defensive process that prevents an individual from being overwhelmed by the emotional consequences of adversity and stress (Brown and Reuber, 2016a). Although this may stem from previous adverse life events (see earlier), it may also arise from an incapacity to deal with 'normal adversity'. Indeed, dysfunctional family relationships, including poor communication or support, insecure attachment styles, and interpersonal conflict, are more frequent in patients with PNES than in those with epileptic seizures (Reuber, 2008). PNES may also represent an avoidant or defensive response to acute anxiety, rather than to adversity per se. Although anxiety symptoms do not appear to be more common in PNES, compared with epilepsy, autonomic arousal is present before, during, and after PNES, resulting in physiological symptoms that are not accompanied by fear or distress (Brown and Reuber, 2016a). Related to this, deficits in emotion processing have been identified in patients with PNES. Patients have high levels of alexithymia, which is a deficit in the recognition and verbal expression of emotional states, and instead a tendency to the physical expression of emotion. Consequently, they also have difficulty in recognizing emotional factors as possible triggers for their episodes (Baslet et al., 2016). This may be underpinned by preconscious, interictal emotional and fear hypersensitivity and maladaptive ways of regulating this intensity, including use of avoidance, rather than effective behavioural strategies (Bakvis et al., 2011). This model is given further credence by the defence mechanisms used by patients with PNES (Brown and Reuber, 2016a) and the high levels of medically

unexplained symptoms reported by patients with PNES (Dixit et al., 2013). Indeed, a subgroup of patients exhibit a 'conversion V' profile on the MMPI (i.e. elevations on the hypochondriasis and hysteria sub-scales, coupled with a smaller elevation on the depression sub-scale), compared to patients with epilepsy (Brown and Reuber, 2016a).

PNES as a learnt behaviour

In this model, PNES represents a learnt, involuntary behaviour, which affords both primary (relief from emotional conflict or tension) and secondary (deriving advantages such as attention, relief from responsibilities, or attaining disability benefits) gain (Brown and Reuber, 2016a). The fact that the prevalence of epilepsy among patients with PNES is greater than in the general population and always precedes the development of PNES in these patients supports this model (Reuber, 2009). Rates of concurrent epilepsy among patients with PNES range from 5% to 50%, due to variability in the diagnostic criteria for epilepsy (Asadi-Pooya and Sperling, 2015). Epilepsy may contribute to the risk of developing PNES because the experience or observation of epileptic seizures in others or the media may provide a basis for model learning (Reuber, 2009).

Treatment of PNES

The ILAE has published clear guidance on the management of patients with PNES (LaFrance et al., 2013b). The first step in management after securing the diagnosis of PNES is effective communication of the diagnosis with the patient. In some instances, structured communication of the diagnosis of PNES alone may effect a significant reduction in the frequency of episodes (Hall-Patch et al., 2010). However, most patients will continue to have frequent episodes and need further intervention. Before any specific treatment recommendations are made, patients should have a formal psychiatric assessment, so that treatment can be tailored to individual patients. Treatment recommendations are based mainly on observational studies, and there are few randomized trials available.

Cognitive behavioural treatment

CBT based on a fear avoidance model has been studied in two RCTs and may be useful in patients in whom PNES acts as a dissociative response in stressful circumstances (Goldstein et al., 2010; LaFrance et al., 2014). Both studies demonstrated significant reductions in seizure frequency, though complete seizure remission was less common and long-term outcomes unknown. In addition, only one of the trials demonstrated a positive effect on depression, anxiety, quality of life, and global functioning (LaFrance et al., 2014), while the other showed no effect of treatment on psychosocial function, health service use, or employment (Goldstein et al., 2010). Other forms of psychotherapy, such as group or family therapy, mindfulness, and psychodynamic psychotherapy, also may be useful in specific circumstances, though the evidence for them is based on observational studies and case series (LaFrance et al., 2013b). It is now becoming evident that multiple psychotherapeutic approaches tailored on the individual patient are needed (Agrawal et al., 2014).

Pharmacotherapy

Pharmacological treatment of patients should begin with early tapering and discontinuation of AEDs, unless a specific AED has a documented beneficial psychopharmacological effect (LaFrance et al., 2013b). Antidepressants and anxiolytics should be prescribed on an individualized basis to address specific psychiatric comorbidities in patients with PNES. One blinded, randomized controlled study demonstrated a non-significant reduction in PNES frequency when sertraline was prescribed alone (LaFrance et al., 2010), while another study showed that when it was combined with CBT, it reduced seizures by 59%, compared to 51% when CBT was used alone (LaFrance et al., 2014).

Prognosis

Although the treatments described above may be effective in the short term, long-term outcomes in event frequency and functional status are less promising. At a mean of 11 years after seizure onset, two-thirds of patients continue to have seizures and more than half may be dependent on social security, while only a minority are seizure-free and economically active despite some form of therapeutic intervention (Reuber et al., 2003). Poor prognostic indicators include comorbid epilepsy, concurrent psychiatric diagnoses, violent hypermotor seizures, high accident and emergency attendance rates, and being in receipt of social security benefits, while good prognostic indicators include higher educational levels, young age of onset and diagnosis, acceptance of diagnosis, good social support, employment at baseline, and lower somatization and depersonalization scores (Baslet et al., 2016). Ultimately, the heterogenous nature of this patient population means that a 'one-size-fits-all' treatment plan is unlikely to be successful.

KEY LEARNING POINTS

- Psychiatric disorders occur more frequently in epilepsy than in the general population and can deeply affect quality of life and increase morbidity and mortality.
- Mood and anxiety disorders represent the most frequently reported psychiatric comorbidities.
- Psychiatric complications of epilepsy treatment, such as surgery, and treatment-emergent adverse events of AEDs need to be considered.
- SSRIs are reasonably safe in patients with epilepsy, while only clozapine, among antipsychotics, pose a risk.
- PNES need a multidisciplinary approach and psychotherapeutic interventions should be tailored to the individual patient.
- PNES represent a heterogenous construct, and multiple psychological and cognitive variables need to be considered.

REFERENCES

Adachi, N., et al. (2000). Predictive variables of interictal psychosis in epilepsy. *Neurology*, 55, 1310–14.

Adachi, N., et al. (2007). Duration of postictal psychotic episodes. *Epilepsia*, 48, 1531–7.

Adachi, N., et al. (2013). Basic treatment principles for psychotic disorders in patients with epilepsy. *Epilepsia, 54 Suppl 1*, 19–33.

Adelow, C., et al. (2012). Hospitalization for psychiatric disorders before and after onset of unprovoked seizures/epilepsy. *Neurology*, 78, 396–401.

Agrawal, N., Gaynor, D., Lomax, A., Mula, M. (2014). Multimodular psychotherapy intervention for nonepileptic attack disorder: an individualized pragmatic approach. *Epilepsy & Behavior*, 41, 144–8.

Alper, K., et al. (2007). Seizure incidence in psychopharmacological clinical trials: an analysis of Food and Drug Administration (FDA) summary basis of approval reports. *Biological Psychiatry*, 62, 345–54.

Asadi-Pooya, A.A., Sperling, M.R. (2015). Epidemiology of psychogenic nonepileptic seizures. *Epilepsy & Behavior: E&B*, 46, 60–5.

Ashidate, N. (2006). [Clinical study on epilepsy and psychosis]. *Seishin Shinkeigaku Zasshi = Psychiatria Et Neurologia Japonica*, 108, 260–5.

Avbersek, A., Sisodiya, S. (2010). Does the primary literature provide support for clinical signs used to distinguish psychogenic nonepileptic seizures from epileptic seizures? *Journal of Neurology, Neurosurgery, and Psychiatry*, 81, 719–25.

Baker, G.A., et al. (1996). The associations of psychopathology in epilepsy: a community study. *Epilepsy Research*, 25, 29–39.

Bakvis, P., et al. (2011). Automatic avoidance tendencies in patients with psychogenic non-epileptic seizures. *Seizure*, 20, 628–34.

Barry, J.J., et al.; Advisory Group of the Epilepsy Foundation as part of its Mood Disorder. (2008). Consensus statement: the evaluation and treatment of people with epilepsy and affective disorders. *Epilepsy & Behavior: E&B, 13 Suppl 1*, S1–29.

Baslet, G., et al. (2016). Psychogenic Non-Epileptic Seizures: An Updated Primer. *Psychosomatics*, 57, 1–17.

Bear, D., Fedio, P. (1977) Quantitative analysis of interictal behaviour in temporal lobe epilepsy. *Archives of Neurology*, 34, 454–67.

Bell, G.S., et al. (2009). Suicide in people with epilepsy: how great is the risk? *Epilepsia*, 50, 1933–42.

Blanchet, P., Frommer, G.P. (1986). Mood change preceding epileptic seizures. *Journal of Nervous and Mental Disease*, 174, 471–6.

Bleuler, E. (2013). *Lehrbuch der Psychiatrie*. Springer-Verlag.

Blumer, D. (2000). Dysphoric disorders and paroxysmal affects: recognition and treatment of epilepsy-related psychiatric disorders. *Harvard Review of Psychiatry*, 8, 8–17.

Brandt, C., Mula, M. (2016). Anxiety disorders in people with epilepsy. *Epilepsy & Behavior*, 59, 87–91.

Brown, R.J., Reuber, M. (2016a). Psychological and psychiatric aspects of psychogenic non-epileptic seizures (PNES): A systematic review. *Clinical Psychology Review*, 45, 157–82.

Brown, R.J., Reuber, M. (2016b). Towards an integrative theory of psychogenic non-epileptic seizures (PNES). *Clinical Psychology Review*, 47, 55–70.

Bruton, C.J., et al. (1994). Epilepsy, psychosis, and schizophrenia: clinical and neuropathologic correlations. *Neurology*, 44, 34–42.

Chen, D.K., et al.; Therapeutics and Technology Assessment Subcommittee of the American Academy of Neurology. (2005). Use of serum prolactin in diagnosing epileptic seizures: report of the Therapeutics and Technology Assessment Subcommittee of the American Academy of Neurology. *Neurology*, 65, 668–75.

Chiesa, V., Gardella, E., Tassi, L., et al. (2007). Age-related gender differences in reporting ictal fear: analysis of case histories and review of the literature. *Epilepsia*, 48, 2361–4.

Christensen, J., et al. (2007). Epilepsy and risk of suicide: a population-based case–control study. *The Lancet Neurology*, 6, 693–8.

de Boer, H.M., et al. (2008). The global burden and stigma of epilepsy. *Epilepsy & Behavior*, 12, 540–6.

Devinsky, O., et al. (1991). Clozapine-related seizures. *Neurology, 41*, 369–71.

Dickinson, P., Looper, K.J. (2012). Psychogenic nonepileptic seizures: a current overview. *Epilepsia, 53*, 1679–89.

Dixit, R., et al. (2013). Medical comorbidities in patients with psychogenic nonepileptic spells (PNES) referred for video-EEG monitoring. *Epilepsy & Behavior, 28*, 137–40.

Duncan, J.S., et al. (2006). Adult epilepsy. *Lancet, 367*, 1087–100.

Feichtinger, M., et al. (2001). Ictal fear in temporal lobe epilepsy: surgical outcome and focal hippocampal changes revealed by proton magnetic resonance spectroscopy imaging. *Archives of Neurology, 58*, 771–7.

Fiseković, S., Burnazović, L. (2007). Epileptic psychoses—evaluation of clinical aspects. *Bosnian Journal of Basic Medical Sciences, 7*, 140–3.

Fisher, R.S., et al. (2014). ILAE official report: a practical clinical definition of epilepsy. *Epilepsia, 55*, 475–82.

Fiszman, A., et al. (2004). Traumatic events and posttraumatic stress disorder in patients with psychogenic nonepileptic seizures: a critical review. *Epilepsy & Behavior, 5*, 818–25.

Flor-Henry, P. (1983). Determinants of psychosis in epilepsy: laterality and forced normalization. *Biological Psychiatry, 18*, 1045–57.

Gaitatzis, A., et al. (2004). The psychiatric comorbidity of epilepsy. *Acta Neurologica Scandinavica, 110*, 207–20.

Galtrey, C.M., et al. (2016). Stress and epilepsy: fact or fiction, and what can we do about it? *Practical Neurology, 16*, 270–8.

Gatzonis, S.D., et al. (2000). Acute psychosis and EEG normalisation after vagus nerve stimulation. *Journal of Neurology, Neurosurgery, and Psychiatry, 69*, 278–9.

Geschwind, N. (1997). *Norman Geschwind: Selected Publications on Language, Epilepsy, and Behavior*. Butterworth-Heinemann.

Getz, K., et al. (2003). Negative symptoms and psychosocial status in temporal lobe epilepsy. *Epilepsy Research, 53*, 240–4.

Gilliam, F.G., et al. (2006). Rapid detection of major depression in epilepsy: a multicentre study. *The Lancet Neurology, 5*, 399–405.

Gloor, P., et al. (1982). The role of the limbic system in experiential phenomena of temporal lobe epilepsy. *Annals of Neurology, 12*, 129–44.

Goldstein, L.H., et al. (2010). Cognitive-behavioral therapy for psychogenic nonepileptic seizures: a pilot RCT. *Neurology, 74*, 1986–94.

Gowers, W.R. (2015). *Epilepsy, and Other Chronic Convulsive Diseases*—Scholar's Choice Edition. Scholar's Choice.

Guimond, A., et al. (2008). Ictal fear depends on the cerebral laterality of the epileptic activity. *Epileptic Disorders, 10*, 101–12.

Gutierrez-Galve, L., et al. (2012). Cortical abnormalities and their cognitive correlates in patients with temporal lobe epilepsy and interictal psychosis. *Epilepsia, 53*, 1077–87.

Hall-Patch, L., et al.; NEST collaborators. (2010). Acceptability and effectiveness of a strategy for the communication of the diagnosis of psychogenic nonepileptic seizures. *Epilepsia, 51*, 70–8.

Hecimovic, H., et al. (2012). Depression but not seizure factors or quality of life predicts suicidality in epilepsy. *Epilepsy & Behavior, 24*, 426–9.

Hesdorffer, D.C., et al. (2012). Epilepsy, suicidality, and psychiatric disorders: a bidirectional association. *Annals of Neurology, 72*, 184–91.

Hesdorffer, D.C., et al. (2016). Occurrence and Recurrence of Attempted Suicide Among People With Epilepsy. *JAMA Psychiatry, 73*, 80–6.

Hubsch, C., et al. (2011). Clinical classification of psychogenic non-epileptic seizures based on video-EEG analysis and automatic clustering. *Journal of Neurology, Neurosurgery, and Psychiatry, 82*, 955–60.

Jackson, J.H. (1958). *Selected Writings: On Epilepsy and Epileptiform Convulsions*. Staples Press.

Janz, D. (2002) The psychiatry of idiopathic generalized epilepsy. In: Trimble, M.R., Schmitz, B. (eds.) *The Neuropsychiatry of Epilepsy*. Cambridge University Press, Cambridge, pp. 41–61.

Jones, J.E., et al. (2005). Clinical assessment of Axis I psychiatric morbidity in chronic epilepsy: a multicenter investigation. *Journal of Neuropsychiatry and Clinical Neurosciences, 17*, 172–9.

Kanemoto, K., Kawasaki, J., Kawai, I. (1994). Postictal psychoses: in comparison with acute interictal psychoses. *Japanese Journal of Psychiatry and Neurology, 48*, 209–11.

Kanemoto, K., et al. (2010). Violence and postictal psychosis: a comparison of postictal psychosis, interictal psychosis, and postictal confusion. *Epilepsy & Behavior, 19*, 162–6.

Kanner, A.M., et al. (2000). The Use of Sertraline in Patients with Epilepsy: Is It Safe? *Epilepsy & Behavior, 1*, 100–5.

Kanner, A.M., et al. (2004). Prevalence and clinical characteristics of postictal psychiatric symptoms in partial epilepsy. *Neurology, 62*, 708–13.

Kerr, M.P., et al.; International League of Epilepsy (ILAE) Commission on the Neuropsychiatric Aspects of Epilepsy. (2011). International consensus clinical practice statements for the treatment of neuropsychiatric conditions associated with epilepsy. *Epilepsia, 52*, 2133–8.

Koch-Stoecker, S., et al. (2013). Treatment of postsurgical psychiatric complications. *Epilepsia, 54 Suppl 1*, 46–52.

Kraepelin, E., Johnstone, T. (2015). *Lectures on Clinical Psychiatry*. BiblioLife.

Kuyk, J., et al. (1999). Hypnotic recall: a positive criterion in the differential diagnosis between epileptic and pseudoepileptic seizures. *Epilepsia, 40*, 485–91.

LaFrance, W.C., et al. (2010). Pilot pharmacologic randomized controlled trial for psychogenic nonepileptic seizures. *Neurology, 75*, 1166–73.

LaFrance, W.C., Jr, et al. (2013a). Minimum requirements for the diagnosis of psychogenic nonepileptic seizures: A staged approach: A report from the International League Against Epilepsy Nonepileptic Seizures Task Force. *Epilepsia, 54*, 2005–18.

LaFrance, W.C., et al. (2013b). Management of psychogenic nonepileptic seizures. *Epilepsia, 54*, 53–67.

LaFrance, W.C., et al.; NES Treatment Trial (NEST-T) Consortium. (2014). Multicenter pilot treatment trial for psychogenic nonepileptic seizures: a randomized clinical trial. *JAMA Psychiatry, 71*, 997–1005.

Landolt, H. (1962). [Psychic disorders in epilepsy. Clinical and electroencephalographic research]. *Deutsche Medizinische Wochenschrift (1946), 87*, 446–52.

Lawton, G., et al. (2008). Comparison of two types of dissociation in epileptic and nonepileptic seizures. *Epilepsy & Behavior, 13*, 333–6.

Leander, J.D. (1992). Fluoxetine, a selective serotonin-uptake inhibitor, enhances the anticonvulsant effects of phenytoin, carbamazepine, and ameltolide (LY201116). *Epilepsia, 33*, 573–6.

Logsdail, S.J., Toone, B.K. (1988). Post-ictal psychoses. A clinical and phenomenological description. *British Journal of Psychiatry, 152*, 246–52.

Mendez, M.F., et al. (1993). Schizophrenia in epilepsy: seizure and psychosis variables. *Neurology, 43*, 1073–7.

Mula, M. (2010). The Landolt's phenomenon: an update. *Epileptologia, 18*, 39–44.

Mula, M. (2013). The interictal dysphoric disorder of epilepsy: a still open debate. *Current Neurology and Neuroscience Reports, 13*, 355.

Mula, M. (2014). Epilepsy-induced behavioral changes during the ictal phase. *Epilepsy & Behavior, 30*, 14–16.

Mula, M. (2016). *Neuropsychiatric Symptoms of Epilepsy*. Springer.

Mula, M. (2016a). The interictal dysphoric disorder of epilepsy: legend or reality? *Epilepsy & Behavior, 58*, 7–10.

Mula, M. (2016b). The pharmacological management of psychiatric comorbidities in patients with epilepsy. *Pharmacological Research, 107*, 147–53.

Mula, M., Kanner, A.M. (2013). Introduction–Treatment of psychiatric disorders in adults with epilepsy: what every epileptologist should know. *Epilepsia, 54 Suppl 1*, 1–2.

Mula, M., Sander, J.W. (2007). Negative effects of antiepileptic drugs on mood in patients with epilepsy. *Drug Safety, 30*, 555–67.

Mula, M., Sander, J.W. (2015). Suicide and epilepsy: do antiepileptic drugs increase the risk? *Expert Opinion on Drug Safety, 14*, 553–8.

Mula, M., et al. (2008a). Clinical correlates of schizotypy in patients with epilepsy. *Journal of Neuropsychiatry and Clinical Neurosciences, 20*, 441–6.

Mula, M., et al. (2008b). Clinical and psychopathological definition of the interictal dysphoric disorder of epilepsy. *Epilepsia, 49*, 650–6.

Mula, M., et al. (2010). Interictal dysphoric disorder and periictal dysphoric symptoms in patients with epilepsy. *Epilepsia, 51*, 1139–45.

Mula, M., et al. (2013). Antiepileptic drugs and suicidality: an expert consensus statement from the Task Force on Therapeutic Strategies of the ILAE Commission on Neuropsychobiology. *Epilepsia, 54*, 199–203.

Mula, M., et al. (2016). Validation of rapid suicidality screening in epilepsy using the NDDIE. *Epilepsia, 57*, 949–55.

Ngugi, A.K., et al. (2011). Incidence of epilepsy: a systematic review and meta-analysis. *Neurology, 77*, 1005–12.

Nishida, T., et al. (2006). Postictal mania versus postictal psychosis: differences in clinical features, epileptogenic zone, and brain functional changes during postictal period. *Epilepsia, 47*, 2104–14.

Pacia, S. V., Devinsky, O. (1994). Clozapine-related seizures: experience with 5,629 patients. *Neurology, 44*, 2247–9.

Park, S.-J., et al. (2015). Identifying clinical correlates for suicide among epilepsy patients in South Korea: A case-control study. *Epilepsia, 56*, 1966–72.

Penfield, W. (1946). Psychical Seizures. *British Medical Journal, 2*, 639–41.

Perucca, P., Mula, M. (2013). Antiepileptic drug effects on mood and behavior: molecular targets. *Epilepsy & Behavior, 26*, 440–9.

Petramfar, P., et al. (2009). Serum creatine phosphokinase is helpful in distinguishing generalized tonic-clonic seizures from psychogenic nonepileptic seizures and vasovagal syncope. *Epilepsy & Behavior, 15*, 330–2.

Qin, P. (2005). Risk for schizophrenia and schizophrenia-like psychosis among patients with epilepsy: population based cohort study. *BMJ, 331*, 23.

Quiske, A., et al. (2000). Depression in patients with temporal lobe epilepsy is related to mesial temporal sclerosis. *Epilepsy Research, 39*, 121–5.

Reuber, M. (2008). Psychogenic nonepileptic seizures: answers and questions. *Epilepsy & Behavior, 12*, 622–35.

Reuber, M. (2009). The etiology of psychogenic non-epileptic seizures: toward a biopsychosocial model. *Neurologic Clinics, 27*, 909–24.

Reuber, M., et al. (2002a). Diagnostic delay in psychogenic nonepileptic seizures. *Neurology, 58*, 493–5.

Reuber, M., et al. (2002b). Interictal EEG abnormalities in patients with psychogenic nonepileptic seizures. *Epilepsia, 43*, 1013–20.

Reuber, M., et al. (2002c). Evidence of brain abnormality in patients with psychogenic nonepileptic seizures. *Epilepsy & Behavior, 3*, 249–54.

Reuber, M., et al. (2003). Outcome in psychogenic nonepileptic seizures: 1 to 10-year follow-up in 164 patients. *Annals of Neurology, 53*, 305–11.

Reuber, M., et al. (2011). Psychogenic nonepileptic seizure manifestations reported by patients and witnesses. *Epilepsia, 52*, 2028–35.

Ring, H.A., et al. (1998). A prospective study of the early postsurgical psychiatric associations of epilepsy surgery. *Journal of Neurology, Neurosurgery, and Psychiatry, 64*, 601–4.

Robertson, M.M., Trimble, M.R. (1985). The treatment of depression in patients with epilepsy. A double-blind trial. *Journal of Affective Disorders, 9*, 127–36.

Sander, J.W., Shorvon, S.D. (1996). Epidemiology of the epilepsies. *Journal of Neurology, Neurosurgery, and Psychiatry, 61*, 433–43.

Scaramelli, A., et al. (2009). Prodromal symptoms in epileptic patients: clinical characterization of the pre-ictal phase. *Seizure, 18*, 246–50.

Smith, P.E.M. (2012). Epilepsy: mimics, borderland and chameleons. *Practical Neurology, 12*, 299–307.

Stone, J., et al. (2002). What should we say to patients with symptoms unexplained by disease? The 'number needed to offend'. *BMJ, 325*, 1449–50.

Syed, T.U., et al. (2011). Can semiology predict psychogenic nonepileptic seizures? A prospective study. *Annals of Neurology, 69*, 997–1004.

Taylor, D.C. (1971). Ontogenesis of chronic epileptic psychoses: a reanalysis. *Psychological Medicine, 1*, 247–53.

Tebartz Van Elst, L., et al. (2002). Amygdala pathology in psychosis of epilepsy: A magnetic resonance imaging study in patients with temporal lobe epilepsy. *Brain, 125*(Pt 1), 140–9.

Tellenbach, H. (1965). Epilepsie als anfallsleiden und als psychose. Uber alternative psychosen paranoider pragung bei 'forcierter normalisierung' (Landolt) des elektroenzephalogramms epileptischer. *Nervenarzt 36*, 190–202.

Tellez-Zenteno, J. F., et al. (2007). Psychiatric comorbidity in epilepsy: a population-based analysis. *Epilepsia, 48*, 2336–44.

Temkin, O. (2010). *The Falling Sickness: A History of Epilepsy from the Greeks to the Beginnings of Modern Neurology*. JHU Press.

Thomé-Souza, M.S., et al. (2007). Sertraline and fluoxetine: safe treatments for children and adolescents with epilepsy and depression. *Epilepsy & Behavior, 10*, 417–25.

Trimble, M. (2013). Treatment issues for personality disorders in epilepsy. *Epilepsia, 54*(Suppl 1), 41–5.

Trimble, M.R. (1991). *The Psychoses of Epilepsy*. New York, NY: Raven Press.

Trimble, M.R., Schmitz, B. (1998). *Forced Normalization and Alternative Psychoses of Epilepsy*. Wrightson Biomedical Pub.

Trimble, M.R., Schmitz, B. (2011). *The Neuropsychiatry of Epilepsy*. Cambridge: Cambridge University Press.

Varma, S., et al. (2011). Clozapine-related EEG changes and seizures: dose and plasma-level relationships. *Therapeutic Advances in Psychopharmacology*, *1*, 47–66.

Wandschneider, B. (2012) Frontal lobe function and structure in juvenile myoclonic epilepsy: a comprehensive review of neuropsychological and imaging data. *Epilepsia*, *53*, 2091–8.

Wasserman, D., Wasserman, C. (2009). *Oxford Textbook of Suicidology and Suicide Prevention*. Oxford: Oxford University Press.

Waxman, S.G., Geschwind, N. (1975) The interictal behaviour syndrome of temporal lobe epilepsy. *Archives of General Psychiatry*, *32*, 1580–6.

Willment, K., et al. (2015). Cognitive impairment and evaluation in psychogenic nonepileptic seizures: an integrated cognitive-emotional approach. *Clinical EEG and Neuroscience*, *46*, 42–53.

Woollacott, I.O.C., et al. (2010). When do psychogenic nonepileptic seizures occur on a video/EEG telemetry unit? *Epilepsy & Behavior*, *17*, 228–35.

18

Neuropsychiatric aspects of movement disorders

Andrea E. Cavanna and Hugh Rickards

Introduction

Within the last 30 years, starting with the publication of Alexander, de Long, and Strick's description of parallel circuits through the striatum (Alexander et al., 1986), there has been a change in the way that motor and postural phenomena have been seen in medicine. Human beings have evolved motor functions to serve survival behaviours, and so it should not be surprising to see that our motor systems are deeply integrated, in terms of both neuroanatomy and phenomenology, with our mood, cognitive state, volition, and arousal. The anatomy of this integration and 'cross-talk' has been described beautifully in primates (Haber, 2003). However, the traditional cultural and linguistic separation between the worlds of 'mind' and 'brain' does not fit this model well and has held back our understanding of these conditions. In this chapter, we attempt to bring together these ideas to develop a shared understanding of a variety of brain conditions that include motor, postural, affective, volitional, and cognitive aspects.

Parkinson's disease

PD is a heterogenous neurodegenerative illness, characterized clinically by slowness, rigidity, and emergent (4–6 Hz) resting tremor (Parkinson, 1817). Parkinsonism is a syndrome with those features, but with a specific cause (for instance, it can be induced by antipsychotic medications). Related disorders, often referred to as 'Parkinson plus' conditions, include the basic triad of features but have additional features; these are multisystem atrophy (MSA) which has cerebellar and autonomic variants, corticobasal degeneration (CBD) associated with limb apraxias, asymmetry, and cognitive impairment, and progressive supranuclear palsy (PSP), a tauopathy characterized by 'Mona Lisa' stare, growling speech, paralysis of upgaze, falling backwards, and alien hand phenomenon.

The classical pathology of PD is loss of dopamine-producing cells in the *pars compacta* of the substantia nigra. The characteristic micropathology is the Lewy body. Accumulation of Lewy bodies often starts in the brainstem and olfactory cortex, progresses to the midbrain, and, later in the illness, can become diffuse in the cortex.

PD is also characterized by a range of changes in mental state and behaviour. These are described commonly under the current rubric of 'non-motor symptoms', which is a poorly validated term, implying that motor behaviours are independent of the mental state and that motor function is *regarded as the 'primary problem'* in terms of symptoms. In fact, depression causes the greatest impairment in quality of life in PD (Schrag et al., 2000), and psychosis is the primary cause of family breakdown and nursing home placement (Goetz and Stebbins, 1993). For many, the first clinical symptom is REM sleep behaviour disorder, which can occur many years prior to the onset of clear motor signs, and probably indicates Lewy body pathology affecting the reticular activating system in the brainstem (Boeve, 2013).

Depression and anxiety are common in PD, with some studies suggesting that anxiety is considerably more common in the period before obvious motor onset (Lin et al., 2015), which may reflect the pathology of the disease. Diagnosing depression in PD can be difficult, as much classical depressive phenomenology is shared with PD phenomenology (sleep and appetite disturbance, weight loss, loss of concentration, hypomimia, and bradyphrenia). This can lead to both under- and over-diagnosis. Mood state can also vary with motor state, and so depressive and anxiety symptoms can occur as 'end-of-dose' effects. The key discriminating features for a diagnosis of depression in PD are pervasive low mood with marked anhedonia and early morning wakening with diurnal variation in mood (Leentjens et al., 2003). This should be seen in the context of the overall rate of deterioration of the underlying PD. If function declines more quickly than before, depression should be suspected. Depression in PD is treated no differently to current treatment for major depression, although concurrent use of SSRIs and dopamine replacement therapies can produce nausea. Sexual dysfunction, inherent in some parkinsonian conditions (such as MSA), needs to be carefully distinguished from that caused by antidepressant treatment. Evidence for psychological treatments for depression in PD is lacking, but CBT for depression has been found useful, especially in older patients on polypharmacy (Dobkin et al., 2011). A full range of anxiety disorders can occur in PD, but care is needed to exclude anxiety as an 'end-of-dose' effect (in which case the treatment would be to try and even out the plasma level of dopamine replacement therapy). Psychosis is common in PD and is characterized by visual hallucinations, especially of people and animals, which are often small and can be non-threatening. Pareidolic illusions (the interpretation of random images or patterns of light and shadow as faces or other non-random phenomena) are also common. All these visual symptoms can be preceded by vivid dreams and nightmares. Initially, the hallucinations may be hypnopompic or hypnogogic (Diederich et al., 2009). They may also be the cause of secondary delusions (often of infidelity or self-reference). In patients with abnormal visual perceptions, the diagnosis of delirium needs to be considered and the usual causes excluded or treated. Dopamine replacement drugs commonly worsen hallucinosis and should be rationalized and minimized. Anticholinergic drugs should be stopped where possible. If the symptoms are functionally impairing, then the use of antipsychotic medication should be considered. The best evidence supports the use of clozapine, and the more recently developed drug pimavanserin shows promise (Jethwa and Onalaja, 2015). Hallucinations may be the first sign of dementia in PD. The typical clinical picture of dementia related to PD is of a fluctuating mental state and consciousness, hallucinations, bradyphrenia, and generalized impairment of cognition. Evidence to support the idea that 'dementia in PD' and 'Lewy body dementia' are distinct biological entities is lacking, and it may be more useful to consider these as a broad spectrum of disorders caused by Lewy body pathology, which include problems with movement, agency, mood, perception, and general cognition. Treatment trials of cholinesterase inhibitors in Lewy body diseases suggest a statistically significant improvement in symptoms, but it remains unclear whether this is clinically meaningful when balanced against the possibility of adverse events. Impulse control disorders can occur in PD, with the major risk factor being dopamine replacement, particularly, but not exclusively, dopamine agonists. Impulsive behaviours commonly include Internet gambling, playing scratch cards, TV shopping, playing fruit machines, and engaging in compulsive online sex. Patients should be routinely warned of these potential adverse events prior to the initiation of dopamine replacement, as the consequences can be economically and personally catastrophic. Treatment is by reduction in the dose of dopamine replacement medication and pragmatic management of risk. Patients may deliberately overuse dopaminergic drugs to maintain a 'hyper-rewarded' state (Voon et al., 2011). 'Punding' is a form of compulsive behaviour usually seen later in the illness and consists of repetitive behaviours of fascination with, and dismantling of, objects (often mechanical). It is associated with dementia. Therapy for PD radically changed with the advent of deep brain stimulation (DBS), which is usually indicated for the treatment of excessive motor fluctuations and dyskinesias. The standard target for DBS is the subthalamic nucleus bilaterally. DBS often enables dopamine replacement therapy to be reduced and has not been found generally deleterious to mental health. The excess in suicide following DBS which was initially reported (Voon et al., 2008) may, in fact, be due to an increased suicide risk in all PD patients eligible for surgery, compared to PD patients in general (Veck et al., 2018).

What is currently described as PD is a heterogenous group of conditions, and the core hope is that further research will probably see its deconstruction and replacement with a more accurate classification system based on pathology and aetiology. This will likely lead to more specific therapies and a clearer delineation of precise psychopathology.

Huntington's disease

HD is a genetic degenerative brain disorder, which has a prevalence of up to 15 per 100,000 (Rawlins et al., 2016) and an incidence (in the UK) of around seven cases per million patient-years (Wexler et al., 2016). Incidence is stable, but prevalence is rising in Western countries, indicating better case ascertainment, less stigma, and longevity. HD is inherited in an autosomal dominant fashion. The most obvious features are abnormalities of motor behaviour and posture, but the most disabling features are changes in mental state and behaviour, particularly irritability, apathy, and social cognitive change (Eddy et al., 2016).

The gene is located in the IT15 region on the short arm of chromosome 4 and is generally fully penetrant (The Huntington's Collaborative Research Group, 1993). An area of CAG repeats becomes expanded, producing a larger polyglutamine chain, which leads to protein misfolding (the creation of the mutant huntingtin protein, or mHtt) and cell toxicity. This protein tends to aggregate in all cells and is toxic to cells of the nervous system, particularly medium spiny neurones in the striatum. mHtt is produced from conception and is relatively well dealt with in the early stages of life. However, it gradually accumulates in cells throughout life. Age at the development of obvious symptoms is commonly in the forties, but it can be at any age. At a population level, age at motor onset is inversely proportional to CAG repeat length (long repeats signify earlier development of symptoms). However, this is a poor predictor at an individual level and recent GWAS have indicated at least five other genes which significantly contribute to the speed and timing of progression (Genetic Modifiers of Huntington's Disease (GEM-HD) Consortium, 2015). Typically, CAG repeat lengths of 40 and above are regarded as a 'positive genetic test'. Higher CAG lengths (for instance, 55 and over) can lead to juvenile HD, which is characterized by a more akinetic, bradyphrenic, dysphonic, rigid condition (previously called the 'Westphal variant'). CAG lengths of between 36 and 39 are called 'reduced penetrance alleles'. These are often associated with later age of onset and a prodrome characterized by mental and behavioural changes (particularly affective disorders). The idea of 'age of onset' in HD is misleading, as it is clear that the pathology is present from conception and that brain changes are measurable 20 years or more prior to the onset of more specific clinical signs such as chorea or dystonia (Tabrizi et al., 2013) In addition, non-specific symptoms, such as irritability, apathy, and social cognitive changes often develop insidiously and can be significantly disabling, many years prior to what is currently called onset. From a pathological point of view, the most obvious changes are seen in the striatum, with a tenfold rate of striatal shrinkage, compared to non-HD brains, which is obvious for many years prior to 'onset'. Functional imaging has shown that the brain utilizes compensatory strategies to maintain function from an early stage. Early pathology is often seen in the striatum and posterior white matter and spreads throughout the brain (Tabrizi et al., 2013).

Reproductive strategies (prenatal testing and pre-implantation genetic diagnosis) can be used to prevent the expanded allele from being inherited. Individuals may also be tested themselves, either in a predictive manner (which involves a genetic counselling protocol) or diagnostically (in those people who already have clear symptoms and signs). Fewer than 20% of those at risk will take a predictive test, and fewer still avail themselves of reproductive technology (International Huntington Association and World Federation of Neurology, 1994).

In line with many other brain disorders, there is a paradigm shift away from their conception as 'movement disorders' and towards 'neuropsychiatric disorders'. The most disabling symptoms for patients and carers are usually psychiatric and include irritability, apathy, depression, anxiety, and social cognitive deficit. Chorea and dystonia, the hallmark changes in motor state, are diagnostically specific but tend to occur late in the pathological process and are usually not disabling until the later stages of the illness. The diagnostic specificity of the motor picture has been superseded by a much more specific and sensitive marker—the presence of the gene.

Mental disorders are common in HD. The commonest is organic personality disorder. Factor analyses of mental and behavioural symptoms in HD tend to show three factors: an affective/anxiety factor, an executive/social cognitive factor, and a psychosis factor (although the psychosis factor is small) (Rickards et al., 2011). Affective and anxiety disorders are common, with lifetime prevalences of around 20% for anxiety disorders and between 20% and 56% for affective disorders (De Souza, 2015). Suicidal ideation is common, as is suicide (Hubers et al., 2013). Many patients have an idea of suicide as an 'insurance policy' against inevitable deterioration. In other countries where euthanasia is legal, this is freely discussed in medical settings. Depression in HD is commonly classified as 'major depressive episode NOS (not otherwise specified)'—the clinical symptoms are often classical for major depression, but symptoms can relapse and remit much more quickly than in MDD. In addition, the age of onset for depression in HD is, on average, 14 years later than that for MDD. Depression in HD is relatively evenly distributed between men and women, unlike MDD (De Souza, 2015). Depressive syndromes are commonest in the premotor disorder phase and in the early stages, and tend to become less frequent as the disease progresses. There are no well-designed trials of treatment for depression in HD, but the most commonly prescribed drugs for HD-related depression in Europe are citalopram, paroxetine, and mirtazapine (Mestre et al., 2010).

Obsessive–compulsive disorder (OCD) is rare in HD, but perseveration is extremely common.

Irritability is very common and usually occurs in relation to task overload, mental inflexibility, or social cognitive deficit. Later in the illness, as dementia develops, irritability may be caused by a variety of factors such as pain, constipation, infection, and, rarely, psychosis.

Social cognitive deficit is common, disabling, and relatively understudied in HD. There are clear and progressive deficits in theory of mind, future envisioning, empathy, and understanding of irony (Eddy et al., 2016). Although not usually regarded as a problem by those who carry the gene, these are often highly distressing for carers and family members who grieve for the person they knew. Typically, the types of problems encountered include misunderstanding of subtle social signals, difficulty in picking up emotional signals from body language or tone of voice, problems with conscious reasoning about other peoples' mental states, and reduced (or changed) emotional reaction to environmental stimuli

(Eddy et al., 2016). Apathy is common in HD and not well understood. The pathway that leads to apathy may be a combination of failure of future envisioning and problems with behavioural initiation. A number of cognitive processes related to executive function are impaired in HD. In particular, the ability to multitask and consciously problem-solve can be particularly impaired. This often leads to problems in function at work and in the home. Impairments in problem-solving abilities might be a risk factor for depression, anxiety, and irritability. Psychosis is relatively rare and may fall into two broad groups; earlier in the illness, some patients may manifest overvalued ideas which border on the delusional. In the latter stages of the illness, hallucinations characteristic of the failing brain may appear (van Duijn et al., 2014). Although some patients with HD have a schizophrenia-like illness, it is not clear if this occurs any more frequently than would be expected in the non-HD population.

The essence of management of people with HD is holistic, team-based rehabilitation. Key players in well-structured HD teams include speech therapists, dieticians, physiotherapists, and occupational therapists. Weight loss and dysphagia are common problems in HD and need careful management.

Treatment for HD is currently symptomatic, with a poor evidence base. Traditionally, treatment has been focused on chorea. Drugs that block or deplete dopamine can improve chorea, but often at the expense of dysphoria and worsening cognition. Tetrabenazine, a drug used to treat chorea, appears to be particularly likely to induce these adverse effects. Other dopamine-blocking drugs, such as risperidone, sulpiride, tiapride, and olanzapine, are more commonly used in specialist HD practice, with olanzapine particularly favoured in people who are liable to lose weight. Clonazepam may be used to treat both dystonia and myoclonus that can occur later in the illness. The most commonly prescribed drugs for irritability (Groves et al., 2011), anxiety, and depression are SSRIs, with the addition of mirtazapine as second line, especially for those patients with sleep disturbance. Other than this, practice is idiosyncratic. There is increasing evidence from animal and human studies that physical activity can improve health in people with HD and possibly delay obvious onset (Quinn et al., 2016). With the advent of gene suppression therapies, the first huntingtin-lowering treatments are being tested in humans. Molecules that bind to the huntingtin RNA to prevent its expression can be administered intrathecally and could, in theory, lead to restoration of function of some cells. In the field of HD, psychiatrists encounter a range of psychiatric problems which often result in institutional care, with the presence of a clear biomarker, and potentially disease-modifying treatment.

Tourette syndrome

Tic disorders are hyperkinetic movement disorders characterized by the presence of tics (involuntary, sudden, rapid, recurrent, non-rhythmic movements or vocalizations) (Ganos and Martino, 2015). Tourette syndrome is a complex tic disorder characterized by the presence of both motor and vocal/phonic tics, with onset in childhood and a chronic course. Other tic disorders include persistent (chronic) motor or vocal tic disorder diagnosed when either motor or vocal/phonic tics (but not both) are present as part of the chronic condition and criteria for Tourette syndrome are not fully met. The diagnostic category of a provisional tic disorder is used for patients with single or multiple motor and/or vocal/phonic tics that have been present for <1 year since onset (Black et al., 2016).

Tourette syndrome (or, more appropriately, Gilles de la Tourette syndrome) was named after Georges Gilles de la Tourette (see Fig. 18.1), a French physician who published the first complete description of this condition in 1885 (de la Tourette, 1885), a few years after a previous report on the 'tic non-douloureux' by another French physician Armand Trousseau (Rickards et al., 2010). Tourette syndrome is no longer considered a rare medical condition, as large epidemiological studies and meta-analyses have shown that 0.3–1% of school-age children fulfil established diagnostic criteria for this disorder (Robertson et al., 2009; Scharf et al., 2015). In the UK, it is estimated that as many as 200,000–330,000 individuals have symptoms consistent with Tourette syndrome, with different degrees of severity (Stern et al., 2005).

Tics are characterized by an average age at onset of 6 years and are 3–4 times more common in boys than in girls (Cavanna and Seri, 2013; Ganos and Martino, 2015; Stern, 2018). The commonest tic reported at onset is eye blinking (Martino et al., 2012), followed by other simple motor tics (such as eye rolling, mouth opening, facial grimacing, shoulder shrugging, neck stretching, kicking, and others) and vocal/phonic tics (most commonly sniffing, grunting, and throat clearing. Complex motor tics usually develop a few years after tic onset and involve multiple muscle groups, resulting in whole body movements such as jumping, squatting, abnormal gait, etc. Complex vocal/phonic tics include palilalia (repetition of the patient's own words), echolalia (repeating other people's words), and coprolalia (involuntary swearing as a tic). Although coprolalia invariably features in media portrayals of Tourette syndrome, this complex tic is relatively rare, as it has been documented in about 10% of patients with Tourette syndrome in the community and in up to 30% of patients in specialist clinics, and is not included among the diagnostic criteria (Eddy and Cavanna, 2013a).

Importantly, most patients report that their tics are preceded by a subjective feeling of mounting inner tension, which is temporarily relieved by tic expression (Rajagopal et al., 2013). The presence of these 'premonitory urges' is particularly useful for the differential diagnosis between tics and other repetitive behaviours such as mannerisms and stereotypies. Tics are characterized by a spontaneous waxing and waning course, with significant variations in frequency, severity, and distribution throughout life. The peak in tic severity usually occurs during early teenage years, and the majority of patients report varying degrees of improvement

after adolescence/early adulthood (Hassan and Cavanna, 2012). In general, tic severity is aggravated by environmental factors such as stress, anxiety, and self-consciousness, as well as excitement. Alleviating factors include relaxation and engagement in non-stressful mental and physical tasks requiring active concentration such as playing sports and musical instruments. Social interactions are also known to modulate tic expression, including the expression of particular socially inappropriate behaviours (Eddy and Cavanna, 2013b).

Converging evidence shows that specific behavioural problems are present in the vast majority (90%) of patients with Tourette syndrome (Cavanna, 2018a and b; Cavanna and Rickards, 2013). The commonest psychiatric comorbidities are OCD/behaviours (approximate comorbidity rate 30% each) (Lombroso and Scahill, 2008) and ADHD (60%) (Simpson et al., 2011). Differentiating complex tics from compulsions can pose significant challenges—from a clinical perspective, unlike tics, the compulsions reported by patients with OCD are often purposeful, ritualistic, and routine-like in nature. Moreover, compulsive behaviours are performed as a method to reduce psychological anxiety caused by intrusive (obsessional) thoughts, while tics are mainly driven by premonitory urges that are more physical in nature and are described as feelings of somatic discomfort, pain, or tension (Worbe et al., 2010). Intriguingly, patients with Tourette syndrome report a significantly higher prevalence of concerns for symmetry, evening-up behaviours, obsessional counting (arithmomania), ordering, and 'just-right' perceptions, whereas patients with primary OCD have a higher rate of concerns for contamination and cleaning/washing rituals. Since young patients with tics are invariably described as inattentive, restless, and hyperactive, specialist diagnostic skills are often required to disentangle the motor dyscontrol and the difficulties in sustaining attention, due to the constant efforts produced to actively suppress tics, from the presence of comorbid attention-deficit and hyperactivity symptoms. Collateral history from parents and teachers plays an important part in the clinical assessment of comorbid ADHD in children with Tourette syndrome (Simpson et al., 2011). Other comorbid conditions include autism spectrum disorders (Canitano and Vivanti, 2007), affective disorders (Robertson, 2006), and impulse control disorders (Wright et al., 2012). The recent development of disease-specific health-related quality of life measures for patients with Tourette syndrome (Cavanna et al., 2013) has allowed a more accurate assessment of the differential impact of tics and psychiatric comorbidities on patients' well-being, thus providing treating clinicians with useful indications for the prioritization of management strategies (Evans et al., 2016). Treatment interventions for tics include behavioural approaches (habit reversal therapy and exposure and response prevention), pharmacotherapy (mainly antidopaminergic agents and α-2 agonists), and, in the most severe and refractory cases, DBS (targeting the thalamus or the globus pallidus) (Cavanna and Seri, 2013; Pringsheim et al., 2019; Waldon et al., 2013).

Both antidopaminergic and serotonergic agents have been found to be potentially useful in patients with obsessive–compulsive symptoms, and there is no absolute contraindication to the use of CNS stimulants in patients with comorbid ADHD. Finally, the importance of psychoeducation should not be underestimated, as accurate information on Tourette syndrome should be extended to include

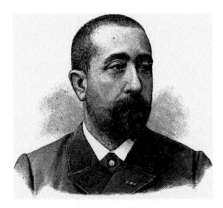

Fig. 18.1 Georges Gilles de la Tourette (1857–1904).

the patient's family, teachers, employers, and other professionals involved (Cavanna and Seri, 2013).

Dystonia

Dystonia is a movement disorder characterized by sustained or intermittent muscle contractions that cause abnormal motor patterns and/or postures (Marsden, 1976). The first description of this condition dates back to 1911 when Hermann Oppenheim (see Fig. 18.2) reported four young patients and coined the term 'dystonia musculorum deformans' to indicate that 'muscle tone was hypotonic at one occasion and in tonic muscle spasm at another, usually, but not exclusively, elicited upon voluntary movements' (Oppenheim, 1911). Oppenheim's terminology has persisted until now. However, since his first account, there has been continuous controversy about the classification and aetiology of dystonia syndromes, reflecting developments in the understanding of the various clinical manifestations and underlying pathophysiological mechanisms. Although the exact brain alterations responsible for the different forms of dystonia are not fully understood, basal ganglia structures and their connections with cortical areas have been implicated in shared pathophysiological mechanisms (Conte et al., 2016).

The term dystonia encompasses a heterogenous group of clinically diverse phenotypes which share the common denominator of abnormal and sustained muscular contractions. Specifically, some forms of dystonia are focal and affect isolated body parts, whereas others are generalized, impacting virtually every movement; some have onset in early childhood, while others become manifest later in life. Focal dystonias (e.g. blepharospasm, oromandibular dystonia, torticollis) are the most frequent forms of dystonia in adult patients. Historically, primary focal dystonias were often categorized as cramps, task-specific, or occupational spasms (e.g. writer's cramp) or labelled as psychogenic (Munts and Koehler, 2010; Stahl and Frucht, 2017). In general, several features were traditionally regarded as supportive of a 'functional' basis for focal dystonias, including the bizarre nature of the movements, a female preponderance, relief of

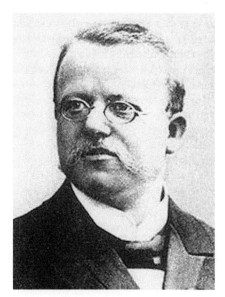

Fig. 18.2 Hermann Oppenheim (1858–1919).

dystonic postures by use of a sensory trick ('geste antagoniste'), improvement of dystonia through relaxation, sensitivity of symptoms to psychological stress, occurrence of spontaneous remissions, and, most importantly, absence of any identifiable structural abnormalities that explain the symptoms (Oppenheim, 1911). It was at the International Symposium on Dystonia (1975) that the movement disorder community recognized focal dystonia as a product of basal ganglia dysfunction, rather than a psychological conflict, thus emphasizing the organic nature of this condition.

In 1984, an ad hoc committee assembled by the Dystonia Medical Research Foundation provided the first consensus statement on dystonia as a syndrome consisting 'of sustained muscle contractions, frequently causing twisting and repetitive movements, or abnormal postures', a definition that has been retained to date as the classic description of dystonia (Fahn et al., 1987). According to the European Federation of Neurological Societies guidelines, the aetiology of dystonia syndromes is classified as primary, heredodegenerative, and secondary (or symptomatic) (Albanese et al., 2011). The classification of dystonia has evolved over time, until a recent revision of the classification scheme identified two different axes: clinical features (five phenomenological descriptors: age at onset, body distribution, temporal pattern, comorbid movement disorders, and other neurological manifestations) and aetiology (based on identifiable anatomical changes and pattern of inheritance) (Albanese et al., 2013). This scheme has been proposed to improve the current classification system, which is based on the three main axes of aetiology, age at onset, and body distribution (Fahn, 2011). Likewise, a recently proposed revision of the definition of dystonia focuses on the presence of sustained or intermittent muscle contractions causing abnormal, often repetitive, movements or postures, or both (Albanese et al., 2013). Dystonic movements are recognized as being typically patterned, twisting, and possibly tremulous, and are often initiated or worsened by voluntary action and associated with overflow muscle activation.

Focal dystonia with onset in adulthood is the most thoroughly investigated form of dystonia from the psychiatric perspective (Berman et al., 2017; Jahanshahi et al., 2005; Zurowski et al., 2013). It has been consistently shown that the various focal dystonia syndromes are not uniform in their manifestations of psychiatric symptoms (Fabbrini et al., 2010). A high prevalence of psychiatric disturbances, particularly of depression and anxiety, has been found in patients with cervical dystonia. Similarly, patients with blepharospasm appear to be more likely to suffer from mood disorders than controls. There is also evidence for increased rates of psychiatric comorbidity in generalized forms of dystonia, specifically OCD in patients with myoclonus dystonia and recurrent depression in patients with a genetic vulnerability to dystonia (*DYT1* mutation). The assessment of the frequency and type of psychiatric comorbidity in rarer forms of focal dystonia (e.g. arm dystonia), as well as other generalized and inherited forms of dystonia, needs further investigation.

Although psychiatric symptoms are often secondary to the presence of dystonia, a number of observations suggest that psychiatric disorders can be an intrinsic part of the clinical spectrum of dystonia. For example, several studies have shown that psychiatric disorders, such as depression and anxiety, can precede the motor manifestations of dystonia (Lencer et al., 2009; Moraru et al., 2002; Wenzel et al., 1998). Moreover, the severity of depression does not appear to correlate with the severity of dystonia (Stamelou et al., 2012), suggesting that affective symptoms have multiple causes, in addition to reaction to the motor disability. In fact, in a 5-year follow-up study on patients with cervical dystonia, it was shown that psychiatric disorders were stable in spite of a reduction in the severity of the motor dysfunction (Berardelli et al., 2015). It is possible that dysfunction in the cortico-limbic-striatal pathways is a common pathophysiological substrate of neuropsychiatric disturbances in the context of dystonia. Psychiatric disorders have a major impact on the health-related quality of life of patients with dystonia, with depression and anxiety not only affecting mental health, but also having a larger effect on physical aspects of quality of life than dystonia severity (Ben-Shlomo et al., 2002). Treatment trials of psychiatric illness in the context of dystonia are lacking. Current psychotherapeutic approaches are symptom-based and time-limited, and target affective and anxiety disorders (Zurowski et al., 2013). Moreover, psychiatric comorbidities can influence the assessment of dystonia treatment effects, including patients' response to muscle relaxants. Increased awareness of the effects of psychiatric treatment on both mental and motor/physical aspects of quality of life is needed to implement multidimensional approaches to improve the objective and subjective well-being of patients with dystonia.

Functional movement disorders

The concepts underpinning the idea of functional neurological disorders are shaky. However, it is clear that there are a range of impairments to movement, balance, and coordination that do not conform to standard neuropathological models. Different mechanisms have been postulated to explain these phenomena, including a symbolic response to psychological trauma, cultural ideas of what it is to be ill, over- and under-focus on symptoms, or an exaggeration of normal physiological responses (such as shivering). The deliberate production of symptoms is referred to as factitious disorder or malingering, although assessing 'deliberateness' is not an easy, or a binary, process. Language serves us poorly in our understanding of these conditions, particularly as the language of movement regularly contains the subtext of agency and mental state, and vice versa. Nevertheless, this group of processes have been amalgamated into a group called functional movement disorders (FMDs). In the 1960s, the British psychiatrist Eliot Slater (Slater, 1965) stated that all these disorders were 'a snare, a delusion'. He believed that, if the patients were followed up for long enough, they all developed other illnesses (mostly neurological ones). However, Crimlisk et al. (1998), in a follow-up study, clearly showed that the majority of diagnoses of functional neurological disorders were stable over time. However, this high reliability does not clearly speak for the validity of the 'organic/functional' dichotomy. Some groups of stable conditions, such as the paroxysmal dystonias, have been moved wholesale from the functional to the organic, with the discovery of the relevant ion channel pathology (Gardiner et al., 2015). This highlights the need for positive diagnostic tests for functional disorders based on the mechanism, rather than diagnoses of exclusion in those patients with psychiatric histories. It is important to remember that the dichotomous 'organic/functional' model is just a model, and not a biological fact. In most cases, there do appear to be two different processes leading to similar symptoms (organic versus functional

tremor being a good example). However, there are other cases where the dichotomous model may not work so well (such as dystonia). Cases of FMD may have a variety of risk factors, including biological and psychological. The relationship between FMDs and early adverse environmental experiences is complex; in common with other somatoform disorders, early trauma is a clear risk factor but is neither necessary nor sufficient to cause symptoms.

In motor terms, the commonest functional movement disorders are tremor, dystonia, and myoclonus. Tremor and dystonia together make up around 70% of FMDs. Functional gait disturbance has been traditionally included in the movement disorder group. The idea of a functional tic disorder is more complex still and outside the scope of this textbook.

Features in the clinical history that would suggest a diagnosis of FMD are: a sudden onset and quick progression to maximum severity, periods of relapse and remission, lack of consistency over time, and brief paroxysms of movement. Functional tremor tends to be of variable frequency and amplitude and is distractible. Patients with FMD may also have a history of other functional symptoms. The entrainment test (Roper et al., 2013) is the best method for positively diagnosing functional tremor and involves the patient tapping out specific rhythms with the least tremulous hand. Functional tremors normally worsen while under a load, in contrast to organic tremors. Restraint of a shaking limb may lead to more violent shaking or transfer of the tremor to other body parts (Deuschl et al., 1998). Accelerometry studies of functional tremor suggest that, for the most part, the tremor is not present, but the patient only becomes aware of it when it is suggesting a problem with selective attention. The presence of *Bereitschaftpotentials* can be used to more accurately diagnose functional myoclonus, as they do not occur with 'organic' myoclonus (Esposito et al., 2009). Fixed-flexion dystonic disorders (usually involving a flexed elbow and wrist or ankle flexion and inversion) are regarded as functional and can often occur in response to a relatively minor trauma in the affected area. People with this disorder (and all functional motor disorders) commonly have other functional neurological symptoms and psychopathology. (Schrag et al., 2004). Hoover's sign (Ziv et al., 1998) may be positive in functional motor disorders in the absence of the subjective complaint of muscle weakness. Treatment of fixed-flexion deformities of this type is notoriously difficult, and the affected limbs can develop complex regional pain syndrome. Recent evidence suggests that therapeutic examination under sedation can lead to improvement in some cases (Stone et al., 2014).

Functional gait disorder may occur alongside other functional motor disorders and can include 'give-way' weakness at the knees, hesitation or 'walking on ice' gait, and exaggerated swaying without falling during the Romberg test. The base of the gait is often narrow, unlike standard ataxias.

Evidence on treatment of functional motor disorders is sparse. Most authors in the field agree that diagnostic consultation is a key part of therapy (Carson et al., 2016). Clinicians should explain what is known about functional disorders, including that they are not 'done on purpose' and that they are not 'going mad'.

The best evidence points to 'psychologically minded rehabilitation' by a skilled interdisciplinary team. Novel physiotherapy interventions based on the idea of manipulation of attention have shown early promise (Neilsen et al., 2015). In cases of clear, unresolved psychological trauma, more exploratory approaches may be appropriate, but their efficacy is unclear. Once the diagnosis of FMD is made, there is a need to prevent unnecessary investigation and medication, as well as to reduce any secondary disability. Coexisting psychopathology should be treated in the usual way (the presence of additional psychiatric diagnoses, such as depression or anxiety, is a good prognostic factor). Otherwise, prognosis for these disorders is unclear. Early work suggested that many cases were self-limiting in the early stages (Ljunberg, 1957). It is, however, clear that, once people with FMD present to secondary care (either neurology or psychiatry), the prognosis is significantly worse. A number of studies looking at outcome have been based in specialist centres, which may have negatively biased outcomes. Early diagnosis, short duration of symptoms, and 'overall satisfaction with care' appear to be the strongest predictors of good outcome (Gelauff et al., 2014). There is a renaissance of neurological interest in functional disorders, and this is a historic opportunity to share language, skills, and understanding between professions in order to help these patients.

Drug-induced movement disorders

The introduction of the antidopaminergic agent chlorpromazine in 1952 marked a milestone in modern psychiatry—in addition to its antipsychotic properties, psychiatrists soon became aware of the potential of this drug to cause major adverse effects, including akathisia, parkinsonism, and acute dystonia (Mehta et al., 2015). By the late 1950s, the existence of a more persistent, late-appearing form of dyskinesia was recognized, and since then, considerable clinical experience has accumulated on the use of antidopaminergic agents and the range of drug-induced movement disorders. From a clinical point of view, it is useful to categorize induced movement disorders caused by psychiatric drugs into acute and chronic conditions.

Acute dystonia is characterized by orofacial dystonia, opisthotonus (back arching), and neck extension (Mehta et al., 2015). Dystonic reactions can occur 2–5 days after the administration or uptitration of antidopaminergic drugs, usually neuroleptics, although atypical antipsychotics, including clozapine, have also been associated with these adverse effects. Risk factors include male gender (male:female ratio 2:1), young age (below 30 years), high potency and dose of antidopaminergic agent, familial predisposition, learning disability, substance abuse (cocaine), and medical comorbidities (AIDS). Proposed pathophysiological mechanisms for acute dystonia include dopaminergic hypofunction as a result of relative overactivity of cholinergic pathways, and paradoxical dopaminergic hyperactivity induced by blockade of presynaptic dopamine receptors. Management strategies include (injectable) anticholinergic drugs, antihistamine drugs (diphenhydramine), and occasionally benzodiazepines (diazepam). Iatrogenic laryngospasm can be severe enough to warrant tracheostomy.

The term akathisia in ancient Greek literally means 'inability to sit still' and was first used in the medical literature at the beginning of the twentieth century (Haskovec, 1902). Patients with akathisia report a subjective feeling of restlessness, mainly affecting their legs and resulting in limb movements and a tendency to shift body position in the chair while sitting or to march while standing (Mehta et al., 2015). Acute akathisia usually develops within the first 2 weeks of antidopaminergic drug administration or uptitration, although reactions within hours or after up to 6 weeks have been reported. Higher rates of akathisia are seen with the use of high-potency D2-blocking agents, supporting the D2 antagonism hypothesis, although this does not explain why anticholinergic (benztropine, trihexyphenidyl, procyclidine, biperiden, orphenadrine) and β-adrenergic-blocking agents (propranolol) are the most effective treatments. Other potentially useful agents for acute akathisia include the α-2 adrenergic presynaptic agonist clonidine, as well drugs modulating serotonergic neurotransmission (mirtazapine and trazodone).

Drug-induced parkinsonism (rigidity, bradykinesia, and resting tremor) is a relatively frequent adverse effect of antidopaminergic drugs, especially neuroleptics and most atypical antipsychotics, with the exception of clonidine and possibly low-dose quetiapine (Mehta et al., 2015). Although drug-induced parkinsonism tends to be symmetrical, up to one-third of patients present with asymmetrical motor features resembling idiopathic PD (Sethi and Zamrini, 1990). The co-occurrence of a hyperkinetic movement disorder (e.g. oro-buccal dyskinesia) in the absence of levodopa treatment suggests a diagnosis of drug-induced parkinsonism over PD (which is also characterized by the presence of non-motor features). However, in some cases, drug-induced parkinsonism can unmask subclinical PD. Dopamine transporter imaging (DAT scan) is helpful in differentiating true nigrostriatal dysfunction seen in idiopathic PD from iatrogenic conditions. Most cases resolve within 6 months of discontinuation of the antidopaminergic agent. There seems to be a complex interplay between the dose and potency of the antidopaminergic agent and individual susceptibility (older age, female gender, pre-existing cerebral atrophy, and possibly genetic susceptibility) in the pathogenesis of drug-induced parkinsonism (Erro et al., 2015). Management starts with prevention, by aiming at the lowest efficacious dose of atypical antipsychotics, rather than neuroleptics. The usefulness of prophylactic treatment with anticholinergic drugs is controversial and possibly limited to patients at higher risk treated with high-dose and high-potency dopamine blockers. Treatment of clinically manifest drug-induced parkinsonism is challenging and involves gradual withdrawal of the causative agent and replacement with a less offending agent. Although mild conditions are often left untreated, symptoms can be managed with amantadine and anticholinergic and antihistaminergic drugs.

Drug-induced parkinsonism can sometimes occur in a delayed fashion; however, the most commonly seen tardive (late-appearing) movement disorders caused by psychiatric drugs are antidopaminergic drug-induced tardive dyskinesia (with its variants), tardive dystonia, and tardive akathisia (Mehta et al., 2015). Classic tardive dyskinesia is characterized by repetitive, coordinated, seemingly purposeful movements, mainly affecting the orofacial area, following exposure to antidopaminergic agents for at least 1–3 months. Rarer tardive dyskinesia variants include tardive tourettism, tardive myoclonus, and tardive tremor. Old age, female gender, cumulative drug exposure, coexisting affective disorder, substance abuse, and diabetes are consistently reported as the main risk factors. The exact pathophysiology of tardive dyskinesia is not fully understood. However, converging lines of evidence point towards (D2) dopamine receptor hypersensitivity, caused by iatrogenic blockade and possibly leading to maladaptive plasticity in striato-cortical transmission. GABAergic depletion has been proposed as an alternative/complementary pathophysiological model.

Tardive dystonia most commonly involves the hands and the jaw, often resembling primary focal dystonia syndromes (Mehta et al., 2015). Compared to tardive dyskinesia, tardive dystonia is more severe and common in young patients, with no preponderance in female gender. The clinical presentation of tardive akathisia is similar to that of acute akathisia, with the exception of increased leg and trunk repetitive movements. The clinical course of tardive dyskinesia is characterized by remission in up to 40% of patients who discontinue the antidopaminergic drug (Mehta et al., 2009). Tardive dystonia tends to be more persistent than classic tardive dyskinesia, whereas tardive akathisia does not disappear on discontinuation of the offending agent.

Management strategies for tardive syndromes include prevention of iatrogenic harm, downtitration and replacement/withdrawal of antidopaminergic drugs, and symptomatic treatment of the movement disorder (Mehta et al., 2015). Presynaptic dopamine depletors (tetrabenazine and reserpine) are among the most commonly used medications for classic tardive dyskinesia. Use of other pharmacological agents (including amantadine, benzodiazepines, baclofen, valproate, donepezil, lithium, and zonisamide) is not supported by high levels of evidence. Tetrabenazine, benzodiazepines, and baclofen are the agents most commonly used in the symptomatic treatment of tardive dystonia. Anticholinergic drugs, which are beneficial in tardive dystonia, tend to worsen classic tardive dyskinesia. Tardive akathisia does not consistently respond to pharmacotherapy, although tetrabenazine and reserpine can sometimes be helpful.

Movement disorders caused by psychiatric drugs, other than antidopaminergic agents, are more commonly seen in patients with abnormal development or brain injury and usually remit on discontinuation of the causative drug (Mehta et al., 2015). AEDs are known to potentially cause or exacerbate both postural and resting tremor (especially valproate), akathisia (especially carbamazepine), chorea, and myoclonus. Lithium can cause or exacerbate akathisia and chorea, while serotonergic agents (tricyclic antidepressants and SSRIs) have been associated with all the above-mentioned iatrogenic movement disorders.

Conclusion

Movement and posture are an integral part of what it is to be alive. Traditionally, the elucidation of patterns of movement and posture was essential to the specific diagnosis of a variety of nervous system disorders. We are now undergoing a paradigm shift; we have come to realize that movement, posture, affect, cognition, and volition all interact to produce human behaviour. This is true, both in terms of neuroanatomy and phenomenology. The utility of motor symptoms as an aid to diagnosis has diminished with the advent of more clearly delineated molecular pathology (a good example being HD). Finally, focus on the lived experience of patients and their carers has shown that problems with pure movement, if such things exist, are rarely the major cause of disability. However, because of their visibility and 'otherness', abnormal movements have probably distracted from the profoundly disabling mental and behavioural symptoms of many brain disorders and led to errors in relation to both research and treatment. In the future, there is likely to be further clarification on the molecular pathologies of a range of brain disorders which include changes in affect, volition, cognition, sensation, perception, movement, and posture—a truly neuropsychiatric approach.

KEY LEARNING POINTS

- PD is characterized by the triad of tremor, bradykinesia, and rigidity.
- 'Parkinson plus' syndromes include MSA, PSP, and CBD.
- REM sleep behaviour disorder and anxiety may precede obvious motor symptoms.
- Depression and anxiety disorders are common and should be distinguished from end-of-dose effects. Initial treatment is similar to that of MDD.
- Psychosis is characterized by visual hallucinations and illusions. Dopamine replacement therapy is a clear risk factor.
- Psychosis should be treated by reducing dopamine therapy and, if needed, clozapine.
- Impulse control disorders are common and are related to dopamine agonists.
- Cognitive impairment is common in PD, and many patients develop dementia eventually, which is characterized by subcortical cognitive changes, fluctuant attention, and hallucinations.
- Cholinesterase inhibitors may help improve cognition, but it is not clear if the effect is clinically significant.
- DBS to the subthalamic nucleus may be helpful for dyskinesias in PD and do not appear to be psychiatrically harmful. Increased suicide rates in those for whom surgery is indicated highlight the need for careful monitoring post-surgery.
- HD is an autosomal dominant disorder which is neurodegenerative.
- The characteristic symptoms of HD are apathy, irritability, and social cognitive loss. Chorea and dystonia are common, but not usually disabling until the later stages.
- There is a single genetic change (an expansion of CAG repeats on chromosome 4) that leads to symptoms of HD, usually obvious from middle age, but which can present at any age.
- The commonest psychiatric complications of HD are organic personality disorder, followed by depression, anxiety, and later dementia.
- Social cognitive deficit is common and disabling in HD and can manifest as apathy, irritability, and lack of empathy.
- Management of HD requires experienced multidisciplinary teams and should address function, cognition, swallow, weight maintenance, mood, irritability, and movement disorder.
- Depression, anxiety, and irritability may benefit by environmental interventions and pharmacotherapy.
- Drugs for chorea may lead to worsening mental state (apathy and dysphoria).
- More recently, disease-modifying treatments of HD have been trialled in human subjects for the first time, offering promise for possible disease prevention and better symptom control.
- Tourette syndrome is characterized by multiple motor and vocal/phonic tics.

- Coprolalia (involuntary swearing as a complex tic) is reported by a minority of patients.
- The commonest psychiatric comorbidities of Tourette syndrome are OCD and ADHD.
- Treatment options for tics include behavioural interventions and pharmacotherapy.
- Use of DBS for severe, treatment-refractory cases is still in its pioneering stage.
- Dystonia is a movement disorder characterized by sustained or intermittent muscle contractions, either isolated (focal dystonia) or diffuse (generalized dystonia).
- Psychiatric disorders are highly prevalent in patients with dystonia (especially focal dystonia) and have a profound effect on quality of life.
- Patients with dystonia frequently meet criteria for anxiety and affective disorders.
- Psychiatric disorders appear to be related to the underlying disease processes of many dystonia syndromes.
- Reactive elements exacerbate psychiatric distress and may be a result of the visible and painful nature of the motor symptoms.
- The concept of 'functional motor disorders' and the language that surrounds the concept are still problematic, as they rely on the model of an 'organic/functional' dichotomy which is not universally applicable.
- The aetiology of functional motor disorders is unknown but may be related to attentional biases, exaggeration of physiological responses, and more rarely, symbolism.
- People with existing brain diseases are more likely to suffer from functional symptoms, including functional motor disorders.
- Functional motor disorders are a relatively stable group of conditions temporally.
- The diagnosis of functional motor disorders should be made by utilizing positive signs (such as Hoover's sign or the entrainment test), rather than by excluding organic pathology, which is likely to increase diagnostic validity.
- Treatment of functional motor disorders begins with careful explanation of the diagnosis and psychoeducation.
- Psychologically minded rehabilitation is the best treatment for functional motor disorders.
- The presence of other mental disorders (such as depression or anxiety) may be a good prognostic sign, and these should be treated as part of overall management.
- Prognosis of functional motor disorders in the early weeks after onset is good but deteriorates quickly with time.
- Drug-induced movement disorders include acute and chronic conditions.
- Drug-induced movement disorders are most commonly associated with antidopaminergic drugs.
- The commonest clinical presentations of drug-induced movement disorders encompass dyskinesia, dystonia, akathisia, and parkinsonism.
- At low doses, most atypical antipsychotics carry a lower risk of causing tardive dyskinesia than neuroleptics.
- Tardive dyskinesia can occur following a minimum of 3 months of antidopaminergic drug exposure (1 month in patients older than 60 years).

REFERENCES

Albanese, A., Asmus, F., Bhatia, K.P., et al. (2011). EFNS guidelines on diagnosis and treatment of primary dystonias. *European Journal of Neurology*, 18, 5–18.

Albanese, A., Bhatia, K., Bressman, S.B., et al. (2013). Phenomenology and classification of dystonia: A consensus update. *Movement Disorders*, 28, 863–73.

Alexander, G.E., DeLong, M.R., Strick, P.L. (1986). Parallel Organization of functionally Segregated Circuits linking basal ganglia and cortex. *Annals of Reviews in Neuroscience*, 9, 357–81.

Ben-Shlomo, Y., Camfield, L., Warner, T. (2002). What are the determinants of quality of life in people with cervical dystonia? *Journal of Neurology Neurosurgery and Psychiatry*, 72, 608–14.

Berardelli, I., Ferrazzano, G., Pasquini, M., Berardelli, A., Biondi, M., Fabbrini, G. (2015). Clinical course of psychiatric disorders in patients with cervical dystonia. *Psychiatry Research*, 229, 583–5.

Berman, B.D., Junker, J., Shelton, E., et al. (2017). Psychiatric associations of adult-onset focal dystonia phenotypes. *Journal of Neurology Neurosurgery and Psychiatry*, 88, 595–602.

Black, K.J., Black, E.R., Greene, D.J., Schlaggar, B.L. (2016). Provisional tic disorders: What to tell parents when their child first starts ticcing. *F1000Research*, 5, 696.

Boeve, B.F. (2013). idiopathic REM Sleep behaviour disorder in the development of Parkinson disease. *Lancet Neurology*, 12, 469–82.

Canitano, R., Vivanti, G. (2007). Tics and Tourette syndrome in autism spectrum disorders. *Autism*, 11, 19–28.

Carson, A., Lehn, A., Ludwig, J., Stone, J. (2016). Explaining functional disorders in the neurology clinic: a photo story. 16, 56–61.

Cavanna, A.E. (2018a). Gilles de la Tourette syndrome as a paradigmatic neuropsychiatric disorder. *CNS Spectrums*, 23, 213–18.

Cavanna, A.E. (2018b). The neuropsychiatry of Gilles de la Tourette syndrome: The état de l'art. *Revue Neurologique*, 174, 621–7.

Cavanna, A.E., Rickards, H. (2013). The psychopathological spectrum of Gilles de la Tourette syndrome. *Neuroscience and Biobehavioral Reviews*, 37, 1008–15.

Cavanna, A.E., Seri, S. (2013). Tourette's syndrome. *British Medical Journal*, 347, f4964.

Cavanna, A.E., David, K., Bandera, V., et al. (2013). Health-related quality of life in Gilles de la Tourette syndrome: A decade of research. *Behavioural Neurology*, 27, 83–93.

Conte, A., Berardelli, I., Ferrazzano, G., Pasquini, M., Berardelli, A., Fabbrini, G. (2016). Non-motor symptoms in patients with adult-onset focal dystonia: Sensory and psychiatric disturbances. *Parkinsonism and Related Disorders*, 22, S111–14.

Crimlisk, H.L., Bhatia, K., Cope, H., David, A., Marsden, C.D., Ron, M.A. (1998). Slater revisited: 6 year follow-up study of patients with medically unexplained motor symptoms. *British Medical Journal*, 316, 582–6.

De Souza, J. (2015). *The Psychiatric Phenotype of Huntington's Disease*. PhD Thesis. Birmingham, University of Birmingham.

Deuschl, G., Coster, B., Lucking, C.H., Scheidt, C. (1998). Diagnostic and pathophysiological aspects of psychogenic tremors. *Movement Disorders*, 13, 294–302.

Diederich, N.J., Fenelon, G., Stebbins, G, Goetz, C.G. (2009). Hallucinations in Parkinson disease. *Nature Reviews Neurology*, 5, 331–42.

Dobkin, R.D., Menza, M., Allen, L.A., et al. (2011). Cognitive-Behavioural Therapy for depression in Parkinson's disease: A randomised, controlled trial. *American Journal of Psychiatry*, 168, 1066–74.

Eddy, C.M., Cavanna, A.E. (2013a). 'It's a curse!': Coprolalia in Tourette syndrome. *European Journal of Neurology*, 20, 1467–70.

Eddy, C.M., Cavanna, A.E. (2013b). On being your worst enemy: An investigation of socially inappropriate symptoms in Tourette syndrome. *Journal of Psychiatric Research*, 47, 1259–63.

Eddy, C.M., Parkinson, E.G., Rickards, E.H.G. (2016). Changes in Mental state and behaviour in Huntington's disease. *Lancet Psychiatry*, 3, 1079–86.

Erro, R., Bhatia, K.P., Tinazzi, M. (2015). Parkinsonism following neuroleptic exposure: A double-hit hypothesis? *Movement Disorders*, 30, 780–5.

Esposito, M., Edwards, M.J., Bhatia, K.P., et al., (2009). Idiopathic spinal myoclonus: a clinical and neurophysiological assessment of a movement disorder of uncertain origin. *Movement Disorders*, 24, 2344–9.

Evans, J., Seri, S., Cavanna, A.E. (2016), The effects of Gilles de la Tourette syndrome and other chronic tic disorders on quality of life across the lifespan: A systematic review. *European Child and Adolescent Psychiatry*, 25, 939–48.

Fabbrini, G., Berardelli, I., Moretti, G., et al. (2010). Psychiatric disorders in adult-onset focal dystonia: A case-control study. *Movement Disorders*, 25, 459–65.

Fahn, S. (2011). Classification of movement disorders. *Movement Disorders*, 26, 947–57.

Fahn, S., Marsden, C.D., Calne, D.B. (1987). Classification and investigation of dystonia. In: Marsden, C.D. and Fahn, S. (eds.) *Movement Disorders*, pp. 332–58. London, Butterworths.

Ganos, C., Martino, D. (2015). Tics and Tourette syndrome. *Neurologic Clinics*, 33, 115–36.

Gardiner, A.R., Jaffer, F., Dale, R.C., et al. (2015). The clinical and genetic heterogeneity of paroxysmal dyskinesias. *Brain*, 138, 3567–80

Gelauff, J., Stone, J., Edwards, M., Carson, A. (2014). The prognosis of functional (psychogenic) motor symptoms: a systematic review. *Journal of Neurology, Neurosurgery and Psychiatry*, 85, 220–6.

Genetic Modifiers of Huntington's disease (GEM-HD) Consortium. (2015). Identification of genetic factors that modify clinical onset of Huntington's disease. *Cell*, 162, 516–26.

Gilles de la Tourette, G. (1885). Etude sur une affection nerveuse caracterisée par de l'incoordination motrice accompagnée d'écholalie et de coprolalie. *Archives de Neurologie*, 9, 19–42, 158–200.

Goetz, C.G., Stebbins, G.T. (1993). Risk factors for nursing home placement in advanced Parkinson's disease. *Neurology*, 43, 2227–9.

Groves, M., van duijn, E., Anderson, K., et al. (2011). An international Survey-based algorithm for the pharmacological treatment of irritability in Huntington's disease. *PLoS Currents Huntington Disease*. Edition 1. doi:10.1371/currents.RRN1259.

Haber, S.N. (2003), The primate basal ganglia: parallel and integrative networks. *Journal of Chemical Neuroanatomy*, 26, 317–30.

Haskovec, L. (1902). Akathisie. *Archives Bohemes de Medecine Clinique*, 17, 704–8.

Hassan, N., Cavanna, A.E. (2012). The prognosis of Tourette syndrome: Implications for clinical practice. *Functional Neurology*, 27, 23–7.

Hubers, A.A., van Duijn, E., Roos, R.A.C., et al.; The REGISTRY investigators of the European Huntington Disease Network. (2013). Suicidal ideation in a European Huntington's disease population. *Journal of Affective Disorders* 151, 248–58.

International Huntington Association (IHA) and World Federation of Neurology (WFN) Resarch Group on Huntington's disease (1994). Guidelines for the molecular genetics predictive test in Huntington's disease. *Neurology*, 44, 1533–66.

Jahanshahi, M. (2005). Behavioral and psychiatric manifestations in dystonia. *Advances in Neurology*, 96, 291–319.

Jethwa, K.D., Onalaja, O.A. (2015). Antipsychotics for the management of Parkinson's disease: a systematic review and meta-analysis. *British Journal of Psychiatry Open*, 1, 27–33.

Leentjens, A.F.G., Marinus, J., Van Hilten, J.J., Lousberg, R., Verhey, F.R.J. (2003). The contribution of somatic symptoms to the diagnosis of depressive disorder in Parkinson's disease. *Journal of Neuropsychiatry and Clinical Neurosciences*, 15, 74–7.

Lencer, R., Steinlechner, S., Stahlberg, J., et al. (2009). Primary focal dystonia: Evidence for distinct neuropsychiatric and personality profiles. *Journal of Neurology Neurosurgery and Psychiatry*, 80, 1176–9.

Lin, C.H., Lin, J.-W., Liu, Y.-C., Chang, C.-H, Wu, R.-M. (2015). Risk of Parkinson's disease following anxiety disorders: a nationwide population-based cohort study. *European Journal of Neurology*, 22, 1280–7.

Ljungberg, L. (1957). Hysteria: a clinical, prognostic and genetic study. *Acta Psychiatrica Neurologica Scandinavica*, 112, 1–162.

Lombroso, P.J., Scahill, L. (2008). Tourette syndrome and obsessive-compulsive disorder. *Brain and Development*, 30, 231–7.

Marsden, C.D. (1976). The problem of adult-onset idiopathic torsion dystonia and other isolated dyskinesias in adult life (including blepharospasm, oromandibular dystonia, dystonic writer's cramp, and torticollis, or axial dystonia). *Advances in Neurology*, 14, 259–76.

Martino, D., Cavanna, A.E., Robertson, M.M., Orth, M. (2012). Prevalence and phenomenology of eye tics in Gilles de la Tourette syndrome. *Journal of Neurology*, 259, 2137–40.

Mehta, S.H., Morgan, J.C., Sethi, K.D. (2009). Paroxysmal dyskinesias. *Current Treatment Options in Neurology*, 11, 170–80.

Mehta, S.H., Morgan, J.C., Sethi, K.D. (2015). Drug-induced movement disorders. *Neurologic Clinics*, 33, 153–74.

Mestre, T., Coelho, M., Ferreira, J.J. (2010). Prescription patterns for Huntington's disease in Europe: results from the REGISTRY observational study. *Journal of Neurology, Neurosurgery and Psychiatry*, 81(Suppl 1), A48.

Moraru, E., Schnider, P., Wimmer, A., et al. (2002). Relation between depression and anxiety in dystonic patients: Implications for clinical management. *Depression and Anxiety*, 16, 100–3.

Munts, A.G., Koehler, P.J. (2010). How psychogenic is dystonia? Views from past to present. *Brain*, 133, 1552–64.

Neilsen, G., Stone, J., Matthews, A., et al. (2015). Physiotherapy for functional motor disorders: a consensus recommendation. *Journal of Neurology Neurosurgery and Psychiatry*, 86, 1113–19.

Oppenheim, H. (1911). About a rare spasm disease of childhood and young age (Dysbasia lordotica progressiva, dystonia musculorum deformans). *Neurologische Centralblatt*, 30, 1090–107.

Parkinson, J. (1817). *An essay on the shaking palsy*. London, Whittingham and Rowland for Sherwood, Neely and Jones.

Pringsheim, T., Holler-Managan, Y., Okun, M.S., et al. (2019). Comprehensive systematic review summary: Treatment of tics in people with Tourette syndrome and chronic tic disorders. *Neurology*, 92, 907–15.

Quinn, L., Hamana, K., Kelson, M., et al. (2016). A randomised controlled trial of a multimodal exercise intervention in Huntington's disease. *Parkinsonism and Related Disorders*, 31, 46–52.

Rajagopal, S., Seri, S., Cavanna, A.E. (2013). Premonitory urges and sensorimotor processing in Tourette syndrome. *Behavioural Neurology*, 27, 65–73.

Rawlins, M.D., Wexler, N.S., Wexler, A.R., et al. (2016). The Prevalence of Huntington's disease. *Neuroepidemiology*, 46, 144–53.

Rickards, H., De Souza, J., van Walsem, M., et al.; The European Huntington's disease Network. (2011). Factor analysis of behavioural symptoms in Huntington's disease. *Journal of Neurology, Neurosurgery and Psychiatry*, 82, 411–12.

Rickards, H., Woolf, I., Cavanna, A.E. (2010). Trousseau's disease: A description of Gilles de la Tourette syndrome 12 years before 1885. *Movement Disorders*, 25, 2285–9.

Robertson, M.M. (2006). Mood disorders and Gilles de la Tourette's syndrome: An update on prevalence, etiology, comorbidity, clinical associations, and implications. *Journal of Psychosomatic Research*, 61, 349–58.

Robertson, M.M., Eapen, V., Cavanna, A.E. (2009). The international prevalence, epidemiology and clinical phenomenology of Tourette syndrome: A cross-cultural perspective. *Journal of Psychosomatic Research*, 67, 475–83.

Roper, L.S., Saifee, T.A., Parees, I., Rickards, H., Edwards, M.J. (2013). How to use the entrainment test in the diagnosis of functional tremor. *Practical Neurology*, 13, 396–8.

Scharf, J.M., Miller, L.L., Gauvin, C.A., Alabiso, J., Mathews, C.A., Ben-Shlomo, Y. (2015). Population prevalence of Tourette syndrome: A systematic review and meta-analysis. *Movement Disorders*, 30, 221–8.

Schrag, A., Jahanshahi, M., Quinn, N. (2000). What contributes to Quality of Life in patients with Parkinson disease? *Journal of Neurology, Neurosurgery and Psychiatry*, 69, 308–12.

Schrag, A., Trimble, M., Quinn, N., Bhatia, K. (2004). The syndrome of fixed dystonia: an evaluation of 103 patients. *Brain*, 127, 2360–72.

Sethi, K.D., Zamrini, E.Y. (2015). Asymmetry in clinical features of drug-induced parkinsonism. *Journal of Neuropsychiatry and Clinical Neurosciences*, 2, 64–6.

Simpson, H.A., Jung, L., Murphy, T.K. (2011). Update on attention-deficit/hyperactivity disorder and tic disorders: A review of the current literature. *Current Psychiatry Reports*, 13, 351–6.

Slater, E. (1965). Diagnosis of 'hysteria'. *British Medical Journal*, 1, 1395–9.

Stahl, C.M. and Frucht, S.J. (2017). Focal task specific dystonia: A review and update. *Journal of Neurology*, 264, 1536–41.

Stamelou, M., Edwards, M.J., Hallett, M., Bhatia, K.P. (2012). The non-motor syndrome of primary dystonia: Clinical and pathophysiological implications. *Brain*, 135, 1668–81.

Stern, J.S. (2018). Tourette's syndrome and its borderland. *Practical Neurology*, 18, 262–70.

Stern, J.S., Burza, S., Robertson, M.M. (2005). Gilles de la Tourette's syndrome and its impact in the UK. *Postgraduate Medical Journal*, 81, 12–19.

Stone, J., Hoeritzauer, I., Brown, K., Carson, A. (2014). Therapeutic sedation for functional (psychogenic) symptoms. *Journal of Psychosomatic Research*, 76, 165–8.

Tabrizi, S.J., Scahill, R.A., Owen, G., et al.; TRACK HD Investigators. (2013). Predictors of phenotypic progression and disease onset in pre-manifest and early-stage Huntington's disease in the TRACK-HD study: analysis of 36-month observational data. *The Lancet Neurology*, 12, 637–49.

The Huntington's Collaborative Research Group. (1993). A novel gene containing a trinucleotide repeat that is expanded and unstable on Huntington's disease chromosomes. *Cell*, 72, 971–83.

Van Duijn, E., Craufurd, D., Hubers, A.M., et al.; The European Huntington's Disease Network Behavioural Phenotype Working Group. (2014). Neuropsychiatric symptoms in a European Huntington's disease cohort (REGISTRY). *Journal of Neurology, Neurosurgery, and Psychiatry*, 85, 1411–18.

Veck, H.K., Rickards, H. (2018). A systematic review of the Risk of Suicide after deep brain stimulation for Parkinson's disease. (abstract. 14. BNPA Winter Meeting 2018).

Voon, V., Krack, P., Lang, AE., et al. (2008). A multicentre study on suicide outcomes following subthalamic stimulation for Parkinson's disease. *Brain*, 131, 2720–8.

Voon, V., Mehta, A.R., Hallett, M. (2011). Impulse control disorders in Parkinson's disease: recent advances. *Current Opinion in Neurology*, 24, 324–30.

Waldon, K., Hill, S., Termine, C., Balottin, U., Cavanna, A.E. (2013). Trials of pharmacological interventions for Tourette syndrome: A systematic review. *Behavioural Neurology*, 26, 265–73.

Wenzel, T., Schnider, P., Wimmer, A., Steinhoff, N., Moraru, E., Auff, E. (1998). Psychiatric comorbidity in patients with spasmodic torticollis. *Journal of Psychosomatic Research*, 44, 687–90.

Wexler, N.S., Collett, L., Wexler, A.R., et al. (2016). Incidence of adult Huntington's disease in the UK: A UK-based primary care study and systematic review. *British Medical Journal Open*, 6, e009070.

Worbe, Y., Mallet, L., Golmard, J.L., et al. (2010). Repetitive behaviours in patients with Gilles de la Tourette syndrome: Tics, compulsions, or both? *PLoS One*, 5, e12959.

Wright, A., Rickards, H., Cavanna, A.E. (2012). Impulse control disorders in Gilles de la Tourette syndrome. *Journal of Neuropsychiatry and Clinical Neurosciences*, 24, 16–27.

Ziv, I., Djaldetti, R., Zoldan, Y., Avraham, M., Melamed, E. (1998). Diagnosis of 'non-organic' limb paralysis by a novel objective motor assessment: the quantitative Hoover's test. *Journal of Neurology*, 245, 797–802.

Zurowski, M., McDonald, W.M., Fox, S., Marsh, L. (2013). Psychiatric comorbidities in dystonia: Emerging concepts. *Movement Disorders*, 28, 914–20.

19

Neuropsychiatry of stroke and transient ischaemic attack

Yvonne Chun, Laura McWhirter, and Alan Carson

Stroke and transient ischaemic attack

Stroke is defined as 'a clinical syndrome characterized by an acute loss of focal cerebral function with symptoms lasting more than 24 hours or leading to death, and which is thought to be due to either spontaneous haemorrhage into the brain substance (haemorrhagic stroke) or inadequate cerebral blood supply to a part of the brain (ischaemic stroke) as a result of low blood flow, thrombosis or embolism associated with diseases of the blood vessels (arteries or veins), heart or blood' (Warlow et al., 2008)[1].

A transient ischaemic attack (TIA), often referred to as a 'mini-stroke', is 'an acute loss of focal cerebral function or ocular function with symptoms lasting less than 24 hours, thought to be due to inadequate cerebral or ocular blood supply as a result of low blood flow, thrombosis or embolism' (Hankey et al., 1994).

In practice, TIA and stroke are clinically indistinguishable within the first few hours of symptom onset and should therefore be considered as an 'acute stroke syndrome'.

Stroke is a sudden, potentially fatal and disabling illness. It is one of the leading causes of death and disability, both globally and in the UK. In the UK, stroke affects around 150,000 people a year (Townsend et al., 2012). A quarter of strokes are fatal within a year, and over a third of stroke survivors are living with severe disability. While primarily a disease affecting older people (over 65 years), about one in four strokes occurs in those under the age of 65 (Hall et al., 2012). Hypertension, atrial fibrillation, carotid artery stenosis, diabetes, and smoking are the main modifiable risk factors for stroke and TIA.

Stroke represents a significant health and economic burden to the UK. Stroke costs the UK £9 billion a year, including expenditure on health and social care (49%), informal care (27%), loss of productivity (15%), and benefit payments (9%) (Saka et al., 2009). In a survey of 500 25- to 59-year olds, nearly 70% reported they were unable to return to work following a stroke (Clarke and de Bruin, 2012).

About 20% of ischaemic strokes are preceded by a TIA (Rothwell et al., 2005). Although its symptoms are only temporary, TIA carries a high risk of stroke, with the greatest risk being within the first few days of TIA onset. This elevated risk of stroke begins to level off 3 months following symptom onset.

Clinical presentation

Symptoms of a stroke usually occur abruptly and reach maximum severity rapidly at onset. Stroke syndromes present with a wide array of symptoms, depending on the site of the vascular lesion. The Oxfordshire Community Stroke Project (OCSP) classification broadly classifies stroke syndromes into those arising from the anterior circulation, i.e. the carotid territory and its branches, e.g. the middle cerebral artery, and those from the posterior circulation, i.e. the vertebrobasilar territory (see Table 19.1). A total anterior circulation syndrome (TACS) presents with a 'full-house' combination of unilateral motor weakness, a higher cortical deficit, e.g. dysphasia, neglect, and a homonymous visual field defect. A partial anterior circulation syndrome (PACS) presents with any two of the three features of TACS. Lacunar strokes (LACS) are generally deep-seated subcortical infarcts, e.g. in structures within the basal ganglia, the centrum semiovale, and within a territory supplied by one of the perforating arteries coming off the middle cerebral artery. Posterior circulation stroke syndromes (POCS) have varied presentations, depending on the location of the vascular lesion, e.g. cerebellum, brainstem (sites of the nuclei of cranial nerves III–XII), occipital cortex, and thalamus.

Good history taking and neurological examination are usually sufficient in making the diagnosis of a stroke or to raise suspicion of a stroke mimic, e.g. space-occupying lesion, seizure, migraine, or functional neurological disorder. In the absence of typical stroke symptoms, such as motor weakness or speech disturbance, diagnosis and the time of onset may be unclear. Non-dominant hemispheric syndromes can present with isolated visuospatial dysfunction with anosognosia, an unawareness of one's own impairment, resulting in the individual coming across as behaving 'oddly' or confused to the observer. An isolated visual field defect, such as homonymous

---

[1] Reproduced from C. P. Warlow, et al. (2008). *Stroke Practical Management*, 3rd Edition. Wiley-Blackwell.

Table 19.1 The OCSP classification of stroke syndromes

Total anterior circulation syndrome (TACS)	*1. Motor:* Hemiplegia and/or facial weakness or severe hemiparesis ± hemisensory deficit *2. Higher cerebral:* Dysphasia (dominant hemisphere) Visuospatial deficit or neglect (non-dominant hemisphere) *3. Visual field:* Homonymous hemianopia
Partial anterior circulation syndrome (PACS)	Two of (1), (2), and (3)
Lacunar syndrome (LACS)	*Pure motor stroke:* Unilateral weakness must involve at least two out of three areas of the face, whole arm, and leg *Pure sensory stroke* *Ataxic hemiparesis* *Sensorimotor stroke* (NB No visual field defect, no impairment in higher cerebral function)
Posterior circulation syndrome (POCS)	*Any of the following:* Ipsilateral cranial nerve (III–XII) palsy with contralateral motor and/or sensory deficit Bilateral motor and/or sensory deficit Disorder of conjugate eye movement Cerebellar dysfunction Isolated hemianopia or cortical blindness

Source data from C. P. Warlow, et al. (2008). *Stroke Practical Management*, 3rd Edition. Wiley-Blackwell.

hemianopia due to an occipital infarct, may not become immediately apparent to the patient. A thalamic stroke can present with disturbed consciousness and neuropsychological disturbances, e.g. apathy, disorientation, and memory dysfunction, with or without motor sensory dysfunction, thus making diagnosis challenging (Warlow et al., 2008). POCS can present in a stuttering course, contrary to the typical presentation of maximal symptom severity at onset. The National Institute of Health Stroke Scale (NIHSS) is a 15-item neurological examination which enables rapid, standardized neurological assessment and scoring of stroke severity (Brott et al., 1989).

Role of brain imaging

Brain imaging using CT or MRI is mandatory in all acute stroke presentations, predominantly for excluding intracranial haemorrhage (ICH) or other pathologies, e.g. brain tumours, for which thrombolytic or antithrombotic therapy is contraindicated. MRI diffusion-weighted sequence is a sensitive test in detecting acute ischaemia within 12 hours of onset (Brazzelli et al., 2009). Angiographic imaging (CT or MR angiogram) are sometimes performed to look for underlying vascular pathology, e.g. intracranial aneurysm in ICH, or carotid or vertebral artery dissection.

Stroke aetiology

Approximately 85% of strokes are ischaemic, 10% ICH, and 5% subarachnoid haemorrhage (Sudlow et al., 1997). The commonest pathophysiological mechanisms underlying ischaemic strokes are: (i) large vessel-to-vessel thromboembolism (50%) originating from atheromatous large vessels such as the carotid arteries and aortic arch; (ii) cardioembolism (20%) frequently related to atrial fibrillation or other cardiac conditions, e.g. infective endocarditis, prosthetic heart valve, atrial myxoma; and (iii) small vessel disease (lacunar strokes) (25%) related to hypertension and diabetes (Warlow et al., 2008). Giant cell arteritis, e.g. temporal arteritis, can give rise to a thromboembolic stroke and is suspected in the elderly presenting with headache, monocular blurred vision, and raised inflammatory markers. Younger strokes tend to occur in the absence of conventional cardiovascular risk factors and may be caused by rarer causes such as carotid or vertebral artery dissection, paradoxical embolism through a patent foramen ovale, recreational drug use, inflammatory vascular disorders, hereditary disorders, e.g. cerebral autosomal dominant arteriopathy with subcortical infarcts and leukoencephalopathy (CADASIL), Fabry's disease, mitochondrial myopathy encephalopathy, lactic acidosis, and stroke-like episodes (MELAS), and coagulation disorders, e.g. autophospholipid syndrome. Strokes caused by cerebral venous thrombosis ('venous strokes') can occur in individuals with risk factors for venous thromboembolism, e.g. oral contraceptives, thrombophilia conditions associated with a history of deep vein thrombosis or pulmonary embolism, recurrent miscarriages, and malignancies.

Primary ICH most commonly occurs in hypertensive individuals. In the elderly, a lobar ICH suggests underlying cerebral amyloid angiopathy. ICH can also occur secondary to an underlying vascular abnormality, e.g. intracranial aneurysm, arteriovenous malformation, cavernoma, brain tumour, or septic emboli. Subarachnoid haemorrhage can occur secondary to rupture of an intracranial aneurysm or vascular malformation.

Acute stroke management

Hyperacute stroke management focuses on the timely delivery of evidence-based interventions to revascularize a blocked artery within the first few hours of onset of an ischaemic stroke.

Intravenous thrombolysis with a tissue plasminogen activator (tPA), such as alteplase, should be given as early as possible to patients with acute ischaemic strokes presenting within 4.5 hours of symptom onset to reduce disability by 3–6 months (Emberson et al., 2014).

In a subset (about 10%) of acute ischaemic stroke patients who demonstrate radiographic evidence of a proximal anterior circulation large-vessel occlusion (proximal middle cerebral or distal internal carotid artery) within 6 hours of symptom onset, mechanical thrombectomy using a stentriever device offers a remarkable benefit in reducing disability at 3 months (number needed to treat = 3) (Goyal et al., 2016).

The modified Rankin scale (mRS) is a measure of stroke outcome and is widely used in clinical practice and as a primary outcome in clinical trials evaluating the effectiveness of stroke interventions. An mRS grade of 0–2 denotes a good outcome or a non-disabling stroke, whereas an mRS grade of 3–5 represents increasing severity of functional dependence and a poor outcome (van Swieten et al., 1988).

All stroke patients should be admitted to an acute stroke unit equipped to provide organized stroke unit care, delivered by a multidisciplinary team of stroke physicians, nurses, and therapists specialized in looking after stroke patients. This model of care reduces mortality and disability after a stroke (Stroke Unit Trialists' Collaboration, 2013).

Secondary prevention

Ischaemic stroke and TIA broadly share similar risk factors and pathogenesis. While short-term prognosis and hyperacute treatment slightly differ, the two diagnoses share the same long-term secondary prevention approach, encompassing antiplatelet therapy, statins, antihypertensives, oral anticoagulation for atrial fibrillation, diabetic management, and lifestyle modifications, e.g. smoking cessation and weight loss. Owing to the very high risk of stroke within the first few days of a TIA, all suspected TIAs are referred urgently for specialist assessment at emergency TIA clinics.

Neuropsychiatric sequelae of stroke

Stroke is a disorder of the brain and it is inevitable that some patients should experience neuropsychiatric impairments, just as they would somatosensory or autonomic dysfunctions. In spite of this, neuropsychiatric manifestations of stroke are underappreciated in clinical settings. Independent of stroke severity, post-stroke psychiatric comorbidities are associated with a decreased likelihood of returning to work, poorer quality of life, and long-term disability (Glozier et al., 2008, Maaijweeet al., 2016). This chapter covers the commonest and important post-stroke neuropsychiatric manifestations: anxiety, depression, cognitive impairment and delirium, fatigue, emotional lability, psychosis, and apathy.

Anxiety disorders after stroke

Stroke is a life-changing illness that potentially threatens the individual's survival, independence, and ability to participate in occupational and social activities. Patients with disabling strokes face uncertainties surrounding the likelihood of recovery and prognosis, while patients with non-disabling strokes are warned of an ongoing threat of a recurrence, or worse—that of a severely debilitating stroke. It is not yet clear which factors determine the development of an anxiety disorder after stroke, when anxiety becomes intense, disproportionate, or difficult to control, impacting on daily functioning. Anxiety disorders may present in the acute setting or during rehabilitation or become apparent only after discharge (Campbell Burton et al., 2013).

Phobic anxiety disorders

Phobia is a fear that is disproportionate to the danger of well-defined situations or stimuli.

Exposing the individual to a feared situation leads to an unpleasant emotional state, ranging from mild nervousness and tension to autonomic symptoms such as palpitations, sweating, or a full-blown panic attack. This phobic anxiety state is so unpleasant that the individual may endure the situation with considerable distress, feels an intense desire to escape, or avoid encounter with the situation altogether (avoidant behaviour). Anticipatory anxiety may be evident simply by thinking about the feared situation. Persistent avoidant behaviour may prevent the individual from participating in usual activities. Individuals feel relieved once away from their feared stimulus. We found, in our series of over 200 stroke survivors, phobic fears were often centred on agoraphobic and social situations (see Case study 1).

It may be difficult to ascertain whether someone's fear amounts to a phobic disorder when the individual attributes his anxiety and avoidant behaviour to the restrictions resulting from his physical impairments. For example, fears of falling, travelling alone, and social interaction in patients with leg weakness, ataxia, dysarthria, or dysphasia may be entirely reasonable and proportionate, ensuring that the individual does not endanger themselves in certain situations. In others, however, the anxiety and avoidance may exceed what is beyond reasonable and becomes maladaptive, causing distress or severe restriction in activities. Adaptive fear and maladaptive phobic fear may be considered on a continuum, with the distinction of one from the other made by clinical judgement, taking into account the individual's biological, psychological, and social factors.

Generalized anxiety disorder

In generalized anxiety disorder (GAD), the experience of anxiety is poorly defined and unremitting, sometimes described as 'free-floating'. It is characterized by persistent worries about multiple daily life events and difficulty in controlling the worrying. In addition, the individual needs to have three or more of the following associated symptoms for more days than not: feeling tense or 'keyed up', fatigue, difficulty concentrating, irritability, muscle tension, or sleep disturbance. In diagnosing GAD post-stroke, the DSM criterion of symptoms being present for at least 6 months is often omitted.

A *panic attack* can happen in the context of any anxiety disorder. It refers to a discrete period in which there is a sudden onset of intense apprehension and fearfulness and associated feelings of an impending catastrophe. During a panic attack, individuals commonly experience autonomic symptoms such as palpitations, sweating, shaking, chest discomfort, and the feeling of detachment or of losing control. Phobic anxiety is often accompanied by panic symptoms.

Aetiology

Studies of association between lesion location and stroke severity have been inconsistent (Menlove et al., 2015). In non-stroke patients, the amygdala and insula consistently exhibit heightened activity on functional neuroimaging in specific phobia, social anxiety, and PTSD, and the same areas are associated with fear conditioning in healthy individuals (Etkin et al., 2007). However, no similar studies have been conducted in stroke patients with anxiety.

Epidemiology

Anxiety affects around a quarter of stroke survivors (Campbell Burton et al., 2013). Phobic disorders, e.g. agoraphobia, specific phobias, and GAD were the commonest anxiety diagnoses elicited in clinical psychiatric interviews of stroke survivors (Burvill et al., 1995; Sagen et al., 2010). Anxiety after a stroke can last as long as 10 years and reduces quality of life (Ayerbe et al., 2014).

There are consistent associations between post-stroke anxiety and pre-stroke depression and early anxiety after a stroke (Menlove et al., 2015). There is conflicting evidence for associations with younger age and female sex, the conventional risk factors for anxiety disorders in the general population.

Treatment

There is limited RCT evidence to guide treatment of anxiety disorders after stroke (Knapp et al., 2017). Treatments for stroke patients follows what is standard and evidence-based for phobic disorders and GAD in the general adult population. CBT using exposure techniques forms the mainstay of treatment for panic and phobic disorders, e.g. agoraphobia, specific phobia. However, clinicians should be aware that many stroke patients are unable to comply with CBT and find the rigour of psychotherapy treatment too demanding and drop out of therapy. SSRIs and self-help CBT-based therapy may also be considered.

Once identified, GAD should follow a stepped-care model, offering first lower-intensity psychological interventions, e.g. non-facilitated self-help, guided self-help, and psychoeducational groups, followed by high-intensity psychological intervention or drug treatment such as SSRIs or serotonin–noradrenaline reuptake inhibitors (SNRIs). Patients should be informed of possible side effects of any psychotropic medications. Refractory cases of anxiety disorders are best managed in specialist neuropsychiatry or liaison psychiatry services.

CASE STUDY 1

Mr LH, a 45-year-old self-employed builder, suffered a left partial anterior circulation stroke 3 months ago, with no residual physical deficits.

'I walked into a side street that was very crowded. I felt like a sardine and thought I was going to freak out. I started to feel short of breath, sweaty, my chest felt funny and there was tingling down my arms. I managed to step out of the crowd into a quieter street. I was glancing around to make sure nobody was looking at me. I was afraid that people would think I was going nuts and needed to go to a psychiatric ward!'

'I used to be very confident at speaking to my clients, but now I get anxious about meeting them. One time, I caught myself avoiding eye contact when I was talking to a client. I was really worried that the client was not going to hire me. I am definitely getting less work because of this anxiety.'

'I feel like I am being judged when people look at me and I hate it!'

Depression after stroke

Depression after stroke interferes with rehabilitation (Gillen et al., 1999) and may be associated with increased mortality in the long term (Bartoli et al., 2013). The diagnosis of a depressive episode requires the presence and persistence of either or both of the two key features—(i) depressed mood and (ii) anhedonia (the loss of pleasure or interests)—along with at least four of the additional symptoms—weight loss or gain, insomnia, psychomotor agitation or retardation, fatigue, feelings of worthlessness, lack of concentration, and suicidal ideation (American Psychiatric Association, 2013). Symptoms have to be present nearly every day, for at least 2 weeks, and be sufficient to interfere with daily, social, or occupational functioning.

Patients with a history of anhedonia exhibit a genuine loss of interest or pleasure in activities, rather than the loss of ability to take part due to physical limitations resulting from their stroke. Further enquiry by the clinician may reveal that the individual retains a great deal of interest or pleasure in learning about, or watching, the activities, even if he or she is, for the time being, unable to participate in these activities. Phrasing questions properly is key in history taking, making sure the patient understands the question is about enjoyment in activities he or she is still capable of, and not the degree of upset and frustration at their limitations. Many somatic features of depression are also symptoms of stroke or other post-stroke neuropsychiatric manifestations, e.g. fatigue, poor sleep, loss of appetite. Loss of concentration and psychomotor agitation or retardation are often observed in stroke patients, especially in the context of coexisting post-stroke cognitive impairment or delirium. Hypoactive delirium, in particular, can mimic an apathetic presentation of depression. A change in sleeping pattern is common after stroke, particularly on a hospital ward. Loss of appetite may be related to being on a diet with modified consistency or supplemental tube feeding in cases of dysphagia or due to a change in taste as a result of damage to structures along the gustatory pathway, e.g. lesions to the pons, thalamus, or insula cortex (Dutta et al., 2013). Eliciting suicidal ideation is important, as depression increases the risk of suicidal ideation and attempts and completed suicides in stroke patients (Fuller-Thomson et al., 2012). Inpatient therapists will comment that some patients are just not making progress in their rehabilitation, but for no apparent reason. Such comments should always lead to a careful enquiry about possible depression.

Aetiology

The neurobiological basis of mood regulation is complex. Key structures, including the prefrontal cortex, amygdala, and hippocampus, function within a wider neurocircuit, interacting with other areas, e.g. the thalamus, striatum, hypothalamus, and brainstem (Palazidou, 2012). Neurotransmission, neuroendocrine function (hypothalamic–pituitary–adrenal axis), inflammatory cytokines, and neurogenesis are potentially implicated in the regulation of mood. Studies of post-stroke depression have not yielded any dominant pathogenic mechanism, and no consistent association with lesion location has been found (left versus right; anterior versus posterior circulation) (Carson et al., 2000).

Epidemiology

Depression affects a third of stroke survivors (Hackett et al., 2014). Consistent predictors of depression after stroke are pre-stroke depression, increased stroke severity, and physical disability (Kutlubaev et al., 2014). No consistent association has been found for age, sex, lesion location, or cognitive impairment. In a Swedish nationwide cohort of post-stroke suicides, the incidence of completed suicides (30 suicides per 100,000 person-years) was nearly twice that of the general population (Eriksson et al., 2015). Younger age, being male, severe stroke, living alone at stroke onset, a lower level of education, and self-reported depression at 3 months post-stroke were associated with an increased risk of suicidal attempts, with the risk being highest within the first 2 years of stroke (Eriksson et al., 2015).

Treatment

The latest Royal College of Physicians (RCP) stroke guidelines recommend information provision, support, and advice for people with mild depressive symptoms (Royal College of Physicians, 2016). Social interaction, exercise, or other psychosocial interventions, e.g. psychoeducational groups, should be considered. There is a modest benefit with the use of antidepressants, e.g. SSRI, in reducing depression symptoms after stroke, but this may be offset by a significant increase in side effects, e.g. gastrointestinal disturbance, sedation, confusion (Hackett et al., 2008). Response to antidepressants should be reviewed in the first 2–4 weeks, and changes made according to clinical response. Aim to continue antidepressants for at least 4 months beyond initial recovery of depressive symptoms. Brief, structured psychological therapy may also be considered.

Post-stroke fatigue

Post-stroke fatigue (PSF) is defined as the experience of significant fatigue, a lack of energy, or an increased need to rest every day or nearly every day, leading to difficulty in taking part in everyday activities for at least 2 weeks in community patients or a need to terminate an activity or therapy early in hospital stroke patients (Lynch et al., 2007).

Clinical features

Patients with PSF may report a level of unprecedented tiredness or a feeling of exhaustion following little or no activity (see Case study 2). A subjective need for greater effort to complete what were previously less taxing tasks or activities may be present. Fatigue does not necessarily improve with rest, and patients may or may not report adequate sleep. Therapists often report having to shorten rehabilitation sessions due to profound fatigue on the acute stroke unit. Fatigue scales, e.g. the Fatigue Assessment Scale and Fatigue Severity Scale, are useful for quantifying fatigue severity. PSF can affect patients following a stroke of any severity. It can present early or within the first 3 months of a stroke or later, and can persist for up to 36 months (Duncan et al., 2012). An assessment for a concurrent depressive illness and anxiety disorder should be carried out. PSF can be debilitating and adversely impact on survival and occupational functioning (Glader et al., 2002).

Aetiology

The pathophysiology of PSF is not well established. Data extrapolated from other neurological conditions in which fatigue is prevalent suggest a likely complex interplay among biological, psychological, personal, social, and environmental factors. The striatal–thalamic–frontal neurocircuitry may have a role in fatigue, based on functional neuroimaging studies of multiple sclerosis, TBI, PD, and chronic fatigue syndrome (Mead et al., 2015). Studies of lesion location have not established any convincing evidence for an association with PSF, and data from functional neuroimaging studies of PSF are lacking in stroke (Ponchel et al., 2015). The roles of inflammatory

biomarkers, reduced corticospinal output, and motor cortex excitability have been suggested as possible mechanisms (Kuppuswamy et al., 2015; Kutlubaev et al., 2012).

Epidemiology

Between 30% and 90% of all stroke patients have experienced PSF (Duncan et al., 2012). PSF may be associated with a higher risk of death and lower quality of life (Glader et al., 2002).

Management

A formulation-based approach to understanding fatigue in neurological disorders, proposed by Mead et al. (2015), may be useful in helping clinicians address any potential contributory factors to PSF (see Fig. 19.1) (Mead et al., 2015). A review of sleep, nutrition, concurrent medical conditions, medication side effects, and basic investigations should be undertaken to identify other causes of fatigue, e.g. infections, anaemia, hypothyroidism, metabolic disturbance. Concurrent psychiatric illnesses, such as depression or anxiety disorder, should be treated. Graded exercise may be helpful in building exercise tolerance and reducing fatigue (Mead et al., 2015). RCTs of interventions to treat PSF have so far been uninformative (Wu et al., 2015).

> ### CASE STUDY 2
>
> A 68-year-old man, diagnosed with right partial anterior circulation stroke 3 months ago. Residual right leg dragging.
>
> *'I am just really tired for no reason. It seems like I need to rest even when I have done very little. I feel quite annoyed with myself that I can't get anything done. I don't feel that confident yet on going out alone or taking the buses with my current level of fatigue.'*

Emotionalism after stroke

Emotionalism, or emotional lability, after a stroke refers to the sudden-onset episodes of crying or, less commonly, laughter that appear disproportionately intense to the provoking stimulus and are beyond the individual's control (Cummings et al., 2006). Emotionalism tends to present within the first 4–6 weeks of a stroke (House et al., 1989). Typically, patients report being more 'emotional' than prior to their stroke and an increased frequency in crying which is provoked by stimuli that would not have previously prompted an emotional response of such intensity. The pathological crying rarely occurs completely unprovoked. It typically occurs in response to emotionally congruent or sentimental stimuli, e.g. depressing thoughts of illness, death in the family or friends, watching a sad or touching story on television, seeing the grandchildren, being asked about well-being or the symptom of tearfulness. The intensity of symptoms varies and can cause embarrassment in social situations when severe. The phenomenon of uncontrollable laughing or mirthless laughter occurring completely unprovoked with no relevant context, sometimes reported in other neurological conditions, e.g. multiple sclerosis, gelastic seizures, is rare in stroke.

There is no standardized assessment for emotionalism. It is thought to affect 8–30% (Hackett et al., 2010). Association with

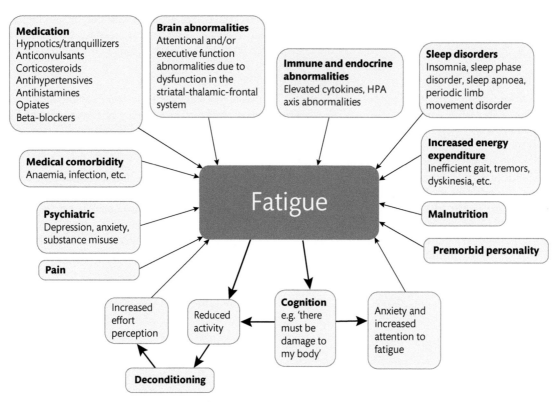

Fig. 19.1 Formulation-based approach to understanding fatigue in neurological conditions.
Reproduced with permission from Mead, G., Welch, K. The impact of fatigue on neurorehabilitation. In *Oxford Textbook of Neurorehabilitation*. V. Dietz and N. Ward (Eds.). Oxford, UK: Oxford University Press. Copyright © 2015, Oxford University Press. DOI: 10.1093/med/9780199673711.001.0001. Reproduced with permission of the Licensor through PLSclear.

frontal lobe lesions has been suggested but is not well established. Patients should be given reassurance. There is currently weak evidence supporting the use of antidepressants to reduce the frequency and severity of abnormal crying associated with stroke, but definitive trials are warranted.

Psychosis after stroke

The commonest cause of psychotic symptoms in the period immediately following a stroke is delirium, in which hallucinations may be visual or auditory and delusions are usually fleeting and persecutory in nature. In delirium, psychotic symptoms usually fluctuate in severity on a background of fluctuating consciousness and inattention. Treatment of delirium consists of identifying and treating underlying contributory conditions, optimizing hydration and nutrition, adjusting the environment, and reducing or removing exacerbating medications such as anticholinergics, opiates, and benzodiazepines. Low-dose antipsychotic medication (e.g. haloperidol) may shorten the duration of delirium but should only be used on a short-term basis. When delirium occurs in the first 2–3 days after a stroke, the possibility of alcohol withdrawal delirium should be considered, which, in contrast to delirium due to other causes, requires treatment with benzodiazepines and intravenous thiamine.

Pre-existing psychosis is perhaps the next commonest cause of psychosis after a stroke.

Lifestyle factors and cardiovascular and metabolic side effects of antipsychotic medication place individuals with schizophrenia at

an increased risk of stroke, compared with the general population. However, people with psychosis who have a stroke may be less likely to receive appropriate treatment (Kisely et al., 2009).

New-onset schizophrenia-like psychotic disorders occur rarely after a stroke. It has been suggested that they are most often associated with right-sided lesions (Rabins et al., 1991), but given the low numbers in this report, we would suggest this is treated with caution until there is more robust replication of the findings. There may also be an association with post-stroke epilepsy (Levine and Finklestein, 1982).

Peduncular hallucinosis is a rare syndrome of complex visual hallucinations associated with infarcts involving the pons and the midbrain. It does seem to be occurring at a slightly increased frequency as a complication of interventional neuroradiologic procedures; in these circumstances, it is usually self-limiting.

Circumscribed delusions sometimes arise in individuals with anosognosia after a stroke and are almost always associated with right hemisphere brain damage (see Case study 3). In somatoparaphrenia, affected individuals develop delusional beliefs that they do not own the limbs of the affected (usually left) side of the body. Individuals with somatoparaphrenia have unilateral spatial and body neglect and usually also have motor and somatosensory deficits (Vallar and Ronchi, 2009). There is not only denial of hemiparesis with confabulation, but also delusion of non-ownership. Patients believe that the arm or leg is truly not their own or that it has been amputated, and may state confidently that it belongs to a nearby person or another specific person or that it is a foreign body such as an artificial arm or leg. There is no established effective treatment for somatoparaphrenia, although in research settings, use of mirrors to create an illusion of normal movement in the affected hand seems to transiently restore a sense of limb ownership (Fotopoulou et al., 2011).

CASE STUDY 3

Mr AJ, a 54-year-old man with a right partial anterior circulation stroke, started to report to nursing staff that he was being treated on a cruise liner. On assessment, this was a firmly held belief. He was oriented to time and date and his sleep–wake cycle and attention were preserved. When he was asked to look outside the window and he saw hospital porters delivering goods, he surmised that the ship must be in 'dry dock', adding that ' … *with the state of the place, the liner was in need of a good refit*'. Mr AJ was felt to have a delusional interpretation of correctly perceived stimuli and a diagnosis of a reduplicative paramnesia was made. It settled over a week without the need for antipsychotics.

Cognitive impairment after stroke

Cognitive disorders after a stroke can be broadly divided into three groups: delirium, strategic infarctions, and dementia. Delirium presents acutely and is no different after a stroke to any other delirium presentation, except that in aphasic strokes, diagnoses may depend more on observation. The presentation is of disorientation, fluctuating conscious levels, disturbance of sleep–wake activity, altered motor activity, hallucinations, and illusions. The neuropsychological hallmark is disruption of attention. While the hyperactivity variant comes to clinical attention very quickly, the more common hypoactive variant is easily overlooked. As delirium affects 30–40% of patients during the first week after a stroke, all patients should be routinely screened (Gustafson et al., 1991; Langhorne et al., 2000; Rahkonen et al., 2000). The Confusion Assessment Method or Delirium Rating Scale may be a useful aid. (McManus et al., 2009a). Differentials include focal cognitive deficits affecting declarative memory, dementia, depression, and apathy. Delirium is more common where there is pre-existing dementia, old age, impaired vision, impaired swallow, and inability to raise both arms (McManus et al., 2009b; Sheng et al., 2006). The diagnosis is important, as it is associated with poorer prognosis, longer duration of hospitalization, increased mortality, increased risk of dementia, and institutionalization (Gustafson et al., 1991; Henon et al., 1999; Reitz et al., 2008). Management follows standard strategies.

Strategic infarction refers to the occurrence of unexpectedly severe cognitive impairment consequent to small areas of infarct, in which classic signs, such as hemiplegia, will often be absent. The medial thalamus, the inferior genu of the internal capsule, the basal ganglia, the left angular gyrus (causing Gerstmann's syndrome of agraphia, acalculia, left–right disorientation, and finger agnosia), and the territory of the posterior cerebral arteries are among sites where apparently small infarcts can have devastating cognitive consequences (Kumral et al., 1999; Rockwood et al., 1999; Tatimichi et al., 1992, 1995).

Dementia after a stroke is a common occurrence, affecting around 30% of subjects, depending on the definition used (Douiri et al., 2013, Schaapsmeerders et al., 2013). Aphasia syndromes are well recognized and common after dominant hemisphere total anterior circulation and partial anterior circulation infarcts and may occur in isolation, but more commonly with other impairments. Less overt presentations with impairment of attention, speed of processing, working memory, and executive function are common in milder presentations (Hurford et al., 2013), and the site of infarct does not always correlate well with neuropsychological function, showing the complexity of cognitive networks and their adaptation after stroke. Disorders of memory tend to show less improvement than disorders of processing speed and attention (Douiri et al., 2013; Schaapsmeerders et al., 2013). Of note, cognitive impairment appears, if anything, to be slightly more common after lacunar strokes and such patients tend to deteriorate over time, suggesting small vessel disease, rather than the fact that the actual lacunar infarct may be the problem (Makin et al., 2013).

Cognitive tests, such as the MoCA and ACE-3, perform well against a more detailed neuropsychological assessment (Pendlebury et al., 2012), but the MMSE and Abbreviated Mental Test are limited and probably should not be used. The Visual Cognitive Assessment Test (VCAT) is a good option in aphasic patients (Kandiah et al., 2016). None of these measures have a timed test of processing speed, except for a limited digit–symbol task in the VCAT, and further testing may be required where this is an isolated problem that is a concern to the patient. Clinicians should be alert to anxiety and depression as alternate explanations and be aware they commonly contaminate testing results.

Apathy

Relatives often get distressed at a lack of volition following a stroke, although the patient themselves is often blithely unconcerned. Apathy affects approximately 25% of patients and appears to be distinct from depression (Matsuzaki et al., 2015; van Dalen et al., 2013). Disruption to fronto-subcortical circuits has been implicated, although there is no coherent picture of key structures (Yang et al., 2015). Patients with apathy show little spontaneous action or speech; their responses may be delayed, short, slow, or absent (Fisher et al., 1995). Apathy is frequently associated with hypophonia, perseveration, grasp reflex, compulsive motor manipulations, cognitive impairment, and older age. It is associated with poor functional outcomes (Hama et al., 2007). Therapeutic trials have been few and are generally disappointing (Starkstein et al., 2016).

Conclusion

Neuropsychiatric complications are common, but underappreciated by stroke health professionals. These complications overlap substantially and can impact adversely on rehabilitation and functioning. Neuropsychiatric care post-stroke should be incorporated into routine stroke care pathways.

KEY LEARNING POINTS

- Symptoms of a stroke usually occur abruptly and reach maximum severity rapidly at onset. Approximately 85% of strokes are ischaemic; 10% are ICH, and 5% are subarachnoid haemorrhage.
- The two commonest anxiety disorders after a stroke are thought to be phobic disorders and GAD.
- Depression affects a third of stroke survivors. Consistent predictors of depression after a stroke are pre-stroke depression, increased stroke severity, and physical disability.
- Emotionalism, or emotional lability, after a stroke refers to sudden-onset episodes of crying or, less commonly, laughter that appear disproportionately intense to the provoking stimulus and are beyond the individual's control. Emotionalism tends to present within the first 4–6 weeks of a stroke.
- Cognitive disorders after a stroke can be broadly divided into three groups: delirium, strategic infarctions, and dementia.
- The commonest cause of psychotic symptoms in the period immediately following a stroke is delirium; by contrast, new-onset schizophrenia-like psychotic disorders are rare. Circumscribed delusions sometimes arise in individuals with anosognosia after a stroke, and peduncular hallucinosis seems to be occurring with a slightly increased frequency as a complication of interventional neuroradiologic procedures.

REFERENCES

American Psychiatric Association. (2013). *Diagnostic and Statistical Manual of Mental Disorders*, fifth edition. Arlington, VA, American Psychiatric Association.

Ayerbe, L., S. A. Ayis, S. Crichton, C. D. Wolfe, A. G. Rudd (2014). Natural history, predictors and associated outcomes of anxiety up to 10 years after stroke: the South London Stroke Register. *Age Ageing* 43: 542–7.

Bartoli, F., N. Lillia, A. Lax, et al. (2013). Depression after Stroke and Risk of Mortality: A Systematic Review and Meta-Analysis. *Stroke Research and Treatment* 2013: 862978.

Brazzelli, M., P. A. Sandercock, F. M. Chappell, et al. (2009). Magnetic resonance imaging versus computed tomography for detection of acute vascular lesions in patients presenting with stroke symptoms. *Cochrane Database of Systematic Reviews* 4: CD007424.

Brott, T., H. P. Adams, Jr., C. P. Olinger, et al. (1989). 'Measurements of acute cerebral infarction: a clinical examination scale. *Stroke* 20: 864–70.

Burvill, P. W., G. A. Johnson, K. D. Jamrozik, C. S. Anderson, E. G. Stewart-Wynne, T. M. Chakera (1995). Anxiety disorders after stroke: results from the Perth Community Stroke Study. *British Journal of Psychiatry* 166: 328–32.

Campbell Burton, C. A., J. Murray, J. Holmes, F. Astin, D. Greenwood, P. Knapp (2013). Frequency of anxiety after stroke: a systematic review and meta-analysis of observational studies. *International Journal of Stroke* 8: 545–59.

Carson, A. J., S. MacHale, K. Allen, et al. (2000). Depression after stroke and lesion location: a systematic review. *The Lancet* 356: 122–6.

Clarke, A., de Bruin, D. (2012). *Short-changed by stroke. The finanacial impact of stroke on people of working age.* London, Stroke Association.

Cummings, J., Arciniegas, D., Brooks, B., et al. (2006). Defining and Diagnosing Involuntary Emotional Expression Disorder. *CNS Spectrums* 11(S6): 1–11.

Douiri, A., A. G. Rudd, C. D. A. Wolfe. (2013). Prevalence of poststroke cognitive impairment South London stroke register 1995–2010. *Stroke* 44: 138–45.

Duncan, F., S. Wu, G. E. Mead. (2012). Frequency and natural history of fatigue after stroke: A systematic review of longitudinal studies. *Journal of Psychosomatic Research* 73: 18–27.

Dutta, T. M., A. F. Josiah, C. A. Cronin, G. F. Wittenberg, J. W. Cole. (2013). Altered taste and stroke: a case report and literature review. *Topics in Stroke Rehabilitation* 20: 78–86.

Emberson, J., K. R. Lees, P. Lyden, et al. (2014). Effect of treatment delay, age, and stroke severity on the effects of intravenous thrombolysis with alteplase for acute ischaemic stroke: a meta-analysis of individual patient data from randomised trials. *The Lancet* 384: 1929–35.

Eriksson, M., E.-L. Glader, B. Norrving, K. Asplund. (2015). Poststroke suicide attempts and completed suicides: A socioeconomic and nationwide perspective. *Neurology* 84: 1732–8.

Etkin, A., T. D. Wager. (2007). Functional Neuroimaging of Anxiety: A Meta-Analysis of Emotional Processing in PTSD, Social Anxiety Disorder, and Specific Phobia. *American Journal of Psychiatry* 164: 1476–88.

Fisher, C.M. (1995). Abulia. In: Bogousslavsky, J., Caplan, L. (eds). *Stroke Syndromes*. Cambridge, Cambridge University Press, pp. 182–7.

Fotopoulou, A., P. M. Jenkinson, M. Tsakiris, P. Haggard, A. Rudd, M. D. Kopelman (2011). Mirror-view reverses somatoparaphrenia: dissociation between first- and third-person perspectives on body ownership. *Neuropsychologia* 49: 3946–55.

Fuller-Thomson, E., M. J. Tulipano, M. Song (2012). The association between depression, suicidal ideation, and stroke in a population-based sample. *International Journal of Stroke* 7: 188–94.

Gillen, R., T. L. Eberhardt, H. Tennen, G. Affleck, Y. Groszmann. (1999). Screening for depression in stroke: relationship to rehabilitation efficiency. *Journal of Stroke and Cerebrovascular Disease* 8: 300–6.

Glader, E. L., B. Stegmayr, K. Asplund. (2002). Poststroke fatigue: a 2-year follow-up study of stroke patients in Sweden. *Stroke* 33: 1327–33.

Glozier, N., M. L. Hackett, V. Parag, C. S. Anderson. (2008). The influence of psychiatric morbidity on return to paid work after stroke in younger adults: the Auckland Regional Community Stroke (ARCOS) Study, 2002 to 2003. *Stroke* 39: 1526–32.

Goyal, M., B. K. Menon, W. H. van Zwam, D. W. J., et al. (2016). Endovascular thrombectomy after large-vessel ischaemic stroke: a meta-analysis of individual patient data from five randomised trials. *The Lancet* 387: 1723–31.

Gustafson, Y.A, Olsson, T.B., Eriksson, S.A., Asplund, K.B., Bucht, G. (1991). Acute Confusional States (Delirium) in Stroke Patients. *Cerebrovascular Diseases* 1: 257–64.

Hackett, M. L., C. S. Anderson, A. House, J. Xia. (2008). Interventions for treating depression after stroke. *Cochrane Database of Systematic Reviews* 4: CD003437.

Hackett, M. L., K. Pickles. (2014). Part I: Frequency of Depression after Stroke: An Updated Systematic Review and Meta-Analysis of Observational Studies. *International Journal of Stroke* 9: 1017–25.

Hackett, M. L., M. Yang, C. S. Anderson, J. A. Horrocks, A. House. (2010). Pharmaceutical interventions for emotionalism after stroke. *Cochrane Database Systematic Reviews* 2: CD003690.

Hall, M., S. Levant, C. J. DeFrances. (2012). Hospitalization for stroke in U.S. Hospitals, 1989–2009. *NCHS Data Brief* 95: 1–8.

Hama, S., H. Yamashita, M. Shigenobu, et al. (2007). Depression or apathy and functional recovery after stroke. *International Journal of Geriatric Psychiatry* 22: 1046–51.

Hankey, G., C. P. Warlow. (1994). Clinical features and differential diagnosis. In: Warlow, C. P., van Gijn, J. (eds). *Transient Ischaemic Attacks*, pp. 79–127. London, W.B. Saunders Co Ltd.

Henon, H., Lebert, F., Durieu, I., et al. (1999). Confusional state in stroke: relation to preexisting dementia, patient characteristics, and outcome. *Stroke* 30: 773–9.

House, A., M. Dennis, A. Molyneux, C. Warlow, K. Hawton, (1989). Emotionalism after stroke. *BMJ* 298: 991–4.

Hurford, R., A. Charidimou, Z. Fox, L. Cipolotti, D. J. Werring (2013). Domain-specific trends in cognitive impairment after acute ischaemic stroke. *Journal of Neurology* 260: 237–41.

Kandiah, N., Zhang, A., Bautista, D.C., et al. (2016). Early detection of dementia in multilingual populations: Visual Cognitive Assessment Test (VCAT). *Journal of Neurology, Neurosurgery, and Psychiatry* 87, 156–60.

Kisely, S., L. A. Campbell, Y. Wang. (2009). Treatment of ischaemic heart disease and stroke in individuals with psychosis under universal healthcare. *British Journal of Psychiatry* 195: 545–50.

Knapp, P., C. A. Campbell Burton, J. Holmes, et al. (2017). Interventions for treating anxiety after stroke. *Cochrane Database of Systematic Reviews* 5: CD008860.

Kumral, E., Evyapan, D., Balkir, K. (1999). Acute caudate vascular lesions. *Stroke* 30: 100–8.

Kuppuswamy, A., E. V. Clark, I. F. Turner, J. C. Rothwell, N. S. Ward. (2015). Post-stroke fatigue: a deficit in corticomotor excitability? *Brain* 138(Pt 1): 136–48.

Kutlubaev, M. A., F. H. Duncan, G. E. Mead. (2012). Biological correlates of post-stroke fatigue: a systematic review. *Acta Neurologica Scandinavica* 125: 219–27.

Kutlubaev, M. A., M. L. Hackett. (2014). Part II: Predictors of Depression after Stroke and Impact of Depression on Stroke Outcome: An Updated Systematic Review of Observational Studies. *International Journal of Stroke* 9: 1026–36.

Langhorne, P., Stott, D.J., Robertson, L., et al. (2000). Medical complications after stroke: a multicenter study. *Stroke* 31: 1223–9.

Levine, D. N., S. Finklestein. (1982). Delayed psychosis after right temporoparietal stroke or trauma: relation to epilepsy. *Neurology* 32: 267–73.

Lynch, J., G. Mead, C. Greig, A. Young, S. Lewis, M. Sharpe. (2007). Fatigue after stroke: The development and evaluation of a case definition. *Journal of Psychosomatic Research* 63: 539–44.

Maaijwee, N. A., I. Tendolkar, L. C. Rutten-Jacobs, et al. (2016). Long-term depressive symptoms and anxiety after transient ischaemic attack or ischaemic stroke in young adults. *European Journal of Neurology* 23: 1262–8.

Makin, S. D. J., S. Turpin, M. S. Dennis, J. M. Wardlaw. (2013). Cognitive impairment after lacunar stroke: systematic review and meta-analysis of incidence, prevalence and comparison with other stroke subtypes. *Journal of Neurology, Neurosurgery, and Psychiatry* 84: 893–900.

Matsuzaki, S., Hashimoto, M., Yuki, S., Koyama, A., Hirata, Y., Ikeda, M. (2015). The relationship between post-stroke depression and physical recovery. *Journal of Affective Disorders* 176, 56–60.

McManus, J., R. Pathansali, H. Hassan, et al. (2009a). The course of delirium in acute stroke. *Age Ageing* 38: 385–9.

McManus, J., R. Pathansali, H. Hassan, et al. (2009b). The evaluation of delirium post-stroke. *International Journal of Geriatric Psychiatry* 24: 1251–6.

Mead, G., Welch, K. (2015). The impact of fatigue on neurorehabilitation. In: Dietz, V., Ward, N. (eds). *Oxford Textbook of Neurorehabilitation*, pp. 328–40. Oxford, Oxford University Press.

Menlove, L., E. Crayton, I. Kneebone, R. Allen-Crooks, E. Otto, H. Harder. (2015). Predictors of Anxiety after Stroke: A Systematic Review of Observational Studies. *Journal of Stroke and Cerebrovascular Diseases* 24: 1107–17.

Palazidou, E. (2012). The neurobiology of depression. *British Medical Bulletin* 101: 127–45.

Pendlebury, S.T., J. Mariz, L. Bull, Z. Mehta, P.M. Rothwell. (2012). MoCA, ACE-R, and MMSE versus the National Institute of Neurological Disorders and Stroke–Canadian Stroke Network vascular cognitive impairment harmonization standards neuropsychological battery after tiA and stroke. *Stroke* 43: 464–9.

Ponchel, A., S. Bombois, R. Bordet, H. Henon. (2015). Factors Associated with Poststroke Fatigue: A Systematic Review. *Stroke Research and Treatment* 2015: 347920.

Rabins, P. V., S. E. Starkstein, R. G. Robinson. (1991). Risk factors for developing atypical (schizophreniform) psychosis following stroke. *Journal of Neuropsychiatry and Clinical Neuroscience* 3: 6–9.

Rahkonen, T., Makela, H., Paanila, S., et al. (2000). Delirium in elderly people without severe predisposing disorders: etiology and 1-year prognosis after discharge. *International Psychogeriatrics* 12: 473–81.

Royal College of Physicians. (2016). *Royal College of Physicians National Clinical Guideline for Stroke*, fifth edition. Available from: https://www.rcplondon.ac.uk/guidelines-policy/stroke-guidelines.

Reitz, C., Bos, M. J., Hofman, A., Koudstaal, P. J., Breteler, M. M. (2008). Prestroke Cognitive Performance, Incident Stroke, and Risk of Dementia The Rotterdam Study. *Stroke* 39, 36–41.

Rockwood, K., Bowler, J., Erkinjuntti, T., et al. (1999). Subtypes of vascular dementia. *Alzheimer Disease and Associated Disorders* 13 (suppl 3): S59–65.

Rothwell, P. M., C. P. Warlow. (2005). Timing of TIAs preceding stroke: time window for prevention is very short. *Neurology* 64: 817–20.

Sagen, U., A. Finset, T. Moum, et al. (2010). Early detection of patients at risk for anxiety, depression and apathy after stroke. *General Hospital Psychiatry* 32: 80–5.

Saka, O., A. McGuire, C. Wolfe. (2009). Cost of stroke in the United Kingdom. *Age Ageing* 38: 27–32.

Schaapsmeerders, P., N. A. M Maaijwee, E. J. van Dijk, et al. (2013). Long-term cognitive impairment after first-ever ischemic stroke in young adults. *Stroke* 44: 1621–8.

Sheng, A. Z., Shen, Q., Cordato, D., Zhang, Y. Y., Yin Chan, D. K. (2006). Delirium within three days of stroke in a cohort of elderly patients. *Journal of American Geriatric Society* 54: 1192–8.

Starkstein, S. E., Brockman, S., Hatch, K. K., et al. (2016). A Randomized, Placebo-Controlled, Double-Blind Efficacy Study of Nefiracetam to Treat Poststroke Apathy. *Journal of Stroke and Cerebrovascular Diseases* 25, 1119–27.

Stroke Trialists' Collaboration. (2013). Organised inpatient (stroke unit) care for stroke. *Cochrane Database of Systematic Reviews* **9**: CD000197.

Sudlow, C. L., C. P. Warlow. (1997). Comparable studies of the incidence of stroke and its pathological types: results from an international collaboration. *Stroke* **28**: 491–9.

Tatimichi, T. K., Desmond, D. W., Prohovnik, I., et al. (1992). Confusion and memory loss from capsular genu infarction: a thalamocortical disconnection syndrome? *Neurology* **42**: 1966–79.

Tatimichi, T. K., Desmond, D. W., Prohovnik, I. (1995). Strategic infarcts in vascular dementia: a clinical and brain imaging experience. *Arzneimittelforschung* **54**: 371–85.

Townsend, N., Wickramasinghe, K., Bhatnagar, P., et al. (2012). *Coronary heart disease statistics 2012 edition*. London, British Heart Foundation.

Vallar, G., R. Ronchi. (2009). Somatoparaphrenia: a body delusion. A review of the neuropsychological literature. *Experimental Brain Research* **192**: 533–51.

van Dalen, J. W., E. P. Moll van Charante, P. J. Nederkoorn, W. A. van Gool, E. Richard. (2013). Poststroke apathy. *Stroke* **44**: 851–60.

van Swieten, J. C., P. J. Koudstaal, M. C. Visser, H. J. Schouten, J. van Gijn. (1988). Interobserver agreement for the assessment of handicap in stroke patients. *Stroke* **19**: 604–7.

Warlow, C. P., M. S. Dennis, J. van Gijn, et al. (2008). *Stroke Practical Management*, third edition. Oxford, Blackwell Publishing.

Wu, S., M. A. Kutlubaev, H. Y. Chun, et al. (2015). Interventions for post-stroke fatigue. *Cochrane Database Systematic Reviews* **7**: CD007030.

Yang, S. R., X. Y. Shang, , J. Tao, et al. (2015). Voxel-based analysis of fractional anisotropy in post-stroke apathy. *PLoS One* **10**: e116168.

20

Infections of the central nervous system

Guleed Adan, Sam Nightingale, Christine Burness, and Tom Solomon

Introduction

Central nervous system (CNS) infections, caused by various pathogens, can lead to a wide range of neuropsychiatric sequelae, including acute psychosis, mood disorders, and chronic dementias. Early recognition is critical as brain infections are often treatable and consequent neuropsychiatric illness can be reversed if diagnosed in a timely fashion.

In addition to psychiatric symptoms, CNS infections may present with other features such as fever, meningism, cranial nerve deficit, and seizures. Although the presence of these additional features can often provide a clue to an underlying CNS infection, they are not always present; hence CNS infections should be considered in the differential diagnosis of psychiatric patients in certain situations.

In this chapter, CNS infections that have psychiatric manifestations or have psychiatric sequelae are discussed, in particular HIV, neurosyphilis, meningitis, and encephalitis.

Neurosyphilis

See Box 20.1 for a summary of the neuropsychiatric manifestations of neurosyphilis.

Epidemiology

It is estimated that 25–30% of all admissions to psychiatric institutions were due to syphilis in the pre-antibiotic era (Gatchel et al., 2015). Although rates have dramatically decreased since the advent of penicillin in the 1940s, there has been a steep increase in infections since 2000 (Ghanem, 2010). In 2012, there were thought to be 18 million cases of syphilis, with 6 million new cases among adults (Newman et al., 2015). The new infections are mainly in men who have sex with men (MSM) and individuals co-infected with HIV (Hook, 2017; Stamm, 2010).

Aetiology

Syphilis is caused by the pathogenic organism *Treponema pallidum*. Treponemes are spirochaetes and visualized as thin, delicate, helically coiled organisms that measure 5–20 μm in length (Gray and Powles, 2013). Once considered a late manifestation of syphilis, CNS involvement may happen at any stage of infection. Neurosyphilis was first described in the late nineteenth century and identified as a cause of dementia and psychosis.

Clinical features

Asymptomatic neurosyphilis

Patients have serological or clinical evidence of systemic syphilis, combined with abnormal CSF findings due to *T. pallidum*: increased white cell count, elevated protein, and reactive CSF Venereal Disease Research Laboratory (VDRL) test, in the absence of neurological symptoms or signs.

Meningitis

Patients generally present with meningitis within a year of infection (Carmo et al., 2001). Findings include signs of meningism, papilloedema, cranial nerve palsies, nausea, vomiting, and convulsions. Syphilitic meningitis has been common in the antibiotic era (Seeley and Venna, 2004).

Meningovascular syphilis

This manifestation presents, on average, 7 years after primary infection (Gray and Powles, 2013). Syphilitic meningitis can lead to endarteritis of small, medium, and large blood vessels. This can result in ischaemia, thrombosis, or infarction. Middle cerebral artery territory strokes are the commonest clinical finding, given the propensity for this vessel to be affected.

Tabes dorsalis

This is seen, on average, 21 years following infection and is the result of degeneration of the posterior roots and columns of the spinal cord. Commonly occurring features include pupillary abnormalities, dorsal column sensory dysfunction, 'lightening' pains, and ataxia.

Parenchymal neurosyphilis

An acute encephalitis syndrome with a presentation similar to that of viral encephalitis has been described as a result of neurosyphilis (Szilak et al., 2001). Affected individuals are often younger and present with seizures and impaired consciousness, together with radiological abnormalities.

Personality change—often the earliest presenting feature of neurosyphilis and noted by relatives of the patient. Characterized by a change in temperament, emotional lability, or socially disinhibited actions.

Grandiosity—grandiose delusions that revolve around power, money, and social superiority are typical of the condition. As the disease progresses, the delusions are succeeded by feelings of apathy and generalized disinterest.

Dementia—gradual impairment of memory, slowed thinking, and loss of insight. Can be complicated by persecutory delusions that are often short-lived. The cognitive decline can also be interspersed by episodes of euphoria or delirium.

Depression—patients can present with symptoms of a depressive illness, often against a background of a dementing process caused by the disease. Delusions are a prominent feature of the mood disorders seen in neurosyphilis.

General paresis

Otherwise known as 'general paresis of the insane', this is a neuropsychiatric disorder that presents 10–24 years after infection and was seen in 5% of patients in the pre-antibiotic era (Marra, 2015). It begins with an insidious change in personality, such as temperament, but in half of cases, the initial presentation is abrupt, with a dramatic and out-of-character action that brings the patient to the attention of medical professionals (Marra, 2015). Whether insidious or more rapid in onset, a change in personality is a common and important presenting neuropsychiatric feature of neurosyphilis (Hutto, 2001).

Several distinct forms of paresis have been described that focus on the mental state of the patient. Abnormal cognition is the commonest psychiatric disorder associated with neurosyphilis, but patients can also present with mania, schizophrenia, and depression (Hutto, 2001). Dementia involves impairment of memory, loss of insight, and deterioration in cognitive abilities such as calculation and recall. It is associated with recurrent episodes of impaired consciousness which exacerbates confusion. Fleeting persecutory delusions, together with transient episodes of euphoria, further complicate the condition.

Early in the disease, the patient can be neurologically intact. However, the most frequent neurological findings include pupillary abnormalities, tremor, dysarthria, brisk reflexes, and incoordination.

Assessment

Diagnosis of symptomatic neurosyphilis is based on clinical features, supported by the presence of pleocytosis and reactive CSF-VDRL test. CSF white cell concentration in neurosyphilis is normally >10 cells/µL, with lymphocytosis. Diagnosis of asymptomatic neurosyphilis is entirely dependent on CSF abnormalities. Neuroimaging can be used to support a diagnosis but cannot be used alone to make a diagnosis. Findings visible on MRI brain can include cerebral infarction, arteritis, and non-specific white matter lesions (Peng et al., 2008).

Prior to a lumbar puncture (LP), patients should have serological testing for systemic syphilis. Serological tests can be divided into non-treponemal and treponemal tests:

- Non-treponemal tests:
  - VDRL.
  - Rapid plasma reagin (RPR).
  - Toluidine red unheated serum test (TRUST).

These tests are quantitative, and therefore, titres can indicate the severity of disease. As levels fall with treatment, they can be used to monitor disease response. Non-treponemal tests can, however, miss early primary infection, and as levels also naturally fall with time, reactivity can decrease. These tests measure IgM and IgG antibody and are not specific for *T. pallidum*.

- Treponemal tests:
  - Fluorescent treponemal antibody absorption (FTA-Abs).
  - *T. pallidum* particle agglutination (TPPA).
  - Enzyme immunoassay (EIA).
  - Chemiluminescence immunoassay (CIA).
  - Microbead immunoassay (MBIA).
  - *T. pallidum* haemagglutination assay (TPHA).
  - *T. pallidum* immobilization (TPI).

These tests are qualitative, so they cannot be used to measure disease response. They are, however, useful in detecting early primary and treated infection as the reactivity persists.

Both treponemal and non-treponemal serology should be used in combination due to limitations of each test, including false positives and the inability for treponemal tests to distinguish between recent and distant infection (CDC, 2008).

All patients diagnosed with neurosyphilis should be tested for other sexually transmitted infections, particularly HIV, as co-infection is common.

Management

Penicillin remains the treatment of choice for neurosyphilis, with intravenous adminstration preferred due to assumed higher treponemicidal levels in the CSF. Updated UK guidelines to treatment can be found at: https://www.bashhguidelines.org/current-guidelines/genital-ulceration/syphilis-2015/.

In addition to penicillin, antipsychotic drugs are indicated for the symptoms of agitation, delusions, and hallucinations. Antidepressants should also be used for depressive symptoms, but ECT should be avoided due to the risk of sudden clinical deterioration with worsening of symptoms.

Prognosis

Prognosis was poor in the pre-antibiotic era, with patients diagnosed with severe neurocognitive dysfunction as a result of general paresis only having an average survival of 2.5 years (Marra, 2015). The extent of the resolution of symptoms varies, depending on the clinical subtype of neurosyphilis the patient had before treatment. Patients with syphilitic meningitis often recover fully, yet those with paresis rarely regain full cognitive function.

For key points to remember from this chapter, see Box 20.2.

- Neurosyphilis can present in so many different ways that it is prudent to consider serological testing in all patients admitted to psychiatric services.
- Due to high rates of co-infection with HIV, if testing for syphilis, always consider a test for HIV, and vice versa.
- Always consider a diagnosis of general paresis prior to making a diagnosis of primary dementia in patients presenting with a decline in cognitive ability suggestive of a dementing process.
- Early treatment with penicillin in the initial stages of neurosyphilis prevents the development of general paresis at a later stage.

Box 20.3 Neuropsychiatric manifestations of HIV

- Cognitive impairment:
  - HIV-associated dementia—marked cognitive impairment that produces severe interference with activities of daily living. A subcortical phenotype with variable motor involvement.
  - MCI—milder forms of cognitive impairment occur despite effective antiretroviral therapy. A cortical phenotype with impaired abstraction and executive function.
- Psychiatric disorders:
  - Depression—up to twice as common in HIV-infected populations.
  - Anxiety—can be related to issues around the illness and its stigma.
  - OCD—a specific condition around issues of HIV infection has been described.
  - 'AIDS mania'—with key features of irritability and agitation, rather than elation and euphoria.
  - 'AIDS lethargy'—apathy, tiredness, and lack of emotional engagement.

Human immunodeficiency virus

For a summary of the neuropsychiatric manifestations of HIV, see Box 20.3.

Epidemiology

The World Health Organization (2018) estimates that 36.9 million people globally are infected with HIV, with 2 million new infections per year occurring in 2014. The disease is seen worldwide, with the highest prevalence in sub-Saharan Africa and an increasingly significant impact in Eastern Europe, India, and China (Fettig et al., 2014).

Psychiatric disorders are more common in populations with HIV. For example, HIV-positive individuals are twice as likely to be diagnosed with MDD than HIV-negative individuals (Ciesla and Roberts, 2001).

Cognitive disorders are also seen. In the pre-antiretroviral therapy (ART) era, HIV-associated dementia (HAD) was prevalent and affected up to 50% of patients prior to death (Brew and Chan, 2014). This decreased with the introduction of ART (Nightingale et al., 2014) and is now only described in around 2% of populations with ready access to modern ART. Despite this, milder forms of cognitive impairment persist. These impairments have a different phenotype—more cortical dysfunction than subcortical, with deficits in learning, memory, and executive function predominating (Heaton et al., 2011). The prevalence of these milder forms of cognitive impairment in treated populations is debated, and estimates range from 5% to 50%, depending on the definitions and methods used (Nightingale et al., 2014).

Aetiology

HIV can be found in the CNS early in infection (Ellis et al., 2009). HIV enters the brain via activated infected macrophages and monocytes. Toxic viral products and cell-derived toxins lead to breakdown of the BBB, loss of white matter density, neuronal loss, and astrocyte and oligodendrocyte injury (Ellis et al., 2009). This can lead to HAD in advanced infection.

Clinical features

Cognitive

HIV-associated dementia

HAD is a progressively disabling subcortical dementia that is characterized by loss of attention and concentration, forgetfulness, marked psychomotor retardation, social withdrawal, apathy, and increased irritability (Brew and Chan, 2014). The commonest early symptoms are said to be impaired memory and deficits in concentration.

Although, early in the disease, there may be little to find on neurological examination, as the condition progresses, there may be positive signs such as hyperreflexia, ataxia, bradykinesia, spasticity, and pyramidal signs. Motor abnormalities become more pronounced with disease progression, especially slowing and impairment of fine movements (e.g. fastening buttons and handwriting). Gait disturbances worsen and can be seen alongside tremor and lower limb weakness. Late-stage features of the disease may include tremor, seizures, weakness, and incontinence. Later stages may also be complicated by painful peripheral neuropathy that contributes to the diminishing quality of life in these patients.

Prior to widespread use and availability of ART, HAD was common, occurring in up to 50% of patients prior to death (Nightingale et al., 2014). In developed nations with access to effective ART, the incidence of HAD has drastically decreased, mirroring the trend seen with other AIDS-related pathologies (Garvey et al., 2011). HAD now occurs in <2% of individuals with HIV, and this is usually associated with treatment failure, late diagnosis, or undiagnosed advanced disease (Heaton et al., 2010). HAD continues to be a significant issue in the developing world due to poor access to ART.

Mild cognitive impairment

Although HAD is now less common, milder forms of cognitive impairment persist in ART-treated populations. MCI is phenotypically different to HAD. It is characterized by deficits in cortical and executive functions, as opposed to the subcortical dementing process of HAD. Estimates of prevalence vary considerably, based on the methods and definitions used (Nightingale et al., 2014).

The causes of this milder impairment are often multifactorial and include compartmentalized HIV, ART neurotoxicity, alcohol and substance abuse, cerebrovascular disease, hepatitis C co-infection, and comorbid psychiatric illness (Saylor et al., 2016). Many patients with MCI in the context of HIV often have a combination of factors that all contribute to their cognitive deficits. Thus, the direct impact of HIV on cognition can be difficult to determine (Nightingale and Winston, 2017). All potentially contributing factors and predisposing conditions should be considered when presented with these patients in clinical practice.

Psychiatric

Depression

Depression in the HIV-positive population is common. HIV-positive individuals are twice as likely to be diagnosed with MDD than HIV-negative individuals (Ciesla and Roberts, 2001). Subcohorts that have been found to be more at risk of developing depression include those with advanced HIV at presentation or a previous history of psychiatric disease (Atkinson et al., 2008). Depression is well recognized as a cause of poor outcome in many chronic medical conditions. In HIV, it can be underdiagnosed, and thus undertreated (Asch et al., 2003).

There can be overlap between the somatic features of depression and symptoms that are commonly seen in the advanced stages of HIV infection. Features such as fatigue, insomnia, malaise, and loss of appetite are common to both disease processes. Anhedonia and cyclical mood variation as the day progresses, as seen in depression, have been shown to be useful discriminating features between the two conditions (Treisman et al., 2001). Improved access to effective ART has decreased the number of patients developing advanced HIV and AIDS; hence this diagnostic difficultly is now less of an issue in developed countries.

Early recognition and treatment of depression in HIV are important for reducing morbidity and mortality (Leserman, 2008). Patients with HIV should be screened for depressive symptoms, allowing for early diagnosis and treatment. Management of HIV is heavily reliant on compliance to antiretroviral medication, and depression has been shown to have a significantly negative impact on the ability of the individual to cope with their condition and subsequent management (Antoni et al., 2005; Tucker et al., 2003). There is no consensus on the most effective class of antidepressant to use in depression (Cavalcante et al., 2010).

There is a higher prevalence of mania in HIV-positive individuals, compared to the general population, and the rate increases with progression of HIV. Early in infection, the rate of mania (1–2%) appears only marginally higher than that seen in the general population (Lyketsos and Treisman, 2001). With progression to AIDS, prevalence is higher, with between 4% and 8% of patients being found to be manic (Venugopal et al., 2001). The timing of the symptoms of mania are found to be closely correlated to the neurocognitive degeneration that is associated with advanced disease (Carroll and Brew, 2017). The condition is termed 'AIDS mania', but it is phenotypically different and less severe from the stereotypical mania seen in psychiatric clinical practice. Classically, the syndrome is characterized by an overarching feature of agitation and irritability, rather than a feeling of elation (Martínez et al., 2017).

Psychosis

Psychosis is less common than mood disorders in HIV and is typically associated with advanced disease. Psychosis seen in HIV is characterized by delusions, hallucinations, bizarre behaviour, formal thought disorder, and emotional lability. In the early antiretroviral era, HIV-positive individuals with psychosis were shown to have greater degrees of neurocognitive impairment, when compared with a HIV-positive cohort without psychosis (Evans et al., 2002). Risk factors for the development of new-onset psychosis in HIV-positive patients include a past history of psychiatric illness, poor cognitive performance, and not being on ART (Ronchi et al., 2000). In addition, there have been case reports of new-onset psychosis following the initiation of antiretrovirals. Although several agents have been implicated, this is most commonly seen following initiation of the non-nucleoside reverse transcriptase inhibitor (NNRTI) drug efavirenz.

Obsessive–compulsive disorder

An OCD related to issues around HIV has been reported in the literature (McDaniel and Johnson, 1995), which can involve repeated checking for progression of the illness, as well as an incessant and obsessive desire to recall previous sexual partners.

Assessment

Cognitive testing

The HIV Dementia Scale has been validated in HIV-positive cohorts. This test includes tests of motor speed, as well as cognitive ability, and was designed to assess HAD. It is insensitive for milder cognitive impairments seen in ART-treated cohorts (Heaton et al., 2011). In patients presenting with milder cognitive symptoms, the most useful assessment is formal neuropsychometric testing by an experienced neuropsychologist. Estimates of premorbid function are important and a collateral history from relatives or those close to the patient is useful to assess premorbid status.

Imaging

Neuroimaging in HIV is most useful in excluding other conditions and CNS complications of HIV-1 infection such as progressive multifocal leukoencephalopathy, toxoplasmosis, or lymphoma (Masters and Ances, 2014). In HAD, MRI shows white matter hyperintensity and cortical atrophy with ventricular dilatation. In MCI, MRI can show hazy white matter hyperintensity, with or without diffuse atrophy, or can be normal.

Cerebrospinal fluid

CSF analysis is useful to exclude the presence of opportunistic infection and to measure CSF HIV viral load. In the pre-ART era, raised CSF HIV viral load was associated with HAD. The association between CSF HIV viral load and milder cognitive deficits in patients receiving ART is less clear. HIV can be found at higher levels in the CSF, the so-called CSF escape. CSF escape can be due to compartmentalized virus in the CNS, and CSF virus can show resistance mutations not seen in blood (Nightingale et al., 2014).

There are currently no other CSF markers that have been shown to reliably correlate with the cognitive or neuropsychiatric manifestations of HIV. However, this is an area of ongoing study.

Management

Cognitive impairment in HIV is an indication to start ART. In ART-treated patients with cognitive problems, first consideration must be given to whether HIV is adequately controlled in the blood and whether there are any comorbidities or drug toxicities that could be contributing to cognitive problems. If CSF escape is present and resistant virus identified in the CSF, medications can be adjusted according to the resistance profile of the CSF virus. Otherwise ART can be adjusted according to estimates of effectiveness in the CNS. Which ART drugs are more effective in the CNS is a subject of ongoing research (Nightingale et al., 2014).

Some ART agents can lead to neuropsychiatric side effects. In particular, efavirenz, an NNRTI, is of particular importance. It can cause symptoms of dizziness, agitation, hallucinations, amnesia, insomnia, and nightmares and can lead to worsening and relapse of existing psychiatric illness. Mild symptoms often settle if the drug is continued.

There is no consensus on the optimal antidepressant or antipsychotic medications for use in patients with HIV. When prescribing these treatments, it is important to consider ART interactions. For detailed information on potential drug interactions, see http://www.HIV-druginteractions.org

Prognosis

The prognosis for HIV-positive individuals has dramatically improved since the beginning of the epidemic due to the widespread availability of combination ART. Psychiatric illness can negatively impact outcomes of people living with chronic HIV infection.

Box 20.4 Points to remember

- HIV-1 infection should always be considered as a possible diagnosis in those presenting with cognitive impairment. It is common, preventable, and treatable if a diagnosis is made.
- Although advanced cognitive deficits such as HAD are now much less common, milder forms of cognitive deficit still persist despite effective ART.
- MCI can be subtle, and detailed neuropsychometric testing with comparison to premorbid estimates is required for assessment.
- Some ART can be associated with neurotoxicity, in particular efavirenz which commonly causes anxiety, nightmares, amnesia, and agitation.
- When prescribing psychiatric medication, it is always important to consider potential pharmacological interactions with antiretrovirals.
- Untreated psychiatric disease in HIV is associated with increased morbidity and mortality; therefore, it must be diagnosed and treated at the earliest opportunity.

Depression has been associated with HIV disease progression and higher rates of mortality (Leserman et al., 2002). Studies have demonstrated that if psychiatric symptoms, particularly depression, are treated adequately, it can lead to improved psychosocial functioning and quality of life (Elliott et al., 2002).

As HAD is an AIDS-defining condition associated with advanced infection, prognosis can be poor. Some improvement in cognitive function can be seen following initiation of effective ART, and long-term survival can be achieved with adequate immune reconstitution. Milder forms of cognitive impairment in people receiving ART carries a much better prognosis. Progression depends on the underlying cause but, in most cases, is not rapidly progressive. The degree to which such cognitive deficits interact with ageing is a subject of ongoing research.

For key points to remember from this chapter, see Box 20.4.

Meningitis

Tuberculous meningitis

Tuberculous meningitis (TBM) is an important diagnosis that should not be missed due to its high mortality and morbidity. If diagnosed appropriately, it is readily treatable. Often the diagnosis is delayed due to a non-specific presentation which can include neuropsychiatric features. The onset of TBM is often insidious; pyrexias can be low-grade and often lag behind the other clinical symptoms, and there is often little to no meningism (Thwaites and Hien, 2005).

Epidemiology

Extrapulmonary tuberculosis (TB) makes up 10% of all cases of symptomatic disease, and of these, TB is found in the CNS in 5% of cases. Rates of TBM are higher in HIV-positive individuals (Jarvis et al., 2010), with the highest rates found within the most immunocompromised cohorts (Nelson and Zunt, 2011).

Aetiology

TBM is caused by *Mycobacterium tuberculosis*. The bacteria is passed on via inhalation of particles known as droplet nuclei, following coughing or sneezing from an infected individual.

Psychiatric features

The early stage of the illness is often defined by subtle personality change or changes in behaviour that are often first noticed by those closest to the patient. Changes include apathy, irritability, and low mood. These gradual changes then lead to a state of reduced awareness to external stimuli. TBM can also make patients hallucinate or even delirious to the extent seen in alcohol withdrawal (Jebaraj et al., 2005). This can further complicate the diagnosis, and these patients have also previously been misdiagnosed with alcohol-related encephalopathies such as Wernicke's, particularly if there are cranial nerve palsies, in addition to the confused state (Chou et al., 2012). Once treatment has been started, patients with TBM can progress from the confusional state to one of amnesia, which can persist for weeks. A characteristic feature in this phase of the illness is that the patients are found to be in a state of euphoria despite their extreme memory difficulties (Henn, 2014). Neurosyphilis is an important differential in the TBM subgroup who display neuropsychiatric features. Even after completed treatment, memory is slow to recover and can take some time to return to baseline function.

Investigation and treatment

CSF analysis is key and findings often include a raised opening pressure, with a lymphocytosis of 100–1000 cells/mm³. CSF protein is increased in most cases, while CSF glucose, when compared to a paired serum sample, is reduced in the vast majority. Typical CSF findings in meningitis of different causes can be seen in Table 20.1.

Antituberculous treatment should be started as soon as the diagnosis is made on a clinical basis. Treatment typically includes isoniazid, rifampicin, pyrazinamide, and streptomycin (Mai and Thwaites, 2017).

Prognosis

TBM without treatment can lead to hydrocephalus and eventual coma (30–60%). This can be prevented with early neurosurgical intervention which involves insertion of an extraventricular shunt (Chatterjee, 2011).

Bacterial and viral meningitis

Bacterial and viral meningitis are not classically associated with neuropsychiatric presentations or the development of subsequent

Table 20.1 Typical CSF findings in meningitis

Cause	White cell count (×106 cells/L)	Cell type	CSF:serum glucose (normal ≥0.5)	Protein (g/L) (normal 0.2–0.4)
Viral	0–1000	Mononuclear	>0.5	0.4–0.8
Bacterial	100–5000	Neutrophilic	<0.5	0.5–2.0
Tuberculous	50–300	Mononuclear	<0.3	0.5–3.0

psychiatric disease. There have been, however, studies that have found neurocognitive deficits following infection.

There have been reports of mild cognitive deficit after viral meningitis in adults (Sittinger et al., 2002). Deficits were found in non-verbal memory functions, in addition to decreased levels of attention and speed of cognitive performance. This supports the findings of similar studies that found that sleep was affected (Schmidt et al., 2006), as well as concentration in tasks (Forsgren et al., 2002). This area has been the subject of much debate, and there are those who consider the mild cognitive deficits to be as a result of a severe infection, rather than the meningitis itself.

Cognitive deficiencies have been reported in children who have had bacterial meningitis. Children are most affected with persistent difficulties in learning, deficits in short-term memory, behavioural problems, and poor academic performance (Grimwood et al., 2000). Similar cognitive deficits have been demonstrated in adults, with short-term memory and executive functions as the domains that are affected most often and most severely after bacterial meningitis (Schmidt et al., 2006).

For key points to remember from this chapter, see Box 20.5.

Encephalitis

Epidemiology

There is an estimated incidence of encephalitis in the tropical world of 6.3 per 100,000 (Jmor et al., 2008). In the UK, the Health Protection Agency identified an annual incidence of 1.5 cases per 100,000 (Granerod et al., 2013). The epidemiology of encephalitis can be classified broadly into non-geographically restricted sporadic causes and geographically restricted endemic causes (Solomon et al., 2007). Infectious causes must be distinguished from autoimmune causes, which have many overlapping clinical features (Venkatesan et al., 2019).

Aetiology

The pathogen most commonly responsible for sporadic encephalitis is herpes simplex virus (HSV) type 1 (Solomon et al., 2012). The commonest cause of epidemic viral encephalitis is Japanese encephalitis virus (Granerod et al., 2010). In many cases, the cause is unknown, with reports of only 40–70% of cases having an aetiological agent identified (Glaser et al., 2003).

Box 20.5 Points to remember

- TBM has a non-specific presentation which is not always typical of a CNS infection.
- Often subtle psychiatric symptoms may be the only thing that will allude to the diagnosis of TBM.
- Always consider TBM in patients with non-specific neurological symptoms and changes in consciousness, together with personality changes that may be apparent to relatives.
- TBM as a diagnosis should often be considered in parallel with other conditions such as neurosyphilis.
- The incidence of TBM is much higher in immunocompromised individuals, hence the need to have a low threshold to consider this diagnosis.
- Bacterial and viral meningitis are not frequently associated with neuropsychiatric disorders at presentation but can both result in subtle cognitive deficits after acute illness.

Clinical features

Patients often present with headache, altered mental status, and fever, following a prodromal flu-like illness. The fever is not a universal feature and can often be low-grade or fluctuating (Granerod et al., 2010; Solomon et al., 2012). The impairment in consciousness level and mental state classically associated with encephalitis can manifest as mild somnolence, delirium or disorientation and behavioural change, or coma (Raschilas et al., 2002). The presence of focal neurological deficit or seizures reflects parenchymal inflammation and are thus more supportive of a diagnosis of encephalitis, rather than meningitis.

Psychiatric features

Cases of encephalitis can present with psychiatric features, in addition to the more classical features of parenchymal inflammation. In a review of 62 cases of encephalitis, psychiatric symptoms were found at presentation with hallucinations (60%), delusions (54%), and mood disorders (27%) (Caroff et al., 2001). Often, prior to impaired consciousness, patients go through a period of marked delirium, sometimes with hallucinations. This combination of acute confusion and hallucinations can lead to a misdiagnosis of delirium tremens or a metabolic encephalopathy.

The psychiatric features are highly dependent on the parenchymal structures that are most affected. Patients can present with features of aggression and socially inappropriate behaviour in the case of frontal lobe involvement or memory loss and emotional lability in the case of limbic system involvement (Solomon et al., 2012).

Often psychiatric symptoms are the dominant features at presentation, especially for immune-mediated encephalitis, such as that due to NMDA antibodies, when more classical clinical symptoms associated with encephalitis are entirely absent.

Psychiatric symptoms are common after encephalitis, with reports of anxiety (67%), mood disorder (59%), and depression (58%) (Dowell et al., 2001). One study found a prevalence of personality disorder of 45% in survivors of HSV encephalitis (McGrath et al., 1997). There have also been reports of psychoses and emotional lability persisting after treatment and discharge from hospital (Gaber et al., 2003).

Assessment and management

Following bedside neurological assessment, which includes full assessment of consciousness level, a timely LP should be carried out for analysis of the CSF (Solomon et al., 2007). Polymerase chain reaction (PCR) to detect viral DNA in the CSF is essential, with sensitivities of 98% and specificities of 99% in detecting HSV-1 (Kleinschmidt-DeMasters and DeBiasi, 2001). LP may be normal early in the condition. Five to 10% of adults with proven HSV encephalitis can present with initial CSF findings which are normal, with no pleocytosis, and a negative HSV PCR (Solomon et al., 2012).

In HSV encephalitis, a CT scan may be normal early in the disease but can go on to reveal the classical finding of low attenuation in the temporal lobes (Chaudhuri and Kennedy, 2002). MRI is more sensitive in detecting changes earlier on in the condition (Solomon et al., 2012).

Timely treatment is imperative due to poor prognosis associated with delayed therapy. The patient should be stabilized initially with good seizure control with AEDs and definitive airway management, if needed. Aciclovir should be commenced as soon as possible

> **Box 20.6** Points to remember
>
> - Encephalitis can present with psychiatric features preceding classical features of parenchymal inflammation such as seizures, coma, or other focal neurology.
> - The psychiatric symptoms that manifest are highly dependent on the area of the brain affected.
> - Prompt diagnosis and treatment with aciclovir has a significant effect on reducing mortality and morbidity; therefore, atypical psychiatric presentations of encephalitis should not be missed.
> - Psychiatric symptoms can persist even after treatment.
> - Patients should be counselled for neuropsychological sequelae that can persist long after treatment and can be debilitating.

where there is a convincing case based on clinical assessment alone. Although neuroimaging and initial CSF analysis can be useful, they should not delay treatment (Solomon et al., 2007).

Prognosis

Prior to aciclovir, mortality stood at 70% and there was significant morbidity, with 50% of survivors being left with severe sequelae (Raschilas et al., 2002). With antiviral treatment now more common, mortality rates have reduced to between 3% and 15% (Raschilas et al., 2002). Following treatment, patients can, however, be left with quite significant cognitive dysfunction, the most debilitating of which can be severe anterograde amnesia in 25–75%, in addition to a less severe retrograde memory impairment (Hokkanen and Launes, 2000). Even patients who make a good clinical recovery after treatment can be left with debilitating neuropsychological dysfunction and thus require careful counselling regarding this and follow-up with specialist cognitive services.

For key points to remember from this chapter, see Box 20.6.

Other CNS infections

Subacute sclerosing panencephalitis

Subacute sclerosing panencephalitis (SSPE) is a rare condition that presents many years after an acute measles infection. The initial symptoms include subtle cognitive deterioration, typically in older children. The intellectual decline is gradual and manifests as poor educational performance. It is associated with personality and behavioural change. Motor features can present at any time of the illness and classically include myoclonic jerking of the head, trunk, and limbs. In the more advanced stages of the disease, the patient can develop various degrees of visual impairment and significant neurological dysfunction, including quadraparesis and eventual coma. EEG findings can be characteristic and typically show stereotyped bilateral (asymmetrical) synchronous, periodic complexes, present in the absence of myoclonic jerks. An important finding in the CSF is raised IgG, while CT and MRI imaging can show white matter lesions and eventual atrophy in the brainstem and other structures (Praveen-Kumar et al., 2007).

SSPE is a highly devastating and progressive CNS infection, which results in death in almost 95% of patients, with the remaining 5% going into spontaneous remission. Patients who survive do not generally regain their cognitive functioning, but some with a milder phenotype develop a relapsing–remitting pattern of cognitive

dysfunction after the acute phase of the illness. Measles rates are once again increasing, because of growing vaccine hesitancy (World Health Organization, 2019), and we can expect to see more cases of SSPE in the future.

Neurocysticercosis

The causative organism of neurocysticercosis is *Taenia solium*, a cestode parasite. Humans act as hosts for the *cysticercus*, the larval form of the parasite that is typically found in the faecal matter of pigs (Serpa et al., 2006). Infection with the larvae leads to the formation of multiple cysts within the brain, and the majority of clinical features manifest themselves when the larvae die. The consequent inflammation leads to the classical presentation of acute seizures, which can then progress to epilepsy as the cysts calcify. There have been reports of depression and psychosis with neurocysticercosis, both in the acute phase and as a longer-term complication of infection (Verma and Kumar, 2013). Diagnosis involves a combination of clinical assessment, brain imaging, and serological testing. Management involves AEDs, anti-parasitic agents, anti-inflammatory drugs, and rarely surgery in the case of significant hydrocephalus. Prevention is the preferred method of eradication, involving vaccination of pigs and improved sanitation.

Whipple's disease

Whipple's disease is a rare, systemic infectious disease, classically affecting the gastrointestinal (GI) system, caused by the bacterium *Tropheryma whipplei*. The main feature is malabsorption when the GI system is involved, but it can also affect the brain (Ratnaike, 2000). The CNS is involved in approximately half of cases, with cognitive changes being the commonest feature (75%) (Ratnaike, 2000). A significant proportion of patients with CNS involvement display psychiatric features, including anxiety, depression, hypomania, and psychosis (Anderson, 2000). Eye movement abnormalities are very common in neuro-Whipple's, with a vertical supranuclear gaze palsy being the commonest finding (Gerard et al., 2002). In addition to the ocular abnormalities, a pathognomonic sign of neuro-Whipple's is oculomasticatory myorhythmia (Anderson, 2000). Oculomasticatory myorhythmia involves continuous smooth, pendular convergent and divergent oscillations of the eyes at the primary position, with saccades, with fixation, and even during sleep. Concurrent synchronous contraction of masticatory muscles, but not palatal muscles, characterizes this condition (Baizabal-Carvallo et al., 2015).

Lyme disease

Lyme disease is caused by *Borrelia burgdorferi*, a spirochaete that is transmitted to humans via tick bites. The condition is particularly prevalent in North America, with over 30,000 cases reported annually to the Centers for Disease Control and Prevention (CDC). Following a tick bite, the characteristic erythema migrans rash develops some days or weeks later. It is normally accompanied by a number of systemic symptoms, including fever, headache, and myalgia. Neurological symptoms include subacute meningitis, painful radiculitis, and transverse myelitis. Rarely, CNS Lyme disease can present with acute psychiatric disorders, with a study describing two patients presenting with panic disorder and another presenting with acute mania (Fallon et al., 1993). Neuropsychiatric symptoms include difficulty with concentration and recall in particular, as well as some reports of chronic fatigue syndrome. Depression as a late complication of Lyme disease is common, with rates of 26–66% reported in the literature (Fallon and Nields, 1994). It is worth noting that other studies have found that psychiatric comorbidity is higher in patients with chronic Lyme disease, compared to healthy controls (Hassett et al., 2008). Diagnosis is made with *Borellia* antibody testing of the CSF and serum. The antibody response takes several weeks to reach a detectable level, so antibody tests in the first few weeks of infection may be negative. Laboratory diagnosis in the UK follows a two-step approach. Firstly, sensitive screening tests are used initially because they can detect low levels of antibodies, but they have the disadvantage of producing occasional false-positive results in samples from some patients with other conditions, including glandular fever, syphilis, other infections, rheumatoid arthritis, and other autoimmune conditions. Samples giving reactive or indeterminate screening test reactions are then tested with a western blot, which is more specific. The ratio of CSF antibody level to serum antibody level can aid in making a diagnosis, and an index of <1 is suggestive of CNS Lyme disease. Treatment of Lyme disease is with the oral antibiotics doxycycline, amoxicillin, or cefuroxime for 2 weeks for erythema migrans. Facial palsy and other neurological complications need longer treatment (typically 3–4 weeks). For updated UK guidance on diagnosis and treatment, see https://www.nice.org.uk/guidance/ng95.

Human African trypanosomiasis

Trypanosomiasis, or sleeping sickness, is due to the protozoans *Trypanosoma brucei gambiense* and *T. brucei rhodesiense*. Bites from the tsetse fly transmit the disease, which classically results in an initial fever which then progresses into the sleeping sickness stage. Alongside somnolence, there may be seizures, incoordination, and hemiplegia. Psychiatric features are common, with rates of 80–95% reported in all cases (Bédat-Millet et al., 2000). Patients can present with personality change, psychosis, affective disorder, and cognitive decline. In *T. brucei gambiense*, there is rapid progression and death usually occurs within months, but sometimes weeks. *T. brucei rhodesiense* symptoms are more slowly progressive and some patients have been known to survive with treatment.

Typhus fever

The commonest cause of typhus *Rickettsia prowazekii* is transmitted by the body louse. It is thought that there is direct CNS invasion, with resulting neurological and psychiatric symptoms, both being a prominent feature of the condition. Psychosis has been the most commonly reported psychiatric feature, and other symptoms include fever, headache, cough, myalgia, rash, and delirium (Sejvar et al., 2012). CNS symptoms become more profound towards the later stages of the febrile period.

Conclusion

CNS infections cause a wide spectrum of neuropsychiatric disorders, from acute psychosis to chronic dementing illnesses. Symptoms suggestive of an underlying psychiatric condition may occur, alongside other features of CNS infection such as fever,

meningism, cranial neuropathy, and seizures. These may provide a clue to an infectious aetiology. However, in many cases, these features are absent and investigation for CNS infections should not be limited to psychiatric patients exhibiting these features. It is important for psychiatrists to be proficient in neurological examination to help aid the detection of any focal neurological deficit which may help point to an alternative diagnosis. CNS infections should be considered in the differential diagnoses of any patient with neuropsychiatric pathology, especially those who are immunocompromised or may have travelled to, or reside in, tropical locations. They are important to recognize, as in many cases, they are readily treatable and a timely diagnosis can prevent cognitive decline; in some cases, established neuropsychiatric disease can be reversed by appropriate treatment.

KEY LEARNING POINTS

- CNS infections, caused by various pathogens, can lead to a wide range of neuropsychiatric sequelae, including acute psychosis, mood disorders, and chronic dementias. Early recognition is critical, as brain infections are often treatable and possible neuropsychiatric illness can be reversed if the diagnosis is timely.
- In addition to psychiatric symptoms, CNS infections may also present with other signs such as fever, meningism, cranial nerve deficit, and seizures. Although the presence of these additional features can often provide a clue to an underlying CNS infection, they are not always present; hence CNS infections should be considered in the differential diagnosis of psychiatric patients in certain situations.

REFERENCES

Anderson, M., 2000. Neurology of Whipple's disease. *Journal of Neurology, Neurosurgery, and Psychiatry*. Available from: http://jnnp.bmj.com/content/68/1/2.short.

Antoni, M. et al., 2005. Increases in a marker of immune system reconstitution are predated by decreases in 24-h urinary cortisol output and depressed mood during a 10-week stress. *Journal of Psychomatic Research*. Available from: http://www.sciencedirect.com/science/article/pii/S0022399904005252.

Asch, S.M. et al., 2003. Underdiagnosis of depression in HIV: who are we missing? *Journal of General Internal Medicine*, 18(6), pp. 450–60.

Atkinson, J.H. et al., 2008. Two-year prospective study of major depressive disorder in HIV-infected men. *Journal of Affective Disorders*, 108(3), pp. 225–34.

Baizabal-Carvallo, J.F., Cardoso, F. & Jankovic, J., 2015. Myorhythmia: Phenomenology, etiology, and treatment. *Movement Disorders*, 30(2), pp. 171–9.

Bédat-Millet, A.L. et al., 2000. [Psychiatric presentation of human African trypanosomiasis: overview of diagnostic pitfalls, interest of difluoromethylornithine treatment and contribution of magnetic resonance imaging]. *Revue Neurologique*, 156(5), pp. 505–9.

Brew, B. & Chan, P., 2014. Update on HIV dementia and HIV-associated neurocognitive disorders. *Current Neurology and Neuroscience Reports*. Available from: http://link.springer.com/article/10.1007/s11910-014-0468-2.

Carmo, R.A. et al., 2001. Syphilitic meningitis in HIV-patients with meningeal syndrome: report of two cases and review. *Brazilian Journal of Infectious Diseases*, 5(5), pp. 280–7.

Caroff, S. et al., 2001. Psychiatric manifestations of acute viral encephalitis. *Psychiatric Annals*. Available from: http://www.healio.com/psychiatry/journals/psycann/2001-3-31-3/%7B107f277f-9d7a-493b-be6c-e5c4f74365c0%7D/psychiatric-manifestations-of-acute-viral-encephalitis.

Carroll, A. & Brew, B., 2017. HIV-associated neurocognitive disorders: recent advances in pathogenesis, biomarkers, and treatment. *F1000Research*, 6, p.312. Available from: http://www.ncbi.nlm.nih.gov/pubmed/28413625.

Cavalcante, G.I.T. et al., 2010. Implications of Efavirenz for Neuropsychiatry: A Review. *International Journal of Neuroscience*, 120(12), pp. 739–45.

Centers for Disease Control and Prevention. 2008. Syphilis testing algorithms using treponemal tests for initial screening: four laboratories, New York City, 2005–2006. *MMWR Morb Mortality Wkly Rep* 57: 872–5.

Chatterjee, S., 2011. Brain tuberculomas, tubercular meningitis, and post-tubercular hydrocephalus in children. *Journal of Pediatric Neurosciences*. Available from: http://pediatricneurosciences.com/article.asp?issn=1817-1745;year=2011;volume=6;issue=3;spage=96;epage=100;aulast=Chatterjee.

Chaudhuri, A. & Kennedy, P., 2002. Diagnosis and treatment of viral encephalitis. *Postgraduate Medical Journal*. Available from: http://pmj.bmj.com/content/78/924/575.short.

Chou, P.-S. et al., 2012. Central Nervous System Tuberculosis. *The Neurologist*, 18(4), pp. 219–22.

Ciesla, J. & Roberts, J., 2001. Meta-analysis of the relationship between HIV infection and risk for depressive disorders. *American Journal of Psychiatry*. Available from: http://ajp.psychiatryonline.org/doi/abs/10.1176/appi.ajp.158.5.725.

Dowell, E., Easton, A. & Solomon, T., 2001. *The Consequences of Encephalitis, Report of a Postal Survey, 2000*. Malton: The Encephalitis Society.

Elliott, A., Russo, J. & Roy-Byrne, P., 2002. The effect of changes in depression on health related quality of life (HRQoL) in HIV infection. *General Hospital Psychiatry*. Available from: http://www.sciencedirect.com/science/article/pii/S0163834301001748.

Ellis, R.J., Calero, P. & Stockin, M.D., 2009. HIV infection and the central nervous system: a primer. *Neuropsychology Review*, 19(2), pp. 144–51.

Evans, D., Have, T. Ten & Douglas, S., 2002. Association of depression with viral load, CD8 T lymphocytes, and natural killer cells in women with HIV infection. *American Journal of Psychiatry*. Available from: http://ajp.psychiatryonline.org/doi/abs/10.1176/appi.ajp.159.10.1752.

Fallon, B. & Nields, J., 1994. Lyme disease: a neuropsychiatric illness. *American Journal of Psychiatry*. Available from: http://ajp.psychiatryonline.org/doi/abs/10.1176/ajp.151.11.1571.

Fallon, B.A. et al., 1993. Psychiatric manifestations of Lyme borreliosis. *Journal of Clinical Psychiatry*, 54(7), pp. 263–8.

Fettig, J. et al., 2014. Global epidemiology of HIV. *Infectious Disease Clinics of North America*, 28(3), 323–37.

Forsgren, M., Sköldenberg, B. & Aurelius, E., 2002. Neurologic morbidity after herpes simplex virus type 2 meningitis: a retrospective study of 40 patients. *Scandinavian Journal of Infectious Diseases*. Available from: http://www.tandfonline.com/doi/abs/10.1080/00365540110080485.

Gaber, T., Eshiett, M. & Kennedy, P., 2003. Resolution of psychiatric symptoms secondary to herpes simplex encephalitis. *Journal of Neurology*. Available from: https://www.ncbi.nlm.nih.gov/pmc/articles/PMC1738621/.

Garvey, L. et al., 2011. HIV-associated central nervous system diseases in the recent combination antiretroviral therapy era. *European Journal of Neurology*. Available from: http://europepmc.org/abstract/med/21159073.

Gatchel, J. et al., 2015. Neurosyphilis in psychiatric practice: a case-based discussion of clinical evaluation and diagnosis. *General Hospital Psychiatry*, 37(5), pp. 459–63.

Gerard, A. et al., 2002. Neurologic presentation of Whipple disease: report of 12 cases and review of the literature. *Medicine*. Available from: http://journals.lww.com/md-journal/Abstract/2002/11000/Neurologic_Presentation_of_Whipple_Disease__Report.5.aspx.

Ghanem, K.G., 2010. REVIEW: Neurosyphilis: A Historical Perspective and Review. *CNS Neuroscience & Therapeutics*, 16(5), pp. e157–68.

Glaser, C., Gilliam, S. & Schnurr, D., 2003. In search of encephalitis etiologies: diagnostic challenges in the California Encephalitis Project, 1998—2000. *Clinical Infectious*. Available from: http://cid.oxfordjournals.org/content/36/6/731.short.

Granerod, J. et al., 2013. New estimates of incidence of encephalitis in England. *Emerging Infectious Diseases*, 19(9), p. 1455.

Granerod, J., Ambrose, H. & Davies, N., 2010. Causes of encephalitis and differences in their clinical presentations in England: a multicentre, population-based prospective study. *The Lancet Infectious Diseases*. Available from: http://www.sciencedirect.com/science/article/pii/S147330991070222X.

Gray, T.G. & Powles, E., 2013. Understanding and managing syphilis. *InnovAiT*, 6(12), pp. 781–9.

Grimwood, K. et al., 2000. Twelve year outcomes following bacterial meningitis: further evidence for persisting effects. *Archives of Disease in Childhood*. Available from: http://adc.bmj.com/content/83/2/111.short.

Hassett, A., Radvanski, D. & Buyske, S., 2008. Role of psychiatric comorbidity in chronic Lyme disease. *Arthritis & Rheumatology*. Available from: http://onlinelibrary.wiley.com/doi/10.1002/art.24314/full.

Heaton, R. et al., 2010. HIV-associated neurocognitive disorders persist in the era of potent antiretroviral therapy CHARTER Study. *Neurology*. Available from: http://www.neurology.org/content/75/23/2087.short.

Heaton, R. et al., 2011. HIV-associated neurocognitive disorders before and during the era of combination antiretroviral therapy: differences in rates, nature, and predictors. *Journal of Neurovirology*. Available from: http://link.springer.com/article/10.1007/s13365-010-0006-1.

Henn, F.A., 2014. *Contemporary Psychiatry*. Volume 1, Foundations of Psychiatry, Springer.

Hokkanen, L. & Launes, J., 2000. Cognitive outcome in acute sporadic encephalitis. *Neuropsychology Review*. Available from: http://link.springer.com/article/10.1023/A:1009079531196.

Hook, E.W., 2017. Syphilis. *The Lancet*. 389, 1550–7.

Hutto, B., 2001. Syphilis in Clinical Psychiatry: A Review. *Psychosomatics*, 42(6), pp. 453–60.

Jarvis, J., Meintjes, G. & Williams, A., 2010. Adult meningitis in a setting of high HIV and TB prevalence: findings from 4961 suspected cases. *BMC Infectious Diseases*. Available from: https://bmcinfectdis.biomedcentral.com/articles/10.1186/1471-2334-10-67.

Jebaraj, P., Oommen, M. & Thopuram, P., 2005. Tuberculous meningitis masked by delirium in an alcohol-dependent patient: a case report. *Acta Psychiatrica*. Available from: http://onlinelibrary.wiley.com/doi/10.1111/j.1600-0447.2005.00606.x/full.

Jmor, F., Emsley, H. & Fischer, M., 2008. The incidence of acute encephalitis syndrome in Western industrialised and tropical countries. *Virology*. Available from: https://virologyj.biomedcentral.com/articles/10.1186/1743-422X-5-134.

Kleinschmidt-DeMasters, B. & DeBiasi, R., 2001. Polymerase chain reaction as a diagnostic adjunct in herpesvirus infections of the nervous system. *Brain*. Available from: http://onlinelibrary.wiley.com/doi/10.1111/j.1750-3639.2001.tb00414.x/abstract.

Leserman, J., 2008. Role of depression, stress, and trauma in HIV disease progression. *Psychosomatic Medicine*. Available from: http://journals.lww.com/psychosomaticmedicine/Abstract/2008/06000/Role_of_Depression,_Stress,_and_Trauma_in_HIV.4.aspx.

Leserman, J., Petitto, J. & Gu, H., 2002. Progression to AIDS, a clinical AIDS condition and mortality: psychosocial and physiological predictors. *Psychological Medicine*. Available from: http://journals.cambridge.org/article_S0033291702005949.

Lyketsos, C. & Treisman, G., 2001. Mood disorders in HIV infection. *Psychiatric Annals*. Available from: http://www.healio.com/psychiatry/journals/psycann/2001-1-31-1/%7B07459c88-2fa9-4147-b455-65ee57a1605f%7D/mood-disorders-in-hiv-infection.

Mai, N.T. and Thwaites, G.E., 2017. Recent advances in the diagnosis and management of tuberculous meningitis. *Current Opinion in Infectious Diseases*, 30, pp. 123–8.

Marra, C.M., 2015. Neurosyphilis. *CONTINUUM Lifelong Learning in Neurology*, 21(6), pp. 1714–28.

Martínez, L. et al., 2017. Mood disorders in HIV infection. *European Psychiatry*, 41, p. S482.

Masters, M. & Ances, B., 2014. Role of Neuroimaging in HIV-Associated Neurocognitive Disorders. *Seminars in Neurology*, 34(1), pp. 89–102.

McDaniel, J. & Johnson, K., 1995. Obsessive-compulsive disorder in HIV disease: response to fluoxetine. *Psychosomatics*. Available from: https://scholar.google.co.uk/scholar?q=Obsessive-Compulsive+Disorder+in+HIV+Disease+McDaniel%2C+J.+Stephen+et+al.+1995&btnG=&hl=en&as_sdt=0%2C5.

McGrath, N., Anderson, N. & Croxson, M., 1997. Herpes simplex encephalitis treated with acyclovir: diagnosis and long term outcome. *Journal of Neurology*. Available from: http://jnnp.bmj.com/content/63/3/321.short.

Nelson, C. & Zunt, J., 2011. Tuberculosis of the central nervous system in immunocompromised patients: HIV infection and solid organ transplant recipients. *Clinical Infectious Diseases*. Available from: https://academic.oup.com/cid/article-abstract/53/9/915/345757.

Newman, L. et al., 2015. Global Estimates of the Prevalence and Incidence of Four Curable Sexually Transmitted Infections in 2012 Based on Systematic Review and Global Reporting Z. Meng, ed. *PLoS One*, 10(12), p. e0143304.

Nightingale, S. et al., 2014. Controversies in HIV-associated neurocognitive disorders. *The Lancet*. Available from: http://www.sciencedirect.com/science/article/pii/S1474442214701371.

Nightingale, S. & Winston, A., 2017. Measuring and managing cognitive impairment in HIV. *AIDS*, 31 Suppl 2, pp. S165–72.

Peng, F. et al., 2008. CT and MR findings in HIV-negative neurosyphilis. *European Journal of Radiology*, 66(1), pp. 1–6.

Praveen-Kumar, S. et al., 2007. Electroencephalographic and imaging profile in a subacute sclerosing panencephalitis (SSPE) cohort: a correlative study. *Clinical Neurophysiology*. Available from: http://www.sciencedirect.com/science/article/pii/S1388245707002982.

Raschilas, F., Wolff, M. & Delatour, F., 2002. Outcome of and prognostic factors for herpes simplex encephalitis in adult patients: results of a multicenter study. *Clinical Infectious Diseases*. Available from: http://cid.oxfordjournals.org/content/35/3/254.short.

Ratnaike, R., 2000. Whipple's disease. *Postgraduate Medical Journal*. Available from: http://pmj.bmj.com/content/76/902/760.short.

Ronchi, D. De, Faranca, I. & Forti, P., 2000. Development of acute psychotic disorders and HIV-1 infection. *International Journal of Psychiatry Medicine*. Available from: http://journals.sagepub.com/doi/abs/10.2190/PLGX-N48F-RBHJ-UF8K.

Saylor, D. et al., 2016. HIV-associated neurocognitive disorder — pathogenesis and prospects for treatment. *Nature Reviews Neurology*, 12(4), pp. 234–48.

Schmidt, H. et al., 2006. Neuropsychological sequelae of bacterial and viral meningitis. *Brain*. Available from: http://brain.oxfordjournals.org/content/129/2/333.short.

Seeley, W.W. & Venna, N., 2004. Neurosyphilis presenting with gummatous oculomotor nerve palsy. *Journal of Neurology, Neurosurgery, & Psychiatry*, 75(5), p. 789.

Sejvar, J. et al., 2012. Neurologic Manifestations Associated with an Outbreak of Typhoid Fever, Malawi—Mozambique, 2009: An Epidemiologic Investigation. *PLoS One*, 7(12), p. e46099.

Serpa, J.A., Yancey, L.S. & White Jr, A.C., 2006. Advances in the diagnosis and management of neurocysticercosis. *Expert Review of Anti-infective Therapy*, 4(6), pp. 1051–61.

Sittinger, H. et al., 2002. Mild cognitive impairment after viral meningitis in adults. *Journal of Neurology*. Available from: http://www.springerlink.com/index/M3T04V6BP2APNXED.pdf.

Solomon, T. et al., 2012. Management of suspected viral encephalitis in adults–association of British Neurologists and British Infection Association National Guidelines. *Journal of Infection*. Available from: http://www.sciencedirect.com/science/article/pii/S0163445311005639.

Solomon, T., Hart, I. & Beeching, N., 2007. Viral encephalitis: a clinician's guide. *Practical Neurology*. Available from: http://pn.bmj.com/content/7/5/288.short.

Stamm, L. V, 2010. Global challenge of antibiotic-resistant Treponema pallidum. *Antimicrobial agents and chemotherapy*, 54(2), pp. 583–9.

Szilak, I. et al., 2001. Neurosyphilis Presenting as Herpes Simplex Encephalitis. *Clinical Infectious Diseases*, 32(7), pp. 1108–9.

Thwaites, G.E. & Hien, T.T., 2005. Tuberculous meningitis: many questions, too few answers. *The Lancet Neurology*, 4(3), pp. 160–70.

Treisman, G., Angelino, A. & Hutton, H., 2001. Psychiatric issues in the management of patients with HIV infection. *JAMA*. Available from: http://jamanetwork.com/journals/jama/fullarticle/194450.

Tucker, J., Burnam, M. & Sherbourne, C., 2003. Substance use and mental health correlates of nonadherence to antiretroviral medications in a sample of patients with human immunodeficiency virus infection. *American Journal of Medicine*. Available from: http://www.sciencedirect.com/science/article/pii/S0002934303000937.

Venkatesan, A., Michael, B.D., Probasco, J.C., Geocadin, R.G., and Solomon, T., 2019. Acute encephalitis in immunocompetent adults. *The Lancet*, 393, pp. 702–16.

Venugopal, D. et al., 2001. Mania in HIV infection. *Indian Journal of Psychiatry*, 43(3), pp. 242–5.

Verma, A. & Kumar, A., 2013. Neurocysticercosis presenting as acute psychosis: A rare case report from rural India. *Asian Journal of Psychiatry*. Available from: http://www.sciencedirect.com/science/article/pii/S1876201813001809.

World Health Organization, 2018. *Number of people newly infected with HIV*. Available from: http://www.who.int/gho/hiv/epidemic_status/incidence/en/

World Health Organization, 2019. *Over 100 000 people sick with measles in 14 months: with measles cases at an alarming level in the European Region, WHO scales up response*. Available from: http://www.euro.who.int/en/media-centre/sections/press-releases/2019/over-100-000-people-sick-with-measles-in-14-months-with-measles-cases-at-an-alarming-level-in-the-european-region,-who-scales-up-response.

21

Neuropsychiatric aspects of CNS tumours in adults

Alex J. Mitchell and Audrey Hopwood

Introduction

A brain tumour is the most feared cancer diagnosis by the general public because of its morbidity and mortality (YouGov Poll, 2011). Primary brain tumours account for about 1.5% of all new cases of cancer, and 2.5% of all cancer deaths. However, most brain tumours are, in fact, metastases from other cancer sites. Brain tumours cause considerable psychological and psychiatric complications, as well as a burden for caregivers, and reductions in overall quality of life (QoL) (Baker et al., 2015) Around 90% of patients will suffer neuropsychiatric complications, and in around 20%, these are the presenting symptoms (Keschner et al., 1983). As presentation varies enormously across all ages, tumour sites, and tumour types, establishing the correct clinical diagnosis is not always straightforward, and hence diagnostic delays are not uncommon. Most patients living with a brain tumour have unmet supportive care needs and this is often felt in equal measure by their family members. Common unmet needs include a lack of prognostic information, the need for financial advice, problems maintaining independence, and difficulty coping with emotional symptoms (Long et al., 2016). Neuropsychiatric complications can often improve following brain tumour treatment but can also deteriorate. Indeed cognitive deterioration is an important prognostic marker. New therapeutic techniques have improved survival and are gradually improving QoL. However, these are only effective if neuropsychiatric complications are recognized and addressed.

Classification and epidemiology of brain tumours

Intracranial brain tumours are neoplasms that arise within the CNS (about 15% of cases) or spread from other tumour sites (metastatic) (about 85% of cases). Primary brain tumours arise from the brain parenchyma, supporting structures, cranial and spinal nerves, and other specialized structures. However, most are of neuroepithelial origin. Lymphomas can also occur in the brain as the primary site. The World Health Organization (WHO) classification has recently been revised (see Box 21.1), according to differentiation,

anaplasia, and aggressiveness (Louis et al., 2016). Tumours of the CNS include tumours of neuroepithelial tissue, tumours of cranial and paraspinal nerves, tumours of the meninges, lymphomas and haematopoietic neoplasms, germ cell tumours, tumours of the sellar region, and metastatic tumours (see Box 21.1). This chapter will focus on primary brain tumours, particularly high-grade glioblastoma, as there is relatively little research on neuropsychiatry of cerebral metastases.

There are three main types of gliomas; astrocytoma, oligodendroglioma, and ependymoma. Each of these can be benign (grades I and II) or aggressive (grades III and IV) tumours. Grade I tumours are uncommon, comprising about 2% of brain tumours, grade II 8%, and grade III 20%. High-grade gliomas (grade IV) have cells that vary in size and shape, and for this reason, they were also known as glioblastoma multiforme (GBM). This is the commonest type, accounting for 70% of astrocytomas. Meningeal-derived meningiomas are the other common tumour type, comprising up to 30% of brain tumours. Ninety-five per cent of meningiomas are benign and tend to cause less morbidity than gliomas. Primary tumours represent only about 15% of all brain tumours; most are metastatic tumours from other sites. Metastases may arise from various different primary tumour sites such as lung (which is the source of about half of all metastases—especially the non-small cell type), breast cancer (20% of all metastases), melanoma (10% of all metastases), colorectal (8%), and less commonly, kidney, gall bladder, liver, thyroid, testicle, prostate, uterus or ovary, and pancreas (all <5%). Systemic lymphoma (especially non-Hodgkin's type) and leukaemia may also metastasize to the brain. Two-thirds of metastases involve the brain parenchyma (frontal, parietal, occipital, and temporal lobes), and one-third involves the leptomeninges or dura. It is thought that of those patients with cancer about one in ten will suffer a brain metastasis but many are undetected (Schouten et al., 2002).

About 80,000 people in the United States and 10,000 in the UK are diagnosed with a primary brain tumour each year, and about 60% are malignant. The incidence of tumours of the CNS increases with advancing age, but there is an important peak in young children. In children, brain tumours primarily arise in

Box 21.1 WHO grades of select CNS tumours

Diffuse astrocytic and oligodendroglial tumours	
Diffuse astrocytoma, IDH-mutant	II
Anaplastic astrocytoma, IDH-mutant	III
Glioblastoma, IDH-wildtype	IV
Glioblastoma, IDH-mutant	IV
Diffuse midline glioma, H3 K27M-mutant	IV
Oligodendroglioma, IDH-mutant and 1p/19q-codeleted	II
Anaplastic oligodendroglioma, IDH-mutant and 1p/19q-codeleted	III
Other astrocytic tumours	
Pilocytic astrocytoma	I
Subependymal giant cell astrocytoma	I
Pleomorphic xanthoastrocytoma	II
Anaplastic pleomorphic xanthoastrocytoma	III
Ependymal tumours	
Subependymoma	I
Myxopapillary ependymoma	I
Ependymoma	II
Ependymoma, *RELA* fusion-positive	II or III
Anaplastic ependymoma	III
Other gliomas	
Angiocentric glioma	I
Choroid glioma of third ventricle	II
Choroid plexus tumours	
Choroid plexus papilloma	I
Atypical choroid plexus papilloma	II
Choroid plexus carcinoma	III
Neuronal and mixed neuronal-glial tumours	
Dysembryoplastic neuroepithelial tumour	I
Gangliocytoma	I
Ganglioglioma	I
Anaplastic ganglioglioma	III
Dysplastic gangliocytoma of cerebellum (Lhermitte–Duclos)	I
Desmoplastic infantile astrocytoma and ganglioglioma	I
Papillary glioneuronal tumour	I

Rosette-forming glioneuronal tumour	I
Central neurocytoma	II
Extraventricular neurocytoma	II
Cerebellar liponeurocytoma	II
Tumours of the pineal region	
Pineocytoma	I
Pineal parenchymal tumour of intermediate differentiation	II or III
Pineoblastoma	IV
Papillary tumour of the pineal region	II or III
Embryonal tumours	
Medulloblastoma (all subtypes)	IV
Embryonal tumour with multi-layered rosettes, C19MC-altered	IV
Medulloepithelioma	IV
CNS embryonal tumour, NOS	IV
Atypical teratoid/rhabdoid tumour	IV
CNS embryonal tumour with rhabdoid features	IV
Tumours of the cranial and paraspinal nerves	
Schwannoma	I
Neurofibroma	I
Perineurioma	I
Malignant peripheral nerve sheath tumour (MPNST)	II, III, or IV
Meningiomas	
Meningioma	I
Atypical meningioma	II
Anaplastic (malignant) meningioma	III
Mesenchymal, non-meningothelial tumours	
Solitary fibrous tumour/haemangiopericytoma	I, II, or III
Haemangioblastoma	I
Tumours of the sellar region	
Craniopharyngioma	I
Granular cell tumour	I
Pituicytoma	I
Spindle cell oncocytoma	I

the brainstem and cerebellum, but in adults, they mostly arise from the cortex or meninges. Long-term survival of 10 or more years in those with grade I and II astrocytomas is about 40%, but only 25% of those with grade III astrocytomas and 6% with grade IV survive 5 years. However, the disease course is very variable and the latest therapeutic regimens offer improvements in survival. New genetic markers, including *IDH1/IDH2* gene mutations, chromosome 1p and 19q co-deletion, *TP53* mutation, and MGMT promoter methylation status have been established more recently as important diagnostic and prognostic markers in patients with glioma (Cohen and Colman, 2015). Altogether it is estimated that 700,000 people in the United States and 30,000 in the UK are living with a brain tumour. The actual number is probably higher because of undiagnosed cases. In the population, 1–2% of MRIs and routine autopsies reveal undiagnosed primary brain tumours, most often slow-growing meningiomas (Vernooij et al., 2007). Given this increase in brain tumour survivors, it is vitally important neuropsychiatric complications are addressed and QoL emphasized in the form of appropriate rehabilitation and support.

Clinical features of brain tumours

Presenting symptoms

Brain tumours cause local tissue destruction and/or compression of surrounding areas of the cortex and, rarely, distant metastasis outside the brain. As such, patients may have non-focal signs and symptoms or focal manifestations related to the specific area of the brain occupied by the tumour. About 80% of tumours are localized at the time of presentation; 16% are regional, and 2% metastasized. It is important to recognize that many neurological and psychiatric presentations cannot be confidently linked with lesion location. In 10% of cases, the presentation is an acute stroke-like episode, and in about a third, the first presentation is a seizure. However, in one carefully studied series of 75 patients with high-grade gliomas, seizures were present at diagnosis in half of cases and occurred later in a further 30% (Van Breemen et al., 2009). Seizures are often focal or focal with secondary generalization. Headache is the commonest initial presenting symptom in half of cases (Forsyth and Posner, 1993). Common presenting symptoms are shown in Fig. 21.1. Early morning brain

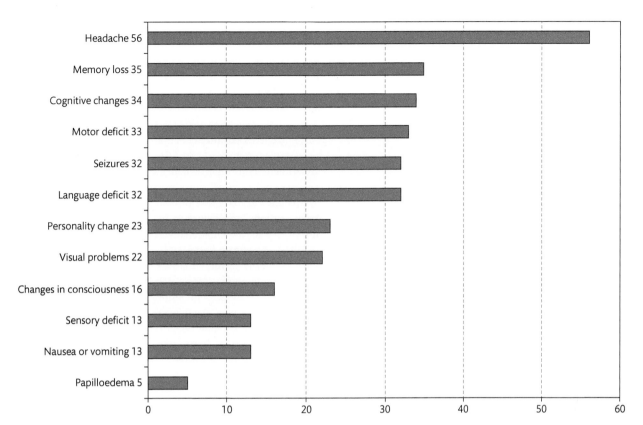

Fig. 21.1 Presenting symptoms in adults with brain tumours.
Source data from Chang SM, Parney IF, Huang W, et al., for the Glioma Outcomes Project Investigators. Patterns of care for adults with newly diagnosed malignant glioma. *JAMA.* 2005;293(5):557–564.

tumour headache and postural headache (classically linked with raised intracranial pressure) appear less common than expected, as most are described as tension-type (77%), migraine-type (9%), and other types (14%) (Forsyth and Posner, 1993). Clinically, progressive severity, unilateral localization, and new onset after 50 years are red flags. In up to a third of patients presenting with a brain tumour, the first symptom is cognitive impairment (Chang et al., 2005) and a small number present with miscellaneous neuropsychiatric symptoms as their first presentation, which are often misdiagnosed or attributed to depression alone. Patients with benign meningioma may have an occult diagnosis and chronic neuropsychiatric symptoms; indeed meningioma appears to be over-represented in psychiatric series (Gupta and Kumar, 2004). Many patients have had signs and symptoms of their disease for many months before a radiologic or histologic diagnosis is made (Singh et al., 2014). Regarding the presenting symptoms of metastases, signs and symptoms are similar but evolve more rapidly, typically over days to weeks. Neuropsychiatric complications, particularly involving mood or cognition, occur in the majority of patients with metastases (Chang et al., 2009).

Important localizing symptoms and signs

Most primary brain tumours occur in the posterior fossa (30%), frontal lobe (25%), temporal lobe (20%), and less often the parietal lobe (12%), pituitary (10%), or occipital lobes (4%) (American Brain Tumor Association, 2014; Lohr and Cadet, 1987). Regarding the site of metastases, small cell carcinoma of the lung most commonly metastasizes to the frontal lobe, cerebellum, and parietal lobes; malignant melanoma tends to metastasize to the frontal and temporal lobes, breast carcinoma to the cerebellum and basal ganglia, large cell carcinoma of the lung to the occipital lobe, and squamous cell carcinoma of the lung to the cerebellum (Graf et al., 1988). Metastases to the hippocampi are extremely rare. It is important to note that half of patients with metastases have involvement of two or more sites and, as such, presentation may be complex.

A summary of localizing neuropsychiatric symptoms and signs is shown in Box 21.2. Frontal tumours may cause classic neurological complications, including: weakness contralateral to the motor cortex, apraxia and mild rigidity without weakness in premotor frontal lesions, expressive dysphasia with dominant Broca's lesions, and primitive frontal 'release' signs, including abnormal grasp, suck, snout, and palmomental reflexes. Frontal lobe lesions have been associated with three kinds of neuropsychiatric presentation: orbitofrontal syndrome, dorsolateral prefrontal syndrome, and medial frontal syndrome. Orbitofrontal syndrome usually presents with disinhibition, irritability, and lability, and patients' families may report a 'change in personality'. In the dorsolateral prefrontal syndrome, patients have difficulty with sustained attention and/or sequencing and may show perseverative behaviour. In the medial frontal (anterior cingulate) presentation, patients have abulia, apathy, indifference, and psychomotor retardation and, in extreme cases, may be akinetic with mutism. Tumours of the temporal lobes cause a variety of neurological and neuropsychiatric complications. Dominant temporal lobe syndromes include auditory hallucinations, dysnomia, receptive (Wernicke's) dysphasia, and various memory deficits (e.g. anterograde amnesia), as well as contralateral homonymous quadrantanopsia (inferior anterior temporal lobe

Box 21.2 Summary of localizing neuropsychiatric symptoms

Frontal lobe tumour

Orbitofrontal Disinhibition, poor judgement (risk-taking) and empathy, lack of insight.

Dorsolateral prefrontal cortex Executive dysfunction (planning and set-shifting).

Mediofrontal Apathy, akinetic mutism.

Precentral Contralateral monoplegia or hemiplegia, apraxia.

Paracentral Incontinence.

Broca's area Expressive (motor) dysphasia, transcortical motor aphasia.

Frontal middle gyrus Saccadic gaze abnormality.

Poorly localized Motor perseveration, primitive reflexes, utilization/imitation behaviour, inattention.

Frontal lobe seizures

Eye deviation, amnesia.

Parietal lobe tumour

Post-central gyrus Sensory loss (astereognosis, sensory inattention).

Optic radiation Lower homonymous quadrantanopia.

Non-dominant hemisphere Dressing apraxia, anosognosia, constructional apraxia, geographical agnosia, spatial neglect.

Dominant hemisphere Finger or body agnosia, agraphia, acalculia, alexia, left–right disorientation (Gerstmann's syndrome).

Parietal lobe seizures

Somatic (haptic) hallucinations.

Temporal lobe tumour

Wernicke's area Receptive dysphasia, transcortical sensory aphasia.

Insula (superior gyrus) Cortical deafness and amusia.

Medial temporal Amnesia (episodic memory).

Dominant inferior lateral Semantic amnesia (semantic if left-sided; faces if right-sided).

Non-dominant inferior lateral Facial amnesia.

Limbic area Hyperorality, hypersexuality, visual agnosia, metamorphosis (Klüver–Bucy syndrome).

Optic radiation Upper homonymous quadrantanopia.

Temporal lobe seizures

Forced thinking, forced recall, déjà vu, jamais vu.

Occipital lobe tumour

Cortical lesion Homonymous hemianopia.

Pole Central (macular) hemianopia.

Striate Cortical blindness, Anton's syndrome.

Occipitotemporal (non-dominant) Prosopagnosia (failure to recognize familiar faces).

Association cortex Alexia without agraphia, palinopsia (after-effects).

Occipital lobe seizures

Elementary visual hallucinations.

Basal ganglia tumour

Dominant hemisphere Impaired verbal fluency, impaired motor programming, poor concentration.

Non-dominant hemisphere Impaired visuospatial memory, impaired visuospatial fluency.

Basal ganglia seizures

Obsessive–compulsive disorder (?)

Corpus callosum tumour

With occipital lobe involvement Alexia without agraphia.

Without occipital lobe involvement Left-hand agraphia and anomia, alien hand syndrome.

Adapted with permission from Mitchell, A. (2004). *Neuropsychiatry and Behavioural Neurology Explained*. Published by Saunders, an imprint of Elsevier.

lesions). Non-dominant temporal lobe lesions cause spatial disorientation and problems with perception of taste, hearing, vision, or movement. Posterior temporal lobe tumours that extend posteriorly cause dyslexia and anomia.

Neurological features of lesions in the parietal lobes are typically contralateral cortical sensation, including inability to localize body parts, defects in two-point discrimination, and inability to recognize letters or numbers traced on the skin (graphesthesia) or objects placed in the hand (astereognosia), apraxia, and neglect. Gerstmann syndrome, which includes agraphia, acalculia, finger agnosia, and right–left disorientation, is a dominant parietal lobe syndrome. Occipital lobe tumours cause visual field deficits, visual hallucinations, and failure to recognize familiar faces (prosopagnosia). Visual hallucinations caused by occipital lobe lesions usually manifest as uniform flashes of lights of various shapes, as opposed to the typically formed images noted with temporal lobe lesions. Contralateral homonymous hemianopia is possible with severe tissue loss. Rarely bilateral lesions may cause Anton syndrome, in which the patient is blind but is not aware of his/her blindness. Thalamic tumours may cause obstructive hydrocephalus, giving headache, nausea and vomiting, dizziness, diplopia, gait abnormality, contralateral hemisensory loss or hemiparesis, pain syndromes, and reduced arousal. Basal ganglia lesions usually cause movement disorder such as choreoathetosis. Tumours that extend into the optic chiasm can cause visual field defects, loss of visual acuity, papilloedema, and optic atrophy. Tumours of the cerebellum cause ipsilateral ataxia, hypotonia, nystagmus, and coordination, falls, and gait problems. Brainstem involvement usually causes cranial nerve and long-tract signs. Pituitary adenomas may cause headache and a large number of endocrine disturbances, including Cushing's disease. Lesions of the hypothalamus produce endocrine dysfunction, anorexia/hyperphagia, acromegaly, Cushing's syndrome, precocious puberty, infertility, loss of libido, amenorrhoea and galactorrhoea, diabetes insipidus, and syndrome of inappropriate antidiuretic hormone secretion (SIADH).

Psychiatric complications in patients with brain tumours

Patients with brain tumours have an appreciably higher rate of organic psychiatric disorders, neuropsychiatric diagnoses, and, in particular, cognitive deficits. However, it is very important not to overlook more basic aspects such as distress, anxiety, and QoL/survivorship issues.

Distress and impaired quality of life in patients with brain tumours

Of all cancers, brain tumours usually impose the highest emotional burden for the patient and family (Janda et al., 2007; Kvale et al., 2009). Several studies have used the simple, but highly acceptable, Distress Thermometer (DT) to screen for distress in brain tumour patients. On this tool, 28–52% suffer from elevated current distress in the first year after diagnosis (Keir et al., 2008; Ostrom et al., 2014; Rooney et al., 2013). It is important to recognize that distress (and anxiety) is often persistent and up to 60% of long-term survivors of brain tumour have distress (Keir et al., 2008), as do 75% at

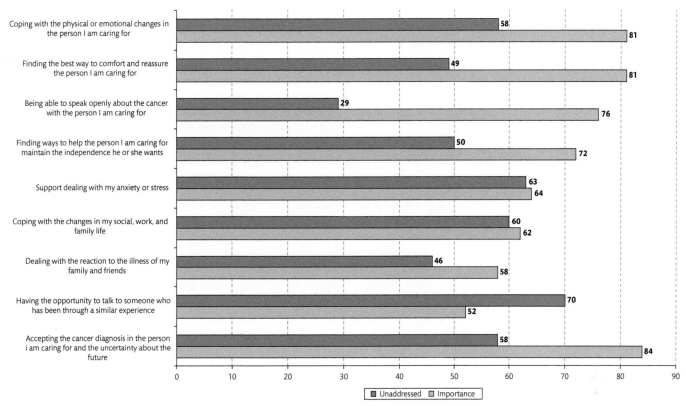

Fig. 21.2 Unaddressed issues for caregivers of adults with brain tumours.
Source data from Rupa Parvataneni, Mei-Yin Polley, Teresa Freeman, Kathleen Lamborn, Michael Prados, Nicholas Butowski, Raymond Liu, Jennifer Clarke, Margaretta Page, Jane Rabbitt, Anne Fedoroff, Emelia Clow, Emily Hsieh, Valerie Kivett, Rebecca DeBoer, Susan Chang Identifying the needs of brain tumor patients and their caregivers *Journal of Neuro-Oncology* September 2011, Volume 104, Issue 3, pp 737–744.

the time of recurrence (Trad et al., 2015). In caregivers, distress is common and often untreated, with one study showing 78% of caregivers screened positive for distress (Tomita and Raimondi, 1981). Issues for caregivers are often unaddressed, as shown in Fig. 21.2. Predictors of distress include degree of functional impairment, uncertainty about disease progression, loss of employment/role, financial problems, confidence about future treatment options and trust in clinicians, and perceived support (Halkett et al., 2015; Rooney et al., 2013).

Regarding QoL, reductions may occur as a result of the brain tumour, cancer treatment, and psychiatric complications (Baker et al., 2015). Regarding tumour location and QoL, some studies reported that left-sided (dominant) tumours were associated with reductions in QoL, while others reported that right-sided (non-dominant) tumours caused lower health-related QoL (HRQoL) reductions (Hahn et al., 2003; Salo et al., 2002). However, laterality on its own probably has a modest effect. Indeed once histopathology and tumour volumes are matched, effects on QoL are often similar (Drewes et al., 2016). Tumour site may be more important than laterality, e.g. poor QoL has been recorded in patients with frontal lobe tumours (Dehcordi et al., 2012) or diencephalon (Halkett et al., 2015). However, negative studies exist regarding lesion location, highlighting that function, independence, support, unmet needs, and distress should be assessed on a case-by-case basis (Porter et al., 2014; Rooney et al., 2013).

Several brain tumour-specific instruments have been developed, including the European Organisation for Research and Treatment of

Cancer (EORTC) QLQ-BN20 which consists of 20 items assessing visual disorder, motor dysfunction, various disease symptoms, treatment toxicity, and future uncertainty (Aaronson et al., 1993). A FACT module (FACT-Br) has been developed as an alternative brain cancer-specific module (Weitzner et al., 1995). Compared with the EORTC questionnaires, the FACT is more focused on psychosocial aspects than medical items.

Patients often struggle to maintain their premorbid function and role. One in four patients has major interference of symptoms with ability to work or perform social activities (Armstrong et al., 2016). In one study as few as one in five returned to work (Mackworth et al., 1992) but in another 75% successfully returned to work (Feuerstein et al., 2007a). Return to work is strongly related to residual injury; predictors of failure to return to work include cognitive impairment, depression, fatigue, sleep problems, and problem-solving limitations (Feuerstein et al., 2007b). Many patients lose their role at work and at home, and hence rehabilitation in brain tumour survivors is of key importance. Unfortunately, only a minority of patients are offered formal rehabilitation (Pace et al., 2016).

Cognitive impairment in patients with brain tumours

Cognitive impairment is one of the most important complications in those with primary or metastatic brain tumours, impacting directly on the independence of the patient, as well as on caregiver burden. Cognitive functioning is related to the patient's ability to perform activities of daily living, manage daily tasks and finances, recognizing unsafe behaviour, and remaining engaged with treatment decision-making and informed consent (Wietzner and Meyers, 1997). Understanding cognitive dysfunction is a challenge because deficits may be caused by the tumour, tumour-related seizures, radiotherapy or chemotherapy effects, surgical complications, psychological distress/depression, or indeed any combination of these. Risk factors for severe deficits include large lesions, left-hemisphere localization, and GBM and/or high-grade tumours (Cheng et al., 2010).

The type of cognitive deficit, particularly when tested with expert neuropsychological testing, can help identify the extent and location of the lesion (Brown et al., 2006). Yet, a surprising finding from the literature is that cognitive deficits are often not restricted to the area of the brain where the tumour is located (Bergo et al., 2015). Focal neuropsychological deficits are more common than global impairment, but delirium and dementia can follow any form of brain tumour where tissue loss is significant. Delirium and dementia are classically linked with tumours of the frontal cerebral cortex, medial temporal lobe, and corpus callosum, but they can result from a variety of subcortical lesions as well. Specific forms of amnesia are seen with lesions in the medial temporal lobe (hippocampus), frontal lobe, fornix, mammillary bodies, and thalamus. Broadly it is estimated 10% of patients develop dementia after a brain tumour diagnosis and up to 90% show specific neuropsychological deficits (Klein et al., 2003; Zucchella et al., 2013). As such, cognition should be routinely assessed in all brain tumour patients who are struggling with daily function. Even in long-term glioblastoma survivors of 6 years or more, cognitive deficits are found in up to half of patients (Scott et al., 1999). Using self-reported data, the 2010 Livestrong Foundation survey found that of all cancers, brain tumours posed the highest risk for subjective cognitive impairment (Schmidt et al., 2016) (Fig. 21.3).

Cognitive deficits most commonly affect executive functions, verbal memory, visuospatial memory, verbal fluency, information processing speed, and sustained attention. Frontal tumours are associated with deficits in working memory, inhibition of interference on ongoing actions, social cognition, risk assessment, decision-making, use of external feedback, initiative, abstraction, flexibility, planning, cognitive flexibility, verbal fluency, and ability to solve complex problems. Temporal tumours may affect naming, verbal fluency, comprehension, verbal (dominant) or non-verbal (non-dominant) memory, semantic competence, and social cognition. Occipital–parietal tumours may impair visuospatial recognition, semantic competence, and social cognition. Tumours of the cerebellum may compromise the capacity to modulate several connected areas (executive dysfunction, spatial memory, and language such as prosody). Tumours of the diencephalon and corpus callosum often cause memory problems, and some subcortical tumours can produce a subcortical dementia picture characterized by general slowing of thought processes and apathy, without dysphasia or dyspraxia.

Tuche and colleagues examined 139 patients neuropsychologically and found 90% of patients had test performances below the tenth percentile in at least one area of cognition, especially in executive function (78%), memory, and attention (60% of patients) (Tucha et al., 2000). Zucchella et al. (2013) found 54% presented with multidomain cognitive impairments, while 46% of the patients revealed specific cognitive deficits in language (16%), memory (14%), attention (9%), executive functions (6%), and visuospatial abilities (1%).[49] Age, lesion location, and receipt of chemotherapy were predictors. Talacchi et al. (2011) documented cognitive impairment in glioma patients and 79% of patients had cognitive deficit in at least one test. Verbal memory, visuospatial memory, and word fluency were the most frequently affected functions.

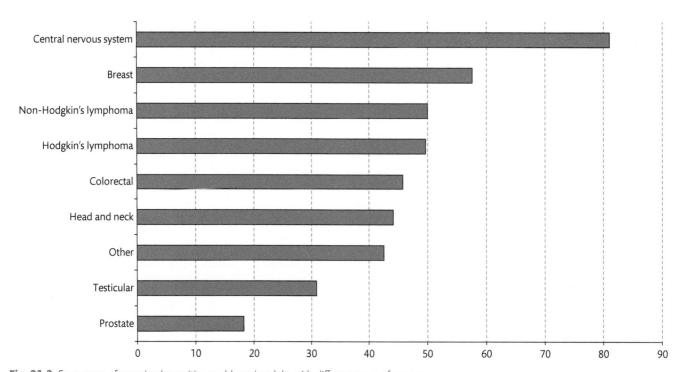

Fig. 21.3 Frequency of perceived cognitive problems in adults with different types of cancer.
Source data from Schmidt, J.E., Beckjord, E., Bovbjerg, D.H. et al. Prevalence of perceived cognitive dysfunction in survivors of a wide range of cancers: results from the 2010 LIVESTRONG survey *J Cancer Surviv* (2016) 10: 302. doi:10.1007/s11764-015-0476-5.

Given the high prevalence of cognitive problems, regular screening and holistic/functional assessment are recommended, particularly after acute treatment has been completed. Bedside cognitive tools, such as the MMSE, are commonly used as an initial screening approach and have the advantage of high acceptability but should rarely be relied upon alone. Instruments such as the Addenbrooke's Cognitive Examination-Revised (ACE-R), Montreal Cognitive Assessment (MoCA), and Cambridge Cognition Examination (CAMCOG) are more sophisticated, but tailored neuropsychological testing remains the gold standard (Olson et al., 2011). In a head-to-head comparison in 36 brain tumour patients 2 months after surgical resection, it was found that 31% of patients were impaired on the MoCA, compared with 70% on neuropsychological testing (Robinson et al., 2015). Fifty per cent of the MoCA-intact patients were impaired on tests of executive function, including abstraction, and a quarter of these patients were impaired in the domains of attention and memory. Becker et al. examined 58 brain tumour patients using three 'bedside' methods and found accurate detection of cognitive impairment was 37% using the Brief Cognitive Status Exam, 93% using the MoCA, and 44% using the MMSE, as compared to neuropsychological testing (Becker et al., 2016).

Mood disorder in patients with brain tumours

About one in three unselected general cancer patients have a distinct mood disorder often in the context of an adjustment disorder, but also as major depression, minor depression, or GAD (Mitchell et al., 2011). Psychologically, anger, dysphoria, irritability, and intrusive thoughts about disease progression are common symptoms. Somatic symptoms, such as fatigue, poor concentration, and insomnia of depression, are usually amplified by a cancer diagnosis, but they appear to retain their diagnostic role in depression (Mitchell et al., 2012). Depression and anxiety are often unrecognized and undertreated. For example, among 598 patients with high-grade glioma, 93% of patients self-reported depression and yet physicians noted depression in only 15% (Litofsky et al., 2004).

Only a minority of mood studies in patients with brain tumours have used formal operational criteria. In a review of diagnostic interview studies, Rooney et al. found the prevalence of clinical depression to be 15% (range 6–28%) (Rooney et al., 2011). Although this is similar to the rate found in other cancers (Olson et al., 2011), a recent meta-analysis found that patients with brain tumours may have higher rates of clinical depression on structured interviews (Krebber et al., 2014). Clinical depression was found in 28% (20%–38%) in those with a brain tumour, compared with 11% (8%–16%) for patients with breast cancer. Rates of depression on self-report scales are considerably higher. In one of the largest studies using PHQ-9 and Generalized Anxiety Disorder-7 item (GAD-7), 41% had current depression and 48% current GAD (Arnold et al., 2008). Major risk factors are degree of functional impairment, impairment in QoL, and lack of support (Litofsky et al., 2004; Rooney et al., 2011). Increasingly, lesion location is downplayed as a predictor of depression, in favour of a more personalized functional approach (Litofsky et al., 2004). Mood disorder can follow complications of radiotherapy, chemotherapy, and surgery, as well as steroid use such as dexamethasone (see Neuropsychiatric complications of brain tumour treatments, p.236) (Fardet et al., 2012). In several studies, depression is the strongest independent predictor of QoL (Mainio et al., 2006) and has been shown to have an adverse impact on survival in some, but not all, studies. For example, in 1052 patients with astrocytoma, preoperative depression was independently associated with decreased survival (relative risk 1.41) after adjustment for degree of disability, tumour grade, and treatment (Gathinji et al., 2009).

Regarding choice of self-report depression scales, Rooney et al. (2013) compared the DT, the HADS (depression sub-scale) HADD, and the PHQ-9 in 155 patients, of whom 21 had major depression on the Structured Clinical Interview for DSM-IV (SCID). Results are shown in Table 21.1. None of the tools were adequate at confirming depression, but DT ≥7, HADS-D ≥7, and PHQ-9 ≥10 were all excellent at ruling out depression. For example, 96% of those without depression scored DT <7 and of those who did score DT <7, the negative predictive value was 92.8%. Some clinicians prefer a rapid initial screening with a very brief measure. The PHQ-2 (Bunevicius et al., 2013) is better than a single question on depression, but an alternative is the Emotion Thermometers tool (http://www.emotionthermometers.com) which measures several emotional domains.

Anxiety in patients with brain tumours

When considering anxiety in adults with a brain tumour, only a small number of studies have examined self-reported anxiety. From studies using the HADS (anxiety sub-scale) (HADS-A), anxiety was present in 13–35% of patients (e.g. Bao et al., 2016). For example, in a study of 109 patients seen before biopsy or resection of an intracranial tumour performed 7 days after radiological diagnosis, Pringle et al. found that 30% of patients with brain tumours suffered from anxiety, compared with 16% with depression, using the HADS (Pringle et al., 1999). Using the GAD-7 in 348 patients in a follow-up clinic, Litofsky and colleagues found 48% had significant anxiety (Litofsky et al., 2004). Gender, tumour grade, and previous psychiatric history are significant predictors of a diagnosis of anxiety; coping style also has an influence (Keeling et al., 2013). Irle et al. (1994) compared the psychiatric symptoms in 141 patients following brain tumour surgery with that of 29 patients who had undergone surgery for a slipped disc.[68] Patients with lesions of the ventral frontal and temporo-parietal cortex reported more post-operative anxiety and depression, irritability, anger, and fatigue. As with depression, lesion location is rarely a useful pointer towards anxiety because fear of progression and complications is so dominant (Arnold et al., 2008). Nevertheless, Mainio et al. found that preoperative patients with right hemisphere tumours had higher anxiety scores, compared with those with left hemisphere involvement (Mainio et al. 2003). Mainio et al. (2005) also found obsessionality scores were higher with left anterior region tumours, measured 3 months post-operatively. However, these are weak influences, compared to worries about disease progression or lack of social support.

Mania in patients with brain tumours

Mania is an important complication that is poorly studied. Belyi (1987) noted an association of right frontal lesions and euphoria, whereas left frontal lesions tended to present with akinesia, abulia, and dysphoria.[72] Case series of patients who have sustained a head injury or stroke also suggest an association between mania and cortical or subcortical right-sided lesions. Other associations in the literature are with the basotemporal region, the parathalamic structures, the cingulate gyrus, and the inferior medial frontal lobe.

Table 21.1 Accuracy of three screening methods for depression in patients with brain tumours

Test	Sensitivity	Specificity	PPV	NPV	Clinical utility (+)	Clinical utility (−)	Likelihood ratio (LR+)	Likelihood ratio (LR−)
Distress Thermometer								
DT ≥4	90.5% (77.9–100)	71.6% (64–79.3)	33.3% (21.1–45.6)	98.0% (95.2–100.0)	0.302 (0.115–0.488) Very poor	0.702 (0.643–0.761) Good	3.19 (2.36–4.32)	0.13 (0.04–0.50)
DT ≥5	81.0% (64.2–97.7)	84.3% (78.2–90.5)	44.7% (28.9–60.5)	96.6% (93.3–99.9)	0.362 (0.149–0.576) Poor	0.814 (0.769–0.860) Excellent	5.17 (3.31–8.05)	0.23 (0.09–0.55)
DT ≥6	61.9% (41.1–82.7)	90.3% (85.3–95.3)	50.0% (30.8–69.2)	93.8% (89.6–98.0)	0.310 (0.064–0.555) Very poor	0.847 (0.807–0.887) Excellent	6.38 (3.45–11.81)	0.42 (0.24–0.73)
Hospital Depression and Anxiety Scale								
HADS-D ≥7	95.2% (86.1–100.0)	91.0% (86.2–95.9)	62.5% (45.7–79.3)	99.2% (97.6–100.0)	0.595 (0.405–0.786) Fair	0.903 (0.870–0.936) Excellent	10.63 (6.15–18.40)	0.05 (0.01–0.35)
HADS-D ≥8	76.2% (58.0–94.4)	92.5% (88.1–97.0)	61.5% (42.8–80.2)	96.1% (92.8–99.5)	0.469 (0.240–0.698) Poor	0.890 (0.855–0.924) Excellent	10.21 (5.37–19.41)	0.26 (0.12–0.55)
HADS-D ≥9	71.4% (52.1–90.8)	95.5% (92.0–99.0)	71.4% (52.1–90.8)	95.5% (92.0–99.0)	0.510 (0.274–0.747) Fair	0.912 (0.882–0.943) Excellent	15.95 (6.97–36.49)	0.30 (0.15–0.59)
Patient Health Questionnaire								
PHQ-9 ≥9	95.2% (86.1–100.0)	75.4% (68.1–82.7)	37.7% (24.7–50.8)	99.0% (97.1–100.0)	0.359 (0.173–0.546) Very poor	0.746 (0.692–0.800) Good	3.87 (2.83–5.28)	0.06 (0.01–0.43)
PHQ-9 ≥10	81.0% (64.2–97.7)	85.8% (79.9–91.7)	47.2% (30.9–63.5)	96.6% (93.4–99.9)	0.382 (0.167–0.598) Poor	0.829 (0.786–0.873) Excellent	5.71 (3.58–9.09)	0.22 (0.09–0.54)
PHQ-9 ≥11	71.4% (52.1–90.8)	87.3% (81.7–92.9)	46.9% (29.6–64.2)	95.1% (91.3–98.9)	0.335 (0.106–0.564) Very poor	0.831 (0.788–0.873) Excellent	5.63 (3.35–9.47)	0.33 (0.17–0.65)

NPV, negative predictive value; PPV, positive predictive value. Clinical utility from http://clinicalutility.co.uk/.

Adapted wih permission from data in Rooney AG, et al. Screening for major depressive disorder in adults with cerebral glioma: an initial validation of 3 self-report instruments. *Neuro Oncol.*, 15(1):122–9. Copyright © 2012, Oxford University Press. https://doi.org/10.1093/neuonc/nos282.

Mania is a recognized complication of steroid use. Less common emotional problems sometimes seen with frontal or temporal lobe lesions include irritability and anger, emotionalism, affective lability, and episodic behavioural dyscontrol.

Psychotic symptoms in patients with brain tumours

There has been no systematic study of psychosis in this field, but a review of 148 case reports found 22% had psychotic symptoms (Madhusoodanan et al., 2010). Psychosis can be caused by seizures, delirium, dementia, and steroid use. Although psychosis remains rare, simple olfactory or gustatory hallucinations or visual hallucinations can occur with temporal lobe tumours, and occasionally more complex patterns can occur. Very simple visual hallucinations (flashes, zigzags) are normally linked with occipital tumours. Rarely, parietal lobe tumours cause localized tactile and kinaesthetic hallucinations. Peduncular hallucinosis, originally described by Lhermitte (1922), are bizarre hallucinations that may have an amusing quality (e.g. Lilliputian hallucinations). They may occur in those with upper midbrain posterior fossa tumours. Delusions are rare, without cognitive impairment, and may be mixed with confabulation, typically poorly elaborated and not held with great conviction. There are case reports of patients with temporo-parietal lesions resulting in delusions, but more common is the delusion-like syndrome of anosognosia (denial of disability) that typically follows a parietal lesion. Pure delusions (such as in Capgras misidentification syndrome) may be slightly more common in patients with right-sided lesions.

Neuropsychiatric complications of brain tumour treatments

Adverse effects of surgery

For most patients, the ideal treatment for a brain tumour is complete surgical resection, but this is indicated only for well-circumscribed tumours (typically, this is possible for meningioma, acoustic neuroma, and pituitary adenoma). However, older age and mental health should not be a contraindication to surgery. An alternative is debulking, which aims to reduce local and diffuse symptoms and usually improves survival. Surgery, followed by radiation, has been shown to increase the duration of life (40 versus 15 weeks) and to prolong the period of functionally independent survival (38 versus 8 weeks), compared to biopsy plus radiation. Cognition and QoL often improve after surgery, but rarely completely (Klein et al.,

2001). Extensive surgery involving the dominant hemisphere can cause dysphasia, although it frequently improves. Patients often do not anticipate that cognitive problems will not fully resolve after initial cancer treatment is completed. That said, cognitive change can be an early warning sign of disease extension or recurrence (Armstrong et al., 2003). Talacchi found 79% were impaired before surgery (especially in memory and some executive function), compared to 38% of patients post-operatively (Talacchi et al., 2011). In 38% of patients, deficits were unchanged, 24% improved, and 38% worsened. This is not uncommon; in another study, before meningioma surgery, 69% scored low in one or more cognitive domains, and post-operatively, 44% were still impaired (Meskal et al., 2015).

Adverse effects of supportive medications

High-grade glial tumours, metastatic tumours, and some meningiomas are surrounded by oedema which usually responds to dexamethasone (Dietrich et al., 2011). However, high doses of dexamethasone over a long period causes well-known adverse effects, including Cushingoid weight gain, immunosuppression, proximal myopathy, hyperglycaemia, hypertension, increased gastric acid secretion, and osteoporosis. Psychiatric symptoms include agitation, depression, dysphoria, mania, europhoria, insomnia, and cognitive impairment. Mania has been found in 28%, psychosis 14%, and delirium 10% (Wolkowitz et al., 1990). The severity of memory impairment with steroids approximately correlates with dose/time duration of use (Brown, 2009). Steroids bind the glucocorticoid receptors in the hippocampus. Brown et al. compared hippocampal volumes in patients treated with ≥10 mg/day of prednisone for >6 months to those who had no recent prednisone exposure, and found a 9% decrease in volume, along with memory impairment and depressive symptoms, in the exposed group (Brown et al., 2008).

Adverse effects of radiation therapy

Whole brain radiotherapy is an important treatment modality in the management of CNS tumours, helping to control tumour growth and improve survival. However, only one in five patients experience improvement in neurologic function and frail patients have poor tolerance for radiation. Cognitive deficits are the hallmark of post-radiotherapy encephalopathy, which are sometimes irreversible, and therefore influence treatment decisions, including the dose and type of radiotherapy (Crossen et al., 1994; Meyers and Brown, 2006). Radiotherapy for high-grade tumours improves QoL in eight out of ten patients, but even when treatment is successful, then global cognitive deficits are documented in 12–28% at 1 year post-radiotherapy on the MMSE (Talet et al., 2012). Further, on a more sensitive battery of neurocognitive tests, 48–85% have deficits at 1 year (Talet et al., 2012). Impairment in processing speed, attention, executive function, and memory is commonly seen in brain tumour survivors previously treated with radiation therapy, although the extent is variable.

Radiation encephalopathy has been classified into three phases: acute, early-delayed, and late-delayed. Acute encephalopathy develops within days (up to a month) with nausea, headache, and worsening of neurological deficits. Early-delayed effects occur 1–6 months later with lethargy, resurgence of neurological signs, and a transient decline in cognitive functioning. Late-delayed complications occur 6 months later, possibly caused by vascular abnormalities, demyelination, and ultimately white matter necrosis and

features of cognitive problems with verbal memory, spatial memory, attention, and novel problem-solving ability. Some patients may develop irreversible focal encephalopathy and/or dementia usually accompanied by ataxia and urinary incontinence (Vigliani et al., 1999). Radiation-induced dementia is rare with fraction sizes of <3 Gy (Klein et al., 2002). However, patients who survive >2 years after radiotherapy have a continually increasing risk of developing dementia over time (DeAngelis et al., 1989). Unfortunately, these complications can occur without radiographic or clinical evidence of demyelination or white matter necrosis.

Given the significant issue of radiotherapy-induced cognitive decline, there is great effort to find the best regimen in terms of not only survival, but also QoL and preserved cognition. There is some evidence of a dose–response relationship between radiation to the bilateral hippocampal region and memory function (Gondi et al., 2013). As a result, hippocampal-avoidance whole brain radiotherapy is a technique that involves conformal sparing of the hippocampal stem cell compartments, using intensity-modulated radiotherapy, which helps preserve cognition (Gondi et al., 2014) In those with cerebral metastases, there is a possibility that use of stereotactic radiosurgery alone, compared with stereotactic radiosurgery, plus whole brain radiotherapy produces less cognitive deterioration (Brown et al., 2016). Proton beam therapy is also an option for those with cerebral metastases, which often results in greater sparing of healthy brain tissue, a more targeted delivery of radiation, smaller penetration of tissue beyond the tumour, and less deteriorated cognition (Blomstrand et al., 2012). Stereotactic radiosurgery delivers a single high-precision radiation dose and can be a promising alternative to traditional whole brain radiotherapy, particularly for brain metastasis of <3 cm in diameter. Whole brain radiotherapy delivers between five and 25 low doses of ionizing radiation to the whole brain, while stereotactic radiosurgery delivers high-dose radiation only to the visible brain metastases.

Adverse effects of chemotherapy

The role of chemotherapy is mainly for those with malignant gliomas and primary CNS lymphomas, but focus should be on QoL, not just extension of life. Older drugs such as methotrexate, cytosine arabinoside, cisplatin, vincristine, asparaginase, procarbazine, 5-fluorouracil, high-dose nitrosoureas, and high-dose etoposide have been linked with encephalopathy/delirium and were often CNS-toxic. Typical presentation generally begins with insomnia, agitation, clouding of consciousness, and cognitive decline, possibly with seizures and/or myoclonus. New drugs such as the DNA-alkylating agent temozolomide and the vascular endothelial growth factor monoclonal antibody bevacizumab (Avastin®) offer promise alone or, more recently, in combination with radiotherapy (followed by adjuvant temozolomide post-radiotherapy) (Stupp et al., 2005). Patients receiving temozolomide have more than double the possibility of survival at 2 years versus radiation alone. The effect on metastatic brain tumours, however, is modest (Ma et al., 2016). In general, cognition and QoL improve with temozolomide monotherapy, whereas no change, or even deterioration, is more likely on procarbazine (Gallego et al., 2011). However, adverse effects can occur; for example, in one study, 25% of patients developed substantial cognitive dysfunction and 10% developed leukoencephalopathy (Brandes et al., 2009). Trials for patients with perceived and/or objective cognitive impairment after chemotherapy (chemo-brain) have been lacking (see Interventions to help with cognitive impairment), but many drug trials are now measuring QoL. For example, in one study, the addition of temozolomide during and after radiotherapy produced a significantly longer survival time without a long-lasting negative effect on HRQoL (Taphoorn et al., 2010).

Supportive care for patients with brain tumours

Supportive care should be part of a rehabilitation package which promotes independence and quality of life. Patients' value nurse specialists and other allied health professionals who are available to answer everyday concerns (National Cancer Action Team, 2010). In June 2006, the National Institute for Health and Care Excellence (NICE) produced guidance for treating adults with CNS tumours (National Institute for Health and Care Excellence, 2006). NICE (2006) said 'The psychological and social well-being of the patient, their relatives and carers should be considered throughout the course of the illness' and recommends that 'clinical neuropsychologists, with specialist training and expertise in the assessment and management of cognitive impairment and personality change, and neuropsychiatrists, with specialist training and expertise in the management of patients with severe mental health problems in the context of organic brain disease, have a key contribution to the care of patients with CNS tumours.' A recent meta-analysis of patients with brain tumours undergoing inpatient physical rehabilitation showed 36% improvement in functional status (Formica et al., 2011). Areas likely to improve the most include mobility, self-care, communication, and social interaction. Recent quality standards for brain tumour treatment have been introduced in the UK (NHS England, 2020).

Most patients living with a brain tumour have unmet supportive care needs, as do their family members (Janda et al., 2008; Madsen and Poulsen, 2011) (see Fig. 21.2). In one study, 63% of relatives said they were not satisfied with the degree of support dealing with anxiety or stress (Parvataneni et al., 2011). Several complications pose particular difficulties for caregivers; these include disinhibition, loss of insight, aggression, loss of social awareness, low motivation, and depression. Compared with controls, brain tumour sufferers are more likely to underestimate their psychological and interpersonal problems (Andrewes et al., 2013). Problems are often complex and interrelated. Fifty per cent of brain tumour patients report ten concurrent symptoms, most notably: fatigue, drowsiness, difficulty remembering, disturbed sleep, and distress (Armstrong et al., 2016). Fatigue is a major issue in recovery from a brain tumour and is linked with depression, distress, and lesion location (Valko et al., 2015) but will often respond to a rehabilitation approach.

The NICE guidelines above recommend that ongoing training (especially communication skills) should be provided for all staff providing psychological support to patients with CNS tumours. To help patients and their caregivers cope with a brain tumour, it is important to provide education and promote autonomy (Langbecker et al., 2015). Self-help materials, group therapy, and peer support are increasingly seen as important supplements to traditional psychological and psychiatric care (Boele et al., 2014a; Ozier and Cashman 2016). These interventions can help promote positive experiences of living with a brain tumour. National guidelines suggest that depression in patients with a chronic physical condition should, where possible, be treated with a combination of medication

and an effective psychological treatment such as CBT or mindfulness (Hart et al., 2012). However, this is unlikely to be sufficient alone. Exercise-based programmes are often extremely valuable at promoting QoL after cancer (Mishra et al., 2012). Specific supportive care interventions for patients with brain tumours are being developed and show promise for supporting patients and families (Ownsworth et al., 2015). In an early report, Locke et al. (2008) recruited 19 dyads and trialled a combined cognitive rehabilitation and positive problem-solving intervention but found little effect. Ownsworth et al. (2014) found that a customized programme improved QoL (but not anxiety) and well-being, and reduced depressive symptoms up to 6 months post-intervention. Fundamentally, patients should be offered the same quality of psychiatric care as medical care. Indeed, prompt medical treatment should not be prejudiced by a psychiatric diagnosis (Boele et al., 2014b). If there are problems with mental health interfering with adherence and uptake of medical care, then clinical nurse specialists, liaison psychiatrists, or psycho-oncologist can have an important role.

Interventions to help with cognitive impairment

Everyday practical tips are shown in Box 21.3 and include a number of potentially useful apps for those with memory problems (Independent Living Centre NSW, 2007).

Formal therapeutic interventions include drug trials and trials of rehabilitation approaches, most of which have been published in the last 5 years. Meyers et al. (1998) conducted neuropsychologic assessments in 30 patients with primary brain tumours before and during treatment with 10 mg methylphenidate. Significant improvements in cognitive function occurred, as well as improved gait and motivation to perform activities, but a second study found little effect and an open-label study found small effects (Butler et al., 2007; Gehring and Patwardhan, 2012). In a much larger study, Brown et al. (2013) examined the effects of memantine on cognitive function in 508 patients receiving whole brain radiotherapy. Memantine was started within 3 days of radiotherapy and continued for 24 weeks without undue side effects. The memantine arm had significantly longer time before cognitive decline and there was significant impairment in the placebo arm (53.8% versus 64.9%, respectively), with benefits in executive function, processing speed, and delayed recognition. Shaw

---

> **Box 21.3** Practical strategies to cope with memory problems
>
> 1 Modification of the environment to simplify demanding tasks, e.g. use of home delivery service.
> 2 Keep a weekly planner of upcoming events.
> 3 Keep an activity list of enjoyable activities.
> 4 Use reminders on mobile/tablet.
> 5 Keep a daily diary to refer to later, if needed.
> 6 Use repetition to aid memory.
> 7 Write down prompts/reminders manually or electronically.
> 8 Ask family and friends to send reminder texts.
> 9 Put labels around the house.
> 10 Consider locator lost and found apps.
> 11 Use clear, large-letter clocks.
> 12 Develop routines for regular tasks.
> 13 Use apps such as: 'Did I turn it off', 'Apple reminder', 'Timehop', 'Anydo', 'Medisafe'.

et al. (2006) trialled 5 mg donepezil per day for 6 weeks, then 10 mg per day for 18 weeks in 34 patients (of whom 24 completed 18 weeks), with patients mostly having low-grade glioma. Scores significantly improved between baseline (pre-treatment) and week 24 on measures of attention/concentration, verbal memory, and figural memory, with a trend for verbal fluency. HRQoL also improved. Rapp et al. (2013) conducted an RCT of donepezil and found no significant improvement on cognitive function in brain tumour survivors following radiation, compared to placebo, but secondary analysis of severely impaired patients showed an improvement in verbal memory. Rapp et al. (2015) re-examined donepezil in 198 adult brain tumour survivors 6 months after partial or whole brain irradiation. Patients took 5 mg donepezil for 6 weeks, then 10 mg for 18 weeks, or placebo. A cognitive test battery showed donepezil did not significantly improve the overall score, but it did result in modest improvements in several cognitive functions, especially among patients with greater pre-treatment impairments. These results seem to suggest cognitive interventions are most effective in those with more severe deficits, but nevertheless patients with mild to moderate deficits are likely to benefit too.

Regarding cognitive rehabilitation, there have been five RCTs to date (Gehring et al., 2009; Locke et al., 2008; Richard et al., 2016; Yang et al., 2014; Zucchella et al., 2013). Yang examined 38 brain tumour patients and found superior improvements in visual and auditory continuous performance scores, digit and visual span tests, and verbal and visual learning tests. Lock et al. examined 19 patients/caregiver dyads before or upon initiation of radiation therapy, but results were unclear in this trial as only 13 dyads completed. However, the intervention was described as 'very helpful' or 'somewhat helpful' by 88% of study participants (Lock et al., 2008). Gehring et al. recruited 140 patients (117 low-grade) to a trial of multifaceted rehabilitation programme versus a waiting-list control group (Gehring et al., 2009). The intervention incorporated both computer-based attention retraining and compensatory skills training of attention, memory, and executive functioning. Participants completed a battery of neuropsychological tests and QoL scales. Cognition improved and improvement was sustained at 6-month follow-up, especially in tests of attention and verbal memory. Younger patients with more education experienced greater improvements. There was also an improvement in mental fatigue. Zucchella et al. (2013) examined 58 patients (25 with high-grade tumours) who were randomized after surgery to neurocognitive rehabilitation or a control group. They found a statistically significant difference in visual attention and verbal memory, but not in logical executive functioning or QoL. Richard et al. (2016) conducted a study comparing two cognitive rehabilitation programmes—mindfulness goal management training and the Brain Health psychoeducation workshop. They found that significant improvement in executive functions and greater attainment of pre-training functional goals in the goal management training group, while the psychoeducation workshop group showed an significant improvement in mood and behavioural regulation. It is important to note that even when cognitive rehabilitation does not improve cognition, there may be benefits in fatigue and QoL, while helping patients understand better the nature and degree of their impairment or disability and helping introduce problem-solving and social skills.

Conclusion

Of all cancers, brain tumour causes the highest rates of distress, depression, and cognitive impairment. Neuropsychiatric symptoms are an important red flag for future deterioration but should be addressed in their own right. Patients often have complex overlapping symptoms, and often localization of the site of the brain tumour is not possible. Nevertheless, neuropsychiatric symptoms disproportionately influence QoL. Patients given high-quality supportive and rehabilitation care have better satisfaction, improved QoL, and better physical outcomes.

KEY LEARNING POINTS

- A brain tumour is the most feared cancer diagnosis by the general public.
- Primary brain tumours account for about 1.5% of all new cases of cancer, and 2.5% of all cancer deaths; however, most brain tumours are, in fact, metastases from other cancer sites.
- Brain tumours cause considerable psychological and psychiatric complications, as well as a burden for caregivers, and hence reductions in overall QoL.
- Around 90% will suffer neuropsychiatric complications, and in around 20%, these are the presenting symptom. Neuropsychiatric complications often improve following brain tumour treatment such as radiotherapy, but they can also deteriorate.
- New therapeutic techniques offer improved survival and also benefit QoL. However, this is only effective if neuropsychiatric complications are recognized and addressed.

REFERENCES

American Brain Tumor Association. Available from: http://www.abta.org/resources/health-care-provider/final-adult-clinical-practice.pdf

Aaronson NK, Ahmedzai S, Bergman B. The European Organization for Research and Treatment of Cancer QLQ-C30: A quality of life instrument for use in international clinical trials in oncology. J Natl Cancer Inst, 1993; 85: 365–76.

Andrewes HE, Drummond KJ, Rosenthal M, Bucknill A, Andrewes DG. Awareness of psychological and relationship problems amongst brain tumour patients and its association with carer distress. Psychooncology, 2013; 22: 2200–5.

Armstrong CL, Goldstein B, Shera D, Ledakis GE, Tallent EM. The predictive value of longitudinal neuropsychologic assessment in the early detection of brain tumor recurrence. Cancer, 2003; 97: 649–56.

Armstrong TS, Vera-Bolanos E, Acquaye AA, et al. The symptom burden of primary brain tumors: evidence for a core set of tumor- and treatment-related symptoms. Neurooncol, 2016; 18: 252–60.

Arnold SD, Forman LM, Brigidi BD, Carter KE, Schweitzer HA, Quinn HE, Guill AB, Herndon JE, Raynor RH. Evaluation and characterization of generalized anxiety and depression in patients with primary brain tumors Neuro Oncol, 2008; 10: 171–81.

Baker PD, Bambrough J, Fox JRE, Kyle SD. Health-related quality of life and psychological functioning in patients with primary malignant brain tumors: a systematic review of clinical, demographic and mental health factors. Neuro Oncol Pract, 2016; 3: 211–21.

Bao, Y, Li L, Guan Y, et al. Prevalence and associated positive psychological variables of anxiety and depression among patients with central nervous system tumors in China: a cross-sectional study. Psycho-Oncology, 2017; 26: 262–9.

Belyi BI. Mental impairment in unilateral frontal tumours: role of the laterality of the lesion. Int J Neurosci, 1987; 32: 799–810.

Bunevicius A, Deltuva V, Tamasauskas S, Tamasauskas A, Bunevicius R. Screening for psychological distress in neurosurgical brain tumor patients using the Patient Health Questionnaire-2. Psychooncology, 2013; 22: 1895–900.

Becker J, Steinmann E, Könemann M. Cognitive screening in patients with intracranial tumors: validation of the BCSE. J Neurooncol, 2016; 127: 559.

Bergo E, Lombardi G, Guglieri I, Capovilla E, Pambuku A, Zagonel V. Neurocognitive functions and health-related quality of life in glioblastoma patients: a concise review of the literature. Eur J Cancer Care, 2019; 28: e12410.

Blomstrand M, Brodin NP, Munck AF, et al. Estimated clinical benefit of protecting neurogenesis in the developing brain during radiation therapy for pediatric medulloblastoma. Neuro-oncology, 2012; 14: 882–9.

Boele FW, Klein M, Reijneveld JC, Verdonck-de Leeuw IM Heimans. Symptom management and quality of life in glioma patients. JJ CNS Oncol, 2014b; 3: 37–47.

Boele FW, Verdonck-de Leeuw IM, Cuijpers P, Reijneveld JC, Heimans JJ, Klein M. Internet-based guided self-help for glioma patients with depressive symptoms: design of a randomized controlled trial. BMC Neurol, 2014a; 14: 81.

Brandes AA, Franceschi E, Tosoni A. Temozolomide concomitant and adjuvant to radiotherapy in elderly patients with glioblastoma: correlation with MGMT promoter methylation status. Cancer, 2009; 115: 3512–18.

Brown ES. Effects of glucocorticoids on mood, memory, and the hippocampus. Treatment and preventive therapy. Ann N Y Acad Sci, 2009; 1179: 41–55.

Brown PD, Jaeckle K, Ballman KV, et al. Effect of Radiosurgery Alone vs Radiosurgery With Whole Brain Radiation Therapy on Cognitive Function in Patients With 1 to 3 Brain Metastases: A Randomized Clinical Trial. JAMA, 2016; 316: 401–9.

Brown PD, Jensen AW, Felten SJ. Detrimental effects of tumour progression on cognitive function of patients with high-grade glioma. J Clin Oncol, 2006; 24: 5427–33.

Brown PD, Pugh S, Laack NN, et al. Radiation Therapy Oncology Group (RTOG). Memantine for the prevention of cognitive dysfunction in patients receiving whole-brain radiotherapy: a randomized, double-blind, placebo-controlled trial. Neuro Oncol, 2013; 15: 1429–37.

Brown SE, Woolston DJ, Alan B. Frol Amygdala Volume in Patients Receiving Chronic Corticosteroid Therapy. Biol Psychiatry, 2008; 63: 705–9.

Butler JM, Case LD, Atkins J, et al. A phase III, double-blind, placebo controlled prospective randomized clinical trial of d-threomethylphenidate HCl in brain tumor patients receiving radiation therapy. Int J Radiat Oncol Biol Phys, 2007; 69: 1496–501.

Chang SM, Parney IF, Huang W, et al., for the Glioma Outcomes Project Investigators. Patterns of care for adults with newly diagnosed malignant glioma. JAMA, 2005; 293: 557–64.

Chang EL, Wefel JS, Hess KR, et al. Neurocognition in patients with brain metastases treated with radiosurgery or radiosurgery plus whole-brain irradiation: a randomised controlled trial. Lancet Oncol, 2009; 10: 1037–44.

Cheng JX, Liu BL, Zhang X. Health-related quality of life in glioma patients in China. BMC Cancer, 2010; 10: 305.

Cohen AL, Colman H. Glioma Biology and Molecular Markers Current Understanding and Treatment of Gliomas. Cancer Treat Res, 2015; 163: 15–30.

Crossen JR, Garwood D, Glatstein E, Neuwelt EA. Neurobehavioral sequelae of cranial irradiation in adults: a review of radiation-induced encephalopathy. J Clin Oncol, 1994; 12: 627–42.

DeAngelis LM1, Delattre JY, Posner JB. Radiation-induced dementia in patients cured of brain metastases. Neurology, 1989; 39: 789–96.

Dietrich J, Rao K, Pastorino S, Kesari S. Corticosteroids in brain cancer patients: benefits and pitfalls. Expert Rev Clin Pharmacol, 2011; 4: 233–42.

Drewes C, Sagberg LM, Jakola AS, Solheim O. Quality of life in patients with intracranial tumors: does tumor laterality matter? J Neurosurg, 2016; 25: 1–8.

Fardet L, Petersen I, Nazareth I. Suicidal behaviour and severe neuropsychiatric disorders following glucocorticoid therapy in primary care. Am J Psychiatry, 2012; 169: 491–7.

Feuerstein M, Hansen JA, Calvio LC, Johnson L, Ronquillo JG. Work productivity in brain tumor survivors. J Occup Environ Med, 2007a; 49: 803–11.

Feuerstein M, Hansen JA, Calvio LC, Johnson L, Ronquillo JG. Work Productivity in Brain Tumor Survivors. J Occup Environ Med, 2007b; 7: 803–11.

Formica V, Del Monte G, Giacchetti L, Giaquinto S, Fini M, Roselli M. Rehabilitation in neuro-oncology: A meta-analysis of published data and a mono-institutional experience. Integr Cancer Ther, 2011; 10: 119–26.

Forsyth PA, Posner JB. Headaches in patients with brain tumors: a study of 111 patients. Neurology, 1993; 43: 1678.

Gallego Perez-Larraya J, Ducray F, Chinot O, et al. Temozolomide in elderly patients with newly diagnosed glioblastoma and poor performance status: an ANOCEF phase II trial. J Clin Oncol, 2011; 29: 3050–5.

Gathinji M, McGirt MJ, Attenello FJ. Association of preoperative depression and survival after resection of malignant brain astrocytoma. Surg Neurol, 2009; 71: 299–303.

Gehring K, Patwardhan SY, Collins R. A randomized trial on the efficacy of methylphenidate and modafinil for improving cognitive functioning and symptoms in patients with a primary brain tumor. J Neurooncol, 2012; 107: 165.

Gehring K, Sitskoorn MM, Gundy CM, et al. Cognitive rehabilitation in patients with gliomas: a randomized, controlled trial. J Clin Oncol, 2009; 27: 3712–22.

Gondi V, Hermann BP, Mehta MP, Tomé WA. Hippocampal dosimetry predicts neurocognitive function impairment after fractionated stereotactic radiotherapy for benign or low-grade adult brain tumors. Int J Radiat Oncol Biol Phys, 2013; 85: 348–54.

Gondi V, Pugh SL, Tome WA. Preservation of memory with conformal avoidance of the hippocampal neural stem-cell compartment during whole-brain radiotherapy for brain metastases (RTOG 0933): a phase II multi-institutional trial. J Clin Oncol, 2014; 32: 3810–16.

Graf AH, Buchberger W, Langmayr H, Schmid KW. Site preference of metastatic tumours of the brain. Virchows Arch A Pathol Anat Histopathol, 1988; 412: 493–8.

Gupta RK1, Kumar R. Benign brain tumours and psychiatric morbidity: a 5-years retrospective data analysis. Aust N Z J Psychiatry, 2004; 38: 316–19.

Hahn CA, Dunn RH, Logue PE, King JH, Edwards CL, Halperin EC. Prospective study of neuropsychological testing and quality-of-life assessment of adults with primary malignant brain tumours. Int J Radiation Oncol, 2003; 55: 992–9.

Halkett GK, Lobb EA, Rogers MM, et al. Predictors of distress and poorer quality of life in High Grade Glioma patients. Patient Educ Couns, 2015; 98, 525–32.

Hart SL, Hoyt MA, Diefenbach M, et al. Meta-analysis of efficacy of interventions for elevated depressive symptoms in adults diagnosed with cancer. J Natl Cancer Inst, 2012; 104: 990–1004.

Independent Living Centre NSW. 2007. *Helpful Handbook for Memory Loss.* Available from: http://ilctas.asn.au/client-assets/info-sheets/HelpfulHandbookForMemoryLoss.pdf

Irle E, Peper M, Wowra B. Mood changes after surgery for tumors of the cerebral-cortex. Arch Neurol, 1994; 51: 164–74.

Janda M, Steginga S, Dunn J, Langbecker D, Walker D, Eakin E. Unmet supportive care needs and interest in services among patients with a brain tumour and their carers. Patient Educ Couns, 2008; 71: 251–8.

Janda M, Steginga S, Langbecker D, Dunn J, Walker D, Eakin E. Quality of Life among patients with a brain tumour and their carers. J Psychosom Res, 2007; 63: 617–23.

Keeling M, Bambrough J, Simpson J. Depression, anxiety and positive affect in people diagnosed with low-grade tumours: the role of illness perceptions. Psycho-Oncology, 2013, 22: 1421–7.

Keir ST, Calhoun-Eagan RD, Swartz JJ, Saleh OA, Friedman HS. Screening for distress in patients with brain cancer using the NCCN's rapid screening measure. Psychooncology, 2008; 17: 621–5.

Keir ST, Farland MM, Lipp ES, Friedman HS. Distress persists in long-term brain tumor survivors with glioblastoma multiforme. J Cancer Surviv, 2008; 2: 269–74.

Keschner M, Bender MB, Strauss I. Mental symptoms associated with brain tumour: a study of 530 verified cases. JAMA, 1983; 110: 714–18.

Klein M, Heimans JJ, Aaronson NK, et al. Effect of radiotherapy and other treatment-related factors on mid-term to long-term cognitive sequelae in low-grade gliomas: a comparative study. Lancet, 2002; 360: 1361–8.

Klein M, Postma TJ, Taphoorn MJ, et al. The prognostic value of cognitive functioning in the survival of patients with high-grade glioma. Neurology, 2003; 61: 1796–8.

Klein M, Taphoorn MJ, Heimans JJ, et al. Neurobehavioral status and health-related quality of life in newly diagnosed high-grade glioma patients. J Clin Oncol, 2001; 19: 4037–47.

Krebber AM, Buffart LM, Kleijn G, Riepma IC, de Bree R, Leemans CR. Prevalence of depression in cancer patients: a meta-analysis of diagnostic interviews and self-report instruments. Psychooncology, 2014; 23: 121–30.

Kvale EA, Murthy R, Taylor R, Lee JY, Nabors LB. Distress and Quality of Life in primary high-grade brain tumor patients. Support Care Cancer, 2009; 17: 793–9.

Langbecker D, Janda M. Systematic review of interventions to improve the provision of information for adults with primary brain tumors and their caregivers. Front Oncol, 2015; 5: 1.

Lhermitte J. Syndrome de la calotte pédonculaire. Les troubles psychosensorielles dans les lésions du mésencéphale. Rev Neurol (Paris), 1922; 38:1359–65.

Litofsky NS, Farace E, Anderson F, Meyers CA, Huang W, Laws ER. Glioma Outcomes Project Investigators. Depression in patients with high-grade glioma: results of the Glioma Outcomes Project. Neurosurgery, 2004; 54: 358–67.

Locke DE, Cerhan JH, Wu W, Malec JF, Clark MM, Rummans TA. Cognitive rehabilitation and problem-solving to improve quality of life of patients with primary brain tumours: a pilot study. J Support Oncol, 2008; 6: 383–91.

Lohr JB, Cadet JL. Neuropsychiatric aspects of brain tumors. In: Hales RE & Yudofsky SC (eds). *The American Psychiatric Press Textbook of Neuropsychiatry.* Washington, DC, American Psychiatric Press, 1987; pp. 351–64.

Long A, Halkett GKB, Lobb EA, Shaw T, Hovey E, Nowak AK. Carers of patients with high-grade glioma report high levels of distress, unmet needs, and psychological morbidity during patient chemoradiotherapy. Neuro Oncol Pract, 2016; 3: 105–12.

Louis, D.N., Perry, A., Reifenberger, G. et al. The 2016 World Health Organization Classification of Tumors of the Central Nervous System: a summary Acta Neuropathol, 2016; 131: 803.

Ma W, Li N, An Y, Zhou C, Bo C, Zhang G. Effect of Temozolomide and Radiotherapy on Brain Metastatic Tumor: A Systematic Review and Meta-analysis. World Neurosurg, 2016; 16: 30084–5.

Mackworth N, Fobair P, Prados MD. Quality of life self-reports from 200 brain tumor patients: comparisons with Karnofsky performance scores. J Neurooncol, 1992; 14: 243–53.

Madhusoodanan S, Opler MG, Moise D, et al. Brain tumor location and psychiatric symptoms: is there any association? A meta-analysis of published case studies. Expert Rev Neurother, 2010; 10: 1529–36.

Madsen K, Poulsen HS. Needs for everyday life support for brain tumour patients' relatives: systematic literature review. Eur J Cancer Care, 2011; 20: 33–43.

Mainio A, Hakko H, Niemela A, Tuurinkoski T, Koivukangas J, Rasanen P. The effect of brain tumour laterality on anxiety levels among neurosurgical patients. J Neurol, 2003; 74: 1278–82.

Mainio, A., Hakko, H., Niemela, A., Salo, J., Koivukangas, J. & Rasanen, P. Level of obsessionality among neurosurgical patients with a primary brain tumor. J Neuropsychiatry Clin Neurosci, 2005; 17: 399–404.

Mainio A, Tuunanen S, Hakko H, Niemela A, Koivukangas J, Rasanen P. Decreased quality of life and depression as predictors for shorter survival among patients with low-grade gliomas: a follow-up from 1990 to 2003. European Arch Psychiatry Clin Neurosci, 2006; 256: 516–21.

Meskal I, Gehring K, van der Linden SD. Cognitive improvement in meningioma patients after surgery: clinical relevance of computerized testing. J Neurooncol, 2015; 121: 617.

Meyers CA, Brown PD. Role and relevance of neurocognitive assessment in clinical trials of patients with CNS tumors. J Clin Oncol, 2006; 24: 1305–9.

Meyers CA, Weitzner MA, Valentine AD, Levin VA. Methylphenidate therapy improves cognition, mood, and function of brain tumor patients. J Clin Oncol, 1998; 16: 2522–7.

Mishra SI, Scherer RW, Snyder C, Geigle PM, Berlanstein DR, Topaloglu O. Exercise interventions on health-related quality of life for people with cancer during active treatment. Cochrane Database of Systematic Reviews, 2012; 8: CD008465.

Mitchell AJ, Chan M, Bhatti H, Halton M, Grassi L, Johansen C, Meader N. Prevalence of depression, anxiety, and adjustment disorder in oncological, haematological, and palliative-care settings: a meta-analysis of 94 interview-based studies. Lancet Oncol, 2011; 12: 160–74.

Mitchell AJ, Lord K, Symonds P. Which symptoms are indicative of DSMIV depression in cancer settings? An analysis of the diagnostic significance of somatic and non-somatic symptoms. J Affect Disord, 2012; 138: 137–48.

National Cancer Action Team. 2010. *Excellence in cancer care: the contribution of the clinical care nurse specialist.* Available from: http://www.macmillan.org.uk/documents/aboutus/commissioners/excellenceincancercarethecontributionoftheclinicalnursespecialist.pdf

National Institute for Health and Care Excellence. 2006. *Improving Outcomes for People with Brain and Other CNS Tumours.* Available from: http://www.nice.org.uk/csgbraincns.

NHS England. Commissioning for quality and innovation. 2020. https://www.england.nhs.uk/nhs-standard-contract/cquin/

Olson R, Tyldesley S, Carolan H, Parkinson M, Chhanabhai T, McKenzie M. Prospective comparison of the prognostic utility of the Mini Mental State Examination and the Montreal Cognitive Assessment in patients with brain metastases. Support Care Cancer, 2011; 19: 1849–55.

Ostrom QT, Gittleman H, Liao P. CBTRUS statistical report: primary brain and central nervous system tumors diagnosed in the United States in 2007–2011. Neuro Oncol, 2014; 16 Suppl 4: iv1–63.

Ownsworth T, Chambers S, Damborg E, Casey L, Walker DG, Shum DH. Evaluation of the making sense of brain tumor program: a randomized controlled trial of a home-based psychosocial intervention. Psychooncology, 2015; 24: 540–7.

Ozier D, Cashman R. A mixed method study of a peer support intervention for newly diagnosed primary brain tumour patients. Can Oncol Nurs J, 2016; 26: 104–11.

Pace, A., Villani, V., Parisi, C. Rehabilitation pathways in adult brain tumor patients in the first 12 months of disease. A retrospective analysis of services utilization in 719 patients. Support Care Cancer, 2016; 24: 4801–6.

Parvataneni R, Polley MY, Freeman T, et al. Identifying the needs of brain tumor patients and their caregivers. J Neurooncol, 2011; 104: 737–44.

Porter KR, Menon U, Vick NA, Villano JL, Berbaum ML, Davis FG. Assessment of clinical and nonclinical characteristics associated with health-related quality of life in patients with high-grade gliomas: a feasibility study. Support Care Cancer, 2014; 22: 1349–62.

Pringle AM, Taylor R, Whittle IR. Anxiety and depression in patients with an intracranial neoplasm before and after tumour surgery. Br J Neurosurg, 1999; 13: 46–51.

Rapp S, Case D, Peiffer A. Donepezil for irradiated brain tumor survivors: A phase III, randomized, placebo-controlled clinical trial. J Clin Oncol, 2015; 33: 1653–9.

Raysi Dehcordi S, De Paulis D, Marzi S. Survival prognostic factors in patients with glioblastoma: our experience. J Neurosurg Sci, 2012; 56: 239–45.

Richard NM, Bernstein LJ, Mason WP, et al. Cognitive rehabilitation for brain tumor survivors: a pilot randomized controlled trial. J Neurooncol, 2019; 142: 565–75.

Robinson GA, Biggs V, Walker DG. Cognitive Screening in Brain Tumors: Short but Sensitive Enough? Front Oncol, 2015; 5: 60.

Rooney A, Carson A, Grant R. Depression in cerebral glioma patients: a systematic review of observational studies. J Natl Cancer Inst, 2011; 103: 61–76.

Rooney AG, McNamara S, Mackinnon M, Fraser M, Rampling R, Carson A. The frequency, longitudinal course, clinical associations, and causes of emotional distress during primary treatment of cerebral glioma. Neuro Oncol, 2013; 15: 635–43.

Rooney AG, et al. Screening for major depressive disorder in adults with cerebral glioma: an initial validation of 3 self-report instruments. Neuro Oncol, 2013;15(1):122–9.

Salo J, Niemela A, Joukamaa M, Koivukangas J. Effect of brain tumour laterality on patients' perceived quality of life. J Neurol Neurosurg Psychiatry, 2002; 72: 373–7.

Schmidt JE, Beckjord E, Bovbjerg DH. Prevalence of perceived cognitive dysfunction in survivors of a wide range of cancers: results from the 2010 LIVESTRONG survey. J Cancer Surviv, 2016; 10: 302.

Schouten LJ, Rutten J, Huveneers HA, Twijnstra A. Incidence of brain metastases in a cohort of patients with carcinoma of the breast, colon, kidney, and lung and melanoma. Cancer, 2002; 94: 2698–705.

Scott JN, Rewcastle NB, Brasher PM. Which glioblastoma multiforme patient will become a long-term survivor? A population-based study. *Ann Neurol*, 1999; 46: 183–8.

Shaw EG, Rosdhal R, D'Agostino RB Jr. Phase II study of donepezil in irradiated brain tumor patients: effect on cognitive function, mood, and quality of life. J Clin Oncol, 2006; 24: 1415–20.

Singh D, Kapoor A, Khadda S, et al. Psychotic manifestations as an initial presentation in glioma: two case reports and review of literature. Neuropsychiatria i Neuropsychologia 2014; 9: 1–3.

Stupp R, Mason WP, van den Bent MJ, et al. Radiotherapy plus concomitant and adjuvant temozolomide for glioblastoma. N Engl J Med, 2005; 352: 987–96.

Talacchi A, Santini B, Savazzi S, Gerosa M. Cognitive effects of tumour and surgical treatment in glioma patients. J Neurooncol, 2011; 103: 541–9.

Tallet AV, Azria D, Barlesi F, et al. Neurocognitive function impairment after whole brain radiotherapy for brain metastases: actual assessment. Radiat Oncol, 2012; 7: 77.

Taphoorn MJ, Sizoo EM, Bottomley A. Review on quality of life issues in patients with primary brain tumors. Oncologist, 2010; 15: 618–26.

Trad W, Koh ES, Daher M, et al. Screening for Psychological Distress in Adult Primary Brain Tumor Patients and Caregivers: Considerations for Cancer Care Coordination. Front Oncol, 2015; 5: 203.

Tucha O, Smely C, Preier M, Lange KW. Cognitive deficits before treatment among patients with brain tumors. Neurosurgery, 2000; 47: 324–34.

Valko PO, Siddique A, Linsenmeier C, Zaugg K, Held U, Hofer S. Prevalence and predictors of fatigue in glioblastoma: a prospective study. Neuro Oncol, 2015;17: 274–81.

van Breemen MS, Rijsman RM, Taphoorn MJ. Efficacy of anti-epileptic drugs in patients with gliomas and seizures. J Neurol, 2009; 256: 1519.

Vernooij MW, Ikram MA, Tanghe HL, et al. Incidental findings on brain MRI in the general population. N Engl J Med, 2007; 357: 1821–8.

Vigliani MC, Duyckaerts C, Hauw JJ, Poisson M, Magdelenat H, Delattre JY. Dementia following treatment of brain tumors with radiotherapy administered alone or in combination with nitrosourea-based chemotherapy: a clinical and pathological study. J Neurooncol, 1999; 41: 137–49.

Weitzner MA, Meyers CA. Cognitive functioning and quality of life in malignant glioma patients: a review of the literature. Psychooncology, 1997; 6: 169–77.

Weitzner MA, Meyers CA, Gelke CK. The Functional Assessment of Cancer Therapy (FACT) scale. Development of a brain subscale and revalidation of the general version (FACT-G) in patients with primary brain tumors. Cancer, 1995; 75: 1151–61.

Wolkowitz OM, Rubinow D, Doran AR, Breier A, Berrettini WH, Kling MA. Prednison effects on neurochemistry and behaviour—reliminary findings. Arch Gen Psychiatry, 1990; 47: 963–8.

Yang S, Chun MH, Son YR. Effect of virtual reality on cognitive dysfunction in patients with brain tumor. Ann Rehabil Med, 2014; 38: 726–33.

YouGov. 2011. *YouGov Survey Results*. http://cdn.yougov.com/today_uk_import/yg-archives-life-cancerresearch-diseases-150811.pdf

Zucchella C, Bartolo M, Di Lorenzo C, Villani V, Pace A. Cognitive impairment in primary brain tumors outpatients: a prospective cross-sectional survey. J Neurooncol, 2013; 112: 455–60.

Zucchella C, Capone A, Codella V, et al. Cognitive rehabilitation for early post-surgery inpatients affected by primary brain tumor: a randomized, controlled trial. J Neurooncol, 2013; 114: 93–100.

22

Inflammatory and autoimmune disorders in neuropsychiatry

Thomas A. Pollak, Ester Coutinho, Emma Palmer-Cooper, and Angela Vincent

Introduction

Accumulating evidence suggests a close link between the immune system and the central nervous system in neuropsychiatric disorders. Systemic or neurological autoimmune disorders can have marked neuropsychiatric manifestations, sometimes as first disease manifestation, while immune abnormalities have been recognized for many years in association with primary psychiatric disorders. Moreover, the clinical interface between psychiatry and neurology has undergone significant change in the last decade, in large part driven by the rise in awareness of the autoimmune encephalitides that are caused by antibodies to specific neuronal surface membrane proteins such as the NMDA receptor (NMDAR), leucine-rich glioma inactivated 1 (LGI1), or contactin-associated protein-like 2 (CASPR2). These disorders were, until recently, considered to be rarities on the neurologist's list of differential diagnoses but are now familiar to even most general adult neurologists and psychiatrists.

After a brief introduction to the concepts of autoimmunity, we describe recent findings in three sections: (1) those well-known autoimmune disorders in which psychiatric presentations are common; (2) psychiatric presentations associated with autoimmune forms of encephalitis; and (3) evidence that supports a role for autoantibodies in some patients with primary psychiatric disorders.

Autoimmunity

A disease is termed autoimmune if an abnormal adaptive immune response to a self-antigen, either by auto-reactive T cells or autoantibodies, causes, or is associated with, the observed pathology. A practical approach to establish the diagnosis of autoimmune diseases, invoked many times, is based on the Koch/Witebsky postulates: (1) demonstration of circulating or cell-bound antibodies; (2) identification of the specific antigen against which this antibody is directed; (3) the production of antibodies against the same antigen in experimental animals; (4) the appearance of pathological changes in the corresponding tissues of animals immunized against

the antigen, or injected with serum from actively immunized animals, similar to those in the human disease (Witebsky et al., 1957); and, one might also add, (5) similar findings in animals injected with the patient's serum or IgG; and (6) improvement of the condition or prevention of disease progression with elimination or suppression of the autoimmune response (i.e. with immunotherapies). Analogous criteria can be applied to autoimmunity driven by self-reactive T cells. Autoimmune disorders are designated as either systemic or organ-specific, depending on the extent and location of tissue damage.

Autoimmune disorders with marked neuropsychiatric manifestations

Many, if not all, systemic or neurological autoimmune disorders can have a profound impact on the patient's mental health. A primary psychiatric dysfunction in the context of autoimmunity can be directly caused by a brain-directed immune response. However, the clinician (either a psychiatrist or a neuroimmunologist) when assessing the patient with new-onset psychiatric symptoms must first exclude other aetiologies, such as infectious illnesses, adverse drug reactions, or metabolic abnormalities, before establishing a diagnosis of autoimmune psychiatric dysfunction. Likewise, psychiatric symptoms can result from the impact of the chronic disability caused by the autoimmune condition, and this possibility needs to be considered and addressed. Further complicating the picture, psychiatric disorders can occur independently of the autoimmune condition, and several epidemiological studies and a meta-analysis (Benros et al., 2011; Benros et al., 2014; Cullen et al., 2019) suggest that the risk of diagnosis of an independent psychiatric disorder is higher in a patient with an autoimmune disorder, and vice versa.

In this section, we focus on three disorders that, due to their prevalence and/or relevance of the associated psychiatric manifestations, are more likely to be seen by the psychiatrist in routine clinical practice: systemic lupus erythematosus (SLE), multiple sclerosis (MS), and autoimmune encephalopathies (AEs).

Systemic lupus erythematosus

SLE is a complex, chronic relapsing–remitting autoimmune inflammatory disorder. The aetiology is still not fully understood, but the pathophysiological mechanisms include loss of immune tolerance, production of autoantibodies, and formation of immune complexes that can deposit in tissues and promote systemic inflammation. Any body system can be affected, including the central and peripheral nervous systems. Criteria for CNS-associated neuropsychiatric SLE, sometimes also designated neurolupus, cover a wide spectrum of psychiatric and neurological dysfunction, from diffuse psychiatric manifestations (cognitive deficit, mood and anxiety disorders, acute confusional state, headache, and psychosis) to focal neurological dysfunction (cerebrovascular disease, seizures, myelopathy, aseptic meningitis, movement disorder, and demyelinating syndromes). Epidemiological data on neuropsychiatric SLE lack consistency, with frequency rates ranging from 12% to 95% (Unterman et al., 2011), possibly because of the inclusion of non-specific symptoms such as headache, mild cognitive dysfunction, and mild mood and anxiety disorders. Further complicating the diagnosis, diffuse psychiatric symptoms develop slowly and fluctuate in severity, often independently from the systemic disease activity. Furthermore, MRI studies have poor sensitivity and specificity for neuropsychiatric lupus (reviewed in Jeltsch-David and Muller, 2014). As a consequence, the diagnosis of neuropsychiatric SLE remains essentially clinical since, despite several efforts, there are no reliable biomarkers. Several reports suggested that anti-double-stranded DNA (dsDNA) antibodies cross-reacting with a short peptide sequence of the NR2 subunit of the NMDAR had a role in the pathogenesis of neuropsychiatric SLE (DeGiorgio et al., 2001, Kowal et al., 2006), but the association of these antibodies with neurocognitive or other deficits was variable in different cohorts of lupus patients (reviewed in Lauvsnes and Omdal, 2012). It is possible that CSF levels of NR2 antibodies would be more helpful, but the evidence is lacking (discussed in Gulati et al., 2016). Recent evidence has implicated an abnormal type 1 interferon response in neuropsychiatric SLE, which, in turn, may mediate microglial-dependent synaptic pruning (Bialas et al., 2017).

Psychiatric presentations of neuropsychiatric SLE

Four presentations are of particular relevance to the psychiatrist.

Lupus psychosis is a rare (1.5%) (Hanly et al., 2019), but serious, presentation of neuropsychiatric SLE that usually presents early in the course of the disease, and usually in the context of other manifestations of disease activity (Pego-Reigosa and Isenberg, 2008). It can be indistinguishable from a psychotic episode in a patient with a schizophrenia-spectrum disorder. The largest study to date suggested that it is overwhelmingly a single-episode disorder (Hanly et al., 2019), although smaller studies using different ascertainment criteria have described chronic mild psychotic symptoms in a minority of patients (Pego-Reigosa and Isenberg, 2008). Anti-ribosomal P protein antibodies show some promise as a biomarker for lupus psychosis, but results are inconsistent (e.g. Haddouk et al 2009; Hanly et al., 2019).

Treatment involves antipsychotic agents, and if there is evidence of generalized SLE activity, steroids and immunosuppressive therapy (cyclophosphamide, followed by maintenance with azathioprine) are warranted (Bertsias et al., 2010). Up to 80% of patients show complete remission early on in the course of treatment (Appenzeller et al., 2008; Hanly et al., 2019).

Mood and anxiety disorders are common among SLE patients, and it is often difficult to determine whether they result from the disease activity or from a reactive process in a patient with a severe, debilitating chronic condition. Manifestations include major depression, mood disorders with depressive, manic or mixed features, generalized anxiety, specific phobias, panic disorder, or OCD (Bachen et al., 2009). There is no strong evidence to support the use of serological markers or brain imaging. Antidepressants and biofeedback-assisted cognitive behavioural therapy are the treatments of choice, but immunosuppressive treatment to control generalized activity might also lead to improvement of major depression (Bertsias et al., 2010).

Mild to moderate cognitive dysfunction is also common in patients with SLE, while severe cognitive dysfunction occurs in approximately 6% of patients (Unterman et al., 2011). Risk factors for the latter are generalized SLE activity, evidence of CNS changes on MRI (cortical atrophy or focal lesions), positive antiphospholipid antibodies, and hypertension (Tomietto et al., 2007). Attention, visual and verbal memory, executive function, and psychomotor speed are the most commonly affected domains. Young-onset (<60 years of age), rapid-onset, or moderate to severe cognitive deterioration, preceding head trauma, new-onset neurological symptoms, and recent initiation of immunosuppressive or antiplatelet/anticoagulation therapy warrant brain MRI in a patient with cognitive decline. Management aims at treating exacerbating causes and controlling vascular risk factors (Bertsias et al., 2010).

Finally, an *acute confusional state*, defined by fluctuating levels of consciousness and decreased attention of acute onset, occurs in approximately 5% of SLE patients. As in all cases of acute confusional state, regardless of the comorbid neurological diagnosis, other predisposing factors such as infections or metabolic dysfunctions need to be excluded, and both CSF analysis and brain MRI are useful investigations. If other underlying causes are excluded, a combination of steroids and immunosuppressive drugs have been found to be effective in a high proportion of patients (Bertsias et al., 2010).

Of note, corticosteroid-induced psychiatric disease occurs in approximately 5% of SLE patients treated with steroids and might be associated with hypoalbuminaemia. It manifests primarily as a mood disorder, rather than as psychosis. It is important to consider this entity in the assessment of an SLE patient, since immunosuppressive treatment aiming at controlling a primary psychiatric dysfunction might worsen the condition. Symptoms usually resolve with discontinuation of corticosteroid medication (Appenzeller et al., 2008).

Multiple sclerosis

MS is a demyelinating disorder of the CNS and is the most frequent cause of chronic neurological disability in young adults. MS is associated with a wide range of neuropsychiatric syndromes (Feinstein, 2007). A practical approach can distinguish the psychiatric manifestations seen in MS patients into two broad categories: psychiatric syndromes that can occur at any stage of the disease (major depression, bipolar disorder, and psychosis) and psychiatric syndromes more common at later stages of the disease, usually in the context of cognitive impairment (euphoria, pseudobulbar affect, and personality changes). Despite marked differences in the psychiatric manifestations, they all impact significantly on morbidity and, particularly in the case of major depression and bipolar disorder, on mortality.

Depressive symptoms are common among patients with MS, with lifetime prevalence rates of MDD as high as 25% (Patten et al., 2003). It is unclear whether depression in MS is related to the degree of disability or years of disease, as studies have reported conflicting results (reviewed in Chwastiak and Ehde, 2007), but it is clear that depressive syndromes occur throughout the natural history of disease. Patients present with similar phenomenology to primary major depression, but neurovegetative symptoms (fatigue, sleep or appetite disorders) can confuse the diagnosis. Importantly, suicide risk in MS patients was shown to be twice that of the general population (particularly in females during the first year of diagnosis) (Bronnum-Hansen et al., 2005). Predictors of suicidal intent, in another population study, included severity of major depression, alcohol abuse, and isolation (Feinstein, 2002). The biology of depression in MS is not fully understood, and according to some studies, both psychosocial determinants (disability, uncertainty, hope, and emotion-centred coping) and specific lesion locations (left medial inferior prefrontal cortex T2 lesion volume and left anterior temporal CSF volume) each account for 40% of depression variance (Feinstein et al., 2004; Lynch et al., 2001). Few studies have addressed the efficacy of antidepressants and cognitive behavioural therapy specifically in MS patients.

Elevated rates of *bipolar disorder* have been identified among MS patients, with a prevalence of around 5% (Marrie et al., 2015). The cause for bipolar disorder in the context of MS is unknown, but a biological inflammatory mechanism is postulated. Presentations at disease onset are not uncommon, which argue against an exclusive role for emotional distress due to diagnosis or disability. There are no specific treatment studies for MS-associated bipolar disorder. Mood-stabilizing medication (e.g. lithium carbonate, valproic acid) and sedation (benzodiazepines) are used in routine clinical practice.

A *psychotic episode* occurs in approximately 4% of MS patients during the course of their disease (Marrie et al., 2015). The phenomenology of MS-related psychosis is variable, with schizophreniform presentations somewhat more common than affective psychosis (Camara-Lemarroy et al., 2017; Gilberthorpe et al., 2017). Some authors have suggested the association represents comorbidity, rather than a common pathophysiology; indeed population studies have suggested an increased risk of schizophrenia in up to a third in people with MS (Eaton et al., 2010). Nonetheless, little is known about the biological basis of psychosis in MS and there are no specific treatment trials. Small-dose atypical antipsychotics are usually preferred due to a reduced risk of extrapyramidal side effects.

A series of *mood, affect, and behavioural symptoms* can develop in more advanced cases. These conditions manifest in patients with higher disability, cognitive dysfunction, and heavier total lesion load on MRI. Euphoria is defined as a fixed state of well-being, which reveals the patient's lack of insight, even in the presence of marked physical morbidity. Although this might cause distress to the caregivers, the patient does not suffer and there is no treatment. Pseudobulbar affect is a disorder in which expressions of affect are not representative of the underlying emotion, occurring in 10% of MS patients. Patients with pseudobulbar affect have uncontrollable laughing and/or crying episodes, often in the absence of an appropriate stimulus or the corresponding emotion. The biological mechanisms are poorly understood. This condition causes significant distress for both patient and family, and first-line therapy usually involves SSRIs. Other personality changes, such as irritability, apathy, or disinhibition, are also frequent in late-stage MS and might correlate with lesion location.

Lastly, the psychiatric effects of MS treatment should also be taken into consideration. As in SLE, corticosteroid treatment in MS patients might be associated with affective disorders, particularly mania, and rarely psychotic symptoms. Early reports suggested that treatment with interferon β-1b could be linked to increased rates of depression and suicidal ideation, but there is currently no evidence to link this medication with mood disorders in MS patients (Mirsky et al., 2016).

Autoimmune encephalopathies

In 1960, Brierley and colleagues described three cases of 'subacute encephalitis of later adult life mainly affecting the limbic areas' and presenting with psychiatric symptoms, mainly affective symptoms (Brierley et al., 1960); later the syndrome was recognized as occurring in association with a carcinoma (Corsellis et al., 1968). While Brierley remained agnostic as to a potential immune aetiology, the concept of limbic encephalitis (LE) has remained central to neurology. Not long after, cases of encephalopathy associated with specific autoantibodies were reported in 1966 by Lord Brain and colleagues (Brain et al., 1966). The initial description of Hashimoto's encephalopathy (now also called steroid-responsive encephalopathy associated with autoimmune thyroiditis, or SREAT) suggested that not all encephalopathies were cancer-related, although the role of thyroid antibodies in this syndrome is still debated (Litmeier et al., 2016).

Thus, until this century, LE has largely been recognized as a paraneoplastic phenomenon. Further evidence and characterization of so-called 'onconeural' antibodies which were directed against tumour antigens also expressed by the nervous system supported the relationship and definition of paraneoplastic LE (Dalmau et al., 1999). Initially, the antibodies were demonstrated by binding to different cell types on brain slices, but multiple antigenic targets have now been described. These targets are intracellular, strongly suggesting that the antibodies are not pathogenic *in vivo*; instead, they are useful biomarkers of an (incompletely understood) cytotoxic T-cell-mediated process (Graus and Dalmau, 2012). These conditions tend to be subacute with progressive neurological impairment and are not considered further here.

The modern era of autoimmune encephalitis (AIE) studies was inaugurated by the discovery of encephalopathy syndromes associated with antibodies targeting extracellular neuronal proteins (henceforth neuronal surface antibodies, or NSAbs). The most important feature of these syndromes is that, whether associated with a tumour or not, the patients almost always respond to immunotherapies and make good recoveries of most cognitive and other problems, highlighting the importance of early diagnosis.

In parallel, gene cloning and expression of membrane proteins led to the development of live cell-based assays (CBAs) which, unlike the traditional immunological assays, maintain the antigenic protein in its native conformation and can detect antibodies to extracellular targets (those having 'pathogenic potential') (Rodriguez Cruz et al., 2015). Unfortunately, for distribution, commercial

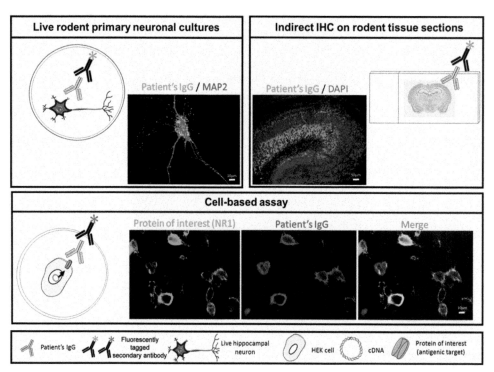

Fig. 22.1 Overview of three antibody detection techniques and representative fluorescent photomicrographs from an NMDAR antibody-positive sample. Left upper panel: schematic representation and photomicrograph of live rodent primary neuronal cultures. Rodent hippocampal neurons at 12–14 DIV are incubated with the patient's serum (or CSF) and antibody binding is detected by visual fluorescence using a secondary antibody (patient's IgG, green). Neurons are then permeabilized and counterstained with a neuronal marker (MAP2, red). Right upper panel: schematic representation and photomicrograph of indirect immunohistochemistry on rodent tissue sections. Rodent brain sections are incubated with the patient's serum (or CSF) and antibody binding is detected by visual fluorescence using a secondary antibody (patient's IgG, green). Sections are then counterstained with 4′,6-diamidino-2-phenylindole (DAPI, blue) to visualize cell nuclei. Bottom panel: schematic representation and photomicrographs of routine diagnostic CBA. Human embryonic kidney (HEK) cells are transfected with an EGFP-tagged cDNA of the protein of interest, which is expressed at the cell surface (NR1; green). Afterwards, HEK-transfected cells are incubated with the patient's serum (or CSF) and antibody binding is then detected by visual fluorescence using a secondary antibody (patient's IgG, red). IHC, immunohistochemistry.

assays have to use fixed cells in which sensitivity could be lost and the distinction between extracellular and intracellular binding may be less clear. For research purposes and for finding new antigenic targets in patients with a suspected AIE, staining of live rodent primary neuronal cultures *in vitro* or immunohistochemistry of rodent sections are useful first steps (see Fig. 22.1).

AEIs are of importance to the psychiatrist for three reasons.

Firstly, AIE commonly presents with psychiatric symptoms, although usually alongside neurological features. (Red flags for the possibility of AIE in patients presenting with psychiatric symptoms are listed in Box 22.1.) The psychiatric features can be acute and severe and require intensive and specialized psychiatric management (Irani et al., 2010b). Secondly, AIE can present with 'isolated' psychiatric symptoms which, in some cases, may represent a 'phenocopy' of a primary psychiatric disorder with few, if any, overt red flags for organicity (Kayser et al., 2013). Thirdly, the antigenic target in AIE is frequently a neurotransmitter receptor or an associated protein; these proteins are often implicated in the aetiologies of primary psychiatric disorders through pharmacological models or genetic associations (Pollak et al., 2016).

Here, the different antibody-associated forms of AIE will be briefly described. It should be appreciated that in a field led by neurologists, a detailed description of psychiatric symptomatology beyond broad descriptors such as 'personality change', 'mood problems', and 'psychosis' is often lacking.

Box 22.1 Clinical red flags for the possibility of autoimmune encephalitis in a patient presenting with psychiatric symptoms

- Subacute onset (<3 months)
- Speech dysfunction
- Seizures
- Catatonia
- Movement disorder
- Decreased conscious level
- Significant cognitive impairment
- Autonomic instability
- Neuroleptic sensitivity/NMS
- Hyponatraemia
- Headache

Supportive paraclinical features

- MRI abnormality (T2/FLAIR hyperintensities in medial temporal lobe; atrophy)
- EEG abnormalities (slowing, focal epileptiform activity, extreme delta brush)
- CSF lymphocytic pleocytosis
- PET/SPECT regional hypermetabolism

Source data from Al-Diwani et al., 2017, Herken and Prüss, 2017, Rickards et al., 2014

NMDAR-antibody encephalitis

This is now the commonest and best known form of AIE and of direct relevance to psychiatry. First described in 2007 in young women with ovarian teratoma who presented with psychosis, seizures, and catatonia, NMDAR-antibody encephalitis is a severe multi-stage disorder with a characteristic symptomatic progression in the majority of cases (Dalmau et al., 2007). The commonest psychiatric phenomena in isolated psychiatric presentations include delusions, visual and auditory hallucinations, and aggression. A viral or 'viral-like' prodrome occurs in approximately 20% of patients who then progress to prominent psychiatric and behavioural disturbance, cognitive dysfunction, and seizures of variable semiology (Irani et al., 2010b). These features are usually followed by movement disorder (including catatonia), dysautonomia, and coma. Patients are often children or younger adult females, but affected males are not uncommon. The formal diagnosis of 'definite NMDAR-antibody encephalitis' (Graus et al., 2016) rests on the presence of CSF or serum NMDAR antibodies, although a positive serum result requires evidence of additional confirmatory immunoassays which are usually restricted to research settings. Retrospective encephalitis case series suggest that the prevalence may be greater than that of herpes simplex encephalitis (Gable et al., 2012) and approximates to 1–2 per million per year.

Around 80% of patients initially presented to mental health services (Dalmau et al., 2008), although this proportion has reduced with time and increasing awareness of the disorder among physicians. In terms of psychiatric symptomatology, NMDAR encephalitis appears to have a particularly close association with psychosis and catatonia. Case series suggest that the psychotic presentation is polymorphic, with predominant affective components, rather than schizophreniform in nature—indeed there appears to be no one-to-one correspondence with specific psychosis-spectrum diagnostic constructs in current use (Al-Diwani et al., 2019; Warren et al., 2018).

In the largest observational case series, 4% of presentations of NMDAR encephalitis were with isolated psychiatric symptoms (mainly psychosis), but this increased to 28% if patients relapsed (Kayser et al., 2013). Psychiatric phenomenology in isolated psychiatric presentations was broadly similar to the more common fulminant presentation, with delusions, visual and auditory hallucinations, and aggression common. The demarcation between AIE presenting with isolated psychiatric symptoms and a primary psychiatric disorder associated with neuronal autoantibodies is discussed further below.

Encephalitis associated with antibodies to voltage-gated potassium channel-complexed proteins

First described in 2001, voltage-gated potassium channel (VGKC)-antibody encephalitis tends to present with memory deficits, disorientation, and temporal lobe seizures, although psychiatric features, including psychosis, depression, and anxiety, have all been described (Buckley et al., 2001; Prüss and Lennox, 2016; Somers et al., 2011). It is largely a disorder of later life (median incidence around 60 years), with a male-to-female ratio of approximately 3:2.

Although the antibodies were initially thought to bind the VGKC itself, they bind mainly to one of two proteins that are tightly complexed with the VGKC—CASPR2 or LGI1 (Irani et al., 2010a). LGI1 antibodies are predominantly associated with classical LE, usually non-paraneoplastic; this is often preceded by a distinctive seizure semiology termed faciobrachial dystonic seizures (FBDS) which presents as brief dystonic posturing of one arm and the ipsilateral side of the face. CASPR2 antibodies can also be found with LE, but this antibody more typically associates with insomnia, confusion and hallucinations, autonomic dysfunction, and, when noticed, evidence of peripheral nervous system hyperexcitability causing muscle fasciculations and cramps (Liguori et al., 2001). This rare syndrome, called Morvan's syndrome, can be misdiagnosed as a primary psychiatric disease if the peripheral and systemic features are not recognized (Spinazzi et al., 2008).

Encephalitis associated with antibodies to other neuronal antigens

Other antibodies associated with an autoimmune form of LE are directed against the AMPA receptor (AMPAR) (Lai et al., 2009) or GABA-B receptor (Lancaster et al., 2010). These conditions are frequently associated with tumours (often breast, lung, or thymomas) but, like non-paraneoplastic LE, tend to do well with immunotherapies, although the prognosis when tumour-associated is never so good, relapses are common and long-term recovery more limited.

Dopamine D2 receptor antibodies have been described in paediatric dyskinetic encephalitis lethargica, Tourette syndrome, and paediatric psychosis (Dale et al., 2012; Pathmanandavel et al., 2015), although there have been few confirmatory studies and other antibodies may also play a role in those in whom immunotherapy responses appear to be good.

New antigens associated with AE are reported every few months, although the number of patients described in each report is often small and the phenotype of the associated encephalopathy relatively non-specific (notable exceptions include IgLON5 antibodies, which associate with an encephalopathy syndrome featuring prominent non-REM and REM parasomnia with breathing dysfunction and gait disorder (Sabater et al., 2014)).

Mechanisms and aetiology

Pathogenic autoantibodies in AIE often have a common mechanism of action—divalent binding of antibodies to their targets on the surface of a neuronal membrane leads to internalization of the target protein. The best studied example is the NMDAR. On neurones cultured *in vitro*, the antibodies bind, which, over hours, leads to internalization of NMDARs. This causes receptor hypofunction and is assumed to result in systems-level brain dysfunction due to reduced glutamate-mediated currents and synaptic plasticity (Dalmau et al., 2008; Hughes et al., 2010). Since the effects of NMDAR antagonists, such as ketamine, recapitulate positive, negative, and psychomotor features of psychotic disorders (Javitt et al., 2012), the psychosis and catatonia in NMDAR encephalitis may represent a remarkable *in vivo* confirmation of the NMDAR hypofunction model of psychosis. AMPAR antibodies also internalize their targets, but GABA-B receptor antibodies appear to inhibit directly receptor function (Nibber et al., 2017). LGI1 antibodies act by displacing LGI1 from its location that forms a complex between presynaptic VGKCs and post-synaptic AMPARs in central synapses (Ohkawa et al., 2013).

NMDAR encephalitis was initially described in association with ovarian teratoma (Dalmau et al., 2007), although estimates of teratoma prevalence in the disorder are currently around 30%, with the highest proportion in young women. Teratoma tissue expresses the NMDAR in both NMDAR encephalitis patients and those without neurological disease (Clark et al., 2014), suggesting that ectopic expression of the receptor is the initiator of autoimmunity. AIE associated with other antigens have neoplastic associations to varying degrees (e.g. GABA-B encephalitis is commonly associated with small-cell lung carcinoma, but dopamine-2 receptor (D2R) encephalitis is reported mainly in children, and not in association with any cancer), but as a whole the disorder is not thought to be paraneoplastic in the majority of cases. This raises the question of what initiates autoimmunity in non-paraneoplastic cases.

In recent years, serum and CSF NMDAR antibodies have been noted in patients experiencing symptomatic relapse following HSV encephalitis, including small children (Armangue et al., 2014; Hacohen et al., 2014). Previously thought to be a recurrence of viral encephalitis, many of these cases show no evidence of ongoing viral infection and it is now understood that these patients are likely suffering from a post-infectious AE. Whether it is the viral infection itself or the neuronal damage (and subsequent exposure of neuronal antigens to the immune system) that initiates autoimmunity in these patients is not known. On the one hand, NSAbs have been described in association with an increasing number of neurotropic viral infections, including cytomegalovirus (CMV), Ebstein–Barr virus (EBV), varicella-zoster virus (VZV), and influenza (Linnoila et al., 2016, Prüss et al., 2014)—as well as non-encephalitic HSV infection (Salovin et al., 2018). On the other hand, they have also been described very occasionally in conditions where the primary pathology is understood to be neurodegenerative or characterized by neuronal tissue damage such as CJD, AD, or even peripheral nerve injury (Busse et al., 2014; Doss et al., 2014; Mackay et al., 2012; Prüss et al., 2014).

'Atypical' presentations

Many patients with atypical manifestations of NSAb-associated CNS disease have been described, resulting in a 'phenotype spread' phenomenon for most antigens (Irani et al., 2014). Atypical neurological manifestations include isolated seizure syndromes (Dubey et al., 2017), dementia and cognitive syndromes (Doss et al., 2014; Pruss et al., 2012), and movement disorders (Damato et al., 2018). The relevance or pathogenicity of NSAbs in such cases is not always clear, however, particularly if an immunotherapy response was not demonstrated.

NSAbs have been described in non-encephalitic neurological disorders with unknown aetiology (e.g. idiopathic or cryptogenic epilepsy), as well as in disorders where the likely aetiology is known such as dementia. Therefore, when NSAbs are found in primary psychiatric disorders (see Neuronal surface antibodies in psychiatry, p. 251), it is not always clear whether these antibodies are relevant to the clinical presentation. There are some emerging data, however, to suggest that when found in neurological disorders, such as epilepsy or dementia, or even some cancers, NSAbs predispose an individual towards a clinical presentation with more severe psychiatric symptomatology or cognitive impairment (Bartels et al., 2019; Busse et al., 2014; Ekizoglu et al., 2014); whether these patients respond to immunotherapies has not yet been studied systematically.

Treatment and outcome

Treatment for AIE involves immunotherapies to suppress antibody production. As such, first-line therapies include high-dose (usually intravenous) corticosteroids, intravenous immunoglobulins, or plasma exchange. Second-line immunosuppressive treatments include cyclophosphamide, mycophenolate mofetil, or B-cell-depleting therapies such as rituximab. Timely initiation of treatment is essential and associated with reduced mortality and better functional and cognitive outcomes (Irani et al., 2013; Titulaer et al., 2013). Given the turnaround time for laboratory testing of NSAbs in some locations, immunotherapy is frequently initiated empirically before a positive test is returned. In recognition of this necessity, diagnostic guidelines for 'probable AE' have been developed (Graus et al., 2016) alongside more recently developed guidelines aimed at recognising 'autoimmune psychosis' in mental health contexts (Pollak et al., 2020).

Beyond immunological treatments, there is often significant need for psychiatric input in the management of patients with AIE who can be highly agitated while on medical wards, presenting risk to themselves and others. No trials of psychiatric medications in AIE have been attempted, but a consensus on principles of best treatment practice may be emerging. Management of acute behavioural disturbance is probably best attempted initially with non-neuroleptic medications such as benzodiazepines. In NMDAR and some other encephalitides, these may have a special role in the treatment of catatonia, in which case large doses may be required.

There is emerging evidence that AIE may be associated with increased sensitivity to antipsychotic medication, resulting in an NMS-type clinical picture and even rhabdomyolysis (Lejuste et al., 2016; Lim et al., 2016). The diagnosis is complicated by overlap of the presenting features of NMS (catatonia, agitation, confusion, rigidity, autonomic instability) and of AE; indeed, there exist case reports where an NMS-type presentation was the presenting feature of AIE in patients who had previously received a psychiatric diagnosis (Punja et al., 2013). The mechanism behind this sensitivity remains unclear but is likely to be related to the dopamine-blocking effects of antipsychotics. For this reason, most authors recommend the use of second-generation sedating antipsychotics in patients who cannot be adequately managed with benzodiazepines alone.

Reports of successful use of ECT in cases of AIE raise the intriguing possibility that ECT has a hitherto uncharacterized immunological mechanism of action. Successful use of ECT has been described in patients refractory to first- and second-line immunotherapies, and improvement of neurological and psychiatric symptoms alike have been noted (Gough et al., 2016) alongside more recently developed guidelines aimed at recognising 'autoimmune psychosis' in mental health contexts (Pollak et al., 2020).

Recovery from AIE can be impressive, with even comatose patients returning to premorbid or near-premorbid function. However, initial widespread optimism has been tempered somewhat, as quantitative neuropsychological and neuroimaging studies have demonstrated that brain damage and cognitive dysfunction may persist for years after the acute illness, even in cases in which recovery is felt to be good on coarser measures of functioning (Butler et al., 2014; Finke et al., 2012; Irani et al., 2013). Scant attention has been paid to psychiatric outcomes following AIE—what little information there is suggests that psychiatric sequelae and even emergence of *de novo* psychiatric disorders of varying severity may occur more commonly than is currently recognized (Sarkis et al., 2014) and may represent a considerable area of unmet clinical need.

Neuronal surface antibodies in psychiatry

A more recent and emerging focus at the interface of neuroimmunology and psychiatry concerns the prevalence and possible pathogenicity of NSAbs in patients with a primary psychiatric diagnosis. There have been a number of published case studies detailing the clinical presentation and treatment response of these patients (summarized in Table 22.1), in addition to a modest, but expanding, list of studies of NSAb prevalence in patient groups in a number of psychiatric disorders. Two meta-analyses have attempted to summarize the literature on NSAbs in psychiatric patient groups, focusing on NMDAR antibodies in psychiatric disorders (Pearlman and Najjar, 2014; Pollak et al., 2014). The focus on psychotic disorders reflects the dominance of psychotic symptoms in the psychiatric presentation of encephalopathies associated with NSAbs, particularly NMDAR antibodies. This focus may owe more to the fact that the psychotic symptoms have a clinical impact which often surpasses that of other psychiatric symptoms. Psychotic symptoms are not so common in the non-NMDAR encephalopathies, and testing for antibodies to NMDAR and other targets in a wider range of psychiatric disorders may be worthwhile.

Overall, it appears that antibodies against neuronal cell surface membrane proteins (or associated proteins) are detectable in the blood of a small proportion of patients with primary psychiatric diagnoses. However, whether the prevalence of antibody positivity is significantly different to that of healthy adults who are not symptomatic is still uncertain. Typically, studies restrict themselves to measuring serum antibodies using CBAs. Relatively few studies have attempted confirmatory antibody testing with other kinds of immunoassay (Bergink et al., 2015; Pathmanandavel et al., 2015) or assessed the functional impact of NSAbs found in the serum of patients with psychiatric disorders (Castillo-Gomez et al., 2016; Choe et al., 2013; Hammer et al., 2014). Importantly, few CSF samples have been available for study. A recent series of studies from Bordeaux have demonstrated that serum NMDAR antibodies from individuals with psychosis *can* have profound effects on receptor dynamics and neuronal function, suggesting pathogenic *potential* (Jezequel et al., 2017a,b, 2018).

Psychotic disorders

Most research published to date on NSAbs in psychiatric disorders has focused on NMDAR antibodies. The largest prospective study published to date in a first-episode psychosis population reported NMDAR antibodies in 3% of 228 patients with a first episode of psychosis and none in an age-matched control group (Lennox et al., 2017); GABA-A receptor antibodies were also present in another 3.5% of patients and in the control group. Other studies indicate that controls are not always negative for NMDAR antibodies and possibly other NSAbs, and an earlier review and meta-analysis of smaller studies indicated, more conservatively, that patients with a psychotic disorder were around three times more likely to test positive for these antibodies (Pearlman and Najjar, 2014). It is likely that differences in the assays used to detect NSAbs contribute significantly to the heterogeneity in the prevalence in psychiatric populations. In general, studies using CBAs that use live, non-permeabilized cells (Jezequel et al., 2017a; Lennox et al., 2017;

Pathmanandavel et al., 2015; Zandi et al., 2011) have found patient–control differences more consistently than have studies using fixed and permeabilized cells (Dahm et al., 2014; Hammer et al., 2014; Masopust et al., 2015).

The occurrence and significance of other NSAbs have been investigated in psychosis populations, albeit in fewer studies (see Table 22.1). Prevalence estimates in patients with psychosis vary between 2% and 7% (Dahm et al., 2014; Endres et al., 2015; Lennox et al., 2017; Schou et al., 2016), with some studies finding no evidence of NSAbs in patient groups (de Witte et al., 2015; van Mierlo et al., 2015). Dopamine receptor antibodies have also been identified, with reports of between 0% and 9.5% prevalence, including children (Muller et al., 2014; Pathmanandavel et al., 2015; Tanaka et al., 2003), and GABA-A receptor antibodies were found in 4% of psychotic patients (Endres et al., 2015; Haussleiter et al., 2012; Lennox et al., 2017). In general, AMPAR antibodies have not been reported at significant rates (Haussleiter et al., 2012; Lennox et al., 2017; Steiner et al., 2013).

Initially, data suggested that NSAbs were more prevalent in the early stages of a psychotic disorder, compared to later, chronic, or treatment-refractory stages of the disorder (Pollak et al., 2014). However, this has been challenged by more recent studies that have reported seropositivity in patients, even in the chronic stages of a psychotic disorder (Beck et al., 2015).

Non-psychotic disorders

NMDAR antibody prevalence in affective disorders ranges between 2.6% and 10.5%, with no clear difference compared to healthy adults (Dahm et al., 2014; Pearlman and Najjar, 2014; Steiner et al., 2013), although there is some evidence that acute mania may be associated with an elevated NMDAR antibody titre (Dickerson et al., 2012).

There is converging evidence to suggest that some neuropsychiatric disorders featuring tics and/or obsessions and compulsions have an autoimmune component, and attention has accordingly focused on establishing associations with NSAbs. Somewhat divergent from the literature described up to this point, which has mainly relied on CBAs, reactivity to the dopamine D2R was described using enzyme-linked immunosorbent assay (ELISA) and western blot assays on antibodies from patients with basal ganglia disorders associated with streptococcal infection, including Sydenham's chorea and paediatric autoimmune neuropsychiatric disorders associated with streptococcal infections (PANDAS) (Brimberg et al., 2012). Studies that have used CBAs to detect D2R antibodies have been less consistent, with antibodies detected in Sydenham's chorea, Tourette syndrome, and paediatric dyskinetic encephalitis lethargica, but not PANDAS (Dale et al., 2012). One study has reported seropositivity for NMDAR antibodies in four out of 21 children with Tourette syndrome (Dua et al., 2014), although a larger, more recent paper found negligible rates of NMDAR antibodies in children with tic disorders (Baglioni et al., 2019).

Maternal antibodies to neuronal proteins, transferred to the fetus during neurodevelopment, have been postulated to cause damage to developing neuronal circuits and neurodevelopmental disorders in the offspring. A first pilot study (Dalton et al., 2003) reported antibodies binding to neuronal proteins in one mother of two consecutive children, one with autism and one with a speech disorder, and showed that pregnant mouse dams injected with that sera had pups that displayed deficits in neuromotor coordination and changes in cerebellar metabolites, assessed by MRS. A specific antibody target was not found at the time. Since then, several publications have assessed the presence of antibodies towards fetal antigens in the sera

Table 22.1 Neurological and psychiatric associations of neuronal surface antibodies

Antigen	Main encephalopathy syndrome; which psychiatric features?	Other associated neurological disorders	Antigen description/epitope	Antibodies in isolated psychiatric syndromes
NMDAR	Encephalopathy (usually extralimbic). Psychiatric features include anxiety, agitation, bizarre behaviour, catatonia, delusional or paranoid thoughts, and visual or auditory hallucinations. Also movement disorder, seizures, autonomic instability (Irani et al., 2010b; Kayser et al., 2013; Titulaer et al., 2013)	Post-herpes simplex encephalitis relapse with chorea; idiopathic epilepsy; immunotherapy-responsive dementia (Doss et al., 2014; Prüss et al., 2012)	Ligand-gated ion channel. Antibodies bind to ATD of NR1 subunit (Gleichman et al., 2012). Antibodies to NR2 subunit reported in some patients with neuropsychiatric SLE, but not diagnostic (Lauvsnes and Omdal, 2012)	Case reports and series: psychosis, autism, BPAD, and eating disorders (Choe et al., 2013; Creten et al., 2011; Heresco-Levy et al., 2015; Mechelhoff et al., 2015; Perogamvros et al., 2012; Zandi et al., 2014) Prevalence: meta-analyses: schizophrenia 7% (IgG, A + M), only FEP greater than controls (Pollak et al., 2014); odds ratio of seropositivity in schizophrenia, schizoaffective disorder, BPAD, or MDD versus controls = 3.1 (Pearlman and Najjar, 2014), but note subsequent studies show, variously, zero prevalence (de Witte et al., 2015; Masopust et al., 2015), no difference from controls (Dahm et al., 2014; Steiner et al., 2014) or 3% prevalence in FEP (Lennox et al., 2017) Treatment-refractory psychosis 7% (Beck et al., 2015); post-partum psychosis 2% (Bergink et al., 2015); paediatric psychosis 14% (Pathmanandavel et al., 2015); borderline personality disorder 2.4% (Dahm et al., 2014)
LGI1	LE with or without faciobrachial dystonic seizures. Psychiatric features include confusion, hallucinations, and depression (Irani et al., 2010a)	Morvan's syndrome, NMT, epilepsy, REM sleep behaviour disorder (Irani et al., 2010a)	VGKC- and AMPAR-associated secreted molecule	Prevalence: schizophrenia 0.1%; not found in affective disorders or borderline PD (Dahm et al., 2014). FEP 1% (Lennox et al., 2017)
CASPR2	Morvan's syndrome. Psychiatric features include confusion, hallucinations, agitation, and delusions (Irani et al., 2011)	LE, NMT, epilepsy (Irani et al., 2010a). Autonomic dysfunction	VGKC-associated axonal/nodal and synaptic protein. Multiple epitopes in extracellular domain (Olsen et al., 2015; Pinatel et al., 2015)	Prevalence: schizophrenia 1.5%; affective disorder 0.6%, not found in borderline PD (Dahm et al., 2014). FEP 1% (Lennox et al., 2017)
AMPAR	LE. Psychiatric features include confusion, personality change, psychosis, apathy, agitation, and confabulation (Dogan Onugoren et al., 2014; Hoftberger et al., 2015; Lai et al., 2009)	n/a	Ligand-gated ion channel Bottom lobe of ATD (Gleichman et al., 2014)	Case reports: psychosis associated with LE (Elamin et al., 2015; Graus et al., 2010) Prevalence: not found in schizophrenia, FEP, affective disorders, or borderline PD (Dahm et al., 2014; Lennox et al., 2017)
GABA-A receptor	LE with refractory seizures. Psychiatric features include confusion, affective changes (including depression), and hallucinations (Petit-Pedrol et al., 2014)	Varied presentations (Pettingill et al., 2015)	Ligand-gated ion channel α_1 or β_3 subunits (Petit-Pedrol et al., 2014) α_1 and γ_2 subunits (Pettingill et al., 2015)	Cases described with predominant anxiety and catatonia (Pettingill et al., 2015). Case report of seropositive schizophrenia (Haussleiter et al., 2017) Prevalence: 4% FEP (Lennox et al., 2017)
GABA-B receptor	LE with refractory status epilepticus. Psychiatric features include psychosis, agitation, and catatonia (Dogan Onugoren et al., 2014; Lancaster et al., 2010)	Opsoclonus-myoclonus; cerebellar ataxia; PERM (Hoftberger et al., 2013; Lancaster et al., 2010)	Ligand-gated ion channel	No relevant case reports Prevalence: 0.3% of affective disorder (Dahm et al., 2014)

D2R	'Basal ganglia encephalitis' with prominent movement disorder (dystonia, parkinsonism, chorea, tics). Psychiatric features include agitation, depression, psychosis, and emotional lability	SC, PANDAS (Cox et al., 2013)	Metabotropic receptor. IgG from SC, but not PANDAS, patients binds to extracellular epitope at ATD (Cox et al., 2013)	No relevant case reports Prevalence: paediatric psychosis 7% (Pathmanandavel et al., 2015); Tourette syndrome 9% (Dale et al., 2012); not found in acute exacerbation of established schizophrenia (Muller et al., 2014)
DPPX	LE with enteropathy. Psychiatric features include amnesia, delirium, psychosis, and depression (Boronat et al., 2013; Tobin et al., 2014)	PERM (Balint et al., 2014)	Auxiliary subunit of Kv4.2 potassium channels	Prevalence: 0.1% of schizophrenia (Dahm et al., 2014)
MGluR5	'Ophelia syndrome': LE in association with Hodgkin's lymphoma. One case of LE without lymphoma. Psychiatric features include depression, anxiety, delusions, visual and auditory hallucinations, and anterograde amnesia (Lancaster et al., 2011)	n/a	Metabotropic receptor	Prevalence: 0.1% of schizophrenia (Doss et al., 2014)

ATD, amino terminal domain; BPAD, bipolar affective disorder; CBA, cell-based assay; ELISA, enzyme-linked immunosorbent assay; FEP, first-episode psychosis; LE, limbic encephalitis; MDD, major depressive disorder; NMT, neuromyotonia; PD, personality disorder; PERM, progressive encephalomyelitis with rigidity and myoclonus; RIA, radioimmunoassay; SC, Sydenham's chorea; PANDAS, paediatric autoimmune neuropsychiatric disorders associated with streptococcal infections.

Adapted from Pollak, T. A., et al. Autoantibodies to central nervous system neuronal surface antigens: psychiatric symptoms and psychopharmacological implications. *Psychopharmacology*, 233: 1605–21. Copyright © 2015, The Author(s). https://doi.org/10.1007/s00213-015-4156-y.

of mothers of autistic children (reviewed in Estes and McAllister, 2015). Until recently, none of these studies had demonstrated the presence of a specific antibody to a known neuronal target that had the potential to be pathogenic, and none validated a specific antibody as pathogenic by passive immunization in an animal model. A recent publication (Brimberg et al., 2016), however, reported CASPR2 antibodies in 37% of mothers of autism cases whose sera were found to bind to brain extracts on a western blot, but also in 8–12% of controls. These findings were not replicated by us in another cohort of mothers of children with autism, but maternal CASPR2 antibodies were raised in mothers of children with intellectual and motor disabilities (Coutinho et al., 2017a). Further studies assessing the clinical phenotype of children born to mothers with CASPR2 antibodies and standardization of antibody detection methods are necessary. Despite these divergent results, long-lasting changes in brain histology and behaviour were identified in mice exposed to CASPR2 antibodies *in utero* (Brimberg et al., 2016; Coutinho et al., 2017b), confirming the pathogenic potential of CASPR2 antibodies in neurodevelopmental disorders.

Implications of NSAbs in psychiatric disorders

There are a number of considerations regarding the possible pathogenicity of anti-neuronal antibodies in psychiatric populations and their implications for clinical practice. Nosologically, there is ample room for confusion. It is incorrect to state, as some authors have, that the presence of potentially pathogenic NSAbs in blood or the CSF of a psychiatric patient means that, diagnostically, that patient should be considered to have autoimmune encephalitis. Others have preferred terms such as 'attenuated syndromes', 'monosymptomatomic presentations' or '*formes frustes*' to convey the idea that, in essence, the patient has a 'mild' form of encephalopathy. Nonetheless, these terms are still inadequate, as they presuppose a pathogenic, disease-relevant role for the NSAb in question, a role that has not been decisively demonstrated.

The Koch/Witebsky postulates, outlined at the start of this chapter, place strict demands on the establishment of causality in any putatively autoimmune disorder. A full discussion of whether any of the postulates have been met with regard to NSAbs and psychiatric symptoms is beyond the scope of this chapter (see Coutinho et al., 2014 for an in-depth analysis), but it is clear that further mechanistic studies are required. Furthermore, these mechanistic studies must be clear in distinguishing patients seropositive for NSAbs with autoimmune encephalitis from patients with psychiatric disorders who do not have these autoantibodies.

Al-Diwani and colleagues have proposed the pragmatic category of 'synaptic and neuronal autoantibody-associated psychiatric syndromes' (SNAps) to delineate this patient group (Al-Diwani et al., 2017). Clearly, they argue, SNAps should not be considered as AIE since the majority of these patients do not go on to develop the full symptom spectrum of encephalitis (there will, of course, be rare cases of 'encephalitis caught early'). On the other hand, it is premature, at a scientific and at a clinical level, to dismiss NSAbs in psychiatric patients as 'epiphenomenal' or 'false-positive results'. On the contrary, the possibility that NSAbs may represent a marker of immunotherapy response in these patients mandates an expanding agenda of mechanistic and clinical studies of these patients.

There are an increasing number of case reports and series documenting symptom improvement when NSAb-positive patients with psychiatric disorders are treated with immunotherapy. Yoshimura and Takaki reviewed the case report literature for presentations of NMDAR antibody-associated syndromes presenting without seizures, involuntary movements, hypoventilation, or tumours. Twelve patients presented with psychiatric or cognitive symptoms, with few or no neurological or motor symptoms—every one of these patients responded well to immunotherapy (Yoshimura and Takaki, 2017). Clearly, however, case reports are highly subject to publication bias in that a patient who showed no immunotherapy response is less likely to be considered worthy of submission to, or publication by, a journal. In the largest case series to date, Zandi and colleagues reported the response to immunotherapy of nine patients with acute psychosis and NMDAR antibodies; eight responded to treatment, with six achieving symptomatic remission (Zandi et al., 2014). Nonetheless, while open-label, these exciting data must be treated with caution. RCTs of immunotherapy in the treatment of NSAb-positive psychiatric patients are currently under way and may show promise yet as an example of the shift towards *personalized medicine* in an area where biological treatments have, for decades, been broadly similar, in terms of both mechanisms of action and clinical efficacy.

Clinical implications

NSAb testing in clinical psychiatric practice is increasingly commonplace in Europe and the United States, but given that the significance of a positive serum sample is still unclear, who should clinicians test and what should they make of a positive result? One approach may be to preferentially screen psychiatric patients who present with so-called 'red flag' signs. These are 'encephalopathy-like' features that might indicate a higher index of suspicion for organic disease with a psychiatric presentation. They include focal neurological signs, significant speech disorder, seizures, movement disorder or catatonia, decreased conscious level, autonomic instability, or neuroleptic sensitivity (Al-Diwani et al., 2017; Herken and Prüss, 2017). An associated tumour should always be considered particularly if the patients have NMDAR (teratoma), CASPR2 (thymoma), or GABA-B receptor (lung, breast, or thymoma) antibodies.

Additionally, paraclinical supportive evidence for the relevance of a positive serum NSAb result (even in the absence of the *clinical* red flag signs described above) would include MRI abnormalities (particular T2 or FLAIR high signal in medial temporal areas), an encephalopathic EEG or the presence of focal epileptiform discharges, and CSF abnormalities, including lymphocytic pleocytosis or unmatched oligoclonal bands (and in areas where it is routine, regional hypermetabolism on PET or SPECT) (Pollak et al., 2020). Early involvement of neurology colleagues is crucial, both at the assessment stage and, if relevant, in consideration of immunotherapies. In the UK, specialist psychiatry–neurology joint clinics for patients with suspected autoimmune psychiatric involvement have been developed, with the aim of providing comprehensive assessment, investigation, and neuroimmunological expertise to this complex patient group.

In a field that is rapidly evolving, best practice is likely to change equally rapidly. Of some note is the fact that, at a clinical population level, studies have failed to demonstrate clinically meaningful differences between NSAb-positive and NSAb-negative patients with psychiatric disorders (Hammer et al., 2014; Lennox et al., 2017). That is, when clinical psychiatric patients are screened 'blindly' for NSAbs, those who are seropositive *do not* appear more encephalopathic or more 'organic' nor do they have appreciable differences in presenting psychopathology. It is apparent, then, that if randomized trials demonstrate that NSAb seropositivity is indeed an indicator of immunotherapy response in a particular psychiatric population, the above notion of red flag signs will clearly be superseded by the requirement to screen all such patients for NSAbs of interest.

KEY LEARNING POINTS

- Evidence continues to be found to suggest the close link of the CNS and the immune system in neuropsychiatric disorders.
- As interest in AIEs, produced by the interaction of NSAbs with proteins such as the NMDAR and LGI1, increased over the last decade, the clinical interface between psychiatry and neurology underwent significant advances.
- This chapter provides a basic overview of autoimmunity, before discussing recent findings. Firstly, autoimmune disorders which commonly present with psychiatric comorbidities are explored such as SLE and MS. Then, the psychiatric presentations of various autoimmune forms of encephalitis are discussed, along with their treatment and outcomes. Finally, the relevance of NSAbs to psychiatry is discussed in greater detail.

REFERENCES

Al-Diwani, A., et al. 2017. Synaptic and neuronal autoantibody-associated psychiatric syndromes (SNAps): Controversies and Hypotheses. *Frontiers in Psychiatry*, 8, 13.

Al-Diwani, A., et al. 2019. The psychopathology of NMDAR-antibody encephalitis in adults: a systematic review and phenotypic analysis of individual patient data. *Lancet Psychiatry*, 6, 235–46.

Appenzeller, S., et al. 2008. Acute psychosis in systemic lupus erythematosus. *Rheumatol Int*, 28, 237–43.

Armangue, T., et al. 2014. Herpes simplex virus encephalitis is a trigger of brain autoimmunity. *Ann Neurol*, 75, 317–23.

Bachen, E. A., et al. 2009. Prevalence of mood and anxiety disorders in women with systemic lupus erythematosus. *Arthritis Rheum*, 61, 822–9.

Baglioni, V., et al. 2019. Antibodies to neuronal surface proteins in Tourette Syndrome: Lack of evidence in a European paediatric cohort. *Brain, Behavior, and Immunity*, 81, 665-9. doi:10.1016/j.bbi.2019.08.008.

Balint, B., et al. 2014. Progressive encephalomyelitis with rigidity and myoclonus: a new variant with DPPX antibodies. *Neurology*, 82, 1521–8.

Bartels, F., et al. 2019. Neuronal Autoantibodies Associated with Cognitive Impairment in Melanoma Patients. *Ann Oncol*, 30, 823–9.

Beck, K., et al. 2015. Prevalence of serum N-methyl-D-aspartate receptor autoantibodies in refractory psychosis. *Br J Psychiatry*, 206, 164–5.

Benros, M. E., et al. 2011. Autoimmune diseases and severe infections as risk factors for schizophrenia: a 30-year population-based register study. *Am J Psychiatry*, 168, 1303–10.

Benros, M. E., et al. 2014. A nationwide study on the risk of autoimmune diseases in individuals with a personal or a family history of schizophrenia and related psychosis. *Am J Psychiatry*, 171, 218–26.

Bergink, V., et al. 2015. Autoimmune Encephalitis in Postpartum Psychosis. *Am J Psychiatry*, appiajp201514101332.

Bertsias, G. K., et al. 2010. EULAR recommendations for the management of systemic lupus erythematosus with neuropsychiatric manifestations: report of a task force of the EULAR standing committee for clinical affairs. *Ann Rheum Dis*, 69, 2074–82.

Bialas, A. R., et al. 2017. Microglia-dependent synapse loss in type I interferon-mediated lupus. *Nature*, 546, 539–43.

Boronat, A., et al. 2013. Encephalitis and antibodies to dipeptidyl-peptidase-like protein-6, a subunit of Kv4.2 potassium channels. *Ann Neurol*, 73, 120–8.

Brain, L., et al. 1966. Hashimoto's and encephalopathy. *Lancet*, 288, 512–14.

Brierley, J. B., et al. 1960. Subacute encephalitis of later adult life. Mainly affecting the limbic areas. *Brain*, 83, 357–68.

Brimberg, L., et al. 2012. Behavioral, pharmacological, and immunological abnormalities after streptococcal exposure: a novel rat model of Sydenham chorea and related neuropsychiatric disorders. *Neuropsychopharmacology*, 37, 2076–87.

Brimberg, L., et al. 2016. Caspr2-reactive antibody cloned from a mother of an ASD child mediates an ASD-like phenotype in mice. *Mol Psychiatry*, 21, 1663–71.

Bronnum-Hansen, H., et al. 2005. Suicide among Danes with multiple sclerosis. *J Neurol Neurosurg Psychiatry*, 76, 1457–9.

Buckley, C., et al. 2001. Potassium channel antibodies in two patients with reversible limbic encephalitis. *Ann Neurol*, 50, 73–8.

Busse, S., et al. 2014. Seroprevalence of N-methyl-D-aspartate glutamate receptor (NMDA-R) autoantibodies in aging subjects without neuropsychiatric disorders and in dementia patients. *Eur Arch Psychiatry Clin Neurosci*, 264, 545–50.

Butler, C. R., et al. 2014. Persistent anterograde amnesia following limbic encephalitis associated with antibodies to the voltage-gated potassium channel complex. *J Neurol Neurosurg Psychiatry*, 85, 387–91.

Camara-Lemarroy, C. R., et al. 2017. The varieties of psychosis in multiple sclerosis: A systematic review of cases. *Mult Scler Relat Disord*, 12, 9–14.

Castillo-Gomez, E., et al. 2017. All naturally occurring autoantibodies against the NMDA receptor subunit NR1 have pathogenic potential irrespective of epitope and immunoglobulin class. *Mol Psychiatry*, 22, 1776–84.

Choe, C. U., et al. 2013. A clinical and neurobiological case of IgM NMDA receptor antibody associated encephalitis mimicking bipolar disorder. *Psychiatry Res*, 208, 194–6.

Chwastiak, L. A. & Ehde, D. M. 2007. Psychiatric issues in multiple sclerosis. *Psychiatr Clin North Am*, 30, 803–17.

Clark, R. M., et al. 2014. The N-methyl-D-aspartate receptor, a precursor to N-methyl-D-aspartate receptor encephalitis, is found in the squamous tissue of ovarian teratomas. *Int J Gynecol Pathol*, 33, 598–606.

Corsellis, J. A. N., et al. 1968. 'Limbic encephalitis' and its association with carcinoma. *Brain*, 91, 481–96.

Coutinho, E., et al. 2014. Do neuronal autoantibodies cause psychosis? A neuroimmunological perspective. *Biol Psychiatry*, 75, 269–75.

Coutinho, E., et al. 2017a. CASPR2 autoantibodies are raised during pregnancy in mothers of children with mental retardation and disorders of psychological development but not autism. *J Neurol Neurosurg Psychiatry*, 88, 718–21.

Coutinho, E., et al. 2017b. Persistent microglial activation and synaptic loss with behavioral abnormalities in mouse offspring exposed to CASPR2-antibodies in utero. *Acta Neuropathol*, 134, 567–83.

Cox, C. J., et al. 2013. Brain human monoclonal autoantibody from sydenham chorea targets dopaminergic neurons in transgenic mice and signals dopamine D2 receptor: implications in human disease. *J Immunol*, 191, 5524–41.

Creten, C., et al. 2011. Late onset autism and anti-NMDA-receptor encephalitis. *Lancet*, 378, 98.

Cullen, A. E., et al. 2019. Associations Between Non-neurological Autoimmune Disorders and Psychosis: A Meta-analysis. *Biol Psychiatry*, 85, 35–48.

Dahm, L., et al. 2014. Seroprevalence of autoantibodies against brain antigens in health and disease. *Ann Neurol*, 76, 82–94.

Dale, R. C., et al. 2012. Antibodies to surface dopamine-2 receptor in autoimmune movement and psychiatric disorders. *Brain*, 135, 3453–68.

Dalmau, J., et al. 2008. Anti-NMDA-receptor encephalitis: case series and analysis of the effects of antibodies. *Lancet Neurol*, 7, 1091–8.

Dalmau, J., et al. 1999. Paraneoplastic neurologic syndromes: pathogenesis and physiopathology. *Brain Pathol*, 9, 275–84.

Dalmau, J., et al. 2007. Paraneoplastic anti-N-methyl-D-aspartate receptor encephalitis associated with ovarian teratoma. *Ann Neurol*, 61, 25–36.

Damato, V., et al. 2018. The clinical features, underlying immunology, and treatment of autoantibody-mediated movement disorders. *Mov Disord*, 33, 1376–89.

Dalton, P., et al. 2003. Maternal neuronal antibodies associated with autism and a language disorder. *Ann Neurol*, 53, 533–7.

De Witte, L. D., et al. 2015. Absence of N-Methyl-D-Aspartate Receptor IgG Autoantibodies in Schizophrenia: The Importance of Cross-Validation Studies. *JAMA Psychiatry*, 72, 731–3.

Degiorgio, L. A., et al. 2001. A subset of lupus anti-DNA antibodies cross-reacts with the NR2 glutamate receptor in systemic lupus erythematosus. *Nat Med*, 7, 1189–93.

Dickerson, F., et al. 2012. Antibodies to the glutamate receptor in mania. *Bipolar Disord*, 14, 547–53.

Dogan Onugoren, M., et al. 2015. Limbic encephalitis due to GABAB and AMPA receptor antibodies: a case series. *J Neurol Neurosurg Psychiatry*, 86, 965–72.

Doss, S., et al. 2014. High prevalence of NMDA receptor IgA/IgM antibodies in different dementia types. *Ann Clin Transl Neurol*, 1, 822–32.

Dua, P., et al. 2014. Detection of antibodies against the N-methyl-d-aspartate receptor in a sub-group of patients diagnosed with Tourette's syndrome. *Journal of Neuroimmunology*, 275, 98.

Dubey, D., et al. 2017. Predictive models in the diagnosis and treatment of autoimmune epilepsy. *Epilepsia*, 58, 1181–9.

Eaton, W. W., et al. 2010. Autoimmune diseases, bipolar disorder, and non-affective psychosis. *Bipolar Disord*, 12, 638–46.

Ekizoglu, E., et al. 2014. Investigation of neuronal autoantibodies in two different focal epilepsy syndromes. *Epilepsia*, 55, 414–22.

Elamin, M., et al. 2015. Posterior cortical and white matter changes on MRI in anti-AMPA receptor antibody encephalitis. *Neurol Neuroimmunol Neuroinflamm*, 2, e118.

Endres, D., et al. 2015. Immunological findings in psychotic syndromes: a tertiary care hospital's CSF sample of 180 patients. *Front Hum Neurosci*, 9, 476.

Estes, M. L. & McAlllister, A. K. 2015. Immune mediators in the brain and peripheral tissues in autism spectrum disorder. *Nat Rev Neurosci*, 16, 469–86.

Feinstein, A. 2002. An examination of suicidal intent in patients with multiple sclerosis. *Neurology*, 59, 674–8.

Feinstein, A. 2007. Neuropsychiatric syndromes associated with multiple sclerosis. *J Neurol*, 254 Suppl 2, II73–6.

Feinstein, A., et al. 2004. Structural brain abnormalities in multiple sclerosis patients with major depression. *Neurology*, 62, 586–90.

Finke, C., et al. 2012. Cognitive deficits following anti-NMDA receptor encephalitis. *J Neurol Neurosurg Psychiatry*, 83, 195–8.

Gable, M. S., et al. 2012. The frequency of autoimmune N-methyl-D-aspartate receptor encephalitis surpasses that of individual viral etiologies in young individuals enrolled in the California Encephalitis Project. *Clin Infect Dis*, 54, 899–904.

Gilberthorpe, T. G., et al. 2017. The spectrum of psychosis in multiple sclerosis: a clinical case series. *Neuropsychiatr Dis Treat*, 13, 303–18.

Gleichman, A. J., et al. 2014. Antigenic and mechanistic characterization of anti-AMPA receptor encephalitis. *Ann Clin Transl Neurol*, 1, 180–9.

Gleichman, A. J., et al. 2012. Anti-NMDA receptor encephalitis antibody binding is dependent on amino acid identity of a small region within the GluN1 amino terminal domain. *J Neurosci*, 32, 11082–94.

Gough, J. L., et al. 2016. Electroconvulsive therapy and/or plasmapheresis in autoimmune encephalitis? *World J Clin Cases*, 4, 223–8.

Graus, F., et al. 2010. The expanding clinical profile of anti-AMPA receptor encephalitis. *Neurology*, 74, 857–9.

Graus, F. & Dalmau, J. 2012. Paraneoplastic neurological syndromes. *Curr Opin Neurol*, 25, 795–801.

Graus, F., et al. 2016. A clinical approach to diagnosis of autoimmune encephalitis. *Lancet Neurol*, 15, 391–404.

Gulati, G., et al. 2016. Anti-NR2 antibodies, blood-brain barrier, and cognitive dysfunction. *Clin Rheumatol*, 35, 2989–97.

Hacohen, Y., et al. 2014. NMDA receptor antibodies associated with distinct white matter syndromes. *Neurol Neuroimmunol Neuroinflamm*, 1, e2.

Haddouk, S., et al. 2009. Clinical and diagnostic value of ribosomal P autoantibodies in systemic lupus erythematosus. *Rheumatology (Oxford)*, 48, 953–7.

Hammer, C., et al. 2014. Neuropsychiatric disease relevance of circulating anti-NMDA receptor autoantibodies depends on blood-brain barrier integrity. *Mol Psychiatry*, 19, 1143–9.

Hanly, J. G., et al. 2019. Psychosis in Systemic Lupus Erythematosus: Results From an International Inception Cohort Study. *Arthritis Rheumatol*, 71, 281–9.

Haussleiter, I. S., et al. 2012. Investigation of antibodies against synaptic proteins in a cross-sectional cohort of psychotic patients. *Schizophr Res*, 140, 258–9.

Haussleiter, I. S., et al. 2017. A case of GABAR antibodies in schizophrenia. *BMC Psychiatry*, 17, 9.

Heresco-Levy, U., et al. 2015. Clinical and electrophysiological effects of D-serine in a schizophrenia patient positive for anti-N-methyl-D-aspartate receptor antibodies. *Biol Psychiatry*, 77, e27–9.

Herken, J. & Pruss, H. 2017. Red Flags: Clinical Signs for Identifying Autoimmune Encephalitis in Psychiatric Patients. *Front Psychiatry*, 8, 25.

Hoftberger, R., et al. 2013. Encephalitis and GABAB receptor antibodies: novel findings in a new case series of 20 patients. *Neurology*, 81, 1500–6.

Hoftberger, R., et al. 2015. Encephalitis and AMPA receptor antibodies: Novel findings in a case series of 22 patients. *Neurology*, 84, 2403–12.

Hughes, E. G., et al. 2010. Cellular and synaptic mechanisms of anti-NMDA receptor encephalitis. *J Neurosci*, 30, 5866–75.

Irani, S. R., et al. 2010a. Antibodies to Kv1 potassium channel-complex proteins leucine-rich, glioma inactivated 1 protein and contactin-associated protein-2 in limbic encephalitis, Morvan's syndrome and acquired neuromyotonia. *Brain*, 133, 2734–48.

Irani, S. R., et al. 2010b. N-methyl-D-aspartate antibody encephalitis: temporal progression of clinical and paraclinical observations in a predominantly non-paraneoplastic disorder of both sexes. *Brain*, 133, 1655–67.

Irani, S. R., et al. 2014. Cell-surface central nervous system autoantibodies: clinical relevance and emerging paradigms. *Ann Neurol*, 76, 168–84.

Irani, S. R., et al. 2011. Faciobrachial dystonic seizures precede Lgi1 antibody limbic encephalitis. *Ann Neurol*, 69, 892–900.

Irani, S. R., et al. 2013. Faciobrachial dystonic seizures: the influence of immunotherapy on seizure control and prevention of cognitive impairment in a broadening phenotype. *Brain*, 136, 3151–62.

Javitt, D. C., et al. 2012. Has an angel shown the way? Etiological and therapeutic implications of the PCP/NMDA model of schizophrenia. *Schizophr Bull*, 38, 958–66.

Jeltsch-David, H. & Muller, S. 2014. Neuropsychiatric systemic lupus erythematosus: pathogenesis and biomarkers. *Nat Rev Neurol*, 10, 579–96.

Jezequel, J., et al. 2017a. Dynamic disorganization of synaptic NMDA receptors triggered by autoantibodies from psychotic patients. *Nat Commun*, 8, 1791.

Jezequel, J., et al. 2017b. Cell- and Single Molecule-Based Methods to Detect Anti-N-Methyl-D-Aspartate Receptor Autoantibodies in Patients With First-Episode Psychosis From the OPTiMiSE Project. *Biol Psychiatry*, 82, 766–72.

Jezequel, J., et al. 2018. Molecular Pathogenicity of Anti-NMDA Receptor Autoantibody From Patients With First-Episode Psychosis. *Am J Psychiatry*, 175, 382–3.

Kayser, M. S., et al. 2013. Frequency and characteristics of isolated psychiatric episodes in anti-N-methyl-d-aspartate receptor encephalitis. *JAMA Neurol*, 70, 1133–9.

Kowal, C., et al. 2006. Human lupus autoantibodies against NMDA receptors mediate cognitive impairment. *Proc Natl Acad Sci U S A*, 103, 19854–9.

Lai, M., et al. 2009. AMPA receptor antibodies in limbic encephalitis alter synaptic receptor location. *Ann Neurol*, 65, 424–34.

Lancaster, E., et al. 2010. Antibodies to the GABA(B) receptor in limbic encephalitis with seizures: case series and characterisation of the antigen. *Lancet Neurol*, 9, 67–76.

Lancaster, E., et al. 2011. Antibodies to metabotropic glutamate receptor 5 in the Ophelia syndrome. *Neurology*, 77, 1698–701.

Lauvsnes, M. B. & Omdal, R. 2012. Systemic lupus erythematosus, the brain, and anti-NR2 antibodies. *J Neurol*, 259, 622–9.

Lejuste, F., et al. 2016. Neuroleptic intolerance in patients with anti-NMDAR encephalitis. *Neurol Neuroimmunol Neuroinflamm*, 3, e280.

Lennox, B. R., et al. 2017. Prevalence and clinical characteristics of serum neuronal cell surface antibodies in first-episode psychosis: a case-control study. *Lancet Psychiatry*, 4, 42–8.

Liguori, R., et al. 2001. Morvan's syndrome: peripheral and central nervous system and cardiac involvement with antibodies to voltage-gated potassium channels. *Brain*, 124, 2417–26.

Lim, J. A., et al. 2016. Frequent rhabdomyolysis in anti-NMDA receptor encephalitis. *J Neuroimmunol*, 298, 178–80.

Linnoila, J. J., et al. 2016. CSF herpes virus and autoantibody profiles in the evaluation of encephalitis. *Neurol Neuroimmunol Neuroinflamm*, 3, e245.

Litmeier, S., et al. 2016. Initial serum thyroid peroxidase antibodies and long-term outcomes in SREAT. *Acta Neurol Scand*, 134, 452–7.

Lynch, S. G., et al. 2001. The relationship between disability and depression in multiple sclerosis: the role of uncertainty, coping, and hope. *Mult Scler*, 7, 411–16.

Mackay, G., et al. 2012. NMDA receptor autoantibodies in sporadic Creutzfeldt-Jakob disease. *J Neurol*, 259, 1979–81.

Marrie, R. A., et al. 2015. The incidence and prevalence of psychiatric disorders in multiple sclerosis: a systematic review. *Mult Scler*, 21, 305–17.

Masopust, J., et al. 2015. Anti-NMDA receptor antibodies in patients with a first episode of schizophrenia. *Neuropsychiatr Dis Treat*, 11, 619–23.

Mechelhoff, D., et al. 2015. Anti-NMDA receptor encephalitis presenting as atypical anorexia nervosa: an adolescent case report. *Eur Child Adolesc Psychiatry*, 24, 1322–4.

Mirsky, M. M., et al. 2016. Antidepressant Drug Treatment in Association with Multiple Sclerosis Disease-Modifying Therapy: Using Explorys in the MS Population. *Int J MS Care*, 18, 305–10.

Muller, U. J., et al. 2014. Absence of dopamine receptor serum autoantibodies in schizophrenia patients with an acute disease episode. *Schizophr Res*, 158, 272–4.

Nibber, A., et al. 2017. Pathogenic potential of antibodies to the GABAB receptor. *Epilepsia Open*, 2, 355–9.

Ohkawa, T., et al. 2013. Autoantibodies to epilepsy-related LGI1 in limbic encephalitis neutralize LGI1-ADAM22 interaction and reduce synaptic AMPA receptors. *J Neurosci*, 33, 18161–74.

Olsen, A. L., et al. 2015. Caspr2 autoantibodies target multiple epitopes. *Neurol Neuroimmunol Neuroinflamm*, 2, e127.

Pathmanandavel, K., et al. 2015. Antibodies to surface dopamine-2 receptor and N-methyl-D-aspartate receptor in the first episode of acute psychosis in children. *Biol Psychiatry*, 77, 537–47.

Patten, S. B., et al. 2003. Major depression in multiple sclerosis: a population-based perspective. *Neurology*, 61, 1524–7.

Pearlman, D. M. & Najjar, S. 2014. Meta-analysis of the association between N-methyl-d-aspartate receptor antibodies and schizophrenia, schizoaffective disorder, bipolar disorder, and major depressive disorder. *Schizophr Res*, 157, 249–58.

Pego-Reigosa, J. M. & Isenberg, D. A. 2008. Psychosis due to systemic lupus erythematosus: characteristics and long-term outcome of this rare manifestation of the disease. *Rheumatology (Oxford)*, 47, 1498–502.

Perogamvros, L., et al. 2012. The role of NMDA receptors in human eating behavior: evidence from a case of anti-NMDA receptor encephalitis. *Cogn Behav Neurol*, 25, 93–7.

Petit-Pedrol, M., et al. 2014. Encephalitis with refractory seizures, status epilepticus, and antibodies to the GABAA receptor: a case series, characterisation of the antigen, and analysis of the effects of antibodies. *Lancet Neurol*, 13, 276–86.

Pettingill, P., et al. 2015. Antibodies to GABAA receptor alpha1 and gamma2 subunits: clinical and serologic characterization. *Neurology*, 84, 1233–41.

Pinatel, D., et al. 2015. Inhibitory axons are targeted in hippocampal cell culture by anti-Caspr2 autoantibodies associated with limbic encephalitis. *Front Cell Neurosci*, 9, 265.

Pollak, T. A., et al. 2016. Autoantibodies to central nervous system neuronal surface antigens: psychiatric symptoms and psychopharmacological implications. *Psychopharmacology (Berl)*, 233, 1605–21.

Pollak, T. A., et al. 2014. Prevalence of anti-N-methyl-D-aspartate (NMDA) receptor [corrected] antibodies in patients with schizophrenia and related psychoses: a systematic review and meta-analysis. *Psychol Med*, 44, 2475–87.

Pollak, T. A. et al. 2020. Autoimmune psychosis: an international consensus on an approach to the diagnosis and management of psychosis of suspected autoimmune origin. *Lancet Psychiatry*, 7, 93–108. doi:10.1016/S2215-0366(19)30290-1.

Pruss, H., et al. 2014. A case of inflammatory peripheral nerve destruction antedating anti-NMDA receptor encephalitis. *Neurol Neuroimmunol Neuroinflamm*, 1, e14.

Pruss, H., et al. 2012. IgA NMDA receptor antibodies are markers of synaptic immunity in slow cognitive impairment. *Neurology*, 78, 1743–53.

Pruss, H. & Lennox, B. R. 2016. Emerging psychiatric syndromes associated with antivoltage-gated potassium channel complex antibodies. *J Neurol Neurosurg Psychiatry*, 87, 1242–7.

Punja, M., et al. 2013. Anti-N-methyl-D-aspartate receptor (anti-NMDAR) encephalitis: an etiology worth considering in the differential diagnosis of delirium. *Clin Toxicol (Phila)*, 51, 794–7.

Rodriguez Cruz, P. M., et al. 2015. Use of cell-based assays in myasthenia gravis and other antibody-mediated diseases. *Exp Neurol*, 270, 66–71.

Sabater, L., et al. 2014. A novel non-rapid-eye movement and rapid-eye-movement parasomnia with sleep breathing disorder associated with antibodies to IgLON5: a case series, characterisation of the antigen, and post-mortem study. *Lancet Neurol*, 13, 575–86.

Salovin, A., et al. 2018. Anti-NMDA receptor encephalitis and nonencephalitic HSV-1 infection. *Neurol Neuroimmunol Neuroinflamm*, 5, e458.

Sarkis, R. A., et al. 2014. Neuropsychiatric and seizure outcomes in nonparaneoplastic autoimmune limbic encephalitis. *Epilepsy Behav*, 39, 21–5.

Schou, M., et al. 2016. Prevalence of serum anti-neuronal autoantibodies in patients admitted to acute psychiatric care. *Psychol Med*, 1–11.

Somers, K. J., et al. 2011. Psychiatric manifestations of voltage-gated potassium-channel complex autoimmunity. *J Neuropsychiatry Clin Neurosci*, 23, 425–33.

Spinazzi, M., et al. 2008. Immunotherapy-reversed compulsive, monoaminergic, circadian rhythm disorder in Morvan syndrome. *Neurology*, 71, 2008–10.

Steiner, J., et al. 2014. Prevalence of N-methyl-D-aspartate receptor autoantibodies in the peripheral blood: healthy control samples revisited. *JAMA Psychiatry*, 71, 838–9.

Steiner, J., et al. 2013. Increased prevalence of diverse N-methyl-D-aspartate glutamate receptor antibodies in patients with an initial diagnosis of schizophrenia: specific relevance of IgG NR1a antibodies for distinction from N-methyl-D-aspartate glutamate receptor encephalitis. *JAMA Psychiatry*, 70, 271–8.

Tanaka, S., et al. 2003. Autoantibodies against four kinds of neurotransmitter receptors in psychiatric disorders. *J Neuroimmunol*, 141, 155–64.

Titulaer, M. J., et al. 2013. Treatment and prognostic factors for long-term outcome in patients with anti-NMDA receptor encephalitis: an observational cohort study. *Lancet Neurol*, 12, 157–65.

Tobin, W. O., et al. 2014. DPPX potassium channel antibody: frequency, clinical accompaniments, and outcomes in 20 patients. *Neurology*, 83, 1797–803.

Tomietto, P., et al. 2007. General and specific factors associated with severity of cognitive impairment in systemic lupus erythematosus. *Arthritis Rheum*, 57, 1461–72.

Unterman, A., et al. 2011. Neuropsychiatric syndromes in systemic lupus erythematosus: a meta-analysis. *Semin Arthritis Rheum*, 41, 1–11.

Van Mierlo, H. C., et al. 2015. No evidence for the presence of neuronal surface autoantibodies in plasma of patients with schizophrenia. *Eur Neuropsychopharmacol*, 25, 2326–32.

Warren, N., et al. 2018. Refining the psychiatric syndrome of anti-N-methyl-d-aspartate receptor encephalitis. *Acta Psychiatr Scand*, 138, 401–8.

Witebsky, E., et al. 1957. Chronic thyroiditis and autoimmunization. *J Am Med Assoc*, 164, 1439–47.

Yoshimura, B. & Takaki, M. 2017. Anti-NMDA Receptor Antibody Positivity and Presentations Without Seizure, Involuntary Movement, Hypoventilation, or Tumor: A Systematic Review of the Literature. *J Neuropsychiatry Clin Neurosci*, 29, 267–74.

Zandi, M. S., et al. 2011. Disease-relevant autoantibodies in first episode schizophrenia. *J Neurol*, 258, 686–8.

Zandi, M. S., et al. 2014. Immunotherapy for patients with acute psychosis and serum N-Methyl D-Aspartate receptor (NMDAR) antibodies: a description of a treated case series. *Schizophr Res*, 160, 193–5.

23

Neuropsychiatry of demyelinating disorders

Anthony Feinstein and Bennis Pavisian

Introduction

Any chapter on demyelinating disorders will be dominated by discussion of multiple sclerosis (MS). This is true from a neuropsychiatry perspective as well. For the sake of completeness, however, reference will be made briefly to neuromyelitis optica (NMO), central pontine myelosis, and Marchiava-Bignami syndrome. Beginning with MS, one approach has been to divide the behavioural syndromes into two broad categories, namely disorders of cognition and mood/affect. This will be followed here. The mood section will be further subdivided into depression, bipolar affective disorder, euphoria, and pseudobulbar affect (PBA). For each of these conditions, data pertaining to prevalence, phenomenology, imaging correlates, and treatment will be reviewed.

Multiple sclerosis

MS is the commonest cause of neurological disability in young and middle-aged adult. It is an autoimmune disease of the CNS, characterized by inflammatory changes and neurodegeneration, the proportion of which depends on the disease course. The prevalence rate for MS is highest in northern countries. The female-to-male sex ratio is 3:1. MS typically begins with a relapsing–remitting (RRMS) course, characterized by waxing and waning in symptoms, with recovery between episodes. Over time, most people with RRMS progress to secondary progressive MS (SPMS), in which relapses give way to a steadily progressive physical decline. Approximately 10% of people with MS present with a primary progressive disease course (PPMS), notable for a progressive neurological decline, rather than relapses and remissions from disease onset. Neurological disability is typically quantified by the Expanded Disability Status Scale (EDSS), with scores ranging from 0 (no disability) to 10 (death). There are currently 15 disease-modifying therapies, all but two (ocrelizumab and siponimod) limited to people with RRMS.

Disorders of cognition

Charcot observed that people with MS (PwMS) may show (marked enfeeblement of memory, conceptions are formed slowly, and intellectual and emotional faculties are blunted in their totality) (Charcot, 1868). Notwithstanding this perceptive observation, little attention, with a couple of notable exceptions, was directed towards cognitive difficulties in this population over the next 100 years. It was only with the advent of MRI in the mid-1980s that behavioural scientists looked anew at the possibility of cognitive deficits in this disorder. The reason for this was the marked superiority of MRI over CT when it came to viewing the brain changes associated with demyelination and atrophy.

Prevalence

A seminal paper by Rao et al. (1991a) revealed the degree to which PwMS were cognitively impaired. The sample comprised 100 individuals with MS who underwent a detailed neuropsychological battery that included 31 tests. Results were compared to a group of healthy controls. PwMS failed, on average, 4.64 (SD = 4.9) tests versus 1.13 (SD = 1.8) in the controls. Taking failure on four or more cognitive indices as a marker of overall cognitive impairment, the authors arrived at a prevalence of 43%. This figure has remained relatively constant over time, providing the sample is essentially limited to individuals with RRMS. The prevalence rises in progressive disease, with figures of 50% and 60% reported for people with PPMS (Wachowius et al., 2005) and SPMS (Planche et al., 2016), MS respectively.

Of note is that cognitive difficulties may be present, even before individuals progress to the full MS diagnosis. The data here come from people with clinically isolated syndromes (CIS), namely those affecting the optic nerve, brainstem, and spinal cord, which are frequently a harbinger of MS (Feinstein et al., 1992). Furthermore, more recent research has indicated that cognitive impairment may even be present in up to 30% of individuals with radiologically isolated syndrome (Amato et al., 2012). The clinical significance of these results is that cognitive impairment discernable in individuals with CIS predicts earlier conversion to full MS (Zipoli et al., 2010) and, if present in early relapsing–remitting disease, is indicative of progression to greater neurological disability (Deloire et al., 2010).

Nature of cognitive impairment

The quintessential cognitive abnormality in PwMS is impaired information processing speed which is present in approximately 50%

of PwMS (Benedict et al., 2006). Charcot noted this, and contemporary neuropsychology has confirmed it. Here the Symbol Digit Modalities Test (SDMT) has emerged as the most sensitive and patient-friendly method of detecting impairment (Benedict et al., 2012) and is slowly replacing the Paced Auditory Serial Addition Test (PASAT) as the test of choice in this regard. The SDMT is relatively resistant to practice effects, making it a useful measure in clinical trials.

Other cognitive domains commonly affected are visual learning and memory, verbal memory, complex attention, and executive functioning (Benedict et al., 2006). Memory deficits are thought to primarily involve encoding, rather than retrieval (DeLuca et al., 2013). On the other hand, agnosia, apraxia, and aphasia are rare, which helps explain why the Mini Mental State Examination is insensitive in detecting cognitive abnormalities in this group (Beatty and Goodkin, 1990).

Detecting cognitive impairment

There are numerous neuropsychological approaches to the detection of cognitive impairment in PwMS. The choice will depend on factors such as duration of assessment, availability of neuropsychological expertise, and the questions being asked of the assessment. The most widely used screening battery is the Brief Repeatable Neuropsychological Battery (BRNB) (Rao, 1990), which contains the SDMT and PASAT as markers of processing speed and attention, the Selective Reminding Test (SRT) and the 10/36 Spatial Memory Recall Test as indicators of verbal and visual memory, respectively, and the Controlled Oral Word Association Test (COWAT), which measures multiple aspects of cognition such as verbal fluency, attention, executive function, vigilance, and semantic memory. The battery takes approximately 40 minutes to complete, is available in multiple languages, and has serial versions for repeat testing. A more comprehensive battery—the Minimal Assessment of Cognitive Function in MS (MACFMS) (Benedict et al., 2002)—has been devised by consensus opinion and includes seven tests encompassing five cognitive domains. Once more, the SDMT, PASAT, and COWAT appear alongside different tests of memory [California Verbal Learning Test (CVLT), Brief Visual Memory Test (BVMT)] and tests of executive (D-KEFS) and visual–spatial (Judgement of Line Orientation) function. The battery takes 90 minutes to complete. Should the clinician require a shorter assessment, the Brief International Cognitive Assessment in MS (BICAMS) (Langdon et al., 2012) has been developed, which includes the SDMT, CVLT, and BVMT. The BICAMS takes 10 minutes, has been validated in multiple languages, and contains serial versions. All three batteries mentioned above do require a degree of psychometric expertise in administering the tests. This has prompted a move towards standardized, easy-to-administer, computerized testing, of which various programs are now available (Lapshin et al., 2013).

Clinical correlates of cognitive dysfunction

There is a modest correlation between the degree of neurological disability, as captured on the EDSS, and cognitive dysfunction (Rao et al., 1991a). This reflects the limitations of the EDSS, which is heavily biased towards pyramidal dysfunction. Gender differences in cognition have also been reported, with males showing greater dysfunction linked to more extensive brain imaging abnormalities (Schoonheim et al., 2012a,b). If female gender is relatively

protective, so too is cognitive reserve. This refers to the individual's premorbid intellectual abilities, which are the product of innate intelligence, an intellectually enriched environment, and active leisure pursuits. High cognitive reserve, as measured by premorbid intelligence quotient (IQ), lessens the likelihood of developing cognitive impairment, even in the presence of brain atrophy (Sumowski et al., 2009).

Imaging correlates of cognition

Cognitive dysfunction correlates with numerous indices of structural brain pathology elicited by MRI. These include total and regional lesion volumes, atrophy (Filippi et al., 2010), and indices derived from normal-appearing brain tissue using diffusion tensor and magnetization transfer imaging (Cercignani et al., 2001). A particularly robust marker of impaired cognition is increased third ventricular width (Benedict et al., 2004), which reflects the presence of thalamic atrophy (Houtchens et al., 2007). These imaging parameters are known to deteriorate as the disease progresses from CIS through to a secondary progressive stage and therefore account for the concomitant cognitive decline (Deloire et al., 2011).

Functional brain changes indicate the degree to which neuroplasticity is at play in cognitive processes. Irrespective of the chosen cognitive parameter, fMRI findings illustrate a pattern of altered activation during completion of a cognitive task. This may take a form of extraneous and excessive activation, as in the SDMT (Genova et al., 2009), or reduced activation when tasks increase in complexity (Mainero et al., 2004). This suggests the presence of a threshold effect in PwMS beyond which attempts at cognitive compensatory mechanisms fail. fMRI studies also reveal the presence of resting state changes that are predictive of cognitive dysfunction (Rocca et al., 2010). In a study of 24 PwMS with progressive MS and 24 healthy control subjects, differences emerged with respect to default mode network activity which correlated significantly not only with abnormalities on the PASAT and word list generation (COWAT), but also diffusion tensor imaging indices derived from the corpus callosum and cingulum.

Cannabis and cognition in MS

Approximately 18% of PwMS smoke or ingest cannabis on a regular basis (Chong et al., 2006). Evidence suggests that use may further effect cognition, leading to more marked memory, processing speed, and executive function deficits (Honarmand et al., 2011) In addition, fMRI findings reveal a pattern of dysfunctional brain activation that accompanies the increased cognitive deficits (Pavisian et al., 2014). The potentially deleterious effect of smoked or ingested cannabis on cognition should be weighed up against benefits pertaining to pain and spasticity. However, to date, empirical data attesting to these benefits await confirmation. The situation differs with respect to pharmaceutically manufactured cannabis derivatives such as nabiximols, the use of which has been endorsed for pain relief by an AAN taskforce (Koppel et al., 2014).

Treatment

Pharmacotherapy of cognitive dysfunction in MS offers little benefit. Medications known to be helpful in Alzheimer's Disease, such as donepezil, have no proven efficacy in PwMS (Krupp et al.,

2011). While there are some tentative data indicating modest benefits from L-amphetamine when it comes to improvement on the SDMT, the use of stimulant medication, in general, has proved disappointing (Amato et al., 2013). If there are cognitive benefits from disease-modifying treatments, these are more likely to become apparent with long-term use, given the beneficial effects of treatment on brain atrophy (Sormani et al., 2014).

A more rewarding area of treatment is cognitive rehabilitation, which may be divided into two categories. The first is compensatory, which implies assisting cognitively impaired PwMS in working around their deficits while maximizing residual strengths. Such an approach does not lead to cognitive improvement, but rather mitigates the dysfunction associated with deficits. Potentially more rewarding are treatments geared towards remediation of deficits. Notwithstanding, a lukewarm Cochrane review on the subject (das Nair et al., 2012), there are now consistent data that speak of treatment benefits. A double-blind, placebo-controlled RCT of 86 PwMS revealed that ten sessions of therapy geared towards facilitating learning led to significant memory improvement in the treatment, but not placebo, group (Chiaravalloti et al., 2013). Furthermore, these benefits were still evident 6 months post-treatment. A subsequent study reported equally impressive cognitive benefits following 15 weeks of domain-specific training (Mattioli et al., 2016). Benefits endured for up to 2 years following treatment cessation. Imaging data add construct validity to these results by showing increased cerebral activation in neural circuits implicated in specific cognitive tasks, but only in the treatment group (Chiaravalloti et al., 2012). Finally, there are some preliminary data suggesting that aerobic exercise may have beneficial cognitive effects, even in PwMS with progressive disease (Briken et al., 2014).

Importance of cognitive dysfunction

Cognitive deficits exert a deleterious effect on numerous aspects of daily functioning in PwMS, including employment, relationships, leisure pursuits, and activities of daily living (Rao et al., 1991b). As such, it is important that deficits are not overlooked and, when present, treated. The latter can prove challenging in the absence of access to cognitive rehabilitation. At the very least, PwMS should be provided with compensatory strategies to maximize their existing abilities.

Disorders of mood and affect

Depression

Prevalence

The rates of major depression in PwMS attending neurological clinics approach 50% (Sadovnick et al., 1996). Epidemiologic data confirm this elevated prevalence. Using population-based administrative health data, Marrie et al. (2015) identified 44,452 PwMS and 220,849 healthy control subjects matched demographically and geographically. The annual incidence of depression was 979/100,000 persons with MS, well above that in the control group. Supporting data come from the Canadian Community Health Survey (of 115,071 subjects), which revealed that the 12-month prevalence rate of depression in PwMS aged 18–45 years was 25.7% (Patten et al., 2003). The rate of depression in PwMS is also higher than that found in most other neurological disorders (Siegert and Abernethy, 2005).

Assessing depression

The assessment of depression in PwMS can present a clinical challenge, given the potential overlap in symptoms between depression on the one hand and MS on the other. Examples include fatigue, insomnia, and impaired concentration. Self-report psychometric scales have been developed with this in mind. The Hospital Anxiety and Depression Scale (HADS) and the Beck Fast Screen for Medically Ill Patients have both been validated for use in PwMS (Benedict et al., 2003; Honarmand and Feinstein, 2009). Both these scales have removed these potential somatic confounders and focus on the core depressive features of sadness accompanied by depressive cognitions or core negative beliefs such as poor self-esteem, hopelessness, and pessimism over the future, to give a few examples. There is no clear association between depression and disease type or degree of physical disability, as determined by the EDSS. The association with sex is equivocal, with some studies supporting an association and others not (Patten et al., 2003; Theaudin et al., 2016).

Aetiology

There is now a small, but compelling, literature linking depression in PwMS to indices of structural brain damage. Pujol et al. (1997) were the first to report an association between hyperintense lesion areas and symptoms of depression, as elicited on the Beck Depression Inventory. However, the imaging data could account for only 17% of the depression variance. In a more wide-ranging study, Feinstein et al. (2004) demonstrated the importance of hyper- and hypointense lesions and regional atrophy in the pathogenesis of MS-related depression. A subsequent diffusion tensor imaging (DTI) study revealed that depressed MS individuals were more likely to have structural abnormalities in normal-appearing brain tissue (Feinstein et al., 2009). The DTI data, in combination with lesion volume and markers of atrophy, accounted for approximately 45% of the depression variance. DTI tractography has also shown a pattern of abnormal connectivity in limbic regions in depressed versus non-depressed PwMS (Nigro et al., 2014). The importance of brain pathology in depressed PwMS was further underscored in a study that examined medial temporal lobe changes (Gold et al., 2010). Atrophy of the hippocampus, in particular the dentate gyrus, was found to correlate with depression and moreover was linked to alterations in the circadian rhythm of cortisol secretion, suggestive of HPA axis dysfunction. A similar change in serial cortisol levels was reported in a study that also demonstrated the increased presence of contrast-enhancing lesions, indicative of an inflammatory response, in depressed PwMS (Fassbender et al., 1998). These structural MRI data are supported by an fMRI study that revealed dysfunctional connectivity between the hippocampus on the one hand and the orbitofrontal and DLPFC on the other. The functional connectivity between the amygdala and the DLPFC was also found to be abnormal (Riccelli et al., 2015).

The complexities of brain imaging changes in the context of emotional distress is illustrated by an RCT of stress reduction therapy in PwMS. Participants were randomized into two groups, namely those receiving 24 weeks of therapy and those on a waitlist. Both groups underwent gadolinium (Gd)-enhanced brain imaging every 8 weeks over a 24-week period. A significantly higher percentage of Gd-free lesions was found in the treatment group, a finding that quickly dissipated when the treatment ended (Mohr et al., 2012).

There was, however, no difference in depression scores between the treatment and waitlist groups.

The brain imaging findings are complemented by psychosocial inquiry. Depression has been associated with the uncertainty inherent in the disease course of MS, poor coping strategies, helplessness, poor social relationships, loss of recreational activities, and high levels of stress. A constellation of some of these variables was shown to account for approximately 40% of the depression variance (Lynch et al., 2001), indicating that psychosocial factors are no less important than the MRI data when looking for the origin of depressive symptomology. Of these numerous variables, coping mechanisms are considered particularly important. Numerous studies have shown that problem-focused approaches to dealing with disability are more beneficial from a mood perspective than emotion-based or avoidance strategies (Arnett et al., 2002).

There are a number of other miscellaneous factors that have been associated with depression in PwMS. Early findings from studies of disease-modifying treatments suggested that depression was a side effect of interferon beta-1β treatment (The IFNB Multiple Sclerosis Study Group, 1993). The risk, however, is now known to be low (Schippling et al., 2016) and linked to the presence of depression prior to treatment and unrealistic expectations associated with treatment (Mohr et al., 1997). To date, there are no compelling genetic data on depression in PwMS. In addition, putative links with immune system abnormalities have yet to be explored in detail despite some preliminary findings suggestive of a causative relationship (Feinstein et al., 2014).

Treatment

Despite the frequency with which depression occurs in PwMS, there are only two trials of antidepressant medication that are deemed methodologically robust by the Cochrane reviews (Koch et al., 2011). One of these involved the tricyclic drug desipramine and the other the SSRI paroxetine. Both found that the medication was modestly effective in reducing symptom frequency and severity, but that anticholinergic side effects made it difficult for a number of individuals to tolerate the medication and reach therapeutic dosages. While there are numerous other open-label and anecdotal trials supporting the use of antidepressant medication in this group, the American Academy of Neurology concluded that medication was not the treatment of choice for depressed PwMS (Minden et al., 2014). Instead cognitive behavioural therapy (CBT) was considered more effective and endorsed as the treatment of choice. In addition, CBT can be effectively administered over the telephone to PwMS, a significant advantage in a disease in which immobility will influence clinic attendance (Mohr et al., 2005). More recently, a self-administered CBT programme has been trialled in an RCT and found to be effective in PwMS (Fischer et al., 2015).

A variant of CBT, namely mindfulness-based therapy, has also been shown to offer benefits to PwMS with depression (Grossman et al., 2010). The jury, however, is still out on the effectiveness of exercise as a treatment for depression in PwMS (Dalgas et al., 2015). Finally, in the case of intractable, treatment-resistant depression, ECT is a safe and effective intervention, based on a series of case reports. Data relating to TMS and tDCS are more equivocal (Palm et al., 2014).

Importance of depression

In a disease without cure, symptom management takes on added importance. In the case of depression, this importance is magnified by a number of clinically relevant factors. Depression is a major determinant of quality of life (Fernández-Jiménez and Arnett, 2014), can add to the cognitive burden associated with MS (Demaree et al., 2003), and helps explain why rates of suicide are elevated in PwMS, relative to the general population and most other neurological disorders (Stenager et al., 1992). In relation to the latter, data show that suicidal intent is present at some point and up to one in three PwMS and is associated with the presence of major depression, the severity of the depression, social isolation, and increased alcohol consumption (Feinstein, 2002). These observations take on added salience, given that depression in PwMS is often missed in a neurology clinic and, even when detected, is frequently undertreated (Mohr et al., 2006).

Anxiety

The literature pertaining to anxiety in PwMS is small. Epidemiological data reveal high comorbidity, with an incidence of 638/100,000, second only to depression (Marrie et al., 2015) with which it is often comorbid. There is no clear association with disease type, duration of disease, or degree of physical disability. The prevalence of generalized anxiety disorder, panic disorder, and obsessive compulsive disorder is thought to be three times that found in the general population (Korostil and Feinstein, 2007). As with depression, somatic confounders can lead to false-positive diagnoses. Teasing out symptom attribution can prove challenging, and it is here that psychometric inquiry with the HADS can prove helpful. There are no MRI studies devoted to anxiety in MS. Treatment data are few, with some promising CBT findings (Askey-Jones et al., 2013).

Bipolar affective disorder

The annual incidence of bipolar disorder per 100,000 PwMS has been estimated at 328 (Marrie et al., 2015). Epidemiological data from Monroe County, New York indicate that the prevalence in PwMS is twice what it is in the general population (Schiffer et al., 1986). Reasons for this elevated risk are unclear, given the paucity of research on the topic. Some early tentative data pointed towards a possible genetic link, but no replication studies were forthcoming (Schiffer et al., 1986). Steroid use may also precipitate a manic episode in PwMS, most notably in those with a history of depression, either before or after the diagnosis of MS, and a family history of depression, alcoholism, or both (Minden et al., 1988). There are no brain MRI data nor randomized control treatment studies in this population. As such, clinicians have to borrow from the general psychiatry literature when it comes to management, but with certain practical caveats. For example, a person with MS and a neurogenic bladder could have difficulty tolerating lithium carbonate, an effective mood-stabilizing agent, but one associated with diuresis as a side effect.

Euphoria

This may be described as a fixed mental state characterized by a cheerful optimism in relation to future physical functioning, notwithstanding the presence of major neurological compromise. The syndrome occurs in approximately 9% of PwMS (Fishman et al., 2004) and is generally limited to those with an extensive lesion burden, marked brain atrophy, significant physical limitations, and a progressive disease course (Rabins et al., 1986). There is no treatment for the condition, which is best viewed as a fixed mental state akin to a personality change.

Pseudobulbar affect

PBA has also been called pathological laughing and crying, emotional incontinence, and intermittent involuntary explosive disorder (Cummings et al., 2006). The behavioural changes reflect the presence of crying in the absence of sadness, or laughter without mirth, or a combination of the two emotional states. It can occur in up to 10% of PwMS (Feinstein et al., 1997) and is associated with a progressive disease course and more extensive cognitive dysfunction relative to PwMS without the syndrome (Hanna et al., 2016). MRI findings are sparse but do point towards bilateral cerebral involvement in inferior parietal and medial frontal brain regions (Ghaffar et al., 2008). A single case report of PBA, albeit in an individual with a stroke affecting the cerebellum, highlighted the importance of this brain region in modifying affect according to social cues (Parvizi et al., 2001). Finally, the brainstem has also been implicated, given the central role played by the bulbar nuclei in regulating affective displays. The syndrome responds well to treatment with low-dose amitriptyline, an SSRI, or a combination of dextromethorphan and quinidine (Pioro, 2014).

Psychosis

The epidemiologic data relating to psychosis in PwMS are equivocal with findings for (Patten et al., 2005) and against (Marrie et al., 2015) an elevated rate relative to the general population. In an exhaustive review of schizophrenia-like psychosis linked to disorders of the CNS, Davison and Bagley (Davison et al., 1969) failed to find an increased rate of psychosis in PwMS. As with most of the syndromes described above, there are no randomized controlled treatment studies. Antipsychotic medication is the mainstay of treatment, with case reports favouring the newer agents such as risperidone (Hussain and Belderbos, 2008) and ziprasidone (Davids et al., 2004).

Neuromyelitis optica

NMO is a severe inflammatory demyelinating disease of the CNS that differs from MS. It can present with recurrent attacks that are not limited to the optic nerve and spinal cord. The behavioural literature on NMO is small and inconsistent in relation to cognitive dysfunction and brain correlates. This is illustrated by cognitive comparisons between people with MS and NMO which reveal the latter to be either less (Kim et al., 2016), equally (Moore et al., 2016), or more (Saji et al., 2013) impaired. This uncertainty extends to the brain imaging data. Whereas Blanc et al. (2012) found an association between cognitive deficits and a loss of global and focal white matter volume, others have implicated grey matter changes only. Thus, associations have been reported between impaired cognition and cortical neuronal loss (Saji et al., 2013) and regional brain atrophy that includes the thalamus (Wang et al., 2015). The

imaging–cognition data highlight the multifocal nature of this disease, an observation further underscored by the presence of reduced hippocampal volume in cognitively impaired people with NMO (Liu et al., 2015). In addition to the cognitive changes, elevated rates of anxiety and depression have been documented, the latter linked closely to impaired cognition and more extensive neurological disability (Moore et al., 2016).

Central pontine myelinosis

Central pontine myelinosis is an acute, and often fatal, complication of alcoholism. Low sodium and undernutrition are frequently associated with the condition. Clinical features include obtundation, bulbar palsy, quadriplegia, and loss of pain sensation in the limbs and trunk (Louis et al., 2015). Impaired cognition has been reported in a number of case reports and may represent the most enduring clinical feature in people who recover neurologically (Odier et al., 2010).

Marchiafava-Bignami disease

Marchiafava-Bignami disease is characterized by demyelination of the corpus callosum without inflammation. Other white matter regions and rarely the grey matter may also be involved. The cause is unknown. There is no systematic neuropsychiatric literature on the condition. Isolated case reports describe cognitive impairment with visual hallucinations (Augusto et al., 2015) and delusions (Shi Hui et al., 2015) as part of the clinical course.

Conclusion

Behavioural difficulties are common in people with MS and all, except euphoria, are amenable to treatment. Evidence from brain imaging, in particular, highlights the close association between cognitive dysfunction, depression, and PBA on the one hand and cerebral change, both structural and functional, on the other. In a disease without cure, good symptom management takes on an even greater importance. It therefore behoves clinicians to be on the lookout for the neuropsychiatric manifestations of the disease, given that treatment can significantly enhance the quality of life in those affected.

KEY LEARNING POINTS

- MS is the commonest cause of neurological disability in young and middle-aged adults.
- Cognitive impairment affects between 40 and 60% of PwMS. It is not responsive to medication. Cognitive rehabilitation can prove beneficial.
- Almost one in two PwMS will develop a clinically significant depression. Abnormalities on brain MRI account for close to 50% of the depression variance. Cognitive behaviour therapy is the treatment of choice.

- Pseudobulbar affect occurs in approximately 10% of PwMS and responds well to amitriptyline, an SSRI or a combination of dextromethorphan and quinidine.

REFERENCES

Amato, M.P. et al., 2012. Association of MRI metrics and cognitive impairment in radiologically isolated syndromes. *Neurology*, 78(5), pp.309–14.

Amato, M.P. et al., 2013. Treatment of cognitive impairment in multiple sclerosis: Position paper. *Journal of Neurology*, 260(6), pp.1452–68.

Arnett, P.A. et al., 2002. Relationship between coping, cognitive dysfunction and depression in multiple sclerosis. *The Clinical Neuropsychologist*, 16(3), pp.341–55.

Askey-Jones, S. et al., 2013. Cognitive behaviour therapy for common mental disorders in people with multiple sclerosis: a bench marking study. *Behaviour research and therapy*, 51(10), pp.648–55.

Augusto, L. et al., 2015. Marchiafava-Bignami disease as a cause of visual hallucinations. *Revista Brasileira de Psiquiatria*, 37(1), p.82.

Beatty, W.W. & Goodkin, D.E., 1990. Screening for cognitive impairment in multiple sclerosis: an evaluation of the Mini-Mental State Examination. *Archives of Neurology*, 47(3), pp.297–301.

Benedict, R.H.B. et al., 2002. Minimal neuropsychological assessment of MS patients: a consensus approach. *The Clinical Neuropsychologist*, 16(3), pp.381–97.

Benedict, R.H.B. et al., 2004. Prediction of neuropsychological impairment in multiple sclerosis: comparison of conventional magnetic resonance imaging measures of atrophy and lesion burden. *Archives of Neurology*, 61(2), pp.226–30.

Benedict, R.H.B. et al., 2012. Reliability and equivalence of alternate forms for the Symbol Digit Modalities Test: implications for multiple sclerosis clinical trials. *Multiple Sclerosis*, 18(9), pp.1320–5.

Benedict, R.H.B. et al., 2003. Validity of the beck depression inventory-fast screen in multiple sclerosis. *Multiple Sclerosis*, 9(4), pp.393–6.

Benedict, R.H.B. et al., 2006. Validity of the minimal assessment of cognitive function in multiple sclerosis (MACFIMS). *Journal of the International Neuropsychological Society*, 12(04), pp.549–58.

Blanc, F. et al., 2012. White matter atrophy and cognitive dysfunctions in neuromyelitis optica. *PLoS One*, 7(4), p.e33878.

Briken, S. et al., 2014. Effects of exercise on fitness and cognition in progressive MS: a randomized, controlled pilot trial. *Multiple Sclerosis*, 20(3), pp.382–90.

Cercignani, M. et al., 2001. Magnetisation transfer ratio and mean diffusivity of normal appearing white and grey matter from patients with multiple sclerosis. *Journal of Neurology, Neurosurgery & Psychiatry*, 70(3), pp.311–17.

Charcot, J.-M., 1868. Histologie de le sclerose en plaques. *Gazette Hospital Paris*, 141, pp.554–8.

Chiaravalloti, N.D. et al., 2013. An RCT to treat learning impairment in multiple sclerosis. The MEMREHAB trial. *Neurology*, 81(24), pp.2066–72.

Chiaravalloti, N.D. et al., 2012. Increased cerebral activation after behavioral treatment for memory deficits in MS. *Journal of Neurology*, 259(7), pp.1337–46.

Chong, M.S. et al., 2006. Cannabis use in patients with multiple sclerosis. *Multiple Sclerosis*, 12, pp.646–51.

Cummings, J.L. et al., 2006. Defining and diagnosing involuntary emotional expression disorder. *CNS spectrums*, 11(6), pp.1–7.

Dalgas, U., Stenager, E. & Sloth, M., 2015. The effect of exercise on depressive symptoms in multiple sclerosis based on a meta-analysis and critical review of the literature. *European Journal of Neurology*, 22(3), pp.443–e34.

Davids, E., Hartwig, U. & Gastpar, M., 2004. Antipsychotic treatment of psychosis associated with multiple sclerosis. *Progress in Neuro-Psychopharmacology and Biological Psychiatry*, 28(4), pp.743–4.

Davison, K., Bagley, C. & Herrington, R.N., 1969. Schizophrenia-like psychoses associated with organic disorders of the central nervous system: a review of the literature. In: Herrington, R.N. (ed). Current Problems in Neuropsychiatry. *British Journal of Psychiatry Special Publication No. 4*. Headley Brothers, Ashford.

Deloire, M. et al., 2010. Early cognitive impairment in multiple sclerosis predicts disability outcome several years later. *Multiple Sclerosis*, 16(5), pp.581–7.

Deloire, M.S.A. et al., 2011. MRI predictors of cognitive outcome in early multiple sclerosis. *Neurology*, 76(13), pp.1161–7.

DeLuca, J. et al., 2013. Memory impairment in multiple sclerosis is due to a core deficit in initial learning. *Journal of Neurology*, 260(10), pp.2491–6.

Demaree, H. a, Gaudino, E. & DeLuca, J., 2003. The relationship between depressive symptoms and cognitive dysfunction in multiple sclerosis. *Cognitive Neuropsychiatry*, 8(3), pp.161–71.

Fassbender, K. et al., 1998. Mood disorders and dysfunction of the hypothalamic-pituitary-adrenal axis in multiple sclerosis: association with cerebral inflammation. *Archives of Neurology*, 55(1), pp.66–72.

Feinstein, A., 2002. An examination of suicidal intent in patients with multiple sclerosis. *Neurology*, 59(5), pp.674–8.

Feinstein, A. et al., 2009. Diffusion tensor imaging abnormalities in depressed multiple sclerosis patients. *Multiple Sclerosis*, 16(2), pp.189–96.

Feinstein, A. et al., 1997. Prevalence and neurobehavioral correlates of pathological laughing and crying in multiple sclerosis. *Archives of Neurology*, 54(9), pp.1116–21.

Feinstein, A. et al., 2004. Structural brain abnormalities in multiple sclerosis patients with major depression. *Neurology*, 62(4), pp.586–90.

Feinstein, A. et al., 2014. The link between multiple sclerosis and depression. *Nature Reviews Neurology*, 10(9), pp.507–17.

Feinstein, A., Youl, B. & Ron, M., 1992. ACUTE OPTIC NEURITIS. *Brain*, 115(5), pp.1403–15.

Fernández-Jiménez, E. & Arnett, P.A., 2014. Impact of neurological impairment, depression, cognitive function and coping on quality of life of people with multiple sclerosis: A relative importance analysis. *Multiple Sclerosis*, 21(11), pp.1468–72.

Filippi, M. et al., 2010. The contribution of MRI in assessing cognitive impairment in multiple sclerosis. *Neurology*, 75(23), pp.2121–8.

Fischer, A. et al., 2015. An online programme to reduce depression in patients with multiple sclerosis: a randomised controlled trial. *The Lancet Psychiatry*, 2(3), pp.217–23.

Fishman, I. et al., 2004. Construct validity and frequency of euphoria sclerotica in multiple sclerosis. *Journal of Neuropsychiatry and Clinical Neurosciences*, 16(3), pp.350–6.

Genova, H.M. et al., 2009. Examination of processing speed deficits in multiple sclerosis using functional magnetic resonance imaging. *Journal of the International Neuropsychological Society*, 15(3), pp.383–93.

Ghaffar, O., Chamelian, L. & Feinstein, A., 2008. Neuroanatomy of pseudobulbar affect. *Journal of Neurology*, 255(3), pp.406–12.

Gold, S.M. et al., 2010. Smaller cornu ammonis 2–3/dentate gyrus volumes and elevated cortisol in multiple sclerosis patients with depressive symptoms. *Biological Psychiatry*, 68(6), pp.553–9.

Grossman, P. et al., 2010. MS quality of life, depression, and fatigue improve after mindfulness training. A randomized trial. *Neurology*, 75(13), pp.1141–9.

Hanna, J., Feinstein, A. & Morrow, S.A., 2016. The association of pathological laughing and crying and cognitive impairment in multiple sclerosis. *Journal of Neurological Sciences*, 361, pp.200–3.

Honarmand, K. et al., 2011. Effects of cannabis on cognitive function in patients with multiple sclerosis. *Neurology*, 76(13), pp.1153–60.

Honarmand, K. & Feinstein, A., 2009. Validation of the Hospital Anxiety and Depression Scale for use with multiple sclerosis patients. *Multiple Sclerosis*, 15(12), pp.1518–24.

Houtchens, M.K. et al., 2007. Thalamic atrophy and cognition in multiple sclerosis. *Neurology*, 69(12), pp.1213–23.

Hussain, A. & Belderbos, S., 2008. Risperidone depot in the treatment of psychosis associated with multiple sclerosis-a case report. *Journal of Psychopharmacology*, 22(8), pp.925–6.

Kim, S.-H. et al., 2016. Cognitive impairment differs between neuromyelitis optica spectrum disorder and multiple sclerosis. *Multiple Sclerosis*, 22(14), pp.1850–8.

Koch, M.W. et al., 2011. Pharmacologic treatment of depression in multiple sclerosis. *The Cochrane Library*.

Koppel, B.S. et al., 2014. Systematic review: Efficacy and safety of medical marijuana in selected neurologic disorders: Report of the Guideline Development Subcommittee of the American Academy of Neurology. *Neurology*, 82(17), pp.1556–63.

Korostil, M. & Feinstein, a, 2007. Anxiety disorders and their clinical correlates in multiple sclerosis patients. *Multiple Sclerosis*, 13(1), pp.67–72.

Krupp, L.B. et al., 2011. Multicenter randomized clinical trial of donepezil for memory impairment in multiple sclerosis. *Neurology*, 76(17), pp.1500–7.

Langdon, D. et al., 2012. Recommendations for a Brief International Cognitive Assessment for Multiple Sclerosis (BICAMS). *Multiple Sclerosis*, 18(6), pp.891–8.

Lapshin, H. et al., 2013. Assessing the validity of a computer-generated cognitive screening instrument for patients with multiple sclerosis. *Multiple Sclerosis*, 19(14), pp.1905–12.

Liu, Y. et al., 2015. Structural MRI substrates of cognitive impairment in neuromyelitis optica. *Neurology*, 85(17), pp.1491–9.

Louis, E.D., Mayer, S.A. & Rowland, L.P., 2015. *Merritt's Neurology.* Lippincott Williams & Wilkins.

Lynch, S.G., Kroencke, D.C. & Denney, D.R., 2001. The relationship between disability and depression in multiple sclerosis: the role of uncertainty, coping, and hope. *Multiple Sclerosis*, 7(6), pp.411–16.

Mainero, C. et al., 2004. fMRI evidence of brain reorganization during attention and memory tasks in multiple sclerosis. *Neuroimage*, 21(3), pp.858–67.

Marrie, R.A. et al., 2015. Differences in the burden of psychiatric comorbidity in MS vs the general population. *Neurology*, 85(22), pp.1972–9.

Mattioli, F. et al., 2016. Two Years Follow up of Domain Specific Cognitive Training in Relapsing Remitting Multiple Sclerosis: A Randomized Clinical Trial. *Front Behav Neurosci*, 10, p.28.

Minden, S.L. et al., 2014. Evidence-based guideline: Assessment and management of psychiatric disorders in individuals with MS Report of the Guideline Development Subcommittee of the American Academy of Neurology. *Neurology*, 82(2), pp.174–81.

Minden, S.L., Orav, J. & Schildkraut, J.J., 1988. Hypomanic reactions to ACTH and prednisone treatment for multiple sclerosis. *Neurology*, 38(10), p.1631.

Mohr, D.C. et al., 2012. A randomized trial of stress management for the prevention of new brain lesions in MS. *Neurology*, 79(5), pp.412–19.

Mohr, D.C. et al., 2005. Telephone-administered psychotherapy for depression. *Archives of General Psychiatry*, 62(9), pp.1007–14.

Mohr, D.C. et al., 2006. Treatment of depression for patients with multiple sclerosis in neurology clinics. *Multiple Sclerosis*, 12(2), pp.204–8.

Mohr, D.C. et al., 1997. Treatment of depression improves adherence to interferon beta-1b therapy for multiple sclerosis. *Archives of Neurology*, 54(5), pp.531–3.

Moore, P. et al., 2016. Cognitive and psychiatric comorbidities in neuromyelitis optica. *Journal of the Neurological Sciences*, 360, pp.4–9.

das Nair, R., Martin, K. & Lincoln, N.B., 2012. Memory rehabilitation for people with multiple sclerosis. *The Cochrane Library*.

Nigro, S. et al., 2014. Structural 'connectomic' alterations in the limbic system of multiple sclerosis patients with major depression. *Multiple Sclerosis*, 21(8), pp. 1003–12.

Odier, C., Nguyen, D.K. & Panisset, M. 2010. Central pontine and extrapontine myelinolysis: from epileptic and other manifestations to cognitive prognosis. *Journal of Neurology*, 257(7), pp.1176–80.

Palm, U. et al., 2014. Non-invasive brain stimulation therapy in multiple sclerosis: a review of tDCS, rTMS and ECT results. *Brain Stimulation*, 7(6), pp.849–54.

Parvizi, J. et al., 2001. Pathological laughter and crying. *Brain*, 124(9), pp.1708–19.

Patten, S.B. et al., 2003. Major depression in multiple sclerosis: a population-based perspective. *Neurology*, 61(11), pp.1524–7.

Patten, S.B., Svenson, L.W. & Metz, L.M., 2005. Psychotic disorders in MS: population-based evidence of an association. *Neurology*, 65(7), pp.1123–5.

Pavisian, B. et al., 2014. Effects of cannabis on cognition in patients with MS: A psychometric and MRI study. *Neurology*, 82(21), pp.1879–87.

Pioro, E.P., 2014. Review of dextromethorphan 20 mg/quinidine 10 mg (NUEDEXTA˚) for pseudobulbar affect. *Neurology and Therapy*, 3(1), pp.15–28.

Planche, V. et al., 2016. Cognitive impairment in a population-based study of patients with multiple sclerosis: differences between late relapsing– remitting, secondary progressive and primary progressive multiple sclerosis. *European Journal of Neurology*, 23(2), pp.282–9.

Pujol, J. et al., 1997. Lesions in the left arcuate fasciculus region and depressive symptoms in multiple sclerosis. *Neurology*, 49(4), pp.1105–10.

Rabins, P. V et al., 1986. Structural brain correlates of emotional disorder in multiple sclerosis. *Brain*, 109(4), pp.585–97.

Rao, S.M., 1990. *A Manual for the Brief Repeatable Battery of Neuropsychological Tests in Multiple Sclerosis.* New York, NY: National Multiple Sclerosis Society.

Rao, S.M., Leo, G.J., Bernardin, L.M., et al., 1991a. Cognitive dysfunction in multiple sclerosis: frequency, patterns, and predictions. *Neurology*, 41(5), pp.685–91.

Rao, S.M., Leo, G.J., Ellington, L., et al., 1991b. Cognitive dysfunction in multiple sclerosis: Impact on employment and social functioning. *Neurology*, 41(5), pp.692–6.

Riccelli, R. et al., 2015. Individual differences in depression are associated with abnormal function of the limbic system in multiple sclerosis patients. *Multiple Sclerosis*, 22(8), pp.1094–105.

Rocca, M. a. et al., 2010. Default-mode network dysfunction and cognitive impairment in progressive MS. *Neurology*, 74(16), pp.1252–9.

Sadovnick, A.D. et al., 1996. Depression and multiple sclerosis. *Neurology*, 46(3), pp.628–32.

Saji, E. et al., 2013. Cognitive impairment and cortical degeneration in neuromyelitis optica. *Annals of Neurology*, 73(1), pp.65–76.

Schiffer, R.B., Wineman, N. & Weitkamp, L., 1986. Association between bipolar affective disorder and multiple sclerosis. *Am J Psychiatry*, 143, pp.94–5.

Schippling, S. et al., 2016. Incidence and course of depression in multiple sclerosis in the multinational BEYOND trial. *Journal of Neurology*, pp.1–9.

Schoonheim, M.M. et al., 2012a. Gender-related differences in functional connectivity in multiple sclerosis. *Multiple Sclerosis*, 18(2), pp.164–73.

Schoonheim, M.M. et al., 2012b. Subcortical atrophy and cognition Sex effects in multiple sclerosis. *Neurology*, 79(17), pp.1754–61.

Shi Hui, P. et al., 2015. A Rare Case Of Sub-Acute Form Of Marchiafava-Bignami Disease Presenting Predominantly With Psychotic Symptoms. *ASEAN Journal of Psychiatry*, 16(2), pp.245–8.

Siegert, R.J. & Abernethy, D. 2005. Depression in multiple sclerosis: a review. *Journal of Neurology, Neurosurgery, and Psychiatry*, 76, pp.469–75.

Sormani, M.P., Arnold, D.L. & De Stefano, N., 2014. Treatment effect on brain atrophy correlates with treatment effect on disability in multiple sclerosis. *Annals of Neurology*, 75(1), pp.43–9.

Stenager, E.N. et al., 1992. Suicide and multiple sclerosis: an epidemiological investigation. *Journal of Neurology, Neurosurgery & Psychiatry*, 55(7), pp.542–5.

Sumowski, J.F., Chiaravalloti, N. & DeLuca, J., 2009. Cognitive reserve protects against cognitive dysfunction in multiple sclerosis. *Journal of Clinical and Experimental Neuropsychology*, 31(8), pp.913–26.

Theaudin, M, Romero, C, Feinstein, A. 2016. In multiple sclerosis anxiety, not depression, is related to gender. *Multiple Sclerosis*, 22(2), pp.239–44.

The IFNB Multiple Sclerosis Study Group, 1993. Interferon beta-1b is effective in relapsing-remitting multiple sclerosis: I. Clinical results of a multicenter, randomized, double-blind, placebo-controlled trial. *Neurology*, 43(4), pp.655–5.

Wachowius, U. et al., 2005. Cognitive impairment in primary and secondary progressive multiple sclerosis. *Journal of Clinical and Experimental Neuropsychology*, 27(1), pp.65–77.

Wang, Q. et al., 2015. Gray matter volume reduction is associated with cognitive impairment in neuromyelitis optica. *American Journal of Neuroradiology*, 36(10), pp.1822–9.

Zipoli, V. et al., 2010. Cognitive impairment predicts conversion to multiple sclerosis in clinically isolated syndromes. *Multiple Sclerosis*, 16(1), pp.62–7.

24

Functional neurological disorders

Mark Edwards, Sarah R. Cope, and Niruj Agrawal

Introduction

Over most of recorded medical history, it has been recognized that a group of patients present with neurological symptoms that are incongruent and at odds with symptoms caused by typical neurological disease. The nature of these symptoms and the clinical signs that accompany them suggest that normal function is possible, but that the patient cannot (or will not) access this normal function. The debate regarding the voluntariness or otherwise of such symptoms is a key reason why considerable conflict often arises in the interaction between such patients and healthcare providers. It also accounts for why diagnostic and treatment services for patients with functional neurological symptoms, one of the commonest diagnoses made in neurological practice, are very poorly developed, compared to other causes of neurological symptoms.

The ancient Greeks used the term 'Hysteria' for this condition and related it to the uterus wandering within the (woman's) body. Hippocrates described this to be related to women remaining unfruitful for too long, and Galen thought this was a disease caused by sexual deprivation in particularly passionate women. Over the following centuries, aetiological theories placed the origin of Hysteria in the brain and recognized its occurrence in both men and women. In the late nineteenth century, an explosion of interest in the condition occurred, in conjunction with the 'clinico-anatomic' methodological approach to neurological illness pioneered by Charcot. The concept of 'functional' neurological illness emerged at that time—a broad term to describe causes of neurological symptoms that were not associated with a structural lesion at autopsy. Freud and Breuer's approach to such patients, later considerably developed by Freud alone, formed the basis for the development of psychoanalysis and crystallized key concepts regarding aetiology in such patients, especially the role of (repressed) emotional trauma and the symbolic nature of the neurological symptoms. With the separation of neurology and psychiatry that occurred around this time, Hysteria found its uncomfortable place in medical practice as a condition presenting to neurologists, but where management was seen as belonging to psychiatrists, psychologists, and psychotherapists.

Given this unusual position, Hysteria missed out on the revolution that occurred in biomedical understanding of illness over the twentieth century. This situation was not aided by a perception that Hysteria was a diagnosis that was often incorrect and that it was common for such patients to be found to have an organic disease at a later stage, a perception fuelled, in part, by Eliot Slater's influential paper *The Diagnosis of Hysteria* (Slater, 1965). Slater's conclusions were proven to be inaccurate in a study carried out decades later at the same centre (Crimlisk et al., 1998). Since the latter part of the twentieth century, there has been increasing scientific interest in this area, pioneered by epidemiological work showing the high prevalence of such patients in neurological practice and the stability of the diagnosis over time (Stone et al., 2005). A new approach to, and interest in, diagnosis and management among neurologists and neuropsychiatrists has begun to translate into specific services for patients and a growing body of scientific work on aetiology and pathophysiology.

Terminology and classification

A number of diagnostic labels have been used to describe this condition historically, many of which still remain in clinical use. This causes confusion among patients and clinicians. Box 24.1 lists some of the commonly used labels over the years. Still there is no clear consensus on the best terminology for this condition that is universally accepted. Lots of these labels are unsatisfactory for different reasons. Many of these are now obsolete and not in common use, such as Hysteria—rightly so. Many others such as psychogenic or psychosomatic suggest underlying psychological mechanisms, which may or may not be present or apparent. Non-diagnoses such as non-epileptic attack tell a patient what they do not have, but not what they do have.

The commonly used terms (included in ICD-10 and DSM-5) somatoform, conversion, or dissociation are based on psychodynamic theories and may not be accurate. The term 'medically unexplained symptoms' is used widely, but this, in our opinion, is an unhelpful and inaccurate term. Stone et al. (2002) found that, among patients with neurological illness, the term 'functional neurological symptoms' caused the least offence. There has been general (but certainly not universal) recognition among neurologists and neuropsychiatrists that this is a therapeutically useful diagnostic label (Edwards et al., 2014). DSM-5 has moved towards adopting this term. Clinicians can also commonly refer separately to three broad groups of functional neurological disorder (FND) as functional non-epileptic attacks (FNEAs), functional motor disorder (FMD), and functional cognitive disorder (FCD), although a number of other functional presentations, including visual loss, deafness, sensory disturbances, etc., are also seen.

Box 24.2 describes DSM-5 classification, and Box 24.3 describes ICD-10 classification for FND, though the terminology differs slightly. It is expected that ICD-11 will move closer to DSM-5 and adopt the term 'functional'. DSM-5 now has greater emphasis on making a positive clinical diagnosis, with less emphasis on both ruling out all the possible organic neurological explanation and providing a convincing psychological formulation at the time of diagnosis.

Epidemiology

In primary care settings, 20–30% of patients present with symptoms that do not have clear organic explanation and can be broadly defined as somatoform (Fink, 1999). These include symptoms that affect various different organs of body. One-third of new referrals in neurological settings have been estimated to be poorly explained by identifiable organic disease (Carson et al., 2000). Another study (Snijders et al., 2004) noted 35% of new neurology referrals were neurologically unexplained and represented functional disorders. Specialist neurology clinics, such as epilepsy clinics or movement disorder clinics, will commonly come across patients with FND. Approximately 20% of accident and emergency (A&E) presentations with status epilepticus are not epileptic and are functional in nature. Approximately half of refractory status presentations in A&E are non-epileptic in nature.

Functional neurological symptoms can be disabling. Carson et al. (2011) noted that at 1 year follow-up, at least 50% had stopped working and over a quarter were receiving illness-related financial benefits. Yearly costs associated with this condition in the UK are estimated to be approximately £18 billion, which is more than the annual cost associated with dementia in the UK (Bermingham et al., 2010).

Aetiology and pathophysiology

Aetiological studies have identified higher rates than control populations of childhood adversity, recent adverse life events, personality disorder, and mood disorders in people with FND (Kranick et al., 2011; Roelofs et al., 2005). However, the proportion of patients with such aetiological factors is very variable between studies, with all studies reporting some patients without any obvious predisposing factor to the development of the FND, and many finding only a minority of patients have such factors. There is an obvious issue regarding the method of assessment of such factors in epidemiological studies and whether such factors may be present, but not recognized by the patient. Despite this, it is clear that the tendency to assume that there must be a causative emotionally traumatic event in the background in every patient and that treatment must always focus on identifying this is not only incorrect but also can be damaging to patients. Higher levels of dissociative experiences have been described in FND and exploration of these may be helpful during clinical assessment. Often people with FND may have other somatoform spectrum disorders, including chronic pain, fatigue, or cardiac or gastrointestinal symptoms. Their illness belief system, behavioural avoidance, excessive attention, excessive autonomic arousal, and their past experiences of illness may be aetiologically linked either as precipitating or perpetuating factors. As functional neurological symptoms commonly co-occur, there is likely to be common routes to development in terms of underlying mechanisms.

Patients commonly report physical health events (which, of course, have both a physical and a psychological dimension) just prior to the onset of functional symptoms, something also reflected in the common co-occurrence of typical neurological illness with functional neurological symptoms (about 15% of patients with neurological disease diagnoses have functional neurological symptoms too) (Parees et al., 2014; Stone et al., 2012a, b).

Cognitive and neurobiological models for the development of functional symptoms have highlighted the importance of body-focused attention and of beliefs/expectations regarding symptoms (Brown, 2004). In one approach, a Bayesian hierarchical model of brain function has been used to conceptualize how strong predictions/expectations regarding particular symptoms might be established by the interaction between physical precipitating events and predisposing psychological factors (Edwards et al., 2012). When combined with self-directed attention, such predictions can manifest without an associated sense of agency or will for the symptoms produced.

Considering predisposing, precipitating, and perpetuating factors of a biological, psychological, and social nature provides a useful and rich framework to understand the development and maintenance of functional neurological symptoms. This approach can be useful for planning treatment and for improving patients' understanding of the interacting factors that may be contributing to their symptoms.

In FNEA, Rusch et al. (2001) suggest there are six categories of patients, based on aetiology, psychosocial history, and psychotherapy response: anxiety/panic; impaired affect regulation and interpersonal skills; PTSD; somatization/conversion; depression; and reinforced behaviour patterns. Brown (2013) proposes two clusters. Cluster 1 includes people who have difficulty identifying, accepting, and talking about their feelings (alexithymia) and difficulties with emotion regulation. This is congruent with the idea that FNEAs develop as a mechanism in response to overwhelming distress (Reuber et al., 2004; Uliaszek et al., 2012; Urbanek et al., 2014) and that alexithymia may be an important factor in the development of FND (Demartini et al., 2014; Lumley et al., 2007; Urbanek et al., 2014). The group of Cluster 2 patients was characterized by higher somatization and depression scores than a control epilepsy group, but generally minimal psychiatric difficulties, and Brown suggests this group's experience of FNEA can be explained by the difficulty in disengaging attention from symptoms and distortions in perception of somatosensory symptoms, as proposed by a model of somatization (Brown, 2004; Brown, 2013). The latter explanation is also in line with the framework proposed by Edwards and colleagues for FMD (Edwards et al., 2013). Recently, an integrative theory of FNEA has been proposed (Brown and Reuber, 2016b).

Diagnosis

Diagnosis of FND is primarily clinical. It has often been considered a diagnosis of exclusion, but this is incorrect and can lead to significant harm from endless rounds of tests and delaying a proper explanation of the diagnosis and access to appropriate treatments. However, it is important to recognize that many patients with FND have both physical and mental health comorbidities, and these need proper assessment (including investigation in some cases)

and treatment. There has been an increasing recognition of the triggering of FND by physical health problems and how commonly FND co-occurs with neurological disease. Thus, a comprehensive neurological assessment is very important in ensuring a correct diagnosis of all current problems, including FND, and to consider their appropriate investigation and treatment.

Conceptually, functional neurological symptoms represent abnormal function in a system that can be demonstrated to be capable of normal function. This concept is easiest to understand in reference to functional motor symptoms. For example, in unilateral functional leg weakness, Hoover's sign can be demonstrated—power of hip extension is weak when tested directly by asking the patient to push their leg down, but power returns to normal when activity in the same muscle is triggered by flexion at the opposite hip. Thus, abnormal function exists (the weak leg), but one can demonstrate that normal function is possible (normal power in the leg when the movement is triggered 'automatically'). In functional tremor, the patient cannot stop their tremor voluntarily, but when they are asked to make a distracting, competing movement with the other hand, the tremor pauses. Thus, abnormal function exists (the arm is shaking), but the possibility of normal function can be demonstrated (the arm stops shaking when attention is diverted away). This same concept can be applied to sensory symptoms—in functional hemianaesthesia of the body, sensory evoked potentials are normal, showing abnormal function (loss of sensation), but the possibility of normal function is demonstrated (normal electrophysiological markers of sensory conductance from limb to brain). Similarly, in functional non-epileptic attacks, the abnormal function of limb shaking and loss of awareness occurs in the presence of documented normal function of the brain (EEG showing rhythms associated with normal wakefulness). When testing people with functional memory impairment, tests of implicit memory are normal despite often severely abnormal function in basic explicit memory tests.

Functional symptoms also often break basic 'rules' of neuroanatomy, physiology, and physics. For example, patients may report tubular visual field defects (a field defect that is the same size when measured close to the patient or far away), something that breaks the rules of optics. Patients may report massive variability in symptom severity, including times when symptoms are completely absent—something rarely seen in neurological disease. Patients may have 'curative' placebo effects with treatment, e.g. an immediate response of functional dystonia to botulinum toxin injections (which take 2–3 days to begin to work physiologically). There is often a clear attentional element to symptoms where deficits are maximal when attention is focused by the patient onto their body (e.g. during physical examination), compared to normal function when distracted (putting their coat on, getting something out of their bag). One can see this in eye movements where normal saccadic eye movements are made during conversation, but then during eye movement examination, eye movements are dramatically abnormal.

Occasionally specific investigations can be helpful in supporting the diagnosis of FND. For example, in functional myoclonus, combined EEG and EMG recordings can show a pre-movement potential in the EEG prior to the myoclonic jerk, something not seen in organic myoclonus. In functional tremor, a battery of electrophysiological tests have been found to separate functional from organic tremor with high specificity and sensitivity. In non-epileptic attacks, an EEG during an attack is very helpful in proving the diagnosis—particularly helpful when a group of patients have both epileptic and non-epileptic attacks. However, often tests are not needed, as the diagnosis is clear on clinical grounds.

As mentioned previously, careful clinical assessment is needed to identify comorbidities in both physical and mental health, and the finding of a clear functional symptom should not stop consideration of additional illnesses that may be present. This is also true in the follow-up of patients with FND where new symptoms should not be automatically dismissed as being 'just' part of FND, but should be subject to normal clinical assessment in their own right.

Diagnostic explanation

There is no hiding from the fact that many doctors find consultations with patients with FND frustrating and difficult, and that attitudes towards these patients are frequently negative. Much of this negativity may come from a belief that symptoms are faked, and also from negative experiences occurring when trying to explain symptoms to patients. In turn, patients with FND often report very negative encounters with doctors and other health professionals, reporting that the explanations given made them feel as though they were making up their symptoms and should just 'snap out of it'.

One reason why diagnostic explanation goes so badly wrong is that it is often performed in a way that is completely different from how other medical diagnoses are explained (Stone, 2016; Stone and Edwards, 2012). Normal practice in diagnostic explanation is to validate symptoms and their associated impact, to give the diagnosis a name, to explain *how* the diagnosis has been made, and to give an idea of treatment and prognosis. Explaining *why* symptoms have occurred is not generally part of this process, and if it is, it reflects the variability of aetiological risk factors between individuals with a particular illness and the many unknowns about why illness develops. In patients with FND, this process is turned on its head. Patients may be told only that their tests are normal, with no explanation offered for the symptoms they have. If the diagnosis is explained, it is often done so on an aetiological level—'these symptoms are not physical symptoms but are due to stress/trauma', which is an explanation that is hard to follow at best, and at worst translates into symptoms being not real or 'all in the mind'. Patients are often given no advice on treatment or prognosis, or if they are referred to treatment services (physiotherapy, neuropsychiatry, psychology), no rationale is given for why these treatments might work. Given this state of affairs, it is perhaps not surprising that patients often seek further medical opinions and request more tests. This behaviour, often suggested to be 'doctor shopping' or 'abnormal illness behaviour', can be interpreted in many patients as a normal response to having disabling symptoms with no clear explanation or plan for treatment being offered.

One approach to diagnostic explanation is simply to follow the normal process of explanation for other illnesses. It is often helpful to validate the symptoms (given that the patient may have had negative experiences previously in healthcare encounters) by saying that you believe the symptoms and do not think they are imagined or 'put on'. A clear diagnostic label can be given, e.g. 'you have a functional neurological disorder' or 'you have functional weakness'. An explanation of how the diagnosis has been made can then be given. This is easier for motor symptoms where by demonstrating the physical signs such as Hoover's sign or distractibility of tremor, one can show how the diagnosis has been made while at the same time demonstrating the possibility of normal function (and hence the possibility of recovery or improvement). It is then reasonable to discuss risk factors for the development of FND that include both physical and mental health problems, as well as past emotional trauma. However, as one would expect with any risk factor, such problems are not present in everyone, or may be present but not relevant. Presented in this way, it promotes an open-minded discussion of the relevance, or not, of such factors (and therefore whether they need to be considered as part of treatment), rather than a surety that childhood trauma (for example) must be present, and if the patient says it is not, it can only be because they are repressing the memory of it or are not prepared to 'confess'. When handled correctly, this way of explaining the diagnosis provides the patient with an explanation that is understandable, surety that they are being believed, and the opportunity for a holistic discussion about risk factors, triggers, and maintaining factors, including psychological, emotional, and social factors.

The process of diagnosis (including investigation and consideration of comorbid illness) and diagnostic explanation is one that really needs to be complete before moving forward to consider treatment planning. It is a process that largely falls into the remit of neurologists, as they will be the person to whom the patient is referred and it is within their skill set to make a positive diagnosis of an FND and to consider alternative or additional diagnoses that might be present. It is also reasonable for the patient to expect an explanation of the diagnosis from a neurologist. Without this process being complete, it is much less likely that treatment services will be able to engage successfully with the patient. In an ideal world, there should be a joined-up approach and an overlap between neurologists, neuropsychiatrists, psychologists, and other treating professionals such as physiotherapists where communication of the diagnosis and psychoeducation are done jointly, along with giving a rationale for the proposed treatment.

Treatment planning in FND

The foundation of successful treatment is a good diagnostic explanation that is understood and accepted by the patient and is shared among the treating health professionals. Given the disparate nature of the services that might be involved in treating a patient with FND, this is difficult to achieve and speaks to an urgent need for organized care of patients with FND within mixed neurological and neuropsychiatric teams. Comprehensive multidisciplinary assessment should take place after initial neurological assessment. This could include neuropsychiatric assessment and other assessments to inform treatment, including psychological and physiotherapy assessments.

Patients with FND are hugely diverse in their symptomatology, symptom severity, and comorbidities. It is logical therefore that treatment needs diversity too. There is, unfortunately, little high-quality evidence to guide treatment decisions. In a group of patients, there is a very complex interaction between functional neurological symptoms, physical health problems, mental health problems, and social and financial problems caused by disability, and a suitably composed rehabilitation team would seem best placed to make treatment suggestions. Communication with other involved services is often necessary in order to avoid different (potentially unhelpful) messages being given to patients about their symptoms, as well as to reduce unnecessary or duplicate interventions. In other patients, good diagnostic explanation, signposting to online sources of information, and the offer of follow-up, if needed, are all that is necessary. In many patients, chronic pain and fatigue are dominant symptoms, and involvement of chronic pain and fatigue management programmes can be very helpful. This 'stratified' approach to treatment services is supported by a recent consensus proposal from Healthcare Improvement Scotland (2012).

The main specific treatments for FND are psychological and physiotherapy-based, either alone or in combination as a multi-disciplinary (including inpatient) treatment programme. There is growing evidence that a specific approach, based on an understanding of the specific nature of FND, is needed, whereas generic psychological or physical treatment often does not help and may be counterproductive.

Treatments for FND

As one of the main explanations for FND is underlying psychological distress, many patients will be referred to a psychiatrist, a clinical psychologist, or a CBT therapist (Gaynor et al., 2009; Hopp and LaFrance, 2012; Nielsen et al., 2015). However, while psychological treatment may be the desired intervention, it is not always available, as demonstrated by a survey conducted in the UK and Ireland which revealed that while 93% of their respondents wanted to refer patients with FNEA for psychological treatment, only 35% could refer all of their patients and 15% were unable to refer any patients (Mayor et al., 2011).

The evidence base for psychological treatments of FND specifically is limited, due to a lack of large RCTs. A Cochrane review (Ruddy and House, 2005) reviewing psychosocial interventions for conversion disorder (FND) found 43 relevant papers, but only three papers met the inclusion criteria (the RCTs). Of those reviewed, one study examined paradoxical injunction therapy (Ataoglu et al., 2003) and the other two studies examined the efficacy of hypnosis (Moene et al., 2002, 2003). The review concluded that the studies were of poor methodological quality and that benefits and/or harm of psychosocial interventions are not fully known. In the UK, NHS Scotland (2012) (Health Improvement Scotland, 2012) recommends that treatment for FND should include the following: (1) FND diagnosed, and the diagnosis explained by a neurologist; (2) brief treatments offered when explanation alone is unsuccessful, e.g. brief guided self-help programme; (3) services for patients with severe and intractable functional neurological symptoms.

The heterogeneity of the overall FND population, in terms of presentation and responses to treatment, makes generalizations regarding treatment difficult. Within FNEA, it has been highlighted that variable results found in studies are likely to be due to the heterogeneity of patients (Brown and Reuber, 2016a). Research tends to examine treatment of FNEA, FMD, and FCD separately, with the majority of research on psychological treatments for FND being carried out on the FNEA population. Each of these sub-categories of FND will be examined in turn.

Functional non-epileptic attacks

A Cochrane review published in 2014 concluded there was little reliable evidence to support any treatment for FNEA, including CBT (Martlew et al., 2014). Nevertheless, CBT has been the most rigorously examined treatment and has the strongest evidence base. Psychodynamic approaches have been found to be effective in uncontrolled studies. Other interventions that have been studied are paradoxical intention (Ataoglu et al., 2003), hypnosis (patient sample included a subset of those with FNEA) (Moene et al., 2002, 2003), inpatient multidisciplinary treatment (Demartini et al., 2014), and eye movement desensitization and reprocessing (EMDR) (Kelley and Benbadis, 2007; van Rood and de Roos, 2009). Carlson and Nicholson Perry (2017) carried out a meta-analysis of psychological treatment for FNEA and found that after psychological intervention, 47% of patients were seizure-free and 82% of people had a frequency reduction of 50%. Their results also indicated that a flexible and patient-centred, rather than a manualized, approach may produce better outcomes. People presenting with FNEA may have a range of underlying psychological processes and it is debated that one treatment approach rigidly applied may not be applicable to all. A multi-modular approach has been proposed to deal with the heterogeneity of presentations necessitating different psychological treatments more tailored to an individual patient (Agrawal et al., 2014).

Cognitive behavioural therapy

CBT has been found to be effective as a treatment for other somatoform disorders (Kroenke, 2007). In pilot RCTs examining CBT (Goldstein et al., 2010; LaFrance et al., 2014), it has been found that individual CBT significantly reduced the number of fits experienced by patients. LaFrance and colleagues randomized 38 patients to receive either medication only (sertraline hydrochloride), CBT alone (12 sessions), CBT with medication, or treatment-as-usual (TAU). They found that CBT with or without sertraline achieved significantly greater seizure reduction and improvement in comorbid symptoms and overall functioning. The medication-only and TAU groups showed no improvements. Goldstein and colleagues randomized 66 patients with FNEA to receive either CBT (12 sessions) plus standard medical care (SMC) or SMC alone. They found that the CBT group achieved significantly greater seizure reduction at the end of treatment. This pilot study was followed by a large multi-centre RCT in the UK. They found that CBT (plus SMC) had no statistically significant advantage, in terms of the primary outcome of seizure reduction, when compared with SMC alone. However, they report significant group differences for clinically relevant secondary outcomes, including longest period of seizure freedom in the previous 6 months, improved psychosocial functioning, reduced psychological distress, and higher patient and clinician ratings of improvement (Goldstein et al., 2020).

Goldstein and colleagues proposed CBT, based on a fear avoidance model, whereby FNEA are considered to be dissociative responses to heightened arousal (without necessarily being aware of this heightened arousal—so-called 'panic without panic') (Goldstein and Mellers, 2006). Attacks can then be interpreted as dangerous, which generates feelings of fear and leads to avoidance of associated activities and developing 'safety-seeking behaviours' such as only going out with another person. This can have a negative impact on a person's mood and confidence, as they are no longer engaging in activities that are important to them. Other maintaining factors could be seeking reassurance from others and potential benefits of the 'sick role' such as being given greater support (Goldstein et al., 2004). Treatment based on this model includes an individual formulation of onset and maintenance completed for each patient, which then guides treatment. Treatment can include strategies that interrupt FNEA, supporting patients to reduce avoidance behaviour, teaching relaxation strategies, and identifying and modifying responses to any unhelpful thoughts that may be contributing to maintenance of attacks, low self-esteem, low mood, or anxiety. LaFrance and colleagues' CBT intervention is based on a treatment manual developed by the team. Treatment focuses on identifying and challenging cognitive distortions, identifying triggers for FNEA, changing unhelpful behaviour, training in healthy communication with others, and learning relaxation strategies.

CBT-based psychoeducational group treatment has been found to significantly improve well-being (Conwill et al., 2014) and functioning (Chen et al., 2014) in uncontrolled studies. An RCT of guided self-help CBT for FND (127 patients with FNEA and FMD included) has been evaluated and found to significantly improve subjective health (Sharpe et al., 2011). A self-help book based on this treatment has been published (Williams et al., 2011).

Psychodynamic approaches

Psychodynamic or psychoanalytic approaches have been examined in uncontrolled studies. De Oliveira Santos et al. (2014) examined data from 37 patients who completed 48 sessions of psychoanalytic treatment over a period of 12 months; 29.7% stopped having FNEA, 51.4% experienced a reduction in attacks, and 18.9% did not improve. Barry et al. (2008) report on group psychodynamic psychotherapy carried out over 32 weeks. Twelve patients attended, and seven patients attended 75% or more of sessions. They reported a decrease in seizure frequency and improvement in terms of BDI and the Global Severity Index on the Symptoms Checklist-90.

Psychodynamic interpersonal therapy (PIT), a variant of psychodynamic therapy emphasizing the interpersonal process, was originally developed by Robert F. Hobson and has been adapted to treat patients with functional symptoms (Reuber et al., 2007). Mayor et al. (2010) reported on the outcome of 47 patients with FNEA who were treated with up to 20 sessions of augmented PIT. At follow-up (12–61 months after the end of treatment), 25.5% of patients were no longer experiencing FNEA and 40% reported an improvement in terms of frequency. PIT has been examined in an RCT evaluating its efficacy for improving the QoL of patients with multiple 'medically unexplained' symptoms such as pain, dizziness, fatigue, and bowel dysfunction. Researchers found that 12 sessions of PIT, based on a manual they developed, versus enhanced medical care, resulted in significant improvements in physical QoL and somatization at 9-month follow-up (Sattel et al., 2012).

These studies indicate a possible benefit of psychodynamic or psychoanalytic psychotherapy, but as they are uncontrolled, it is not possible to determine whether the improvement in some patients was due to the therapy specifically or another factor such as regular contact with a caring professional. PIT appears to be a promising intervention for FNEA, but controlled studies are needed.

Functional motor disorder

Physiotherapy

Physiotherapy has clear face validity as a treatment for patients with functional motor symptoms. There is a growing evidence base to support the usefulness of specific physiotherapy treatment. A systematic review of physiotherapy for FMD found 29 papers reporting on treatment and observed that improvements were noted in 60–70% of patients (Nielsen et al., 2013). Many of the studies reviewed were small cohort studies, but larger studies have now been performed. A 5-day intensive physiotherapy programme that includes movement retraining, as well as examining unhelpful expectations and identifying physical and psychological triggers, has demonstrated significant improvements on physical domains, but not mental health measures (Nielsen et al., 2015). A randomized feasibility study including 60 patients provided additional support for the approach with over 70% of those in the intervention group reported a good outcome, compared to <20% of the control group. Encouragingly, this treatment effect was found even though most patients had symptom duration of over 5 years and had all received physiotherapy previously (Nielsen et al., 2017). A multicentre RCT of this intensive physiotherapy approach is underway (Nielsen et al., 2019). Intensive physiotherapy (twice daily for 5 consecutive days) has also been found to be a successful treatment for FMD by Czarnecki et al. (2012). They reported that after treatment, around 70% of patients were markedly improved or in remission, as rated on patient- and clinician-rated measures. Additionally, compared to a control group, they found that the treatment group were significantly more likely to rate themselves as being markedly improved or in remission at long-term follow-up. An RCT evaluating a 3-week inpatient rehabilitation programme for functional gait disorder, compared to waiting list control, obtained significant improvements in walking ability and QoL. Treatment included adapted physical activity within a cognitive behavioural paradigm, and there were three main aspects: symptom explanation, positively reinforcing normal function and improvements, and not positively reinforcing dysfunction (Jordbru et al., 2014). Consensus guidelines for physiotherapy have been developed to help guide physiotherapy provision and service development (Nielsen et al., 2014).

The effect of physiotherapy is sometimes ascribed to 'face saving'—in other words, providing patients with a 'way out' of symptoms that does not involve them acknowledging a psychological dimension to symptoms. However, a number of studies now show a benefit of specific physiotherapy for people who had previously had physiotherapy without benefit. This suggests that there is a specific component to physiotherapy that is of benefit over and above its general acceptability as a treatment. As with many non-psychological treatments, specialist physiotherapy for FMD has a psychological and an educational dimension that is likely to help symptom improvement through validation, explanation, and challenging of unhelpful beliefs.

Cognitive behavioural therapy

As described in the FNEA section, CBT psychoeducation for FND in both guided self-help and group format has been found to improve subjective health and well-being, respectively (Conwill et al., 2014; Sharpe et al., 2011). CBT has been examined as part of inpatient treatment packages (see below). In a study of 15 patients with functional tremor, Espay et al. (2019) report significant improvements of tremor severity, following CBT, and those who improved also showed associated changes on fMRI images in areas associated with emotional processing (anterior cingulate/paracingulate regions). Dallocchio et al. (2016) carried out a small randomized study evaluating CBT alone and CBT plus adjunctive physical activity, compared with standard medical care as a control group. Both treatment groups improved over time, compared with control, with no significant differences between treatment groups.

Multidisciplinary inpatient treatment

Multidisciplinary inpatient treatment for severe FMD has been examined in several studies. Saifee and colleagues reported on patients with severe refractory symptoms who had attended an inpatient treatment programme that included neuro-physiotherapy, occupational therapy, CBT, support from mental health nurses, neuropsychiatry assessment and input, and input from neurologists. Thirty-two patients were contacted for follow-up and 26 patients responded. Fifty-eight per cent reported that they had improved after treatment, but patients were unlikely to have returned to work, even if they reported improvement (Saifee et al., 2012). A retrospective study reported on patients admitted over a 5-year period (33 cases) to a neuropsychiatry unit. Treatment on the unit included neuropsychiatry, CBT delivered by a clinical psychologist if the patient was assessed as suitable, physiotherapy, and occupational therapy. They found that patients significantly improved on the Modified Rankin Scale (MRS), which is a measure that grades symptoms on a scale where 0 is 'no symptoms at all' and 5 is 'severe disability: bedridden, incontinent, and requiring constant nursing care and attention', as well as significant improvements on mobility and activities of daily living (ADLs) (McCormack et al., 2014). Demartini et al. (2014) assessed the outcomes of 66 patients with FND (predominantly functional motor symptoms) admitted to an inpatient multidisciplinary team unit. At discharge, patients reported improvements in terms of their mood and the extent their symptoms bothered them. On the clinician-rated Health of the Nation Outcome Scale (HoNOS), there were also significant improvements. Fifty-five per cent (n = 36) were assessed at 12-month follow-up, with significant improvements maintained.

Due to the multiple modalities of treatment on these inpatient programmes, it is not possible to know the relative contributions of different aspects of the treatments to the treatment effect observed. Indeed it is likely to be different between different patients. However, these studies do suggest that for some very disabled patients, inpatient specialist rehabilitation can lead to long-term benefit. As such, treatment will always be limited in availability, due to its intensive and expensive nature, a key priority is to identify patients who are most likely to benefit.

Hypnosis

Moene et al. (2003) carried out an RCT of a hypnosis-based outpatient treatment for FMD. Forty-nine patients were randomly assigned to either hypnosis (one explanation session plus ten treatment sessions) or waiting list control. Five patients dropped out (four from the treatment group, one from waiting list control), and data were analysed for the remaining 44 patients. Of those in the treatment group, 12 out of the 20 patients received extra treatment

sessions (mean number of extra sessions = 6.3). They found that the hypnosis group had a significant reduction in symptoms and impairments in daily life, physical, and social activities. This was maintained at 6-month follow-up. Moene and colleagues also evaluated hypnosis as an add-on in an RCT based on an inpatient unit where they compared inpatient treatment-as-usual (TAU), which included multidisciplinary team input, and TAU plus hypnosis. The hypnosis component included an introductory session plus 8-weekly sessions. They found that the addition of the hypnosis component did not significantly improve treatment outcome (Moene et al., 2002).

Psychodynamic approaches

Hinson et al. (2006) reported on a single-blind clinical trial of 12 sessions of psychodynamic psychotherapy for FMD delivered to nine patients. Seven patients improved in terms of movement disorder severity, with two patients worsening. Six patients improved on measures of depression and anxiety, and three worsened. Augmented PIT has been evaluated as a treatment for FND generally (Reuber et al., 2007). In a sample of 91 patients (many of whom had multiple functional neurological symptoms), most were experiencing FNEA (68%), but the sample also included patients with FMD (around 30%). For the total sample, significant improvements, after therapy and at 6-month follow-up, were obtained on measures of mood and functioning. The therapy was also calculated to be cost-effective.

Functional cognitive disorder

In this section, FCD refers to functional neurological symptoms, such as subjectively poor memory and concentration, and does not refer to dissociative amnesia or dissociative fugue states. Despite FCD being a relatively common presentation (Pennington et al., 2015), and often a long-term problem (Schmidtke et al., 2008), treatment for FCD has been infrequently studied. Patients frequently experience functional cognitive symptoms, alongside other more dominant functional neurological symptoms, and other functional somatic syndromes such as fibromyalgia (Teodoro et al., 2018) and this could be why FCD has not been researched more often. Also, in clinical practice, functional cognitive symptoms co-occurring with other functional neurological symptoms can resolve when these other symptoms are targeted. Nevertheless, for some patients, this is not the case, and research into effective treatments for FCD is needed.

High memory-related achievement motivation or memory-related perfectionism and low memory-related self-efficacy have been found in patients with FCD (Metternich et al., 2008), and this points towards possible treatment targeting these areas. It has been proposed that FCD could be considered a neurocognitive hypochondriasis, whereby a person is hypervigilant to cognitive failures, views them as evidence of problematic dysfunction, and finds them distressing (Brauer Boone, 2009). It seems that in line with other FND, heightened attention to cognitive errors, and over-interpretation of the meaning of the errors, contribute to the maintenance of functional cognitive symptoms (Teodoro et al., 2018). Treatment targeting memory-related anxiety, using evidence-based treatment for health anxiety, such as CBT (Warwick et al., 1996), may be beneficial, but this is purely hypothetical and has not been established.

Pennington et al. (2015) recommend a management strategy that includes relevant medical investigations (e.g. EEG, neuroimaging, blood tests) and neuropsychological testing to rule out disease and degeneration. Patients can often remain worried about their memory, despite investigations coming back normal, and a 1-year follow-up can be a helpful method of reducing doubt about diagnosis. They recommend framing the diagnosis, by explaining that subjective experience of cognition is influenced by internal (e.g. distress, pain) and external factors (e.g. stressful environment) and that functional cognitive symptoms are common. They suggest emphasizing performance on neuropsychological tests being as expected for their age and pointing out factors that may be contributing to memory-related anxiety such as memory-related perfectionism and focusing on insignificant cognitive errors. Referral to neuropsychiatry is necessary for those with persistent symptoms and/or significant mental health problems. Additionally, the authors suggest that offering a neuropsychology feedback session is beneficial, as an opportunity to identify possible precipitating factors and explore how they cope with their experience of cognitive difficulties (Pennington et al., 2015).

A pilot RCT of group therapy for FCD (referred to as functional memory disorder by the authors) has been trialled, targeting memory-related self-efficacy. Forty patients with FCD were allocated to either the 13-week intervention group or waiting list control. The intervention group focused on improving patients' stress management skills and reducing memory-related anxiety using cognitive restructuring of unhelpful cognitions related to their memory. They found that the treatment group had significantly increased memory-related self-efficacy post-treatment (3 months) and at 6-month follow-up (Metternich et al., 2008).

Prognosis

Prognosis in patients with FND is very variable. In one meta-analysis of over 10,000 patients with functional motor symptoms, about 40% were the same or worse at long-term follow-up (Gelauff et al., 2014). The majority of the remaining patients had continued symptoms. Certain groups (severe pain, fatigue, fixed dystonic postures) appear to do worse than others. The presence of depression or anxiety has been reported to be a good prognostic factor, presumably because it represents a treatable comorbidity. It is currently not known what the impact might be of organized treatment services for people with FND on long-term outcome.

Conclusion

FND is one of the commonest diagnoses made in neurology clinics. Early and accurate diagnosis and clear communication of the diagnosis by a neurologist are an essential part of the treatment pathway. Further treatment should be individually tailored to the clinical presentation and underlying risk factors and may include, where appropriate (and where available), neuropsychiatric assessment and management and/or interventions from clinical psychologists, physiotherapists, occupational therapists, and speech and language therapists. Patients with severe symptoms may be referred for intensive multidisciplinary inpatient treatment.

KEY LEARNING POINTS

- FND is a common diagnosis in neurological practice.
- Functional neurological symptoms represent abnormal function in a system that can be demonstrated to be capable of normal function.
- Many patients with FND have both physical and mental health comorbidities, and these need proper assessment (including investigation in some cases) and treatment.
- Higher rates of childhood adversity, mood disorders, personality disorders, dissociative tendencies, somatization, emotional regulation difficulties, and alexithymia have been found in the FND population (but not invariably), when compared to controls, and may be predisposing factors.
- Common precipitating factors are experiencing a physical illness or stressful life events. Important maintaining factors in FND are illness beliefs and expectations and attention towards the unwanted symptoms.
- Clear communication of the diagnosis is an important part of treatment.
- The main treatment for FNEAs is psychological treatment, with the strongest evidence supporting the use of FNEA-specific CBT.
- Specialist physiotherapy is a well-supported treatment for FMDs, and there is a small amount of evidence for psychological approaches.
- Multidisciplinary inpatient treatment is used for severe and intractable cases of FND.

REFERENCES

Agrawal, N., Gaynor, D., Lomax, A. and Mula, M., 2014. Multimodular psychotherapy intervention for nonepileptic attack disorder: An individualized pragmatic approach. *Epilepsy & Behavior*, 41, pp.144–8.

Alberto J. et al., 2019. Clinical and neural responses to cognitive behavioral therapy for functional tremor. *Neurology*, 93(19), e.1787–98.

Ataoglu, A. et al., 2003. Paradoxical Therapy in Conversion Reaction. *Journal of Korean Medical Science*, 18(4), pp.581–4.

Barry, J.J. et al., 2008. Group therapy for patients with psychogenic nonepileptic seizures: a pilot study. *Epilepsy & Behavior*, 13(4), pp.624–9.

Bermingham SL, Cohen A, Hague J, Parsonage M. 2010. The cost of somatisation among the working-age population in England for the year 2008–2009. *Ment Health Fam Med*, 7, 71–84.

Brauer Boone, K., 2009. Fixed belief in cognitive dysfunction despite normal neuropsychological scores: Neurocognitive hypochondriasis? *The Clinical Neuropsychologist*, 23, pp.1016–36.

Brown, R.J., 2013. Emotional dysregulation, alexithymia, and attachment in psychogenic nonepileptic seizures. *Epilepsy & Behavior*, 29(1), pp.178–83.

Brown, R.J., 2004. Psychological mechanisms of medically unexplained symptoms: an integrative conceptual model. *Psychological Bulletin*, 130(5), pp.793–812.

Brown, R.J. & Reuber, M., 2016a. Psychological and psychiatric aspects of psychogenic non-epileptic seizures (PNES): A systematic review. *Clinical Psychology Review.* Available at: http://linkinghub.elsevier.com/retrieve/pii/S0272735815301446.

Brown, R.J. & Reuber, M., 2016b. Towards an integrative theory of psychogenic non-epileptic seizures (PNES). *Clinical Psychology Review,* 47, pp.55–70.

Carlson, P. & Nicholson Perry, K. 2017. Psychological interventions for psychogenic non-epileptic seizures: A meta-analysis. *Seizure,* 45, pp.142–50.

Carson AJ, Ringbauer B, Stone J, McKenzie L, Warlow C, Sharpe M,. 2000. Do medically unexplained symptoms matter? A prospective cohort study of 300 new referrals to neurology outpatient clinics. *J Neurol Neurosurg Psychiatry,* 68, pp.207–10.

Carson A, Stone J, Hibberd C, et al. 2011. Disability, distress and unemployment in neurology outpatients with symptoms 'unexplained by organic disease'. *J Neurol Neurosurg Psychiatry,* 82, pp.810–13.

Chen, D. et al., 2014. Brief group psychoeducation for psychogenic nonepileptic seizures: A neurologist-initiated program in an epilepsy center. *Epilepsia,* 55(1), pp.156–66.

Conwill, M. et al., 2014. CBT-based group therapy intervention for nonepileptic attacks and other functional neurological symptoms: A pilot study. *Epilepsy and Behavior,* 34, pp.68–72.

Crimlisk, H.L., Bhatia, K., Cope, H., David, A., Marsden, C.D., Ron, M.A. 1998. Slater revisited: 6 year follow up study of patients with medically unexplained motor symptoms. *BMJ,* 316, p.582.

Czarnecki, K. et al., 2012. Functional movement disorders: Successful treatment with a physical therapy rehabilitation protocol. *Parkinsonism.Relat Disord,* 18, pp.247–51.

Dallocchio, C., Tinazzi, M., Bombieri, F., Arno, N. & Erro, R, 2016. Cognitive behavioural therapy and adjunctive physical activity for functional movement disorders (conversion disorder): a pilot, single-blinded, randomized study. *Psychother Psychosom,* 85(6), pp. 381–3.

Demartini, B., Batla, A., et al., 2014. Multidisciplinary treatment for functional neurological symptoms: a prospective study. *Journal of Neurology,* 261(12), pp.2370–7.

Demartini, B., Petrochilos, P., et al., 2014. The role of alexithymia in the development of functional motor symptoms (conversion disorder). *J Neurol Neurosurg Psychiatry,* 85, pp.1132–7.

Edwards, M.J., Adams, R.A., Brown, H., Pareés, I. and Friston, K.J., 2012. A Bayesian account of 'hysteria'. *Brain,* 135(11), pp.3495–512.

Edwards, M.J., Fotopoulou, A. & Pareés, I., 2013. Neurobiology of functional (psychogenic) movement disorders. *Current Opinion in Neurology,* 26(4), pp.442–7.

Edwards, M.J., Stone, J., Lang, A.E. 2014. From psychogenic movement disorder to functional movement disorder: it's time to change the name. *Mov Disord.* 29(7), pp.849–52.

Stone, J., Edwards, M. 2012. Trick or treat? Showing patients with functional (psychogenic) motor symptoms their physical signs. *Neurology,* 79, 282–4.

Fink, P., Sørensen, L., Engberg, M., Holm, M., Munk-Jørgensen, P. 1999. Somatization in primary care. Prevalence, health care utilization, and general practitioner recognition. *Psychosomatics,* 40(4), 330–8.

Gaynor, D., Cock, H. & Agrawal, N., 2009. Psychological treatments for functional non-epileptic attacks: A systematic review. *Acta Neuropsychiatrica,* 21, pp.158–68.

Gelauff, J., Stone, J., Edwards, M., Carson, A. 2014 The prognosis of functional (psychogenic) motor symptoms: a systematic review. *J Neurol Neurosurg Psychiatry,* 85(2), 220–6.

Goldstein, L.H. et al., 2004. An evaluation of cognitive behavioral therapy as a treatment for dissociative seizures: a pilot study. *Cogn Behav Neurol,* 17(1), pp.41–9.

Goldstein, L.H. et al., 2010. Cognitive-behavioral therapy for psychogenic nonepileptic seizures: a pilot RCT. *Neurology,* 74(24), pp.1986–94.

Goldstein, L.H. & Mellers, C., 2006. Ictal symptoms of anxiety, avoidance behaviour, and dissociation in patients with dissociative seizures. *J Neurol Neurosurg Psychiatry,* 77, pp.616–21.

Goldstein, L. et al., 2020. Cognitive behavioural therapy for adults with dissociative seizures (CODES): a pragmatic, multicentre, randomised controlled trial. *Lancet Psychiatry,* 7, pp.491–505.

Healthcare Improvement Scotland, 2012. *Stepped care for functional neurological symptoms.* Available at: http://www.healthcareimprovementscotland.org.

Hinson, V.K. et al., 2006. Single-blind clinical trial of psychotherapy for treatment of psychogenic movement disorders. *Parkinsonism Relat Dis,* 12, pp.177–80.

Hopp, J.L. & LaFrance, W.C., 2012. Cognitive Behavioral Therapy for Psychogenic Neurological Disorders. *The Neurologist,* 18(6), pp.364–72.

Jordbru, A. et al., 2014. Psychogenic gait disorder: A random ized controlled trial of physical rehabilitation with one-year follow -up. *J Rehabil Med,* 46(2), pp.181–7.

Kelley, S.D.M. & Benbadis, S., 2007. Eye Movement Desensitization and Reprocessing in the Psychological Treatment of Trauma-Based Psychogenic Non-Epileptic Seizures. *Clin Psychol Psychother,* 14, pp.135–44.

Kranick S, Ekanayake V, Martinez V, Ameli R, Hallett M, Voon V. 2011. Psychopathology and psychogenic movement disorders. *Mov Disord,* 26(10), 1844–50.

Kroenke, K., 2007. Efficacy of Treatment for Somatoform Disorders: A Review of Randomized Controlled Trials. *Psychosomatic Med,* 69, pp.881–8.

LaFrance, W.C. et al., 2014. Multicenter Pilot Treatment Trial for Psychogenic Nonepileptic Seizures. *JAMA Psychiatry,* 71(9), p.997.

Lumley, M. a, Neely, L.C. & Burger, A.J., 2007. The Assessment of Alexithymia in Medical Settings: Implications for Understanding and Treating Health Problems. *Journal of Personality Assessment,* 89(3), pp.230–46.

Martlew, J., Pulman, J. & Marson, A.G. 2014. Psychological and behavioural treatments for adults with non- epileptic attack disorder. *Cochrane Database of Systematic Reviews,* 2, CD006370.

Mayor, R., Howlett, S., Grünewald, R., Reuber, M. 2010. Long-term outcome of brief augmented psychodynamic interpersonal therapy for psychogenic nonepileptic seizures: seizure control and health care utilization. *Epilepsia ,* 51, 1169–76.

Mayor, R., Smith, P.E. & Reuber, M., 2011. Management of patients with nonepileptic attack disorder in the United Kingdom: a survey of health care professionals. *Epilepsy & Behavior,* 21(4), pp.402–6.

Mccormack, R. et al., 2014. Specialist inpatient treatment for severe motor conversion disorder: a retrospective comparative study. *J Neurol Neurosurg Psychiatry,* 85, pp.893–8.

Metternich, B. et al., 2008. A pilot group therapy for functional memory disorder. *Psychother Psychosomatics,* 77(4), pp.259–60.

Moene, F.C. et al., 2002. A randomised controlled clinical trial on the additional effect of hypnosis in a comprehensive treatment programme for in-patients with conversion disorder of the motor type. *Psychother Psychosomatics,* 71(2), pp.66–76.

Moene, F.C. et al., 2003. A Randomized Controlled Clinical Trial of a Hypnosis-Based Treatment for Patients with Conversion Disorder, Motor Type. *Int J Clin Exp Hypn*, 51(1), pp.29–50.

Nielsen, G. et al., 2019. Physio4FMD: protocol for a multicentre randomised controlled trial of specialist physiotherapy for functional motor disorder. *BMC Neurol*, 19, p.242.

Nielsen, G. et al., 2017. Randomised feasibility study of physiotherapy for patients with functional motor symptoms. *Journal of Neurology, Neurosurgery and Psychiatry*, 88, pp.484–90.

Nielsen, G. et al., 2015. Outcomes of a 5-day physiotherapy programme for functional (psychogenic) motor disorders. *Journal of Neurology*, 262(3), pp.674–81.

Nielsen, G. et al., 2014. Physiotherapy for functional motor disorders: a consensus recommendation. *Journal of Neurology, Neurosurgery, and Psychiatry*, pp.1–7.

Nielsen, G., Stone, J. & Edwards, M.J., 2013. Physiotherapy for functional (psychogenic) motor symptoms: A systematic review. *Journal of Psychosomatic Research*, 75, pp.93–102.

De Oliveira Santos, N. et al., 2014. Psychogenic non-epileptic seizures and psychoanalytical treatment: Results. *Revista da Associação Médica Brasileira*, 60(6), pp.577–84.

Pareés I, Kojovic M, Pires C, et al. 2014. Physical precipitating factors in functional movement disorders. *Journal of Neurological Science*, 338, 174–7.

Pennington, C. et al., 2015. Functional cognitive disorder: what is it and what to do about it? *Practical Neurology*, 15, pp.436–44.

Reuber, M. et al., 2004. Multidimensional assessment of personality in patients with psychogenic non-epileptic seizures. *Journal of Neurology, Neurosurgery, and Psychiatry*, 75, pp.743–8.

Reuber, M. et al., 2007. Tailored psychotherapy for patients with functional neurological symptoms: A pilot study. *Journal of Psychosomatic Research*, 63, pp.625–32.

Roelofs K, Spinhoven P, Sandijck P, Moene FC, Hoogduin KA. 2005. The impact of early trauma and recent life-events on symptom severity in patients with conversion disorder. *Journal of Nervous and Mental Disease*, 193(8), 508–14.

van Rood, Y.R. & de Roos, C., 2009. EMDR in the Treatment of Medically Unexplained Symptoms: A Systematic Review. *Journal of EMDR Practice and Research*, 3(4), pp.248–63.

Ruddy, R. & House, A., 2005. Psychosocial interventions for conversion disorder. *Cochrane Database of Systematic Reviews*, 4, CD005331.

Rusch, M.D. et al., 2001. Psychological Treatment of Nonepileptic Events. *Epilepsy & Behavior*, 2(3), pp.277–83.

Saifee, T.A. et al., 2012. Inpatient treatment of functional motor symptoms: A long-term follow-up study. *Journal of Neurology*, 259(9), pp.1958–63.

Schmidtke, K., Pohlmann, S. & Metternich, B., 2008. The syndrome of functional memory disorder: definition, etiology, and natural course. *American Journal of Geriatric Psychiatry*, 16(12), pp.981–8.

Sharpe, M. et al., 2011. Guided self-help for functional (psychogenic) symptoms: A randomized controlled efficacy trial. *Neurology*, 77(6), pp.564–72.

Slater, E. 1965. Diagnosis of Hysteria. *Br Med J*, 1(5447), pp.1395–9.

Snijders, T.J., Leeuw, F.E., Ursula, M., Klumpers, H. 2004. Prevalence and predictors of unexplained neurological symptoms in an academic neurology outpatient clinic *Journal of Neurology*, 251, p.66.

Stone, J., Wojcik, W., Durrance, D., et al. 2002. What should we say to patients with symptoms unexplained by disease? The 'number needed to offend'. *BMJ*, 325, pp.1449–50.

Stone, J., Smyth, R., Carson, A., et al. 2005. Systematic review of misdiagnosis of conversion symptoms and 'hysteria'. *BMJ*, 331, pp.989–94.

Stone, J., Carson, A., Duncan, R., et al. 2012a. Which neurological diseases are most likely to be associated with 'symptoms unexplained by organic disease'. *Journal of Neurology*, 259(1), pp.33–8.

Stone, J. 2016. Functional neurological disorders: the neurological assessment as treatment. *Practical Neurology*, 16(1), pp.7–17.

Stone, J., Warlow, C., Sharpe, M. 2012b. Functional weakness: clues to mechanism from the nature of onset. *Journal of Neurology, Neurosurgery, and Psychiatry*, 83(1), pp.67–9.

Teodoro, T., Edwards, M.J &, Isaacs, J.D.J, 2018. A unifying theory for cognitive abnormalities in functional neurological disorders, fibromyalgia and chronic fatigue syndrome: systematic review. *Journal of Neurology, Neurosurgery and Psychiatry*, 89(12), pp.1308–19.

Uliaszek, A.A., Prensky, E. & Baslet, G., 2012. Emotion regulation profiles in psychogenic non-epileptic seizures. *Epilepsy & Behavior*, 23(3), pp.364–9.

Urbanek, M. et al., 2014. Regulation of emotions in psychogenic nonepileptic seizures. *Epilepsy and Behavior*, 37, pp.110–15.

Warwick, H.M.C. et al., 1996. A controlled trial of cognitive-behavioural treatment of hypochondriasis. *British Journal of Psychiatry*, 169, pp.189–95.

Williams, C. et al., 2011. *Overcoming Functional Neurological Symptoms: A Five Areas Approach*, London: Hodder Arnold.

25

Memory disorders and dementias

Thomas E. Cope, Jeremy D. Isaacs, and Michael D. Kopelman

Introduction

Memory disorders can be classified as either transient or persistent, and have underlying neurological or psychological causes. Table 25.1 shows examples of disorders across the four quadrants that arise in this classification (Kopelman, 2002). Not all of these disorders will be considered in this chapter, but there will be examples from all four quadrants with particular emphasis on the dementias.

Any neuropsychiatrist should be familiar with some basic concepts that psychologists and neuropsychologists have developed in investigating memory and its disorders. 'Primary' or 'working' memory refer to memory lasting a few seconds or as long as rehearsed—what William James called the 'specious present' (James, 1886). It can be subdivided by modality and is most commonly expressed as a visuospatial sketchpad and a phonological loop, coordinated by a central executive (Baddeley and Hitch, 1974). This is characteristically preserved in the amnesic syndrome but can be selectively impaired in some dementias (e.g. catastrophic failure of the phonological loop is seen in non-fluent variant primary progressive aphasia (nfvPPA), as articulatory control difficulties prevent rehearsal). Note that the term 'short-term memory' is best avoided, as it is used in very different ways by different disciplines and the lay public. 'Episodic' or 'autobiographical' memory refers to a person's recollection of past incidents and events, which occurred at a specific time and place, such that the individual can 'travel back mentally in time' (Tulving, 1972). By definition, this is severely impaired in the amnesic syndrome. 'Semantic' memory refers to knowledge of concepts, facts, and language that do not have a specific location in time and place. This is variably affected in the amnesic syndrome but can be disproportionately affected in certain other disorders, most notably in semantic dementia (SD). Implicit memory refers to learning without awareness, e.g. procedural (perceptuo-motor) skills, which can be preserved in (episodic) memory disorders. Finally, anterograde amnesia refers to impairment of new learning, i.e. in recall and recognition memory for episodes and facts arising after the onset of an illness or injury, whereas retrograde amnesia refers to loss of memory for episodes and facts that occurred before the onset of an illness or injury.

Transient neurological amnesias

Discrete episodes of amnesia can arise from various aetiologies such as delirium, traumatic brain injury, seizures induced by epilepsy or electroconvulsive therapy, alcoholic 'blackout', or cerebral hypoglycaemia. We will consider here two prototypical syndromes in this category: transient global amnesia (TGA) and transient epileptic amnesia (TEA).

Transient global amnesia

TGA is a syndrome characterized by an isolated temporary amnesia for a period of a few hours (Fisher, 1958). During an attack, patients are frequently disoriented in time, place, and person, and ask repetitive questions on these topics (Bolwig, 1968). Past autobiographical memories are variably affected. After an attack, there is a total loss of episodic memory for the period of confusion and usually a period of time beforehand. The syndrome is commoner in men than in women and often occurs in the sixth or seventh decade of life. The mean duration of an episode is approximately 4 hours but can be very variable. It can follow strenuous exercise, a stressful life event, or a medical, surgical, or dental procedure (Hodges and Ward, 1989). Unlike TEA (see Transient epileptic amnesia, p. 278), there is usually just a single episode, with approximately 6% of patients experiencing a second attack (Melo et al., 1992). Recurrent attacks should prompt a search for a structural (Shuping et al., 1980b) or embolic (Shuping et al., 1980a) cause. Approximately 25% of cases are associated with migraine and probably represent a 'migrainous variant' (Hodges and Warlow, 1990; Quinette et al., 2006), and approximately 7% of cases subsequently turn out to have an epileptic basis. In approximately 65% of cases, the aetiology is unknown. Some studies have observed that vascular risk factors are over-represented in patients with TGA, compared to controls (Shuping et al., 1980a), but under-represented, compared to patients with TIA (Melo et al., 1992). However, other studies have reported no association with vascular factors, other than migraine. Some individuals display diffusion-weighted imaging changes in medial temporal regions during and after an attack, consistent with the memory disorder, but the evidence for an ischaemic cause is somewhat conflicted (see Huber et al., 2002 for a review).

Table 25.1 A simple classification of memory disorders by chronicity and aetiology

	Discrete Episode	Persistent
Neurological	Toxic confusional state	Mild/moderate momory disorder
	Head injury	Amnesic syndrome – episodic
	Alcoholic 'black-out'	Alzheimer dementla-global
	Cerebral hypoxla	Mild cognitive impairment (MCI)
	Transient Global Amnesia (TGA)	Other dementias; see text,
	Post-ECT	
Psychogenic:	Situation - specific (e.g. offence, PTSD)	Depressive Pesudodementia
	Fugue states	'Focal retrograde amnesia'

Adapted with permission from Kopelman, M. D.. Amnesia: organic and psychogenic. *The British Journal of Psychiatry*, 150(4): 428–442. Copyright © 1987 The Royal College of Psychiatrists. https://doi.org/10.1192/bjp.150.4.428.

Transient epileptic amnesia

TEA is a syndrome of recurrent, brief attacks of amnesia due to focal temporal lobe seizures. It often occurs on waking and is most common in middle-aged men (Zeman and Butler, 2010). Like TGA, repetitive questioning is common, but the attacks are recurrent (averaging 14 a year) and briefer, characteristically lasting 30–60 minutes. The amnesia for the attack may be less dense (Zeman et al., 1998). The EEG is abnormal during an attack but is commonly normal between attacks. However, patients often report interictal memory complaints. A loss of remote autobiographical knowledge (Butler et al., 2007) and accelerated long-term forgetting (Muhlert et al., 2010) have been claimed in some cases. One study involved patients and their spouses or friends visiting the stately homes of Britain while wearing video cameras. When quizzed on the same day about what they had seen, patients performed as well as controls, but recall across a number of modalities (images, thoughts, events, and sensory information) was much poorer after a delay of days to weeks. While the seizures, and consequently the discrete amnestic attacks, may respond well to small doses of anticonvulsant medication, it has been claimed that the interictal difficulties are less tractable (Butler, 2006).

Persisting memory disorders: the amnesic syndrome

The amnesic syndrome (Whitty and Zangwill, 1966) can be defined as 'an abnormal mental state in which memory and learning are affected out of all proportion to other cognitive functions in an otherwise alert and responsive patient' (Victor et al., 1971). Conditions giving rise to an amnesic syndrome or a mild/moderate memory disorder include: herpes encephalitis, cerebral hypoxia/ischaemia, thiamine deficiency in Korsakoff syndrome, limbic encephalitis (resulting from, for example, voltage-gated potassium channel antibodies), head injury, certain types of vascular pathology (thalamic

infarction, posterior cerebral infarct, some subarachnoid haemorrhages), deep-lying tumours (third ventricle, large pituitary adenomas), and tuberculous meningitis. Such a wide variety of individual aetiological categories means that the International Classification of Diseases (ICD) fails to indicate the true incidence, prevalence, and morbidity of non-dementia memory disorders.

In this chapter, we will consider three examples in more detail and then say a few words about the very interesting phenomenon of memory confabulation. Other information on disorders that can affect memory is covered in the chapters on traumatic brain injury (see Chapter 16), infections of the central nervous system (see Chapter 20), tumours (see Chapter 21), inflammatory and autoimmune disorders (see Chapter 22), demyelinating disorders (see Chapter 23), mitochondrial disorders (see Chapters 12 and 26), alcohol-related disorders (see Chapter 27), side effects of drugs and toxins (see Chapter 28), obstructive sleep apnoea (see Chapter 29), nutritional deficiencies (see Chapter 33), and delirium (see Chapter 35).

Korsakoff syndrome

CASE STUDY 1

Case AB (Kopelman et al., 1997) was a 43-year-old woman, who had grown up in a northern industrial town and worked in a paramedical profession. She was admitted to hospital in mid summer. Upon arrival, she was agitated, disorientated, and forgetful, and showed considerable confusion. In the week before her admission, work colleagues had become increasingly worried about her behaviour. She had a history of previous alcohol-related problems. At the time of her admission, she denied heavy drinking, but half a bottle of vodka was found in her handbag.

On neurological examination at admission, AB showed confusion, ataxia, and horizontal nystagmus on both left and right lateral gaze, with partial ophthalmoplegia. There was no evidence of peripheral neuropathy. A diagnosis of Wernicke's encephalopathy was made, and AB received intravenous thiamine and multivitamins. As her confusion settled, her memory emerged as severely and disproportionately impaired.

We learnt from her brother that AB's father had also been a heavy drinker and had fallen in front of a train 20 years earlier. AB had been very close to her father, and her own alcohol consumption was said to have increased dramatically following his death.

From admission, AB confabulated floridly. For example, when first seen by our team, she told us that she was suffering from measles. She often believed that she was in the hospital where she used to work. She mistook doctors or researchers for family members, close and trusted friends, or other people she had never known. She described how she had recently been home to the north of England with both her parents, and that her father had suffered a stroke (they had both been dead for many years).

Clinical features

In 1889, Korsakoff described over 30 alcoholic cases and 14 non-alcoholic cases (the latter almost certainly all had nutritional/thiamine depletion) of this disorder (Korsakoff, 1889a; Victor and Yakovlev, 1955). It commonly, but not always, follows

Wernicke's syndrome of ophthalmoplegia, nystagmus, ataxia, and confusion (which are, in turn, commonly accompanied by peripheral neuropathy). It consists of an abnormal mental state in which memory and learning are affected out of all proportion to other cognitive functions (Victor et al., 1971), resulting from thiamine depletion. Korsakoff himself wrote (Korsakoff, 1889b): 'At first during conversation with such a patient (he or she) gives the impression of a person in complete possession of his (or her) faculties; he (she) reasons about everything perfectly well, draws correct deductions from given premises, makes witty remarks, plays chess or a game of cards, in a word comports himself (herself) as a mentally sound person.'[1] However, '... the patient constantly asks the same questions and repeats the same stories ... may read the same page over and again sometimes for hours ... is unable to remember those persons whom he (she) met only during the illness, for example, the attending physician or nurse.'[2]

Aside from severe anterograde amnesia, there is invariably severe retrograde amnesia with a 'temporal gradient' (relative sparing of early memories). This can be demonstrated in neuropsychological investigations and appears to be related to the degree of executive dysfunction and frontal and thalamic atrophy (Kopelman, 1989; Kopelman et al., 2003). Although 'spontaneous' confabulation is common in the early confusional state of Wernicke's encephalopathy, it is relatively rare in the more chronic stages (see Confabulation, p. 280).

Aetiology

The underlying pathology in the Wernicke–Korsakoff syndrome consists of loss of neurones, gliosis, and microhaemorrhages in periventricular and para-aqueductal brain regions. The critical damage, causing anterograde amnesia, probably consists of pathology in the pathways connecting the mammillary bodies, the mammillo-thalamic tract, and the anterior thalamus (the circuit of Papez). There is very commonly associated frontal cortical atrophy, loss of large neurones in the superior frontal cortex, hypothalamus, and cerebellum, loss of prefrontal white matter, and neuronal dendritic shrinkage (Harding et al., 2000; Harper, 2009; Harper et al., 1987; Mair et al., 1979; Torvik, 1982; Victor et al., 1971). Sullivan and Pfefferbaum (2009) have published images showing signal alteration in the thalamus, fornix, mammillary bodies, and periventricular grey matter in the earliest stages of the disease.

Epidemiology and prognosis

Because alcoholics seldom get properly assessed, there is a dearth of epidemiological studies. However, two investigations reported that the classical neuropathology was found in 12–15% of alcoholics at autopsy, compared with clinical diagnostic rates of only 2–3%.

Victor et al. (1971) reported that 25% of Korsakoff patients 'recovered'; 50% showed improvement over time, and 25% of Korsakoff patients showed no change over time.

---

[1] Korsakoff S. Etude médico-psychologique sur une forme des maladies de la mémoire. *Revue Philosophique*. 1889b; 28: 501–530.
[2] Korsakoff S. Etude médico-psychologique sur une forme des maladies de la mémoire. *Revue Philosophique*. 1889b;28(501):e530.

Herpes encephalitis

CASE STUDY 2

CW (Wilson et al., 2008) was an outstanding musician and a gifted musical scholar. At the age of 46, he developed an influenza-type illness with headache and fever. He was admitted to hospital some days later, and the diagnosis of herpes simplex encephalitis was made. Initially, his level of consciousness fluctuated, but when alertness improved, a profound amnesia remained. CW could converse normally, but he would greet his wife as if he had not seen her for weeks, even after being separated for only a couple of hours.

On formal testing, CW was impaired across tests of anterograde memory, autobiographical memory, and naming, but relatively preserved at measures of IQ and executive function. He showed relative preservation of semantic knowledge, retaining much of his knowledge about Renaissance composers. There was a striking dissociation between his procedural memory (retained skill at playing the piano or organ) and his (explicit memory) awareness that he had played recently.

MRI brain scans in 1991 and 2006 were similar, demonstrating extensive loss of the left temporal lobe and, similarly, severe loss of right medial temporal lobe tissue, with some degree of generalized cortical atrophy.

Clinical features

The disorder commonly commences with high fever, headache, nausea, and vomiting, followed by an impaired level of consciousness, coma, and seizures. These symptoms may initially be fluctuant, resulting in a delayed diagnosis, as occurred in CW's case. Moreover, there are other cases with a more insidious onset, including lethargy, bizarre behaviour, hallucinations, and confusion, which precede the symptom of fever. Such cases may be referred to psychiatrists, and, again, diagnosis may be delayed. Examples of bizarre behaviour include dressing at night to go to an imagined funeral or failure to recognize relatives.

Following recovery from coma, there may be additional non-amnestic symptoms. These include restless hyperactivity, confusion, anosmia, olfactory and gustatory hallucinations, psychotic or strange behaviour, disinhibition and personality change, and naming and reading disorders. There may also be seizures.

CW exhibited characteristic features of an 'amnesic syndrome', including relative preservation of intelligence and immediate (primary/working) memory, very severe impairment of everyday or episodic memory, extensive retrograde amnesia for past personal events, and relative preservation of semantic knowledge and perceptuomotor (procedural) skills (such as how to play the piano or organ). He also showed repetitive questioning and some degree of irritability.

Neuroimaging showed extensive loss of volume and signal alteration in the medial temporal lobes, sometimes extending into the medial frontal regions, and this may be accompanied by more widespread cortical atrophy. PET tends to show pronounced changes in the temporal lobes, either unilaterally or bilaterally.

Aetiology and epidemiology

Possibly 50% of cases represent primary infections, and another 50% consist of 'reactivation' of the virus. Reactivation of herpes simplex virus type 1 (HSV-1) is not well understood and can be triggered by stress, trauma, sunlight, or fever. It is thought that the virus may spread along the olfactory nerves to the base of the brain and temporal lobes, or from the trigeminal ganglia within the brainstem via sensory nerves to the dura at the base of the brain and thence to the temporal lobes.

Herpes encephalitis is estimated to affect one per 400,000 people in the UK per annum.

Treatment and prognosis

Treatment is with antiviral agents, such as aciclovir, which significantly improve prognosis if administered promptly following initial symptoms. Various studies have reported good outcome at 6 months in terms of degree of impairment and social functioning, including return to employment (McGrath et al., 1997; Raschilas et al., 2002). If not administered promptly, severe cognitive and neuropsychiatric disorders can be lifelong.

Cerebral hypoxia/ischaemia

CASE STUDY 3

A (Kopelman and Morton, 2015) was an actor of considerable accomplishments. At 66, he suffered a myocardial infarction and cardiac arrest, while speaking at a public meeting. He was resuscitated at the scene and later received two coronary stents and a cardioverter–defibrillator.

A's recovery was slow. He was initially very confused, disorientated in time and place, and frequently confabulating, often with grandiose content. He was profoundly amnestic and anosognosic. It took 2 months before he was able to recognize reliably family members.

Five months after his initial illness, he was partially orientated and was confabulating much less floridly. However, he was still severely amnesic and was completely unaware of his heart attack or cardiac arrest. He still suffered intermittent confabulations and confusions, thinking, for example, that he was supposed to attend a court case, which had taken place 20 years earlier, and being surprised to learn that his mother was deceased.

When tested, he showed a deficit, relative to healthy controls, in learning of both new lines and past lines, but he showed relative sparing in re-learning the past lines, despite not having any awareness of having performed these plays before (implicit memory).

A CT brain scan showed widening of the frontotemporal sulci, including the temporal horns of the lateral ventricles, consistent with medial temporal lobe atrophy. An 18-fluoro-deoxy-glucose PET scan showed reduced glucose uptake in the thalami bilaterally, the retrosplenium, and the medial and ventromedial frontal cortex.

Clinical features and aetiology

Acute cerebral hypoxia/ischaemia can give rise to a number of cognitive profiles, including an amnesic syndrome very similar to that of Korsakoff syndrome or herpes encephalitis, as described in Korsakoff syndrome and Herpes encephalitis. It can arise from heroin overdoses, suicide attempts by hanging or with the exhaust pipe of a car, cardiac arrests, or surgical and anaesthetic accidents.

Caine and Watson (2000) reported that 70–74% of cases showed cell loss in the cerebral cortex, basal ganglia, or hippocampi, and 56% showed thalamic changes; only 18.5% showed changes confined to the hippocampi. Likewise, their report described widespread cognitive deficits that involved memory, visuospatial, or visual recognition problems and changes in personality or behaviour; approximately 20% had an isolated amnestic syndrome.

Consistent with this, autopsy studies have commonly described hippocampal atrophy (Rempel-Clower et al., 1996), but PET investigations have reported changes elsewhere in the limbic circuits, including the thalami and retrosplenium (Markowitsch et al., 1997; Reed et al., 1999).

Management consists of treatment of the underlying cause, followed by appropriate neuropsychological rehabilitation. Although the long-term prognosis of the severely brain-damaged is often assumed to be poor, gradual improvements through time are often discernible.

Confabulation

Confabulation consists of false or erroneous memories arising unintentionally in the context of neurological amnesia. The memories may be false in themselves or 'real' memories jumbled and confused in temporal context and retrieved inappropriately. Many authors distinguish between 'spontaneous confabulation', in which there is a persistent unprovoked outpouring of erroneous memories, and 'momentary' or 'provoked' confabulation, which consists of fleeting intrusion errors or distortions when memory is challenged (Kopelman, 1987b). The former is a pathological phenomenon, often secondary to ventromedial or orbitofrontal pathology (Gilboa et al., 2006), whereas the latter is a normal response to a weak or failing memory. In neither case is confabulation the deliberate 'filling in' of gaps, as is commonly believed. Other authors have proposed more elaborate taxonomies of confabulation (Schnider, 2008).

Confabulation is sometimes assumed to be pathognomonic of Korsakoff syndrome, but this is inaccurate. As already stated, it appears to be secondary to specific frontal pathology (Gilboa et al., 2006; Toosy et al., 2008). There are various competing theories of how confabulation arises. One theory is that it consists of real memories confused in temporal sequence—a confusion of 'old recollections with present impressions' (Korsakoff, 1889a). This view is sometimes expressed as a disorder in 'reality monitoring' (Schnider, 2008). A variant is that, in confabulation, temporal consciousness is intact, but malfunctioning, such that the patient returns recurrently to a period of the most 'stable' long-term memories. Another theory is that the problem resides in specifying the trace to be retrieved and, in particular, in filtering out errors, perhaps because of a defective 'feeling of rightness' (Gilboa et al., 2006). Other theorists place emphasis on motivational accounts, suggesting that confabulation performs a 'self-serving' role in the context of the patient's situation (Fotopoulou et al., 2008). Yet others have proposed a combination of factors.

The dementias: introduction

The dementias are persistent disorders of the mental processes affecting more than one cognitive domain, which are generally, but not universally, progressive. They must be of sufficient severity to interfere with an individual's ability to function at work or home, and represent a decline from a previous level of function (McKhann et al., 2011). The dementias can be classified either by their cognitive phenotype or by their aetiological origin, and there is not necessarily a linear mapping between the two.

The assessment of dementia is a multidisciplinary pursuit, with clinical and diagnostic assessments undertaken by psychiatrists, psychologists, neurologists, geriatricians, and, increasingly, specialist nurses, occupational therapists, and other allied health professionals. A general clinical approach to cognitive impairment is discussed in Chapters 2 and 11, complemented by appropriate neurological examination (see Chapter 3) and focused investigation (see Chapters 7, and 8). Here we outline the core conditions in terms of their clinical features, epidemiology, and aetiology, followed by a brief discussion of management and prognosis. For illustrative purposes, the structural investigations presented will usually be MRI, but in many cases CT would be clinically sufficient, as the primary purpose of the scan is usually to exclude structural causes of the clinical syndrome (i.e. tumours, bleeds, infarcts, and abscesses) (Cole, 1978). Assessment of cognitive symptoms is often aided by administration of a brief standardized neuropsychometric instrument that provides quantitative and qualitative data on cognitive performance. For illustrative purposes here, we use the Addenbrooke's Cognitive Examination, third edition (ACE-III) (Hsieh et al., 2013) due to its simplicity of administration and favourable sensitivity and specificity (Larner, 2007, 2015), but similar clinical tools are available that might be more appropriate in particular practice settings. These supplement, but do not replace, a more detailed neuropsychological assessment.

Core progressive dementias

Alzheimer's disease—amnestic

CASE STUDY 4

A 70-year-old retired engineer presents to clinic, accompanied by his wife and daughter. His relatives tell you that, over the past 2 years, he has been becoming increasingly forgetful, especially for recent events. He has missed a number of appointments and recently became lost while driving an unfamiliar route. The patient himself feels that his relatives are over-emphasizing his difficulties but admits to his memory not being as good as it once was. He is still able to manage all of his activities of daily living but is unable to recall what he had for dinner yesterday. There are no abnormalities on physical or general neurological examination. He scores 72 on the ACE-III (attention 12/18, memory 14/26, fluency 10/14, language 24/26, visuospatial 12/16), with a notable impairment of both recall memory and recognition memory. After sensitively informing him of the likely diagnosis, you organize an MRI scan, which is illustrated in Fig. 25.1.

Clinical features

A number of diagnostic criteria are available for the diagnosis of Alzheimer's disease, but the most commonly used are those jointly proposed by the National Institute of Neurological and Communicative Disorders and Stroke and the Alzheimer's Disease and Related Disorders Association (now known as the Alzheimer's Association) in 1984 (McKhann et al., 1984). These have stood the test of time, but there have been attempts to update them with more modern imaging techniques for both research (Dubois et al., 2007) and clinical (McKhann et al., 2011) purposes. The condition is characterized by an insidious onset over months or years of an amnestic syndrome, without the core features of another of the conditions discussed later in this chapter.

Aetiology

In its canonical form, Alzheimer's disease is a progressive disorder of episodic memory, reflecting the typical early involvement of the hippocampal formation. Histologically, this initially manifests as abnormal tau lesions (non-argyrophilic pretangle material, argyrophilic neuropil threads, neurofibrillary tangles), and β-amyloid deposition (Braak and Braak, 1995; Braak and Del Tredici, 2015). Accumulating evidence suggests that this pathological process begins decades before clinical onset (Bateman et al., 2012; Braak and Del Tredici, 2015). As the disease progresses, the accumulation of pathology accelerates and spreads to involve other cortical areas and therefore cognitive domains. Less commonly, the predominant burden of tau and amyloid pathology is outside of the hippocampal formation, resulting in the rarer forms of Alzheimer's disease discussed later.

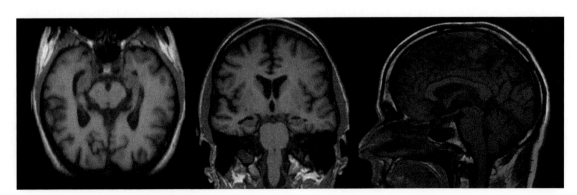

Fig. 25.1 MRI images for amnestic Alzheimer's disease in Case study 4. Radiological convention. T1-weighted axial, coronal, and sagittal projections. Disproportionate bilateral atrophy of the hippocampi can be seen.

Alzheimer's disease is predominantly a sporadic disease, but risk and age of onset are influenced by a number of genetic polymorphisms (Harold et al., 2009). The strongest association is with the apolipoprotein E allele ε4 (Saunders et al., 1993), the presence of which leads to a younger age of onset (Meyer et al., 1998). It is unclear whether this risk is primarily mediated by congenital alterations in brain activity and connectivity (Filippini et al., 2009) or a direct effect on β-amyloid (Bales et al., 1997). Around 2% of cases result from autosomal dominant mutations in genes coding for either the amyloid precursor protein (APP) or the γ-secretase complex components presenilin 1 (PSEN1) and 2 (PSEN2) (Brouwers et al., 2008). Duplication of APP due to trisomy 21, and consequent overexpression of APP, is the cause of early-onset Alzheimer's disease in Down's syndrome (Rumble et al., 1989).

Management

At the time of writing, no effective disease-modifying therapies are available for Alzheimer's disease. By 2013, >200 drug candidates had been evaluated unsuccessfully (Becker and Greig, 2013). It has been proposed that one or more of these candidates might still prove efficacious in presymptomatic disease, but clinical trials in this group are difficult because high-risk case selection is complex and measurement of progression in the absence of validated biomarkers requires long and expensive clinical trials (Fitzgerald, 2014). As well as drugs that specifically target Alzheimer-type pathology, novel agents are in development that target more general cellular stress response or neuroinflammatory pathways to prevent toxic protein accumulation (Halliday and Mallucci, 2014; Moreno et al., 2013).

Therefore, at present, the aim of treatment is to manage symptoms. The mainstay of management for all of the diseases discussed in this chapter is to provide information and guidance to patients and their family about support available and the likely course of the disease to enable future planning. Assessment and information exchange should be holistic and, as a minimum, should cover: advanced planning of decision-making arrangements for health and finances (e.g. lasting power of attorney in English law); financial matters and available benefits; housing and social arrangements and future plans; cognitive stimulation; carer support; and opportunities for pharmacological intervention.

Initial symptomatic treatment in mild to moderate disease is usually with a cholinesterase inhibitor (and, if possible, the cessation of anticholinergic medications) (Lu and Tune, 2003). On average, these result in small improvements in cognitive test scores and measures of activities of daily living and behaviour (Birks, 2006). The three drugs in this class (donepezil, rivastigmine, and galantamine) have similar efficacy (Bullock et al., 2005). Which to initiate is therefore a clinical judgement based on practical concerns, side effect profile, and cost. Donepezil and long-acting galantamine have once-daily dosing, while rivastigmine has a patch preparation that can be useful in late disease if swallowing is impaired (this can be particularly useful in Lewy body disorders). Donepezil seems to have a more tolerable side effect profile than rivastigmine (Bullock et al., 2005), but there is no difference in serious adverse effects. Common side effects include nausea, vomiting, and diarrhoea—these effects can be dose-dependent, and it is therefore common practice to begin at a low dose and to slowly titrate upwards to the highest tolerable level. Serious

adverse events are very rare, but caution should be exercised in the presence of cardiac rhythm abnormalities and patients with peptic ulcer disease (Schachter and Davis, 1999). In the absence of side effects, it is recommended to continue these medications lifelong because of the risk of cognitive relapse on their cessation (Rainer et al., 2001).

Where dementia is moderate to severe (or in milder disease where cholinesterase inhibitors cannot be tolerated), the NMDA receptor antagonist memantine should be considered (Raina et al., 2008). This has a small, but robustly demonstrable, benefit to measures of cognition, activities of daily living, behaviour, and overall performance status (Tariot et al., 2004).

Pharmacological intervention for other specific neuropsychiatric symptoms should be addressed with caution. Memantine is now advocated as the drug of choice for behavioural disturbance but is not always effective. While there is sometimes a role for low doses of antipsychotics in managing difficult behaviours that might have significant negative sequelae (such as jeopardizing an otherwise successful residential placement), the side effect profile of these drugs means that it is normally preferable to address these issues with social interventions and targeted carer support. When the potential benefit of these medications is felt to outweigh the harms, particular consideration should be given to minimizing cardiovascular risk (Banerjee, 2009) and monitoring for neuroleptic-induced parkinsonism (Caligiuri et al., 1999).

Low mood is a frequent complaint in dementia. Unfortunately there is converging evidence that commonly used antidepressant medications are broadly ineffective at treating low mood in Alzheimer's disease, while carrying a side effect burden (Banerjee et al., 2011). Mirtazapine can improve carer quality of life, primarily by improving appetite and sleep, while high-dose citalopram was effective for agitation (Porsteinsson et al., 2014). The specific indication for treatment should therefore be carefully considered.

Epidemiology

Alzheimer's disease is the commonest dementia in the Western world, representing approximately 70% of the 4.6 million global annual incident cases (Ferri et al., 2005). Prevalence is felt to be rising especially rapidly in the developing world, as life expectancy increases (Reitz et al., 2011). While age-for-age dementia incidence is falling in the UK (Matthews et al., 2013, 2016), the ageing population means that dementia continues to rise in both prevalence and incidence. Prevalence increases rapidly with age, from <5% of those aged below 75 to 10% at age 80–84, 20% at age 85–89, and 30% over age 90.

Prognosis

Alzheimer's disease is a relentlessly progressive condition that alters behaviour (Reisberg et al., 1996), induces dependency, and shortens life expectancy. The most powerful predictors of life expectancy from diagnosis are age, sex, the degree of cognitive impairment at diagnosis, and the magnitude of cognitive decline over the first year (Larson et al., 2004). Median life expectancy for 70-year-old women with Alzheimer's disease is 8 years, compared to 16 years for those without. For men at age 70, it is 4.4 years, compared to 12.4 years without. Diagnosis at an older age has less impact on survival—prognosis for Alzheimer's sufferers at age 90 is 2–3 years, compared to 3–4 years without. MMSE scores below 24/30 at diagnosis predict poorer prognosis, with scores below 17 having a particularly high hazard ratio for death (2.6 times that of an MMSE score of >24). A decline of >5 points in the MMSE score over the first year results in a hazard ratio of 1.6. Recent suggestions of multi-modal prognostication using quantitative neuroimaging and CSF analysis have not yet found clinical utility but hold promise for research applications (Perrin et al., 2009).

Alzheimer's disease–posterior cortical atrophy (Benson's syndrome)

CASE STUDY 5

A 58-year-old man presents to clinic with his wife. Two years ago, he noticed difficulty with using money, being unable to easily distinguish between coins without feeling them. A year later, he began to have problems noticing hazards while driving. His wife describes him as 'looking, but not seeing'. He has been assessed by an optician and an ophthalmologist, both of whom simply said that his visual acuity was normal. On examination, you note simultagnosia, bilateral dyspraxia, dyscalculia, dysarithmetria, and visual working memory difficulties. His speech is also slightly hesitant, and he displays some anomia, with preserved semantic knowledge, during confrontational naming. There are no abnormalities on neurological examination, and specifically there is no movement disorder. The ACE-III score was 82/100 (attention 18/18, memory 22/26, fluency 12/14, language 22/26, visuospatial 8/16). His MRI scan demonstrated global atrophy, especially severe in the parietal lobes (see Fig. 25.2).

Clinical features

Reflecting the biparietal predominance of pathological damage (Ossenkoppele et al., 2015b), posterior cortical atrophy is a primary disorder of the dorsal 'where' visual stream (McMonagle et al., 2006; Ungerleider and Mishkin, 1982), leading to visuospatial disorientation, with or without a broader biparietal syndrome of ideomotor and gesture copy apraxia, Gerstmann syndrome (dysgraphia, dyscalculia, finger agnosia, and left–right confusion), and Balint's syndrome (optic ataxia, ocular apraxia, and simultagnosia). An associated occipitotemporal syndrome of alexia and apperceptive agnosia (including prosopagnosia) is also common, as is the later emergence of a parietal, Alzheimer-type language deficit (see Alzheimer's disease—logopenic and mixed primary progressive aphasia).

Epidemiology and management

There have been no robust epidemiological or prevalence studies of focal presentations of Alzheimer's disease. The clinical perception is that even if all of the focal subtypes are combined, they are still far less common than typical Alzheimer's disease. There is also a perception that focal presentations tend to present at an earlier age than typical Alzheimer's disease. Medical management is generally similar to that for typical Alzheimer's disease, as the symptoms become more phenotypically similar as the disease progresses. The additional consideration in posterior cortical atrophy is management of the visual symptoms, which can be very disabling. Driving should cease at an early stage. It has been our experience that some patients have found it beneficial to become registered as legally blind, as in the UK, this facilitates access to a number of benefits and concessions, as well as practical support from charitable bodies. This application can require careful wording, as patients with cortical blindness of this type will have good visual acuity and the visual field might appear normal to single-target confrontation. An ophthalmologist's report will be required, and the criterion that can usually be applied is that which states: 'If you have a good visual acuity, you will usually have had to have lost a large part of your visual field to be certified as severely sight impaired (blind) or sight impaired (partially sighted).' It should be stressed that, while detection of single targets can be intact, analysis of the visual field as a whole is catastrophically impaired.

Prognosis

Although there is a clinical perception that the prognosis of posterior cortical atrophy is better than that of amnestic Alzheimer's disease, this seems to be a result of the generally younger age of presentation and the often shorter duration of symptoms before coming to medical attention. When age-matched groups were studied, there was no significant difference between typical and focal Alzheimer's disease in time from first symptoms to death (mean 9.7 years) (Alladi et al., 2007).

Alzheimer's disease–logopenic and mixed primary progressive aphasia

CASE STUDY 6

A 59-year-old right-handed man presents to clinic with an 18-month history of subjective speech disturbance. He describes difficulty in finding words, such that he becomes derailed halfway through a sentence. He is clear that he can bring to mind the object

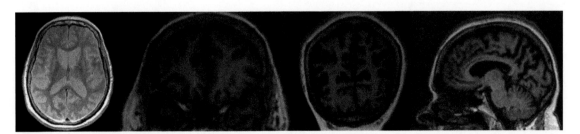

Fig. 25.2 MRI images for posterior cortical atrophy in Case study 5. Radiological convention. Proton density-weighted axial projection; T1-weighted coronal projections through frontal and then parietal regions; and T1-weighted sagittal projection. Disproportionate bilateral parietal lobe atrophy can be seen.

or concept and give a description of it, but feels as if the word it-self is stuck 'at the tip of his tongue'. He has given up work because of this difficulty, although his managers had not felt that his performance had deteriorated. Conversationally he is fluent and his speech is contentful, but there are pauses as he gropes for words, and sometimes the train of thought is lost. There are some problems with confrontational naming, but he is able to give a semantically detailed description of these items. He finds it difficult to repeat long sentences, giving close approximations that carry the gist and are grammatically correct. He scores 89/100 on the ACE-III (attention 18/18, memory 19/26, fluency 10/14, language 26/26, visuospatial 16/16). His MRI scan demonstrates mild global atrophy, with a parietal predominance (see **Fig. 25.3**).

Clinical features

Aphasia is very common in typical Alzheimer's disease (Cummings et al., 1985), but in rare cases, it can be the leading or only clinical feature. The core clinical feature of this condition is a deficit in responsive and confrontational naming, with preserved semantic knowledge. This can often be subtle at presentation, as patients notice the problem early, frustrated by pauses in their speech as they find themselves groping for words. The diagnostic criteria for logopenic variant primary progressive aphasia are the presence of impaired single-word retrieval in both spontaneous speech and naming, together with impaired repetition of sentences and phrases in a length-dependent manner, as well as three out of the following: phonological errors, spared single-word comprehension and object knowledge, spared motor speech, and absence of agrammatism (Gorno-Tempini et al., 2011). These features are strongly supportive of Alzheimer's pathology involving the left parietal lobe (Gorno-Tempini et al., 2004). In recent years, it has been suggested that these diagnostic criteria are too narrow. There is converging evidence that any primary progressive aphasia that does not meet the diagnostic criteria for SD or progressive non-fluent aphasia (i.e. a mixed aphasia) is also likely to represent Alzheimer's pathology in the left parietal lobe (Sajjadi et al., 2012a, 2014), especially if confrontational anomia or amnesia is present (Alladi et al., 2007).

Alzheimer's disease–behavioural/dysexecutive ('frontal') variant

Clinical features

It can be very difficult to clinically distinguish between a variant of Alzheimer's disease with prominent behavioural or dysexecutive features and the behavioural variant of frontotemporal dementia (bvFTD). Presentations can be very similar (see vignette and clinical features of bvFTD below) (Woodward et al., 2010). The clinical syndrome reflects the distribution of neuronal loss, rather than its aetiology, with distinct regional atrophy patterns found in syndromes characterized by disinhibition, apathy, or aberrant motor behaviours (Rosen et al., 2005). In common with typical variants of Alzheimer's disease, the burden of atrophy is still in temporoparietal regions, so the term 'frontal Alzheimer's disease' has fallen out of favour in recent years (Ossenkoppele et al., 2015a). The presence of significantly impaired episodic memory is not sufficient evidence that one is dealing with a dementia of the Alzheimer's type, as there is now converging evidence for memory involvement in a significant proportion of bvFTD (Hornberger and Piguet, 2012; Hornberger et al., 2010), but should prompt the clinician to consider further investigation with detailed neuropsychological, neuroimaging, and/or neuropathological assessment (Larner, 2006). While an educated guess as to the likely aetiology can be made, it should be borne in mind that without pathological or biomarker confirmation, at least 5–10% of seemingly typical cases are misclassified (Alladi et al., 2007; Graham et al., 2005; Rascovsky et al., 2011).

Management

While cholinesterase inhibitors have some efficacy in managing the neuropsychiatric manifestations of Alzheimer's disease (Wynn and Cummings, 2004), they have been reported to worsen behavioural symptoms in frontotemporal dementia (Kimura and Takamatsu, 2013; Mendez et al., 2007). Similarly, while memantine had promising initial anecdotal reports of efficacy in bvFTD (Swanberg, 2007), two RCTs proved negative (Boxer et al., 2013; Vercelletto et al., 2011). Given the practical difficulties in distinguishing these two syndromes, circumspection and careful assessment of response should be employed in prescribing.

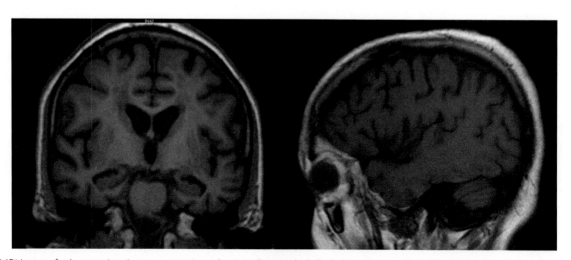

Fig. 25.3 MRI images for logopenic primary progressive aphasia in Case study 6. Radiological convention. T1-weighted coronal and sagittal projections. Subtle atrophy of the hippocampi and parietal lobe can be seen, with left-sided predominance.

Strategies for the management of bvFTD are discussed in the next section.

Frontotemporal dementia–behavioural variant

CASE STUDY 7

A 77-year-old right-handed woman is referred to clinic by her family. They report that she has become progressively more 'childish' over the past 2 years. She is inappropriately familiar with strangers and displays total disregard for etiquette such as table manners. You notice that her clothes are dirty and that she is wearing three scarves, two pairs of trousers, and two bras. Her husband, who is well kempt, reports that she insists on re-wearing dirty clothes and that he is unable to intervene. The patient tells you that there is a man living in her attic; she has never seen him but she knows that he is there. On examination, you note the presence of primitive reflexes (grasp, palmomental, pout), as well as deltoid fasciculations, thinning of the first dorsal interosseous and thenar eminence bilaterally, slow tongue movements, and hyperreflexia. The ACE-III score is 85/100 (attention 16/18, memory 21/26, fluency 10/14, language 21/26, visuospatial 16/16). Her language deficits are in naming, and you note that she has some mild semantic impairment for these items.

Clinical features

The most recent diagnostic criteria allow for the diagnosis of 'possible' bvFTD on clinical grounds in the presence of three of the following six features: disinhibition, apathy, loss of empathy, perseverative behaviours, hyperorality (an excessively sweet tooth), and dysexecutive neuropsychological profile (Rascovsky et al., 2011). The level of certainty is increased to 'probable' in the presence of functional disability and characteristic neuroimaging, while 'definite' diagnosis requires either histopathological confirmation or a pathogenic mutation. It is especially important to assess for progression of symptoms and neuroimaging changes, as a significant proportion of cases diagnosed on clinical features alone fail to progress in terms of clinical syndrome or atrophy (Hornberger et al., 2009; Kipps et al., 2010). It is unclear whether these cases represent atypical late-onset neuropsychiatric disease (Belin et al., 2015) or exacerbation of lifelong personality traits due to normal ageing. When progression is established (Mioshi and Hodges, 2009), these criteria have a sensitivity of 72–95% and a specificity of 82–95% (Harris et al., 2013), with the majority of misclassifications being with frontal Alzheimer-type pathology, as discussed earlier.

Over time, the evolution of the syndrome to include semantic deficits is common (Coyle-Gilchrist et al., 2016), reflecting a shared aetiology with SD. A proportion of patients with bvFTD will go on to develop progressive supranuclear palsy (PSP) (Kaat et al., 2007) or, as here, motor neurone disease.

Aetiology

The clinical syndrome of FTD represents several histopathological patterns of frontotemporal lobar degeneration (FTLD) (a wider term encompassing frontotemporal dementia, PSP, and corticobasal syndrome (CBS) due to their overlapping neuropathological features). Forty to 50% of cases display inclusions of the microtubule-binding protein tau (Mackenzie et al., 2010) with either three or four microtubule-binding repeats (Cairns et al., 2007). Approximately 40–50% of cases have inclusions of TDP-43 (43-kDa TAR DNA-binding protein) (Piguet et al., 2011) and 5% inclusions of FUS (fused in sarcoma) (Seelaar et al., 2010a). These proteins are both involved in RNA processing, but their pathogenic mechanisms are not yet known. The remaining 5% of cases with typical phenotype and distribution of neuronal loss (and without Alzheimer-type or Lewy body pathology) are negative for tau, TDP-43, and FUS, suggesting an as yet unknown pathogenic mechanism (Mackenzie et al., 2008).

bvFTD is highly heritable, with up to 50% of patients having a family history of the disorder (a far higher proportion than the other FTD syndromes, which do not generally run in families) (Rosso et al., 2003). A single causative gene can be demonstrated in approximately half of these cases, with the proportion rising in clear autosomal dominant inheritance patterns with multiple family members affected (Rohrer et al., 2009). It is now possible to test for most of the common exon mutations on a single chip; *MAPT* and *GRN* each account for 5–11% of frontotemporal dementia, while *TARDBP, FUS, TBK1, CHMP2B, VCP, SQSTM1, UBQLN1,* and *hnRMP1a* account for progressively fewer cases and tend to be associated with additional clinical features (Seelaar et al., 2010b). At least as common as any of these is a hexanucleotide repeat expansion in the intron C9ORF72. This must be separately tested and is particularly suggested by the presence of motor neurone disease (DeJesus-Hernandez et al., 2011; Renton et al., 2011) or prominent psychiatric features in the proband or family members (Arighi et al., 2012; Snowden et al., 2012). While C9ORF72 has autosomal dominant inheritance, it is incompletely penetrant and manifests differently within a family as motor neurone disease, psychiatric disorders, and bvFTD, alone or in combination. In the vignette, the combination of bvFTD, motor neurone disease, and delusions would strongly suggest C9ORF72, even in the absence of a family history.

Management

As discussed in Alzheimer's disease—behavioural/dysexecutive ('frontal') variant, there is no role for cholinesterase inhibitors or memantine in bvFTD.

The only medication for which significant benefit for the behavioural symptoms of bvFTD has been demonstrated is trazodone (Lebert et al., 2004), from which sustained benefit can often be obtained (Lebert, 2006). These benefits are not always observed, and the decision to continue with this medication should be made by the prescriber based on a comprehensive assessment of both patient and carer experience.

The cornerstone of treatment is social. Abnormal behaviours can be challenging, especially for carers. It is important to consider whether any community stakeholders would benefit from being aware of the diagnosis, and to suggest this to patients and their families. It is often appropriate for families to inform local law enforcement services and frequently visited shops.

Driving can be a particularly thorny issue—patients with bvFTD, more than any other group in the dementia clinic, lack insight into their symptoms and the problems they cause in judgement. While it is usual practice in the UK to tell patients that they must inform the DVLA of their diagnosis, in bvFTD, it is often necessary to firmly advise against driving and directly inform the Driver and Vehicle

Licensing Agency (DVLA) of this advice. Family members can be a useful guide towards the necessity of taking such action.

Hyperorality and dietary changes are often a significant issue. Overeating can represent a simple utilization behaviour, in which case it can be fairly easily addressed by selective purchasing and locking cupboards. In some individuals, however, obtaining sweet foods becomes an overarching goal-directed behaviour and weight gain can be dramatic. Social interventions are often insufficient in these cases, and pharmacological intervention is required. Diabetes is often comorbid, and metformin can be a useful suppressor of appetite. Similarly, if myoclonus, tremor, or seizures are present, topiramate might be an appropriate choice to reduce weight gain. Limited or repetitive diets can be similarly damaging, and in such cases, potential vitamin deficiencies should be addressed, lest a diet of biscuits and fizzy drinks lead to scurvy.

Epidemiology

bvFTD has a significantly younger age of onset than the other disorders in the FTLD spectrum (Coyle-Gilchrist et al., 2016), with the majority of both genetic and sporadic cases presenting before the age of 65 (peak incidence across FTLD as a whole is between age 65 and 80). The incidence of FTLD in the UK is about 1.6/100,000 person-years, with bvFTD representing approximately a quarter of these cases (SD and nfvPPA together represent another quarter, with the other half being CBS or PSP). When adjusted for higher female life expectancy, there is no significant gender bias in bvFTD or in FTLD as a whole.

Prognosis

Mean survival from symptom onset is approximately 8 years. The clinical syndrome evolves significantly through this period, as overactivity, social inappropriateness, and hypersexuality that can be so distressing in early disease frequently give way to a syndrome of apathy and semantic impairment after the first few years. This should be recognized by dynamic symptom management, with cessation of no-longer-necessary medications and proactive interventions given equal priority.

Frontotemporal dementia–semantic dementia

CASE STUDY 8

A 70-year-old right-handed man is brought to clinic by his wife. He has not noticed any problems and is unsure why he has been brought to clinic. His wife says that she first noticed something wrong a year ago, when they were perusing a restaurant menu and her husband asked her what asparagus was. Since then, his understanding of words and concepts, both written and spoken, has gradually declined. He is still able to drive and route-find and enjoys playing bridge to a relatively high standard. His conversational speech is fluent and grammatical, but empty of content words. He is unable to name lower-frequency animals, nor is he able to tell you which of several model animals is dangerous or edible. When asked to draw animals, he produces images that lack distinctive features, e.g. a camel without a hump and an elephant without a trunk (Bozeat et al., 2003). Similarly, he cannot name or demonstrate the use of some kitchen implements. He is able to repeat long words and sentences without difficulty, but has poor understanding. When reading aloud, he pronounces irregular words phonetically (surface dyslexia) (Woollams et al., 2007). The ACE-III score is 70/100 (attention 18/18, memory 22/26, fluency 2/14, language 12/26, visuospatial 16/16). His MRI scan demonstrates severe selective atrophy of the left temporal lobe (see Fig. 25.4).

Clinical features

SD is a stereotyped syndrome of progressive loss of semantic knowledge associated with left-sided temporal lobe atrophy (Basso et al., 1988; Hodges et al., 1992; Snowden et al., 1989; Warrington, 1975). It is often classified together with the other neurodegenerative aphasias (nfvPPA and logopenic Alzheimer's disease), as fluent, content-less speech is a leading symptom. This is, however, a consequence of a broader loss of semantic knowledge for objects. This can be best conceptualized by an example; if a patient with logopenic Alzheimer's disease is presented with a model lion, they

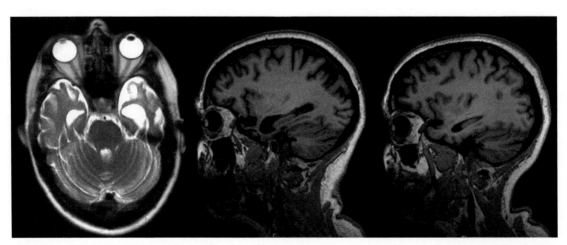

Fig. 25.4 MRI images for semantic dementia in Case study 8. Radiological convention. T2-weighted axial projection; and T1-weighted sagittal projections through the left and right temporal lobes at roughly the same eccentricity. Severe, selective atrophy of the temporal poles can be seen, with significant left-sided predominance.

might not be able to tell you that it is a lion (displaying anomia), but they would be able to give semantic detail about lions, e.g. that they are dangerous and live in Africa. A patient with SD might similarly lack the word 'lion', but in this case, they would also lack all knowledge about lions. Therefore, although they do indeed have agnosia for words, this amodal deficit extends to all semantic domains and is not primarily an aphasia (Bozeat et al., 2000; Fairhall and Caramazza, 2013).

In fact, it is possible that a patient with SD will tell you that what they are looking at is a cat and that they have one at home. This reflects the postulated mechanism for semantic memory, whereby knowledge about objects is stored as a commonly observed 'template', with specific differentiating flags. For example, an elephant might be stored as a commonly observed large quadruped such as a horse, with the additional flags 'has a trunk', 'lives in Africa or Asia', 'has big ears', 'is very large', etc. (Snowden et al., 2001). This can be clinically observed by asking patients with SD to draw animals with distinguishing features. The more unique the feature, the more likely it is to be omitted, e.g. a patient with SD might draw an elephant without a trunk, a camel without a hump, or a duck with four legs (Bozeat et al., 2003).

Behavioural features are common, especially later in the disease course when the right temporal lobe becomes involved. These overlap with bvFTD but are more likely to comprise compulsive, repetitive behaviours and disinhibition than apathy and indiscriminate eating, reflecting a temporal, rather than frontal, predominance of atrophy (Snowden et al., 2001). The syndrome of predominant right-sided temporal atrophy is dominated by this behavioural phenotype, often in combination with prosopagnosia (loss of semantic knowledge of familiar people) (Evans et al., 1995). Similarly, as temporal lobe atrophy becomes bilateral, an additional SD phenotype often develops.

Overall, there can be striking preservation of ability outside of semantic and behavioural domains. It is not uncommon for a patient to demonstrate catastrophic loss of object knowledge but retain complex procedural skills and navigational ability. Schemata can be well preserved but sometimes break down with object substitution, e.g. proficiently making a cup of tea, but then putting the milk in the cupboard and tea bags in the fridge.

Aetiology

SD is almost always associated with TDP-43-related histopathology affecting the temporal lobes, with a left-sided predominance (Hodges et al., 2009). In contrast to bvFTD, it does not show significant heritability, and indeed at least three patients are known to have had SD and an unaffected monozygotic twin (personal communication from Professor Karalyn Patterson).

Frontotemporal dementia–non-fluent variant primary progressive aphasia

CASE STUDY 9

A 63-year-old right-handed woman presents to clinic with a 1-year history of progressively worsening difficulty in getting her words out. She finds this extremely frustrating. She is very clear that she knows what the word is that she wants to say, but she is unable to articulate it. She has not noticed any other problems. Her conversational speech is effortful, with phonological paraphasias being especially noticeable in words requiring articulatory agility. It is also telegraphic, lacking connecting words and some grammatical form. She performs poorly at parsing grammatically complex sentences but demonstrates flawless confrontational naming and semantic knowledge. You ask for a sample of her writing and note that this too contains grammatical errors. She scores 96/100 on the ACE-III (attention 18/18, memory 25/26, fluency 12/14, language 25/26, visuospatial 16/16). Her MRI scan appeared normal (see **Fig. 25.5**).

Clinical features

nfvPPA, previously known as progressive non-fluent aphasia (PNFA), is an adult-onset neurodegenerative aphasia characterized by apraxia of speech and/or agrammatism (Gorno-Tempini et al., 2011). Importantly, patients should not have word-finding difficulties (anomia) in the early stages of the disease; if this is present, a diagnosis of mixed primary progressive aphasia should be made and the underlying neuropathology is almost always of the Alzheimer's type (Sajjadi et al., 2012b, 2014). Sentence repetition is impaired where articulatory agility is required or the grammatical

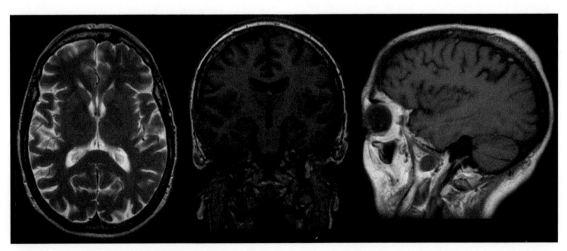

Fig. 25.5 MRI images for non-fluent variant primary progressive aphasia in Case study 9. Radiological convention. T2-weighted axial projection; and T1-weighted coronal and sagittal projections. Normal appearances for age can be seen, with good hippocampal bulk.

structure is complex. Semantic deficits should not be present in early disease, but these and/or behavioural features can evolve later. Yes/no confusion is a common feature in relatively early disease, and digit span can be markedly shortened due to impairment of the phonological loop (Baddeley and Hitch, 1974). Neuroimaging changes can be very subtle in early disease, often appearing normal in the single subject, but predominant atrophy is in the left frontal lobe (Grube et al., 2016; Rogalski et al., 2011).

Although nfvPPA is commonly thought of as an expressive aphasia, the neurodegenerative equivalent of Broca's syndrome, patients also frequently complain that perceiving speech is effortful, even in optimal listening environments. Many have sought hearing aids but been told that they do not have a peripheral deficit. It is thought that this reflects a double-hit to auditory processing, with impairments in basic auditory processing (Goll et al., 2010, Grube et al., 2016) compounded by damage to frontal regions, making predictions to 'fill in' unclear speech (Cope et al., 2017).

The diagnostic criteria require the presence of only one of apraxia of speech and agrammatism. This has led some authors to propose that nfvPPA should be clinically subdivided into an agrammatic variant (agPPA) and an apraxic variant (primary progressive apraxia of speech—PPAOS) (Josephs et al., 2012, 2013). The justification for this division has been the observation that those presenting with PPAOS are more likely to develop a motor syndrome consistent with PSP or CBS later in their illness (Josephs et al., 2005) and have a neuropathological diagnosis of tau, rather than TDP-43 pathology (Josephs et al., 2006a). This subdivision has not gained widespread acceptance for several reasons:

1. There is a clear spectrum to nfvPPA, with some patients displaying predominant apraxia of speech and others having marked difficulties with both expressive and receptive grammar, but all patients displaying deficits in both domains on careful testing.

2. Less than half of patients with PPAOS will develop a movement disorder, and even if this does occur, this transformation often emerges 5 or more years into the illness (Josephs et al., 2012, 2014). Similarly, movement disorders sometimes occur later in the illness of those who present with agrammatism.

3. While there is a statistical trend for symptom type at onset to predict progression and pathology, even in the presence of a movement disorder, predominant TDP-43 pathology, in the absence of Tau, has been observed.

4. Although there are differences in patterns of atrophy between PPAOS and agPPA at the group level (Josephs et al., 2013), these are relatively subtle. Changes in cortical thickness in the inferior frontal gyrus correlate with grammatical processing, while those in the inferior frontal sulcus correlate with fluency (Rogalski et al., 2011). These are neighbouring regions, and the differences are certainly less marked than those between PPAOS and PSP (Whitwell et al., 2013).

5. nfvPPA is already a very rare syndrome, and further subdivision would make clinician education and meaningful research more difficult.

Aetiology

The syndrome of nfvPPA predicts atrophy centred on the left frontal lobe, but not the nature of the causative pathology. The majority of cases represent tauopathies, but a significant minority have TDP-43-related disease (Josephs et al., 2006b; Kertesz et al., 2005; Knibb et al., 2006a, b; Mesulam et al., 2014). Neuropathological series vary markedly (from 0% to 40%) in the proportion of nfvPPA found to have Alzheimer's neuropathology. This likely represents differences in local diagnostic practice, perhaps in terms of the stringency with which anomic patients are excluded from nfvPPA diagnosis.

Management and prognosis

Patients with nfvPPA are intensely frustrated by their symptoms and present early in their disease course (Coyle-Gilchrist et al., 2016). The cornerstone of therapy is explanation of symptoms and practical management of the aphasia; there is no role for medications, unless additional motor or behavioural features emerge later in disease. It is often fruitful to approach nfvPPA in the same way as Broca's aphasia, with the provision of communication aids and explanation cards. Some patients even find it simpler to tell shopkeepers and acquaintances that they have had a stroke, as this encapsulates their problems more quickly than an explanation of an unusual neurodegeneration. Speech therapy can be helpful in teaching strategies to avoid words with challenging articulation or sentences with ambiguous grammar, but attempts at rehabilitation are rarely fruitful.

Yes/no confusion can be challenging and perplexing to carers and should be explicitly acknowledged and explained. Strategies for dealing with this include asking patients to include a gesture, as well as a verbal response (e.g. thumbs up and saying 'yes' together), so that discordance can be more easily recognized, and carers can be trained to present non-binary choices.

Survival from symptom onset averages 9 years (similar to bvFTD), but as symptoms are troublesome, presentation is often earlier. Age of onset is also older than in bvFTD, with peak rates observed between age 65 and 80 (Coyle-Gilchrist et al., 2016). Even when patients present at a young age, a genetic cause is rarely found; while patients with *GRN* mutations often have non-fluent speech, they also have anomia and single-word comprehension problems, not consistent with a diagnosis of nfvPPA (Rohrer et al., 2010).

Vascular cognitive disorder

CASE STUDY 10

A 69-year-old woman attends clinic for review 6 weeks after admission to hospital with acute delirium in the context of community-acquired pneumonia. She is overweight, is a current smoker with a 50-pack year history, and has hypertension and type 2 diabetes, for which she is poorly compliant with treatment. Her daughter says that while the acute inattention, disorientation, and delusions that accompanied the delirium have resolved, she has not returned to baseline and is notably slower in her thinking and unable to organize her daily activities. For 12 months prior to the delirium, there had been some loss of enthusiasm; her flat was not looking quite as tidy as usual, and she had needed help cooking Christmas dinner for the family. Her daughter describes a change in her gait, which looks slower, as though she has 'aged 10 years in 12 months'. She scores 76/100 on the ACE-III [attention 13/18 (with most points lost on serial 7 s), memory 22/26, fluency 4/14, language 23/26, visuospatial 14/16]. CT brain shows extensive confluent periventricular and subcortical low attenuation, suggestive of chronic small vessel ischaemia. There is a mild degree of central brain atrophy, but the hippocampi are of normal volume.

Clinical features

Vascular cognitive disorder (VCD) refers to a heterogenous group of disorders in which progressive cognitive impairment is attributable to cerebrovascular pathology. The term VCD has been proposed to encompass a range of severities (from vascular MCI to vascular dementia) and diverse underlying aetiologies. Diagnostic criteria vary considerably, reflecting the heterogeneity of the disorder. The most specific are the NINDS-AIREN criteria (Erkinjuntti, 1994), which are preferred in research settings (Román et al., 1993). Recently, DSM-5 adopted more pragmatic criteria, for example removing memory impairment as a mandatory feature for the diagnosis of major neurocognitive disorder due to vascular disease (American Psychiatric Association, 2013).

Subcortical small vessel disease (SSVD) typically presents with an insidious onset of impaired attention, cognitive slowing, apathy, and a dysexecutive syndrome, rather than with focal cortical deficits in memory, language, or visuospatial function (Looi and Sachdev, 1999). Indeed, memory can be normal in SSVD or, in contrast to Alzheimer's disease, be characterized by impaired retrieval of information, with preserved retention. Alongside cognitive decline, a range of motor features may be evident, including dyspraxic gait and parkinsonism (Buchman et al., 2013).

Historically, VCD has been characterized as having a 'step-wise' progression; however, clinical experience suggests that this is relatively rare (Cosentino et al., 2004). Depression and apathy are seen more commonly in VCD than in Alzheimer's disease, but delusions and hallucinations are less common (Gupta et al., 2014; Lyketsos et al., 2002).

The diagnosis is based on a consistent clinical picture, accompanied by sufficient cerebrovascular pathology on brain imaging to account for the cognitive decline. However, there is no consensus on the burden of cerebrovascular disease visible on brain imaging that is required to produce dementia. Although some authors have proposed a minimum threshold of 25% of total white matter being affected (Price et al., 2005), in general, white matter lesions should be extensive and confluent (Sachdev et al., 2014). Microhaemorrhages do not robustly predict cognitive impairment (Patel et al., 2013). Brain atrophy, lacunar infarct count, and disruptions to network connectivity, as measured by DTI, are more tightly correlated with cognitive dysfunction (Lawrence et al., 2013, Tuladhar et al., 2016) but are not yet operationalized into clinical diagnostic criteria. Location of lacunar infarcts is also important, with bilateral thalamic lesions and infarcts in the basal ganglia, caudate head, and inferior genu of the anterior capsule being associated with dementia (Jellinger, 2013; Van der Werf et al., 2003).

Aetiology

The commonest cause of VCD is SSVD (Pantoni, 2010). This produces a range of neuropathological changes, most notably lacunar infarcts, leukoaraiosis, and microhaemorrhages in the white and deep grey structures. The other major subtype of VCD is post-stroke dementia. The rate of post-stroke dementia varies widely between studies but broadly affects 15–30% of patients following an ischaemic stroke, the exact phenotype depending on the location of the infarct. A further 20–25% of stroke patients develop dementia after a delay (Pendlebury and Rothwell, 2009). Similar data are seen for haemorrhagic stroke (Biffi et al., 2016). These findings might reflect the contribution of stroke to reducing cognitive reserve in the face of neurodegeneration, or shared risk factors between stroke and Alzheimer's disease such as hypertension (Gorelick, 2004) and cerebral amyloid angiopathy (Ellis et al., 1996). A significant proportion of patients with post-stroke dementia have neuroimaging evidence of cerebral amyloid deposition (Mok et al., 2010).

The vast majority of VCD is sporadic. The principal risk factors include ageing, atrial fibrillation, hypertension, diabetes mellitus, and hyperlipidemia (Gorelick et al., 2011). Some of these risk factors are subtype-specific, e.g. hyperlipidaemia has been associated with a *reduced* burden of white matter hyperintensities in stroke patients, suggesting that it does not lead to small vessel disease, despite its association with large-vessel atherosclerosis (Jimenez-Conde et al., 2010). The extent to which vascular risk factor modulation can prevent VCD is also uncertain. In one study of several thousands of patients with lacunar stroke, intensive blood pressure lowering and/or dual antiplatelet therapy for a median of 3 years did not improve cognitive outcomes (Pearce et al., 2014).

Rarer causes of VCD include cerebral vasculitis and cerebral vasculopathies, as seen in cerebral lupus, antiphospholipid syndrome, or sickle-cell disease. A small proportion of VCD is due to monogenic mutations, the commonest of which is cerebral autosomal dominant arteriopathy with subcortical infarcts and leukoencephalopathy (CADASIL) (Chabriat et al., 2009), which is discussed separately in the next section and is caused by mutations in the *NOTCH3* gene (Joutel et al., 1996). Other genetic causes of VCD include cerebral autosomal recessive arteriopathy with subcortical infarcts and leukoencephalopathy (CARASIL), retinal vasculopathy with cerebral leukodystrophy (RVCL), *COL4A1* mutations, mitochondrial cytopathies, and pseudoxanthoma elasticum (Yamamoto et al., 2011).

Management

Clinical trials of cholinesterase inhibitors and memantine in VCD have demonstrated, at best, marginal improvements in cognitive and functional outcomes (e.g. Birks et al., 2013), and these drugs are not currently recommended for use in the UK.

Epidemiology

The prevalence of vascular dementia is difficult to ascertain because there is no universally agreed definition. Neuropathological cohorts are limited by referral bias, but one large series suggested that 10–15% of dementia cases are due to pure vascular disease in all age groups over the age of 60, while mixed Alzheimer's and vascular disease account for a further 5% in the 60- to 69-years age group, increasing to 30% of the total in the 90 years-plus age group (Jellinger, 2013).

Prognosis

There is some evidence that functional decline in VCD is slower than in AD (Gill et al., 2013). There is a lack of consensus on whether life expectancy in VCD is similar to, or worse than, AD, being between 3 and 5 years (Kua et al., 2014; Wolfson et al., 2001).

Cerebral autosomal dominant arteriopathy with subcortical infarcts and leukoencephalopathy (CADASIL)

CASE STUDY 11

A 68-year-old man presents with a 2-year history of change in personality. Having previously been gregarious and outgoing, he has withdrawn from socializing and, in the words of his wife, has become 'very introverted.' About 6 months after symptom onset, he had a minor stroke, characterized by altered alertness, from which he made a good recovery. Since then, there has been a further gradual decline. He has recently displayed some disorientation in time but, in general, is not forgetful or repetitive. He speaks less, but there has been no major decline in vocabulary and no word-finding difficulties or paraphasias. There has been some decline in empathy. He is more irritable and loses his temper more easily than in the past. He now finds it difficult to use a computer and needs prompting for personal care. In earlier adult life, he had migraine with aura. He is taking clopidogrel, simvastatin, allopurinol, and citalopram. His father had a series of small strokes and, in late life, developed a dementia that was labelled as Alzheimer's disease.

On examination, he is a little slow to stand but walks with a normal stride length. There is very little arm swing, and some tremor emerges in the left arm during walking.

An MRI brain scan (see Fig. 25.6) shows severe ischaemic change in the cerebral white matter and lacunar infarcts in the left frontal lobe, right parietal cortex, basal ganglia, and pons. There is some involvement of the temporal poles, but only partial involvement of the external capsules. There are also microbleeds in the right temporal pole and right external capsule. There is some generalized atrophy, which has progressed a little since a scan 18 months previously. Genetic testing on DNA extracted from blood shows a c.1819C>T mutation in the NOTCH3 gene.

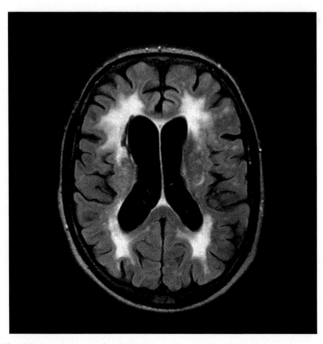

Fig. 25.6 MRI image for CADASIL in Case study 11. Radiological convention. T2 FLAIR-weighted axial projection. Diffuse white matter hyperintensity, with involvement of the corpus callosum, can be seen.

Clinical features

The clinical syndrome of CADASIL typically consists of migraine with aura in young adult life, TIA, and lacunar stroke in early middle age, and VCD from late middle age. The vast majority of carriers have detectable impairments in attention and executive function by the age of 50 (Buffon et al., 2006), and two-thirds of patients have dementia by the age of 65 (Choi, 2010). Psychiatric symptoms are common in CADASIL. In one series, over 40% of CADASIL patients had been treated for depression, which was the single greatest influence on quality of life (Brookes et al., 2013). Apathy is seen in 40% of patients (Reyes et al., 2009).

Epidemiology and aetiology

CADASIL is the commonest genetic form of VCD. It is caused by autosomal dominant mutations in the NOTCH3 gene. Mutation prevalence in the west of Scotland is estimated at 10.7 per 100,000, and disease prevalence at 4.6 per 100,000 (Moreton et al., 2014). NOTCH3 is only expressed in vascular smooth muscle cells; pathogenic mutations cause damage to cerebral arterioles, producing subcortical ischaemia, which, on MRI, manifests as white matter hyperintensities and lacunar infarcts.

Management and prognosis

There is no specific treatment for CADASIL beyond secondary and tertiary prevention of stroke. Smoking particularly increases stroke risk and should be discouraged (Chabriat et al., 2016). Life expectancy is reduced, with median age at death being 70 years for women and 64 years for men (Opherk et al., 2004).

Rapidly progressive dementias

The defining features of rapidly progressive dementias (RPDs) are subacute onset (days or weeks) and progression to death (in untreated or untreatable cases) within 2 years. RPDs can be divided into three main groups.

1. Creutzfeldt–Jakob disease (CJD) and other prion diseases.
2. Chronic neurodegenerative or vascular dementias presenting in an atypically aggressive form.
3. Immune-mediated, infectious, neoplastic, or metabolic encephalopathies where cognitive decline is the lead symptom.

In a US tertiary centre with a specialist interest in prion diseases, 62% of referrals with RPD had prion disease, 15% had a non-prion neurodegenerative disorder (most commonly corticobasal degeneration or frontotemporal dementia), while 8% had an autoimmune encephalopathy (Geschwind et al., 2008). Given that conditions in group 3 are potentially treatable and the particular public health considerations associated with CJD, intensive investigation of RPDs, with neuroimaging and CSF studies in all cases and systemic imaging, specific blood tests, and brain biopsy in some cases, is generally recommended.

Creutzfeldt–Jakob disease and other human prion diseases

Prions are protein-only infectious agents that consist of abnormally folded prion protein. They cause a range of neurodegenerative diseases through as yet incompletely understood mechanisms. This process is, however, reliant on conversion to an abnormal conformation of endogenously expressed cellular prion protein, a highly conserved cell surface glycoprotein of unknown function (Hu et al., 2007; Isaacs et al., 2006). Prion diseases can occur sporadically, through infection with exogenous prions or as a result of mutations in the prion protein gene. All prion diseases are rare; as a group, they occur at a rate of approximately 1–2 cases per million population per year.

Sporadic CJD

> **CASE STUDY 12**
>
> A ward consultation is requested on a 64-year-old woman admitted after a fall. She has been behaving oddly on the ward, reaching out to touch the faces of members of staff who approach her. Her family say that she has appeared vague for the last 3 weeks and forgot to attend a birthday party for her grandson. On examination, she requires assistance to stand and walks with a broad-based gait, bumping into furniture by her bed. Jerky involuntary movements are present intermittently in her outstretched upper limbs, and these are exacerbated by sudden loud sounds such as the slamming of ward bin lids. She is disorientated in time, place, and person and displays higher visual deficits, including difficulty interpreting fragmented letters and objects. There is some evidence of visual neglect affecting the left hemifield. An MRI brain scan is reported to be normal, but on review with a neuroradiologist, it is felt that there is some high signal in the striatum and right parietal cortex on diffusion-weighted imaging.

Clinical features

Sporadic CJD (sCJD) is typically characterized by the triad of rapid cognitive decline, ataxia, and myoclonus. Extrapyramidal and pyramidal signs and ataxia can also be seen. Cortical blindness is a common feature; where it occurs as the initial symptom, this is referred to as the Heidenhain variant (Cooper et al., 2005). Although behavioural and psychological symptoms (BPS) are the presenting symptom in <10% of patients with sCJD, psychotic and mood symptoms eventually affect 43% and 33% of patients, respectively (Thompson et al., 2014). BPS occur more commonly in younger patients (Appleby et al., 2007; Thompson et al., 2014). The commonest psychotic experience is visual hallucinosis, particularly involving animals or human figures, which can occur in isolation or in association with other visual phenomena such as distortions and illusions.

The diagnosis is supported by MRI evidence of high signal in the cerebral cortex (the so-called 'cortical ribbon' sign) and basal ganglia on fluid-attenuated inversion recovery (FLAIR) and diffusion-weighted sequences (Zerr et al., 2009). EEG shows periodic or pseudoperiodic sharp wave complexes in about 60% of cases (Collins et al., 2006a). CSF examination is usually acellular, with normal protein and glucose levels, but shows elevations in biomarkers of rapid neurodegeneration, including 14-3-3, S100, and tau (Sanchez-Juan et al., 2006). A recent innovation is the real-time quaking-induced conversion (RT-QuIC) assay, which detects the ability of abnormal prion protein in the CSF to induce misfolding and aggregation in recombinant prion protein, which can be detected by thioflavin T fluorescence (McGuire et al., 2012). Brain biopsy is occasionally necessary to make a diagnosis and shows spongiform changes, neuronal loss, and astrocytosis. The abnormal prion protein is partially resistant to protease cleavage, producing a series of fragments that can be detected by western blotting of the tissue homogenate.

Aetiology

All acquired prion diseases require host prion protein to convert into an abnormal conformation, but there are genetic polymorphisms in human prion protein that make it more or less resistant to conversion. The most important polymorphism in humans is at codon 129. In the European population, approximately 38% are methionine homozygous (MM), 51% are methionine valine heterozygous (MV), and 11% are valine homozygous (VV). However, homozygotes account for nearly 90% of cases of sCJD, suggesting that heterozygosity confers relative resistance (Puoti et al., 2012).

Epidemiology

sCJD is, by far, the commonest manifestation of human prion diseases, contributing about 85% of all cases. Disease onset is highly unusual below the age of 45; median age at onset is 68 years (Collins et al., 2006b). Clinicians in the UK are asked to report all suspected cases of human prion disease to the National CJD Research and Surveillance Unit in Edinburgh and the National Prion Clinic in London. Similar national surveillance and notification systems exist in other countries.

Prognosis

sCJD progresses rapidly; median time from onset to death is 5 months (Collins et al., 2006b). Currently, there is no available disease-modifying therapy for any prion disease and care is palliative in all cases.

Kuru

Kuru is a human prion disease that reached epidemic levels among the Fore people of Papua New Guinea due to ingestion of infected CNS tissue during endocannibalistic funeral rites (Gibbs et al., 1980). It has not been described in other populations. Kuru probably originated from a case of sporadic CJD in the early twentieth century (Wadsworth et al., 2008). However, it manifests primarily as cerebellar ataxia, with dementia occurring late in the disease course, if at all. This supports experimental findings that the route of transmission can affect the phenotype of prion disease (Langevin et al., 2011). Susceptibility to kuru is strongly influenced by the PRNP codon 129 genotype, with heterozygotes showing resistance to the disease. Occasional cases were still being reported over 50 years after cannibalistic practices were outlawed, suggesting that the incubation period of acquired prion disease in humans can be up to several decades (Collinge et al., 2006).

Variant CJD

Clinical features

Typically, variant CJD (vCJD) presents with a neuropsychiatric prodrome that can include depression, anxiety, insomnia, and apathy (Will et al., 1999). BPS are the presenting symptom in about a quarter of vCJD cases, and psychotic and mood symptoms, respectively, affect half and two-thirds of patients at some point during the disease course (Thompson et al., 2014). The clinical course of vCJD features a wider and less predictable range of features than that of sCJD. Alongside dementia, paraesthesiae and neuropathic pain are commonly seen, and at a later stage, chorea, ataxia, dystonia, myoclonus, and pyramidal signs may emerge. Median survival is 14 months (Will et al., 2000).

Diagnostic criteria for vCJD are based on clinical and investigative findings (World Health Organization, 2002). Supportive features include the so-called 'pulvinar sign' on MRI brain (Collie et al., 2003). Periodic complexes are usually absent on EEG, and CSF biomarker findings are less reliable than in sCJD (Will et al., 2000). Tonsillar biopsy can provide support for the diagnosis, but a definite diagnosis requires neuropathological confirmation.

Aetiology

vCJD has a different distribution of tissue involvement, compared to sCJD, with high concentrations of abnormal prion protein and infectivity found in tonsillar and other lymphoreticular tissues. This facilitates diagnosis via tonsillar biopsy, which is not available for sCJD (Hill et al., 1999). However, the lymphoreticular tropism of vCJD prions also raises the spectre of their secondary transfer via transfusions of blood and blood-derived products. To date, blood transfusions or blood products from donors who later developed vCJD have been linked with three UK cases of vCJD (Wroe et al., 2006) and two cases of asymptomatic splenic vCJD infection in codon 129 MV heterozygotes (Peden et al., 2004, 2010).

Epidemiology

vCJD was first identified in a group of younger people presenting with rapidly progressive dementia in the mid-1990s in the aftermath of the bovine spongiform encephalopathy (BSE) epidemic in the UK. By 2016, there had been 178 cases of vCJD in the UK, 27 in France, and a handful elsewhere in the world. The peak year for vCJD cases in the UK was 2000, with a steady decline since then and only two cases reported since 2012. The most recently reported case in the UK, in 2016, was in a codon 129 MV heterozygote; prior to this, all pathologically confirmed symptomatic cases of vCJD had been MM homozygous at codon 129 of the prion protein (Mok et al., 2017).

Screening of 12,674 appendix samples removed from young adults during the late 1990s revealed three cases of asymptomatic vCJD carriage, two of which were in 129 VV homozygotes (Ironside et al., 2006). These data suggest that subclinical carriage of vCJD prions is present in the UK population and that all three codon 129 genotypes are affected. However, the size of the so-called 'second wave' of vCJD due to primary infection in non-129MM homozygotes and secondary transmission remains uncertain. Epidemiological modelling suggests that the number of affected 129MV and 129VV individuals will be lower than the number of affected MM individuals (Garske and Ghani, 2010). Observations from the kuru epidemic and from modelling prion infection in mice suggest that non-MM genotypes are associated not only with longer incubation times, but also with a lower cumulative incidence (Mead et al., 2009; Takeuchi et al., 2013). Furthermore, current modelling suggests that cases of secondary vCJD will not exceed the number of primary cases and that the likelihood of a self-sustaining epidemic of secondary vCJD is low (Garske and Ghani, 2010).

Genetic CJD

Genetic forms of prion disease are due to mutations in the prion gene *PRNP*. Over 30 pathogenic mutations have been described. All are inherited in an autosomal dominant pattern. The phenotypes associated with genetic prion diseases are highly variable. Age at onset varies from 30 to over 70 years. The commoner point mutations in European populations usually present in the same way as classical sCJD. Other point mutations cause either the relatively slowly progressive cerebellar ataxia of Gerstmann–Sträussler–Scheinker (GSS) syndrome or fatal familial insomnia (FFI), which is characterized by sleep disturbance, alternations in alertness, hallucinations, autonomic disturbances (such as tachycardia, hypertension, hyperhidrosis, and hyperthermia), and dementia. Sporadic cases of FFI have also been reported. Mutations caused by a premature stop codon (thus producing a truncated form of prion protein) can produce Alzheimer-like pathology or, in the case of Y163X, present with chronic diarrhoea and dysautonomia (Mead et al., 2013). BPS are the initial symptom in about half of cases due to the octapeptide repeat insertion (*OPRI*) mutation (Thompson et al., 2014).

There can be considerable phenotypic variability within families, such that the same mutation can manifest in different individuals as classical CJD, GSS, or an atypical picture. Furthermore, the presence of methionine or valine at codon 129 of the mutated allele can influence the phenotype. D178M mutations on a 129V background cause classical CJD, but on a 129M background cause FFI (Goldfarb et al., 1992).

Iatrogenic CJD

Iatrogenic CJD (iCJD) is caused by transfer of infectious prions by tissue grafts or other human-derived products or medical instruments (Brown et al., 1992). Several cases have occurred as a result of dural grafts or administration of growth hormone (GH) derived from cadaveric pituitary glands, with smaller numbers caused by corneal transplants and intracranial EEG electrodes. A total of 1849 people received GH in the UK between 1959 and 1985, of whom 38 were reported to have developed CJD by 2000, with a peak incubation period of 20 years (Swerdlow et al., 2003). Contrasting with the other forms of CJD, among the UK cases of iCJD due to GH treatment, valine–valine homozygosity at the *PRNP* codon 129 is associated with an increased susceptibility and a shorter incubation time, whereas 129MM homozygotes appear more resistant, even compared with 129MV heterozygotes (Rudge et al., 2015).

The phenotype of iCJD is determined by the route of transmission. Cases due to direct inoculation of prions into the brain (e.g. dural grafts) manifest as classical CJD after a relatively short incubation time. Where the infectious prions were initially inoculated outwith the CNS, the incubation period is longer (up to 40 years in some cases), and the clinical syndrome can be closer to that of kuru, starting with cerebellar ataxia and lower limb pain, with dementia as a relatively late feature (Goldfarb et al., 1992).

Lymphomatosis cerebri

Lymphomatosis cerebri is a diffusely infiltrating form of primary CNS lymphoma (PCNSL) that can present with an RPD. The neurological syndrome is variable, depending on the location of disease within the brain. However, unlike other rapidly progressive dementias, seizures, myoclonus, and parkinsonism are rare in

PCNSL (Deutsch and Mendez, 2015). MRI usually shows diffuse white matter T2 hyperintensities (Küker et al., 2005). CSF examination may be normal or show pleocytosis which can, in some cases, be demonstrated to include lymphoma cells on cytological analysis and immunophenotyping (Geschwind et al., 2008).

Subacute sclerosing panencephalitis

Subacute sclerosing panencephalitis (SSPE) is a late complication of measles, typically occurring 6–15 years after the initial infection. It is therefore most commonly seen in children and young adults. The incidence in individuals aged 5 years and over is about one per 100,000 cases of measles (Campbell et al., 2007). It is thought to be due to latent measles infection in neurones, which eventually triggers an inflammatory response, leading to widespread CNS destruction. Four stages of SSPE are recognized, the illness usually progressing to death within 3 years. Stage I is characterized by cognitive decline and behavioural changes, including lethargy, inattention, and irritability. In stage II, cognitive decline progresses to dementia and myoclonus, and seizures emerge. Stage III is characterized by an akinetic rigid syndrome and progressive unresponsiveness. In stage IV, the patient develops akinetic mutism, progressing to coma, accompanied by autonomic instability. A prodromal phase consisting of visual symptoms due to involvement of the visual pathways is recognized and can precede motor and cognitive onset by up to 5 years.

CSF analysis reveals pleocytosis, normal or raised protein levels, and high titres of measles antibody. EEG demonstrates periodic complexes in up to 80% of cases, typically occurring at intervals of 2–20 s. MRI brain reveals the progressive emergence of T2-hyperintense lesions and atrophy in the cerebral cortex, followed by the periventricular white matter and corpus callosum, and then the deep grey nuclei and brainstem (Fisher et al., 2015). Brain biopsy can also be used to confirm the diagnosis. There is no proven treatment for SSPE, although isoprinosine may improve outcomes (Gascon, 2003).

Dementias associated with movement disorders

The neuropsychiatry of movement disorders is covered in detail in Chapter 18, including, for each condition, a description of the epidemiology, semiology of the motor phenotype, aetiology, and management. The discussion here will therefore be restricted to those clinical features that aid the differential diagnosis of these disorders in the cognitive clinic.

Lewy body-related–dementia with Lewy bodies

> **CASE STUDY 13**
>
> A 73-year-old woman is referred by her family doctor because of a 3-year history of hallucinations. These occur when she is tired or the lighting is poor. The commonest manifestation is that she will make three or four coffees for people sitting on the sofa and her husband will have to remind her that it is only the two of them in the house. She also frequently hallucinates individuals in the garden and, on one occasion, thought that they were stealing her furniture. She has good retrospective insight into the fact that these people are not real but finds it very confusing at the time. Her cognition is fluctuant, with good days and bad days. She has REM sleep behaviour disorder. On examination, she has a mild parkinsonian motor syndrome and her sense of smell is poor. Despite only scoring 53/100 on the ACE-III (attention 11/18, memory 12/26, fluency 7/14, language 14/26, visuospatial 9/16), she is still able to travel to and from town alone on the bus once a week where she follows a fixed routine of going to Marks and Spencer's and coming home again. Her MRI scan demonstrated mild global atrophy with preserved hippocampal volume (see Fig. 25.7).

Clinical features

Dementia with Lewy bodies (DLB) is a dementia characterized by fluctuating cognition, attention, and alertness and/or recurrent visual hallucinations. The diagnosis is upgraded from 'possible' to 'probable' by the presence of REM sleep behaviour disorder, severe neuroleptic sensitivity, or abnormal dopamine transporter activity on nuclear imaging (McKeith et al., 2005). Impairments of visuospatial, executive, and attentional function can be particularly prominent. Other supportive features include repeated falls and syncope, transient unexplained losses of consciousness, autonomic dysfunction, delusions, depression, and absence of hippocampal atrophy on structural imaging. DLB is diagnosed when this characteristic cognitive syndrome develops either in the absence of, or within 1 year of, the presentation of a movement disorder typical of idiopathic Parkinson's disease. The evolution of a movement disorder is not inevitable, as a proportion of patients dying with DLB have relative preservation of nigral dopaminergic neurones, and

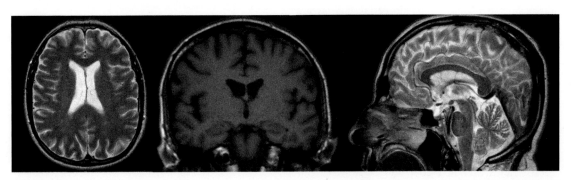

Fig. 25.7 MRI images for dementia with Lewy bodies in Case study 13. Radiological convention. T2-weighted axial projection; T1-weighted coronal projection; and T2-weighted sagittal projection. Mild generalized atrophy can be seen, with good hippocampal bulk and normal brainstem appearances.

consequently normal dopamine transporter imaging (Colloby et al., 2012). It is hypothesized, but not demonstrated, that this group might show less adverse neuroleptic reactions.

Lewy body-related—Parkinson's disease dementia

Parkinson's disease dementia (PDD) is diagnosed when the syndrome of DLB described above evolves >1 year into typical idiopathic Parkinson's disease (McKeith et al., 2005). There is evolving consensus that DLB and PDD represent the same underlying disease, with the phenotypic presentation reflecting a spectrum of relative predominance of Lewy body pathology in the cortex and brainstem (McKeith, 2009; McKeith and Burn, 2000). Patients with Parkinson's disease have quadruple the relative risk of incident dementia of age-matched controls (Hobson and Meara, 2004). Although the severity and duration of parkinsonian symptoms are risk factors in the development of dementia, the strongest risk factor is the patient's current age, with these factors having a multiplicative effect (Levy et al., 2002). Not all dementia developing in Parkinson's disease is PDD—Alzheimer's pathology is found in up to two-thirds of patients with Lewy body disease (Barker et al., 2002), and it is therefore perfectly reasonable to make concomitant diagnoses of idiopathic Parkinson's disease and either Alzheimer's disease or mixed dementia in the presence of a parkinsonian movement disorder and a characteristic amnestic syndrome.

Progressive supranuclear palsy

PSP is a highly protean disease, with only around a quarter of pathologically confirmed cases presenting initially with the classic Richardson's syndrome of falls, postural instability, cognitive dysfunction, and abnormal eye movements (Respondek et al., 2014). Previous diagnostic criteria (Litvan et al., 1996) did not reflect this and consequently suffered from poor sensitivity (Hughes et al., 2002) and specificity (Osaki et al., 2004) at first presentation. Consequently, the Movement Disorder Society has recently published revised criteria that split so-called variant PSP into a new classification, based on the predominant symptomatology, recognizing onsets with movement disorders, cerebellar disorders, primary lateral sclerosis, behavioural features, and abnormal speech (Höglinger et al., 2017; Respondek and Höglinger, 2016). In the context of the cognitive clinic, it is important to remember that up to 20% of PSP cases initially present with a frontal cognitive syndrome that is sometimes indistinguishable from bvFTD until the evolution of the characteristic movement disorder (Kaat et al., 2007). A striking lack of verbal fluency is a frequent finding in PSP and can be especially helpful in distinguishing PSP from idiopathic Parkinson's disease (Rittman et al., 2013). Structural imaging can be helpful in the appropriate clinical context, with the characteristic findings of the 'Mickey Mouse' and 'morning glory' signs on axial sections (Stamelou et al., 2011) and the 'hummingbird' or 'penguin' sign on sagittal sections (Kato et al., 2003; Massey et al., 2012) being formalized in measurements of the midbrain-to-pons ratio (Massey et al., 2013).

Corticobasal syndrome

> ### CASE STUDY 14
>
> A 69-year-old professional organist attends clinic with a friend. For a year or more, he has noticed difficulties with left-sided coordination, which are especially noticeable when playing the organ. He finds that his left hand is less confident and his left foot is hesitant when trying to find the pedals. He has also had some difficulties with walking and generally feels that his left leg is less responsive, but he has never fallen and has no true mobility problems. While he can still sight-read three staves of music, he complains of difficulty integrating this into a single percept. In fact, he initially thought that his difficulties were with his eyes but has now realized there is more going on. Despite this, he is still functioning at an extremely high level and even the choir master at his church has not noticed a problem with his playing. Outside of these domains, he has very few problems. He has no REM sleep behaviour disorder. He has been hyposmic since a sinus washout 15 years ago, but there has been no particular change. He describes normal forgetting, such as going into rooms and forgetting the purpose, but also admits that he is a bit more reliant on his wife to remember appointments. On examination, he has some left-sided difficulties with both ideomotor and gesture copy praxis, and struggles with graphesthesia. Foot tapping is normal and there is no parkinsonism. He scores 95/100 on the ACE-III (attention 18/18, memory 23/26, fluency 13/14, language 25/26, visuospatial 16/16). Given the subtlety of his presentation, a detailed neuropsychological assessment was requested, which revealed impairment across all cognitive domains, dominated by moderate memory and hand-sequencing deficits, with patchy performance across language, visuospatial, and executive functioning tasks. His MRI scan demonstrated subtle biparietal atrophy (see **Fig. 25.8**). His dopamine transporter (DaT) scan demonstrated asymmetrically reduced tracer uptake (see **Fig. 25.9**), and his SPECT scan demonstrated biparietal hypoactivity (see **Fig. 25.8**).

Clinical features and aetiology

It is important to distinguish CBS, which is a clinical diagnosis based on the criteria below, and corticobasal degeneration (CBD), which is a histopathological diagnosis based on a cortical distribution of tau lesions, together with ballooned achromatic neurones and astrocytic plaques (Dickson et al., 2002). There are similarities between the histopathological appearances of CBD and PSP, and some regard them as being opposite ends of a spectrum of cortical versus brainstem involvement (Armstrong et al., 2013). The predictive value of CBS for a post-mortem diagnosis of CBD is poor (Ling et al., 2010; Shelley et al., 2009), and only a small proportion of pathologically confirmed CBD displayed CBS in life (Ling et al., 2010).

A 'possible' diagnosis of CBS can be made in the presence of at least one of the following: limb rigidity or akinesia; limb dystonia; limb myoclonus; and at least one of: orobuccal or limb apraxia; cortical sensory deficit; and alien limb phenomena beyond simple levitation. The diagnosis is upgraded to 'probable' if the presentation is asymmetrical and at least two features from each category are present (Armstrong et al., 2013).

Multiple system atrophy

Dementia is rarer in multiple system atrophy (MSA) than in the other neurodegenerative movement disorders, perhaps reflecting a younger age of onset; severe cognitive decline at presentation should prompt a reconsideration of the diagnosis. ACE score is usually in the normal range, especially if verbal fluency is excluded (Cope et al.,

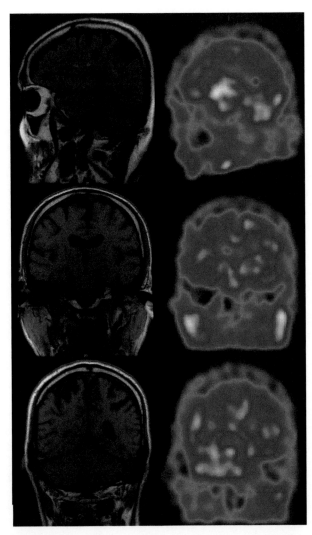

Fig. 25.8 MRI and SPECT images for corticobasal syndrome in Case study 14. Radiological convention. T1-weighted sagittal and coronal projections are shown, next to SPECT images from roughly the same projection. Moderate selective atrophy of parietal lobes can be seen, with a matching reduction in SPECT activity.

2014). Characteristic cognitive deficits can, however, be revealed by detailed neuropsychological testing. Performance is impaired on tests of visuospatial and constructive function (Kawai et al., 2008), executive function (Robbins et al., 1992), and time perception (Cope et al., 2014), especially in the parkinsonian phenotype (MSA-P). Focused intervention for these cognitive deficits can be helpful; for example, impairment of the ability to internally generate a regular beat (Grahn and Rowe, 2012) means that patients with MSA have particularly significant benefits from the use of a metronome to pace their gait (Thaut et al., 1996) and prevent freezing (Okuma, 2006).

Huntington's disease

CASE STUDY 15

A 56-year-old woman presents to clinic with progressively worsening slurred speech and difficulty with coordinating fine hand movements. Tasks like doing buttons, combing her hair, and doing up her bra have become very difficult. Her balance has become poorer,

but she has not fallen. Her husband mentions that she has begun to cram food into her mouth, earning the nickname 'hamster' from family members. You notice choreiform movements, but the patient says that these are not bothersome. Her mood is low; she is visibly anxious, and she becomes tearful while discussing her difficulties. Her maternal grandmother was said to have died from an aggressive form of Parkinson's disease with dementia, while her mother died of cancer in her forties. On examination, you elicit a 'milkmaid grip', an unstable tandem gait, dysdiadochokinesia, symmetrical difficulties with Luria hand movements and finger tapping, impersistence of tongue protrusion, and initiation of saccades with a head thrust. The ACE-III score is 82/100 (attention 16/18, memory 19/26, fluency 7/14, language 24/26, visuospatial 14/16).

Clinical features

While the chorea that characterizes Huntington's disease (HD) is immediately obvious to the observer, it is usually the least disabling of the symptoms. The neuropsychiatric features of HD are significant and can be broadly separated into dementia, executive dysfunction, and affective disorder.

It is a fallacy that the motor disorder develops in advance of the dementia in HD. Even in cohorts with early disease specifically selected for seemingly normal cognition, significant cognitive deficits are revealed, even by screening neuropsychology (Cope et al., 2014). Detailed neuropsychological testing reveals difficulty on tests of executive function, planning, cognitive flexibility, abstract thought, action selection, and time perception (Cope et al., 2014; Montoya et al., 2006; Tabrizi et al., 2009). The affective disorder in HD is heterogenous. Anxiety and irritability are the commonest feature at presentation, often in conjunction with depression, but aggression, compulsive, or addictive behaviours and

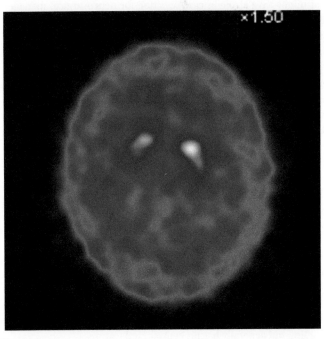

Fig. 25.9 DaT scan summary image for corticobasal syndrome in Case study 14. Radiological convention. Reduced transporter activity can be seen, more marked on the right (in keeping with his predominantly left-sided symptoms).

sometimes inappropriate happiness are observed (Klöppel et al., 2010; Montoya et al., 2006). Psychosis does occur, but in the absence of genetic confirmation of HD, its presence should prompt consideration of the HD mimics dentatorubral-pallidoluysian atrophy (DRPLA) (Adachi et al., 2001) and C9ORF72-related neurodegeneration (Moss et al., 2014). An autosomal dominant family history of a movement disorder or dementia is usually present, but, as here, misdiagnosis in earlier generations is common. At the single-subject level, structural imaging can appear normal in early HD, with the most commonly observed abnormality being flattening of the caudate head (Lang, 1985). The diagnostic genetic test is for an expansion of CAG triplet repeats in the gene encoding the developmental protein huntingtin, which lies on the short arm of chromosome 4. Fewer than 26 repeats is normal, and >40 predicts full penetrance of HD (Walker, 2007).

Normal pressure hydrocephalus

Normal pressure hydrocephalus (NPH) is characterized by an insidious onset of dementia with psychomotor retardation and an apraxic gait, often associated with urinary incontinence, in the presence of ventricular enlargement and normal CSF pressure (Adams et al., 1965). It is a rare condition in younger individuals, but prevalence rises rapidly after the age of 80 (Jaraj et al., 2014). Ventricular enlargement has classically been defined as a ratio of >0.3 between the maximum axial width of the frontal horns of the lateral ventricles and the maximal internal diameter of the skull at the same level (the so-called Evans' index). This is a sensitive measure that lacks specificity, being present in 20% of elderly individuals (Jaraj et al., 2014) and an even greater proportion of those with neurodegenerative disease (Missori et al., 2016). Novel metrics such as the ratio between ventricular and intracranial volumes (Toma et al., 2011) and a reduction in the angle of the corpus callosum on coronal sections (Ishii et al., 2008) have increased specificity and might have a role in case selection for neurosurgical management (Virhammar et al., 2014). NPH is, in many cases, treatable by one of a number of neurosurgical procedures that provide constant drainage of CSF, but case selection remains difficult (Anderson, 1986; Freimann et al., 2012). Gait disturbance commonly responds better than cognitive impairment. At post-mortem, NPH is strongly associated with demyelination of frontal regions in a pattern typical for small vessel disease (Akai et al., 1987). It remains unclear whether this white matter pathology causes the altered CSF dynamics or is a consequence of altered periventricular metabolism (Jeppsson et al., 2013).

Niemann–Pick disease type C

Niemann–Pick disease types A and B are caused by autosomal recessive mutations in *SMPD1* (Schuchman et al., 1992), which cause deficiency or absence of the lysosomal enzyme acid sphingomyelinase (Brady et al., 1966). This leads to a lipid storage disorder characterized by an accumulation of sphingomyelin (Klenk, 1935). Niemann–Pick disease type A is a severe neurodegenerative disease of infancy that leads to death in the first few years of life, while type B causes hepatosplenomegaly, growth retardation, and lung dysfunction but generally has no neurological features.

Niemann–Pick disease type C is caused by autosomal recessive mutations in *NPC1* (95% of cases) or *NPC2*, which respectively encode a large endosomal glycoprotein and a small cholesterol-binding lysosomal protein (Ioannou, 2000). This leads to dysfunctional intracellular transport of cholesterol, leading to its sequestration in lysosomes and/or late endosomes. Age of onset is variable, and while approximately 50% of cases manifest by age 5 years, adult-onset cases make up at least 20% of the total (Vanier and Millat, 2003). Mean age of onset in this subgroup is approximately 25 years, with the oldest reported case presenting at 54 years (Vanier et al., 1991). Presentation is protean, but a progressive dementia is present in approximately 60% of cases. Other clinical features include cerebellar ataxia (76%), vertical supranuclear ophthalmoplegia (75%), dysarthria, (63%), movement disorders (58%), splenomegaly (54%), psychiatric disorders (45%), and dysphagia (37%) (Sevin et al., 2007). Epilepsy and cataplexy are more rarely reported, but the presence of gelastic cataplexy in the absence of a sleep disorder is highly suggestive of Niemann–Pick disease type C.

Psychiatric disturbance is the presenting feature in more than a third of cases and can be manifest for a number of years before visceral or deep brain signs appear. Psychosis is the commonest manifestation, but bipolar disorder, isolated depression, and obsessive–compulsive disorder have been reported (Sullivan et al., 2005). While onset can be progressive, most patients present acutely and have relapsing and remitting disease, leading to an initial diagnosis of schizophrenia before additional clinical features emerge. It is rare but recognised for psychiatric disturbance to complicate later disease in patients initially presenting with motor features.

About a quarter of patients present with isolated cognitive dysfunction. Again, the phenotype is variable, from mild dysexecutive features to aggressive global dementia. Interestingly, neurofibrillary tangles and β-amyloid plaques have been observed in relatively young patients with Niemann–Pick disease type C (Saito et al., 2002), but their presence is the exception, not the rule.

Diagnostic testing for Niemann–Pick disease type C is complex. Classically, the diagnostic cornerstone has been skin biopsy with fibroblast culture and the demonstration of impaired intracellular cholesterol transport with filipin staining (Patterson et al., 2012). This test is strongly positive in about 80% of cases and can also give a clear negative result, but about 20% of patients show only intermediate staining. In recent years, this has been complemented by next-generation sequencing of the *NPC1* and *NPC2* genes, but novel mutations of uncertain significance are commonly found and interpretation can be difficult. Simpler tests, based on mass spectroscopy of plasma biomarkers, have recently become available; validation studies are ongoing, but initial evidence suggests that these tests might prove sensitive, but not specific (Vanier et al., 2016).

Disease modification can be achieved with miglustat, a small-molecule inhibitor of glucosylceramide synthase (Patterson et al., 2007) that has been demonstrated to reduce the rate of disease progression. Current clinical consensus is that all patients with neurological, psychiatric, or cognitive manifestations should be offered this medication. The primary side effects are gastrointestinal and can be partially ameliorated with dietary and anti-propulsive strategies (Belmatoug et al., 2011). There is also a significant role for symptomatic therapy to treat seizures, cataplexy, dystonia, psychiatric disturbance, and sleep disorders.

Spinocerebellar ataxia

Spinocerebellar ataxia (SCA) is a collection of >60 genetic neurodegenerative diseases that are united by their primary manifestation with ataxia and (usually) cerebellar degeneration, but with different associated features. Most are autosomal dominant with adult onset, but X-linked and childhood-onset forms are recognized (Stephen et al., 2016). The SCAs are assigned a number according to the date of discovery of the associated gene, and the classification is consequently confusing and difficult to remember (see Worth, 2004 for a clinically focused review). While even those disorders, such as SCA-6, thought to result in 'pure' cerebellar dysfunction display a subtle 'cerebellar cognitive phenotype' of impairments in cognitive flexibility, response inhibition, verbal reasoning (Cooper et al., 2010), and time interval perception (Grube et al., 2010), many of the SCAs display a broader cognitive phenotype. Cognitive impairment, hallucinations, or depression are especially common as an early or presenting feature in SCA-17, which is caused by a triplet repeat expansion in *TBP* (Rolfs et al., 2003).

Not necessarily progressive cognitive impairments

Mild cognitive impairment

CASE STUDY 16

A 62-year-old mathematics teacher presents to clinic alone. She complains that her memory is generally poorer than it was, and she is finding it especially difficult to learn the names of children in their class. She is not struggling with the mathematical aspect of their work but has found it difficult to adapt to curriculum changes and new information technology. Her mood is stable, and she denies any significant stressors. The ACE-III score is 89 (attention 16/18, memory 20/26, fluency 13/14, language 26/26, visuospatial 16/16).

Clinical features

The primary differentiation between dementia and MCI is one of degree. Generally speaking, a diagnosis of MCI is made when deficits are insufficiently severe to interfere with function at work or in daily activities, but this is not a firm criterion. The distinction is a sensitive clinical judgement that requires a skilled clinician to make a holistic assessment of the patient from primary and secondary sources. In Case study 16's vignette, the patient's work function was affected, but a similar level of difficulty might not have had such a noticeable effect on an individual in a less cognitively demanding role. Clearly, it is not intellectually satisfying for the same constellation of symptoms and signs to lead to different diagnoses dependent solely on work status. Another factor that must weigh on this decision is the level of certainty that one is dealing with a progressive condition. A diagnosis of dementia carries with it the inevitable long-term implications of a neurodegenerative condition; the same is not necessarily true of MCI, from which only a proportion of individuals will progress. Some clinicians might find it appropriate in mild cases to make an initial diagnosis of MCI, pending imaging and longitudinal neuropsychological assessment, while others prefer to refrain from making any diagnosis until progression has been assessed—neither approach is incorrect, and this decision should be made on an individual basis in a patient-centred manner.

Management

Once structural and significant vascular pathology has been excluded with structural imaging, the most important management step in MCI is to monitor for the emergence of a dementia requiring medical or social intervention. It is possible to sub-classify MCI by the cognitive domain or domains affected. It has been proposed by some that those with multidomain symptoms or a predominantly amnestic phenotype are more likely to progress to Alzheimer's disease, and that an individual patient's risk of progression can be more accurately predicted through use of biomarkers of amyloid deposition and neuronal injury, such as CSF tau/phosphorylated tau and Aβ42, PET amyloid imaging, or perfusion imaging with FDG-PET or SPECT (Albert et al., 2011). Others have gone further, suggesting that amnestic MCI with supportive biomarkers should be termed prodromal Alzheimer's disease (Dubois and Albert, 2004). While of undoubted utility in research, where the current focus of therapeutic trials is in early disease, this approach is of limited clinical utility at present and is not currently advocated by the UK National Institute for Health and Care Excellence (National Institute for Health and Care Excellence and Social Care Institute for Excellence, 2006, updated March 2016). Clearly, the emergence of disease-modifying therapeutics will change the balance of this decision.

No drugs are currently licensed for treatment of MCI in the UK and the evidence for any pharmacological intervention in MCI is extremely limited (Cooper et al., 2013; Russ and Morling, 2012). Potentially modifiable factors that influence the progression of MCI to dementia include diabetes, metabolic syndrome, neuropsychiatric symptoms, and low dietary folate (Cooper et al., 2013).

Psychologically based memory disorders

(Transient) psychogenic amnesias

CASE STUDY 17

AT (Kopelman et al., 1994) was a young woman in her thirties who 'came round' on the London Underground, apparently not knowing who or where she was. She was directed to a nearby police station and subsequently admitted to hospital. Various attempts were made to identify her, without initial success. She was an enterprising person and subsequently managed to obtain a job, housing, and a husband. Eventually, she was identified by the Missing Persons Bureau. It emerged she had fled from a stormy marriage abroad. Although there was some evidence that she had made use of her 'convenient' amnesia after arriving in the UK, she consistently maintained that she had complete amnesia for the initial week of her disappearance, consistent with a fugue episode.

Clinical features and aetiology

Psychogenic (dissociative) amnesia can be either global or 'situation-specific' (Kopelman, 2002). In global psychogenic amnesia, there is loss of memories for the entire earlier life, and often loss of the sense of personal identity as well, as in a 'fugue state'. In situation-specific amnesia, there are 'gaps' in memory for specific events, as in post-traumatic stress disorder (PTSD) and as also occur in victims (and sometimes the perpetrators) of offences.

A psychogenic fugue state is a syndrome consisting of a sudden loss of memory, involving autobiographical memories and the sense of personal identity, usually associated with a period of wandering. It normally lasts for a few hours or days (up to about 4 weeks), and there is a subsequent amnesic gap for the period of the 'fugue'. If the amnesia persists, the disorder is better termed 'psychogenic focal retrograde amnesia', but the possibility of simulation should always be considered.

The literature on fugue states indicates that there is always a precipitating stress such as a marital or financial crisis. Previous depressed mood and suicidal ideas are common. Moreover, surprisingly frequently, there has been a past history of a transient neurological amnesia (e.g. from head injury or epilepsy), which may represent a 'learning experience' in this context. Clinical and neuropsychological studies indicate that, during the fugue, there are often 'islands' or 'fragments' of preserved memory, which may appear 'strange and unfamiliar'. In the most persuasive cases, semantic knowledge, verbal learning, and procedural skills remain intact. There are now numerous neuroimaging studies of memory inhibition; although the findings are often inconsistent, the most convincing investigations suggest that there is activation of (inhibitory) centres in the frontal lobes, in parallel with deactivation of medial temporal structures (Anderson et al., 2004; Kikuchi et al., 2010).

While both transient neurological amnesias and transient psychological amnesias can be preceded by a precipitating stress or significant life event, and standard investigations (routine EEG, CT, MRI) can be normal, there are important differences. For example, loss of personal identity is seen in psychogenic cases, but very seldom in neurological amnesia, except for profound dementia. Repetitive questioning is characteristic of the transient neurological amnesias, whereas it is not seen in the psychogenic cases, where there may be 'la belle indifférence' (although this is not, in itself, a useful discriminator) (Stone et al., 2006). Finally, the temporal gradients of retrograde amnesia differ—neurological amnesias show the typical sparing of early memories, whereas psychogenic amnesias may show a 'reversed' temporal gradient.

Situation-specific memory gaps have been reviewed in many papers on PTSD (Brewin et al., 1996), child sexual abuse and rape (Mechanic et al., 1998), and amnesia for offences (Pyszora et al., 2003, 2014).

Subjective memory complaints and memory disorders secondary to a psychiatric syndrome

CASE STUDY 18

A 52-year-old man attends clinic alone. He left school at 16 with three Certificates of Secondary Education (CSEs) and became a planning officer at a telecoms company where he undertook an apprenticeship and several postgraduate qualifications. He describes several years of poor anterograde memory. He has developed elaborate coping mechanisms such as littering his house with Post-It notes and 'quick guides' for new computer programs. He reports poor day-to-day memory but is unable to give concrete examples of this. He presents due to a perceived worsening in symptoms. There have been no concerns from his partner or employer about performance. He reports anxiety at work but ascribes this to his perceived performance difficulties; there is no overt mood disorder. Neurological examination is normal. The ACE-III score is 96 (attention 18/18, memory 23/26, fluency 13/14, language 26/26, visuospatial 16/16). Detailed neuropsychological assessment is undertaken, which reveals normal performance on tests of verbal comprehension, perceptual reasoning, executive function, processing speed, and language, but catastrophic failure on tests of memory. The pattern of failure is a lack of immediate recall of both a story and the Rey complex figure, with consequent impairment of delayed recall. The neuropsychologist reports that he displayed significant anxiety during testing.

Clinical features

Strictly speaking, subjective memory complaints or subjective cognitive impairment (SCI) refer to the presence of cognitive symptoms in the absence of objective evidence of cognitive impairment (Reisberg et al., 2010; Stewart, 2012), characterized by a seeming inconsistency between symptoms and measurable deficit. The aetiological background of SCI is diverse, but there is now some evidence that, in older populations, it can be a predictor of future cognitive decline. Those with SCI do show small differences from controls on neuropsychology and imaging at the group level (Hohman et al., 2011), and SCI sufferers over the age of 65 have a hazard ratio of 2.3 for acquiring dementia within 4 years (Waldorff et al., 2012). However, it should be noted that it is not subjective lapses as such (so-called 'senior moments') that predict imminent dementia, but the onset of lack of awareness of memory impairment (Wilson et al., 2015).

In younger individuals in whom the likelihood of an underlying dementia or other organic disorder is low, the evaluation of subjective cognitive symptoms requires a tailored approach. Analogous to findings in non-epileptic attack disorder, patients with non-organic memory disorders may describe their symptoms in a distinctive way, compared to individuals with organic dementia syndromes (Jones et al., 2016). Typical non-organic subjective cognitive complaints include forgetting of errands prior to their completion, loss of 'train of thought', and temporary inability to recall overlearnt names, words, and PIN numbers (Schmidtke and Metternich, 2009).

It is important to note that (measurable) memory impairments secondary to a psychiatric syndrome (such as clinical depression, anxiety, or transient stress) are common and, in extreme form, can produce a 'pseudodementia' (Ron et al., 1979). Memory symptoms are associated with, and may be a part of, an underlying depression or anxiety disorder. Patients with major depression tend to show overgeneralization in their memory (i.e. they cannot deal with specifics) and have difficulties with accessing positive memories (Nandrino et al., 2003). Fischer et al. (2008) compared depressed and non-depressed individuals without neurological diseases, substance abuse, or psychosis and found that subjective memory complaints were significantly higher in the group diagnosed with a major depressive disorder. Additionally, increased awareness about, or sensitivity towards, memory problems may lead to subjective increase in depression or anxiety symptoms. In order to avoid over-interpretation of cognitive deficits on neuropsychological assessment, symptom validity (effort) testing is recommended for patients with suspected mood-related or functional cognitive symptoms.

Services in the UK specializing in the assessment of younger people with cognitive complaints reported a significant increase in the proportion of referrals with a non-dementia diagnosis in recent years (Stone et al., 2015b). However, there is currently little research, and therefore a lack of consensus, on whether younger individuals who present with SCI in the absence of an organic cause or a major psychiatric disorder are a distinct group. Some authors advocate the use of the term 'functional cognitive disorder' or 'functional memory disorder', analogous to diagnostic labels such as functional movement disorder and sitting in the DSM-5 within the category of Conversion (Functional Neurological) Disorder (Schmidtke et al., 2008; Stone et al., 2015b) and in the ICD-11 as dissociative neurological symptom disorder with cognitive symptoms. Stone and colleagues (2015a) have proposed the following categories of functional cognitive disturbance:

1. Cognitive symptoms as part of anxiety or depression.
2. 'Normal' cognitive symptoms that become the focus of attention.
3. Isolated functional cognitive disorder in which symptoms are outwith 'normal', but not explained by anxiety.
4. Health anxiety about dementia.
5. Cognitive symptoms as part of another functional disorder.
6. Retrograde dissociative (psychogenic) amnesia.

Similarly, Schmidtke and colleagues (2008) have proposed the following criteria for the diagnosis of what they termed functional memory disorder:

1. Complaint of acquired (>6 months) dysfunction of memory that, as perceived by patients, significantly affects their level of functioning in professional and/or private life.
2. Presence of external and/or subjective factors, addressed as psychosocial burden factors, that cause significant psychological stress.
3. Verbal memory and attentional capacity better than 1.5 standard deviations below the mean for age on standardized tests.
4. Absence of a recognizable organic cause of cognitive impairment.
5. Absence of major psychiatric illness, e.g. psychosis, major depression, dissociative disorder, obsessive–compulsive disease, etc. (previous or present).

Management

Appropriate clinical management is usually identification of stressors or underlying psychiatric disorder, and practical suggestions such as list keeping and sleep hygiene. In some patients, over-reliance on lists and notes can become disabling and delay a return to normal utilization of memory with the attendant lapses that are part of normal cognitive fallibility. Providing an explanatory model that includes predisposing, precipitating, and perpetuating factors can be beneficial, in particular identifying hypervigilance and 'catastrophic' reactions to normal cognitive lapses and identifying the centrality of disturbed attentional, rather than mnestic, mechanisms. Subjective memory complaints or functional cognitive disorder do not remit spontaneously in the majority of cases (Schmidtke et al., 2008), and there is some preliminary evidence for psychotherapeutic approaches (Metternich et al., 2008). Common comorbidities in patients with subjective cognitive complaints include chronic fatigue syndrome (CFS), fibromyalgia, chronic pain, and neurotropic polypharmacy; identification of, and specific intervention for, these might help ameliorate the cognitive symptoms.

Aetiology

Subjective lapses of memory and language are extremely common in the healthy adult population (Commissaris et al., 1998; McCaffrey et al., 2006), but it should be noted that people attending memory clinics are not a representative cross-section of the population. They tend to have particular predisposing, precipitating, and perpetuating factors that make them more likely to notice their lapses, interpret their lapses in a particular way, and present to a doctor seeking an explanation. Analogous to other functional neurological disorders, predisposing factors can include psychological trauma earlier in life, perfectionistic expectations of memory performance, past history of psychiatric illness (especially mood disorders), and previous or current somatic complaints such as CFS or fibromyalgia. Precipitating factors include stress, an episode of physical illness (such as minor head trauma or surgery), or a relative with dementia (leading to dementia-specific health anxiety). Perpetuating factors include continuing psychological distress, hypervigilance to cognitive lapses, and catastrophic interpretations of them.

An ongoing controversy is whether SCI following chemotherapy exposure (sometimes referred to as 'chemobrain') is due to an organic or a functional disorder. Large prospective studies have suggested that cognitive symptoms following chemotherapy do not correlate with cognitive deficits but are associated with lower mood and personality traits related to negative affectivity (Hermelink et al., 2010). Certainly, cognitive complaints among breast cancer survivors are no greater than 7–9 years after treatment among women who received chemotherapy than those who did not (Amidi et al., 2015).

One unifying hypothesis underpinning the various functional cognitive disorders (i.e. those occurring in isolation and in association with CFS, fibromyalgia, chemobrain, etc) is of reduced attentional reserve (Teodoro et al., 2018). Thus, individuals can be easily distracted, leading to discontinuities in short-term and working memory that are experienced as 'memory lapses'. The neurobiological underpinnings of functional memory disturbance remain largely unexplored, although one group has reported impaired memory consolidation during sleep (Puetz et al., 2011).

KEY LEARNING POINTS

- Memory disorders are persistent disorders of the mental processes affecting one (amnesic syndrome) or more (the dementias) cognitive domain(s).
- Dementias interfere with an individual's ability to function at work or home, and represent a decline from a previous level of function.
- Dementias can be classified either by their cognitive phenotype or by their aetiological origin, and there is not necessarily linear mapping between the two.
- The assessment of memory disorders and dementias is a multidisciplinary pursuit.

REFERENCES

Adachi N, Arima K, Asada T, et al. Dentatorubral-pallidoluysian atrophy (DRPLA) presenting with psychosis. Journal of Neuropsychiatry and Clinical Neurosciences. 2001;13:258–60.

Adams R, Fisher C, Hakim S, Ojemann R, Sweet W. Symptomatic occult hydrocephalus with normal cerebrospinal-fluid pressure: a treatable syndrome. New England Journal of Medicine. 1965;273:117–26.

Akai K, Uchigasaki S, Tanaka U, Komatsu A. Normal pressure hydrocephalus. Pathology International. 1987;37:97–110.

Albert MS, DeKosky ST, Dickson D, et al. The diagnosis of mild cognitive impairment due to Alzheimer's disease: Recommendations from the National Institute on Aging-Alzheimer's Association workgroups on diagnostic guidelines for Alzheimer's disease. Alzheimer's & Dementia. 2011;7:270–9.

Alladi S, Xuereb J, Bak T, et al. Focal cortical presentations of Alzheimer's disease. Brain. 2007;130(Pt 10):2636–45.

American Psychiatric Association. *Diagnostic and Statistical Manual of Mental Disorders (DSM-5®)*. Washington, DC: American Psychiatric Association; 2013.

Amidi A, Christensen S, Mehlsen M, Jensen A, Pedersen A, Zachariae R. Long-term subjective cognitive functioning following adjuvant systemic treatment: 7–9 years follow-up of a nationwide cohort of women treated for primary breast cancer. British Journal of Cancer. 2015;113:794–801.

Anderson M. Normal pressure hydrocephalus. BMJ. 1986;293:837.

Anderson MC, Ochsner KN, Kuhl B, et al. Neural systems underlying the suppression of unwanted memories. Science. 2004;303:232–5.

Appleby BS, Appleby KK, Rabins PV. Does the presentation of Creutzfeldt-Jakob disease vary by age or presumed etiology? A meta-analysis of the past 10 years. Journal of Neuropsychiatry and Clinical Neurosciences. 2007;19:428–35.

Arighi A, Fumagalli GG, Jacini F, et al. Early onset behavioral variant frontotemporal dementia due to the C9ORF72 hexanucleotide repeat expansion: psychiatric clinical presentations. Journal of Alzheimer's Disease. 2012;31:447–52.

Armstrong MJ, Litvan I, Lang AE, et al. Criteria for the diagnosis of corticobasal degeneration. Neurology. 2013;80:496–503.

Baddeley AD, Hitch G. Working memory. Psychology of Learning and Motivation. 1974;8:47–89.

Bales KR, Verina T, Dodel RC, et al. Lack of apolipoprotein E dramatically reduces amyloid beta-peptide deposition. Nature Genetics. 1997;17:263–4.

Banerjee S. *The use of antipsychotic medication for people with dementia: Time for action*. London: Department of Health; 2009.

Banerjee S, Hellier J, Dewey M, et al. Sertraline or mirtazapine for depression in dementia (HTA-SADD): a randomised, multicentre, double-blind, placebo-controlled trial. The Lancet. 2011;378:403–11.

Barker WW, Luis CA, Kashuba A, et al. Relative frequencies of Alzheimer disease, Lewy body, vascular and frontotemporal dementia, and hippocampal sclerosis in the State of Florida Brain Bank. Alzheimer's Disease Associated Disorders. 2002;16:203–12.

Basso A, Capitani E, Laiacona M. Progressive language impairment without dementia: a case with isolated category specific semantic defect. *Journal of Neurology, Neurosurgery, and Psychiatry*. 1988;51:1201–7.

Bateman RJ, Xiong C, Benzinger TL, et al. Clinical and biomarker changes in dominantly inherited Alzheimer's disease. New England Journal of Medicine. 2012;367:795–804.

Becker RE, Greig NH. Fire in the ashes: Can failed Alzheimer's disease drugs succeed with second chances? Alzheimer's & Dementia. 2013;9:50–7.

Belin C, Maillet D, Pop G, Carpentier A. bvFTD phenocopy syndrome: Myth or reality?(P1. 215). Neurology. 2015;84(14 Supplement):P1. 215.

Belmatoug N, Burlina A, Giraldo P, et al. Gastrointestinal disturbances and their management in miglustat-treated patients. Journal of Inherited Metabolic Disorders. 2011;34:991–1001.

Biffi A, Bailey D, Anderson CD, et al. Risk Factors Associated With Early vs Delayed Dementia After Intracerebral Hemorrhage. JAMA Neurology. 2016;73:969–76.

Birks J, McGuinness B, Craig D. Rivastigmine for vascular cognitive impairment. Cochrane Database of Systematic Reviews. 2013;5:CD004744.

Birks JS. Cholinesterase inhibitors for Alzheimer's disease. Cochrane Database of Systematic Reviews. 2006;25:CD005593.

Bolwig TG. Transient global amnesia. Acta Neurologica Scandinavica. 1968;44:101–6.

Boxer AL, Knopman DS, Kaufer DI, et al. Memantine in patients with frontotemporal lobar degeneration: a multicentre, randomised, double-blind, placebo-controlled trial. The Lancet Neurology. 2013;12:149–56.

Bozeat S, Lambon-Ralph MA, Patterson K, Garrard P, Hodges J. Non-verbal semantic impairment in semantic dementia. Neuropsychologia. 2000;38:1207–15.

Bozeat S, Lambon Ralph MA, Graham KS, et al. A duck with four legs: Investigating the structure of conceptual knowledge using picture drawing in semantic dementia. Cognitive Neuropsychology. 2003;20:27–47.

Braak H, Braak E. Staging of Alzheimer's disease-related neurofibrillary changes. Neurobiology in Aging. 1995;16:271–8.

Braak H, Del Tredici K. The preclinical phase of the pathological process underlying sporadic Alzheimer's disease. Brain. 2015;138:2814–33.

Brady RO, Kanfer JN, Mock MB, Fredrickson DS. The metabolism of sphingomyelin. II. Evidence of an enzymatic deficiency in Niemann-Pick diseae. Proceedings of the National Academy of Sciences of the United States of America. 1966;55:366–9.

Brewin CR, Dalgleish T, Joseph S. A dual representation theory of posttraumatic stress disorder. Psychological Review. 1996;103:670.

Brookes RL, Willis TA, Patel B, Morris RG, Markus HS. Depressive symptoms as a predictor of quality of life in cerebral small vessel disease, acting independently of disability; a study in both sporadic small vessel disease and CADASIL. International Journal of Stroke. 2013;8:510–17.

Brouwers N, Sleegers K, Van Broeckhoven C. Molecular genetics of Alzheimer's disease: an update. Annals of Medicine. 2008;40:562–83.

Brown P, Preece MA, Will RG. ' Friendly fire' in medicine: Hormones, homografts, and Creutzfeldt-Jakob disease. The Lancet. 1992;340:24–7.

Buchman AS, Yu L, Boyle PA, et al. Microvascular brain pathology and late-life motor impairment. Neurology. 2013;80:712–18.

Buffon F, Porcher R, Hernandez K, et al. Cognitive profile in CADASIL. Journal of Neurology, Neurosurgery, and Psychiatry. 2006;77:175–80.

Bullock R, Touchon J, Bergman H, et al. Rivastigmine and donepezil treatment in moderate to moderately-severe Alzheimer's disease over a 2-year period. Current Medical Research and Opinion. 2005;21:1317–27.

Butler CR. Transient epileptic amnesia. Practical Neurology. 2006;6:368–71.

Butler CR, Graham KS, Hodges JR, Kapur N, Wardlaw JM, Zeman AZ. The syndrome of transient epileptic amnesia. Annals of Neurology. 2007;61:587–98.

Caine D, Watson JD. Neuropsychological and neuropathological sequelae of cerebral anoxia: A critical review. Journal of the International Neuropsychological Society. 2000;6:86–99.

Cairns NJ, Bigio EH, Mackenzie IR, et al. Neuropathologic diagnostic and nosologic criteria for frontotemporal lobar degeneration: consensus of the Consortium for Frontotemporal Lobar Degeneration. Acta Neuropathologica. 2007;114:5–22.

Caligiuri MP, Rockwell E, Jeste DV. Extrapyramidal side effects in patients with Alzheimer's disease treated with low-dose neuroleptic medication. American Journal of Geriatric Psychiatry. 1999;6:75–82.

Campbell H, Andrews N, Brown K, Miller E. Review of the effect of measles vaccination on the epidemiology of SSPE. International Journal of Epidemiology. 2007;36:1334–48.

Chabriat H, Hervé D, Duering M, et al. Predictors of Clinical Worsening in Cerebral Autosomal Dominant Arteriopathy With Subcortical Infarcts and Leukoencephalopathy Prospective Cohort Study. Stroke. 2016;47:4–11.

Chabriat H, Joutel A, Dichgans M, Tournier-Lasserve E, Bousser M-G. Cadasil. The Lancet Neurology. 2009;8:643–53.

Choi JC. Cerebral autosomal dominant arteriopathy with subcortical infarcts and leukoencephalopathy: a genetic cause of cerebral small vessel disease. Journal of clinical Neurology. 2010;6:1–9.

Cole G. Intracranial space-occupying masses in mental hospital patients: necropsy study. Journal of Neurology, Neurosurgery, and Psychiatry. 1978;41:730–6.

Collie DA, Summers DM, Sellar RJ, et al. Diagnosing variant Creutzfeldt-Jakob disease with the pulvinar sign: MR imaging findings in 86 neuropathologically confirmed cases. American Journal of Neuroradiology. 2003;24:1560–9.

Collinge J, Whitfield J, McKintosh E, et al. Kuru in the 21st century—an acquired human prion disease with very long incubation periods. The Lancet. 2006;367:2068–74.

Collins S, Sanchez-Juan P, Masters C, et al. Determinants of diagnostic investigation sensitivities across the clinical spectrum of sporadic Creutzfeldt–Jakob disease. Brain. 2006a;129:2278–87.

Collins SJ, Sanchez-Juan P, Masters CL, et al. Determinants of diagnostic investigation sensitivities across the clinical spectrum of sporadic Creutzfeldt-Jakob disease. Brain. 2006b;129(Pt 9):2278–87.

Colloby SJ, McParland S, O'Brien JT, Attems J. Neuropathological correlates of dopaminergic imaging in Alzheimer's disease and Lewy body dementias. Brain. 2012;135(Pt 9):2798–808.

Commissaris C, Ponds R, Jolles J. Subjective forgetfulness in a normal Dutch population: possibilities for health education and other interventions. Patient Educ Couns. 1998;34:25–32.

Cooper C, Li R, Lyketsos C, Livingston G. Treatment for mild cognitive impairment: systematic review. British Journal of Psychiatry. 2013;203:255–64.

Cooper FE, Grube M, Elsegood KJ, et al. The contribution of the cerebellum to cognition in spinocerebellar ataxia type 6. Behavioral Neurology. 2010;23(1-2):3–15.

Cooper S, Murray K, Heath C, Will R, Knight R. Isolated visual symptoms at onset in sporadic Creutzfeldt-Jakob disease: the clinical phenotype of the 'Heidenhain variant'. British Journal of Ophthalmology. 2005;89:1341–2.

Cope TE, Grube M, Singh B, Burn DJ, Griffiths TD. The basal ganglia in perceptual timing: Timing performance in Multiple System Atrophy and Huntington's disease. Neuropsychologia. 2014;52:73–81.

Cope TE, Patterson K, Sohoglu E, et al. Evidence for causal top-down frontal contributions to predictive processes in speech perception. Nature Communications. 2017;8(1):1–16.

Cosentino SA, Jefferson AL, Carey M, et al. The clinical diagnosis of vascular dementia: A comparison among four classification systems and a proposal for a new paradigm. The Clinical Neuropsychologist. 2004;18:6–21.

Coyle-Gilchrist IT, Dick KM, Patterson K, et al. Prevalence, characteristics, and survival of frontotemporal lobar degeneration syndromes. Neurology. 2016;86:1736–43.

Cummings JL, Benson F, Hill MA, Read S. Aphasia in dementia of the Alzheimer type. Neurology. 1985;35:394–7.

DeJesus-Hernandez M, Mackenzie IR, Boeve BF, et al. Expanded GGGGCC hexanucleotide repeat in noncoding region of C9ORF72 causes chromosome 9p-linked FTD and ALS. Neuron. 2011;72:245–56.

Deutsch MB, Mendez MF. Neurocognitive features distinguishing primary central nervous system lymphoma from other possible causes of rapidly progressive dementia. Cognitive and Behavioral Neurology. 2015;28:1.

Dickson DW, Bergeron C, Chin S, et al. Office of Rare Diseases neuropathologic criteria for corticobasal degeneration. Journal of Neuropathology and Experimental Neurology. 2002;61:935–46.

Dubois B, Albert ML. Amnestic MCI or prodromal Alzheimer's disease? The Lancet Neurology. 2004;3:246–8.

Dubois B, Feldman HH, Jacova C, et al. Research criteria for the diagnosis of Alzheimer's disease: revising the NINCDS–ADRDA criteria. The Lancet Neurology. 2007;6:734–46.

Ellis R, Olichney JM, Thal L, et al. Cerebral amyloid angiopathy in the brains of patients with Alzheimer's disease The CERAD experience, part XV. Neurology. 1996;46:1592–6.

Erkinjuntti T. Clinical criteria for vascular dementia: the NINDS-AIREN criteria. Dementia and Geriatric Cognitive Disorders. 1994;5:189–92.

Evans JJ, Heggs A, Antoun N, Hodges JR. Progressive prosopagnosia associated with selective right temporal lobe atrophy. Brain. 1995;118:1–13.

Fairhall SL, Caramazza A. Brain regions that represent amodal conceptual knowledge. Journal of Neuroscience. 2013;33:10552–8.

Ferri CP, Prince M, Brayne C, et al. Global prevalence of dementia: a Delphi consensus study. The Lancet. 2005;366:2112–17.

Filippini N, MacIntosh BJ, Hough MG, et al. Distinct patterns of brain activity in young carriers of the APOE-epsilon4 allele. Proceedings of the National Academy of Sciences of the United States of America. 2009;106:7209–14.

Fischer C, Schweizer TA, Atkins JH, et al. Neurocognitive profiles in older adults with and without major depression. International Journal of Geriatric Psychiatry. 2008;23:851–6.

Fisher C. Transient global amnesia. Transactions of the American Neurological Association. 1958;83:143–6.

Fisher DL, Defres S, Solomon T. Measles-induced encephalitis. QJM. 2015;108:177–82.

Fitzgerald S. Two Large Alzheimer's Trials Fail to Meet Endpoints: What's Next? Neurology Today. 2014;14:12–15.

Fotopoulou A, Conway MA, Solms M, Tyrer S, Kopelman M. Self-serving confabulation in prose recall. Neuropsychologia. 2008;46:1429–41.

Freimann FB, Streitberger K-J, Klatt D, et al. Alteration of brain viscoelasticity after shunt treatment in normal pressure hydrocephalus. Neuroradiology. 2012;54:189–96.

Garske T, Ghani AC. Uncertainty in the tail of the variant Creutzfeldt-Jakob disease epidemic in the UK. PLoS One. 2010;5:e15626.

Gascon GG. Randomized treatment study of inosiplex versus combined inosiplex and intraventricular interferon-α in subacute sclerosing panencephalitis (SSPE): International multicenter study. Journal of Child Neurology. 2003;18:819–27.

Geschwind MD, Shu H, Haman A, Sejvar JJ, Miller BL. Rapidly progressive dementia. Annals of Neurology. 2008;64:97–108.

Gibbs CJ, Amyx HL, Bacote A, Masters CL, Gajdnsek DC. Oral transmission of kuru, Creutzfeldt-Jakob disease, and scrapie to nonhuman primates. Journal of Infectious Diseases. 1980;142:205–8.

Gilboa A, Alain C, Stuss DT, Melo B, Miller S, Moscovitch M. Mechanisms of spontaneous confabulations: a strategic retrieval account. Brain. 2006;129:1399–414.

Gill DP, Hubbard RA, Koepsell TD, et al. Differences in rate of functional decline across three dementia types. Alzheimer's & Dementia. 2013;9:S63–71.

Goldfarb LG, Petersen RB, Tabaton M, et al. Fatal familial insomnia and familial Creutzfeldt-Jakob disease: disease phenotype determined by a DNA polymorphism. Science. 1992;258:806–8.

Goll JC, Crutch SJ, Loo JHY, et al. Non-verbal sound processing in the primary progressive aphasias. Brain. 2010;133:272–85.

Gorelick PB. Risk factors for vascular dementia and Alzheimer disease. Stroke. 2004;35(11 suppl 1):2620–2.

Gorelick PB, Scuteri A, Black SE, et al. Vascular contributions to cognitive impairment and dementia a statement for healthcare professionals from the American Heart Association/American Stroke Association. Stroke. 2011;42:2672–713.

Gorno-Tempini ML, Dronkers NF, Rankin KP, et al. Cognition and anatomy in three variants of primary progressive aphasia. Annals of Neurology. 2004;55:335–46.

Gorno-Tempini ML, Hillis AE, Weintraub S, et al. Classification of primary progressive aphasia and its variants. Neurology. 2011;76:1006–14.

Graham A, Davies R, Xuereb J, et al. Pathologically proven frontotemporal dementia presenting with severe amnesia. Brain. 2005;128:597–605.

Grahn JA, Rowe JB. Finding and Feeling the Musical Beat: Striatal Dissociations between Detection and Prediction of Regularity. Cerebral Cortex. 2012;23:913–21.

Grube M, Bruffaerts R, Schaeverbeke J, et al. Core auditory processing deficits in primary progressive aphasia. Brain. 2016;139:1817–29.

Grube M, Cooper FE, Chinnery PF, Griffiths TD. Dissociation of duration-based and beat-based auditory timing in cerebellar degeneration. Proceedings of the National Academy of Sciences of the United States of America. 2010;107:11597–601.

Gupta M, Dasgupta A, Khwaja GA, Chowdhury D, Patidar Y, Batra A. Behavioural and psychological symptoms in poststroke vascular cognitive impairment. Behavioral Neurology. 2014;2014:430128.

Halliday M, Mallucci GR. Targeting the unfolded protein response in neurodegeneration: a new approach to therapy. Neuropharmacology. 2014;76:169–74.

Harding A, Halliday G, Caine D, Kril J. Degeneration of anterior thalamic nuclei differentiates alcoholics with amnesia. Brain. 2000;123:141–54.

Harold D, Abraham R, Hollingworth P, et al. Genome-wide association study identifies variants at CLU and PICALM associated with Alzheimer's disease. Nature Genetics. 2009;41:1088–93.

Harper C. The neuropathology of alcohol-related brain damage. Alcohol Alcohol. 2009;44:136–40.

Harper C, Kril J, Daly J. Are we drinking our neurones away? BMJ. 1987;294:534–6.

Harris JM, Gall C, Thompson JC, et al. Sensitivity and specificity of FTDC criteria for behavioral variant frontotemporal dementia. Neurology. 2013;80:1881–7.

Hermelink K, Küchenhoff H, Untch M, et al. Two different sides of 'chemobrain': determinants and nondeterminants of self-perceived cognitive dysfunction in a prospective, randomized, multicenter study. Psycho-Oncology. 2010;19:1321–8.

Hill A, Butterworth R, Joiner S, et al. Investigation of variant Creutzfeldt-Jakob disease and other human prion diseases with tonsil biopsy samples. The Lancet. 1999;353:183–9.

Hobson P, Meara J. Risk and incidence of dementia in a cohort of older subjects with Parkinson's disease in the United Kingdom. Movement Disorders. 2004;19:1043–9.

Hodges JR, Mitchell J, Dawson K, et al. Semantic dementia: demography, familial factors and survival in a consecutive series of 100 cases. Brain. 2010;133:300–6.

Hodges JR, Patterson K, Oxbury S, Funnell E. Semantic dementia. Brain. 1992;115:1783–806.

Hodges JR, Ward CD. Observations during transient global amnesia. Brain. 1989;112:595–620.

Hodges JR, Warlow CP. The aetiology of transient global amnesia. Brain. 1990;113:639–57.

Höglinger GU, Respondek G, Stamelou M, et al. Clinical diagnosis of progressive supranuclear palsy: the Movement Disorder Society Criteria. Movement Disorders. 2017;32:853–64.

Hohman TJ, Beason-Held LL, Lamar M, Resnick SM. Subjective cognitive complaints and longitudinal changes in memory and brain function. Neuropsychology. 2011;25:125.

Hornberger M, Piguet O. Episodic memory in frontotemporal dementia: a critical review. Brain. 2012;135:678–92.

Hornberger M, Piguet O, Graham A, Nestor P, Hodges J. How preserved is episodic memory in behavioral variant frontotemporal dementia? Neurology. 2010;74:472–9.

Hornberger M, Shelley BP, Kipps CM, Piguet O, Hodges JR. Can progressive and non-progressive behavioural variant frontotemporal dementia be distinguished at presentation? Journal of Neurology, Neurosurgery, and Psychiatry. 2009;80:591–3.

Hsieh S, Schubert S, Hoon C, Mioshi E, Hodges JR. Validation of the Addenbrooke's Cognitive Examination III in frontotemporal dementia and Alzheimer's disease. Dementia and Geriatric Cognitive Disorders. 2013;36(3-4):242–50.

Hu W, Rosenberg R, Stüve O. Prion proteins: a biological role beyond prion diseases. Acta Neurologica Scandinavica. 2007;116:75–82.

Huber R, Aschoff A, Ludolph A, Riepe M. Transient global amnesia. Journal of Neurology. 2002;249:1520–4.

Hughes AJ, Daniel SE, Ben-Shlomo Y, Lees AJ. The accuracy of diagnosis of parkinsonian syndromes in a specialist movement disorder service. Brain. 2002;125:861–70.

Ioannou YA. The structure and function of the Niemann–Pick C1 protein. Molecular Genetics and Metabolism. 2000;71:175–81.

Ironside JW, Bishop MT, Connolly K, et al. Variant Creutzfeldt-Jakob disease: prion protein genotype analysis of positive appendix tissue samples from a retrospective prevalence study. BMJ. 2006;332:1186–8.

Isaacs J, Jackson G, Altmann D. The role of the cellular prion protein in the immune system. Clinical and Experimental Immunology. 2006;146:1–8.

Ishii K, Kanda T, Harada A, et al. Clinical impact of the callosal angle in the diagnosis of idiopathic normal pressure hydrocephalus. European Radiology. 2008;18:2678–83.

James W. The perception of time. Journal of Speculative Philosophy. 1886;20:374–407.

Jaraj D, Rabiei K, Marlow T, Jensen C, Skoog I, Wikkelsø C. Prevalence of idiopathic normal-pressure hydrocephalus. Neurology. 2014;82:1449–54.

Jellinger KA. Pathology and pathogenesis of vascular cognitive impairment—a critical update. Frontiers in Aging Neuroscience. 2013;5:17.

Jeppsson A, Zetterberg H, Blennow K, Wikkelsø C. Idiopathic normal-pressure hydrocephalus Pathophysiology and diagnosis by CSF biomarkers. Neurology. 2013;80:1385–92.

Jimenez-Conde J, Biffi A, Rahman R, et al. Hyperlipidemia and reduced white matter hyperintensity volume in patients with ischemic stroke. Stroke. 2010;41:437–42.

Jones D, Drew P, Elsey C, et al. Conversational assessment in memory clinic encounters: interactional profiling for differentiating dementia from functional memory disorders. Aging & Mental Health. 2016;20:500–9.

Josephs KA, Boeve BF, Duffy JR, et al. Atypical progressive supranuclear palsy underlying progressive apraxia of speech and nonfluent aphasia. Neurocase. 2005;11:283–96.

Josephs KA, Duffy JR, Strand EA, et al. The evolution of primary progressive apraxia of speech. Brain. 2014;137(Pt 10):2783–95.

Josephs KA, Duffy JR, Strand EA, et al. Syndromes dominated by apraxia of speech show distinct characteristics from agrammatic PPA. Neurology. 2013;81:337–45.

Josephs KA, Duffy JR, Strand EA, et al. Characterizing a neurodegenerative syndrome: primary progressive apraxia of speech. Brain. 2012;135:1522–36.

Josephs KA, Duffy JR, Strand EA, et al. Clinicopathological and imaging correlates of progressive aphasia and apraxia of speech. Brain. 2006a;129:1385–98.

Josephs KA, Duffy JR, Strand EA, et al. Clinicopathological and imaging correlates of progressive aphasia and apraxia of speech. Brain. 2006b;129(Pt 6):1385–98.

Joutel A, Corpechot C, Ducros A, et al. Notch3 mutations in CADASIL, a hereditary adult-onset condition causing stroke and dementia. Nature. 1996;383:707–10.

Kaat LD, Boon A, Kamphorst W, Ravid R, Duivenvoorden H, Van Swieten J. Frontal presentation in progressive supranuclear palsy. Neurology. 2007;69:723–9.

Kato N, Arai K, Hattori T. Study of the rostral midbrain atrophy in progressive supranuclear palsy. Journal of Neurological Sciences. 2003;210:57–60.

Kawai Y, Suenaga M, Takeda A, et al. Cognitive impairments in multiple system atrophy MSA-C vs MSA-P. Neurology. 2008;70(16 Part 2):1390–6.

Kertesz A, McMonagle P, Blair M, Davidson W, Munoz DG. The evolution and pathology of frontotemporal dementia. Brain. 2005;128(Pt 9):1996–2005.

Kikuchi H, Fujii T, Abe N, et al. Memory repression: brain mechanisms underlying dissociative amnesia. Journal of Cognitive Neuroscience. 2010;22:602–13.

Kimura T, Takamatsu J. Pilot study of pharmacological treatment for frontotemporal dementia: risk of donepezil treatment for behavioral and psychological symptoms. Geriatrics & Gerontology International. 2013;13:506–7.

Kipps CM, Hodges JR, Hornberger M. Nonprogressive behavioural frontotemporal dementia: recent developments and clinical implications of the 'bvFTD phenocopy syndrome'. Current Opinion of Neurology. 2010;23:628–32.

Klenk E. Über die Natur der Phosphatide und anderer Lipoide des Gehirns und der Leber bei der Niemann-Pickschen Krankheit. [12. Mitteilung über Phosphatide.]. Hoppe-Seylers Zeitschrift für physiologische Chemie. 1935;235:24–36.

Klöppel S, Stonnington CM, Petrovic P, et al. Irritability in pre-clinical Huntington's disease. Neuropsychologia. 2010;48:549–57.

Knibb JA, Kipps CM, Hodges JR. Frontotemporal dementia. Current Opinion of Neurology. 2006a;19:565–71.

Knibb JA, Xuereb JH, Patterson K, Hodges JR. Clinical and pathological characterization of progressive aphasia. Annals of Neurology. 2006b;59:156–65.

Kopelman MD. Amnesia: organic and psychogenic. British Journal of Psychiatry. 1987a;150:428–42.

Kopelman MD. Two types of confabulation. Journal of Neurology, Neurosurgery, and Psychiatry. 1987b;50:1482–7.

Kopelman MD. Remote and autobiographical memory, temporal context memory and frontal atrophy in Korsakoff and Alzheimer patients. Neuropsychologia. 1989;27:437–60.

Kopelman MD. Disorders of memory. Brain. 2002;125:2152–90.

Kopelman MD, Christensen H, Puffett A, Stanhope N. The great escape: A neuropsychological study of psychogenic amnesia. Neuropsychologia. 1994;32:675–91.

Kopelman MD, Lasserson D, Kingsley D, et al. Retrograde amnesia and the volume of critical brain structures. Hippocampus. 2003;13:879–91.

Kopelman MD, Morton J. Amnesia in an actor: Learning and re-learning of play passages despite severe autobiographical amnesia. Cortex. 2015;67:1–14.

Kopelman MD, Ng N, Brouke OVD. Confabulation extending across episodic, personal, and general semantic memory. Cognitive Neuropsychology. 1997;14:683–712.

Korsakoff S. Etude médico-psychologique sur une forme des maladies de la mémoire. Revue Philosophique. 1889a;28:501–30.

Korsakoff S. Etude médico-psychologique sur une forme des maladies de la mémoire. Revue Philosophique. 1889b;28:e530.

Kua EH, Ho E, Tan HH, Tsoi C, Thng C, Mahendran R. The natural history of dementia. Psychogeriatrics. 2014;14:196–201.

Küker W, Nägele T, Korfel A, et al. Primary central nervous system lymphomas (PCNSL): MRI features at presentation in 100 patients. Journal of Neurooncology. 2005;72:169–77.

Lang C. Is direct CT caudatometry superior to indirect parameters in confirming Huntington's disease? Neuroradiology. 1985;27:161–3.

Langevin C, Andréoletti O, Le Dur A, Laude H, Béringue V. Marked influence of the route of infection on prion strain apparent phenotype in a scrapie transgenic mouse model. Neurobiology of Disease. 2011;41:219–25.

Larner A. Addenbrooke's Cognitive Examination (ACE) for the diagnosis and differential diagnosis of dementia. Clinical Neurology and Neurosurgery. 2007;109:491–4.

Larner AJ. 'Frontal variant Alzheimer's disease': A reappraisal. Clinical Neurology and Neurosurgery. 2006;108:705–8.

Larner AJ. Diagnostic Test Accuracy Studies in Dementia: A Pragmatic Approach. Cham: Springer International Publishing; 2015.

Larson EB, Shadlen MF, Wang L, et al. Survival after initial diagnosis of Alzheimer disease. Annals of Internal Medicine. 2004;140:501–9.

Lawrence AJ, Patel B, Morris RG, et al. Mechanisms of cognitive impairment in cerebral small vessel disease: multimodal MRI results from the St George's cognition and neuroimaging in stroke (SCANS) study. PLoS One. 2013;8:e61014.

Lebert F. Behavioral benefits of trazodone are sustained for the long term in frontotemporal dementia. Therapy. 2006;3:93–6.

Lebert F, Stekke W, Hasenbroekx C, Pasquier F. Frontotemporal dementia: a randomised, controlled trial with trazodone. Dementia and Geriatric Cognitive Disorders. 2004;17:355–9.

Levy G, Schupf N, Tang MX, et al. Combined effect of age and severity on the risk of dementia in Parkinson's disease. Annals of Neurology. 2002;51:722–9.

Ling H, O'Sullivan SS, Holton JL, et al. Does corticobasal degeneration exist? A clinicopathological re-evaluation. Brain. 2010;133:2045–57.

Litvan I, Agid Y, Calne D, et al. Clinical research criteria for the diagnosis of progressive supranuclear palsy (Steele-Richardson-Olszewski syndrome) Report of the NINDS-SPSP International Workshop. Neurology. 1996;47:1–9.

Looi JC, Sachdev PS. Differentiation of vascular dementia from AD on neuropsychological tests. Neurology. 1999;53:670.

Lu C-j, Tune LE. Chronic exposure to anticholinergic medications adversely affects the course of Alzheimer disease. American Journal of Geriatric Psychiatry. 2003;11:458–61.

Lyketsos CG, Lopez O, Jones B, Fitzpatrick AL, Breitner J, DeKosky S. Prevalence of neuropsychiatric symptoms in dementia and mild cognitive impairment: results from the cardiovascular health study. JAMA. 2002;288:1475–83.

Mackenzie IR, Foti D, Woulfe J, Hurwitz TA. Atypical frontotemporal lobar degeneration with ubiquitin-positive, TDP-43-negative neuronal inclusions. Brain. 2008;131:1282–93.

Mackenzie IR, Neumann M, Bigio EH, et al. Nomenclature and nosology for neuropathologic subtypes of frontotemporal lobar degeneration: an update. Acta Neuropathologica. 2010;119:1–4.

Mair W, Warrington E, Weiskrantz L. Memory disorder in Korsakoff's psychosis: a neuropathological and neuropsychological investigation of two cases. Brain. 1979;102:749–83.

Markowitsch HJ, Weber-Luxemburger G, Ewald K, Kessler J, Heiss WD. Patients with heart attacks are not valid models for medial temporal lobe amnesia. A neuropsychological and FDG-PET study with consequences for memory research. European Journal of Neurology. 1997;4:178–84.

Massey LA, Jäger HR, Paviour DC, et al. The midbrain to pons ratio: A simple and specific MRI sign of progressive supranuclear palsy. Neurology. 2013;80:1856–61.

Massey LA, Micallef C, Paviour DC, et al. Conventional magnetic resonance imaging in confirmed progressive supranuclear palsy and multiple system atrophy. Movement Disorders. 2012;27:1754–62.

Matthews F, Stephan B, Robinson L, et al. A two decade dementia incidence comparison from the Cognitive Function and Ageing Studies I and II. Nature Communications. 2016;7:11398.

Matthews FE, Arthur A, Barnes LE, et al. A two-decade comparison of prevalence of dementia in individuals aged 65 years and older from three geographical areas of England: results of the Cognitive Function and Ageing Study I and II. The Lancet. 2013;382:1405–12.

McCaffrey RJ, Bauer L, Palav AA, O'Bryant S. Practitioner's Guide to Symptom Base Rates in the General Population. New York, NY: Springer Science & Business Media; 2006.

McGrath N, Anderson N, Croxson M, Powell K. Herpes simplex encephalitis treated with acyclovir: diagnosis and long term outcome. Journal of Neurology, Neurosurgery, and Psychiatry. 1997;63:321–6.

McGuire LI, Peden AH, Orru CD, et al. Real time quaking-induced conversion analysis of cerebrospinal fluid in sporadic Creutzfeldt-Jakob disease. Annals of Neurology. 2012;72:278–85.

McKeith I. Commentary: DLB and PDD: the same or different? Is there a debate? International Psychogeriatrics. 2009;21:220–4.

McKeith I, Dickson DW, Lowe J, et al. Diagnosis and management of dementia with Lewy bodies third report of the DLB consortium. Neurology. 2005;65:1863–72.

McKeith IG, Burn D. Spectrum of Parkinson's disease, Parkinson's dementia, and Lewy body dementia. Neurologic Clinics. 2000;18:865–83.

McKhann G, Drachman D, Folstein M, Katzman R, Price D, Stadlan EM. Clinical diagnosis of Alzheimer's disease Report of the NINCDS-ADRDA Work Group under the auspices of Department of Health and Human Services Task Force on Alzheimer's Disease. Neurology. 1984;34:939.

McKhann GM, Knopman DS, Chertkow H, et al. The diagnosis of dementia due to Alzheimer's disease: Recommendations from the National Institute on Aging-Alzheimer's Association workgroups on diagnostic guidelines for Alzheimer's disease. Alzheimer's & Dementia. 2011;7:263–9.

McMonagle P, Deering F, Berliner Y, Kertesz A. The cognitive profile of posterior cortical atrophy. Neurology. 2006;66:331–8.

Mead S, Gandhi S, Beck J, et al. A novel prion disease associated with diarrhea and autonomic neuropathy. New England Journal of Medicine. 2013;369:1904–14.

Mead S, Whitfield J, Poulter M, et al. A novel protective prion protein variant that colocalizes with kuru exposure. New England Journal of Medicine. 2009;361:2056–65.

Mechanic MB, Resick PA, Griffin MG. A comparison of normal forgetting, psychopathology, and information-processing models of reported amnesia for recent sexual trauma. Journal of Consulting and Clinical Psychology. 1998;66:948.

Melo T, Ferro J, Ferro H. Transient global amnesia. Brain. 1992;115:261–70.

Mendez MF, Shapira JS, McMurtray A, Licht E. Preliminary findings: behavioral worsening on donepezil in patients with frontotemporal dementia. American Journal of Geriatric Psychiatry. 2007;15:84–7.

Mesulam MM, Weintraub S, Rogalski EJ, Wieneke C, Geula C, Bigio EH. Asymmetry and heterogeneity of Alzheimer's and frontotemporal pathology in primary progressive aphasia. Brain. 2014;137(Pt 4):1176–92.

Metternich B, Schmidtke K, Dykierek P, Hüll M. A pilot group therapy for functional memory disorder. Psychotherapy and Psychosomatics. 2008;77:259–60.

Meyer MR, Tschanz JT, Norton MC, et al. APOE genotype predicts when—not whether—one is predisposed to develop Alzheimer disease. Nature Genetics. 1998;19:321–2.

Mioshi E, Hodges J. Rate of change of functional abilities in frontotemporal dementia. Dementia and Geriatric Cognitive Disorders. 2009;28:404–11.

Missori P, Rughetti A, Peschillo S, et al. In normal aging ventricular system never attains pathological values of Evans' index. Oncotarget. 2016;7:11860–3.

Mok T, Jaunmuktane Z, Joiner S, et al. Variant Creutzfeldt–Jakob disease in a patient with heterozygosity at PRNP codon 129. New England Journal of Medicine. 2017;376:292–4.

Mok V, Leung EYL, Chu W, et al. Pittsburgh compound B binding in poststroke dementia. Journal of Neurological Sciences. 2010;290:135–7.

Montoya A, Price BH, Menear M, Lepage M. Brain imaging and cognitive dysfunctions in Huntington's disease. Journal of Psychiatry and Neuroscience. 2006;31:21.

Moreno JA, Halliday M, Molloy C, et al. Oral treatment targeting the unfolded protein response prevents neurodegeneration and clinical disease in prion-infected mice. Science Translational Medicine. 2013;5:206ra138.

Moreton F, Razvi S, Davidson R, Muir K. Changing clinical patterns and increasing prevalence in CADASIL. Acta Neurologica Scandinavica. 2014;130:197–203.

Moss DJH, Poulter M, Beck J, et al. C9orf72 expansions are the most common genetic cause of Huntington disease phenocopies. Neurology. 2014;82:292–9.

Muhlert N, Milton F, Butler CR, Kapur N, Zeman AZ. Accelerated forgetting of real-life events in transient epileptic amnesia. Neuropsychologia. 2010;48:3235–44.

Nandrino J-L, Pezard L, Posté A, Réveillère C, Beaune D. Autobiographical memory in major depression: A comparison between first-episode and recurrent patients. Psychopathology. 2003;35:335–40.

National Institute for Health and Care Excellence and Social Care Institute for Excellence. *Dementia: Supporting People with Dementia and their Carers in Health and Social Care*. NICE clinical guideline 42; 2006 (updated March 2016).

Okuma Y. Freezing of gait in Parkinson's disease. Journal of Neurology. 2006;253:vii27–32.

Opherk C, Peters N, Herzog J, Luedtke R, Dichgans M. Long-term prognosis and causes of death in CADASIL: a retrospective study in 411 patients. Brain. 2004;127:2533–9.

Osaki Y, Ben-Shlomo Y, Lees AJ, et al. Accuracy of clinical diagnosis of progressive supranuclear palsy. Movement Disorders. 2004;19:181–9.

Ossenkoppele R, Pijnenburg YA, Perry DC, et al. The behavioural/dysexecutive variant of Alzheimer's disease: clinical, neuroimaging and pathological features. Brain. 2015a;138:2732–49.

Ossenkoppele R, Schonhaut DR, Baker SL, et al. Tau, amyloid, and hypometabolism in a patient with posterior cortical atrophy. Annals of Neurology. 2015b;77:338–42.

Pantoni L. Cerebral small vessel disease: from pathogenesis and clinical characteristics to therapeutic challenges. The Lancet Neurology. 2010;9:689–701.

Patel B, Lawrence AJ, Chung AW, et al. Cerebral microbleeds and cognition in patients with symptomatic small vessel disease. Stroke. 2013;44:356–61.

Patterson MC, Hendriksz CJ, Walterfang M, Sedel F, Vanier MT, Wijburg F. Recommendations for the diagnosis and management of Niemann-Pick disease type C: an update. Molecular Genetics and Metabolism. 2012;106:330–44.

Patterson MC, Vecchio D, Prady H, Abel L, Wraith JE. Miglustat for treatment of Niemann-Pick C disease: a randomised controlled study. The Lancet Neurology. 2007;6:765–72.

Pearce LA, McClure LA, Anderson DC, et al. Effects of long-term blood pressure lowering and dual antiplatelet treatment on cognitive function in patients with recent lacunar stroke: a secondary analysis from the SPS3 randomised trial. The Lancet Neurology. 2014;13:1177–85.

Peden A, McCardle L, Head M, et al. Variant CJD infection in the spleen of a neurologically asymptomatic UK adult patient with haemophilia. Haemophilia. 2010;16:296–304.

Peden AH, Head MW, Diane LR, Jeanne EB, James WI. Preclinical vCJD after blood transfusion in a PRNP codon 129 heterozygous patient. The Lancet. 2004;364:527–9.

Pendlebury ST, Rothwell PM. Prevalence, incidence, and factors associated with pre-stroke and post-stroke dementia: a systematic review and meta-analysis. The Lancet Neurology. 2009;8:1006–18.

Perrin RJ, Fagan AM, Holtzman DM. Multimodal techniques for diagnosis and prognosis of Alzheimer's disease. Nature. 2009;461:916–22.

Piguet O, Hornberger M, Mioshi E, Hodges JR. Behavioural-variant frontotemporal dementia: diagnosis, clinical staging, and management. The Lancet Neurology. 2011;10:162–72.

Porsteinsson AP, Drye LT, Pollock BG, et al. Effect of citalopram on agitation in Alzheimer disease: the CitAD randomized clinical trial. JAMA. 2014;311:682–91.

Price C, Jefferson A, Merino J, Heilman K, Libon D. Subcortical vascular dementia Integrating neuropsychological and neuroradiologic data. Neurology. 2005;65:376–82.

Puetz J, Grohmann S, Metternich B, et al. Impaired memory consolidation during sleep in patients with functional memory disorder. Biological Psychology. 2011;86:31–8.

Puoti G, Bizzi A, Forloni G, Safar JG, Tagliavini F, Gambetti P. Sporadic human prion diseases: molecular insights and diagnosis. The Lancet Neurology. 2012;11:618–28.

Pyszora NM, Barker AF, Kopelman MD. Amnesia for criminal offences: a study of life sentence prisoners. Journal of Forensic Psychiatry. 2003;14:475–90.

Pyszora NM, Fahy T, Kopelman MD. Amnesia for violent offenses: factors underlying memory loss and recovery. Journal of the American Academy of Psychiatry and the Law Online. 2014;42:202–13.

Quinette P, Guillery-Girard B, Dayan J, et al. What does transient global amnesia really mean? Review of the literature and thorough study of 142 cases. Brain. 2006;129:1640–58.

Raina P, Santaguida P, Ismaila A, et al. Effectiveness of cholinesterase inhibitors and memantine for treating dementia: evidence review for a clinical practice guideline. Annals of Internal Medicine. 2008;148:379–97.

Rainer M, Mucke H, Krüger-Rainer C, Kraxberger E, Haushofer M, Jellinger K. Cognitive relapse after discontinuation of drug therapy in Alzheimer's disease: cholinesterase inhibitors versus nootropics. Journal of Neural Transmission. 2001;108:1327–33.

Raschilas F, Wolff M, Delatour F, et al. Outcome of and prognostic factors for herpes simplex encephalitis in adult patients: results of a multicenter study. Clinical and Infectious Diseases. 2002;35:254–60.

Rascovsky K, Hodges JR, Knopman D, et al. Sensitivity of revised diagnostic criteria for the behavioural variant of frontotemporal dementia. Brain. 2011;134:2456–77.

Reed L, Marsden P, Lasserson D, et al. FDG-PET analysis and findings in amnesia resulting from hypoxia. Memory. 1999;7:599–614.

Reisberg B, Auer SR, Monteiro IM. Behavioral pathology in Alzheimer's disease (BEHAVE-AD) rating scale. International Psychogeriatrics. 1996;8 Suppl 3:301–8; discussion 51–4.

Reisberg B, Shulman MB, Torossian C, Leng L, Zhu W. Outcome over seven years of healthy adults with and without subjective cognitive impairment. Alzheimer's and Dementia. 2010;6:11–24.

Reitz C, Brayne C, Mayeux R. Epidemiology of Alzheimer disease. Nature Reviews Neurology. 2011;7:137–52.

Rempel-Clower NL, Zola SM, Squire LR, Amaral DG. Three cases of enduring memory impairment after bilateral damage limited to the hippocampal formation. Journal of Neuroscience. 1996;16:5233–55.

Renton AE, Majounie E, Waite A, et al. A hexanucleotide repeat expansion in C9ORF72 is the cause of chromosome 9p21-linked ALS-FTD. Neuron. 2011;72:257–68.

Respondek G, Höglinger G. The phenotypic spectrum of progressive supranuclear palsy. Parkinsonism and Related Disorders. 2016;22:S34–6.

Respondek G, Stamelou M, Kurz C, et al. The phenotypic spectrum of progressive supranuclear palsy: a retrospective multicenter study of 100 definite cases. Movement Disorders. 2014;29:1758–66.

Reyes S, Viswanathan A, Godin O, et al. Apathy A major symptom in CADASIL. Neurology. 2009;72:905–10.

Rittman T, Ghosh BC, McColgan P, et al. The Addenbrooke's Cognitive Examination for the differential diagnosis and longitudinal assessment of patients with parkinsonian disorders. Journal of Neurology, Neurosurgery, and Psychiatry. 2013;84:544–51.

Robbins T, James M, Lange KW, Owen A, Quinn N, Marsden C. Cognitive performance in multiple system atrophy. Brain. 1992;115:271–91.

Rogalski E, Cobia D, Harrison TM, et al. Anatomy of language impairments in primary progressive aphasia. Journal of Neuroscience. 2011;31:3344–50.

Rohrer J, Guerreiro R, Vandrovcova J, et al. The heritability and genetics of frontotemporal lobar degeneration. Neurology. 2009;73:1451–6.

Rohrer JD, Crutch SJ, Warrington EK, Warren JD. Progranulin-associated primary progressive aphasia: a distinct phenotype? Neuropsychologia. 2010;48:288–97.

Rolfs A, Koeppen AH, Bauer I, et al. Clinical features and neuropathology of autosomal dominant spinocerebellar ataxia (SCA17). Annals of Neurology. 2003;54:367–75.

Román GC, Tatemichi TK, Erkinjuntti T, et al. Vascular dementia Diagnostic criteria for research studies: Report of the NINDS-AIREN International Workshop. Neurology. 1993;43:250.

Ron M, Toone B, Garralda M, Lishman W. Diagnostic accuracy in presenile dementia. British Journal of Psychiatry. 1979;134:161–8.

Rosen HJ, Allison SC, Schauer GF, Gorno-Tempini ML, Weiner MW, Miller BL. Neuroanatomical correlates of behavioural disorders in dementia. Brain. 2005;128:2612–25.

Rosso SM, Kaat LD, Baks T, et al. Frontotemporal dementia in The Netherlands: patient characteristics and prevalence estimates from a population-based study. Brain. 2003;126:2016–22.

Rudge P, Jaumuktane Z, Adlard P, et al. Iatrogenic CJD due to pituitary-derived growth hormone with genetically determined incubation times of up to 40 years. Brain. 2015;138:3386–99.

Rumble B, Retallack R, Hilbich C, et al. Amyloid A4 protein and its precursor in Down's syndrome and Alzheimer's disease. New England Journal of Medicine. 1989;320:1446–52.

Russ TC, Morling JR. Cholinesterase inhibitors for mild cognitive impairment. Cochrane Database of Systematic Reviews. 2012;9:CD009132.

Sachdev P, Kalaria R, O'Brien J, et al. Diagnostic criteria for vascular cognitive disorders: a VASCOG statement. Alzheimer's Disease and Associated Disorders. 2014;28:206.

Saito Y, Suzuki K, Nanba E, Yamamoto T, Ohno K, Murayama S. Niemann–Pick type C disease: Accelerated neurofibrillary tangle formation and amyloid β deposition associated with apolipoprotein E ε4 homozygosity. Annals of Neurology. 2002;52:351–5.

Sajjadi S, Patterson K, Arnold R, Watson P, Nestor P. Primary progressive aphasia A tale of two syndromes and the rest. Neurology. 2012a;78:1670–7.

Sajjadi SA, Patterson K, Arnold RJ, Watson PC, Nestor PJ. Primary progressive aphasia: a tale of two syndromes and the rest. Neurology. 2012b;78:1670–7.

Sajjadi SA, Patterson K, Nestor PJ. Logopenic, mixed, or Alzheimer-related aphasia? Neurology. 2014;82:1127–31.

Sanchez-Juan P, Green A, Ladogana A, et al. CSF tests in the differential diagnosis of Creutzfeldt-Jakob disease. Neurology. 2006;67:637–43.

Saunders AM, Strittmatter WJ, Schmechel D, et al. Association of apolipoprotein E allele epsilon 4 with late-onset familial and sporadic Alzheimer's disease. Neurology. 1993;43:1467–72.

Schachter AS, Davis KL. Guidelines for the appropriate use of cholinesterase inhibitors in patients with Alzheimer's disease. CNS Drugs. 1999;11:281–8.

Schmidtke K, Metternich B. Validation of two inventories for the diagnosis and monitoring of functional memory disorder. Journal of Psychosomatic Research. 2009;67:245–51.

Schmidtke K, Pohlmann S, Metternich B. The syndrome of functional memory disorder: definition, etiology, and natural course. American Journal of Geriatric Psychiatry. 2008;16:981–8.

Schnider A. The Confabulating Mind: How the Brain Creates Reality. Oxford: Oxford University Press; 2008.

Schuchman EH, Levran O, Pereira LV, Desnick RJ. Structural organization and complete nucleotide sequence of the gene encoding human acid sphingomyelinase (SMPD1). Genomics. 1992;12:197–205.

Seelaar H, Klijnsma KY, de Koning I, et al. Frequency of ubiquitin and FUS-positive, TDP-43-negative frontotemporal lobar degeneration. Journal of Neurology. 2010a;257:747–53.

Seelaar H, Rohrer JD, Pijnenburg YA, Fox NC, Van Swieten JC. Clinical, genetic and pathological heterogeneity of frontotemporal dementia: a review. Journal of Neurology, Neurosurgery, and Psychiatry. 2011;82:476–86.

Sevin M, Lesca G, Baumann N, et al. The adult form of Niemann-Pick disease type C. Brain. 2007;130(Pt 1):120–33.

Shelley BP, Hodges JR, Kipps CM, Xuereb JH, Bak TH. Is the pathology of corticobasal syndrome predictable in life? Movement Disorders. 2009;24:1593–9.

Shuping JR, Rollinson RD, Toole JF. Transient global amnesia. Annals of Neurology. 1980a;7:281–5.

Shuping JR, Toole JF, Alexander E. Transient global amnesia due to glioma in the dominant hemisphere. Neurology. 1980b;30:88.

Snowden JS, Bathgate D, Varma A, Blackshaw A, Gibbons ZC, Neary D. Distinct behavioural profiles in frontotemporal dementia and semantic dementia. Journal of Neurology, Neurosurgery, and Psychiatry. 2001;70:323–32.

Snowden JS, Goulding P, Neary D. Semantic dementia: a form of circumscribed cerebral atrophy. Behavioral Neurology. 1989;139:578–87.

Snowden JS, Rollinson S, Thompson JC, et al. Distinct clinical and pathological characteristics of frontotemporal dementia associated with C9ORF72 mutations. Brain. 2012;135:693–708.

Stamelou M, Knake S, Oertel W, Höglinger G. Magnetic resonance imaging in progressive supranuclear palsy. Journal of Neurology. 2011;258:549–58.

Stephen C, Sweadner K, Penniston J, Schmahmann J. X-linked spinocerebellar ataxia (SCA) type 1A: a novel late onset phenotype of the ATP2B3 mutation (P5.392). Neurology. 2016;86(16 Supplement):P5.392.

Stewart R. Subjective cognitive impairment. Current Opinion in Psychiatry. 2012;25:445–50.

Stone J, Pal S, Blackburn D, Reuber M, Thekkumpurath P, Carson A. Functional (Psychogenic) Cognitive Disorders: A Perspective from the Neurology Clinic. Journal of Alzheimer's Disease. 2015a;48 Suppl 1:S5–17.

Stone J, Pal S, Blackburn D, Reuber M, Thekkumpurath P, Carson A. Functional (psychogenic) cognitive disorders: A perspective from the neurology clinic. Journal of Alzheimer's Disease. 2015b;48(S1):S5–17.

Stone J, Smyth R, Carson A, Warlow C, Sharpe M. La belle indifférence in conversion symptoms and hysteria. British Journal of Psychiatry. 2006;188:204–9.

Sullivan D, Walterfang M, Velakoulis D. Bipolar disorder and Niemann-Pick disease type C. American Journal of Psychiatry. 2005;162:1021.

Sullivan EV, Pfefferbaum A. Neuroimaging of the Wernicke–Korsakoff syndrome. Alcohol and Alcoholism. 2009;44:155–65.

Swanberg MM. Memantine for behavioral disturbances in frontotemporal dementia: a case series. Alzheimer's Disease and Associated Disorders. 2007;21:164–6.

Swerdlow A, Higgins C, Adlard P, Jones M, Preece M. Creutzfeldt-Jakob disease in United Kingdom patients treated with human pituitary growth hormone. Neurology. 2003;61:783–91.

Tabrizi SJ, Langbehn DR, Leavitt BR, et al. Biological and clinical manifestations of Huntington's disease in the longitudinal TRACK-HD study: cross-sectional analysis of baseline data. The Lancet Neurology. 2009;8:791–801.

Takeuchi A, Kobayashi A, Ironside JW, Mohri S, Kitamoto T. Characterization of variant Creutzfeldt-Jakob disease prions in prion protein-humanized mice carrying distinct codon 129 genotypes. Journal of Biological Chemistry. 2013;288:21659–66.

Tariot PN, Farlow MR, Grossberg GT, et al. Memantine treatment in patients with moderate to severe Alzheimer disease already receiving donepezil: a randomized controlled trial. JAMA. 2004;291:317–24.

Teodoro T, Edwards MJ, Isaacs JD. A unifying theory for cognitive abnormalities in functional neurological disorders, fibromyalgia and chronic fatigue syndrome: systematic review. Journal of Neurology, Neurosurgery, and Psychiatry. 2018;89:1308–19.

Thaut M, McIntosh G, Rice R, Miller R, Rathbun J, Brault J. Rhythmic auditory stimulation in gait training for Parkinson's disease patients. Movement Disorders. 1996;11:193–200.

Thompson A, MacKay A, Rudge P, et al. Behavioral and psychiatric symptoms in prion disease. American Journal of Psychiatry. 2014;171:265–74.

Toma AK, Holl E, Kitchen ND, Watkins LD. Evans' index revisited: the need for an alternative in normal pressure hydrocephalus. Neurosurgery. 2011;68:939–44.

Toosy AT, Burbridge SE, Pitkanen M, et al. Functional imaging correlates of fronto-temporal dysfunction in Morvan's syndrome. Journal of Neurology, Neurosurgery, and Psychiatry. 2008;79:734–5.

Torvik A. Rogde S: Brain lesions in alcoholics. Journal of Neurological Sciences. 1982;56:233–48.

Tuladhar AM, van Uden IW, Rutten-Jacobs LC, et al. Structural network efficiency predicts conversion to dementia. Neurology. 2016;86:1112–19.

Tulving E. Episodic and semantic memory. In: Tulving E, Donaldson W, eds. Organization of Memory. New York, NY: Academic Press; 1972. pp. 381–403.

Ungerleider LG, Mishkin M. Two cortical visual systems. In: Goodale MA, Mansfield RJW, Ingle DJ, editors. Analysis of Visual Behavior. Cambridge, MA: MIT Press; 1982. pp. 549–86.

Van der Werf YD, Scheltens P, Lindeboom J, Witter MP, Uylings HB, Jolles J. Deficits of memory, executive functioning and attention following infarction in the thalamus; a study of 22 cases with localised lesions. Neuropsychologia. 2003;41:1330–44.

Vanier M, Millat G. Niemann–Pick disease type C. Clinical Genetics. 2003;64:269–81.

Vanier MT, Gissen P, Bauer P, et al. Diagnostic tests for Niemann-Pick disease type C (NP-C): A critical review. Molecular Genetics and Metabolism. 2016;118:244–54.

Vanier MT, Rodriguez-Lafrasse C, Rousson R, et al. Type C Niemann-Pick disease: biochemical aspects and phenotypic heterogeneity. Developmental Neuroscience. 1991;13:307–14.

Vercelletto M, Boutoleau-Bretonnière C, Volteau C, et al. Memantine in behavioral variant frontotemporal dementia: negative results. Journal of Alzheimer's Disease. 2011;23:749–59.

Victor M, Adams RD, Collins GH. The Wernicke-Korsakoff syndrome. A clinical and pathological study of 245 patients, 82 with post-mortem examinations. Contemporary Neurology Series. 1971;7:1–206.

Victor M, Yakovlev PI. SS Korsakoff's Psychic Disorder in Conjunction with Peripheral Neuritis A Translation of Korsakoff's Original Article with Brief Comments on the Author and His Contribution to Clinical Medicine. Neurology. 1955;5:394.

Virhammar J, Laurell K, Cesarini KG, Larsson EM. The callosal angle measured on MRI as a predictor of outcome in idiopathic normal-pressure hydrocephalus. Journal of Neurosurgery. 2014;120:178–84.

Wadsworth JD, Joiner S, Linehan JM, Asante EA, Brandner S, Collinge J. Review. The origin of the prion agent of kuru: molecular and biological strain typing. Philosophical Transactions of the Royal Society of London B Biological Sciences. 2008;363:3747–53.

Waldorff FB, Siersma V, Vogel A, Waldemar G. Subjective memory complaints in general practice predicts future dementia: a 4-year follow-up study. International Journal of Geriatric Psychiatry. 2012;27:1180–8.

Walker FO. Huntington's disease. The Lancet. 2007;369:218–28.

Warrington EK. The selective impairment of semantic memory. Quarterly Journal of Experimental Psychology. 1975;27:635–57.

Whitty CWM, Zangwill OL. Amnesia, ed. by CWM Whitty and OL Zangwill. New York, NY: Appleton-Century-Crofts; London: Butterworth; 1966.

Whitwell JL, Duffy JR, Strand EA, et al. Neuroimaging comparison of primary progressive apraxia of speech and progressive supranuclear palsy. European Journal of Neurology. 2013;20:629–37.

Will R, Stewart G, Zeidler M, Macleod M, Knight R. Psychiatric features of new variant Creutzfeldt-Jakob disease. Psychiatric Bulletin. 1999;23:264–7.

Will R, Zeidler M, Stewart G, et al. Diagnosis of new variant Creutzfeldt-Jakob disease. Annals of Neurology. 2000;47:575–82.

Wilson BA, Kopelman M, Kapur N. Prominent and persistent loss of past awareness in amnesia: delusion, impaired consciousness or coping strategy? Neuropsychological Rehabilitation. 2008;18:527–40.

Wilson RS, Boyle PA, Yu L, et al. Temporal course and pathologic basis of unawareness of memory loss in dementia. Neurology. 2015;85:984–91.

Wolfson C, Wolfson DB, Asgharian M, et al. A reevaluation of the duration of survival after the onset of dementia. New England Journal of Medicine. 2001;344:1111–16.

Woodward M, Jacova C, Black SE, Kertesz A, Mackenzie IR, Feldman H. Differentiating the frontal variant of Alzheimer's disease. International Journal of Geriatric Psychiatry. 2010;25:732–8.

Woollams AM, Ralph MAL, Plaut DC, Patterson K. SD-squared: on the association between semantic dementia and surface dyslexia. Psychological Review. 2007;114:316.

World Health Organization. *The revision of the surveillance case definition for variant Creutzfeldt-Jakob disease (vCJD). Report of a WHO consultation. Edinburgh, United Kingdom 17 May 2001.* Geneva: World Health Organization; 2002.

Worth PF. Sorting out ataxia in adults. Practical Neurology. 2004;4:130–51.

Wroe SJ, Pal S, Siddique D, et al. Clinical presentation and pre-mortem diagnosis of variant Creutzfeldt-Jakob disease associated with blood transfusion: a case report. The Lancet. 2006;368:2061–7.

Wynn ZJ, Cummings JL. Cholinesterase inhibitor therapies and neuropsychiatric manifestations of Alzheimer's disease. Dementia and Geriatric Cognitive Disorders. 2004;17:100–8.

Yamamoto Y, Craggs L, Baumann M, Kalimo H, Kalaria R. Review: molecular genetics and pathology of hereditary small vessel diseases of the brain. Neuropathology and Applied Neurobiology. 2011;37:94–113.

Zeman A, Butler C. Transient epileptic amnesia. Current Opinion of Neurology. 2010;23:610–16.

Zeman AZ, Boniface SJ, Hodges JR. Transient epileptic amnesia: a description of the clinical and neuropsychological features in 10 cases and a review of the literature. Journal of Neurology, Neurosurgery, and Psychiatry. 1998;64:435–43.

Zerr I, Kallenberg K, Summers DM, et al. Updated clinical diagnostic criteria for sporadic Creutzfeldt-Jakob disease. Brain. 2009;132(Pt 10):2659–68.

26

Neuropsychiatry of neurometabolic, neuroendocrine, and mitochondrial disorders

Mark Walterfang, Ramon Mocellin, and Dennis Velakoulis

Introduction

Basic cellular metabolic and energy processes, when disrupted, often significantly disrupt the function and development of the CNS, given the highly metabolically active nature of neurones and glia. Marked impairments to these processes often have devastating consequences for the CNS, usually resulting in gross impairments of motor, sensory, and cognitive function, and these are often associated with disruptions to the function of other organ systems. However, when these processes are mild, rather than fulminant, or only emerge during times of significant metabolic stress, these consequences tend to be less severe and these disruptions often then lead to psychiatric illness. Endocrine disorders often affect a number of basic cellular processes, as do mitochondrial disorders, where cellular energy metabolism is often significantly altered. Metabolic disorders, commonly, but not exclusively, related to disordered enzymes involved in basic cellular functions, also cause alterations to neuronal structure and function. In this chapter, we review these groups of disorders, with an emphasis on the disorders that are known to cause psychiatric presentations. The recognition and diagnosis of secondary psychiatric syndromes in neurometabolic, endocrine, and mitochondrial disorders are crucial, given that the majority of these illnesses have specific non-psychiatric treatments that may reverse or attenuate the core pathology, and thus the consequent psychiatric symptoms. This recognition will gain further import over coming years, as new illness, diagnostic, and treatment paradigms emerge for these disorders.

Neurometabolic disorders

The CNS is highly metabolically active, and thus neurones may be highly sensitive to derangements to cellular metabolic processes (Schreiber and Baudry, 1995). An inborn error of metabolism (IEM) occurs when an intrinsic component of a metabolic pathway (most commonly an enzyme) is absent or deficient, leading to impaired synthesis of cellular components or accumulation of toxic end-products. These derangements may disrupt not just normal neuronal functioning, but also affect developmental trajectories in the immature CNS. The severity of metabolic disruption can dictate the nature, severity, and timing of presentation, such as significant neurodevelopmental disruption, motor disturbance, and seizures when severe, ranging from subtle and/or intermittent disruptions to higher functions such as behaviour and cognition when mild. Similarly, severe impairments tend to predict an earlier age of onset, as opposed to milder disruptions that may present later in development or in adulthood (Demily and Sedel, 2014; Walterfang et al., 2013). A list of relevant disorders is shown in Table 26.1.

Disorders that present with neuropsychiatric illness most commonly occur during the period of onset of most psychiatric illnesses—adolescence and young adulthood (Bonnot et al., 2014). As a result, those systems that tend to mature later in the developmental trajectory of the CNS are disrupted—such as systems controlling emotional regulation, reality testing, and higher-order cognitive functioning. However, as many of these disorders are progressive, neuropsychiatric illness may herald, and even precede by many years, more frank motor and cognitive decline as the illness progresses. Onset prior to this period generally leads to intellectual disability associated with significant neurological symptoms such as seizures or motor disturbance (van Karnebeek and Stockler, 2012). Some metabolic disorders, however, cause intermittent (and, if not severe, reversible) disruption to CNS metabolism, particularly during periods of metabolic stress such as pregnancy, acute medical illness, or starvation, particularly in their less fulminant, adult-onset forms.

Metachromatic leukodystrophy (OMIM: 250100)

Metachromatic leukodystrophy (MLD) is an autosomal recessive deficiency of the enzyme aryl-sulfatase A, which results in sulfatide accumulation in myelinated structures, in addition to the kidney and gall bladder. This results in significant leukodystrophy and is seen on MRI as periventricular white matter changes, sparing

Table 26.1 Metabolic disorders associated with psychiatric presentations

Disorder	Inheritance	Location	Gene	Gene product	Stored or altered substance	Prevalence per million
Metachromatic leukodystrophy	AR	22q13.31	ARSA	Arylsulfatase A	Cerebroside sulfate	5–25
Fabry disease	X-linked recessive	Xq22	a-Gal	α-galactosidase A	Globotriaosylceramide	25 (males)
Tay-Sach's disease	AR	15q23-q24	HEXA	β-hexosaminidase A	GM2 gangliosides	150–400 (Jewish), 3 (general population)
Alpha mannosidosis	AR	19q13.1	MANB	α-mannosidase	Oligosaccharides	2
X-linked adrenoleukodystrophy	X-linked recessive	Xq28	ABCD1	ALDP peroxisomal membrane protein	Saturated very long chain fatty acids	50 (males)
Acute intermittent porphyria	AD	11q23.3	HMBS	Porphobilinogen deaminase	Porphobilinogen/aminolevulinic acid	40–100
Phenylketonuria	AR	12q23.2	PAH	Phenylalanine hydroxylase	Phenylketones	50–100
Maple syrup urine disease	AR	19q13.1–13.2, 6p22–p21, 1p31	BCKDHA, BCKDHB, DBT	Branched-chain ketoacid dehydrogenase	Branched-chain amino acids	5
NPC	AR	18q11–12, 14q24.3	NPC1, NPC2	NPC1, NPC2	Cholesterol and gangliosides	10
Cerebrotendinous xanthomatosis	AR	2q33	CYP27A1	Sterol 27 hydroxylase	Cholestanol and cholesterol	300 reported cases
Homocystinuria	AR	21q22.3	CBS	Cystathione synthase	Homocystine and methionine	3–5
Hyperprolinaemia	AR	1p36	ALDH4A1	Pyrroline-5-carboxylate dehydrogenase	Proline	<1
Propionic acidaemia	AR	13q32, 3q21–22	PCCA, PCCB	Propionyl-CoA carboxylase	Propionic acid	10
SSADH deficiency	AR	6p22	ALDH5A1	Succinic semi-aldehyde dehydrogenase	GABA, GHB	<1
Serine deficiency	AR	1p12, 7p11.2, 9q21.2	PHGDH, PSPH, PSAT1	Phosphoglycerate dehydrogenase, phosphoserine phosphatase, phosphoserine aminotransferase	Serine	<1
CFD	AR, autoimmune	11q13.3	FOLR1	FR1	Folate	<1
MELAS	Maternal	mtDNA	MT-TL1	Mitochondrial tRNA leucine 1	n/a	60
Wolfram disease	AR/maternal	4p/mitochondrial	WFS1	Wolframin	n/a	170 reported cases
Wilson's disease	AR	13q14.2-q21	ATP7B	Copper-transporting ATPase	Copper	25

AD, autosomal dominant; AR, autosomal recessive.

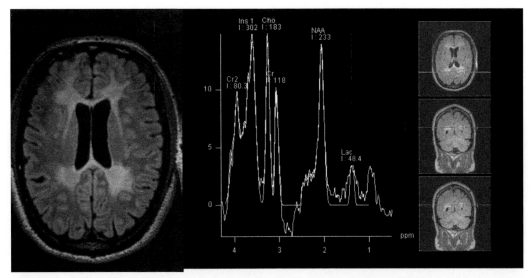

Fig. 26.1 Metachromatic leukodystrophy. On the left, T2-weighted fluid-attenuated inversion recovery (FLAIR) axial image of a 30-year-old male with metachromatic leukodystrophy (MLD), who presented with disinhibition and a frontotemporal dementia-like presentation. Extensive increased signal in the white matter, particularly anteriorly, characteristically spares the subcortical U-fibres. On the right, 1H-MRS of affected white matter, showing elevated myoinositol and choline, without elevated NAA and lactate.

subcortical fibres and with an anterior preponderance (see Fig. 26.1). In its milder adolescent-/adult-onset form, schizophrenia-like psychosis (auditory hallucinations, delusions, formal thought disorder, and catatonia) occurs in up to 40% of patients, particularly those with the I179S mutation, with non-psychotic patients presenting with a predominantly motor (cerebellopyramidal) presentation (Hyde et al., 1992). Cognitively, patients present with executive impairment and reduced speed of processing and attentional dysfunction, consistent with reduced frontal–subcortical connectivity, and ultimately progressing onto dementia (Rosebush et al., 2010). Some adult patients may present with an FTD-like phenotype. Diagnosis is made by examining enzyme levels in peripheral leucocytes. Treatment is usually symptomatic, with bone marrow transplantation useful in some patients, and recombinant enzyme and gene therapies are currently under trial.

Adrenoleukodystrophy (OMIM: 300100)

Adrenoleukodystrophy (ALD) is an X-linked recessive disorder due to mutations to ABCD1, a peroxisomal protein that oxidizes very long-chain fatty acids (VLCFAs). This results in accumulation of VLCFAs in oligodendrocytes, thus affecting CNS white matter, and adrenocortical cells resulting in adrenocortical insufficiency. Males are predominantly affected, although female carriers may show a clinical phenotype due to inactivation of the normal allele. In adults, it can present in a predominantly spinal form, affecting the dorsal columns and corticospinal tract, or in a cerebral form marked by inflammatory demyelination with a posterior predilection, in addition to the thalamus, callosum, and brainstem. On T2-weighted MRI, symmetrical hyperintensity in the posterior callosum then spreads into parieto-occipital regions and may also be seen in anterior zones. The most commonly reported psychiatric presentation is affective illness, with psychosis not uncommon, and may be treatment-resistant. Psychiatric presentations may precede motor changes by a number of years (Rosebush et al., 1999). Mood changes may also be present if adrenocortical insufficiency is not

adequately treated. Diagnosis is made via examination of the serum VLCFA profile. Bone marrow transplantation is the only well-recognized treatment, although autologous haematopoietic stem cell-based gene therapy has shown recent promise.

Cerebrotendinous xanthomatosis (OMIM: 213700)

Cerebrotendinous xanthomatosis (CTX) is a recessive disorder of cholestanol metabolism due to mutations in the *CYP27A1* gene for the enzyme sterol-27-hydroxylase. Cholestanol and its precursors accumulate in white and grey matter, in addition to classical deposition in the extensors, neck, and Achilles tendons, resulting in severe white matter and cerebellar nuclei pathology in the brain. On MRI, this presents as reduced cortical volume and diffuse white matter changes. Neurologically, patients present with ataxia, pyramidal symptoms, seizures, peripheral neuropathy, and dementia. Patients frequently present with psychiatric symptoms, including psychosis, personality change, and agitation, and occasionally depression. Younger patients tend to present with behavioural and personality disturbances associated with learning difficulties, and older patients with mood and psychotic disorders associated with frontal–subcortical dementia. Diagnosis is based on serum cholestanol levels, and treatment is with chenodeoxycholic acid which, when started early, improves neurological and psychiatric symptoms.

Niemann–Pick disease type C (OMIM: 607625)

Niemann–Pick disease type C (NPC) is a progressive neurovisceral recessive disorder of cholesterol trafficking, causing intracellular cholesterol accumulation, particularly in neurones, and resulting in hepatosplenomegaly and cholestasis in children, associated with mental retardation and seizures. However, it is notable for its increasing detection in an adolescent-/adult-onset form, which frequently presents with neuropsychiatric symptoms prior to neurological syndromes, with less clinically significant visceral symptoms. Mutations to *NPC1*, the gene involved in 95% of cases, results in the

(a) (b)

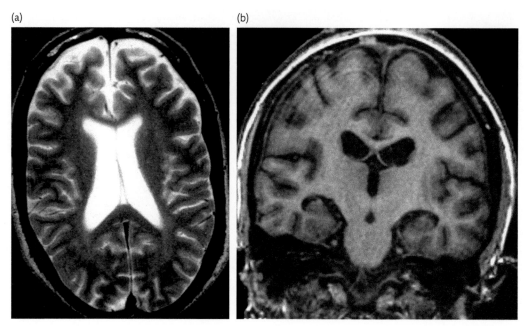

Fig. 26.2 Niemann–Pick type C disease. MRI scans on two individuals with NPC, who presented with major psychotic illness. (a) A T2-weighted axial image of an adult male who presented with schizophrenia at 16, and ataxia and gaze palsy at 25, showing ventricular enlargement and frontal atrophy. (b) A coronal T1-weighted image of a young man who presented with a psychotic bipolar disorder, showing disproportionate hippocampal/ medial temporal atrophy.

accumulation of toxic GM2 and GM3 gangliosides, Alzheimer's-like neurofibrillary tangles, and neuroaxonal dystrophy that affects white matter diffusely and subcortical grey matter in particular, with prominent neuronal loss changes in the cerebellum, thalamus, basal ganglia, and hippocampus (see Fig. 26.2). This results in prominent ataxia, often associated with developing dystonia and executive and memory impairment. Additionally, brainstem changes result in a characteristic vertical supranuclear gaze palsy where vertical saccades, but not pursuit movements, are impaired. Patients can present across the lifespan, and when symptom onset is between the ages of 15 and 30, psychosis is a frequent presentation, often preceding frank neurological symptoms by some years and resulting in a diagnosis of schizophrenia (Walterfang et al., 2006). Diagnosis can be made by assessment of plasma oxysterols or lysosphingomyelin, or *NPC1* genetic analysis. Not infrequently, neurological symptoms are thus attributed to antipsychotic treatment, delaying diagnosis. Treatment with the imino sugar miglustat shows benefit in slowing the disease through the reduction of toxic gangliosides, and intrathecal treatment with cyclodextrin appears to reverse the cholesterol storage deficit and slow neurodegeneration in animal models and human patients. Most psychotic patients respond at least partially to antipsychotic treatment.

GM2 gangliosidosis/Tay–Sach's disease (OMIM: 272800)

Tay–Sach's disease (TSD) is a recessive sphingolipid storage disorder due to impairment in β-hexosaminidase A, which results in accumulation of GM2 gangliosides in neuronal lysosomes. This results in ultrastructural changes to the neuronal body and axons, neuroinflammation, and altered apoptosis, particularly in the cerebellum, thalamus, brainstem, and substantia nigra. In children, it presents with paresis, seizures, cerebellar signs, and rapid degeneration, but a later-onset form associated with some residual enzyme

activity has been described, usually with *G269S* or *W474C* mutations. This form often presents with concomitant psychiatric and neurological symptoms in early adulthood—dysarthria, ataxia, and tremor, and up to half of patients presenting with psychosis marked by auditory and visual hallucinations, disorganization, and catatonia, with affective disorders described less often (Rosebush et al., 1995). Cognitive function may be normal, but patients often have subtle deficits in memory and executive function in processing speed. MRI in these patients often shows cerebellar and cerebral atrophy. Diagnosis is made via demonstration of deficient hexosaminidase activity in peripheral leucocytes. Symptomatic psychiatric treatment is often complicated by partial treatment response.

Alpha mannosidosis (OMIM: 248500)

Alpha mannosidosis (AM) is a recessive lysosomal storage disorder due to mutations on the *MAN2B1* gene that encodes the enzyme α-mannosidase, which catabolizes oligosaccharides; deficiency leads to their accumulation in glia and neurones, impacting myelination initially and later neuronal structure. Usually characterized by moderate mental retardation, hearing loss, and immunodeficiency in children (type I), the indolent adult-onset form (type II) may present initially with schizophrenia-like psychosis prior to the onset of ataxia, hearing loss, and subcortical cognitive decline (Malm et al., 2005). MRI often shows T2-weighted white matter hyperintensity and cerebellar atrophy. Diagnosis is established by reduced enzyme activity in peripheral blood leucocytes and/or altered urinary oligosaccharides. Treatment is limited to bone marrow transplantation currently.

Fabry disease (OMIM: 301500)

Fabry disease (FD) is an X-linked recessive disorder of glycolipid metabolism where mutations to the gene encoding α-galactosidase

A result in accumulation of globotriaosylceramide (Gb3) in blood vessels and some other tissues. Hemizygous males are affected, whereas female carriers vary in the degree of presentation due to variable X-inactivation. Disrupted vascular endothelium results in cutaneous angiokeratomas, hypohydrosis, and corneal opacities. Patients suffer from episodes of pain and acroparaesthesia in the periphery, precipitated by exercise or metabolic demand, which can result in a chronic pain syndrome in adulthood. Vascular disease also causes renal, cardiac, and cerebral vascular events, with MRI of the brain showing subcortical white matter hyperintensity and vascular change in subcortical nuclei and the brainstem. Depressive disorders are over-represented in FD, occurring in up to half of all patients, and are, in part, driven by the burden of pain and disease more generally (Segal et al., 2010). Diagnosis is made through enzyme assay in peripheral leucocytes, and enzyme replacement therapy is available.

Acute intermittent porphyria (OMIM: 176000)

Acute intermittent porphyria (AIP) is an incompletely penetrant and dominant form of the porphyrias where heme biosynthesis defects cause excess urinary porphyrin and precursor secretion. It results from defects in the enzymes that convert and degrade porphobilinogen (PBG), which leads to the accumulation of PBG and amino-levulinic acid (ALA), particularly in situations where an increase in heme biosynthesis is necessary (fasting, fever, menstruation) and with some drugs that induce the P450 system. This may result in alterations to GABAergic and serotonergic transmission. It most commonly presents in women of child-rearing age, often with abdominal pain, peripheral neuropathy (often mimicking Guillain–Barré syndrome), and neuropsychiatric disturbance. Its psychiatric presentation is varied, with psychosis common, but anxiety, agitation, depression, and delirium may be the presenting syndrome (Crimlisk, 1997). Patients in acute crises may be diagnosed with a psychotic or conversion disorder. Coproporphyria, a related dominant disorder affecting a porphyrin oxidase, can present identically. Diagnosis is made when elevations of urinary PBG and ALA are seen in AIP, and coproporphyrin levels in coproporphyria. Gross elevations of urinary porphyrins are known to turn urine amber or purple in direct sunlight. Management relates to avoidance of precipitants (including medications known to trigger an attack), and in acute attacks, fluids, carbohydrate loading, and heme arginate to suppress the heme synthetic pathway. Treatment of psychiatric symptoms involves judicious use of medication that will not worsen the biochemical deficit—chlorpromazine and droperidol for psychosis, lithium for mania, sertraline or fluoxetine for depression, and lorazepam and temazepam for sedation and anxiolysis.

Maple syrup urine disease (OMIM: 248600)

Maple syrup urine disease (MSUD) is a recessive disorder caused by a mutation in one of the four genes that code for the branched-chain α-ketoacid dehydrogenase complex, which alters branched-chain amino acid (BCAA) catabolism. This alters synaptic and glial function and myelination, and induces neuronal apoptosis. Elevations of leucine reduce transport of large neutral amino acids (LNAAs), including most monoamine precursors, which alters monoaminergic transmission; glutamatergic and GABAergic transmission is also altered. Cerebral valine deficiency, secondary to the BCAA-restricted diet used to treat the disease, also impairs neuronal and oligodendrocyte function. MRI shows reductions in cortical volume and T2 signal abnormalities in the white matter. The disorder's name derives from the sweet-smelling bodily fluids that characterize the disease, and affected patients present with ataxia and pyramidal features. Dietary restriction allows patients to survive into adulthood, although often with pyramidal and extrapyramidal signs and subtle executive and attentional impairment. Children may present with attention-deficit disorders, and adults with anxiety and depression, which respond to standard pharmacological treatment (Muelly et al., 2013). Diagnosis rests on analysis of abnormal ketoacids in the urine or an altered serum amino acid profile.

Urea cycle disorders (OMIM: 237300, 311250, 207900, 237310)

The urea cycle eliminates nitrogen through the detoxification of ammonia and comprises six enzymes in the cytoplasm and mitochondria. Most are recessive, although ornithine transcarbamylase (OTC) deficiency is X-linked. Hyperammonaemia alters glutamatergic transmission and glial and axonal function, and presentations usually occur during metabolic stress (fasting, pregnancy, and illness). Acute episodes may show cerebral oedema on MRI, and after chronic illness, gliosis and atrophy may be detectable. Mild urea cycle disorders (UCDs) can present in childhood and adulthood, rather than in infancy, usually as recurrent encephalopathy associated with lethargy, headaches, vomiting, and altered consciousness; this may be accompanied by psychiatric disturbances, particularly psychosis, particularly in post-partum women (Wijburg and Nassogne, 2012). Crises may be worsened by the use of sodium valproate which can exacerbate hyperammonaemia (Chopra et al., 2012).

Phenylketonuria (OMIM: 261600)

Phenylketonuria (PKU) is not an uncommon recessive disorder, caused by mutations in the gene for phenylalanine hydroxylase (PAH), which converts this phenylalanine (Phe) into tyrosine. Reductions of tyrosine, the precursor for monoamines, in the CNS result in depletions of serotonin and dopamine and severely disrupts normal neurodevelopment. Hyperphenylalaninaemia reduces the movement of LNAAs into the CNS, impacting cholesterol and protein synthesis which alters synaptic structure and myelination. Untreated PKU is rare in the Western world, as it is usually detected in newborn screening; however, it results in mental retardation, seizures, and death in childhood without dietary restriction of Phe and supplementation of tyrosine. As a result, severe irreversible cognitive deficits have largely been eliminated, and it is now recommended that most patients continue dietary restrictions lifelong. MRI shows an increased T2 signal in frontal and parieto-occipital zones (see Fig. 26.3), which is at least partially reversible with dietary change. However, even with treatment, patients often have high levels of anxiety, attentional deficits, and depression, reflecting monoaminergic depletion (Brumm et al., 2010). Patients often have subtle executive and attentional impairment which, like PKU-associated psychiatric syndromes, often worsens when dietary control is poor and Phe levels increase (Waisbren et al., 1994). Psychiatric syndromes often respond to tightened dietary control and/or traditional serotonergic antidepressants.

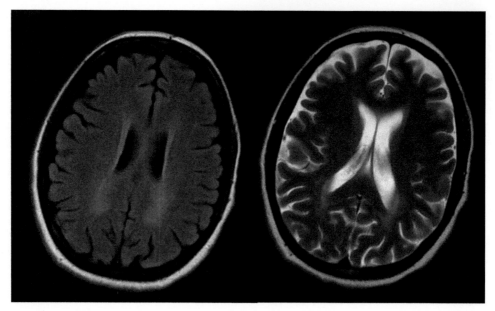

Fig. 26.3 Phenylketonuria. T2-weighted (right) and FLAIR (left) axial images of a 33-year-old woman with PKU who presented with anxiety and subtle executive dysfunction. Bilateral increased signal in the posterior white matter, particularly in the parietal zones, typical for PKU, is seen.

Homocystinurias

Some IEMs lead to elevated serum and urinary homocystine. Defects in cystathione synthase (OMIM: 236200) result in elevated homocystine and methionine, two sulfur-containing amino acids (SCAAs). Elevated SCAAs in the CNS alter NMDA transmission and monoamine release. Disrupted collagen metabolism results in pale, pink skin, lens dislocation and cataracts, arachnodactyly, and scoliosis, in addition to mental retardation, dystonia, seizures, and arteriovenous thromboembolism. Psychosis has been described, although aggression and mood and anxiety disorders are the most frequent (Skovby et al., 2010). MRI scanning often demonstrates strokes and leukodystrophy. Patients are treated with methionine restriction and pyridoxine and cysteine supplementation. An additional pathway for the metabolism of homocystine involving remethylation can be disrupted and involves methionine synthetase (OMIM: 250940) and methylenetetrahydrofolate reductase (MTHFR, OMIM: 236250). Impairment in these enzymes results in high levels of homocystine, but low methionine. Impaired methylation impacts synthesis of myelin basic protein and monoamines and leads to mental retardation, seizures, and hypotonia; MTHFR deficiency has been associated strongly with adolescent and young adult psychosis in its milder form, possibly due to subtle impairments in myelination and dopamine synthesis. The C677T variant, which reduces enzyme activity by 35%, has been described as conferring a 70% increased risk for schizophrenia (Feng et al., 2009).

Serine deficiency

Deficiencies in the L-serine synthesis pathway involve three enzymes: 3-PDGH (OMIM: 601815), 3-PSP (OMIM: 614023), and PSAT (OMIM: 610992). Serine metabolism is crucially involved in phospholipid synthesis, cell proliferation, and NMDA transmission. These patients often present with growth deficiencies, developmental delay, and mental retardation, as well as with behavioural disturbances in childhood (de Koning and Klomp, 2004). Diagnosis is made with low plasma and CSF serine, and some symptoms are improved with treatment with dietary L-serine.

Cerebral folate deficiency

Cerebral folate deficiency (CFD) occurs when CNS levels of 5-MTHF are reduced in the presence of normal extra-CNS levels of folate. This can be both genetic and, rarely, autoimmune in origin. A mutation in the *FOLR1* gene impacts on the folate receptor, causing a reduction in folate transport into the cell; this is known as cerebral folate transport deficiency (CFTD, OMIM: 613068). It presents in young children as psychomotor delay, regression, ataxia, and seizures, with leukodystrophy on MRI due to significantly disrupted myelination. Its autoimmune form is caused by autoantibodies to folate receptors, possibly by sensitization from cow's milk exposure. It may present with autistic features in children and catatonic psychosis in adolescents, or ataxia, seizures, and irritability in infants (Ramaekers et al., 2013). Autoantibodies to folate receptors have been found in autistic and schizophrenia populations, and some of these patients have shown improvement with dietary folinic acid.

Propionic acidaemia (OMIM: 606054)

Propionic acidaemia (PA) is a recessive disorder of a mitochondrial biotin-dependent enzyme which catabolizes the amino acids methionine, valine, threonine, and isoleucine. The build-up of organic acids—particularly propionic acid—in blood and tissues leads to metabolic decompensation during demand and results in acute encephalopathy or a more indolent form delaying psychomotor development and impacting extrapyramidal function. It may present in adulthood and has been associated with psychosis and decompensation in young adults and autism in children (Kolker et al., 2015). Diagnosis rests on organic acid analysis, and treatment is largely symptomatic.

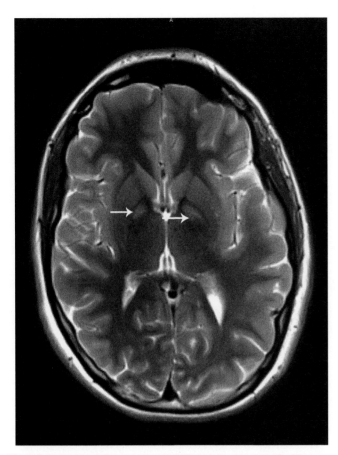

Fig. 26.4 SSADH deficiency. An axial T2-weighted image of a 28-year-old female with SSADH deficiency, who presented with significant psychomotor slowing and obsessive–compulsive phenomena. Significantly increased T2 signal is seen in the globus pallidus (arrows).

Succinic semi-aldehyde dehydrogenase deficiency (OMIM: 271980)

Succinic semi-aldehyde dehydrogenase deficiency (SSADH) deficiency is a rare recessive disorder where the enzyme SSADH, which degrades GABA, results in accumulation of gamma-hydroxybutyric acid (GHB). This alters the balance between excitatory and inhibitory neurotransmission, and appears to particularly affect the basal ganglia, with pallidal hyperintensity on T2 imaging (see Fig. 26.4). Patients present with intellectual disability, extrapyramidal symptoms, and prominent ADHD-like symptoms, autism, and obsessive–compulsive symptoms, with psychosis occurring rarely (Gibson et al., 2003). Most patients present in early childhood, but patients may present in early adulthood. These symptom complexes may respond to stimulants and serotonergic antidepressants. Vigabatrin, which irreversibly inhibits GABA transaminase, has been shown to benefit some patients.

Neuroendocrine disorders

The interaction of psychiatry with endocrinology has passed through a number of phases through history. This includes the use of powdered extracts of endocrine organs in the early twentieth century to treat symptoms such as anhedonia and melancholia and Bernard Carroll's introduction in 1968 of the dexamethasone suppression test as a biological marker for melancholic depression (Shorter and Ink, 2010). Interest in the role of cortisol in other disorders, such as PTSD, has continued to generate interest (Fragkaki et al., 2016). In their seminal systematic study, Dunlap and Moersch characterized the neuropsychiatric features of hyperthyroidism, demonstrating the complexity of the interaction between the hormone and the CNS (Dunlap and Moersch, 1935). Although advances in biochemical detection of endocrine disorders can result in diagnosis prior to the emergence of symptoms, an understanding of the role of endocrine disturbance in the production of neuropsychiatric symptoms remains of significant clinical importance.

Hypothalamic disorders

Abnormalities of the hypothalamus are in the main manifest as pituitary dysfunction. However, the hypothalamus is also involved in the regulation of food intake, energy expenditure, and sleep regulation via the projection of orexinergic neurones to monoaminergic centres in the raphe nuclei and ventral tegmentum and in sleep regulation via links to the circadian pacemaker in the suprachiasmatic nuclei.

Narcolepsy

Narcolepsy is a sleep disorder characterized by excessive daytime somnolence, cataplexy (a sudden loss of muscle tone, often triggered by strong emotional reactions), and REM sleep dysfunction such as hypnagogic hallucinations, automatic behaviour, and sleep paralysis. Orexin levels in the CSF are low or non-existent in 90% of patients and links to the HLA system suggest an autoimmune basis (HLA-DR15 and HLA-DQ6 have been described in up to 85% of patients). Depression has been described in up to 25% of patients in some series, although others have established rates similar to healthy populations (Chow and Cao, 2016). The concept of 'narcoleptic psychosis' is also controversial. Some psychoses in narcolepsy reportedly respond to treatment with stimulants, and REM sleep behaviour disorder may be misdiagnosed as schizophrenia. However, the majority of psychoses associated with narcolepsy relate to stimulant use/misuse, as agents such as dexamphetamine are often used to promote wakefulness in this disorder (Gowda and Lundt, 2014).

Hypothalamic lesions

Lesions of the ventromedial nucleus of the hypothalamus can result in obesity and may initially involve aggressive behaviour and hyperphagia, until a new set weight is reached when reduced appetite and activity are noted. Lateral lesions have been reported to result in an apathetic state. Short-term memory loss has been reported, particularly in lesions of the ventromedial and premamillary areas of the hypothalamus, whereas extensive hypothalamic lesions may produce features of a dementing illness. More rapid or destructive processes present with disturbances of consciousness, temperature, and autonomic dysregulation (Messina et al., 2016).

Childhood tumours involving the anterior and basal hypothalamus, including gliomas, midline cerebellar astrocytomas, and suprasellar ependymomas, may result in the diencephalic syndrome constituting motor hyperactivity, euphoria or inappropriate affect, increased alertness, and emaciation despite normal caloric intake. If death does not ensue, the clinical picture may change to one of obesity and intermittent rage reactions. Slower-growing tumours in adults usually result in a dementia syndrome, endocrine dysfunction, and food intake dysregulation. Predominantly suprasellar tumours, such as craniopharyngiomas, usually present with visual abnormalities and headaches. Hypogonadism, hyperprolactinaemia, diabetes insipidus, and weight gain are common, as are cognitive deterioration and personality change, without evidence of psychosis (Rosenfeld et al., 2014).

Pituitary disorders

Given the complex nature of the hypothalamic–pituitary axis, it is not surprising that neuropsychiatric manifestations of pituitary disease are protean. Pituitary dysfunction may result from pituitary tumours or destructive disease processes.

Pituitary tumours

Pituitary tumours are frequent incidental findings at neuroimaging and are found in up to 20% of adults at autopsy. Symptoms arise from alteration of normal hormone homeostasis or from invasion of surrounding structures.

1. Prolactinomas are the commonest secretory tumours, resulting in amenorrhoea, infertility, and galactorrhoea in women and impotence and occasionally galactorrhoea or gynaecomastia in men. Depression and anxiety symptoms occur with greater frequency and may respond to treatment with the dopamine agonist bromocriptine. Although increased aggression is rarely reported in hyperprolactinaemic human subjects, psychotic symptoms have been described in neuroleptic-naïve patients with hyperprolactinaemia at a case report level. Treatment with antipsychotic agents may then result in further elevation of prolactin. Psychotic symptoms (including delusions and hallucinations) have also been described in bromocriptine-treated patients. The incidental finding of a pituitary adenoma on neuroimaging can complicate the assessment of patients with a psychotic illness stabilized on an antipsychotic agent with hyperprolactinaemia (de Oliveira et al., 2010). Cabergoline (a potent D2 agonist) therapy for pituitary adenomas has been associated with impulse control disorders such as pathological gambling (Almanzar et al., 2013).

2. Growth hormone-secreting tumours are the second commonest functional pituitary adenomas causing acromegaly, which results in soft tissue and bone enlargement, particularly involving the hands, feet, jaw, and tongue, with a typical overall coarsening of facial features. Hypertension, congestive cardiac failure, and obstructive sleep apnoea and hypersomnolence are common associations. Acromegalic patients appear to have a lifetime increased risk of affective disorders when compared with control subjects with and without chronic somatic disease (Sievers et al., 2009). Psychoses are well described when acromegalic patients are treated with bromocriptine, resulting in delusional symptoms, schizophrenia-like presentations, and visual hallucinations. Such symptoms rarely arise in acromegaly without bromocriptine treatment (Martinkova et al., 2011).

3. Adrenocorticotrophic hormone (ACTH)-secreting tumours are the next commonest pituitary tumour type, resulting in excessive cortisol production or Cushing's disease. Neuropsychiatric features of increased cortisol release are discussed in the description of adrenal disease (see Adrenal disorders, p. 318).

4. Other pituitary tumours include luteinizing hormone (LH)- or follicle-stimulating hormone (FSH)-secreting tumours. These are rarely symptomatic. Increased thyroid-stimulating hormone (TSH) may cause hyperthyroidism, the psychiatric aspects of which are discussed later (see Hyperthyroidism, p. 317). Non-secretory pituitary tumours are often larger at diagnosis because of the lack of endocrine symptoms. These tumours may impinge on surrounding structures, resulting in bitemporal hemianopia, oculomotor palsies, headache, and occasionally hypothalamic syndromes (see Hypothalamic disorders). Visual hallucinations have been reported in patients with associated visual field defect resulting from a pituitary tumour impinging on the optic chiasm (Ram et al., 1987). These are more often of the simple, non-formed type and may be exacerbated by bromocriptine (Turner et al., 1984).

Hypopituitarism

Hypopituitarism in adulthood is usually caused by a traumatic (related to head injury), vascular, inflammatory, or immune-mediated destructive process or by compression from an adjacent tumour. Symptoms are determined by the hormone involved. Growth hormone is often first affected, followed by gonadotrophins, with associated amenorrhoea and infertility in women and reduced libido and body hair loss in men. Low TSH can result in hypothyroidism; ACTH deficiency in fatigue, reduced appetite, weight loss, and impaired stress response; and vasopressin deficiency in polyuria and thirst.

A number of neuropsychiatric manifestations have been described in hypopituitarism in the absence of a delirium (Lynch et al., 1994). Symptoms of depression and anxiety are more commonly described than in individuals with chronic disease such as diabetes. Variable degrees of memory impairment, sleep disturbance, and personality change are reported and several observers have reported an absence of affect on mental state examination. Although visual and auditory hallucinations have been described, psychosis is uncommon.

More specific symptoms are attributable to particular hormone deficiencies and may result in specific symptom groups. GH deficiency may result in reduced energy, depressed mood, anxiety, emotional lability, and impulsivity or impaired self-control. Depression, irritability, and insomnia have been associated with low testosterone. Low ACTH can result in fatigue, social withdrawal, and negativism. Classic hypothyroid states (fatigue, depression, insomnia or hypersomnia, and a variety of psychotic symptoms) can result from low TSH. In general, appropriate treatment of the underlying cause and hormone deficiency results in resolution of these features.

Thyroid disorders

Primary thyroid disorders have a much higher incidence in the population. Consequently, psychiatric symptoms that accompany either hypothyroidism or hyperthyroidism have been subject to more systematic studies than those associated with pituitary disorders.

Hyperthyroidism

Hyperthyroidism is the result of excessive activity of thyroid hormones. This may result from a single functioning adenoma or toxic multinodular goitre, or from the presence of a thyroid stimulator (thyroid-stimulating antibody in Graves' disease). Exogenous thyroid hormone and disorders of thyroid hormone storage (related to autoimmune thyroiditis) may result in similar presentations. Depressive symptoms are the commonest psychiatric features seen in hyperthyroidism, occurring in up to 30% of patients, and frequently occur prior to other physical features. This includes not only lowering of mood, but also neurovegetative disturbance such as insomnia, reduced libido, weight loss, and fatigue (Ritchie and Yeap, 2015). However, as distinct from depression, appetite is invariably increased in hyperthyroidism. The severity of the depressive symptoms has not been found to be related to the extent of the biochemical hyperthyroidism or later physical symptoms. Generalized anxiety and agitation are also common, with a prevalence of between 10% and 20%, but panic and agoraphobia are relatively uncommon. Although anxiety may occur prior to the other features of hyperthyroidism, it more often correlates with the severity of the thyrotoxic features. Anxiety and depressive features are often comorbid. Manic symptoms may be difficult to distinguish from psychomotor agitation and anxiety and less common in hyperthyroid states, with a prevalence of between 2% and 5%. Psychotic symptoms, including paranoid delusions and auditory hallucinations, while historically reported as common, have a true prevalence of between 2% and 5%. Depression in hyperthyroidism usually responds to measures which restore the euthyroid state; however, anxiety, fatigue, and loss of function may persist for as long as 12 months after successful treatment (Bunevicius and Prange, 2006). Cognitive dysfunction is less common than in hypothyroidism, with rates of between 5% and 10% described. Presentations include deficits in attention and concentration, slow processing speeds, impairments in immediate memory, defective higher-level problem-solving, or frank delirium. Again, these deficits respond to reversal of the thyrotoxic state. Elderly patients with thyrotoxicosis may present with predominantly apathy, depression, and weight loss, rather than increased psychomotor activity. Typically this presentation is of slower onset and cardiovascular events (angina, cardiac failure, and atrial fibrillation) are more prominent than other clinical features (Feit, 1988).

Hypothyroidism

Primary autoimmune hypothyroidism related to antithyroid antibodies is the commonest cause of hypothyroidism in adults. Treatment for hyperthyroidism, drug-related effects, and iodine deficiency are also common causes, with hypothalamic or pituitary dysfunction accounting for <5% of cases. Hypothyroidism is associated with a variety of psychiatric symptoms, ranging from mild cognitive slowing and depression to frank encephalopathy which often predates other physical features. Cognitive deficits are common, occurring in 50% of cases. Psychomotor speed, memory, and visual–perceptual skills are often impaired. Executive dysfunction is prominent with reduced performance in trail-making and maze tasks. The severity of these disorders correlates with the biochemical abnormality and are usually corrected by return to a euthyroid state. Persistent cognitive deficits are seen in the elderly or those with reduced cognitive reserve.

Depression is less closely related to the severity of biochemical hypothyroidism and reported in approximately 40% of patients. Low mood, fatigue, anhedonia, reduced concentration, and hypersomnolence are the most commonly described features of the depressive syndrome in hypothyroidism. These features predictably respond to treatment of the hypothyroid state (Samuels, 2014). Although manic and hypomanic symptoms have been infrequently reported, hypothyroidism (Khemka et al., 2011) may be a risk factor for the development of bipolar disorder, particularly the rapid cycling form, and treatment of otherwise refractory mood disorders with thyroid hormones can be effective. Generalized anxiety symptoms are described in up to 30% of patients and are strongly correlated with depressive symptoms, but not with biochemical severity.

Psychotic symptoms, including paranoid ideas, misidentification, visual and auditory hallucinations, and thought disorder, were originally thought to be common (and described as 'myxoedematous madness') but likely occur in <5% of all patients with hypothyroidism and tend to emerge after the onset of physical symptoms (Heinrich and Grahm, 2003). Although these symptoms also respond to appropriate thyroid hormone treatment, rapid titration of hormone doses may exacerbate psychosis. Careful addition of a low dose of an antipsychotic to thyroxine has been reported to be well tolerated and result in an earlier remission of psychosis.

Subclinical hypothyroidism refers to scenarios in which thyroid hormone abnormalities occur without overt functional hypothyroidism. Grade II hypothyroidism (elevated TSH without changes in thyroid hormones) has been associated with MDD, treatment resistance, and cognitive dysfunction. Treatment of subclinical hypothyroidism is controversial (Davis et al., 2003).

Parathyroid disorders

The sole function of the parathyroid glands is to maintain calcium homeostasis through the release of parathyroid hormone (PTH). The release of PTH increases serum calcium via stimulating osteoclasts in bone to release calcium and through increasing its absorption in the gut and kidneys.

Hyperparathyroidism

Hyperparathyroidism is usually diagnosed after an incidental finding of hypercalcaemia, with up to 50% of patients being asymptomatic. Increased PTH release is usually caused by a single functioning adenoma, although rarely multiple adenomas may occur as part of multiple endocrine neoplasia syndrome (MENS). Hypercalcaemic symptoms include fatigue, general malaise, proximal muscle weakness, renal colic, abdominal pain, and cognitive decline. Although a number of psychiatric symptoms have been described in hyperparathyroidism (part of the classic tetrad of 'bones, stones, moans, and psychic groans'), the prevalence seems to be <10%. Depressive symptoms with comorbid anxiety are the most commonly reported. Psychotic disorders are less frequent, with persecutory and paranoid delusions predominating (Borer and Bhanot, 1985). Disorders of attention and acute confusional states (with short-term memory dysfunction) often occur. Neuropsychiatric symptoms are often the initial presentation in the elderly. The more severe the hypercalcaemia, the more severe the psychiatric disturbance, but symptoms generally respond to appropriate treatment such as parathyroidectomy.

Hypoparathyroidism

Inadvertent surgical removal during thyroid surgery or excessive removal for hyperparathyroidism is the commonest cause of impaired PTH production in adults. Hypocalcaemia produces symptoms of neuromuscular excitability, including paraesthesiae, muscle cramps, carpopedal spasm, and facial grimacing, progressing to laryngeal spasm and convulsions. Examination may reveal features of tetany, reduced or absent deep tendon reflexes, papilloedema, and QT interval prolongation on ECG. Delirium is now understood to be the commonest neuropsychiatric manifestation. One large study available demonstrated cognitive impairment in 39% of patients, affective or neurotic symptoms in 12%, psychotic symptoms in 11%, and non-specific affective disturbance in 21% of patients (Velasco et al., 1999). Again, the severity of symptoms directly relate to the degree of hypocalcaemia, and appropriate normalization results in resolution of these symptoms, although persistent psychosis has been noted when associated hypomagnesaemia was not addressed.

Adrenal disorders

The adrenal cortex produces glucocorticoids (principally cortisol) and adrenal androgens [predominately dehydroepiandrosterone (DHEA)] under the stimulatory effects of ACTH and aldosterone, a mineralocorticoid, controlled by the renin–angiotensin system. Hyper- or hypofunction of these adrenal systems results in distinct clinical syndromes with complex physical and neuropsychiatric manifestations.

Hyperadrenalism

Excessive production of corticosteroids is usually the result of ACTH overproduction from the anterior pituitary secondary to a pituitary adenoma (Cushing's disease). Other causes include ACTH production from a non-endocrine tumour, an adrenal neoplasm, or, most commonly, exogenous steroids. Hyperadrenalism, or Cushing's syndrome, is characterized by the classic features of hypertension, muscle weakness and fatigue, osteoporosis, cutaneous striae, and easy bruising. A characteristic pattern of obesity is seen involving the upper face (resulting in a 'moon face'), back ('buffalo hump'), and mesentery, resulting in truncal obesity. Women may experience hirsutism, acne, and amenorrhoea, and men decreased libido and impotence. Depression is the most frequently noted psychiatric symptom in up to 70% of patients, with comorbid anxiety in up to 50%. Depressive symptoms may present prior to physical symptoms and respond to treatment of the underlying cause, correlating with lowering of plasma cortisol levels. Elevated mood is reported in <10% in most case series (Starkman, 2013). Delirium is also relatively uncommon and is usually related to supervening infection or other metabolic disorder such as metabolic alkalosis. Although case reports of Cushing's syndrome presenting with florid psychosis exist, this form of presentation is rare. Psychotic symptoms, when present, are almost always mood-congruent delusional beliefs and derogatory auditory hallucinations associated with depressed mood. Cognitive impairment occurs in over 50% of patients, presenting as deficits in verbal memory, attention, and visuomotor and visuospatial function (Sonino et al., 2006). Exogenous administration of steroids is frequently associated with manic symptoms, followed by delirium, depression, and psychotic symptoms (Wolkowitz, 1994). Mixed affective states also appear over-represented. These symptoms may be dose-related and reproducible in the individual, and respond to both cessation of the exogenous steroid and pharmacotherapy with mood-stabilizing agents.

Hypoadrenalism

Hypofunction of the adrenocortical system may result from a primary process at the level of the gland such as destruction by an autoimmune process (Addison's disease), other inflammatory or destructive processes, dysfunction of the hypothalamic–pituitary axis, withdrawal of exogenous steroids, or an inborn failure of enzyme function. Symptom onset is insidious with progressive fatigue, weakness, anorexia, nausea, abdominal pain, weight loss, cutaneous and mucosal pigmentation, hypotension, and hypoglycaemia. Other findings include hyponatraemia, hyperkalaemia, and metabolic acidosis. There are scant reports of neuropsychiatric symptoms in Addison's disease, although depression, reduced motivation, and energy and behavioural changes predominate. Memory dysfunction is the commonest form of cognitive disturbance. Paranoid symptoms and delusions are less common. Auditory and visual hallucinations, changes in conscious state, irritability, insomnia, and nightmares often herald an Addisonian crisis with frank delirium, coma, and seizures. Hyponatraemia and metabolic acidosis may contribute to the delirium and cognitive deficits. As most symptoms resolve with treatment with adequate doses of corticosteroids, use of other psychotropic agents is rarely indicated (Anglin et al., 2006).

Hyperaldosteronism

Excess aldosterone can arise from the adrenal gland (primary aldosteronism) or from an extra-adrenal site (secondary aldosteronism). Primary aldosteronism is usually due to an aldosterone-producing adenoma (Conn's syndrome) or bilateral cortical hyperplasia. Secondary aldosteronism results from renin–angiotensin system dysfunction and hypovolaemia. Conn's syndrome is characterized by hypokalaemia, hypertension, muscle weakness, fatigue, polyuria, and polydipsia. Metabolic alkalosis and hypomagnesaemia may also occur. Historically, depression has been identified as one of the major features, but more recently, generalized anxiety, panic, and features of OCD have been described (Kunzel, 2012).

Untreated primary hyperaldosteronism, and resulting severe hypertension, can result in VaD. Although appropriate treatment (including surgical removal), such as surgical excision of a functioning adenoma, is effective in reversing the physical symptoms of hyperaldosteronism, the effect on anxiety and other symptoms are unknown.

Phaeochromocytoma

Phaeochromocytomas are tumours which secrete catecholamines and most commonly originate in the chromaffin cells of the adrenal medulla, but they may rarely arise from similar cells in sympathetic ganglia. Familial forms are associated with MENS type 2a and 2b and von Recklinghausen's neurofibromatosis. Secretion of catecholamines may be continuous or sporadic, resulting in the characteristic triad of paroxysmal palpitations, headache, and profuse sweating, but also Raynaud's phenomenon, tremor, nausea and vomiting, and abdominal and chest pain. Hypertension (and postural hypotension), pallor, signs of chronic hypertension, such as retinopathy, are usual clinical features. Paroxysmal symptoms occur in 40% of phaeochromocytomas and may present as a phenocopy of anxiety symptoms, particularly a panic episode. These may occur spontaneously or may be precipitated by exercise, postural change, raised intra-abdominal pressure, or emotional excitement or shock. Psychosis and cognitive deficits have not been described, although there are several case reports of a secretory phaeochromocytoma causing relapse of a previously stable psychotic disorder. Location of the underlying tumour and surgical excision with α-adrenergic blockade are effective in resolving most anxiety symptoms if paroxysmal episodes are terminated (Anderson et al., 2013).

Neuroendocrine tumours

The most extensive neuroendocrine system is in the GI tract and associated organs, and when these tissues release excess hormones, a range of neuropsychiatric syndromes can occur. Neoplasms of neuroendocrine cells that secrete serotonin in the respiratory system and GI tract produce carcinoid syndrome, characterized by flushing (often severe facial flushing with bronchial tumours), diarrhoea, wheezing, and hypotension. Neuropsychiatric symptoms include depression (in up to half of patients), anxiety, sleep disorders, and, rarely, psychosis and impulse control disorder (Kohen and Arbouet, 2008). These changes often preceded the other physical symptoms.

Insulinomas

Insulinomas (islet cell tumours of the pancreas which result in unregulated insulin secretion) result in fasting hypoglycaemia (relieved by glucose ingestion) and weight gain. Hypoglycaemia is characterized by hunger, restlessness, palpitations, flushing, and ataxia but may also include malaise, anxiety, depersonalization, and derealization (McCormick et al., 2001). A subacute syndrome characterized by clumsiness and disinhibited or aggressive behaviour (and associated amnesia for these episodes) may mimic alcohol intoxication (Benton, 1988). Global and irreversible cognitive deficits may result if hypoglycaemia is long-standing. Surgical therapy is the most definitive treatment, but hyperglycaemic treatment with the somatostatin analogue octreotide can be helpful.

Glucagonomas

Glucagonomas are rare pancreatic islet cell tumours that secrete glucagon. The presenting features are of impaired glucose tolerance and diabetes and migratory necrolytic erythema (Rodriguez et al., 2016). Anxiety and agitation may accompany these features.

Mitochondrial disorders

Mitochondrial disorders are multisystem disorders that overlap in clinical features and need to be considered as a differential diagnosis across a range of neurological and neuropsychiatric disorders. Diseases caused by defects of mitochondrial oxidative phosphorylation are the commonest IEMs, accounting for one in 5000 live births. Of the 37 genes within mitochondrial DNA, 13 encode polypeptides involved in the respiratory chain/oxidative phosphorylation system. The mitochondrial respiratory chain consists of five enzyme complexes made up of polypeptides encoded by nuclear and mitochondrial genes, except for complex II that is entirely encoded in the cell nucleus. As a result, the mitochondrion is under the genetic control of both nuclear and mitochondrial DNA, and mitochondrial disorders can result from mitochondrial or nuclear DNA mutations.

The genetics of mitochondrial disorders are complex, but the following principles can be applied (Pinto and Moraes, 2014): (1) mitochondrial disorders may be sporadic, maternally inherited, or inherited in an autosomal pattern; (2) due to the polyploid nature of the mitochondrial genome, the one cell may include normal and mutated mitochondrial DNA (heteroplasmy); siblings may show a very broad range of clinical variability due to differences in the inheritance of such heteroplasmic mitochondria; (3) mitochondrial respiratory chain disorders will mostly affect tissues with high metabolic needs, e.g. muscle, central and peripheral nervous systems, the heart, the endocrine system, and the eye; and (4) the clinical expression of mitochondrial disorders may vary widely from individual to individual with the same mutation, depending on the proportion of mitochondria affected in different tissues, the interaction of that individual with the environment, and the differential metabolic energy needs of different tissues within the one individual.

Clinical features common to all mitochondrial disorders include dysfunction of the *endocrine* (short stature, diabetes, thyroid and adrenal disorders), *neurological* (deafness, myopathy, peripheral neuropathy, retinopathy, optic atrophy, ophthalmoplegia, seizures, ataxia, dementia), and *cardiac* (cardiomyopathy, cardiac block) systems. The patterns of clinical presentation vary significantly with regard to age of onset, the temporal order of symptoms and conditions, and progress of the disorders. The combination of a maternal history, multisystem involvement, and a progressive course should arouse clinical suspicion of a mitochondrial disorder. In patients with atypical psychiatric presentations, physical signs, such as muscle weakness, hearing loss, seizures, short stature, diabetes, Wolff–Parkinson–White syndrome, or migraines, should alert clinicians to the possibility of a mitochondrial disorder.

Mitochondrial encephalomyopathy, lactic acidosis, and stroke-like episodes syndrome

Mitochondrial encephalomyopathy, lactic acidosis, and stroke-like episodes syndrome (MELAS), the commonest of the mitochondrial disorders, presents before early adulthood after a period of normal development. About 80% of MELAS cases are due to a mutation in *MT-TL1*, an RNA transfer gene. The characteristic features of MELAS are stroke-like episodes that do not conform to vascular territories and typically occur in temporo-parieto-occipital regions, the basal ganglia, the brainstem, and the cerebellum. Such episodes lead to hemiparesis, hemianopia, and cortical blindness. Vomiting and migraine are often associated clinical symptoms. Lactic acid levels are elevated and have been correlated with the level of neurological symptoms. The course of the disorder is highly variable, ranging from single stroke-like episodes through to a progressive course characterized by one or more of multiple strokes, deafness, diabetes, retinopathy, seizures, and cardiac abnormalities (Pinto and Moraes, 2014). Cases of schizophrenia or schizophrenia-like psychosis associated with MELAS have been reported (Fattal et al., 2006). Such cases typically show an onset in the third decade, years before the clinical diagnosis of MELAS is made. Similar cases of depression and bipolar disorder have been reported, but like the schizophrenia cases, the course of the illness is not typical (Anglin et al., 2012). The development of neurological signs or symptoms, cognitive decline, and evidence of strokes on imaging usually leads to the definitive diagnosis (see Fig. 26.5). The diagnosis of MELAS is based on the clinical syndrome, elevated serum lactic acid levels,

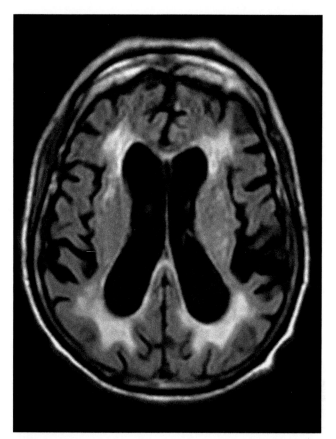

Fig. 26.5 Mitochondrial disease. FLAIR axial images in a 60-year-old woman with MELAS. Extensive subcortical white matter hyperintensity, reflecting marked vascular change, is visible.

and muscle biopsy showing ragged red fibres. Ragged red fibres are muscle fibres exhibiting mitochondrial proliferation in response to mitochondrial failure. MRI scanning typically shows posterior cerebral stroke-like lesions. There is currently no available treatment for MELAS, though antioxidants, respiratory chain substrates, and co-factors have been trialled, with varying results.

Wolfram disease (DIDMOAD)

Wolfram disease is a rare (one per 500,000) autosomal recessive disorder caused by a mutation in the *WFS1* (wolframin) gene on 4p16.1. The disease was initially associated with multiple mito-chondrial deletions but is now considered to be a disease of the endoplasmic reticulum (Urano, 2016), with findings that the *WFS1* gene encodes an endoplasmic reticulum transmembrane protein. Diagnosis is based on clinical suspicion and genetic analysis. Wolfram disease, also known as DIDMOAD (diabetes insipidus, diabetes mellitus, optic atrophy, deafness) is associated with a multisystem disorder. Diabetes in childhood is the com-monest presentation, followed by visual problems and optic at-rophy, diabetes insipidus, and sensorineural deafness. Psychiatric manifestations are relatively common. In one of the original studies, 68 patients with Wolfram disease were reviewed (Swift et al., 1991). Sixty per cent had psychiatric symptoms and 25% were classified as showing severe mental illness. Sixteen per cent of patients had a history of psychotic symptoms. Heterozygous family members exhibited a high rate of psychiatric illness,

approximately eight times greater than for non-carriers of the wolframin gene. A more recent study by the same authors iden-tified that the wolframin mutation was associated with high rates of hospitalization for depression (Swift and Swift, 2005). The prognosis for Wolfram syndrome is poor, as there are no current treatments, though endoplasmic calcium stabilizers may provide a therapeutic option (Urano, 2016).

Conclusion

Neurometabolic, endocrine, and mitochondrial disorders are dis-orders of basic cellular processes that frequently have significant impact on CNS processes, in addition to other organ systems. As our understanding of the molecular biology of neuronal func-tion and of its underpinning by neurogenetic alteration grows, further insights are being developed into how changes to these processes disrupt not only function, but also growth and devel-opment of the brain. When these changes occur during crucial neurodevelopmental periods, or preferentially affect particular neuronal assemblies/populations, psychiatric illness is a frequent presenting or concomitant result. Understanding the nature and particular presentation of these disorders ensures that patients pre-senting with psychiatric illness who may have a metabolic, endo-crine, or mitochondrial component to their presentation will be appropriately and optimally managed.

KEY LEARNING POINTS

- The brain is a highly metabolic organ; hence disorders that affect cellular metabolism or mitochondrial energy function broadly commonly present with central pathology.
- Metabolic disorders that present psychiatrically are most often associated with subtle, rather than gross, changes to cerebral function.
- Some metabolic and endocrine disorders present in an epi-sodic fashion due to acute metabolic derangements.
- A range of other disorders may present initially as a psychi-atric syndrome when pathology is subtle, and as pathology progresses, they then present with cognitive and neurological signs that may assist in the diagnosis of the underlying dis-order, causing a secondary psychiatric syndrome.
- Disruption to late neurodevelopment during the window of onset of most adult psychiatric disorders (young adulthood) appears to significantly increase the likelihood of a secondary psychiatric disorder.

REFERENCES

Almanzar, S., et al. 2013. Dopamine agonist-induced impulse control disorders in a patient with prolactinoma. *Psychosomatics*, 54(4), 387–91.

Anderson, N. E., et al. 2013. Neurological manifestations of phaeochromocytomas and secretory paragangliomas: a reappraisal. *J Neurol Neurosurg Psychiatry*, 84, 452–7.

Anglin, R. E., et al. 2012. The psychiatric manifestations of mitochondrial disorders: a case and review of the literature. *J Clin Psychiatry,* 73, 506–12.

Anglin, R. E., et al. 2006. The neuropsychiatric profile of Addison's disease: revisiting a forgotten phenomenon. *J Neuropsychiatry Clin Neurosci,* 18, 450–9.

Benton, D. 1988. Hypoglycemia and aggression: a review. *Int J Neurosci,* 41, 163–8.

Bonnot, O., et al. 2014. Diagnostic and treatment implications of psychosis secondary to treatable metabolic disorders in adults: a systematic review. *Orphanet J Rare Dis,* 9, 65.

Borer, M. S. & Bhanot, V. K. 1985. Hyperparathyroidism: neuropsychiatric manifestations. *Psychosomatics,* 26, 597–601.

Brumm, V. L., et al. 2010. Psychiatric symptoms and disorders in phenylketonuria. *Mol Genet Metab,* 99 Suppl 1, S59–63.

Bunevicius, R. & Prange, A. J., Jr. 2006. Psychiatric manifestations of Graves' hyperthyroidism: pathophysiology and treatment options. *CNS Drugs,* 20, 897–909.

Chopra, A., et al. 2012. Valproate-induced hyperammonemic encephalopathy: an update on risk factors, clinical correlates and management. *Gen Hosp psychiatry,* 34, 290–8.

Chow, M. & Cao, M. 2016. The hypocretin/orexin system in sleep disorders: preclinical insights and clinical progress. *Nat Sci Sleep,* 8, 81–6.

Crimlisk, H. L. 1997. The little imitator--porphyria: a neuropsychiatric disorder. *J Neurol Neurosurg Psychiatry,* 62, 319–28.

Davis, J. D., et al. 2003. Cognitive and neuropsychiatric aspects of subclinical hypothyroidism: significance in the elderly. *Curr Psychiatry Rep,* 5, 384–90.

De Koning, T. J. & Klomp, L. W. 2004. Serine-deficiency syndromes. *Curr Opin Neurol,* 17, 197–204.

Demily, C. & Sedel, F. 2014. Psychiatric manifestations of treatable hereditary metabolic disorders in adults. *Ann Gen Psychiatry,* 13, 27.

de Oliveira Andrade LJ, Santos França L, Santos França L, Cordeiro de Almeida MA. Double pituitary prolactinoma. *J Clin Endocrinol Metab.* 2010;95:4848–9.

Dunlap, H. & Moersch, F. 1935. Psychic manifestations associated with hyperthyroidism. *Am J Psychiatry,* 91, 1215–38.

Fattal, O., et al. 2006. Review of the Literature on Major Mental Disorders in Adult Patients With Mitochondrial Diseases. *Psychosomatics,* 47, 1–7.

Feit, H. 1988. Thyroid function in the elderly. *Clin Geriatr Med,* 4, 151–61.

Feng, L. G., et al. 2009. Association of plasma homocysteine and methylenetetrahydrofolate reductase C677T gene variant with schizophrenia: A Chinese Han population-based case-control study. *Psychiatry Res,* 168, 205–8.

Fragkaki, I., et al. 2016. Posttraumatic stress disorder under ongoing threat: a review of neurobiological and neuroendocrine findings. *Eur J Psychotraumatol,* 7, 30915.

Gibson, K. M., et al. 2003. Significant behavioral disturbances in succinic semialdehyde dehydrogenase (SSADH) deficiency (gamma-hydroxybutyric aciduria). *Biol Psychiatry,* 54, 763–8.

Gowda, C. R. & Lundt, L. P. 2014. Mechanism of action of narcolepsy medications. *CNS Spectr,* 19 Suppl 1, 25–33; quiz 25–7, 34.

Heinrich, T. W. & Grahm, G. 2003. Hypothyroidism Presenting as Psychosis: Myxedema Madness Revisited. *Prim Care Companion J Clin Psychiatry,* 5, 260–6.

Hyde, T. M., et al. 1992. Psychiatric disturbances in metachromatic leukodystrophy. Insights into the neurobiology of psychosis. *Arch Neurol,* 49, 401–6.

Khemka, D., et al. 2011. Primary hypothyroidism associated with acute mania: case series and literature review. *Exp Clin Endocrinol Diabetes,* 119, 513–17.

Kohen, I. & Arbouet, S. 2008. Neuroendocrine carcinoid cancer associated with psychosis. *Psychiatry (Edgmont),* 5, 29–30.

Kolker, S., et al. 2015. The phenotypic spectrum of organic acidurias and urea cycle disorders. Part 1: the initial presentation. *J Inherit Metab Dis,* 38, 1041–57.

Kunzel, H. E. 2012. Psychopathological symptoms in patients with primary hyperaldosteronism—possible pathways. *Horm Metab Res,* 44, 202–7.

Lynch, S., et al. 1994. Psychiatric morbidity in adults with hypopituitarism. *J R Soc Med,* 87, 445–7.

Malm, D., et al. 2005. Psychiatric symptoms in mannosidosis. *J Intell Dis Res,* 49, 865–71.

Martinkova, J., et al. 2011. Impulse control disorders associated with dopaminergic medication in patients with pituitary adenomas. *Clin Neuropharmacol,* 34, 179–81.

McCormick, J. D., et al. 2001. An obese man with anxiety, sweating, and headache. *Hosp Pract (1995),* 36, 21–2.

Messina, A., et al. 2016. Role of the Orexin System on the Hypothalamus-Pituitary-Thyroid Axis. *Front Neural Circuits,* 10, 66.

Muelly, E. R., et al. 2013. Biochemical correlates of neuropsychiatric illness in maple syrup urine disease. *J Clin Invest,* 123, 1809–20.

Pinto, M. & Moraes, C. T. 2014. Mitochondrial genome changes and neurodegenerative diseases. *Biochim Biophys Acta,* 1842, 1198–207.

Ram, Z., et al. 1987. Visual hallucinations associated with pituitary adenoma. *Neurosurgery,* 20, 292–6.

Ramaekers, V., et al. 2013. Clinical recognition and aspects of the cerebral folate deficiency syndromes. *Clin Chem Lab Med,* 51, 497–511.

Ritchie, M. & Yeap, B. B. 2015. Thyroid hormone: Influences on mood and cognition in adults. *Maturitas,* 81, 266–75.

Rodriguez, G., et al. 2016. Necrolytic migratory erythema and pancreatic glucagonoma. *Biomedica,* 36, 176–81.

Rosebush, P., et al. 2010. Psychosis associated with leukodystrophies. In: Sachdev, P. & Keshavan, M. (eds) *Secondary Schizophrenia.* Cambridge: Cambridge University Press.

Rosebush, P., et al. 1995. Late-onset Tay Sachs disease presenting as catatonic schizophrenia: diagnostic and treatment issues. *J Clin Psychiatry,* 56, 347–53.

Rosebush, P., et al. 1999. The neuropsychiatry of adult-onset adrenoleukodystrophy. *J Neuropsychiatry Clin Neurosci,* 11, 315–27.

Rosenfeld, A., et al. 2014. A review of childhood and adolescent craniopharyngiomas with particular attention to hypothalamic obesity. *Pediatr Neurol,* 50, 4–10.

Samuels, M. H. 2014. Psychiatric and cognitive manifestations of hypothyroidism. *Curr Opin Endocrinol Diabetes Obes,* 21, 377–83.

Scheiber, S. S. & Baudry, M. 1995. Selective neuronal vulnerability in the hippocampus—a role for gene expression? *Trends Neurosci,* 18, 446–51.

Segal, P., et al. 2010. Psychiatric and cognitive profile in Anderson-Fabry patients: a preliminary study. *J Inherit Metab Dis,* 33, 429–36.

Shorter, E. & Ink, M. 2010. *Endocrine Psychiatry: Solving the Riddle of Melancholia.,* New York, NY: Oxford University Press.

Sievers, C., et al. 2009. Prevalence of mental disorders in acromegaly: a cross-sectional study in 81 acromegalic patients. *Clin Endocrinol (Oxf)*, 71, 691–701.

Skovby, F., et al. 2010. A revisit to the natural history of homocystinuria due to cystathionine beta-synthase deficiency. *Mol Genet Metab*, 99, 1–3.

Sonino, N., et al. 2006. Psychological aspects of primary aldosteronism. *Psychother Psychosom*, 75, 327–30.

Starkman, M. N. 2013. Neuropsychiatric findings in Cushing syndrome and exogenous glucocorticoid administration. *Endocrinol Metab Clin North Am*, 42, 477–88.

Swift, M. & Swift, R. G. 2005. Wolframin mutations and hospitalization for psychiatric illness. *Mol Psychiatry*, 10, 799–803.

Swift, R. G., et al. 1991. Psychiatric disorders in 36 families with Wolfram syndrome. *Am J Psychiatry*, 148, 775–9.

Turner, T. H., et al. 1984. Psychotic reactions during treatment of pituitary tumours with dopamine agonists. *BMJ*, 289, 1101–3.

Urano, F. 2016. Wolfram Syndrome: Diagnosis, Management, and Treatment. *Curr Diabetes Rep*, 16, 6.

Van Karnebeek, C. D. & Stockler, S. 2012. Treatable inborn errors of metabolism causing intellectual disability: a systematic literature review. *Mol Genet Metab*, 105, 368–81.

Velasco, P. J., et al. 1999. Psychiatric aspects of parathyroid disease. *Psychosomatics*, 40, 486–90.

Waisbren, S. E., et al. 1994. Review of neuropsychological functioning in treated phenylketonuria: an information processing approach. *Acta Paediatrica*, 407, 98–103.

Walterfang, M., et al. 2013. The neuropsychiatry of inborn errors of metabolism. *J Inherit Metab Dis*, 36, 687–702.

Walterfang, M., et al. 2006. The neuropsychiatry of Niemann-Pick type C disease in adulthood. *J Neuropsychiatry Clin Neurosci*, 18, 158–70.

Wijburg, F. & Nassogne, M.-C. Disorders of the urea cycle and related enzymes. In: Saudubray, J.-M., van den Berghe, G., Walter, J.H. (eds) *Inborn Metabolic Diseases*, fifth edition. Berlin: Springer-Verlag; 2012; pp. 297–310.

Wolkowitz, O. M. 1994. Prospective controlled studies of the behavioral and biological effects of exogenous corticosteroids. *Psychoneuroendocrinology*, 19, 233–55.

27

Neuropsychiatry of alcohol-related brain damage

Ken Wilson

Introduction

Liver disease is recognized as a major 'end-organ disease' related to alcohol misuse. Likewise, the brain is commonly affected by long-term alcohol misuse. Most clinicians will be familiar with the more extreme presentations of neurocognitive dysfunction, such as Wernicke's encephalopathy (WE), and the longer-term manifestation of thiamine deficiency known as Korsakoff's syndrome (KS). However, most clinicians will not be aware that the classical manifestation of these neurocognitive syndromes is relatively rare. Other related manifestations of neurocognitive damage are much more frequent, more subtle, and less easily recognized. This chapter addresses these issues, utilizing the term 'alcohol-related brain damage' (ARBD) to cover the wide spectrum of neurocognitive syndromes that may manifest as a consequence of direct alcohol toxicity and the indirect effects of thiamine deprivation.

Epidemiology

We are confronted with a number of problems when addressing the prevalence and incidence of ARBD. The term itself is problematical as a consequence of its inclusivity and lack of definition. Secondly, epidemiological research into the individual constituent sydromes is sparse. Lastly, simple audits and reviews of clinical notes of patient populations are confounded through a lack of cognitive assessment and recording (Scalzo et al., 2015).

In addressing the longer-term manifestations of ARBD, the term Wernicke–Korsakoff's syndrome (WK) will be used to describe the acute and chronic manifestations of thiamine deficiency. Although WK can be caused by other conditions leading to thiamine deficiency, this chapter focuses on the role of alcohol and related problems. Much of the epidemiological research lies in autopsy examinations. Many of these studies are relatively old and may not reflect current prevalence and incidence. More recently, Galvin and colleagues (2010) combined the data from 20 autopsy studies (*n* = 37,783) and found a prevalence of 1.3%, with an increased prevalence of 9.3% in people with a history of alcohol misuse disorders. A more recent compilation of autopsy studies has been listed

by Scalzo et al. (2015). The 12 studies range from 1961 to 1998 and represent data from the United States, Australia, Brazil, France, Germany, and Norway. There are a number of sampling issues that should be taken into account, but most of the studies examined autopsies (with the exception of two) confined to adult populations. Of the 40,783 autopsies, 1.4% had WK pathology and only 5% had reported a history of alcohol misuse disorders, representing a pervasive underreporting during the patients' lifetime. The authors pointed out that 83% of people with WK did not receive a clinical diagnosis during their lifetime.

DSM-5 employs the term 'alcohol-related neurocognitive disorders (mild and major)' (as opposed to alcohol-related dementia in DSM-IV). These and other definitions, such as ARBD, have been used to explore the prevalence in various clinical populations. Gilchrist and Morrison (2005) estimated that 21% of the Glasgow homeless showed evidence of ARBD. A number of authors have demonstrated that up to 50% of detoxified alcohol dependents demonstrated varying signs of cognitive damage (Zahr et al., 2011). Likewise, Pitel et al. (2011) found that 16% of alcohol dependents had clinical signs of WE and as many as 57% had at least one sign, as defined by the European Federation of Neurological Sciences Criteria (see Box 27.1).

These reports indicate that there is a significant prevalence of ARBD within the general population, with an increased prevalence in high-risk groups and socio-economically deprived populations (MacRae and Cox, 2003). Presentation is usually between the ages of 50 and 60 (MacRae and Cox, 2003), and women may present with a shorter drinking history and at a younger age than their male counterparts (Cutting, 1978).

Aetiology

As illustrated, thiamine deficiency does play a significant role in the aetiology of ARBD and, in particular, WK. Thiamine (a water-soluble vitamin) is a co-enzyme in the metabolism of carbohydrates, lipids, and branched-chain amino acids (Hoyumpa, 1980). Alcohol dependents may frequently neglect a well-balanced diet, with a resultant reduction in thiamine intake. Likewise, there is a reduction in carbohydrates and lipids. The lack of dietary intake is compounded by the direct effect of chronic, excessive alcohol misuse on storage and utilization of thiamine (Thomson, 2000). The neuropathological consequences of thiamine deficiency in the context of alcohol misuse may well be regulated by genetic variables (Ridely and Draper, 2015).

In addition to the effects of thiamine deficiency, recent research has emphasized the direct neuropathological consequences of excessive alcohol ingestion. Inhibitory GABA–benzodiazepine and excitatory glutamatergic systems (Krystal et al., 2003; Ron and Wang, 2009; Tsai and Coyle, 1998) are both boosted. NMDA receptors are increased and there is reduced long-term potentiation (a process key in learning and memory) in rats (White et al., 2000). It is postulated that this process may underlie alcoholic blackouts and amnesia associated with acute or binge drinking. Functional neuroimagery tends to support the potential role of changes in both GABA receptors and glutamate in the context of reduction of activity in the frontal lobes in alcohol dependents (Lingford-Hughes et al., 2005). These studies may lay the foundation for potential therapeutic approaches in the management of withdrawal, so as to reduce the likelihood of future cognitive damage (Mann et al., 2008; Ron and Wang, 2009). Neuroradiological investigations of non-complicated (non-thiamine-deficient) alcohol dependents have consistently demonstrated significant structural brain changes. There is increasing evidence that the frontal lobe is particularly vulnerable to alcohol misuse; post-mortem studies revealed significant neuronal density loss in alcohol dependents (Harper and Mutsumoto, 2005). *In vivo* studies demonstrated reduced blood flow (Gansler et al., 2000) and reduction in event-related potentials in the frontal cortex (Chen et al., 2007).

Thinning of the corpus collosum, frontal dysfunction (Pfefferbaum et al., 1996), and compromise of the cerebellar-pontine-frontal and thalamo-cortical systems have all been documented (Sullivan, 2003). There is generalized cortical reduction, with resultant ventricular enlargement and cortical atrophy (Pfefferbaum et al., 1992). Likewise there is cerebellar neuronal and white matter loss (Sullivan et al., 2000a, b) and hippocampal changes, possibly restricted to the white matter (Harding et al., 1997).

Emerging evidence indicates that the complex interface between the direct effects of chronic alcohol ingestion and thiamine is best modelled as a continuum, rather than a dichotomy. This applies to most parts of the brain, with a number of exceptions. In particular, the mammillary bodies and thalamic radiations seem to be particularly vulnerable to thiamine deficiency, as experienced by patients with WE (Beaunieux et al., 2015; Pitel et al., 2012). The combined effect of thiamine deficiency and direct effects of alcohol toxicity has ramifications for many areas of the cortex and subcortical structures through neuronal depletion and white matter changes, resulting in cortical and subcortical shrinkage (Sullivan and Pfefferbaum, 2009).

Clinical features

Acute/subacute presentation

The wide spectrum of neuropathological changes presenting in long-term alcohol misuse predicates a varied and diverse cognitive presentation. In an acute setting, cognitive problems are evident in acute intoxication and withdrawal states. They are a critical component of WE, associated with acute thiamine deficiency. WE is an acute neurological disorder, consisting of oculomotor abnormalities, cerebellar dysfunction, and altered mental state. It is, of course, important to exclude other frequently encountered conditions such as hepatic encephalopathy and other causes of delirium. Notably, the direct effects of alcohol on the brain (as opposed to indirect through thiamine depletion) may also contribute to the clinical presentation. What evidence there is indicates that alcohol will interfere (in heavy, long-term alcohol misusers) with the aforementioned neurophysiology of cortical and subcortical structures for up to 3 months of abstinence following an acute presentation. Hence the clinical presentation in an acute setting may not be confined to the relatively discrete profile of WK syndrome but may include features of fronto-cerebellar-pontine, limbic system, and general cortical involvement. Indeed, the classical triad of neurological signs of WE is acknowledged as having a low diagnostic sensitivity in an acute presentation (Galvin et al., 2010). To make things more complicated, up to 25% of patients presenting in acute hospital settings also have a history of head injury and/or cerebrovascular disease (Wilson et al., 2012), likely to compromise cognitive performance.

A more common presentation of ARBD is to be experienced in non-acute settings. This presentation is much harder to recognize, more insidious in onset, and consequently rarely treated. It principally manifests as frontal cortex disturbance, presenting with various degrees of dysexecutive syndrome. A number of studies have examined the cognitive profile of people attending alcohol treatment programmes. These include problems in reasoning (Zinn et al., 2004), the ability to understand complex information (Smith and Crady, 1991), understanding risk (Blume 2005), difficulties with abstraction and manipulating memory (Noel et al., 2007), and problems in acquiring novel information (Pitel et al., 2007)—all potentially important problems when the individual is engaged in educational and therapeutic programmes common to alcohol treatment courses.

The acute presentation of neurocognitive problems and WE and the more insidious presentation of dysexecutive syndrome illustrate the extremes of a wide spectrum of differing clinical presentations. Patients will present with varying degrees of cognitive dysfunction across differing intellectual domains as a consequence of both the direct effects of alcohol and the indirect effects of thiamine deficiency. This, in turn, will be influenced by nutritional status, alcohol and withdrawal history (Loeber et al., 2010), genetic variables, and the potential presence of vascular or traumatic brain damage.

In summary, the case of an acute presentation is often florid, representing an acute emergency and warranting immediate intervention and physical stabilization. Malnutrition, neglect, history of frequent admissions, and physical problems, including varying degrees of liver failure, pancreatitis, and neuropathies, all point to the major role of alcohol and potential thiamine deficiency as the primary causation. The more insidious presentation of frontal lobe disturbance may be characterized by less well-defined problems. Such patients may still be in employment, often protected by colleagues. Over time, loss of social awareness, problems in higher-order reasoning, and complex decision management will begin to tell. Memory problems will slowly become more evident, with resultant problems at work and home. This may well be associated with either lack of insight (from a cognitive perspective) or 'denial', characteristic of many alcohol dependents. Domestic relationships are likely to suffer and financial tensions build within the family as employment becomes threatened and social contacts become more circumscribed. The individual is at risk of a downward spiral of social disengagement, domestic isolation, malnutrition, financial impoverishment, increasing cognitive impairment, and long-standing intellectual damage.

Clinical course of ARBD

The acute manifestations of neuronal loss and haemorrhagic lesions in the periventricular and periaqueductal areas (Isenberg-Grzeda et al., 2012) associated with WE will progress to wider involvement of diencephalic and hippocampal mechanisms in the absence of thiamine treatment, resulting in the more chronic KS. However, from a clinical perspective, it is important to acknowledge that the classical presentation of WE is not a prerequisite for the development of KS and related, more permanent cognitive disorders.

KS was first described by Sergi Korsakoff through reporting a series of cases presenting with prodromal confusion, ophthalmoplegia, nystagmus, and ataxia. Kopleman defines KS as 'an abnormal mental state in which memory and learning are affected out of all proportion to other cognitive functions in an otherwise alert and responsive patient, resulting from nutritional depletion, i.e. thiamine deficiency' (Kopelman, 2002; Kopelman et al., 2009).

From a memory perspective, 'working memory' (in this context, the ability of immediate recall of small amounts of information) is usually preserved. Likewise, implicit memory is usually intact (including procedural, perceptuo-motor skills, and priming). Semantic memory can be variably affected (memory of concepts, language, and facts that do not have a 'location 'in time and place). Long-term, biographical (episodic) memory is frequently compromised, resulting in retrograde amnesia that may go back many years. This is often associated with impairment of the contextual aspects of memory (Kessels and Kopleman, 2012), a consequence of damage to the temporal cortices and the hippocampus (Chanraud et al., 2009; Gazdzinski et al., 2005). Memory problems are frequently complicated by confabulations. These false memories are principally of two types—complex, spontaneous confabulations are often characterized by the juxtapositioning of events in the person's life and are characteristic of the WK syndrome. They are associated with orbitofrontal and ventromedial frontal pathology. Momentary confabulations are fleeting intrusion errors or distortions in response to a challenge to the memory.

The direct effects of long-term alcohol misuse on the neurophysiology of the brain may take up to 3 months of abstinence to achieve optimal resolution (Cocchi and Chiavarini, 1997). This period of recovery informs Oslin's diagnostic criteria (Oslin and Carey, 2003) for 'alcohol dementia' which are designed to characterize the more long-standing neurocognitive deficits. This relatively early clinical improvement probably reflects the slowly diminishing direct effects of alcohol on the brain and may well be enhanced by improvement in physical health status, alcohol abstinence, and well-founded nutrition. After this initial period of recovery, the rate of improvement tends to slow down.

There is limited research relating to the long-term outcome of people presenting with ARBD.The most quoted prognostication is that of Smith and Hillman (1999) suggesting that 25% make a complete recovery, 25% make a significant recovery, 25% make a slight recovery, and the remaining 25% make no recovery. More specifically, a small number of follow-up studies had the tendency to confirm the variable prognosis but also hinted at potentially important therapeutic or service issues which may influence outcome.

Assessment and treatment

Acute presentation of ARBD

In the acute presentation of WE, it is important to undertake a full neurological and medical assessment. More specifically, diffusion-weighted MRI imaging is the choice of neuroradiological investigation. Classical WE will present with symmetrical lesions of the thalami, mammillary bodies, tectal plate, and periaqueductal areas. However, atypical widespread lesions are also encountered. These are frequently complicated by ischaemic change or evidence of trauma (Wilson et al., 2012). Notably, a negative MRI does not rule out a diagnosis of WE (Antunez et al., 1998). This emphasizes the relative importance of a detailed neurocognitive assessment.

Thiamine remains the mainstay of treatment in an acute setting. Patients presenting with acute WE should receive intravenous thiamine treatment (2–3 pairs of ampoules three times a day) for at least 2 days. It is self-evident that the patient may well be suffering from other vitamin deficiencies and these will have to be appropriately assessed and treated. There is a small risk of anaphylaxis and appropriate resuscitation facilities should be available. However, this must be balanced against the very real possibility of delay in treatment causing more permanent brain damage (Galvin et al., 2010). Clinical signs and symptoms usually respond within a few days.

Subacute presentation of ARBD

As already mentioned, the subacute presentation of ARBD is common in community settings, presenting with less obvious cognitive dysfunction, including dysexecutive syndrome and varying memory problems—hence the importance of undertaking a full mental health assessment (including cognition) in people presenting to alcohol treatment services (National Institute for Health and Care Excellence, 2011). Those at risk of thiamine deficiency can be identified by the following characteristics (Thomson et al., 2009): weight loss, reduced BMI, history of poor nutrition, recurrent episodes of vomiting, co-occurrence of nutritionally related conditions, polyneuropathy, amblyopia, pellagra, and anaemia.

Such patients may present with a variety of related symptoms: diploplia, giddiness, nausea and vomiting, fatigue, weakness and apathy, insomnia, and lack of concentration. In these situations, prophylactic intramuscular thiamine should be considered, using one pair of ampoules once daily for between 3 and 5 days.

The role of oral thiamine therapy is more contentious, but what guidelines there are suggest 300 mg a day during detoxification and it should also be offered to drinking patients at risk of malnutrition, if they have decompensated liver disease or are in acute or medically assisted withdrawal or before and during a planned medically assisted alcohol withdrawal. Oral thiamine prophylaxis should follow parenteral thiamine treatment (Royal College of Psychiatrists, 2014).

Longer-term psychosocial management

There is some evidence that interventions targeting specific cognitive domains may be of use in terms of improving outcome (Forsberg and Goldman, 1987; Svanberg and Evans, 2013). Such exercises/interventions may have a generic beneficial effect across non-targeted cognitive domains as well (Forsberg and Goldman, 1987). Following this theme, Bates (2002) undertook a comprehensive review of research relating to acquired brain damage and emphasized the importance of an ecologically relevant programme of rehabilitation in which patients are encouraged to acquire skills relevant to their personal functionality and to develop environmental, behavioural, and cognitive processes to accommodate residual areas of deficit. More specifically, in the context of ARBD, Baddeley et al. (2002) advocated memory and orientation aids as playing an important role in rehabilitation.

In the absence of any controlled research into service delivery, any wider therapeutic intervention can only draw on naturalistic follow-up studies of clinical populations. In 1986, Lennane followed up 104 patients for between 8 months and 2 years in the context of a specialized service (Lennane et al., 1986). Approximately half ($n = 53$) were considered to be successful placements; 11 were readmitted to hospital (10.6%), and the remainder were lost to follow-up or presumed dead. However, this rather pessimistic outcome compares favourably with that of Price et al. (1988) who followed up patients in the context of a non-specialized service. In following up 37 patients, only 27% were successfully 'placed'; a further 54% were described as dysfunctional, and the remaining seven died. Based on these two studies, Price made the case for management by a specialized service provision. The potential role of institutions has been examined by a number of authors. Fals-Stewart and Schafer (1992), DeLeon (1984), and DeLeon and Jainhill (1981) noted that outcome appeared to be better when alcohol- and drug-abusing individuals were placed in specialized residential settings, as opposed to generic institutions. Blansjaar et al. (1992) and Ganzelves et al. (1994) found that patients with ARBD performed better in terms of social functioning and of information processing speed in specialized homes compared with those in non-specialized settings. Lastly, Rychtarik et al. (2000) described a better outcome in people with cognitive impairment when treated for alcohol dependency in institutional settings, compared to outpatient clinics.

Subsequently, Wilson et al. (2012) developed a structured intervention informed by Bate's review. The model incorporates aspects of diary keeping, activity scheduling, and graded task assignment, supported by protection from alcohol, nutritional and physical stabilization, and alcohol education. The programme is characterized by five phases of therapeutic engagement:

1. Physical stabilization, thiamine treatment in acute hospital settings.
2. Assessment phase: alcohol protection (in incapacitated patients), nutrition, and physical recovery lasting 3 months.
3. Therapeutic intervention: a 3-year phase of planned and structured intervention, utilizing simple cognitive behavioural techniques to maximize the individual's autonomy and independence.
4. Adjustment phase: provision of psychosocial supportive environment when the patient has reached optimal levels of autonomy and cognitive improvement.
5. Social integration phase: providing the patient with social buffers and support in order to prevent relapse of alcohol misuse.

The intervention was piloted in a consecutive series of 41 patients referred from acute medical inpatient care with severe ARBD. Over 2 years, improvement was demonstrated across a variety of psychosocial domains, including: 'active disturbance of social behaviour', 'problem drinking and drug use', 'cognitive problems', 'physical illness and disability', 'experience of hallucinations, delusions, and confabulation', 'problems with relationships', 'problems with activities of daily living', and 'problems with living conditions and problems with activities'. Most importantly, a comprehensive provision of follow-up, structured intervention (utilizing fairly simple cognitive behavioural techniques), and case management resulted in a marked reduction of acute bed use, a 10% relapse into uncontrolled drinking, and 10% mortality rate. Subsequent reviews have demonstrated that 75% of patients are satisfactorily placed in non-institutional settings (including own domestic homes, supported living, and sheltered accommodation). Even though this study was small, it included extremely ill patients with profound cognitive impairment, significant physical illnesses, and previous multiple hospital admissions.

Options for purposeful intervention also exist for patients presenting with less acute manifestations of ARBD in community settings. Again, there is a relative absence of 'outcome' research. However, relatively simple adaptations to alcohol treatment programmes have been suggested and comprehensively listed in the Royal College of Psychiatrists guidelines (Royal College of Psychiatrists, 2014).

Conclusion

ARBD is a generic term of some clinical relevance in that it subsumes the wide range of presentations caused by the acute and chronic effects of both alcohol and thiamine deficiency on the neurophysiology of the brain. Its presentation may range from the subtleties of frontal lobe dysfunction through to the acute presentation of WE. The diversity and range of presentation make its prevalence difficult to judge, but what research there is indicates that up to 1.5% of the general population have alcohol-related changes in their brain at post-mortem. However, there is evidence that the prevalence may be as much as 30–50% in high-risk communities such as people attending alcohol treatment services. The disproportionate burden on health services is growing (Atkins et al., 2015).

Clinical diagnosis is frequently missed or unrecorded. This is of particular importance as treatment with thiamine will treat the acute presenting syndrome and will prevent longer-lasting damage in people at risk of ARBD. In the absence of commissioned services, patients with ARBD are often considered a nuisance and stigmatized and their cognitive problems rarely addressed. This results in poor prognosis, with evidence of multiple hospital admissions, disproportionate utilization of community services, and a downward spiral of increasing morbidity. Even though there is relatively little evidence of efficacy, what evidence there is suggests that purposeful, structured long-term intervention may be associated with relatively good outcomes, reducing morbidity, reducing alcohol misuse, consequential service utilization, and prevention of the downward spiral of increasing dependency and severity. However, it is important to understand that such structured interventions may only provide a mechanism for clinical intervention, rather than offer claims of a 'curative' nature. Many ARBD sufferers are likely to improve naturally if nutritionally stable, alcohol-free, and supported in their recovery.

KEY LEARNING POINTS

- ARBD is a potentially severe and incapacitating condition, resulting in significant morbidity and utilization of services.
- Its presentation is varied and frequently missed in both acute and community settings.
- There is a paucity of service provision, with patients 'falling between' specialist services and being provided with little care planning or specifically tailored interventions.
- Diagnosis and thiamine treatment are imperative in both acute and non-acute settings in terms of treatment and prevention in at-risk patients.
- Early reports indicate that structured, specialized, and purposeful psychosocial intervention over 2–3 years may play an important role in reducing morbidity, alcohol misuse, and service utilization.

REFERENCES

Antunez E, Estruch R, Cardenal C, Nicolas JM, Fernandez-Sola J, Urbano-Marquez A. (1998) Usefulness of CT and MRI imaging in the diagnosis of acute Wernicke's encephalopathy. *American Journal of Roenterology*, 171, 1131–7.

Atkins S, Rackham K, Acevedo J, Dowman JK, Fowell AJ, Aspinall RJ. (2015) Increasing burden of alcohol related brain injury is disproportionate to hospital admissions with liver disease. *Gut*. Second Digestive Disorders Federation Conference, DDF. London United Kingdom. Conference Publication: 64 (A273),

Baddeley AD, Kopelman MD, Wilson BA. *Handbook of Memory Disorders*, second edition. Chichester: Wiley; 2002.

Bates M, Bowden S, Barry D. (2002) Neurocognitive impairment associated with alcohol use disorders: implications for treatment. *Experimental and Clinical Psychopharmacology*, 10, 193–212.

Beaunieux H, Eustaache F, Pitel A-L. (2015) The relation of alcohol induced brain changes to cognitive function. In: Svanberg J, Withall A, Draper B, Bowden S (eds). *Alcohol and the Adult Brain*. Hove. Psychology Press.

Blansjaar BA, Takens H, Zwinderman AH. (1992) The course of alcohol amnestic disorder: a three-year follow-up study of clinical signs and social disabilities. *Acta Psychiatrica Scandinavica*, 86, 240–6.

Blume AW, Schmaling KB, Marlatt GA. (2005) Memory, executive cognitive function, and readiness to change drinking behaviour. *Addictive Behaviours*, 30, 301–14.

Chanraud S, Leroy C, Martelli C, et al. (2009) Episodic memory in detoxified alcoholics: contribution of grey matter microstructural alteration. *PLoS One*, 4, e6786.

Chen A,C, Porjesz B, Rangaswamy M, et al. (2007) Reduced frontal lobe activity in subjects with high impulsivity and alcoholism. *Alcohol: Clinical and Experimental Research*, 31 156–65.

Cocchi R, Chiavarini M. (1997) Raven's coloured matrices in female alcoholics before and after detoxification: An investigation on 73 cases. *International Journal of Intellectual Impairment*, 11, 45–9.

Cutting J. (1978) A reappraisal of alcoholic psychoses. *Psychological Medicine*, 8, 285–96.

DeLeon G. (1984) Program-based evaluation research in therapeutic communities. *National Institute on Drug Abuse Research Monograph Series*, 51, 69–87.

DeLeon G, Jainhill N. (1981) Male and female drug abusers: Social and psychological status two years after treatment in a therapeutic community. *American Journal of Alcohol Abuse*, 8, 595–600.

Fals-Stewart W. (1992) Using the subtests of the Brain Age Quotientto screen for cognitive deficits among substance abusers. *Perceptual and Motor Skills*, 75, 244–6.

Forsberg LK, Goldman MS. (1987) Experience-dependent recovery of cognitive deficits in alcoholics: Extended transfer of training. *Journal of Abnormal Psychology*, 96, 345–53.

Galvin R, Brathen G. Ivashynka A, Hillbom M, Tanescue R, Leone M. (2010) EFNS guidelines for diagnosis, therapy and prevention of Wernicke Encephalaopathy. *European Journal of Neurology*, 17, 1408–18.

Gansler DA, Harris GJ, Oscar Burman M, et al. (2000) Hypofusion of inferior frontal brain regions in abstinent alcoholics: a pilot SPECT study. *Journal of Studies on Alcohol and Drugs*, 61 32–7.

Ganzelves PGJ, Geus BWJ, Wester AJ. (1994) Cognitive and behavioural aspects of Korsakoff's syndrome: the effect of special Korsakoff wards in a general hospital. *Tijdschriftvoor Alcohol Drugs en AnderePsychotropeStoffen*, 20, 20–31.

Gazdzinski S, Durazzo TC, Studholm C, Song E, Banys P, Meyerhoff DJ. (2005) Quantitative brain MRI in alcohol dependence: preliminary evidence for effects of concurrent chronic cigarette smoking on regional brain volumes. *Alcoholism: Clinical and Experimental Research*, 29, 1482–95.

Gilchrist G, Morrison DS. (2005) Prevalence of alcohol related brain damage among homeless hostel dwellers in Glasgow. *European Journal of Public Health*, 15, 587–8.

Harding AJ, Wong A, Svoboda M, Kril JJ, Halliday GM. (1997) Chronic alcohol consumption does not cause hippocampal neuron loss in humans. *Hippocampus*, 7, 78–87.

Harper CG, Matsumoto I. (2005) Ethanol and brain damage. *Current Opinion in Pharmacology*, 5, 73–8.

Hoyumpa AM. (1980) Mechanism of thiamine deficiency in chronic alcoholism. *American Journal of Clinical Nutrition*, 33, 2750–61.

Isenberg-Grzeda E, Kutner HE, Nicholson SE. (2012) Wernicke-Korsakoff syndrome: under-recognised and under treated. *Psychosomatics*, 53, 507–16.

Kessels RPC, Kopelman MD. (2012) Context memory in Korsakoff's syndrome. *Neuropsychology Review*, 22, 117–31.

Kopelman MD. (2002) Disorders of memory. *Brain*, 125, 2152–90.

Kopelman MD, Thomson A, Guerrini I, et al. (2009) The Korsakoff syndrome: clinical aspects, psychology and treatment. *Alcohol and Alcoholism*, 44, 148–54.

Krystal JH, Petrakis IL, Krupitsky E, et al. (2003) NMDA receptor antagonism and the ethanol intoxication signal: from alcoholism risk to pharmacotherapy. *Annals of the New York Academy of Sciences*, 1003, 176–84.

Lennane KJ. (1986) Management of moderate to severe alcohol related brain damage (Korsakoff's syndrome). *Medical Journal of Australia*, 145, 136–43.

Lingford-Hughes AR, Wilson SJ, Cunningham VJ, et al. (2005) GABA- benzodiazepine receptor function in alcohol dependence: a combined 11C-flumazenil PET and pharmacodynamics study. *Psychopharmacology*, 180, 595–606.

Loeber S, Duka T, Welzel Marquez H, et al. (2010) Effects of repeated withdrawal from alcohol on recovery of cognitive impairment under abstinence and rate or relapse. *Alcohol and Alcoholism*, 45, 541–7.

MacRae S, Cox S. (2003) *Meeting the needs of people with alcohol related brain damage: a literature review on the existing and recommended service provision and models of care.* Stirling: Dementia Services Development Centre, University of Stirling.

Mann K, Kiefer F, Spanagel R, et al. (2008) Acamprosate: recent findings and future research directions. *Alcoholism: Clinical and Experimental Research*, 32, 1105–10.

National Institute for Health and Care Excellence. (2011) *Alcohol-Use Disorders: Diagnosis, Assessment and Management of Harmful Drinking and Alcohol Dependence.* Clinical Guideline [CG115]. London: National Institute for Health and Care Excellence.

Svanberg J, Evans JJ. (2013) Neuropsychological rehabilitation in alcohol-related brain damage: A systematic review. *Alcohol and Alcoholism*, 48, 704–11.

Noel X, Bechara A, Dan B, Hanak C, Verbanck P. (2007) Response inhibition deficit is involved in poor decision making under risk in nonamnesic individuals with alcoholism. *Neuropsychology* 21, 778–86.

Oslin DW, Carey MS. (2003) Alcohol related dementia: validation of diagnostic criteria. *American Journal of Geriatric Psychiatry*, 11, 441–7.

Pfefferbaum A, Lm KO, Zipursky RB, et al. (1992) Brain grey and white matter volume accelerates with ageing in chronic alcoholics: a quantative MRI study. *Alcoholism, Clinical and Experimental Research*, 16, 1078–89.

Pfefferbaum A, Lin KO, Desmond JE, Sullivan EV. (1996) Thinning of the corpus callosum in older alcoholic men: a magnetic resonance imaging study. *Alcoholism: Clinical and Experimental Research*, 20, 752–7.

Pitel AL, Witkowski T, Vabret F, et al. (2007) Effect of episodic and working memory impairments on seamantic and procedural learning at alcohol treatment entry. *Alcoholism: Clinical and Experimental Research*, 31, 238–48.

Pitel AL, Chetalat G, Le Berre AP, Desgranges B, Eustache F, Beaunieux H. (2012) Macrostructural abnormalities in Korsakoff syndrome compared with uncomplicated alcoholism. *Neurology*, 78, 1330–3.

Pitel AL, Zahr Nm, Jackson K, et al. (2011) Signs of preclinical Wernicke's Encephalopathy and thiamine levels as predictors of neuropsychological deficits in alcoholism without Korsakoff's syndrome. *Neuropsychopharmacology*, 36, 580–8.

Price J, Mitchell S, Wiltshire B, et al. (1988) A follow up study of patients with alcohol related brain damage in the community. *Austrailian Drug and Alcohol Review*, 7, 83–7.

Ridely NJ, Draper B. (2015) Alcohol related dementia and brain damage: a fiocus on epidemiology. In: Svanberg J, Whithall A, Draper B, Bowden S (eds). *Alcohol and the Adult Brain.* Hove: Psychology Press.

Ron D, Wang J. (2009) The NMDA receptor and alcohol addiction. In: Van Dongen, AM. *Biology of the NMDA Receptor.* CRC Press.

Royal College of Psychiatrists. (2014) *Alcohol and Brain damage in Adults. With reference to High Risk Groups.* College Report CR185. London: Royal College of Psychiatrists.

Rychtarik RG, Connors GJ, Whitney RB, McGillicuddy NB, Fitterling JM, Wirtz PW. (2000). Treatment settings for persons with alcoholism: Evidence for matching clients to inpatient vs. outpatient care. *Journal of Consulting and Clinical Psychology*, 68, 277–89.

Scalzo S, Bowden S, Hillborn M. (2015) Wernicke-Korsakoff Syndrome in Alcohol and the Adult brain. Current Issues in Neuropsychology. Psychological Press, East Sussex.

Smith DE, McCrady BS. (1991) Cognitive impairment among alcoholics: impact on drink refusal skill acquisition and treatment outcome. *Addictive Behaviours*, 16, 265–74.

Smith I, Hillman A. (1999) Management of Alcohol Korsakoff's syndrome. *Advances in Psychiatric Treatment*, 5, 271–8.

Sullivan EV. (2003) Compromised pontocerebellar and cerebellothalamocortical systems: speculations on theior contributions to cognitive and motor impairment in non amnesic alcoholism. *Alcohol: Clinical and Experimental Research*, 27, 1409–19.

Sullivan EV, Deshmukh A, Desmond JE, Lim K, Pfefferbaum A. (2000a) Cerebellar volume decline in normal aging, alcoholism and Korsakoff's syndrome: relation to ataxia. *Neuropsychology*, 14, 341–52.

Sullivan EV, Pfefferbaum A. (2009) Neuroimaging of the Wernicke Korsakoff Syndrome. *Alcohol and Alcoholism*, 45 155–65

Sullivan EV, Rosenbloom MJ, Lim KO, Pfefferbaum A (2000b) Longitudinal changes in cognition, gait, and balance in abstinent and relapsed alcoholic men: relationship to changes in brain structure. *Neuropsychology*, 14, 178–88.

Thomson A, Guerrini I, Marshall E. (2009) Wernicke's encephalopathy: role of thiamine. *Nutrition Issues in Gastroenterology*, 75, 21–30.

Thomson AD. (2000) Mechanisms of vitamin deficiency in chronic alcohol misusers and the development of the Wernicke-Korsakoff syndrome. *Alcohol and Alcoholism Supplement*, 35, 2–7.

Tsai G, Coyle JT. (1998) The role of glutamatergic neurotransmission in the pathophysiology of alcoholism. *Annual Review of Medicine*, 49, 173–84.

White AM, Matthews DB, Best PJ. (2000) Ethanol, memory, and hippocampal function: a review of recent findings. *Hippocampus*, 10, 88–93.

Wilson K, Halsey A, Macpherson H, et al. The Psycho-Social Rehabilitation of Patients with Alcohol-Related Brain Damage in the Community. *Alcohol and Alcoholism*, 47, 304–11.

Zahr NM, Kaufman KL, Harper CG. (2011) Clinical and pathological features of alcohol related brain damage. *Nature Reviews Neurology*, 7, 284–94.

Zinn S, Stein R, Swartzwelder HS, (2004) Executive functioning early in abstinence from alcohol. *Alcoholism: Clinical and Experimental Research*, 28, 1338–46.

28

Drug use and associated neuropsychiatric conditions

Ashwin Venkataraman, Sam Turton, and Anne Lingford-Hughes

Neurobiology of drug use, abuse, and addiction

Vulnerability to addiction is complex and multifactorial. Risks vary between individuals but include environmental and genetic factors. There is robust evidence to support a role for a genetic risk to addiction, estimated at about 50%, which may underlie aspects such as drug-liking or drug metabolism and vary between different drugs of abuse (Volkow et al., 2011). For example, genes coding for variations in γ-aminobutyric acid A-subtype receptor genes (*GABRA2* and *GABRG2*) are associated with an increased risk of alcohol and heroin dependence (Li et al., 2014). In pre-clinical and clinical models, lower levels of dopamine D2 receptors have been implicated in drug-liking, impulsivity, escalating drug use, and dependence on alcohol or stimulants, but less so for other drugs such as opioids (Badiani et al., 2011; Nutt et al., 2015). Therefore, higher DRD2/D3 receptor levels in non-addicted individuals with a family history of alcoholism have been proposed as protective (Alvanzo et al., 2015). Ongoing epidemiological [e.g. Avon Longitudinal Study of Parents and Children (ALSPAC)] and imaging (IMAGEN, ENIGMA) cohorts are probing mechanisms underpinning drug use that will undoubtedly inform our knowledge and perhaps help to prevent adverse consequences (Schumann et al., 2010; Thompson et al., 2014).

Neurobiology of drug use

Substances of abuse modulate brain systems involved in motivation, reward, decision-making, and memory through interactions with a range of neurotransmitter systems (see Table 28.1). The dopaminergic mesocorticolimbic system has received the most attention due to its role in natural hedonic activities such as food and sex. Substances of abuse modulate activity in the mesolimbic system, though to varying degrees and by different mechanisms (Berridge and Kringelbach, 2015; Koob and Volkow, 2016). For instance, stimulants, such as cocaine and amphetamine, directly target the dopamine system by blocking dopamine reuptake, while amphetamine also increased dopamine release from terminal vesicles (Leyton et al., 2002). Modulation of dopaminergic function by other drugs of abuse, such as alcohol, opioids, and cannabinoids, is more indirect and involves altering the rate of dopaminergic cell firing.

Continued substance use leads to associative pairing between drug-related cues and a rewarding response, reinforcing further drug use and leading to adaptive neuronal and behavioural changes (Koob and Volkow, 2016). In humans, blunted dopaminergic function and low dopamine D2 receptors have been reported in stimulant and alcohol dependence, but less consistently for other drugs of abuse (Nutt et al., 2015). However, more recent data suggest that such reduced dopaminergic function is not always present in these addictions, and interestingly those with less impaired levels of dopamine function have a better prognosis (Martinez et al., 2011). Thus, key brain regions playing an important role in mediating the effects of drugs and implicated in addictive processes include the nucleus accumbens/ventral striatum and their connections with brain regions important in learning (hippocampus), emotional processing (amygdala), and executive function (frontal cortex). It has been proposed that the shift from the ventral to the dorsal striatum is important in habit learning and is associated with a shift from impulsive to compulsive drug use (Everitt and Robbins, 2005). Since dysregulation of the dopaminergic mesolimbic system is implicated in many neuropsychiatric disorders, it may provide a common link with drug abuse.

Other neurotransmitter systems are known to play a key role in mediating the effects of drugs and addiction and its associated processes such as reward and impulsivity. For instance, the pleasurable effects of some drugs, including alcohol, stimulants, and cannabinoids, are associated with increases in endogenous opioids, and dysregulation in the opioid system has been described in several different addictions (Bloomfield et al., 2016; Nutt et al., 2015). Endogenous opioid signalling, similarly to other neurotransmission systems targeted by drugs of abuse such as cannabinoid and GABAergic signalling, modulates dopaminergic mesolimbic activity. Additionally, neuroadaptations of these systems in other brain regions such as the amygdala have been shown to be important in addiction. The amygdala stress-related systems, such as neurokinin 1 (NK1) and the aversive kappa/dynorphin system, may play a more important role than the pleasurable mu/endorphin system. Knowledge of these systems has been key in developing effective medications to treat addiction since those that directly target

Table 28.1 Drugs of abuse: pharmacology and pharmacotherapy

Drug	Primary target	Main effects/ transmitters	Other actions	Clinical pharmacotherapy
Opiates				
Morphine, heroin, codeine, etc.	Mu opioid receptors	? dopamine	Kappa and delta opioid receptors NA	Methadone: full agonist Buprenorphine: partial mu agonist and kappa antagonist Naltrexone: full antagonist Lofexidine and clonidine: α-2 adrenergic receptor agonists
Stimulants				
Cocaine	DAT	↑ dopamine	Local anaesthetic effects by disrupting voltage-gated sodium channels	Lorcaserin 5-HT2C receptor agonist (pre-clinical) (DRD3)
Amphetamine		↑ dopamine	Glutamate, ↑ β-endorphin	(DRD3)
Methamphetamine		↑ dopamine	↑ NA/5HT	
Nicotine	Nicotinic ACh receptor	↑ dopamine		Nicotine replacement Varenicline partial nicotinic agonist
Sedatives				
Alcohol	GABA, glutamate	↑ GABA-A function, ↓ glutamate	↑ β-endorphin Many other systems	Benzodiazepines: GABA-A positive allosteric modulator Baclofen: GABA-B agonist Acamprosate: reduced NMDA and glutamate activity Naltrexone, nalmefene: opioid receptor antagonists
Benzodiazepines	GABA	↑ GABA-A function	↑ dopamine	Flumazenil: GABA-A antagonist
GHB	GABA-B GHB receptor	↑ GABA function		Baclofen: GABA-B agonist
Cannabis	CB1 receptors	? dopamine, ? opioids, ? GABA		
Others				
MDMA/Ecstasy	5-HT transporter (SERT)	↑ 5HT Weak 5HT1 and 5HT2 agonist	↑ dopamine	
Ketamine/PCP	NMDA	↓ glutamate		
LSD	5HT2 receptor	5HT2 agonist	D2 receptor agonist	

↑, increase in levels or function; ↓, decrease in levels or function; DA, dopamine; NA, noradrenaline; DAT, dopamine transporter; LSD, lysergic acid diethylamide; mu, mu opioid; R, receptor; ACh, acetylcholine; GABA, γ-aminobutyric acid; GHB, γ-hydroxybutyrate; NMDA, N-methyl-D-aspartate; DRD3, dopamine D3 receptor; PCP, phencyclidine.

the dopaminergic system have not shown robust clinical efficacy (Lingford-Hughes et al., 2012).

Relief from a negative emotional state, such as anxiety, is a main driver in many individuals for their drug use, rather than wanting to be 'high'. Drug withdrawal can also be a major contributor to continuing drug use, particularly for sedative drugs such alcohol and opioids. Some models of addiction, with the amygdala playing a central role, emphasize these aspects (Koob and Volkow, 2016). With regard to alcohol, the GABA and glutamate systems are implicated in reducing anxiety, sedation, and amnesia. Neuroadaptations in both systems underpin tolerance, and as a consequence, withdrawal-associated neurotoxicity results in seizures, cell loss, and brain atrophy (see Chapter 27).

While many stimulant drugs have a primary effect in the brain by modulating the dopaminergic system, they also affect other neurotransmitter systems such as the serotonergic system. Ecstasy (methylenedioxymethamphetamine), in addition to increasing dopamine, also causes a release of serotonin and blocks the serotonin reuptake transporter. Ecstasy use may induce visual hallucinations, but to lesser degree than drugs with greater hallucinogenic activity such as lysergic acid diethylamide (LSD) and psilocybin.

Neuropsychiatric consequences of substance misuse

For clinicians, substance misuse is frequently seen comorbid with other psychiatric disorders. These individuals are often challenging to engage and treat, which may be compounded by many clinicians' lack of, or limited, training and experience in managing substance misuse. It is important to clinically determine whether the presenting psychiatric symptoms are a consequence of drug intoxication or withdrawal to inform appropriate treatment, as well as educate the patient (Reid et al., 2006) (see Table 28.2). Clinicians may refer to the psychiatric or substance use disorder as primary or secondary, but this may have limited use in the management of the patient. While it is important to establish the relationship between substance use and the psychiatric disorder, both disorders should be treated concurrently, rather than sequentially, as improvement in one condition may not necessarily result in improvement in the other (Lingford-Hughes et al., 2012). There is limited evidence of what the optimal pharmacological or psychological approach to use is for substance misuse comorbid with other psychiatric disorders.

Mood disorders

Mood disorders, including depression, anxiety, and bipolar disorder, are commonly comorbid with substance misuse and dependence (Hasin and Grant, 2015; Hunt et al., 2015).

Depression and anxiety

The association between substance use disorder and depression and anxiety is particularly strong for alcohol. Individuals with a diagnosis of depression have a 16% (range 5–67%) prevalence of current alcohol misuse or a 30% (range 10–60%) prevalence of lifetime alcohol misuse disorder. Alcohol use is associated with worse outcomes in depression, including increased risk of suicide and death, poor social function, and reduced engagement with healthcare (Sullivan et al., 2005). Similarly, there is a 24% lifetime prevalence of alcohol dependence in individuals with an anxiety disorder, and among individuals seeking treatment for an alcohol use disorder, 23% meet the diagnostic criteria for social anxiety disorder (Morris et al., 2005).

The relationship between alcohol use disorder and depression or anxiety is complex and likely to be multifactorial. Psychiatric comorbidity, parental drug and alcohol use, and socio-economic factors are all risks for developing both alcohol dependence and mood disorders (Bonomo et al., 2004; Marmorstein, 2009; Rohde et al., 2001). Clinically, for all patients, a comprehensive history should be taken to understand their relationship, taking into account such factors. Many individuals misusing alcohol cite depression or anxiety as a reason for their drinking. However, many may not realize that alcohol withdrawal is commonly associated with symptoms of depression and anxiety and that these are contributing to their continued drinking. Studies have shown that these symptoms largely subside in the first few weeks of abstinence (Liappas et al., 2002). This is important information for patients and also for clinicians. A substance use history, particularly with regard to alcohol, should be obtained whenever a patient presents with symptoms of depression. Rather than an antidepressant, reducing or stopping drinking, alongside psychosocial support, is likely to result in improved mood.

Similar levels of complexity occur for other drugs of abuse. Depression is also commonly associated with stimulant misuse. Acutely, stimulants have effects that can be characterized as 'antidepressant', including euphoria, increased energy, improved

concentration, and rapid thinking. This period is followed by restlessness, hyperarousal, and insomnia during which users will commonly consume more of the stimulant substance to regain the 'rush'. When stimulant use stops, there is typically a 'crash' which consists of symptoms of hypersomnia, low energy, anxiety, and impaired concentration and cognition (Rounsaville, 2004). This period of depressive-like symptoms contributes to the difficulty in assessing depression in stimulant users in the first 3–5 days following abstinence, and can persist for a number of weeks, depending on the specific drug (McGregor et al., 2005). Such a reduction in mood is also seen for a few days following MDMA (3,4-methylenedioxymethamphetamine or Ecstasy) use, often described as the 'midweek blues' after use at the weekend. Individuals with stimulant dependence (including cocaine and meth/amphetamine) have a lifetime MDD prevalence of 32% (Kosten et al., 1998). While regular cannabis use has been reported to be associated with an increased risk of depression (Degenhardt et al., 2003), there is less of an association with anxiety (Kedzior and Laeber, 2014). A systematic review of longitudinal studies taking into account confounding factors also found that evidence for affective outcomes related to cannabis use was less strong than for psychosis (Moore et al., 2007).

From a neurobiological perspective, there are many features in common between depression and withdrawal in substance use, which likely underpins their overlapping presentations. These include lower dopaminergic function, increased kappa/dynorphin opioid function, and dysregulated serotonergic and stress system function (Green et al., 2003). Additionally, substance misuse is likely to be associated with depression and anxiety indirectly by influencing adverse life events, such as early school leaving and low income, which predispose to mood disorders (Degenhardt et al., 2003).

There have been more trials of comorbid substance use disorder and depression than any other comorbidity and these have been subjected to several meta-analyses (Nunes and Levin, 2004; Riper et al., 2014). Antidepressants are one of the most commonly prescribed medications to people with substance use disorders. However, their effectiveness is not established in improving either depression or substance use disorder. Nevertheless, individuals with substance misuse problems should be regularly assessed for depression and its associated risks, and treatment for depression should be started if symptoms are sufficiently severe or unremitting. Establishing a diagnosis of depression after at least a week of abstinence increases the likelihood of an antidepressant being effective, as individuals with time-limited withdrawal-related depressive symptoms will improve with abstinence without further intervention (Nunes and Levin, 2004). It may also be that serotonergic antidepressants are less effective than mixed antidepressants in improving depression (Nunes and Levin, 2004; Torrens et al., 2005). A reduction in substance use has been reported with antidepressants, but this appears to be neither a robust nor a substantial effect (Nunes and Levin, 2004).

As described earlier, any substance misuse disorder should be treated alongside any other psychiatric disorder. The mainstay of treatment for substance misuse is psychosocial, and a range of therapeutic approaches are available. The evidence is limited to support any specific approach for a particular substance, and typically polydrug use is the norm, so it is more important to focus on therapeutic engagement. Depending on the substance, medication may play an important adjunctive role. For instance, there are a range of medications available for relapse prevention in alcohol dependence,

Table 28.2 Effects of substance use

Drug	Acute effects–intoxication	Chronic effects	Withdrawal
Alcohol	Anxiolytic, sedative, disinhibition, argumentative, aggression, labile mood, impaired attention and judgement, unsteady gait, poor motor control, slurred speech; in severe cases, reduced consciousness to coma	Widespread physical impairments (e.g. liver, cardiac, neurological), psychiatric consequences (e.g. depression, anxiety), cognitive impairment, alcohol-related brain disorder, Korsakoff syndrome (see Box 28.1)	Tremor, shaking, sweating, nausea, psychomotor agitation, insomnia; in severe cases, seizures and delirium tremens
Opioids	Apathy, sedation, disinhibition, psychomotor retardation, impaired attention and judgement, slurred speech, pupillary restriction, drowsiness; in severe cases, reduced consciousness with respiratory depression to coma	Mainly related to physical consequences; few psychiatric consequences, though often associated with depressive disorders	Rhinorrhoea, lacrimation, muscle aches or cramps, abdominal pains, nausea/vomiting, diarrhoea, pupillary dilatation, piloerection (goosebumps), yawning, insomnia
Cannabis	Euphoria, disinhibition, increased appetite, tachycardia, anxiety, agitation, paranoia, altered sense of time, impaired attention and judgement, auditory, visual, and tactile hallucinations, depersonalization, derealization	Chronic intoxication can result in prolonged periods of apathy or amotivational syndrome, which mimics depression; recent evidence suggests increased risk of psychosis, schizophrenia, and possibly cognitive impairment	Anxiety, irritability, tremor of outstretched hands, sweating, muscle aches
Benzodiazepines and other sedatives/hypnotics	Euphoria, apathy, aggression, labile mood, impaired attention, anterograde amnesia, impaired psychomotor performance, unsteady gait, slurred speech, sedation to coma	Uncertain; dysphoria, dysthymia, and insomnia described	Tremor of outstretched hands, nausea/vomiting, tachycardia, postural hypotension, psychomotor agitation, headache, insomnia; in severe cases, transient visual, tactile, or auditory hallucinations, paranoia, seizures
Cocaine	Euphoria, increased energy, hypervigilance, grandiose beliefs, aggression, labile mood, repetitive stereotyped behaviours, auditory, visual, or tactile illusions, paranoia, tachycardia, cardiac arrhythmias, hypertension, sweating, chest pain, pupillary dilatation, psychomotor agitation, weight loss; physical effects include cardiomyopathy, cerebrovascular effects (stroke, haemorrhage), and seizures	Physical effects include cardiomyopathy, cerebrovascular effects (stroke), and weight loss; depressive disorder	Dysphoric mood, anhedonia, lethargy/fatigue, psychomotor retardation or agitation, craving, increased appetite, insomnia or hypersomnia, bizarre or unpleasant dreams
Amphetamines	As for cocaine	As for cocaine	As for cocaine
Ecstasy	Physical effects include anorexia, tachycardia, bruxism, and sweating; hyperthermia, cardiac arrhythmias, and cerebral haemorrhage reported; associated with fatal water intoxication	Concerns that long-term use may result in depression and cognitive impairment	Low mood about 3 days after use ('midweek blues')
LSD	Visual and auditory pseudohallucinations, distortion of sense of time, adverse emotional reactions including fear, anxiety, depression, and paranoia, tachycardia, palpitations, impulsive acts, impaired attention, pupillary dilatation, tremor	Flashbacks; anxiety and depression	None recognized
'Magic mushrooms'	Experience similar to LSD, but milder	Flashbacks possible	
Solvents	Effects similar to drunkenness; delusions, hallucinations, moodiness, convulsions, coma; sudden death can result from airway occlusion and sensitization of the myocardium	Chronic damage to heart, lungs, bone marrow, kidneys, liver; neurological toxicity (e.g. ataxia, neuropathy); cognitive impairment	Unclear
Nitrites	Raised blood pressure, dizziness, headache, and nausea; myocardial infarction possible; raised intraocular pressure	Ulceration around nose and mouth	
Ketamine	Alters perception; euphoria and hallucinations described; nausea and muscle spasms may occur	Sparse literature; flashbacks may occur	
GHB	Euphoria, relaxation, increased sociability and loss of inhibition; has been used as a 'date-rape' drug; can lead to dizziness, blurred vision, hot/cold flushes, excess sweating, confusion, vomiting, loss of consciousness, tremors, blackouts and memory lapses, seizures, agitation, and death	Unclear	Insomnia, anxiety, tremor, confusion, delirium, hallucinations, tachycardia, hypertension, nausea, vomiting, and sweating

Table 28.2 Continued

Drug	Acute effects–intoxication	Chronic effects	Withdrawal
PCP	Hallucinations, altered perception, euphoria or depression, anxiety, paranoia, delirium; respiratory/cardiac failure (rare)	Memory loss, speech difficulties, depression, and weight loss reported	
Khat	Stimulant	Psychological dependence, dental caries and oral cancer; regular use can lead to insomnia, anxiety, and anorexia; users can feel depressed or low if they do not keep taking the drug; rarely, associated with psychosis	

including naltrexone, acamprosate, and disulfiram (Lingford-Hughes et al., 2012). One study has reported that in individuals with alcohol dependence and depression, using an antidepressant and a relapse prevention medication (such as naltrexone) over either drug alone may be the optimal approach in improving both conditions (Petrakis et al., 2012). In opioid dependence, engagement and stabilization with opioid substitution treatment have been shown to result in improved depression, whereas antidepressants have not been shown to have such an effect (Ngo et al., 2011; Nunes et al., 2004). This underlines clinical advice about appropriate prescribing of antidepressants. Higher methadone maintenance doses may be required in patients with depression due to a direct effect of opioid agonism on the reward pathway, as well as the secondary consequences on their chaotic lifestyle (Tenore, 2008). There may be advantages of buprenorphine over methadone in treating depressed opioid addicts due to its kappa antagonism, but this has not been shown consistently (Dean et al., 2004; Gerra et al., 2006).

For other drugs of abuse, there have been fewer studies investigating the management of individuals with comorbid mood disorders. Clinically it is appropriate to focus on supporting the individual to reduce or stop their drug use to improve their mood, and for most remaining drugs of abuse, this will involve psychological approaches (Lingford-Hughes et al., 2012). As described earlier, depressive symptoms will substantially improve for many individuals with this approach, while antidepressants may not work. For instance, managing the mood disorder with standard pharmacological and non-pharmacological treatment may, in turn, lead to a reduction in cannabis use (Baker et al., 2010).

Less is known about optimal management of comorbid anxiety disorder and substance misuse. However, the same approach as for depression can be applied. In PTSD, naltrexone has been shown to reduce drinking in those with comorbid alcohol use disorder (Foa et al., 2013; Petrakis et al., 2012). Importantly, concomitant exposure therapy did not result in exacerbation of drinking.

Bipolar disorder

Bipolar disorder is commonly associated with comorbid substance use disorders. This is particularly evident for alcohol use disorder, with a current diagnosis prevalence of 23.6% and a lifetime prevalence of 58% (Grant et al., 2005). A history of comorbid alcoholism and bipolar disorder is associated with poor outcomes such as occupational status and increased hospitalization (Strakowski et al., 2000). Additionally, comorbid bipolar disorder and drug and

alcohol abuse increase the risk of attempted suicide, although the underpinning mechanisms are not clear (Hawton et al., 2005).

The prevalence range of opiate misuse in bipolar disorder is 3.2–20% (Cassidy et al., 2001) and the prevalence of bipolar disorder in individuals with opiate misuse is 5.4% (Salloum and Thase, 2000). The causality of this relationship is unclear, but the positive mood effects of opiates may contribute to the precipitation of a manic episode (Schaffer et al., 2007). Individuals with a diagnosis of bipolar disorder have increased rates of cannabis use, and there is evidence of cannabis use inducing and exacerbating manic symptoms, although the evidence is limited to a small number of studies with variable quality (Gibbs et al., 2015). Knowledge about the common neurobiology of bipolar and substance use disorders is limited. However, it is interesting that both disorders are associated with higher levels of impulsivity (Strakowski et al., 2010).

There is currently limited evidence to guide clinical practice. Pharmacological approaches for treating bipolar disorder appear to be effective in patients with comorbid substance misuse or dependence. There is evidence that lithium alone may not be as effective as other mood stabilizers (Brown et al., 2003; Brown et al., 2006). As for other psychiatric disorders, appropriate pharmacological and psychological approaches targeted at substance misuse should be applied, alongside management of their bipolar disorder (Lingford-Hughes et al., 2012). Due to the possibility of substances of misuse precipitating or prolonging a manic episode, patients may require medical support during withdrawal, and in particular, medically assisted detoxification from alcohol may be required.

Psychosis

Many drugs of abuse are implicated with psychosis, including alcohol, amphetamine, cannabis, cocaine, hallucinogens, ketamine, and opioids. The link between these and psychosis is more frequently seen in some individuals than others. The diagnostic uncertainty attributing the cause to substance misuse or an underlying psychosis can be challenging in clinical practice. The lack of an objective test clinically available for many substances of abuse, such as the so-called 'novel psychoactive substances', adds further to the challenge. The nature of symptoms varies, depending on the individual, the drug(s) used, the dose, and underlying susceptibilities to the effects of the drug. When dealing with suspected drug-induced psychosis, it is necessary to establish a chronology of substance

Box 28.1 Complications of, and associations with, alcohol misuse

Physical complications

Cardiovascular
- Arrhythmias
- Hypertension
- Cerebrovascular disease
- Coronary heart disease
- Alcoholic cardiomyopathy

Neurological
- Seizures
- Neuropathy
- Marchiafava–Bignami syndrome
- Central pontine myelinosis
- Alcoholic cerebellar degeneration

Gastrointestinal
- Alcoholic liver disease—fatty liver, alcoholic hepatitis, cirrhosis
- Pancreatitis
- Gastric and peptic ulceration
- Mallory–Weiss syndrome

Musculoskeletal
- Gout
- Osteoporosis
- Avascular necrosis
- Acute and chronic skeletal muscle myopathy

Endocrine
- Alcohol-induced pseudo-Cushing's syndrome
- Male hypogonadism
- Increased risk of infertility
- Diabetes

Cancer
- Increased risk of oropharyngeal, laryngeal, oesophageal, liver, breast, and colorectal cancer

Respiratory
- Immune suppression and self-neglect leading to greater incidence of lower respiratory tract infections
- Inhalation of vomit while in stupor may result in pneumonia, with bronchiectasis as a possible sequela

Metabolic
- Hypoglycaemia

Skin
- Psoriasis
- Discoid eczema
- Rosacea

Neuropsychiatric complications
- Transient hallucinatory experiences
- Alcoholic hallucinosis
- Wernicke–Korsakoff's syndrome
- Alcoholic dementia
- Delirium tremens

Comorbid disorders
- Depression
- Anxiety
- Post-traumatic stress disorder
- Psychotic disorders (e.g. schizophrenia)
- Bipolar disorder
- Personality disorder
- Eating disorders
- Other substance abuse

misuse, whether psychosis is occurring during intoxication or withdrawal, as well as the nature of the symptoms, since this will guide the clinician as to which drug may be involved if the patient is unable to say or does not know. The risk associated with their psychosis such as suicide or violence must be ascertained and appropriately managed. It is important to undertake a thorough physical and mental health review to ensure other causes of delirium and other organic illnesses have been ruled out. Treatment should be tailored to the nature of the drug involved; for example, psychotic symptoms associated with alcohol withdrawal (see earlier) is an emergency and should be treated. For more enduring psychotic symptoms, consider the use of dopamine receptor antagonists such as olanzapine.

A proportion of individuals with an underlying psychotic illness misuse drugs, and this can lead to exacerbation of the illness, non-compliance with treatment, and a change in the course of the illness. This is particularly the case in younger users with an early or prodromal psychotic illness (Fiorentini et al., 2011). There are wide variations in reported rates of comorbid substance misuse with psychosis globally, with reports of between 20% and 37% in mental health settings in the UK (Carrà and Johnson, 2009). Up to 5% of individuals presenting with a first episode of psychosis are reported to have substance- or medication-induced psychotic disorder in community settings (Kirkbride et al., 2016). Studies in the United States reported considerably higher estimates, with comorbid substance misuse in 25% of all psychoses overall (American Psychiatric Association, 2013).

Clinically it is important and necessary to identify a clear timeline of the start and progression of the psychotic illness and a chronology of substance misuse; otherwise diagnosis may be difficult. This particularly applies to determining whether the individual has a psychotic disorder independent of their drug misuse. Diagnostic criteria for drug-induced psychosis (DSM and ICD) set time limits. Thus, ICD-10 requires the onset of psychotic symptoms during or within 2 weeks of substance use, that there should be persistence of the psychotic symptoms for >48 hours, and that duration of the disorder should not exceed 6 months. DSM-5 requires that either delusions and/or hallucinations developed during or soon after substance intoxication or withdrawal, and that the substance is capable of producing these symptoms, which are not better explained by a psychotic disorder (American Psychiatric Association, 2013). Further, care should be taken to ensure that these symptoms are not the result of a delirium or other organic causes in all cases.

Alcohol can cause psychosis both acutely during withdrawal as part of delirium tremens, and chronically referred to as alcohol-induced psychotic disorder. Alcohol-induced psychotic disorder is a severe mental illness with poor outcomes such as premature death, with 37% mortality over 8 years, particularly when associated with delirium tremens (Perälä et al., 2010). It has been reported in an inpatient study that up to 3% of patients with alcohol dependence have psychotic symptoms, and of these, approximately a third have alcohol-induced psychotic disorder (Jordaan and Emsley, 2014; Soyka et al., 1988). Clinical features of alcohol-induced psychotic disorder include auditory hallucinations that are often derogatory, persecutory delusions, usually in clear consciousness, and no formal thought disorder (Babor et al., 2015; Jordaan and Emsley, 2014; Soyka et al., 1988).

If not during withdrawal, psychotic symptoms usually occur within a month of intoxication or withdrawal and the patient often is fully orientated and lacks insight that these are alcohol-induced (Babor et al., 2015). Usually these symptoms settle within a few weeks of abstinence, but for others, symptoms become chronic and enduring, a condition also known as alcoholic hallucinosis.

It is important to distinguish alcohol-induced psychotic disorder from schizophrenia. One study showed patients with alcohol-induced psychotic disorder had a significantly lower educational level, later onset of psychosis, higher levels of depressive and anxiety symptoms, fewer negative and disorganized symptoms, better insight and judgement, and less functional impairment, compared to patients with schizophrenia (Jordaan et al., 2009).

Patients with alcohol-induced psychotic disorder often require hospitalization, and treatment is usually with various dopamine receptor antagonist medications. However, there is a paucity of trials and only sporadic case reports comparing the efficacy of each (Jordaan and Emsley, 2014).

The underlying mechanism of how alcohol causes psychosis is unclear, with evidence implicating various mechanisms involving dopamine, 5HT, or GABA (Jordaan and Emsley, 2014). Magnetic resonance neuroimaging studies have shown significant increases in cerebral blood flow to the right calcarine area in alcohol-induced psychotic disorder, compared to healthy volunteers (Jordaan et al., 2010).

Given the ability of stimulants to directly increase dopamine levels, the association with psychosis is unsurprising and likely precipitated acutely by such an increase (Segal and Kuczenski, 1997). Nevertheless, despite this commonality, there are some differences in associated psychotic presentations between the different stimulants. Amphetamine and methamphetamine psychosis has been reported in a wide range (8–46%) of regular users (Bramness et al., 2012; Glasner-Edwards et al., 2008). Clinical features of methamphetamine-induced psychotic disorder are similar to those of paranoid schizophrenia—namely delusions, ideas of reference, and auditory hallucinations, with most symptoms resolving within days or hours of methamphetamine use (Glasner-Edwards et al., 2008; McKetin et al., 2006; Zweben et al., 2004). Symptoms during acute intoxication may be indistinguishable from those of schizophrenia, with only a positive urine drug screen aiding the differential diagnosis (Kaplan and Sadock, 2000). It appears that methamphetamine-induced psychosis may be more enduring than that induced by amphetamine.

There is an increased risk of psychosis in people who use amphetamine who have had previous episodes of amphetamine-induced psychosis and who have an underlying psychotic illness such as schizophrenia (Bramness et al., 2012). There is limited evidence investigating comparative treatments in this group. However,

dopamine receptor antagonists are widely used. Similarly, cocaine can induce a range of psychotic symptoms, most commonly transient paranoia and paranoid delusions in 68–84% of cocaine users (Morton, 1999; Roncero et al., 2013), followed by auditory hallucinations. Formication and stereotyped behaviours, such as picking, along with hypersexuality, have also been associated with cocaine use and intoxication (McClung and Hirsh, 1998; Segal and Kuczenski, 1997). Cocaine-induced psychosis has been associated with greater addiction severity, agitated behaviour, and aggression (Bartlett et al., 1997; Roncero et al., 2014). Those with cocaine-induced psychotic disorder are more likely to be male and have a low BMI and a longer duration of cocaine use with intravenous cocaine (Tang et al., 2014).

There is limited information on the treatment of stimulant-induced psychosis. However, symptoms are usually self-limiting and resolve 3–5 days after cessation of use. Benzodiazepines for associated agitation and dopamine receptor antagonists may be helpful, but there are no specific studies looking at treatment for psychosis, only for treating dependence (Amato et al., 2007; Tang et al., 2014).

Cannabis is one of the most frequently used drugs in most areas of the world, with 20% of young people using it at least weekly (Moore et al., 2007). Current evidence is largely based on cannabis use as an 'illicit' drug. However, recent changes in its legal status and growing use of prescribed cannabis may result in some differences in the associations described. Cannabis can lead to acute transient psychotic episodes during intoxication, persistent psychosis after acute intoxication, and persistent psychosis that is not time-related to use. For example, use in adolescence could increase the relative risk for schizophrenia in adulthood by up to 3 times (D'Souza et al., 2016). There is evidence from multiple studies that regular or heavy cannabis use increases the risk of developing psychotic disorders which persist beyond the half-life of cannabinoids, where if the link was causal, it would mean a lifetime risk of developing schizophrenia of 2% among regular cannabis users (Gage et al., 2016; Moore et al., 2007).

The association of endocannabinoids and psychosis is complex (van Amsterdam et al., 2015). RCTs indicate that delta-9-tetrahydrocannabinol (THC), an agonist at CB1/2 receptors, is the likely active ingredient causing psychosis in pre-clinical and clinical studies (Gage et al., 2016; van Amsterdam et al., 2015). The other active ingredient cannabidiol (CBD) has antipsychotic properties. Various studies have shown that cannabis containing higher THC:CBD ratios results in a greater risk of psychotic outcomes (Iseger and Bossong, 2015; Morgan et al., 2012).

In addition to cannabis, there are over 200 synthetic cannabinoid receptor agonists (SRCAs) such as 'Spice' and 'Black Mamba'. These synthetic compounds have higher affinity for the CB1 receptor than THC, resulting in higher rates of psychosis during intoxication, compared to cannabis. Not all may be detectable by urine drug screens and have gained popularity as a result (Novel Psychoactive Treatment UK Network, 2015). It has been reported that psychosis associated with SRCAs is frequently more agitated and could be related to the sympathomimetic effects of full CB1 agonism. Clinicians should have a low threshold when suspecting toxicity since medical care may be needed due to the possibility of seizures and tachycardia (Novel Psychoactive Treatment UK Network, 2015). While cannabis intoxication is likely to result in transient paranoid ideation (Kaplan and Sadock, 2000), SCRAs are more commonly associated with psychosis (Gunderson et al., 2012).

There is limited evidence investigating comparative treatments for cannabis-induced psychotic disorder. However, dopamine receptor antagonists are widely used. One study of cannabinoid receptor antagonists was discontinued due to side effects, and it is not known whether other antagonists would do the same (Lingford-Hughes et al., 2012).

Hallucinogen persisting perception disorder (HPPD) occurs following cessation of use of a hallucinogen or re-experiencing one or more of the perceptual symptoms that were experienced while intoxicated (American Psychiatric Association, 2013). Prevalence estimates are not known, but initial estimates suggest it is around 4–5% of individuals who use hallucinogens (Abraham et al., 1996). HPPD occurs most frequently after LSD use. However, no correlation with the number of occasions of hallucinogen use has been found.

The mechanisms underpinning hallucinogen-induced psychosis and HPPD are unclear, but it has been suggested that it may arise from excitotoxic destruction of serotonergic inhibitory interneurons at the soma and GABAergic interneurons at the terminals (Abraham and Aldridge, 1993).

Clinically evidence from 20 studies on HPPD showed that what is classified as 'flashbacks' associated with hallucinogen use may also include psychosis, mood changes, panic attacks, depersonalization, dissociation, and experiences of transcendence (Halpern and Pope, 2003). LSD-induced psychosis appears to resemble schizoaffective disorder with visual hallucinations (Abraham et al., 1996). Unlike non-drug-related psychosis, no paranoid misinterpretations of perceptions have been reported in people who have HPPD (Novel Psychoactive Treatment UK Network, 2015).

There are no established treatments for HPPD (Novel Psychoactive Treatment UK Network, 2015). Haloperidol was shown to reduce symptoms. However, it exacerbated flashbacks. In a review of 75 cases of post-LSD psychosis, ECT and lithium were found to be the most effective treatment (Abraham et al., 1996). However, there was significant heterogeneity between these cases, and the last of these studies were in 1983.

There is little evidence linking chronic and heavy use of ketamine and a psychotic disorder. However, it has been used as a pharmacological model of schizophrenia due to its psychosis-like effects in intoxication (Morgan and Curran, 2012). Clinically, daily ketamine use showed a similar pattern of symptoms of prodromal schizophrenia (Morgan et al., 2010). Daily ketamine users scored higher on measures of delusions, dissociation, and schizotypy, compared to infrequent users and polydrug users who do not use ketamine (Curran and Morgan, 2000; Morgan et al., 2010). Ketamine has also been shown to cause a resurgence in psychotic symptoms in stable schizophrenic patients on antipsychotic medication (Lahti et al., 1995). Repeated doses of ketamine in animal models cause abnormal hippocampal neurogenesis and reductions in hippocampal parvalbumin-containing GABAergic interneurons, consistent with 'schizophrenia-like' changes (Keilhoff et al., 2004).

Opiate-induced psychosis is rare, and if present, organic causes must be ruled out (Maremmani et al., 2014). It has been described during ultrarapid opiate detoxification with buprenorphine and also during methadone withdrawal (Weibel et al., 2012); symptoms remit on reintroduction of the opiate substitute medication. Clinically the presentation of opiate withdrawal psychosis has been

commonly characterized by auditory hallucinations and mystical and paranoid delusions during withdrawal.

Catatonia

Catatonia is a motor dysregulation syndrome characterized by a marked inability to move normally. This may be in the context drugs of abuse. However, it is more likely in the context of underlying other psychiatric or general medical disorders. The term catatonia within psychiatry is used to specify a subtype of the underlying illness, rather than a diagnostic entity in itself (American Psychiatric Association, 2013; Fink et al., 2010). Features of catatonia may include mutism, stupor, negativism, posturing, waxy flexibility, stereotypy, automatic obedience, ambitendency, echo phenomena, and mannerisms. Forms of catatonia may include retarded, excited, malignant, and periodic (Fink et al., 2010).

The exact mechanisms causing catatonia are generally not known. However, GABA and dopamine systems have been implicated since benzodiazepines can ameliorate symptoms and dopamine antagonism or depletion may result in motor and autonomic symptoms of catatonia (Brown and Freeman, 2009). There is a paucity of evidence regarding catatonia associated with drugs of abuse, and most is based on case reports.

Catatonia has been described in four clinical case reports during alcohol withdrawal. In some cases, catatonia was difficult to identify due to other predominant symptoms of withdrawal. Also, cessation of benzodiazepines after alcohol detox has precipitated catatonia. Catatonia associated with benzodiazepine withdrawal per se has also been seen but is believed to be rare. Clonazepam withdrawal-induced catatonia has been described in the literature to ameliorate on reinstatement of lorazepam in one case report (Brown and Freeman, 2009). Further cases have been described that support this (Rosebush and Mazurek, 2010). Post-ictal delirium with catatonia occurring after benzodiazepine withdrawal has been described in a case series ($n = 3$) of patients with seizure disorders (Hauser et al., 1989).

Early gamma-hydroxybutyric acid (GHB) withdrawal syndrome resembles alcohol withdrawal associated with autonomic instability, tremor, anxiety, restlessness, nausea, vomiting, and insomnia. This can progress to delirium, hallucinations, and seizures. Cases of GHB withdrawal causing catatonia have been described (Claussen et al., 2014). GHB withdrawal may continue for up to 21 days and can be life-threatening, but treatment with benzodiazepines and baclofen is usually effective (Schep et al., 2012). More severe withdrawal and delirium are seen when GHB is used every 1–8 hours and it is suggested it is as a result of decreased GABA inhibition (van Noorden et al., 2009).

Catatonia associated with synthetic cannabinoids has recently been described in two patients with no previous psychosis. Both patients had catatonic states after chronic, persistent high-dose synthetic cannabinoid use. With abstinence and treatment with benzodiazepines, symptoms rapidly resolved (Khan et al., 2016).

Cocaine use has been associated with stroke. This is the main differential to consider for catatonia in the context of cocaine use. In particular, cocaine use should be considered in younger patients with catatonia and stroke who lack other vascular risk factors (Treadwell and Robinson, 2007).

When presented with suspected drug-induced catatonia, it is necessary to establish the history and chronology of the catatonia and associated neurological symptoms, including the ability of the person to eat and drink. The Bush–Francis Catatonia Rating Scale could be used (Bush et al., 1996). In addition to substance misuse history, medication history should also be obtained. The patient's state of intoxication, withdrawal, or neither should also be established.

A thorough physical (including full neurological) examination should be carried out with investigations, including bloods and urine drug screen, and other causes of delirium ruled out. Malignant catatonia may be associated with raised creatine kinase. Other possible differential diagnoses include NMS, serotonin syndrome, malignant hyperthermia, akinetic mutism, status epilepticus, locked-in syndrome, stiff person syndrome, Parkinson's disease, stroke, and elective mutism (Coffey, 2016). Treatment is generally supportive with benzodiazepines.

Conclusion

Substance misuse may result in a wide range of neuropsychiatric complications. Clinical suspicion of the involvement of substance misuse in psychiatric presentations needs to be high to prevent inappropriate management and enduring adverse consequences. While many presentations commonly seen in clinical practice are with depression or psychosis, rarer presentations can arise but nonetheless are important to recognize and appropriately manage.

KEY LEARNING POINTS

- Neurobiology of addiction:
  - Different substances of abuse have a variety of pharmacological actions on the brain through a range of neurotransmission systems, including dopamine, GABA, and opioid.
  - The pharmacological actions of substances of abuse are important in understanding the acute effects of these drugs and the subsequent neuroadaptation that leads to tolerance and withdrawal symptoms.
  - Substances of abuse have a common effect modulating the mesolimbic dopaminergic pathway, though to varying degrees, and also cause adaptive changes in other neuronal systems such as those important in stress, reward, and impulsivity.
- Mood disorders:
  - There is a strong association between mood disorders and substance abuse and misuse, and it is important to take a clear substance misuse history in all patients presenting with a mood disorder.
  - Substance misuse and mood disorders should be treated in parallel, and improvement in one condition will likely lead to improvement in the other.
  - Antidepressants are not established to improve depression or reduce substance use in individuals with substance addiction. Often engagement in an effective treatment programme for substance misuse/dependence and a reduction in substance use are effective at reducing depression.

- There is evidence of increased effectiveness of antidepressants when used in conjunction with relapse prevention medication at improving depression than either medication alone.
  - Pharmacological treatments for bipolar disorder are effective in individuals with comorbid substance misuse or dependence. Effective treatment for substance misuse problems should be applied alongside treatment for bipolar disorder.
- Psychosis:
  - Many drugs of abuse are implicated in psychosis, and attributing the cause to substance misuse or an underlying psychosis can be challenging in clinical practice.
  - The nature of symptoms varies, depending on the individual, the drug(s) used, the dose, and underlying susceptibilities to the effects of the drug.
  - When dealing with suspected drug-induced psychosis, it is necessary to establish a chronology of substance misuse, whether it is occurring during intoxication or withdrawal, as well as the nature of the symptoms, since this will guide the clinician as to which drug may be involved if the patient is unable to say or does not know.
  - The risk associated with a patient's psychosis, such as suicide and violence, must be ascertained and appropriately managed.
  - It is important to undertake a thorough physical and mental health review to ensure other causes of delirium and other organic illnesses have been ruled out.
  - Treatment should be tailored to the nature of the drug involved; for example, psychotic symptoms associated with alcohol withdrawal are a medical emergency (delirium tremens) and, as such, should be treated. For more enduring psychotic symptoms, consider the use of dopamine receptor antagonists.
- Catatonia:
  - Catatonia has been associated with substance misuse but is rare.
  - When presented with suspected drug-induced catatonia, it is necessary to establish the history and chronology of the catatonia and associated neurological symptoms, including the ability of the person to eat and drink; consider using the Bush–Francis scale.
  - A thorough physical (including full neurology) examination should be carried out with bloods and urine drug screen, and other causes of delirium and stroke should be ruled out.
  - Treatment is generally with benzodiazepines.

REFERENCES

Abraham, H.D. & Aldridge, A.M., 1993. Adverse consequences of lysergic acid diethylamide. *Addiction*, 88(10), pp.1327–34.

Abraham, H.D., Aldridge, A.M. & Gogia, P., 1996. The psychopharmacology of hallucinogens. *Neuropsychopharmacology*, 14(4), pp.285–98.

Alvanzo, A.A.H. et al., 2017. Family history of alcoholism is related to increased D2 /D3 receptor binding potential: a marker of resilience or risk? *Addiction Biology*, 22, 218–28.

Amato, L. et al., 2007. Antipsychotic medications for cocaine dependence. In: L. Amato, ed. *Cochrane Database of Systematic Reviews*. Chichester: John Wiley & Sons, Ltd. Available at: http://doi.wiley.com/10.1002/14651858.CD006306.pub2.

American Psychiatric Association, 2013. *Diagnostic and Statistical Manual of Mental Disorders*. Available at: http://encore.llu.edu/iii/encore/record/C__Rb1280248__SDSM-V__P0,2__Orightresult__X3;jsessionid=ABB7428ECBC4BA66625EDD0E0C5AAFA5?lang=eng&suite=cobalt%5Cnhttp://books.google.com/books?id=EIbMlwEACAAJ&pgis=1.

van Amsterdam, J., Brunt, T. & van den Brink, W., 2015. The adverse health effects of synthetic cannabinoids with emphasis on psychosis-like effects. *Journal of Psychopharmacology*, 29(3), pp.254–63.

Babor, T.F., Hernandez-Avila, C.A. & Ungemack, J.A., 2015. Substance-Related Disorders: Alcohol-Related Disorders. *Psychiatry*, 8(3), pp.1401–33.

Badiani, A. et al., 2011. Opiate versus psychostimulant addiction: the differences do matter. *Nature Reviews Neuroscience*, 12(11), pp.685–700.

Baker, A.L., Hides, L. & Lubman, D.I., 2010. Treatment of Cannabis Use Among People With Psychotic or Depressive Disorders. *Journal of Clinical Psychiatry*, 71(3), pp.247–54.

Bartlett, E. et al., 1997. Selective sensitisation to the psychosis-inducing effects of cocaine: A possible marker for addiction relapse vulnerability? *Neuropsychopharmacology*, 16(1), pp.77–82.

Berridge, K.C. & Kringelbach, M.L., 2015. Pleasure Systems in the Brain. *Neuron*, 86(3), pp.646–64.

Bloomfield, M.A.P. et al., 2016. The effects of Δ9-tetrahydrocannabinol on the dopamine system. *Nature*, 539(7629), pp.369–77.

Bonomo, Y.A. et al., 2004. Teenage drinking and the onset of alcohol dependence: A cohort study over seven years. *Addiction*, 99(12), pp.1520–8.

Bramness, J.G. et al., 2012. Amphetamine-induced psychosis--a separate diagnostic entity or primary psychosis triggered in the vulnerable? *BMC Psychiatry*, 12, p.221.

Brown, E.S. et al., 2006. Lamotrigine for bipolar disorder and comorbid cocaine dependence: A replication and extension study. Journal of Affective Disorders, 93, pp.219–22.

Brown, E.S. et al., 2003. Lamotrigine in patients with bipolar disorder and cocaine dependence. *Journal of Clinical Psychiatry*, 64(2), pp.197–201.

Brown, M. & Freeman, S., 2009. Clonazepam withdrawal-induced catatonia. *Psychosomatics*, 50(3), pp.289–92.

Bush, G. et al., 1996. Catatonia. I. Rating scale and standardized examination. *Acta Psychiatrica Scandinavica*, 93(2), pp.129–36.

Carrà, G. & Johnson, S., 2009. Variations in rates of comorbid substance use in psychosis between mental health settings and geographical areas in the UK. *Social Psychiatry and Psychiatric Epidemiology*, 44(6), pp.429–47.

Cassidy, F., Ahearn, E.P. & Carroll, B.J., 2001. Substance abuse in bipolar disorder. *Bipolar Disorders*, 3(4), pp.181–8.

Claussen, M.C. et al., 2014. Catatonic stupor secondary to gamma-hydroxy-butyric acid (GHB) - dependence and withdrawal syndrome. *Psychiatria Danubina*, 26(4), pp.358–9.

Coffey, M., 2016. Catatonia in adults: Epidemiology, clinical features, assessment, and diagnosis. *UpToDate*. Available at: https://www.uptodate.com/contents/catatonia-in-adults-epidemiology-clinical-features-assessment-and-diagnosis?source=search_result&search=catatonia&selectedTitle=2~58#H6713738.

Curran, H. V & Morgan, C., 2000. Cognitive, dissociative and psychotogenic effects of ketamine in recreational users on the night of drug use and 3 days later. *Addiction*, 95(4), pp.575–90.

D'Souza, D.C. et al., 2016. Cannabinoids and Psychosis. *Current Pharmaceutical Design*. Available at: http://www.ncbi.nlm.nih.gov/pubmed/27568729.

Dean, A.J. et al., 2004. Depressive symptoms during buprenorphine vs. methadone maintenance: Findings from a randomised, controlled trial in opioid dependence. *European Psychiatry*, 19(8), pp.510–13.

Degenhardt, L., Hall, W. & Lynskey, M., 2003. Exploring the association between cannabis use and depression. *Addiction*, 98(11), pp.1493–504.

Everitt, B.J. & Robbins, T.W., 2005. Neural systems of reinforcement for drug addiction: from actions to habits to compulsion. *Nature Neuroscience*, 8(11), pp.1481–9.

Fink, M., Taylor, M.A. & En-, N., 2010. The Catatonia Syndrome. *Archives of General Psychiatry*, 66(11), pp.1173–7.

Fiorentini, A. et al., 2011. Substance-Induced Psychoses: A Critical Review of the Literature. *Current Drug Abuse Reviews*, 4(4), pp.228–40.

Foa, E.B. et al., 2013. Concurrent Naltrexone and Prolonged Exposure Therapy for Patients With Comorbid Alcohol Dependence and PTSD. *JAMA*, 310(5), p.488.

Gage, S.H., Hickman, M. & Zammit, S., 2016. Association between cannabis and psychosis: Epidemiologic evidence. *Biological Psychiatry*, 79(7), pp.549–6.

Gerra, G. et al., 2006. Buprenorphine treatment outcome in dually diagnosed heroin dependent patients: A retrospective study. *Prog Neuropsychopharmacol Biol Psychiatry*, 30(2), pp.265–72.

Gibbs, M. et al., 2015. Cannabis use and mania symptoms: a systematic review and meta-analysis. *Journal of Affective Disorders*, 171, pp.39–47.

Glasner-Edwards, S. et al., 2008. Clinical course and outcomes of methamphetamine-dependent adults with psychosis. *Journal of Substance Abuse Treatment*, 35, 445–50.

Grant, B.F. et al., 2005. Prevalence, correlates, and comorbidity of bipolar I disorder and axis I and II disorders: results from the National Epidemiologic Survey on Alcohol and Related Conditions. *Journal of Clinical Psychiatry*, 66(10), pp.1205–15.

Green, A.R. et al., 2003. The pharmacology and clinical pharmacology of 3,4-methylenedioxymethamphetamine (MDMA, 'ecstasy'). *Pharmacological Reviews*, 55(3), pp.463–508.

Gunderson, E.W. et al., 2012. 'Spice' and 'K2' herbal highs: a case series and systematic review of the clinical effects and biopsychosocial implications of synthetic cannabinoid use in humans. *American Journal on Addictions*, 21(4), pp.320–6.

Halpern, J.H. & Pope, H.G., 2003. Hallucinogen persisting perception disorder: What do we know after 50 years? *Drug and Alcohol Dependence*, 69(2), pp.109–19.

Hasin, D.S. & Grant, B.F., 2015. The National Epidemiologic Survey on Alcohol and Related Conditions (NESARC) Waves 1 and 2: review and summary of findings. *Social Psychiatry and Psychiatric Epidemiology*, 50(11), pp.1609–40.

Hauser, P. et al., 1989. Benzodiazepine withdrawal delirium with catatonic features. Occurrence in patients with partial seizure disorders. *Archives of Neurology*. Available at: http://archneur.jamanetwork.com/article.aspx?doi=10.1001/archneur.1989.00520420118033.

Hawton, K. et al., 2005. Suicide and attempted suicide in bipolar disorder: a systematic review of risk factors. *Journal of Clinical Psychiatry*, 66, pp.693–704.

Hunt, S.A. et al., 2015. Systematic review of neurocognition in people with co-occurring alcohol misuse and depression. *Journal of Affective Disorders*, 179, pp.51–64.

Iseger, T.A. & Bossong, M.G., 2015. A systematic review of the antipsychotic properties of cannabidiol in humans. *Schizophrenia Research*, 162(1), pp.153–61.

Jordaan, G.P. et al., 2009. Alcohol-induced psychotic disorder: a comparative study on the clinical characteristics of patients with alcohol dependence and schizophrenia. *Journal of Studies on Alcohol and Drugs*, 70(6), pp.870–6.

Jordaan, G.P. et al., 2010. Resting brain perfusion in alcohol-induced psychotic disorder: A comparison in patients with alcohol dependence, schizophrenia and healthy controls. *Progress in Neuro-Psychopharmacology and Biological Psychiatry*, 34(3), pp.479–85.

Jordaan, G.P. & Emsley, R., 2014. Alcohol-induced psychotic disorder: a review. *Metabolic Brain Disease*, 29(2), pp.231–43.

Kaplan, H.I. & Sadock, B.J., 2000. *Kaplan & Sadock's Comprehensive Textbook of Psychiatry*. Available at: http://www.amazon.co.uk/Sadocks-Comprehensive-Textbook-Psychiatry-Saddocks/dp/0781768993.

Kedzior, K.K. & Laeber, L.T., 2014. A positive association between anxiety disorders and cannabis use or cannabis use disorders in the general population- a meta-analysis of 31 studies. *BMC Psychiatry*, 14(1), pp.136.

Keilhoff, G. et al., 2004. Increased neurogenesis in a rat ketamine model of schizophrenia. *Biological Psychiatry*, 56(5), pp.317–22.

Khan, M. et al., 2016. Catatonia secondary to synthetic cannabinoid use in two patients with no previous psychosis. *American Journal on Addictions*, 25(1), pp.25–7.

Kirkbride, J.B. et al., 2016. The Epidemiology of First-Episode Psychosis in Early Intervention in Psychosis Services: Findings From the Social Epidemiology of Psychoses in East Anglia [SEPEA] Study. *American Journal of Psychiatry*. Available at: http://ajp.psychiatryonline.org/doi/10.1176/appi.ajp.2016.16010103.

Koob, G.F. & Volkow, N.D., 2016. Neurobiology of addiction: a neurocircuitry analysis. *The Lancet Psychiatry*, 3(8), pp.760–73.

Kosten, T.R., Markou, A. & Koob, G.F., 1998. Depression and stimulant dependence: neurobiology and pharmacotherapy. *Journal of Nervous and Mental Disease*, 186(12), pp.737–45.

Lahti, A.C. et al., 1995. Subanesthetic doses of ketamine stimulate psychosis in schizophrenia. *Neuropsychopharmacology*, 13(1), pp.9–19.

Leyton, M. et al., 2002. Amphetamine-Induced Increases in Extracellular Dopamine, Drug Wanting, and Novelty Seeking A PET/[11C]Raclopride Study in Healthy Men. *Neuropsychopharmacology*, 27(6), pp.1027–35.

Li, D. et al., 2014. Association of Gamma-Aminobutyric Acid A Receptor α2 Gene (GABRA2) with Alcohol Use Disorder. *Neuropsychopharmacology*, 39(4), pp.907–18.

Liappas, J. et al., 2002. Impact of alcohol detoxification on anxiety and depressive symptoms. *Drug and Alcohol Dependence*, 68(2), pp.215–20.

Lingford-Hughes, A. et al., 2012. BAP updated guidelines: evidence-based guidelines for the pharmacological management of substance abuse, harmful use, addiction and comorbidity: recommendations from BAP. *Journal of Psychopharmacology*, 26(7), pp.899–952.

Maremmani, A.G.I. et al., 2014. Substance abuse and psychosis. The strange case of opioids. *European Review for Medical and Pharmacological Sciences*, 18(3), pp.287–302.

Marmorstein, N.R., 2009. Longitudinal associations between alcohol problems and depressive symptoms: Early adolescence through early adulthood. *Alcoholism: Clinical and Experimental Research*, 33(1), pp.49–59.

Martinez, D. et al., 2011. Imaging Dopamine Transmission in Cocaine Dependence: Link Between Neurochemistry and Response to Treatment. *American Journal of Psychiatry*, 168(6), pp.634–41.

McClung, C. & Hirsh, J., 1998. Stereotypic behavioral responses to free-base cocaine and the development of behavioral sensitization in *Drosophila*. *Current Biology*, 8(2), pp.109–12

McGregor, C. et al., 2005. The nature, time course and severity of methamphetamine withdrawal. *Addiction*, 100(9), pp.1320–9.

McKetin, R. et al., 2006. The prevalence of psychotic symptoms among methamphetamine users. *Addiction*, 101(10), pp.1473–8.

Moore, T.H.M. et al., 2007. Cannabis use and risk of psychotic or affective mental health outcomes: a systematic review. *The Lancet*, 370, pp.319–28.

Morgan, C.J.A. et al., 2012. Sub-chronic impact of cannabinoids in street cannabis on cognition, psychotic-like symptoms and psychological well-being. *Psychological Medicine*, 42(2), pp.391–400.

Morgan, C.J.A. & Curran, H.V., 2012. Ketamine use: a review. *Addiction*, 107(1), pp.27–38.

Morgan, C.J.A., Muetzelfeldt, L. & Curran, H.V., 2010. Consequences of chronic ketamine self-administration upon neurocognitive function and psychological wellbeing: a 1-year longitudinal study. *Addiction*, 105(1), pp.121–33.

Morris, E.P., Stewart, S.H. & Ham, L.S., 2005. The relationship between social anxiety disorder and alcohol use disorders: A critical review. *Clinical Psychology Review*, 25(6), pp.734–60.

Morton, W.A., 1999. Cocaine and Psychiatric Symptoms. *Primary Care Companion to the Journal of Clinical Psychiatry*, 1(4), pp.109–13.

Ngo, H.T., Tait, R.J. & Hulse, G.K., 2011. Hospital psychiatric comorbidity and its role in heroin dependence treatment outcomes using naltrexone implant or methadone maintenance. *Journal of Psychopharmacology*, 25(6), pp.774–82.

Novel Psychoactive Treatment UK Network, 2015. *NEPTUNE Guidance on the Clinical Management of Acute and Chronic Harms of Club Drugs and Novel Psychoactive Substances*. Available at: http://www.drugsandalcohol.ie/24292/.

Nunes, E.V. & Levin, F.R., 2004. Treatment of Depression in Patients With Alcohol or Other Drug Dependence. *JAMA*, 291(15), p.1887.

Nunes, E. V., Sullivan, M.A. & Levin, F.R., 2004. Treatment of depression in patients with opiate dependence. *Biological Psychiatry*, 56(10), pp.793–802.

Nutt, D.J. et al., 2015. The dopamine theory of addiction: 40 years of highs and lows. *Nature Reviews Neuroscience*. Available at: http://www.nature.com/doifinder/10.1038/nrn3939.

Perälä, J. et al., 2010. Alcohol-induced psychotic disorder and delirium in the general population. *British Journal of Psychiatry*, 197(3), 200–6.

Petrakis, I.L. et al., 2012. Noradrenergic vs serotonergic antidepressant with or without naltrexone for veterans with PTSD and comorbid alcohol dependence. *Neuropsychopharmacology*, 37(4), pp.996–1004.

Riper, H. et al., 2014. Treatment of comorbid alcohol use disorders and depression with cognitive-behavioural therapy and motivational interviewing: a meta-analysis. *Addiction*, 109(3), pp.394–406.

Reid A., et al., 2006. Neuropharmacology of addiction. Psychiatry, 5(12), pp.449–54.

Rohde, P. et al., 2001. Natural course of alcohol use disorders from adolescence to young adulthood. *Journal of the American Academy of Child and Adolescent Psychiatry*, 40(1), pp.83–90.

Roncero, C. et al., 2013. Cocaine-Induced Psychosis and Impulsivity in Cocaine-Dependent Patients. *Journal of Addictive Diseases*, 32(3), pp.263–73.

Roncero, C. et al., 2014. Neuroticism associated with cocaine-induced psychosis in cocaine-dependent patients: A cross-sectional observational study. *PLoS One*, 9(9), e106111.

Rosebush, P.I. & Mazurek, M.F., 2010. Catatonia and its treatment. *Schizophrenia Bulletin*, 36(2), pp.239–42.

Rounsaville, B.J., 2004. Treatment of cocaine dependence and depression. *Biological Psychiatry*, 56(10), pp.803–9.

Salloum, I.M. & Thase, M.E., 2000. Impact of substance abuse on the course and treatment of bipolar disorder. *Bipolar Disorders*, 2(3 Pt 2), pp.269–80.

Schaffer, C.B. et al., 2007. Mood-Elevating Effects of Opioid Analgesics in Patients With Bipolar Disorder. *J Neuropsychiatry Clin Neurosci*, 19(4), pp.449–52.

Schep, L.J. et al., 2012. The clinical toxicology of gamma-hydroxybutyrate, gamma-butyrolactone and 1,4-butanediol. *Clinical Toxicology*, 50(6), pp.458–70.

Schumann, G. et al., 2010. The IMAGEN study: reinforcement-related behaviour in normal brain function and psychopathology. *Molecular Psychiatry*, 15(12), pp.1128–39.

Segal, D.S. & Kuczenski, R., 1997. An Escalating Dose 'Binge' Model of Amphetamine Psychosis: Behavioral and Neurochemical Characteristics. *Journal of Neuroscience*, 17(7), pp.2551–66.

Soyka, M., Raith, L. & Steinberg, R., 1988. Mean age, sex ratio and psychopathology in alcohol psychoses. *Psychopathology*, 21(1), pp.19–25.

Strakowski, S.M. et al., 2010. Impulsivity across the course of bipolar disorder. *Bipolar Disorders*, 12(3), pp.285–97.

Strakowski, S.M. et al., 2000. The impact of substance abuse on the course of bipolar disorder. *Biological Psychiatry*, 48(6), pp.477–85.

Sullivan, L.E., Fiellin, D.A. & O'Connor, P.G., 2005. The prevalence and impact of alcohol problems in major depression: A systematic review. *American Journal of Medicine*, 118(4), pp.330–41.

Tang, Y., Martin, N.L. & Cotes, R.O., 2014. Cocaine-induced psychotic disorders: presentation, mechanism, and management. *Journal of Dual Diagnosis*, 10(2), pp.98–105.

Tenore, P.L., 2008. Psychotherapeutic benefits of opioid agonist therapy. *Journal of Addictive Diseases*, 27(3), pp.49–65.

Thompson, P.M. et al., 2014. The ENIGMA Consortium: large-scale collaborative analyses of neuroimaging and genetic data. *Brain Imaging and Behavior*, 8(2), pp.153–82.

Torrens, M. et al., 2005. Efficacy of antidepressants in substance use disorders with and without comorbid depression. *Drug and Alcohol Dependence*, 78(1), pp.1–22.

Treadwell, S.D. & Robinson, T.G., 2007. Cocaine use and stroke. *Postgraduate Medical Journal*, 83(980), pp.389–94.

van Noorden, M.S. et al., 2009. Gamma-hydroxybutyrate withdrawal syndrome: dangerous but not well-known. *General Hospital Psychiatry*, 31(4), pp.394–6.

Volkow, N.D. et al., 2011. Addiction: beyond dopamine reward circuitry. *Proceedings of the National Academy of Sciences of the United States of America*, 108(37), pp.15037–42.

Weibel, S. et al., 2012. Case Report: A Case of Acute Psychosis After Buprenorphine Withdrawal. *Journal of Clinical Psychiatry*, 73(6), e756.

Zweben, J.E. et al., 2004. Psychiatric symptoms in methamphetamine users. *American Journal on Addictions*, 13(2), pp.181–90.

29

Neuropsychiatry and sleep disorders

Guy Leschziner, Ivana Rosenzweig, and Brian Kent

Introduction

Sleep and sleep problems have historically largely been ignored by physicians, although psychiatry has long recognized the role of sleep in psychiatric disorders. However, in recent years, there has been an expanding body of evidence more clearly defining the function of sleep and sleep disturbance in a variety of physical and psychiatric conditions such as heart disease, diabetes, dementia, and depression.

From a neuropsychiatric perspective, sleep problems may cause or exacerbate neuropsychiatric disease, influence response to treatment, or be a clinical feature, helpful diagnostic sign, or prognostic indicator of a neuropsychiatric disorder. Insomnia has long been known to be a feature of mania, and early morning waking is a biological hallmark of depressive disorder, but insomnia is also now known to frequently precede a depressive episode, and the presence of insomnia may leave a patient refractory to treatment with antidepressants. Sleep disturbance may lower pain thresholds in chronic pain syndromes and may lower thresholds for seizures or migraine. The presence of dream enactment behaviour may point towards a neurodegenerative disorder related to a synucleinopathy or towards a high risk of cognitive impairment in PD.

Therefore, in view of the complex and extensive relationship between sleep and neuropsychiatry, an understanding of sleep disorders and of their clinical evaluation, investigation, and treatment is of fundamental importance to any practising neuropsychiatrist.

Sleep staging and nomenclature

There are two broad categories of sleep: rapid eye movement (REM) sleep (also known as paradoxical or active sleep) and non-REM (NREM) sleep. The most commonly used sleep staging classification is that of the American Academy of Sleep Medicine (AASM) (Iber et al., 2007), which subdivides NREM sleep into three stages: N1 (transitional sleep), N2 (light sleep), and N3 (deep sleep; also known as slow-wave sleep). The proportion of time spent in each sleep stage alters somewhat across the lifespan, with REM sleep predominating in newborns and infants and then usually comprising 20–25% of total sleep time (TST) thereafter. The proportion of TST spent in N3 sleep peaks in early adolescence, gradually reducing thereafter and accounting for approximately 20–25% of TST throughout adulthood and middle age.

In healthy individuals, sleep is entered via a brief period of N1 sleep, before rapidly transitioning to N3 sleep via N2. The first REM sleep period will usually occur after 60–90 minutes of sleep. This cycle repeats itself 3–4 times in a typical night, with gradually increasing proportions of N2 and REM sleep and diminishing proportions of N3 sleep with each cycle. Thus, N3 sleep predominates in the first third of the night, and N2 and (particularly) REM sleep in the final third of the night. As shall be discussed in greater detail later, the timing and proportion of the different sleep stages can be significantly altered by medication and disease. The characteristics of the different sleep stages are summarized in Table 29.1 and Fig. 29.1.

Insomnia

Insomnia may be primary or related to a variety of underlying pathologies. It is characterized by dissatisfaction with the quality or duration of sleep, and patients will complain of difficulties with sleep initiation or sleep maintenance, of waking up too early in the morning, or of unrefreshing sleep despite adequate sleep opportunity. Impairment of daytime functioning is a mandatory criterion, although the manifestations of this impairment are wide-ranging and include fatigue, impairment of cognition, or mood disturbance.

Insomnia is by far the commonest sleep complaint (Silber, 2005; Winkelman, 2015). Up to one-third of adults report symptoms of insomnia in any year, and approximately 10% of adults have chronic insomnia. While the majority of patients have isolated insomnia, in the absence of any associated physical or psychiatric illness, approximately 40% of patients have comorbid anxiety or depression; indeed, early morning waking is a biological feature of depressive disorder. Insomnia may also coexist with primary sleep disorders such as obstructive sleep apnoea (OSA), restless legs syndrome (RLS), and narcolepsy.

Insomnia is classified into several different types. Acute adjustment insomnia is caused by an obvious stressful event, has a sudden onset, and lasts <3 months. Chronic primary insomnias consist of psychophysiological insomnia, paradoxical insomnia, and idiopathic insomnia. Psychophysiological insomnia is perhaps

Table 29.1 Sleep staging and nomenclature

Sleep stage	Characteristics
NREM sleep	
N1	Transitional sleep from wake
	Low-voltage, mixed-frequency EEG
	Approximately 5% of TST
N2	EEG characterized by K-complexes and sleep spindles
	45–55% of TST
N3	Slow-wave sleep
	EEG characterized by low-frequency, high-voltage delta waves
	20–25% of TST in adults; reduces with increasing age
	Predominates in first third of night
REM sleep	Paradoxical or active sleep
	Phasic bursts of REM
	Peripheral muscle atonia
	EEG resembles wake
	20–25% of TST
	Predominates in final third of night

NREM, non-rapid eye movement sleep; REM, rapid eye movement sleep; TST, total sleep time.

the commonest of these and is characterized by frustration with the process of going to sleep, hyperarousal, rumination, and anxiety and preoccupation regarding the process of going to sleep. The hyperarousal state is often driven by a vicious cycle of anxiety regarding the daytime consequences of poor sleep, resulting in patients trying to actively manage the problem of going to sleep, which worsens the failure of mental relaxation and exacerbates the insomnia. Paradoxical insomnia, previously known as sleep state

misperception, describes the complaint of severe insomnia in the presence of objective evidence of reasonable quality sleep. It is not clear if this is related to unawareness of sleep state or due to underlying unidentified sleep pathology. Idiopathic insomnia refers to a persistent inability to sleep from early life and is thought to be largely of genetic origin.

Secondary insomnias may be due to psychiatric disorders, drugs or substance misuse, or medical conditions. In addition to anxiety and depressive disorder, sleep disturbance is extremely common in psychotic disorders, and irregular sleep/wake syndrome, where there is absence of a well-defined sleep/wake cycle, is frequently associated with schizoaffective disorders.

The management of insomnia depends upon the time course and contributing factors. For acute insomnia, the prescription of short-term hypnotics is an acceptable and standard treatment, but the emphasis has shifted towards non-pharmacological methods for chronic insomnia. It is equally important to address any underlying causes. Non-pharmacological approaches include sleep hygiene advice, stimulus control, and sleep restriction, all tenets of structured cognitive behavioural therapy for insomnia (CBTi), now seen as the gold standard treatment for chronic insomnia (Williams et al., 2013). There is significant evidence for CBTi as an effective long-term treatment for insomnia. However, not all patients respond to this therapy, and other forms of non-pharmacological therapy such as mindfulness-based treatments are now being developed.

Drug treatment in chronic insomnia remains controversial and without specific guidelines. Hypnotic drugs are likely to result in habituation, with resulting risk of dependence. Agents with a longer half-life risk daytime sedation and unwanted cognitive effects; for example, zopiclone has been associated with an increased risk of road traffic accidents in the morning commute. In addition, while hypnotic drugs decrease sleep latency and increase sleep efficiency, most increase the proportion of N2 sleep, rather than deep sleep, which may not be the desired effect. The choice of agent must be based on comorbidities, other medications on which the patient is, and the specific nature of the insomnia being treated (Krystal, 2015). Melatonin is now licensed in the UK for insomnia in patients over 55 years old for up to 13 weeks, although historically it has been used elsewhere in children and adults in a long-term setting. Melatonin is generally extremely well tolerated and habituation is not a frequent problem. Rather than being a sedative, it is viewed as a 'sleep promoter'. While benzodiazepines and tricyclics are still routinely prescribed, the sleep community tends to favour trazodone, a heterocyclic antidepressant that has little potential for tolerance or dependence, or mirtazapine in patients who have comorbid depression. Pregabalin, given at night-time, is also gaining usage, due to its beneficial effects on sleep architecture and its anxiolytic action. Other agents that can be considered in the context of psychiatric disease include agomelatine, which has a melatonin agonist effect, and quetiapine. Novel agents include orexin antagonists (e.g. suvorexant) and melatonin analogues, but long-term experience with these agents is extremely limited.

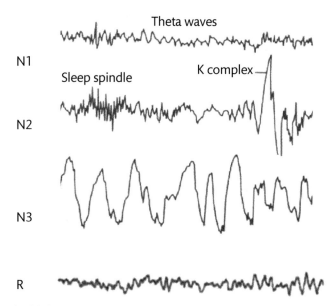

Fig. 29.1 Sleep stages: characteristic EEG traces.

Reproduced with permission from D. Semple and R. Smyth. Sleep Disorders. In *Oxford Handbook of Psychiatry*. Oxford, UK: Oxford University Press. Copyright © 2013, Oxford University Press. DOI: 10.1093/med/9780199693887.001.0001. Reproduced with permission of the Licensor through PLSclear.

Hypersomnias

The central hypersomnias are a group of disorders of presumed CNS origin, the principal symptom of which is that of excessive daytime sleepiness (EDS). These conditions are a diagnosis of exclusion, when alternative explanations for excessive sleepiness, such as sleep restriction, drugs, or other physical sleep pathologies, have been excluded.

Narcolepsy

Narcolepsy is the archetypical central hypersomnia, the pathophysiology of which has been most clearly elucidated in recent years (Leschziner, 2014). First described in the seventeenth century, it is only in the last two decades, through genetic and immunological advances, that this condition has been more precisely defined and understood.

Clinical features

Narcolepsy affects approximately one in 3000 people, although the prevalence varies widely in different geographical regions. The age of onset ranges from early childhood to old age, but there is a bimodal distribution of age of onset, with peaks of onset at around both 15 and 36 years of age (Dauvilliers et al., 2001).

The hallmark of narcolepsy is instability of the transition between sleep and wake, as well as the transition between REM and NREM sleep. This abnormal switching between states of sleep and wake is the basis for features of the classical narcolepsy symptom tetrad of EDS, hypnagogic/hypnopompic hallucinations, sleep paralysis, and cataplexy. Only 10–15% of patients have all four symptoms.

The only mandatory clinical diagnostic feature is persistent EDS (American Academy of Sleep Medicine, 2014). EDS typically presents as discrete sleep episodes but may be more subtle, such as constant sleepiness with occasional exacerbations. It is usually—but not invariably—the earliest manifestation of narcolepsy. Patients characteristically nap for seconds or minutes and find these brief naps refreshing. Dreaming in short naps is another feature of narcolepsy and represents inappropriately early REM sleep. Sleep attacks while standing or eating or during physical exercise particularly suggest narcolepsy.

Patients with narcolepsy have a TST per 24-hour period that is normal or only slightly increased. Indeed, nocturnal insomnia, particularly sleep maintenance insomnia, is another common feature of the condition. Patients often wake at night feeling extremely refreshed, with resultant sleep fragmentation.

Hypnagogic hallucinations affect 30–60% of patients. These may occur at sleep onset or sleep offset, and can be bizarre and frightening; they reflect the onset of REM and dreaming prior to established sleep. They are usually visual, although they may be auditory or sensory. Typical hallucinations are of people standing over the bed or of animals or people in the bedroom, although patients occasionally describe spiritual or other unusual hallucinations such as out-of-body experiences; rarely, they find these comforting and want to avoid ending these experiences with medication. Hallucinations can accompany sleep paralysis (SP), which is especially frightening. This can result in experiences of being physically or sexually assaulted, causing significant anxieties surrounding sleep.

SP, which affects 25–50%, occurs in full consciousness and almost always affects the entire body, with the exception of the eyes; it reflects inappropriate muscle atonia of REM in wakefulness. Patients sometimes report shortness of breath or asphyxiation, presumably due to paralysis of accessory muscles of respiration, contributing further to the terrifying nature of these events. Hypnagogic hallucinations and SP at sleep onset suggest narcolepsy—normal people can experience SP quite commonly, but usually at sleep offset.

The final classical feature is cataplexy, which usually develops within 3–5 years of onset of daytime sleepiness but rarely precedes it. Cataplexy describes the transient and sudden loss of muscle tone in full consciousness, usually precipitated by strong emotion or occasionally spontaneously; it occurs in 60–70% of patients with narcolepsy. Loss of awareness/consciousness is not a feature of cataplexy, although it raises the possibility of loss of tone related to sleep attacks. It may be complete, affecting all muscles, apart from the diaphragm and extraocular muscles, or may be segmental, affecting only the limbs, face, or muscles affecting speech. Onset is usually abrupt, lasting seconds to minutes, although it may wax and wane, and muscle tone returns to normal immediately when the attack ceases. Cataplexy is pathognomonic for narcolepsy, with a few rare exceptions (Leschziner, 2014) and, as such, needs to be carefully discriminated from pseudocataplexy or other forms of drop attacks and startle response. When present, it identifies a subgroup of homogenous patients who are likely to share the same pathophysiological basis for their condition. In fact, the latest iteration of the International Classification of Sleep Disorders (ICSD) divides narcolepsy into type 1 narcolepsy (NT1), defined by the presence of cataplexy or low or absent CSF hypocretin, and type 2 narcolepsy (NT2), defined by the absence of cataplexy or failure to demonstrate low or absent CSF hypocretin.

Other clinical features of narcolepsy include REM sleep behaviour disorder (RBD) (see REM sleep behaviour disorder, p. 350), very vivid or even lucid dreaming, automatic behaviour, and cognitive dysfunction. Depression and anxiety disorders are common (Ohayon, 2013), although it is unclear if these result from the chronic condition or are primary features of narcolepsy.

Pathophysiology

A strong genetic component is suggested by familial studies that showed the risk of developing narcolepsy with cataplexy in a first-degree relative is 1–2%, with a relative risk of 10–40 (Mignot, 2008). There is a strong HLA association, especially with the HLA DQB1*0602 haplotype. Up to 98% of patients with narcolepsy with cataplexy have this haplotype, compared to 25% of the general population. However, concordance rates in monozygotic twins are relatively low, suggesting an important role for environmental factors. The association with the HLA haplotype and subsequent identification of an association with polymorphisms in the T-cell receptor locus in whole-genome association studies imply an autoimmune role in pathophysiology. There are suggestions of infective triggers—the strong seasonal variation in the incidence of narcolepsy suggests a role for winter infections, and patients with recent-onset narcolepsy have high serum titres of anti-streptolysin O antibodies. More recently, the H1N1 swine flu virus and/or vaccination has been linked to narcolepsy (Drakatos and Leschziner, 2014).

Recent work has shown that patients with narcolepsy with cataplexy showed a loss of some or all of the 70,000 hypocretin-producing neurones in the lateral hypothalamus. Low or absent CSF hypocretin-1 levels are consistently found in patients with narcolepsy with cataplexy, although this association is less strong with patients without cataplexy. In humans, it is hypothesized that, in genetically predisposed individuals, immune-mediated destruction of the hypocretin-producing neurones in the lateral hypothalamus is triggered by environmental factors such as infective agents. Recent work has suggested that molecular mimicry of hypocretin by epitopes of the H1N1 swine flu virus may explain the association of NT1 with this virus and the H1N1 vaccine.

The hypocretin-producing locus in the lateral hypothalamus projects widely throughout the brain. Neuronal activity in this locus is highest in wakefulness and is lower in sleep, particularly REM sleep. Loss of these hypocretinergic neurones causes inherent instability in the neural network responsible for maintaining wakefulness and preventing REM sleep.

Diagnosis

The recent third edition of the ICSD has redefined narcolepsy into two entities—NT1 and NT2 (American Association of Sleep Medicine, 2014). NT1 is defined as the presence of cataplexy in the context of a diagnostic multiple sleep latency test (MSLT) or the demonstration of CSF hypocretin deficiency. NT2 defines patients without cataplexy or who demonstrate CSF hypocretin deficiency. In practice, due to infrequent CSF examination in these patients, the MSLT remains the major diagnostic test for narcolepsy. According to the ISCD-3 criteria, a mean sleep latency of ≤8 minutes, with REM sleep occurring in at least two naps, is diagnostic of narcolepsy, provided other conditions have been excluded; REM sleep within 15 minutes of sleep onset on polysomnography (PSG) can replace a sleep-onset REM period (SOREMP) on the MSLT. During the MSLT, patients are given the opportunity to fall asleep on four or five occasions at 2-hourly intervals over a day, with the patient monitored with EEG for sleep-staging purposes.

However, it should be noted that the MSLT is a biological test with high false-positive and lower, but significant, false-negative rates (Baumann et al., 2014). An MSLT diagnostic of narcolepsy is not uncommon in behaviourally induced inadequate sleep syndrome (Marti et al., 2009). Conversely, patients with narcolepsy may have a normal MSLT before the subsequent diagnosis. It is therefore crucial that confounders of the MSLT, such as drugs and prior sleep restriction, are excluded prior to a diagnosis based upon the MSLT (Drakatos et al., 2013), especially in NT2.

Management

The first management step is appropriate sleep hygiene advice. This is to ensure adequate sleep opportunity to rule out an element of chronic sleep deprivation, but also to help control symptoms of EDS. Occasionally patients prefer to manage their symptoms without medication, and if lifestyle permits, planned naps can be sufficient to establish reasonable control in some patients. Planned naps should also be recommended in patients with incomplete control on medication. Daytime naps should be limited to 15–20 minutes, as longer naps risk entering non-REM stage 3 sleep, potentially inducing grogginess or sleep inertia and with possible deleterious consequences for night-time sleep.

For most patients, pharmacotherapy is necessary (Leschziner, 2014). Drug treatment should be focused on the major symptoms the individual is complaining of. Stimulant medications are the mainstay of treatment of EDS. Modafinil and dexamphetamine are licensed agents, but methylphenidate is also commonly prescribed. Modafinil is the best tolerated of these, with a good safety profile, but, unlike the others, is not significantly anti-cataplectic. It has a low risk of addiction but may cause headache, anxiety, palpitations, and rarely hypertension.

Methylphenidate and dexamphetamine have a higher rate of adverse events, especially hypertension and psychiatric effects. They should be used very cautiously in people with a cardiac history. Despite these concerns, these drugs have not been associated with increased serious cardiac events or death, at least in young and middle-aged adults (Habel et al., 2011).

Cataplexy may respond to methylphenidate or dexamphetamine but more usually requires specific anti-cataplectic agents. Clomipramine and venlafaxine are licensed for this indication, and the choice largely depends on other features of narcolepsy. Clomipramine at night may help if there is prominent night-time insomnia, and venlafaxine can provide an additional stimulant effect. Fluoxetine can also be very effective and is usually better tolerated than venlafaxine or clomipramine. These drugs are also extremely effective at treating SP and hypnagogic hallucinations through their REM-suppressing effects.

Sodium oxybate is a relatively new drug for treating cataplexy and EDS. It is a GABA-B agonist, although its mechanism of action is not entirely understood. It is taken as a liquid, and because it has a very short half-life, patients should take one dose immediately before bed, with a second dose 3–4 hours later. There are a number of issues specific to this drug—it is extremely expensive, costing approximately £10,000–15,000 per annum, and because it is extremely sedating, it has been used criminally as a 'date-rape' drug. It also acts as a respiratory depressant, and deaths have occurred in combination with alcohol or other CNS-depressant drugs. If sodium oxybate is not being prescribed, night-time sleep quality should be considered—if the patient is experiencing fragmented sleep, drug options include a sedating tricyclic, melatonin, trazodone, or a Z-drug.

Idiopathic hypersomnia

Idiopathic hypersomnia (IH) is a central hypersomnia related to narcolepsy. Unlike narcolepsy, patients usually complain of unrefreshing sleep, significant sleep drunkenness or other symptoms on waking, a prolonged sleep time, and fewer, but longer and unrefreshing, naps during the day. The epidemiology, natural history, and pathophysiology of this condition is poorly understood (Billiard and Sonka, 2016), but it is thought to be significantly less prevalent than narcolepsy, of the order of 2–20 times rarer. There is thought to be some overlap between NT2 and IH (Šonka et al., 2015), and although the MSLT is used to differentiate IH from narcolepsy, test–re-test reliability of the MSLT is poor, and patients may switch between diagnostic categories with repeated sleep studies (Trotti et al., 2013). Patients with IH frequently have psychiatric comorbidities as a result of the effects of the condition, and this can make discrimination from psychiatric hypersomnolence difficult (Plante, 2016).

Since patients with IH do not experience cataplexy or other features of narcolepsy, treatment is solely with stimulant drugs. More recently, it has been proposed that the underlying pathophysiology of IH is the production of an endogenous substance in the CSF that potentiates GABA transmission and is reversed by flumazenil (Rye et al., 2012). This has led to flumazenil being proposed as a potential treatment for this patient group.

Clarithromycin has also been described as a potential therapeutic agent (Trotti et al., 2014), although the mechanism of action is uncertain and there are concerns regarding cardiac toxicity with long-term treatment.

Episodic hypersomnia

Kleine–Levin syndrome is an extremely rare and poorly understood condition that results in recurrent episodes of profound hypersomnia (Arnulf et al., 2012). It is thought to affect between one and two per million and can occur at any age, although it usually starts in the second decade of life. It is more common in Ashkenazi Jews. Previously thought to be a disorder almost exclusively of males, it is now thought to affect females almost as frequently as males. The condition is characterized by bouts of hypersomnolence, with sufferers sleeping between 15 and 21 hours per day. During bouts, patients will often experience confusion, derealization, megaphagia, and other altered behaviours such as aggression, irritability, and hypersexuality. These bouts tend to last for days to weeks, but in between bouts, individuals are entirely normal, although they may develop mood disturbance due to the impact of the condition. The cause is unknown, but proposed mechanisms include a channelopathy and inflammatory brain conditions. PET and MR perfusion studies suggest thalamic or hypothalamic dysfunction during bouts (Billings et al., 2011). The increased incidence in Ashkenazi Jews implies a genetic predisposition.

Treatment of Kleine–Levin syndrome is challenging. The condition often burns out after a number of years, without treatment. Abortive therapies, such as stimulants, are largely unsuccessful—these drugs may partially address the hypersomnolence but appear to be unhelpful for the associated cognitive symptoms. Treatment often comprises prophylaxis, in an attempt to reduce the frequency and severity of attacks. A number of drugs have been utilized, but treatment is often unsuccessful. The strongest evidence exists for lithium (Leu-Semenescu et al., 2015), which is the standard treatment, but there is some evidence that carbamazepine and lamotrigine may also sometimes be effective. Due to the relative lack of success of treatment, intensive efforts should be undertaken to exclude other more treatable conditions (Nesbitt and Leschziner, 2016).

Restless legs syndrome

RLS is a common neurological disorder characterized by the urge to move the legs, or indeed other body parts, usually accompanied by a range of unpleasant sensations (Leschziner and Gringras, 2012). RLS is a common cause of sleep initiation and sleep maintenance insomnia, unrefreshing sleep, and EDS. However, despite its high prevalence, it is often unrecognized or misdiagnosed, in part due to lack of awareness of the condition, but also as a result of a wide spectrum of symptoms and signs. However, prompt diagnosis and management have a large impact on morbidity and QoL.

Clinical features

RLS is essentially a clinical diagnosis, without specific biological markers. Diagnosis is based upon four essential criteria, as defined by the International Restless Legs Syndrome Study Group (Allen et al., 2014):

- The urge to move the legs, accompanied by uncomfortable or unpleasant sensations. Other body parts can be affected, in addition to the lower limbs.
- The urge to move or unpleasant sensations start during periods of immobility or sleep.
- Movement of the affected limbs results in a partial or transient relief of symptoms.
- Symptoms worsen in the evening or at night—this feature may not persist but should have been present initially.

The nature of the sensory symptoms varies greatly. In some individuals, it presents with a non-specific discomfort, although patients may use a variety of terms to describe their sensations: a sensation of pulling, jittering, worms or insects moving, tingling, itching, aching, bubbling, fidgeting, electric current sensations, tightness, and throbbing (García-Borreguero et al., 2011). In others, the symptoms can be extremely painful. Although the legs are the commonest anatomical site of involvement, the upper limbs, the abdomen, or even the face can be involved. Sleep initiation insomnia may sometimes be the presenting symptom, since patients sometimes do not ascribe the sleep disturbance to the sensory symptoms.

In addition to restlessness, 80–90% of RLS sufferers also experience frank leg movements, which usually arise during sleep but can also occur in wakefulness (Montplaisir et al., 1997). These leg movements are involuntary and typically involve periodic flexion of the hip and knee, dorsiflexion of the foot, and extension of the hallux, although these movements are frequently subtle and may simply manifest as minimal extension of the hallux. These movements, if arising in sleep, may result in frequent arousals from sleep, causing unrefreshing sleep, or complete awakenings, resulting in fragmented sleep and sleep maintenance issues. They may also impact on the sleep quality of the patient's bed partner.

However, periodic limb movements of sleep (PLMS) may occur in isolation, in the absence of symptoms of RLS. The prevalence of periodic limb movement disorder (PLMD) is unknown, as it requires PSG to diagnose, but PLMS are in themselves relatively common, occurring in approximately one-third of patients over 60 years of age. In the context of the sleep clinic setting, frequent PLMS are a common cause of sleep maintenance insomnia and unrefreshing sleep, and the majority of patients with PLMD—the disorder refers to clinical consequences of PLMS—will not have RLS symptoms.

Differential diagnosis

A variety of conditions may mimic RLS. Potential mimics include peripheral neuropathy, cramps, varicose veins, akathisia (a feeling of motor restlessness associated with neuroleptic drugs), fibromyalgia, anxiety, and vascular or neurogenic claudication secondary to spinal stenosis (García-Borreguero et al., 2011). Therefore, it is imperative that a proper history is elucidated, that the symptoms meet all four diagnostic criteria, and that a general and neurological examination is undertaken to exclude these possibilities.

Epidemiology

The prevalence of RLS remains uncertain but is clearly high. On the basis of a single question, prevalence has been estimated at 9–15%, whereas studies that tried to rule out alternative diagnoses estimated the prevalence as 1.9–4.6% (Ohayon et al., 2012b). The prevalence is approximately twice as high in women as in men, and RLS is the commonest movement disorder in pregnancy, affecting between 13.5% and 26.6% of pregnant women.

The majority of patients with RLS have an idiopathic basis. However, a variety of conditions have been associated with a higher prevalence of RLS, although the strength of these associations varies. The most important of these associations are uraemia and iron deficiency (Leschziner and Gringras, 2012).

Pathophysiology

The cause of RLS is not fully understood, although clinical observation has informed our understanding of the condition. Dopaminergic agents improve symptoms, and RLS is frequently triggered or exacerbated by dopaminergic antagonists, implying an important role for dopaminergic transmission. Biochemical studies have largely confirmed evidence of dopaminergic dysregulation in patients with RLS (Leschziner and Gringras, 2012).

Idiopathic RLS appears to have a strong genetic basis. Between 20% and 60% of patients report a positive family history of the condition; twin studies have shown hereditability estimates of 54–83%, and GWAS have shown associations with variants in several genes (Rye, 2015).

Substances and medications exacerbating or triggering RLS

RLS has been associated with a variety of commonly utilized medications, many of which are highly relevant in the management of patients with psychiatric conditions (Winkelman, 2006). Antidepressants, in particular, are exacerbators of RLS, and although data comparing various drugs are scanty, it appears that high-dose tricyclics, venlafaxine, and mirtazapine are the most potent aggravating drugs. Unfortunately, these are agents that are commonly prescribed in unrecognized RLS with a predominant picture of sleep initiation or sleep maintenance insomnia. Other drugs used in psychiatric patients that may have an impact on RLS include β-blockers for anxiety and antipsychotic agents. Antihistamines, often purchased over the counter as sleep-promoting agents, may also exacerbate RLS, resulting in a paradoxical worsening of the insomnia. Other drugs implicated include anti-emetics (with the exception of domperidone which does not cross the BBB), phenytoin, and calcium channel antagonists. Caffeine, alcohol, and nicotine have all been reported to worsen RLS symptoms.

Management

After the diagnosis of RLS has been made, efforts should be made to exclude underlying causes such as an iron deficiency state or uraemia. All patients should have renal function and iron studies, including serum ferritin, checked. Any patient with a serum ferritin level below 50–75 μg/L should be commenced on high-dose oral iron supplementation, either in isolation or in conjunction with treatment for RLS (García-Borreguero et al., 2011). Patients should also be screened for any substances or medications that might exacerbate RLS (Winkelman, 2006), since simple rationalization of medication or a reduction in caffeine, alcohol, or nicotine intake may improve symptoms dramatically.

It is important to point out that only 15% of RLS sufferers require specific treatment (Byrne et al., 2006). The vast majority of patients can be managed using non-pharmacological techniques. Since tiredness or sleep deprivation in themselves can worsen symptoms, considerable effort should be made to optimize sleep hygiene, and indeed for patients with superimposed psycho-physiological insomnia, CBT for insomnia may be helpful. As part of sleep hygiene, stimulating substances should be avoided near bedtime. Many patients also experience significant benefit from relaxation therapy, walking or stretching before bedtime, a warm bath in the evening, or evening massage of the affected limbs.

In the UK, only three agents are licensed for the indication of RLS. These three agents are all dopamine agonists: ropinirole, pramipexole, and rotigotine, the latter as a topical patch. The side effect profile is similar for all the agents (common adverse effects include nausea, headache, and fatigue), with the exception of rotigotine, which also has a frequent adverse effect of skin reaction to the patch. These drugs have certain class-specific issues. Impulse control disorders—compulsive gambling, compulsive eating, problem shopping and hypersexuality—are well documented in patients with PD treated with these drugs, but more recently these adverse effects have also been described in patients with RLS and indeed have been reported in up to 20% of patients (Cornelius et al., 2010). A further issue for dopamine agonists is the phenomenon of augmentation (García-Borreguero and Williams, 2010). Augmentation describes worsening of RLS symptom severity beyond that expected as part of the natural history of the condition. Rates of augmentation are especially high for levodopa, but even with the dopamine agonists, augmentation rates are clinically significant. Augmentation is a dose-related effect and so can be minimized by maintaining as low a dose as possible. Attention should be paid to the serum ferritin, as the likelihood of augmentation increases with low iron stores (Trenkwalder et al., 2008).

Other classes of drugs do not appear to cause augmentation. However, in the UK, all other therapies are off-label, although in the United States, gabapentin enacarbil has been licensed in the last few years. This is a pro-drug of gabapentin, formulated to circumvent issues of poor bioavailability with gabapentin, but is not available in the UK. Gabapentin can, however, be effective in RLS, particularly when pain is a prominent feature. Pregabalin has recently gained increasing use and has better bioavailability, compared to gabapentin. It is also licensed for GAD and therefore is potentially useful in individuals with prominent anxiety symptoms. Other widely used drugs include the opioids—methadone has been demonstrated to be helpful, with no evidence of significant dosage increase despite a 10-year follow-up (Silver et al., 2011), and more recently oxycodone, combined in a prolonged-release formulation with naloxone to prevent GI side effects, has been shown to be effective (Trenkwalder et al., 2013). Clonazepam at low dose can be particularly effective for patients with significant insomnia, although there remain concerns about dependency and the long half-life can potentially result in daytime drowsiness.

From a psychiatric perspective, treatment of depression coexisting with RLS can be problematic. Bupropion, in contrast to other antidepressants, has been reported as being helpful in RLS

(Lee et al., 2009), presumably due to its dopamine reuptake inhibitory effects. A single small RCT of bupropion has at least suggested that it does not seem to worsen RLS severity (Bayard et al., 2011).

Data for the management of isolated PLMD are much more scant, but typically the same therapeutic agents are used as for RLS. A recent meta-analysis has demonstrated evidence for the reduction in the periodic limb movement index for the dopa agonists, oxycodone, pregabalin, gabapentin, and gabapentin enacarbil (Hornyak et al., 2014).

Obstructive sleep apnoea

OSA is a highly prevalent, but markedly underdiagnosed, condition, characterized by collapse of the upper airway during sleep, causing transient interruptions in sleep breathing, with a host of downstream adverse consequences.

Definitions and diagnosis

The presence and severity of OSA are quantified by the assessment of the number of apnoeas (cessations of airflow) and hypopnoeas (reductions of airflow) occurring per hour of sleep—the apnoea–hypopnoea index (AHI). An AHI of <5 events per hour is considered normal, with an AHI of 5–15, 15–30, or >30 events per hour categorized as mild, moderate, or severe sleep apnoea, respectively. Obstructive sleep apnoea syndrome (OSAS) is defined by the presence of OSA on a sleep study, accompanied by significant subjective daytime sleepiness (Iber et al., 2007). The gold standard investigation for the diagnosis of OSA is nocturnal PSG, performed as an inpatient, and incorporating measurement of respiratory effort, airflow, and ECG, with EEG, electro-oculography, and chin and anterior tibialis EMG. On PSG, an apnoea is defined as a reduction of airflow to ≤10% of baseline, lasting >10 s; an apnoeic event is classified as obstructive if respiratory effort persists, or as central if respiratory effort ceases (Iber et al., 2007).

Many definitions of what should constitute hypopnoea have been advanced; the application of these competing definitions to the same sleep study can lead to significant differences in AHI values. However, the most commonly used scoring rule defines hypopnoea as a reduction in airflow of ≥30% from pre-event baseline, lasting ≥10 s, accompanied by 3% arterial oxygen desaturation and/or related arousal from sleep.

While PSG allows the most accurate characterization of sleep breathing, it is a resource-intensive diagnostic tool. The high prevalence of OSA precludes the use of PSG as a routine initial investigation; consequently, a large number of studies have evaluated the ability of other diagnostic modalities to successfully identify clinically significant OSA. These range from full domiciliary PSG to limited cardiorespiratory sleep studies and to home nocturnal oximetry. These alternative testing methods appear to have satisfactory performance characteristics, particularly in patients with a high pre-test probability of OSA, and allow PSG to be reserved for equivocal or complex cases (McEvoy et al., 2016b).

Pathophysiology

The onset of sleep leads to a general reduction in skeletal muscle tone, including a reduction in upper airway muscle tone.

Contingent on a number of anatomical, structural, and functional factors, this can lead to partial or complete collapse of the upper airway during sleep. This, in turn, leads to a marked reduction or complete cessation of airflow, despite ongoing respiratory effort. Airway obstruction is usually relieved by brief arousal from sleep, with a concomitant increase in upper airway muscle tone and restoration of airflow. Ultimately this causes sleep fragmentation, marked intrathoracic pressure swings, and intermittent hypoxia, with consequent nocturnal and daytime symptoms, alongside systemic inflammation, oxidative stress, and sympathetic excitation (Eastwood et al., 2010).

Epidemiology

Sleep apnoea is the commonest physical sleep disorder and is probably also the commonest chronic respiratory disorder (Steier et al., 2014). OSA is significantly commoner in men and has a particularly intimate relationship with obesity, with its prevalence and severity increasing in parallel with increasing BMI (Garvey et al., 2015). The sentinel study of OSA prevalence was the Wisconsin Sleep Cohort study, performed in the early 1990s, in which a large community-based population of middle-aged subjects living in the mid-western United States underwent full PSG (Young et al., 1993). When defined as an AHI of ≥5 events/hour, the prevalence of OSA within this cohort was 24% in men and 9% in women aged 30–60 years. The prevalence of OSA with associated EDS (i.e. OSAS) was estimated at 3–7% in adult men and 2–5% in adult women. Since the early 1990s, however, the world's population has become significantly more obese, and it appears likely that the prevalence of OSA has increased along with this. A recent re-analysis of the Wisconsin Sleep Cohort Study data suggested OSAS could now be found in 14% of men and 5% of women (Peppard et al., 2013), while moderate to severe OSA (AHI ≥15) was found in 49% of middle-aged Swiss men (Heinzer et al., 2015). Subgroups at particularly high risk of OSA include patients with type 2 diabetes mellitus, resistant hypertension, heart failure, and end-stage renal disease, along with—as will be discussed in greater detail in Neurocognitive and psychiatric associations of OSA—those with depression and PTSD.

Clinical features

Patients with OSA and their bed partners may complain of a wide range of nocturnal and daytime symptoms (Gottlieb et al., 2010). Night-time symptoms include domestically disruptive snoring, witnessed apnoeic events, paroxysmal breathlessness, palpitations, nocturia, and night sweats. Patients may wake feeling unrefreshed by sleep, with a sore throat, dry mouth, or frontal headache. While the archetypal daytime symptom of OSA is EDS, this may be absent in a substantial number of individuals with potentially clinically significant sleep apnoea, particularly pre-menopausal women. Other common daytime symptoms include debilitating fatigue, poor concentration, irritability, and memory loss. Reflecting this, patients with OSA have reduced QoL measures and an increased risk of road traffic accidents, when compared with matched controls.

Although OSA may lead to a significant symptom burden in individual patients, of greater concern from a population health perspective is its association, and apparent causative relationship, with a number of medical comorbidities, including hypertension, coronary artery disease (CAD), stroke, type 2 diabetes mellitus, and cancer. Apnoeic and hypopnoeic events occurring during sleep lead to intermittent hypoxia, sympathetic excitation, and rapid and dramatic changes in intra-thoracic pressure. Intermittent hypoxia, in turn, causes systemic inflammation and oxidative stress, with this combination of factors producing a pro-atherogenic microenvironment (Kent et al., 2011). The strongest evidence in this area suggests an important contributory role for OSA in the development of systemic hypertension; data from a community-based North American study of 709 subjects showed that the presence of severe OSA at enrolment conferred a nearly threefold risk of being diagnosed with hypertension over a 4-year follow-up period, independently of the effects of age, obesity, and smoking history, with more recent studies from Europe confirming this apparent relationship (Peppard et al., 2000a). Middle-aged men with severe OSA have a 70% increase in the risk of developing symptomatic CAD, compared with non-apnoeic subjects, while stroke risk was nearly three times higher in men in the most severe OSA quartile enrolled in a large longitudinal study from the United States (Redline et al., 2010). Ultimately, patients with severe OSA seem more likely to die from heart disease, with longitudinal studies suggesting between a threefold and fivefold risk of cardiovascular mortality in these individuals (Garvey et al., 2015).

It also appears that OSA severity has a direct bearing on metabolic health. Cross-sectional data from a large European multicentre study showed a nearly twofold likelihood of concomitant type 2 diabetes mellitus and an increased likelihood of poor glycaemic control among diabetics in subjects with severe OSA (Kent et al., 2014). Similarly, longitudinal data from a large Canadian cohort found that a diagnosis of severe OSA conferred a 37% increase in risk for incident type 2 diabetes mellitus, following statistical adjustment for confounding factors (Kendzerska et al., 2014). This relationship may be mediated through the apparent detrimental effects of OSA and resultant intermittent hypoxia and sympathetic excitation on adipose tissue function, hepatic glucose metabolism, and pancreatic beta-cell survival (Kent et al., 2015).

There is a surprisingly significant degree of overlap between the cellular microenvironment generated by OSA and that required to promote carcinogenesis, with cellular responses to hypoxia, chronic inflammation, and oxidative stress all potential contributors to the development of malignancy (Martínez-García et al., 2016). This observation led to initial animal studies, which examined tumour growth and metastatic potential in murine models of intermittent hypoxia. Cancers in mice exposed to intermittent hypoxia grew faster and were more likely to metastasize, when compared to their normoxic littermates (Martínez-García et al., 2016). Subsequent population level studies in humans have suggested that this may be an effect with clinical relevance—among 1522 subjects enrolled in a community-based longitudinal study in the United States, severe OSA was associated with an almost fivefold risk of cancer death (Nieto et al., 2012). Similarly, in a cohort of nearly 5000 Spanish patients attending sleep clinics, the severity of nocturnal hypoxaemia predicted incident cancer, even following rigorous adjustment for confounding variables (Campos-Rodriguez et al., 2013).

Neurocognitive and psychiatric associations of OSA

Just as it has a detrimental effect on function in other tissue groups and organs, OSA appears to have a significant negative impact upon the brain. Data from animal studies suggest that both intermittent hypoxia and sleep fragmentation lead to significant neuroanatomical

and functional changes within the murine brain. For example, IH-related inflammation and oxidative stress cause injury to sleep–wake-regulating regions of the basal forebrain and brainstem, contributing to marked hypersomnolence in exposed animals. Human imaging studies have demonstrated structural atrophy and functional disturbances in the right basolateral amygdala, the hippocampus, and the right central insula, while clinical studies have found untreated OSA to be associated with impairment in vigilance, attention, executive functioning, and motor coordination (Rosenzweig et al., 2015). Debate continues as to the impact of OSA on memory and language ability, and it remains unclear to what extent nocturnal continuous positive airway pressure (nCPAP) therapy can ameliorate these changes—a recent meta-analysis of published randomized trials in this area found nCPAP use led to a significant improvement in attention, but not in other cognitive domains (Kylstra et al., 2013).

Any effect of OSA on neuroanatomy and cerebral function may be of particular importance in neurodegenerative disorders such as AD. A recent meta-analysis suggested that OSA is five times more likely to be present in subjects with AD than in age-matched controls without cognitive impairment (Emamian et al., 2016), and a number of studies have suggested that treating sleep apnoea in patients with early AD may slow cognitive decline. The mechanisms underpinning this putative relationship have yet to be properly defined, but pre-clinical data showed that intermittent hypoxia promotes cerebral amyloid deposition and tau phosphorylation in the rodent brain (Daulatzai, 2013).

Potential depressive symptoms, such as low mood, irritability, and anxiety, are frequently reported by OSA patients, and its prevalence appears particularly high in patients with MDD and PTSD; there are few data examining its occurrence in patients with schizophrenia, anxiety disorders, or bipolar affective disorder (Gupta and Simpson, 2015). A potential contributory role for OSA in mental health disorders has been suggested by a number of studies, including a large community based study from the United States ($n = 1408$) wherein a dose–response relationship was observed between OSA severity and the likelihood of subsequent depression (Peppard et al., 2006). Similarly, a prospective Australian study of 426 patients attending a sleep clinic found that depressive symptoms were significantly commoner in patients with severe OSA and that these symptoms improved markedly with nCPAP therapy (Edwards et al., 2015). However, there is a lack of prospective randomized trials in this field, and the ability of treatment of OSA to make a meaningful difference to depressive illness remains uncertain.

Management

In obese and overweight individuals, weight loss can significantly ameliorate OSA severity, with a loss of 20% of baseline weight associated with an approximately 50% reduction in AHI (Peppard et al., 2000b). However, in clinical practice, this degree of weight loss is difficult to achieve and maintain, except perhaps in the context of bariatric surgery. Other potential conservative management options include sleeping in a non-supine position and avoidance of alcohol and sedating medications.

The best established treatment for OSA is nCPAP where compressed air is delivered to the patient during sleep from an nCPAP device via a nasal or face mask. The flow of air provides a pneumatic splint, which maintains upper airway patency and permits relatively normal sleep breathing. Daytime sleepiness, QoL measures, and a number of cognitive domains are improved by nCPAP therapy (Sawyer et al., 2011), which also appears to have a significant beneficial effect on blood pressure control in hypertensive patients. Given the relationship between OSA and cardiovascular and metabolic disease, it might be expected nCPAP would also reduce cardiovascular morbidity and mortality in patients with severe OSA, but a number of large randomized studies have failed to affirm this hypothesis (McEvoy et al., 2016a). Patient acceptance of, and adherence to, nCPAP therapy is variable, with up to 50% of patients being non-compliant with treatment after 1 year.

Other treatment options include use of mandibular advancement dental devices, which have been shown to be as efficacious as nCPAP in the management of milder cases of OSA. A subset of patients may also benefit from upper airway surgery, particularly uvulopalatopharyngoplasty with or without tonsillectomy (Browaldh et al., 2013). Growing evidence suggests that electrical stimulation of upper airway muscles—delivered either transcutaneously (Pengo et al., 2016) or via an implantable hypoglossal nerve stimulator (Strollo et al., 2015)—during sleep may lead to significant reductions in AHI in patients who have failed therapy with nCPAP.

Obesity hypoventilation syndrome

Obesity hypoventilation syndrome (OHS) is defined as the presence of daytime hypercapnia ($PaCO_2 \geq 45$ mmHg) in an obese patient (BMI ≥ 30 kg/m^2), occurring in the absence of neuromuscular disease, thoracic deformity, or other mechanical or metabolic causes of hypoventilation. OHS is almost invariably accompanied by OSA, is estimated to occur in approximately 20% of obese OSA patients (Kaw et al., 2009) and increases in prevalence with increasing obesity (Mokhlesi et al., 2007). Clinically, OHS presents with marked hypersomnolence, with or without decompensated hypercapnia, in a morbidly obese patient with severe OSA. Signs of cor pulmonale, due to hypoxia-induced pulmonary hypertension, are significantly commoner in patients with OSA/OHS than those with OSA alone. Medium- to long-term survival is significantly worse in OHS patients than in age- and BMI-matched OSA patients without hypercapnia, with 5-year mortality rates in one study of 15.5% and 4.5%, respectively (Castro-Añón et al., 2015). Much of the excess mortality in OHS appears to be attributable to cardiovascular disease; OHS patients have an adjusted odds ratio of 1.86 for major cardiovascular events, compared to their OSA counterparts (Castro-Añón et al., 2015). OHS may be successfully treated with conventional nCPAP in the majority of cases (Banerjee et al., 2007), but a substantial minority of patients will require non-invasive ventilation, with bilevel positive airway pressure (BiPAP), which may achieve functional improvements above those gained by nCPAP therapy (Masa et al., 2015). Supplemental oxygen may also be required in a proportion of cases, with the rather more drastic step of tracheostomy reserved for highly symptomatic patients intolerant of PAP therapy.

Central sleep apnoea

Central sleep apnoea (CSA) can be differentiated from OSA by the absence of not only airflow, but also of respiratory effort. CSA is by an order of magnitude the less common of the two disorders (Donovan and Kapur, 2016), although it occurs with significant frequency in a number of subgroups of patients, particularly those with severe or suboptimally controlled heart failure (Eckert et al., 2007). Patients with CSA can be classified under several broad headings, including idiopathic CSA, CSA with Cheyne–Stokes respiration (CSA/CSR), high-altitude CSA, CSA due to an underlying neurological or medical disorder, and CSA due to a medication or substance. This latter category is perhaps most relevant in psychiatric cohorts; best characterized in opioid users, significant CSA has been reported to occur in up to 30% of patients receiving methadone maintenance therapy (Wang et al., 2005) and is also significantly commoner in chronic pain patients receiving high-dose opiate analgesia than in matched sleep clinic controls (Rose et al., 2014). A wide range of other CNS-active medications, including benzodiazepines and baclofen, have been reported to contribute to depressed respiratory drive, particularly when used in parallel with opiates. How best to manage CSA remains controversial—in heart failure patients with CSA/CSR, restoring 'normal' sleep breathing with adaptive servo-ventilation (ASV), a form of positive airway pressure therapy, may actually increase mortality risk (Cowie et al., 2015), and while ASV appears capable of abolishing CSA in patients receiving opiate analgesia, it is unclear what impact this has on long-term outcomes (Javaheri et al., 2014).

Parasomnias

The parasomnias are a group of disorders characterized by unwanted and abnormal behaviours or sensory experiences arising from sleep or at sleep onset or offset. They are generally classified according to the sleep stages from which they arise; thus, the ICSD third edition classifies them as non-REM sleep-related, REM-sleep related, or as the enigmatically titled 'other' parasomnias (Sateia, 2014).

Non-REM sleep parasomnias

Typically arising from N3 sleep, the non-REM parasomnias involve a spectrum of abnormal and frequently complex nocturnal behaviours, ranging from confusional arousals to night terrors and sleepwalking. All appear to arise as a result of incomplete transitions between non-REM sleep and wakefulness, and have the potential to lead to significant distress and even injury. They share a number of clinical features which can help to distinguish them from other disorders associated with abnormal nocturnal behaviours. The first of these is their temporal distribution—non-REM parasomnias will usually occur in the first third of the night, rarely occur more than once per night, and will often occur less than nightly. Although the parasomnia events can be associated with congruent dream mentation, patients will often have very limited, if any, recall of the actual events. The majority of adult non-REM parasomnia patients will have a childhood and/or family history of parasomnia behaviours, and may describe their symptoms being triggered by sleep deprivation, stress, and anxiety. A number of medications, including SSRIs, benzodiazepine receptor agonists, and lithium, may also precipitate parasomnia events in susceptible individuals (Zadra et al., 2013).

A diagnosis of non-REM parasomnia can be made from history alone, but video PSG is frequently used to identify any potential contributory sleep-disrupting pathology—such as OSA—and to exclude disorders which may mimic non-REM parasomnia—including RBD and nocturnal frontal lobe epilepsy. PSG findings include sudden spontaneous arousals from N3 sleep, with hypersynchronous delta waves. Sleep deprivation is a useful tool in unmasking parasomnia; for example, sleepwalking episodes are approximately 2.5 times more likely to happen in patients undergoing PSG if they have not slept for the preceding 25 hours (Zadra et al., 2008).

Somnambulism

The archetypal parasomnia is also one of the commonest—sleepwalking has a lifetime prevalence of close to 30% (Ohayon et al., 2012a), with a point prevalence peaking at over 13% in 10-year-old children (Zadra et al., 2013). While sleepwalking behaviours cease over time in the majority of cases, a prevalence of approximately 4% persists into adulthood and is significantly more likely to be seen in subjects with OSA, substance misuse, or psychiatric illness (Ohayon et al., 2012a). Sleepwalking episodes vary significantly in complexity and severity, ranging from simply standing or sitting by the bed to performing complex tasks like cooking, or even to attempting to drive. While the principal indications for treating sleepwalking are reduction of emotional distress and avoidance of physical harm, patients also appear to be more likely to experience EDS and reduced daytime functionality than matched controls (Montplaisir et al., 2011). The majority of cases can be satisfactorily managed by conservative measures—avoidance of precipitating factors and adaptation of the sleeping environment to reduce external stimuli and minimize the risk of physical harm. Scheduled awakenings, whereby a patient is awoken shortly before a sleepwalking episode may be expected to occur, may be highly effective in paediatric sleepwalkers (Galbiati et al., 2015). Pharmacological intervention should be reserved for refractory cases or—particularly—cases where the risk of physical injury is significant. The evidence base in this area is largely limited to case reports and other uncontrolled studies; however, long-term, low-dose benzodiazepine appears to be efficacious and safe, while adjuvant treatment with TCADs may also be of benefit in some patients. A number of behavioural and cognitive therapeutic approaches have also been evaluated, with some apparent success (Galbiati et al., 2015). There is however, a marked paucity of high-quality data in this area (Harris and Grunstein, 2009).

Night terrors

Night terrors ('sleep terrors'; 'pavor nocturnus') may be the most dramatic of the parasomnias, involving sudden distressed arousals from sleep, accompanied by screaming, weeping, and distress, alongside evidence of marked sympathetic activation (Fleetham and Fleming, 2014). A relatively unique clinical characteristic is inconsolability, with any attempts to calm the patient potentially producing a paradoxical worsening of the episode. Although generally confined to the bed, night terrors may nevertheless lead to physical injury to the patient due to associated somnambulism, or to bed partners if the episode precipitates violent behaviour. Highly prevalent in young children (Petit et al., 2015), they are significantly less common in adult populations, occurring in approximately 2% of adults (Ohayon et al., 1999). Treatment of night terrors is similar to that of sleepwalking, involving avoidance of triggering factors and

environmental adaptations, with sedative pharmacotherapy used in severe cases.

Confusional arousal

Probably the commonest non-REM parasomnia, confusional arousal ('sleep drunkenness') occurs at some point in almost all young children and appears to persist in up to 4% of adults (Ohayon et al., 1999). It appears to be particularly common in psychiatric populations and in patients with other sleep-disrupting pathology such as OSA. Episodes are characterized by impaired cognition, following awakenings from N3 sleep, which may be accompanied by abnormal behaviours. Patients will usually have complete amnesia for the events. Use of sedative and other psychoactive substances—including alcohol—has a particularly strong relationship with the risk of confusional arousal, and treatment of the disorder is generally confined to minimization of exposure to these and other potential triggering factors, along with treatment of any concomitant sleep disorders, particularly OSA.

Sleep-related eating disorder

A relatively uncommon variant of sleepwalking, patients with sleep-related eating disorder (SRED) compulsively eat during episodes. SRED is particularly common in patients with other eating disorders and needs to be distinguished from nocturnal eating behaviours and from night eating syndrome wherein patients habitually consume large amounts of food overnight while fully awake (Howell et al., 2009). The principal concern in the management of patients with SRED is harm minimization, avoiding both physical injury and ingestion of potentially hazardous substances. As with the other non-REM parasomnias outlined earlier, the majority of cases can be satisfactorily managed with relatively conservative measures.

Sexsomnia

A rare subtype of non-REM parasomnia, sometimes categorized as a variant of confusional arousal, patients with sexsomnia perform sexual acts during incomplete arousals from N3 sleep, ranging from masturbation to full intercourse (Ariño et al., 2014). They will have complete amnesia for these events, which can lead to marked relationship and forensic issues. Once again, management revolves around avoidance of triggering factors and treatment of any organic sleep disorders, with the option of introducing hypnotic pharmacotherapy (Muza et al., 2016).

REM sleep parasomnias

REM sleep behaviour disorder

Patients with RBD have a loss of the expected peripheral muscle atonia in REM sleep, accompanied by dream enactment behaviours, which are often violent in nature. RBD appears to have a population prevalence of approximately 0.5% (Ohayon et al., 1997) and is substantially commoner in men and with advancing age (Bonakis et al., 2009; Schenck et al., 1993). It is highly prevalent in patients with PD and in other synucleinopathies, narcoleptics, and subjects on antidepressant medication (Bonakis et al., 2009; Frauscher et al., 2010). RBD behaviours are frequently violent and usually confined to the bed, may be associated with aggressive verbalization, and confer a reasonably high risk of physical injury. They can often be clinically distinguished from non-REM parasomnias by their temporal distribution (typically occurring in the second half of the night), later age of onset, and association with violent or threatening dreams (Frauscher et al., 2010).

REM sleep and associated peripheral muscle atonia are mediated via the interaction of a number of pathways in the pons, medulla, and spinal interneurons (España and Scammell, 2011). Lesions at any of these levels can conceptually lead to RBD; data from radiological and autopsy studies suggest that these sites are involved in RBD related to synucleinopathies (Boeve, 2013). RBD may represent a *forme fruste* of PD, DLB, and MSA, with one longitudinal study finding that synucleinopathies were eventually identified in 91% of patients with seemingly idiopathic RBD (Iranzo et al., 2014). Thus, a new diagnosis of RBD without any apparent causative factors should prompt investigation for clinically occult neurodegenerative disease and consideration of initiation of neuroprotective measures.

While a diagnosis of RBD can be made to a significant degree on the basis of the clinical history, current diagnostic criteria mandate the use of PSG to identify the characteristic loss of atonia during REM sleep and to exclude contributory or confounding sleep pathology such as OSA and nocturnal frontal lobe epilepsy (Sateia, 2014). Modification of the sleep environment to minimize risk of harm to patients and their bed partners is a cornerstone of management of RBD, but pharmacotherapy is often indicated—clonazepam and melatonin appear equally efficacious in this respect, with the latter often being better tolerated, particularly in older patients (Jung and St Louis, 2016). While both agents may reduce RBD symptoms, dream enactment behaviours will often persist.

Sleep paralysis

Subjects with SP experience an inability to move at sleep onset or—more commonly—at sleep offset; movement of ocular muscles is almost uniformly preserved. Although particularly common in patients with narcolepsy, isolated SP has a lifetime prevalence of close to 8% in the general population and may occur in over a quarter of university students and a third of psychiatric patients (Sharpless and Barber, 2011). SP is frequently associated with threatening visual and somatic hypnopompic hallucinations, often of seemingly supernatural origin, and patients may seek religious or spiritual assistance prior to presentation to sleep medicine services. Potential contributory or precipitating factors include OSA, sleeping in a supine position, and stress (Ohayon et al., 1999). Reassurance regarding the benign nature of SP, alongside avoidance or treatment of triggering factors, may be the only treatment necessary, but antidepressant therapy may be efficacious in cases where SP refractory to these measures is causing significant distress.

Nightmare disorder

Nightmare disorder may be diagnosed when patients experience recurrent awakenings from sleep with vivid recall of distressing dream mentation, principally arising from REM sleep, without confusion or impaired cognition. Seen in approximately 4% of the general population, it is significantly more common in subjects with psychiatric diagnoses, particularly PTSD (Aurora et al., 2010).

Pharmacotherapy may be indicated where nightmares are associated with significant impairment in sleep quality and QoL measures; the α-adrenergic receptor antagonist prazosin is the agent with the best evidence supporting its use in this area. Second-line agents include clonidine, trazodone, benzodiazepines, and atypical antipsychotic medications (Aurora et al., 2010).

Other parasomnias

Exploding head syndrome

Characterized by the sensation of an explosion, thunderclap, or shock—usually pain-free—occurring in the head at sleep onset or offset, exploding head syndrome is a rather enigmatic entity of uncertain clinical significance (Sharpless, 2014). It appears to occur predominantly at transitions between wakefulness and sleep but does not seem to arise directly from sleep. Important differential diagnoses include nocturnal epilepsy syndromes and headache disorders. Although there is no overarching medical need for treatment of exploding head syndrome, case reports suggest that clomipramine, calcium channel blockers, and anticonvulsants may be of benefit in particularly distressing cases.

Circadian rhythm sleep disorders

Circadian rhythms are 24-hour rhythms in physiology and behaviour generated by molecular clocks, which serve to coordinate internal time with the external world (Jagannath et al., 2017). Circadian rhythm sleep disorders (CRSDs) arise from a misalignment of endogenous circadian rhythms and the 24-hour light–dark cycle of environmental time, resulting in insomnia and/or EDS, impairment of cognitive functioning, increased association with a number of neuropsychiatric disorders, metabolic syndrome, and a reduced QoL (American Academy of Sleep Medicine, 2014; Jagannath et al., 2017; Zee et al., 2013). A bidirectional relationship between mental health issues and circadian disorders is increasingly recognized. The link between neuropsychiatric disorders, including MDD, bipolar affective disorder, and schizophrenia, and the dysregulation of multiple circadian outputs has been suggested by a number of studies to date (Chung et al., 2012, Jagannath et al., 2017, Mondin et al., 2017). Similarly, a number of circadian and clock-controlled gene mutations have recently been identified by GWAS in the aetiology of sleep, mental health, and metabolic disorders (Jagannath et al., 2017). Many clinicians and scientists argue that disruption of the molecular clock is not just a consequence of neuropsychiatric illness, but that it instead forms part of a bidirectional feedback loop (Jagannath et al., 2017), with many disease-relevant processes, such as monoaminergic neurotransmitter synthesis, signalling, and degradation, being under circadian control. Several recent studies also point to a marked disruption in the circadian rhythmicity and phasing of core clock genes across multiple brain regions in patients with neuropsychiatric disorders (Jagannath et al., 2017). Cellular molecular clocks are maintained in synchrony by a master pacemaker located in the suprachiasmatic nuclei (SCN) of the anterior hypothalamus and by a variety of signals that provide temporal cues—so called zeitgebers. The light–dark cycle is the strongest synchronizing agent for the circadian system. However, many other zeitgebers have also been recognized, including feeding, glucocorticoids, temperature, indicators of physiological conditions such as metabolic state, and sleep history (Jagannath et al., 2017).

The pathophysiology of the different types of CRSDs and the exact genetic and neuroendocrine mechanisms underlying these disorders are nonetheless still largely unknown. Similarly, options for the clinical treatment of CRSDs remain limited and are mainly restricted to use of melatonin and light therapy, with the aim of therapeutically re-entraining desynchronized circadian rhythms (Auger et al., 2015). In humans, light exposure before the nocturnal core body temperature minimum produces delays, whereas light pulses after the core body temperature minimum in early morning produces advances (Auger et al., 2015). The human circadian system is most sensitive to short-wavelength blue light (approximately 480 nm) and larger effects are observed with greater intensities and longer durations of light (Auger et al., 2015). In addition to light, the SCN receives internal signals from the pineal gland, via the nocturnal release of melatonin. Endogenous melatonin release begins to increase 2–3 hours before sleep onset and peaks in the middle of the night (Jagannath et al., 2017). In contrast with the effects of light, melatonin during the early morning delays the timing of circadian rhythms, whereas melatonin during the early evening induces advances in this timing (Jagannath et al., 2017).

Among recognized CRSDs, patients with delayed and advanced sleep phase disorder show a chronic or recurrent inability to fall asleep and wake up at socially acceptable times, despite relatively normal sleep quality and structure. An abnormally long or short intrinsic circadian period (tau) is considered to be a critical factor in their pathogenesis, although it is far from clear whether functional changes in the retina, the retinohypothalamic pathway, the SCN, or adjacent hypothalamic nuclei underlie this (Jagannath et al., 2017). In addition, an altered responsiveness to light and alterations in entrainment of the circadian clock to synchronizing factors have all been suggested as possible mechanisms, while a lack of early morning light exposure and exposure to light later in the evening have been proposed to promote delayed sleep phase disorder (DSPD). For diagnostic purposes, symptoms must be present for at least 3 months and schedules need to be documented with sleep diaries and/or wrist actigraphy for a period of at least 7 days (American Academy of Sleep Medicine, 2014; Auger et al., 2015).

Irregular sleep–wake rhythm disorder (ISWRD) is an intrinsic CRSD, characterized by disorganized sleep and wake patterns in affected patients, such that multiple sleep and wake periods occur during the 24-hour cycle (American Academy of Sleep Medicine, 2014). ISWRD is considered to result from dysfunction of the circadian pacemaker itself (Zee et al., 2013), and afflicted individuals experience prolonged periods of wakefulness during the typical nocturnal sleep episode, in addition to excessive sleepiness and prolonged sleep bouts during daytime hours (Auger et al., 2015). Sleep is frequently fragmented and insufficient. ISWRD also appears to more commonly affect patients with neurodevelopmental or neurodegenerative disorders, and it may pose particular challenges for caregivers (Auger et al., 2015). Documentation of multiple non-circadian sleep–wake bouts for a period of at least 7 days is required (American Academy of Sleep Medicine, 2014). Another intrinsic circadian disorder is non-24-hour sleep–wake rhythm disorder (N24SWD), which is characterized by a chronic or recurrent pattern of sleep and wake that is not synchronized to the 24-hour environment (American Academy of Sleep Medicine, 2014).

N24SWD is observed mainly in blind people due to decreased, or lack of, photic reception (Kitamura et al., 2013). Its diagnosis requires an objective record of 14 days of progressively shifting sleep–wake times with sleep diaries and/or actigraphy (Auger et al., 2015). Finally, circadian disorders where extrinsic factors are thought to be the major aetiological cause are jet-lag disorder (JLD) and shift-work disorder (SWD). Both are thought to be due to misalignments between endogenous circadian rhythms and environmental time (Zee et al., 2013). More specifically, 'voluntary' shift of sleep and wake episodes in those disorders are caused by either travelling between time zones or by work schedules, leading to insomnia with excessive sleepiness during wakeful periods.

Therapeutic interventions for CRSDs can be broadly categorized into: (1) prescribed timing of sleep–wake and/or physical activity; (2) strategic exposure and/or avoidance of light; (3) use of medications and/or supplements to phase-shift and/or to promote sleep or wakefulness; and (4) alternating interventions that exert effects by altering bodily functions to impact sleep/wake behaviours (Auger et al., 2015). Most recent clinical practice guidelines for the treatment of intrinsic CRSDs have endorsed appropriately timed melatonin for the treatment of DSPD, blind adults with N24SWD, and children/adolescents with ISWRD with comorbid neurological disorders (Auger et al., 2015). In a similar vein, light therapy with or without accompanying behavioural interventions has been advised for adults with advanced sleep phase disorder, children/adolescents with DSPD, and elderly patients with dementia (Auger et al., 2015).

Sleep and neuropsychiatric conditions

Abnormal sleep patterns and behaviours are extremely common in a range of neuropsychiatric conditions and require recognition, as identification of these patterns may aid the diagnosis of the underlying condition and also permit management of the overall condition to be optimized.

Parkinson's disease and other parkinsonian syndromes

As discussed earlier, RBD is a frequent feature of synucleinopathies, e.g. idiopathic Parkinson's disease (IPD), DLB, MSA, and often precedes the onset of motor or other neurological symptoms by years or even decades (Iranzo et al., 2009). RBD is much rarer in tauopathies such as PSP and FTD, or AD. The presence of RBD is a strong marker for the development of cognitive impairment in IPD. However, patients with PD frequently report other forms of sleep disturbance, roughly 60% in a community-based study (Tandberg et al., 1998).

Insomnia is a commonly reported problem in IPD and is likely to be multifactorial. There remains some controversy as to whether RLS is more frequent in PD, but certainly treatment with levodopa or dopamine agonists during the day may drive augmentation in patients who have an underlying susceptibility to RLS. Furthermore, anxiety is a non-motor feature of PD and may contribute to insomnia. Other factors include nocturnal pain due to dystonia or nocturnal bradykinesia, resulting in difficulty in turning over in bed or getting up to void. Dopamine agonists at bedtime may also influence sleep, either through their stimulant effects or through the generation of impulse control disorders, resulting in compulsive behaviours. In IPD, there are also alterations in nocturnal melatonin secretion that may have a role (Videnovic et al., 2014).

Both patients and their families frequently report EDS. In extreme cases, this can result in a narcolepsy-like picture, with unpredictable sleep attacks throughout the day. Once again, daytime sleepiness is thought to be multifactorial, resulting from disrupted night-time sleep due to PD-related issues or other problems such as sleep apnoea, but in some cases degenerative changes in the brainstem itself may result in central hypersomnia. In addition, dopamine agonists have been demonstrated to result in sleep attacks, and sometimes withdrawal of these agents can result in significant improvement. Another feature of IPD is prolonged confusional arousals that may be mistaken for sleepwalking. These typically occur in patients with significant cognitive impairment or in those being treated with DBS.

In MSA, an important nocturnal issue is nocturnal stridor, thought to be as a result of excessive vocal cord adductor activation (Iranzo, 2007). This is presumed to underlie some cases of sudden death in sleep in MSA, and identification of this condition should precipitate urgent referral for ear, nose, and throat (ENT) evaluation. Treatment options include continuous positive airway pressure (CPAP) and adductor botulinum toxin injections, although evidence for either of these treatments reducing mortality is scant.

Management of these sleep issues in these patients is similar to that in the general population. In this group of conditions, there are specific issues regarding dopaminergic treatment, since a slow-acting preparation of levodopa at night may help nocturnal pain, bradykinesia, and dystonias, and withdrawal of dopamine agonists may improve daytime sleep attacks or nocturnal compulsive behaviour. Due to a higher risk of cognitive dysfunction in these patients, clonazepam should generally not be used as a first-line agent for the management of RBD, and melatonin should be trialled in the first instance. RLS should ideally be treated with alpha–delta ligands, rather than with dopaminergic drugs, and opiates in these patients should be used with caution due to possible neuropsychiatric effects and worsening of constipation.

Alzheimer's disease

Typical patterns of sleep disturbance in AD include sleep initiation insomnia, poor sleep quality, nocturnal hallucinations, nocturnal confusional wanderings, and 'sun-downing' (Ooms and Ju, 2016). These are thought to result from the direct effects of neurodegeneration in sleep-modulating areas of the brain, side effects of medications (acetylcholinesterase inhibitors and memantine can induce insomnia and many antipsychotics are sedating), and associated psychiatric problems such as anxiety or mood disturbance. Management of sleep issues in this patient cohort can be extremely difficult due to competing issues and concerns regarding drug side effects. Melatonin and light therapy may help with circadian rhythm abnormalities and 'sun-downing', but other pharmacological therapies should be carefully considered on a case-by-case basis.

Stroke

Sleep disturbance in stroke patients is both common and of clinical importance. Evidence suggests that sleep problems influence functional outcome, length of inpatient stay, and risk of stroke recurrence (Hermann and Bassetti, 2016), and sleep disturbance affects up to half of all stroke patients (Mims and Kirsch, 2016).

Sleep-disordered breathing is a particular problem, especially in the acute setting, presumably due to alterations in innervation of the oropharyngeal musculature and central apnoea related to brainstem lesions. Other sleep issues include hypersomnia, most frequently seen after striatal, thalamic, or ponto-medullary strokes, insomnia, and occasional symptomatic RLS. Treatment of these problems is similar to that in the general population. CPAP, however, may be challenging to fit and may require proper training of carers, and in general post-stroke hypersomnia is relatively refractory to stimulant therapy.

Traumatic brain injury

This cohort of patients is extremely heterogenous, and the condition is influenced by trauma severity, nature, and localization (Baumann, 2016). However, sleep disturbance is common and not always related to severity or localization. Frequent issues include an increased sleep need, circadian rhythm abnormalities (often a delayed sleep phase or an irregular sleep–wake pattern), and EDS. Insomnia is much less of a problem and can relate to psychological disturbances such as PTSD.

Neuroimmunological disorders

A number of neurological conditions mediated by antibodies result in characteristic sleep disturbances. While patients with MS frequently have insomnia, RLS, PLMD, and hypersomnia, the related condition of neuromyelitis optica (NMO) (previously called Devic's disease) may cause profound hypersomnia or symptomatic narcolepsy (Nishino and Kanbayashi, 2005). NMO is mediated by an antibody directed against the aquaporin-4 water channel protein, which is highly expressed in hypothalamic and periaqueductal areas, and inflammation in these areas may lesion wake-promoting areas.

Two other antibody-mediated conditions merit mention in this context (Vincent et al., 2011). Anti-voltage-gated potassium channel antibodies mediate both central and peripheral nervous system disorders, depending on the antibody subtype. Antibodies directed against LGI1 cause limbic encephalitis, resulting in confusion, memory problems, seizures, hyponatraemia, and insomnia, although occasionally also hypersomnia. Morvan's syndrome, the association of central involvement and peripheral manifestations such as myokymia and autonomic symptoms such as hyperhydrosis, is associated with profound insomnia and, in extreme cases, can result in the complete loss of slow-wave sleep, resulting in a similar sleep architecture as seen in delirium tremens and fatal familial insomnia.

Anti-NMDA receptor antibody encephalitis is frequently driven by ovarian teratoma in young women and presents with behavioural change, agitation, paranoia, and psychosis, with stereotypic bizarre movements of the mouth or limbs. Subsequent development of seizures, catatonia, and autonomic dysfunction can be life-threatening. There is a typical prodrome, and sleep disturbance in the form of insomnia prior to the development of other neuropsychiatric features is a hallmark of this condition.

Low visual acuity

Patients with low visual acuity are frequently referred to the sleep clinic with hallucinations at sleep onset. However, in most cases, careful clinical evaluation reveals that these hallucinations are not associated with drowsiness, but with low lighting levels. Rather than representing a sleep disorder, such as hypnagogic hallucinations, these patients are describing Charles Bonnet hallucinations, resulting from deafferentation of the visual cortex (Lerario et al., 2013). These hallucinations are often vivid, involving people and animals with alterations in size or proportion. Patients will often describe that they continue until the lights are turned on, although they can sometimes be stopped by opening and closing the eyes or looking around. In addition, patients with no vision may develop circadian rhythm disorders due to loss of the role of light in the entrainment of endogenous circadian rhythm (Uchiyama and Lockley, 2015).

Conclusion

Sleep and its disorders have a profound effect on health and well-being. Insufficient or broken sleep has a marked deleterious effect on mental and physical health, while physical sleep disorders, such as narcolepsy and OSA, can have profound psychological, as well as medical, effects. Conversely, psychiatric disease may manifest itself via disturbed nocturnal sleep or EDS. Consequently, primary sleep disorders should be considered in patients presenting with apparent psychiatric or neuropsychiatric symptoms, and mental health needs to be carefully evaluated in those undergoing investigation of sleep-related symptoms.

KEY LEARNING POINTS

- Sleep problems can cause or exacerbate neuropsychiatric disease, influence the course of its treatment, or serve as a diagnostic signpost for a range of neuropsychiatric disorders. For instance, depressive episodes are frequently preceded by insomnia, while dream enactment behaviour may be an indicator of a neurodegenerative disorder.
- This chapter focuses on a number of sleep disorders, from insomnia and various hypersomnias to CRSDs, exploring their clinical features, pathophysiology, and treatment. It begins by delineating the two main types of sleep—REM and NREM—along with their stages, before moving on to examination of specific disorders.
- Finally, neuropsychiatric conditions such as AD and PD are discussed, relating the way in which they present themselves through sleep problems.

REFERENCES

Allen RP, Picchietti DL, García-Borreguero D, et al., Restless legs syndrome/Willis-Ekbom disease diagnostic criteria: updated International Restless Legs Syndrome Study Group (IRLSSG) consensus criteria—history, rationale, description, and significance. *Sleep Med* 2014;**15**:860–73.

American Academy of Sleep Medicine. *International Classification of Sleep Disorders*, third edition. Darien, IL, American Academy of Sleep Medicine, 2014.

Ariño H, Iranzo A, Gaig C, et al. Sexsomnia: parasomnia associated with sexual behaviour during sleep. *Neurologia* 2014;**29**:146–52.

Arnulf I, Rico TJ, Mignot E. Diagnosis, disease course, and management of patients with Kleine-Levin syndrome. *Lancet Neurol* 2012;**11**:918–28.

Auger, R. R., et al. Clinical Practice Guideline for the Treatment of Intrinsic Circadian Rhythm Sleep-Wake Disorders: Advanced Sleep-Wake Phase Disorder (ASWPD), Delayed Sleep-Wake Phase Disorder (DSWPD), Non-24-Hour Sleep-Wake Rhythm Disorder (N24SWD), and Irregular Sleep-Wake Rhythm Disorder (ISWRD). An Update for 2015: An American Academy of Sleep Medicine Clinical Practice Guideline. *J Clin Sleep Med* 2015;**11**:1199–236.

Aurora RN, Zak RS, Auerbach SH, et al., Best practice guide for the treatment of nightmare disorder in adults. *J Clin Sleep Med* 2010;**6**:389–401.

Banerjee D, Yee BJ, Piper AJ, et al. Obesity hypoventilation syndrome: hypoxemia during continuous positive airway pressure. *Chest* 2007;**131**:1678–84.

Baumann CR. Sleep and Traumatic Brain Injury. *Sleep Med Clin* 2016;**11**:19–23.

Baumann CR, Mignot E, Lammers GJ, et al. Challenges in diagnosing narcolepsy without cataplexy: a consensus statement. *Sleep* 2014;**37**:1035–42.

Bayard M, Bailey B, Acharya D, et al. Bupropion and restless legs syndrome: a randomized controlled trial. *J Am Board Fam Med* 2011;**24**:422–8.

Billiard M, Sonka K. Idiopathic hypersomnia. *Sleep Med Rev* 2016;**29**:23–33.

Billings ME, Watson NF, Keogh BP. Dynamic fMRI changes in Kleine-Levin syndrome. *Sleep Med* 2011;**12**:532.

Boeve BF. Idiopathic REM sleep behaviour disorder in the development of Parkinson's disease. *Lancet Neurol* 2013;**12**:469–82.

Bonakis A, Howard RS, Ebrahim IO, et al. REM sleep behaviour disorder (RBD) and its associations in young patients. *Sleep Med* 2009;**10**:641–5.

Browaldh N, Nerfeldt P, Lysdahl M, et al. SKUP3 randomised controlled trial: polysomnographic results after uvulopalatopharyngoplasty in selected patients with obstructive sleep apnoea. *Thorax* 2013;**68**:846–53.

Byrne R, Sinha S, Chaudhuri KR. Restless legs syndrome: diagnosis and review of management options. *Neuropsychiatr Dis Treat* 2006;**2**:155–64.

Campos-Rodriguez F, Martinez-Garcia MA, Martinez M, et al. Association between obstructive sleep apnea and cancer incidence in a large multicenter Spanish cohort. *Am J Respir Crit Care Med* 2013;**187**:99–105.

Castro-Añón O, Pérez de Llano LA, De la Fuente Sánchez S, et al. Obesity-hypoventilation syndrome: increased risk of death over sleep apnea syndrome. *PLoS One* 2015;**10**:e0117808.

Chung JK, Lee KY, Kim SH, et al. 2012. Circadian Rhythm Characteristics in Mood Disorders: Comparison among Bipolar I Disorder, Bipolar II Disorder and Recurrent Major Depressive Disorder. *Clin Psychopharmacol Neurosci* 2012;**10**:110–16.

Cornelius JR, Tippmann-Peikert M, Slocumb NL, et al. Impulse control disorders with the use of dopaminergic agents in restless legs syndrome: a case-control study. *Sleep* 2010;**33**:81–7.

Cowie MR, Woehrle H, Wegscheider K et al., Adaptive Servo-Ventilation for Central Sleep Apnea in Systolic Heart Failure. *N Engl J Med* 2015;**373**:1095–105.

Daulatzai MA. Death by a thousand cuts in Alzheimer's disease: hypoxia--the prodrome. *Neurotox Res* 2013;**24**:216–43.

Dauvilliers Y, Montplaisir J, Molinari N, et al. Age at onset of narcolepsy in two large populations of patients in France and Quebec. *Neurology* 2001;**57**:2029–33.

Donovan LM, Kapur VK. Prevalence and Characteristics of Central Compared to Obstructive Sleep Apnea: Analyses from the Sleep Heart Health Study Cohort. *Sleep* 2016;**39**:1353–9.

Drakatos P, Leschziner GD. Update on hypersomnias of central origin. *Curr Opin Pulm Med* 2014;**20**:572–80.

Drakatos P, Suri A, Higgins SE, et al. Sleep stage sequence analysis of sleep onset REM periods in the hypersomnias. *J Neurol Neurosurg Psychiatry* 2013;**84**:223–7.

Eastwood PR, Malhotra A, Palmer LJ, et al. Obstructive Sleep Apnoea: From pathogenesis to treatment: Current controversies and future directions. *Respirology* 2010;**15**:587–95.

Eckert DJ, Jordan AS, Merchia P, et al. Central sleep apnea: Pathophysiology and treatment. *Chest* 2007;**131**:595–607.

Edwards C, Mukherjee S, Simpson L, et al. Depressive Symptoms before and after Treatment of Obstructive Sleep Apnea in Men and Women. *J Clin Sleep Med* 2015;**11**:1029–38.

Emamian F, Khazaie H, Tahmasian M, et al. The Association Between Obstructive Sleep Apnea and Alzheimer's Disease: A Meta-Analysis Perspective. *Front Aging Neurosci* 2016;**8**:78.

España R, Scammell TE. Sleep neurobiology from a clinical perspective. *Sleep* 2011;**34**:845–58.

Fleetham JA, Fleming JAE. Parasomnias. *CMAJ* 2014;**186**:E273–80.

Frauscher B, Gschliesser V, Brandauer E, et al. REM sleep behavior disorder in 703 sleep-disorder patients: the importance of eliciting a comprehensive sleep history. *Sleep Med* 2010;**11**:167–71.

Galbiati A, Rinaldi F, Giora E, et al. Behavioural and Cognitive-Behavioural Treatments of Parasomnias. *Behav Neurol* 2015;**2015**:786928.

García-Borreguero D, Stillman P, Benes H, et al. Algorithms for the diagnosis and treatment of restless legs syndrome in primary care. *BMC Neurol* 2011;**11**:28.

García-Borreguero D, Williams A-M. Dopaminergic augmentation of restless legs syndrome. *Sleep Med Rev* 2010;**14**:339–46.

Garvey JF, Pengo MF, Drakatos P, et al. Epidemiological aspects of obstructive sleep apnea. *J Thorac Dis* 2015;**7**:920–9.

Gottlieb DJ, Yenokyan G, Newman AB, et al. Prospective study of obstructive sleep apnea and incident coronary heart disease and heart failure: the sleep heart health study. *Circulation* 2010;**122**:352–60.

Gupta MA, Simpson FC. Obstructive sleep apnea and psychiatric disorders: a systematic review. *J Clin Sleep Med* 2015;**11**:165–75.

Habel LA, Cooper WO, Sox CM, et al. ADHD medications and risk of serious cardiovascular events in young and middle-aged adults. *JAMA* 2011;**306**:2673–83.

Harris M, Grunstein RR. Treatments for somnambulism in adults: assessing the evidence. *Sleep Med Rev* 2009;**13**:295–7.

Heinzer R, Vat S, Marques-Vidal P, et al. Prevalence of sleep-disordered breathing in the general population: the HypnoLaus study. *Lancet Respir Med* 2015;**3**:310–18.

Hermann DM, Bassetti CL. Role of sleep-disordered breathing and sleep-wake disturbances for stroke and stroke recovery. *Neurology* 2016;**87**:1407–16.

Hornyak M, Scholz H, Kohnen R, et al. What treatment works best for restless legs syndrome? Meta-analyses of dopaminergic and non-dopaminergic medications. *Sleep Med Rev* 2014;**18**:153–64.

Howell MJ, Schenck CH, Crow SJ. A review of nighttime eating disorders. *Sleep Med Rev* 2009;**13**:23–34.

Iber C, Ancoli-Israel S, Chesson A, et al. *The AASM Manual for the Scoring of Sleep and Associates Events: Rules, Terminology and Technical Specifications*. Westchester, IL, American Academy of Sleep Medicine.

Iranzo A. Sleep and breathing in multiple system atrophy. *Curr Treat Options Neurol* 2007;**9**:347–53.

Iranzo A, Fernández-Arcos A, Tolosa E, et al. Neurodegenerative disorder risk in idiopathic REM sleep behavior disorder: study in 174 patients. *PLoS One* 2014;**9**:e89741.

Iranzo A, Santamaria J, Tolosa E. The clinical and pathophysiological relevance of REM sleep behavior disorder in neurodegenerative diseases. *Sleep Med Rev* 2009;**13**:385–401.

Jaganath, A., Taylore, L., Wakaf, Z., et al. The genetics of circadian rhythms, sleep and health. *Hum Mol Genet* 2017;**26**:R128–38.

Javaheri S, Harris N, Howard J, et al. Adaptive servoventilation for treatment of opioid-associated central sleep apnea. *J Clin Sleep Med* 2014;**10**:637–43.

Jung Y, St Louis EK. Treatment of REM Sleep Behavior Disorder. *Curr Treat Options Neurol* 2016;**18**:50.

Kaw R, Hernandez A V, Walker E, et al. Determinants of hypercapnia in obese patients with obstructive sleep apnea: a systematic review and metaanalysis of cohort studies. *Chest* 2009;**136**:787–96.

Kendzerska T, Gershon AS, Hawker G, et al. Obstructive sleep apnea and risk of cardiovascular events and all-cause mortality: a decade-long historical cohort study. *PLoS Med* 2014;**11**:e1001599.

Kent BD, Grote L, Bonsignore MR, et al. Sleep apnoea severity independently predicts glycaemic health in nondiabetic subjects: the ESADA study. *Eur Respir J* 2014;**44**:130–9.

Kent BD, McNicholas WT, Ryan S. Insulin resistance, glucose intolerance and diabetes mellitus in obstructive sleep apnoea. *J Thorac Dis* 2015;**7**:1343–57.

Kent BD, Ryan S, McNicholas WT. Obstructive sleep apnea and inflammation: relationship to cardiovascular co-morbidity. *Respir Physiol Neurobiol* 2011;**178**:475–81.

Krystal AD. Current, emerging, and newly available insomnia medications. *J Clin Psychiatry* 2015;**76**:e1045.

Kylstra WA, Aaronson JA, Hofman WF, et al. Neuropsychological functioning after CPAP treatment in obstructive sleep apnea: a meta-analysis. *Sleep Med Rev* 2013;**17**:341–7.

Lee JJ, Erdos J, Wilkosz MF, et al. Bupropion as a possible treatment option for restless legs syndrome. *Ann Pharmacother* 2009;**43**:370–4.

Lerario A, Ciammola A, Poletti B, et al. Charles Bonnet syndrome: two case reports and review of the literature. *J Neurol* 2013;**260**:1180–6.

Leschziner G. Narcolepsy: a clinical review. *Pract Neurol* 2014;**14**:323–31.

Leschziner G, Gringras P. Restless legs syndrome. *BMJ* 2012;**344**:e3056.

Leu-Semenescu S, Le Corvec T, Groos E, et al. Lithium therapy in Kleine-Levin syndrome: An open-label, controlled study in 130 patients. *Neurology* 2015;**85**:1655–62.

Marti I, Valko PO, Khatami R, et al. Multiple sleep latency measures in narcolepsy and behaviourally induced insufficient sleep syndrome. *Sleep Med* 2009;**10**:1146–50.

Martínez-García MÁ, Campos-Rodriguez F, Barbé F. Cancer and OSA: Current Evidence From Human Studies. *Chest* 2016;**150**:451–63.

Masa JF, Corral J, Alonso ML, et al. Efficacy of Different Treatment Alternatives for Obesity Hypoventilation Syndrome. Pickwick Study. *Am J Respir Crit Care Med* 2015;**192**:86–95.

McEvoy RD, Antic NA, Heeley E, et al. CPAP for Prevention of Cardiovascular Events in Obstructive Sleep Apnea. *N Engl J Med* 2016a;**375**:919–31.

McEvoy RD, Chai-Coetzer CL, Antic NA. Ambulatory Diagnosis and Management of Obstructive Sleep Apnea: Screening

Questionnaires, Diagnostic Tests, and the Care Team. *Sleep Med Clin* 2016b;**11**:265–72.

Mignot E. Genetic and familial aspects of narcolepsy. *Neurology* 2008;**50**:S16–22.

Mims KN, Kirsch D. Sleep and Stroke. *Sleep Med Clin* 2016;**11**:39–51.

Mokhlesi B, Tulaimat A, Faibussowitsch I, et al. Obesity hypoventilation syndrome: prevalence and predictors in patients with obstructive sleep apnea. *Sleep Breath* 2007;**11**:117–24.

Mondin TC, Cardoso TA, Souza LDM, et al. 2017. Mood disorders and biological rhythms in young adults: A large population-based study. *J Psychiatr Res* 2017;**84**:98–104.

Montplaisir J, Boucher S, Poirier G, et al. Clinical, polysomnographic, and genetic characteristics of restless legs syndrome: a study of 133 patients diagnosed with new standard criteria. *Mov Disord* 1997;**12**:61–5.

Montplaisir J, Petit D, Pilon M, et al. Does sleepwalking impair daytime vigilance? *J Clin Sleep Med* 2011;**7**:219.

Muza R, Lawrence M, Drakatos P. The reality of sexsomnia. *Curr Opin Pulm Med* 2016;**22**:576–82.

Nesbitt AD, Leschziner GD. Migraine with brainstem aura presenting as recurrent hypersomnia (Kleine-Levin syndrome). *Pract Neurol* 2016;**16**:402–5.

Nieto FJ, Peppard PE, Young T, et al. Sleep-disordered breathing and cancer mortality: results from the Wisconsin Sleep Cohort Study. *Am J Respir Crit Care Med* 2012;**186**:190–4.

Nishino S, Kanbayashi T. Symptomatic narcolepsy, cataplexy and hypersomnia, and their implications in the hypothalamic hypocretin/orexin system. *Sleep Med Rev* 2005;**9**:269–310.

Ohayon MM. Narcolepsy is complicated by high medical and psychiatric comorbidities: a comparison with the general population. *Sleep Med* 2013;**14**:488–92.

Ohayon MM, Caulet M, Priest RG. Violent behavior during sleep. *J Clin Psychiatry* 1997;**58**:369–76; quiz 377.

Ohayon MM, Guilleminault C, Priest RG. Night terrors, sleepwalking, and confusional arousals in the general population: their frequency and relationship to other sleep and mental disorders. *J Clin Psychiatry* 1999;**60**:268–76; quiz 277.

Ohayon MM, Mahowald MW, Dauvilliers Y, et al. Prevalence and comorbidity of nocturnal wandering in the U.S. adult general population. *Neurology* 2012a;**78**:1583–9.

Ohayon MM, O'Hara R, Vitiello MV. Epidemiology of restless legs syndrome: a synthesis of the literature. *Sleep Med Rev* 2012b;**16**:283–95.

Ohayon MM, Zulley J, Guilleminault C, et al. Prevalence and pathologic associations of sleep paralysis in the general population. *Neurology* 1999;**52**:1194–200.

Ooms S, Ju Y-E. Treatment of Sleep Disorders in Dementia. *Curr Treat Options Neurol* 2016;**18**:40.

Pengo MF, Xiao S, Ratneswaran C, et al. Randomised sham-controlled trial of transcutaneous electrical stimulation in obstructive sleep apnoea. *Thorax* 2016;**71**:923–31.

Peppard PE, Szklo-Coxe M, Hla KM, et al. Longitudinal association of sleep-related breathing disorder and depression. *Arch Intern Med* 2006;**166**:1709–15.

Peppard PE, Young T, Barnet JH, et al. Increased prevalence of sleep-disordered breathing in adults. *Am J Epidemiol* 2013;**177**:1006–14.

Peppard PE, Young T, Palta M, et al. Prospective study of the association between sleep-disordered breathing and hypertension. *N Engl J Med* 2000a;**342**:1378–84.

Peppard PE, Young T, Palta M, et al. Longitudinal study of moderate weight change and sleep-disordered breathing. *JAMA* 2000b;**284**:3015–21.

Petit D, Pennestri M-H, Paquet J, et al. Childhood Sleepwalking and Sleep Terrors: A Longitudinal Study of Prevalence and Familial Aggregation. *JAMA Pediatr* 2015;**169**:653–8.

Plante DT. Sleep propensity in psychiatric hypersomnolence: A systematic review and meta-analysis of multiple sleep latency test findings. *Sleep Med Rev* 2017;**31**:48–57.

Redline S, Yenokyan G, Gottlieb DJ, et al. Obstructive sleep apnea-hypopnea and incident stroke: the sleep heart health study. *Am J Respir Crit Care Med* 2010;**182**:269–77.

Rose AR, Catcheside PG, McEvoy RD, et al. Sleep disordered breathing and chronic respiratory failure in patients with chronic pain on long term opioid therapy. *J Clin Sleep Med* 2014;**10**:847–52.

Rosenzweig I, Glasser M, Polsek D, et al. Sleep apnoea and the brain: a complex relationship. *Lancet Respir Med* 2015;**3**:404–14.

Rye DB. The Molecular Genetics of Restless Legs Syndrome. *Sleep Med Clin* 2015;**10**:227–33, xii.

Rye DB, Bliwise DL, Parker K, et al. Modulation of vigilance in the primary hypersomnias by endogenous enhancement of GABAA receptors. *Sci Transl Med* 2012;**4**:161ra151.

Sateia MJ. International classification of sleep disorders-third edition: highlights and modifications. *Chest* 2014;**146**:1387–94.

Sawyer AM, Gooneratne NS, Marcus CL, et al. A systematic review of CPAP adherence across age groups: clinical and empiric insights for developing CPAP adherence interventions. *Sleep Med Rev* 2011;**15**:343–56.

Schenck, Hurwitz, Mahowald. Symposium: Normal and abnormal REM sleep regulation: REM sleep behaviour disorder: an update on a series of 96 patients and a review of the world literature. *J Sleep Res* 1993;**2**:224–31.

Sharpless BA. Exploding head syndrome. *Sleep Med Rev* 2014;**18**:489–93.

Sharpless BA, Barber JP. Lifetime prevalence rates of sleep paralysis: a systematic review. *Sleep Med Rev* 2011;**15**:311–15.

Silber MH. Clinical practice. Chronic insomnia. *N Engl J Med* 2005;**353**:803–10.

Silver N, Allen RP, Senerth J, et al. A 10-year, longitudinal assessment of dopamine agonists and methadone in the treatment of restless legs syndrome. *Sleep Med* 2011;**12**:440–4.

Šonka K, Šusta M, Billiard M. Narcolepsy with and without cataplexy, idiopathic hypersomnia with and without long sleep time: a cluster analysis. *Sleep Med* 2015;**16**:225–31.

Steier J, Martin A, Harris J, et al. Predicted relative prevalence estimates for obstructive sleep apnoea and the associated healthcare provision across the UK. *Thorax* 2014;**69**:390–2.

Strollo PJ, Gillespie MB, Soose RJ, et al. Upper Airway Stimulation for Obstructive Sleep Apnea: Durability of the Treatment Effect at 18 Months. *Sleep* 2015;**38**:1593–8.

Tandberg E, Larsen JP, Karlsen K. A community-based study of sleep disorders in patients with Parkinson's disease. *Mov Disord* 1998;**13**:895–9.

Trenkwalder C, Beneš H, Grote L, et al. Prolonged release oxycodone-naloxone for treatment of severe restless legs syndrome after failure of previous treatment: a double-blind, randomised, placebo-controlled trial with an open-label extension. *Lancet Neurol* 2013;**12**:1141–50.

Trenkwalder C, Högl B, Benes H, et al. Augmentation in restless legs syndrome is associated with low ferritin. *Sleep Med* 2008;**9**:572–4.

Trotti LM, Saini P, Freeman A, et al. Improvement in daytime sleepiness with clarithromycin in patients with GABA-related hypersomnia: Clinical experience. *J Psychopharmacol* 2014; 28: 697–702.

Trotti LM, Staab BA, Rye DB. Test-retest reliability of the multiple sleep latency test in narcolepsy without cataplexy and idiopathic hypersomnia. *J Clin Sleep Med* 2013;**9**:789–95.

Uchiyama M, Lockley SW. Non-24-hourour Sleep-Wake Rhythm Disorder in Sighted and Blind Patients. *Sleep Med Clin* 2015;**10**:495–516.

Videnovic A, Noble C, Reid KJ, et al. Circadian melatonin rhythm and excessive daytime sleepiness in Parkinson disease. *JAMA Neurol* 2014;**71**:463–9.

Vincent A, Bien CG, Irani SR, et al. Autoantibodies associated with diseases of the CNS: new developments and future challenges. *Lancet Neurol* 2011;**10**:759–72.

Wang D, Teichtahl H, Drummer O, et al. Central sleep apnea in stable methadone maintenance treatment patients. *Chest* 2005;**128**:1348–56.

Williams J, Roth A, Vatthauer K, et al. Cognitive behavioral treatment of insomnia. *Chest* 2013;**143**:554–65.

Winkelman JW. Considering the causes of RLS. *Eur J Neurol* 2006;**13 Suppl 3**:8–14.

Winkelman JW. Clinical practice. Insomnia disorder. *N Engl J Med* 2015;**373**:1437–44.

Young T, Palta M, Dempsey J, et al. The occurrence of sleep-disordered breathing among middle-aged adults. *N Engl J Med* 1993;**328**:1230–5.

Zadra A, Desautels A, Petit D, et al. Somnambulism: clinical aspects and pathophysiological hypotheses. *Lancet Neurol* 2013;**12**:285–94.

Zadra A, Pilon M, Montplaisir J. Polysomnographic diagnosis of sleepwalking: effects of sleep deprivation. *Ann Neurol* 2008;**63**:513–19.

Zee PC, Attarian H, Videnovic A. Circadian rhythm abnormalities. *Continuum (Minneap Minn)* 2013;**19**:132–47.

30

Child and adolescent neuropsychiatry

Yulia Furlong and Wai Chen

Introduction

Developmental or child neuropsychiatry: past, present, and future

Developmental or child neuropsychiatry encompasses childhood and adolescent psychiatric syndromes of neurobiological origins, yet there is not one single overriding concept of child neuropsychiatry that determines its exact boundary. Inconsistency in the literature can be confusing to a reader new to the field, in particular regarding the exact nature, theories, and practice of this domain. This introduction provides a historical perspective from which different conceptualizations of child neuropsychiatry at different times can be understood and reconciled as a coherent whole.

Within the traditional notion of the brain–mind dichotomy, neurology is conceived to include diseases that have anatomical or structural lesions localized within the brain. Psychiatry, on the other hand, claims the domain of mental illnesses within which 'malfunctioning' of the mind commonly presents without known neurobiological correlates. With recent advances in structural and functional neuroimaging, the brain–mind divide is narrowing; in particular, some psychiatric conditions can be linked to neurocircuitry dysfunction, albeit without focal neurological lesions. Such observations may redraw a new boundary between neurology and psychiatry—neurology can claim disorders of brain lesions, whereas psychiatry can include syndromes caused by aberrant neural networks. For child neuropsychiatry, there are added dimensions to consider, i.e. normative and aberrant developmental trajectories, as well as social ecological contexts, including relationships with family, peers, school, and significant adults. When one evaluates the clinical significance of a child's symptoms and impairments, one must take into account the environmental supports and demands within the context of that child's developmental trajectories of cognitive, language, attentional, emotional, psychological, social/interpersonal, and moral maturity.

Historically, the early foundation for child neuropsychiatry rested upon research in traumatic and infectious brain injuries, when lesion 'localization' was the key objective. In contrast, the current conceptualization acknowledges the complexity and multifactorial origin of all major child neuropsychiatric conditions. There are monogenic disorders due to single-gene defects, such as

di George syndrome—and these are rarer causes of child neuropsychiatric disorders—whereas most are polygenetic conditions. Molecular genetic studies indicate that additive (quantitative trait loci) genes of small effects represent the key genetic substrates for most neurodevelopmental disorders, even though copy number variation (CNV) in genetic structure, as well as polymorphisms of specific genes (which regulate neuronal development, cell division, migration, signalling pathway, and structural organization of neurotransmitter receptors), may play important roles in some cases. Recent findings also identify shared genetic variants across several neurodevelopmental disorders, such as ADHD, autism, schizophrenia, and epilepsy (Williams et al., 2010). In other words, the 'one gene, one disorder' principle does not apply. These neurobiological findings have also begun to challenge the traditional boundaries between psychiatric disorders, given that shared genetic mechanisms have also been found to underline phenotypically distinct diagnostic entities (de Lacy and King, 2013). Such mechanisms have been proposed as relevant in the associations between autism and schizophrenia spectrum disorders, and more specifically between multiple complex developmental disorder and childhood-onset schizophrenia (Buitelaar, 1998; Cheung et al., 2010; Chisholm et al., 2015; Crespi et al., 2010; Rapoport et al., 2009; Sugranyes et al., 2011). The findings suggest the possibility that the comorbid disorders may merely represent phenotypic variants of a common underlying condition.

Gene–environment interaction represents a further mechanism for variance in phenotypic expression beyond the main effects of genes and environmental factors. Imprinting, epigenetic modification, and variable penetrance of genes also influence phenotypic expression. Notably, a 'developmental critical window' represents a sensitive period during which a given phenotype is responsive or malleable to environmental factors, denoting maximum phenotypic plasticity within a discrete period. Overall, the emphasis of 'neurobiological origin' has shifted from the traditional notion of single factor or static neurological lesions to a complex conceptualization of dynamic interaction between genetic factors, environmental insults, protective factors, aberrant neural circuitries, developmental critical windows, life opportunities, and their curtailments—expressed over time, leading to divergent life trajectories—conferring multifinality, rather than biological reductive determinism. We anticipate that further shifts in conceptual frameworks—likely faster and more radical—will occur in the coming decades.

Inevitably, child neuropsychiatry—as demonstrated by its history outlined below—is both an evolving and a heterogenous category, embodying different meanings for different authors at different times.

In the 1980s, Rutter's influential textbook *Developmental Neuropsychiatry* evaluated whether neurological soft signs, drug responses, and neurophysiological and neuropsychological measurements could validate the constructs of brain dysfunction syndromes, hyperkinetic/attentional deficit syndrome, and minimal brain dysfunction. This text also critiqued the application of these objective parameters to clinical settings and nosological validation (Rutter, 1984). This book formed a milestone in demarcating 'developmental neuropsychiatry' from the then mainstream child psychiatry as practised in British child guidance clinics in the 1960s to 1980s, under the predominant influences of family therapy, psychodynamic, and attachment theories.

In the 1990s, the North American publication of Harris' textbook, also entitled *Developmental Neuropsychiatry* (Harris, 1995), marked another key milestone. Notably, Harris included single factorial conditions (such as single-gene disorders and other conditions caused by prenatal insults or toxin exposure). Around the same time, Gillberg published *Clinical Child Neuropsychiatry* (Gillberg, 1995), which included autism spectrum disorders, ADHD, Tourette syndrome, anorexia nervosa, psychosis, behavioural phenotypes, brain injury, epilepsy, and other psychiatric presentations of major neurological conditions. Moreover, he proposed a new category called 'deficits in attention, motor control, and perception' (DAMP) syndrome, which delineated a cluster of children with comorbid ADHD, language and developmental coordination, and autism spectrum disorders. Gillberg proposed DAMP syndrome as a distinct disorder with particularly poor outcomes, representing a 'novel' spectrum disorder which shaded into autism, Asperger, ADHD, OCD, Tourette syndrome, anorexia nervosa, and mental retardation. However, other authors have questioned the validity of DAMP syndrome, which remains a controversial construct and has not been adopted by the DSM or ICD systems. DAMP accordingly has not been widely cited outside publications from Gillberg's group.

In 2006, *Pediatric Neuropsychiatry* was published (Coffey and Edward, 2006). The editors Coffey and Brumback pulled together the expertise of North American neuropsychiatrists, child psychiatrists, paediatricians, and child neurologists. The publication took a fresh approach in combining (1) the neuropsychiatric aspects of traditional child psychiatric disorders with (2) the neuropsychiatric aspects of traditional child neurological disorders. In this unifying approach, child neuropsychiatry claimed the domains of both child psychiatric and child neurological disorders.

Along this continuum, other publications proposed that child neuropsychiatry should include: (1) neurodevelopmental disorders (e.g. autism spectrum disorders, ADHD, tic disorders); (2) neurogenetic behavioural phenotypes (e.g. fragile X, Wlilliams, Lesch–Nyhan, and Prader–Willi syndromes, tuberous sclerosis, and neurofibromatosis); (3) neurobehavioural syndromes caused by prenatal exposure to teratogens (e.g. gestational substance misuse, fetal alcohol syndrome and spectrum disorders); (4) metabolic disorder syndromes (e.g. homocystinuria, OTC deficiency); (5) connective tissue disorder syndromes (e.g. Ehlers–Danlos and Marfan's

syndrome); and (6) psychiatric presentations related to epilepsy, cerebral palsy, tumours, head injuries, or brain injuries due to postnatal environmental insults. More recently, autoimmune diseases have been reported to cause psychiatric presentations, including anti-NMDA receptor encephalitis and 'paediatric autoimmune neuropsychiatric disorders associated with streptococcal infections' (PANDAS); in other words, developmental neuropsychiatry has been extended to include autoimmune disorders. In contrast, for disorders caused by psychological trauma and traditionally regarded as of 'pure psychosocial' origin, neuroimaging research has identified structural changes in the corpus callosum, hippocampus, and prefrontal cortex (PFC) among adults exposed to childhood abuse, including physical, sexual, emotional, and verbal abuse by parents and peers; in other words, there are specificities in neuroanatomical changes in relation to both types of trauma, as well as age exposure windows (Teicher et al., 2002, 2003). The boundaries could therefore be further extended to incorporate the traditionally non-neuropsychiatric disorders of identifiable psychosocial causal factors. In response, some experts have advocated confining child neuropsychiatry to include only behavioural and emotional syndromes caused by organic neurological disorders, thereby re-asserting a narrower and contracted boundary. In other words, they focus only on the neuropsychiatric aspects of traditional child neurological disorders—the second stream defined by Coffey and Brumback. Accordingly, the boundary of child psychiatry can be redrawn—contracting or expanding—depending on whether one takes a 'splitting' ('narrowview') or 'lumping' ('global-view') approach.

This brief historical perspective outlined here provides our readers with a broad overview, within which specific positions taken by different authors can be understood and accommodated. Otherwise, inconsistencies within the literature can confuse a reader new to the field. We thereby avoid taking a specific position with regard to the exact boundary of child neuropsychiatry, as all forms of knowledge are provisional and contingent to changes in the light of emerging evidence. It is therefore our view that the precise boundary of child neuropsychiatry has been changing and will continue to evolve, and it is best therefore to equip our reader with a critical understanding which can facilitate continuous self-directed learning.

We anticipate that future neurodevelopmental research within the National Institute of Mental Health (NIMH) Research Domain Criteria (RDoC) Framework (Cuthbert and Insel, 2013)—as summarized in Table 30.1—will likely yield important advances, further reshaping child neuropsychiatry. Casey, Oliveri, and Insel (Casey et al., 2014) postulated three key concepts which will augment the traction gained in the dimensional approach adopted by the RDoC: (1) developmental trajectory; (2) sensitive period; and (3) dynamic interaction of systems. Firstly, developmental variation can be viewed as neurobiological domains (brain systems) interacting with developmental trajectories which may be linear or non-linear. Secondly, some specific experiences have a strong influence on brain and behaviour only within specific sensitive periods or developmental critical windows. Knowledge of the timing of environmental events impacting the risk of aberrant development not only improves understanding of causality, but also offers opportunities for treatment through the potential manipulation of malleability by extending or reopening these windows themselves. Thirdly, developmental cascades due to a dynamic interaction of systems across development will impact developing (children's)

Table 30.1 Research domain criteria, October 2012 (constructs are listed within each domain)

Negative valence domain	Positive valence systems	Cognitive systems	Systems for social processes	Arousal/modulatory systems
Acute threat ('fear')	Approach motivation	Attention	Affiliation and attachment	Arousal
Potential threat ('anxiety')	Initial responsiveness to reward	Perception	Social communication	Biological rhythms
Sustained threat	Sustained responsiveness to reward	Working memory	Perception and understanding of self	Sleep–wake
Loss	Reward learning	Declarative memory	Perception and understanding of others	
Frustrative non-reward	Habit	Language behaviour		
		Cognitive (effortful) control		

Reproduced from Cuthbert, B.N. and Insel, T.R., Toward the future of psychiatric diagnosis: the seven pillars of RDoC. *BMC Medicine*, 11(1), p. 126. Copyright (2013) Springer Nature. https://doi.org/10.1186/1741-7015-11-126. Distributed under the terms of the Creative Commons Attribution 2.0 Generic (CC BY 2.0). https://creativecommons.org/licenses/by/2.0/.

brains more powerfully than developed (adults') brains. Mapping the sequential and cumulative effects of multiple domains of brain systems intersecting with environmental events and social contextual factors can offer different opportunities for intervention, unique in children and adolescents in altering trajectories at critical windows. RDoC-informed research findings should therefore have a greater impact on neuropsychiatry in children than in adults.

Notwithstanding optimism and potential promises, it must be emphasized that the RDoC framework has not yet created a fully fledged new nosology ready for field trials (Cuthbert, 2014). There are criticisms of the RDoC such as the assumption that a continuous trait must inevitably reflect homogeneity across its range, thus disregarding the roles of discrete causes (Weinberger et al., 2015); our readers should therefore also retain a critical mindset in reviewing RDoC-guided research findings.

Given the limited space, this chapter cannot cover the full corpus of child neuropsychiatry, which would embody a full volume in itself. We therefore aim to focus on key principles which will assist a reader in understanding the practical application of child neuropsychiatry and engaging with further self-directed learning with informed and critical thinking.

The rest of the chapter illustrates some key principles by examples in four sections. The first section focuses on ADHD as an example to illustrate the neuropsychiatric presentation of a diffuse brain disorder. Apart from highlighting the roles of neural circuitry networks, we also review some key changes in DSM-5 in relation to taking a dimensional approach in considering a neurodevelopmental disorder; we also evaluate some recent neuroscience findings relevant to psychopharmacological treatments of ADHD. The second section explores Tourette syndrome as a prototypical neuropsychiatric disorder of developmental origin with characteristic motor and non-motor features—illustrating the merits of the rapprochement of neurology and psychiatry as a combined approach. This section underscores its colourful presentation, phenotypic heterogeneity, distinctive comorbid patterns, involvement of the corticostriato-thalamo-cortical (CSTC) brain circuitry, and treatment strategies specific for children and adolescents. The third section focuses on childhood cranial tumours as an example of localized brain disorders. This section examines how neuroanatomical disruptions and their localization influence the clinical presentations

of cognitive, psychological, and emotional symptoms. The fourth section concerns fetal alcohol spectrum disorders (FASDs) as 'disorders of specific cause', demonstrating how exposure to one specific toxin can disrupt both neurological and somatic development within critical developmental windows during pregnancy, causing brain, behavioural, and cognitive changes, as well as leaving permanent facial and peripheral stigmata. These four conditions are illustrative examples, intended to elucidate some key principles essential in the practice of child neuropsychiatry.

Attention-deficit/hyperactivity disorder as a neuropsychiatric presentation of a diffuse brain disorder

ADHD is one of the commonest childhood neurodevelopmental disorders, characterized by age-inappropriate levels of inattention, hyperactivity, and impulsivity, with impairments across home, school, or social settings. The prevalence rates of ADHD, as defined by the DSM system, vary according to syndromal definition and developmental age, typically ranging between 5% to 7% among school-age children (Polanczyk et al., 2007), while the prevalence of ICD-10-defined hyperkinetic disorder is lower at around 1.5% (Banaschewski et al., 2009).

Research evidence has influenced the DSM-5 revision of ADHD. The notion of 'subtypes of ADHD' (i.e. *combined, predominantly inattentive, predominantly hyperactive/impulsive subtypes*) has been replaced by 'presentations', given research evidence demonstrating temporal and contextual instability of these subtypes. The notion of 'presentation' is more in keeping with the current concept that a disorder arises from the variable and mutable phenotypic expression of a given latent ADHD trait within different developmental and environmental contexts. This contrasts sharply with the idea that a disorder is a fixed entity. As a common pattern, the 'hyperactive/impulsive presentation' tends to occur in younger children and morphs into the 'combined presentation' in mid childhood; when hyperactivity and impulsivity desist with age, the 'combined presentation' frequently transforms into the 'inattentive presentation', which is much commoner in adolescents and adults. This progression, however, is not developmentally deterministic, as individuals progress and regress in a back-and-forth manner along this continuum at different stages of their life.

A dimensional approach is now combined with binary diagnostic categories in the DSM-5, when the clinician can code 'mild', 'moderate', and 'severe' in qualifying the chosen category. Furthermore, in the past, the 'pervasive' criterion required both *impairments* and *symptoms* from ADHD to be *present* across settings, i.e. 'some impairment from the symptoms is present in two or more settings (e.g. at school [or work] and at home)', as in DSM-IV-R whereas in DSM-5, the 'pervasive' criterion now requires symptoms to be present across more than one setting (i.e. Criterion C), but *impairment* present only in one setting (i.e. Criterion D). This is a subtle, but important, change that allows children who have pervasive symptoms across two settings, but impairment only in one setting, to receive a diagnosis and hence treatment. Children with ADHD comorbid with generalized anxiety or social phobia can behave well at school and function adequately without impairments, because they apply enormous efforts to suppress urges at school out of fears or worries. Yet they can unleash their anger and frustrations at home, while expressing their florid ADHD symptoms unchecked at home. Under the DSM-IV system, this group would not meet diagnostic criteria. Moreover, children with ADHD and comorbid autism spectrum disorder can also display impairments only in one setting, when they are disrupted from engaging in activities of their choice or related to their circumscribed interests. This third revision allows children with complex comorbidities to receive diagnosis and treatment.

As research has identified late childhood onset of ADHD, the age of onset has accordingly been raised from 'before 7' to 'before 12'. Finally, the diagnostic threshold has been lowered from 6 to 5 for adolescents of age 17 years or older. These two changes are in line with research evidence that ADHD symptoms exist as a continuous phenotypic trait in the general population, with 'disease' representing one extreme pole of the continuum, rather than ADHD being an 'all-or-none binary entity'. However, clinical decision tends to occur in a binary manner, i.e. to medicate or not to medicate. For this reason, a diagnostic threshold (i.e. symptom count) is based on impairment and dysfunction (i.e. consequences of symptoms) related to a given level of disease burden. As consequences are not invariant, but contingent to environmental support and tolerance, impairments can occur at different ages when environmental demands exceed functional capacity. Environmental expectations change with age; behaviours that were once tolerated in a young child can become objectionable and rejected by peers and adults alike. Parents and schools also vary in their tolerance and acceptance of unruly behaviours. The same level of disease burden embedded within different social environments can therefore express different levels of impairment. The relaxation of age of onset and diagnostic threshold in DSM-5 reflects this more sophisticated approach which takes into account the interplay between the environmental context, the developmental age, and the polythetic symptom dimension.

ADHD as a diffuse brain disorder

There are many comprehensive descriptions of ADHD in standard textbooks and review articles. Given the limited space in this chapter, we focus only on a few specific topics of ADHD which have been less adequately addressed in standard texts: (1) the

issue of emotional dysregulation associated with ADHD; (2) the relevance of neuroscience in understanding the disorder and its pharmacological treatment; and (3) the principles behind specific DSM-5 revisions of ADHD diagnostic criteria and their clinical application.

While DSM-5 characterization of ADHD uses 18 diagnostic criteria based on observable behavioural symptoms (American Psychiatric Association, 2013), ADHD is better conceptualized as a diffuse, rather than localized, brain disorder that affects multiple functional circuitry networks (illustrated in Fig. 30.1) (Purper-Ouakil et al., 2011), in particular those involving the striatum, cerebellum, parietal cortex, and PFC. ADHD is essentially a disorder of self-control affecting cognitive, attentional, behavioural, and emotional domains. Children with ADHD also have higher risks of having language disorders and deficits in higher-order language skills (e.g. making inferences, sequencing, problem-solving, predicting, and determining causes) (Randell et al., 2019), and they also express a higher level of emotional lability, especially those with oppositional defiant disorder and the 'combined presentation' (Liu et al., 2017). Indeed ADHD is a misnomer—it is not a condition of attention deficit, but attention *dysregulation*, as most children with ADHD can concentrate well, or even hyperfocus, when motivated or attending exciting, stimulating, or novel activities, but they cannot activate effortful attention on demand to complete more mundane, but necessary, tasks such as homework or daily chores.

ADHD and emotional dysregulation

Taxonomic systems specifically focus on discriminating features that demarcate ADHD from other disorders, rather than describing

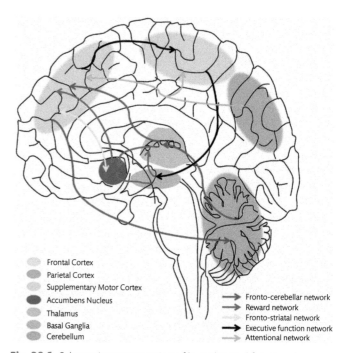

Frontal Cortex
Parietal Cortex
Supplementary Motor Cortex
Accumbens Nucleus
Thalamus
Basal Ganglia
Cerebellum

→ Fronto-cerebellar network
→ Reward network
→ Fronto-striatal network
→ Executive function network
→ Attentional network

Fig. 30.1 Schematic representation of hypothesized functional circuits involved in ADHD, including attention, executive function, frontocerebellar, and reward networks.

all aspects of the full clinical picture. As emotional symptoms are present in other psychiatric disorders, and not unique, necessary, or sufficient to define ADHD, the DSM-5 system does not include the emotional symptoms, despite these symptoms and impairments being integral components of ADHD (Barkley and Fischer, 2010; Merwood et al., 2014). Indeed, many children are referred to neurodevelopmental clinics specifically because of their emotional dysregulation problems. Clinicians therefore must have knowledge and an understanding of the full range of ADHD symptoms, beyond the core symptoms.

About 40% of ADHD children suffer from severe emotional lability problems (Liu et al., 2016). Within this subgroup, the risks of oppositional defiant disorder, conduct disorder, and depression are significantly elevated (Sobanski et al., 2010). ADHD children with comorbid depression are three times more likely to complete suicide (James et al., 2004). As emotional dysregulation mediates the risk between ADHD and depressive symptoms (Seymour et al., 2012), early detection and treatment of emotional symptoms in ADHD may mitigate later risks of self-harm and suicide. Emotional dysregulation or impulsiveness is also one of the most impairing aspects of ADHD, predicting criminality, as well as social, occupational, financial, and interpersonal functional impairments in ADHD adults, above and beyond their core ADHD symptoms (Barkley and Fischer, 2010). This condition in ADHD is commonly expressed in the forms of: (1) proneness to irritability and temper outbursts; (2) emotional lability or instability (mood changes drastically from sadness to anger, elation, or excitability); (3) emotional over-reactivity (feeling overwhelmed, hassled, and despondent, disproportionate to the challenge); and (4) emotional fragility, as in an age-inappropriate tendency to cry easily and often. As such, in our view, neither 'intermittent explosive disorder' nor 'disruptive mood dysregulation disorder' in DSM-5 fully capture or represent the symptom spectrum of ADHD-related emotional dysregulation.

Disrupted amygdalar and subregional connectivities with cortical regions have been reported to correlate with emotional dysregulation symptoms (Hulvershorn et al., 2014; Yu et al., 2016). Two key systems of neural correlates with emotional dysregulation have been identified: the top–down (cortical and paralimbic) and the bottom–up (subcortical and limbic) systems. The bottom–up system is broadly represented as 'reactive', while the top–down system as 'modulating' and 'inhibitory'. Separate orientational, attentional, and cognitive subcircuits are also implicated in emotional dysregulation (details summarized in Shaw et al., 2014). In some ADHD children, their emotional dysregulation symptoms respond well to stimulants, which enhance the orbitofrontal top–down inhibitory control, while others require augmentation with SSRIs. In more severe cases, atypical antipsychotics can be used for D2 blockade. These observations can be understood in relation to functional neural correlates described below.

The hypothesized functional neuroanatomical regions relevant to emotional dysregulation and ADHD symptoms are summarized in Fig. 30.2 (Arnsten and Rubia, 2012). Dopamine (DA), noradrenaline (NA), and serotonin (5HT) are involved in all subregions of the PFC. These subregions and functions are topographically organized along a dorsal–ventral axis. This model is relevant to psychopharmacological treatment in ADHD.

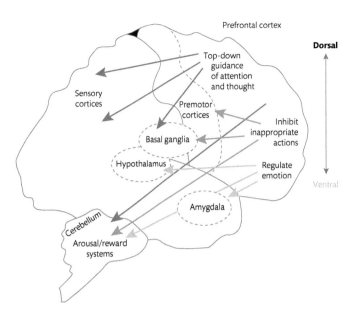

Fig. 30.2 Three key network connections regulating attention, motor inhibition, and emotional control, which correspond with inattention, hyperactivity/impulsivity, and emotional dysregulation aspects of ADHD syndrome.

Adapted with permission from Arnsten, A.F.T. & Rubia, K. Neurobiological Circuits Regulating Attention, Cognitive Control, Motivation, and Emotion: Disruptions in Neurodevelopmental Psychiatric Disorders. *Journal of the American Academy of Child & Adolescent Psychiatry*, 51(4): 356–367. Copyright © 2012 American Academy of Child and Adolescent Psychiatry. Published by Elsevier Inc. All rights reserved. https://doi.org/10.1016/j.jaac.2012.01.008.

Relevance of dynamic network connectivity theory, D1, and α-2A agonism

The relevance of the 'dynamic network connectivity theory' to ADHD, emotional dysregulation, and their psychopharmacological management has been summarized in a recent review (Huss et al., 2016). Briefly, the dynamic network connectivity model (Arnsten, 2009) proposes that the strength of the neural circuitry connection between cortical ('top–down') and subcortical ('bottom–up') regions is dynamically variable, contingent to the state of arousal, conforming to an inverted U-shape relationship in relation to the concentration of neuromodulators, as illustrated in Fig. 30.3.

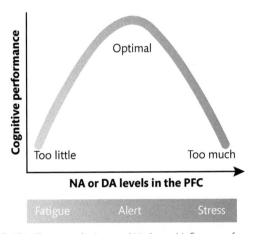

Fig. 30.3 This illustrates the inverted U-shaped influence of noradrenaline (NA) and dopamine (DA) on the prefrontal cortex.

Adapted with permission from Arnsten, A.F.T. Stress signalling pathways that impair prefrontal cortex structure and function. *Nature Reviews Neuroscience*, 10(6): 410–22. Copyright © 2009, Springer Nature. https://doi.org/10.1038/nrn2648.

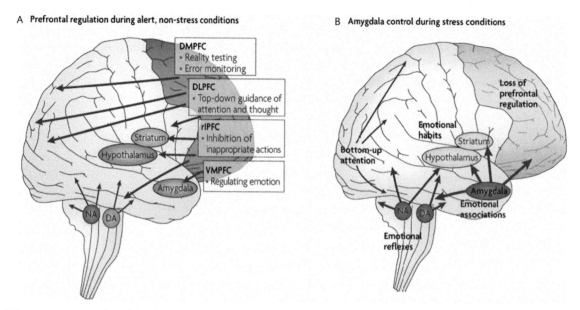

Fig. 30.4 Schematic representation of the dynamic network connectivity model.
Reproduced with permission from Arnsten, A.F.T. Stress signalling pathways that impair prefrontal cortex structure and function. *Nature Reviews Neuroscience*, 10(6): 410–22. Copyright © 2009, Springer Nature. https://doi.org/10.1038/nrn2648.

Under non-stressful and favourable arousal conditions, prefrontal functions and connectivities with other brain regions become optimal (see Fig. 30.4A). Under stress and over-aroused conditions, the functional connectivities become lost, when subcortical regions and functions become autonomous and unregulated by 'top–down' regions (see Fig. 30.4B).

The putative mechanisms for dynamic network connectivity involve the functions of D1 and α-2A receptors and

hyperpolarization-gated cyclic nucleotide-gated (HCN) channels in modulating attentional control, which is briefly summarized in Fig. 30.5. NA and DA modulate the strength of network connections at dendritic spines in the neurones of the PFC. Methylphenidate (MPH) and amphetamine (AMP) inhibit DA reuptake transporters, leading to an increased concentration of DA, which binds with D1 receptors to reduce the 'noise' of neuronal signals by opening HCN channels. Atomoxetine (ATX) and AMP inhibit NA reuptake

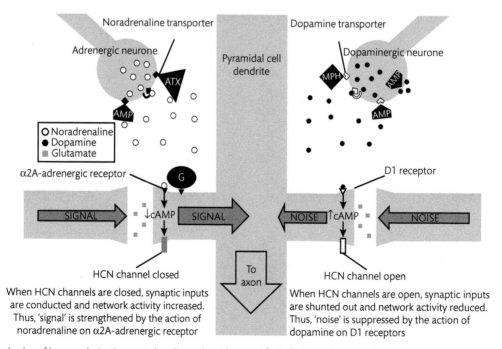

Fig. 30.5 The critical roles of hyperpolarization-gated cyclic nucleotide-gated (HCN) channels in modulating attentional control via D1 and α-2A agonism.
Reproduced with permission from Huss, M., et al. Guanfacine extended release: a new pharmacological treatment option in Europe. *Clinical drug investigation*, 36(1): 1–25. Copyright © 2015, The Author(s). https://doi.org/10.1007/s40261-015-0336-0.

transporters, leading to an increased output of NA, which increases the 'signal' of neuronal transmission, via α-2A agonism, by closing HCN channels. Guanfacine (G) is a direct α-2A agonist that directly stimulates post-synaptic α-2A receptors, rather than indirectly via NA reuptake transporters. This model postulates that the balance and interplay of neural substrates alter the state of neural network connectivity within the brain, thereby influencing cognition, emotion, and downstream behaviour, and it provides an overarching schema to rationalize psychopharmacological strategies for using a specific drug, or a combination of drugs, to manage ADHD and associated emotional dysregulation symptoms.

Summary

In this section, we focus on ADHD as an example of a neuropsychiatric condition due to an underlying neurodevelopmental diffuse brain disorder. In this example, we highlight several key principles. Firstly, the diagnostic criteria stipulated in taxonomic systems are an incomplete description of the syndrome. Some non-core features are not explicitly described but are significantly impairing, and they must not be overlooked in clinical assessment and management. Secondly, most psychiatric disorders represent the extreme pole of a continuous latent trait, shading between 'disorder' and normality. Symptom expression and functional impairment are the results of a dynamic interaction among multiple factors, including developmental maturity, environmental factors (e.g. expectations, support, and tolerance), and the inherent disease burden. The locus of 'diseaseness' for a given individual may shift up and down along this continuum, dependent on the presence of environmental stressors, developmental maturity, and compensatory or mitigating mechanisms. Thirdly, clinical symptoms are the results of dynamic interplay and connectivity of neural networks, rather than fixed aberrant hard-wiring. These considerations reconcile the old dichotomy of 'brain versus mind', epitomizing the evolving rapprochement between neurology and psychiatry. As such, tic disorders co-occur frequently with ADHD, as a quintessential neuropsychiatric disorder of developmental origin, which further illustrates the merits in the rapprochement of neurology and psychiatry as a combined specialty.

Tourette syndrome

Tics are considered the most prevalent movement disorder in childhood, with a range of clinical expression from mild symptoms of simple motor tics to chronic and severe presentations, including the full-blown Tourette syndrome.

History and clinical presentation

In the late nineteenth century, a remarkable period of pioneering discovery and rapid advancement took place in neurology, when Jean-Martin Charcot trained and assembled a group of physicians and scientists in the famous Salpêtrière Hospital in Paris. The group systematically documented and published the descriptions of many brain disorders which still form the foundation of modern neurology. Georges Gilles de la Tourette was one of his students. Around 1884, while still in training under Charcot, Georges Gilles de la Tourette encountered an intriguing disorder characterized by the clinical triad of tics, coprolalia, and echolalia—that has since become known as the syndrome which still bears his name (McNaught, 2010). He first referred to the condition in 1885 as 'maladie des tics' ('disease of tics') in his article in Archives de Neurologie, consisting of a case series of nine patients with the triad of waxing and waning course. Charcot himself later renamed the condition as 'la maladie de Gilles de la Tourette' anglicized to Tourette syndrome (TS), in honour of his student. Tourette was shot in the head (though not killed) by an allegedly psychotic patient and later was admitted to a mental hospital in Switzerland in 1904. He died shortly thereafter, aged 47 (McNaught, 2010).

Around 1920s, the Hungarian psychoanalyst Sandor Ferenczi promoted psychoanalytic views on TS, emphasizing sexual feelings, with their repression and aberrant expression as the underlying drivers. Four decades later, another new paradigm emerged, endorsing a more biologically and empirically based conceptualization; the impetus came broadly from three fronts. The first was derived from psychopharmacology, when Arthur Shapiro demonstrated the effectiveness of haloperidol in treating TS symptoms. The second stemmed from familial studies which identified different shades of milder expression among the relatives of TS patients; the milder expressions ranged from transient to chronic tics in different combinations of motor, vocal, and phonic tics—but without the florid full syndrome. The third impetus came from community survey studies, which showed a prevalence rate of about 1% in schoolchildren, based on the broad phenotype definition. The finding gave support to the view that TS is a spectrum disorder (with varying degree of severity; most prevalent in the school-aged population distributed in the community), rather than as a severe and discrete rare disorder seen only in specialist clinics. These three strands of evidence combined to implicate TS as a condition of genetic and biological aetiologies, rather than aberrant repression of sexuality. Overall, the perceived nature of TS has been transformed from that of a rare neurological disorder to a relatively common neuropsychiatric disorder with a broad spectrum of phenotypic expression, and its aetiology has also been recast as of neurodevelopmental and genetic origin.

Indeed, when the fifth edition of the DSM was published (2013), TS has been regrouped under 'Neurodevelopment Disorders – Movement Disorder', instead of 'Disorders Usually First Diagnosed in Infancy, Childhood or Adolescence', as previously in DSM-IIIR and DSM-IV-TR.

The DSM-5 diagnostic criteria for TS stipulates that both multiple motor and one or more vocal/phonic tics (often tracking a waxing and waning course) should be present, though not necessarily concurrently. The duration is >1 year, with onset before the age of 18 years. The symptoms and impairments are not attributable to the physiological effects of a substance (e.g. cocaine) or another medical condition (e.g. Huntington's disease, post-viral encephalitis) (American Psychiatric Association, 2013). In contrast, 'persistent motor or vocal tic disorder' is defined as either motor or vocal tics (but not both) with a duration of >1 year, and 'provisional tic disorder' is defined as 'less than 1 year since first tic onset'.

Premonitory urges or sensations are relevant to treatment in TS, described as 'the building up of tension', which are distressing and can be briefly relieved by the voluntary execution of tics. Most individuals can suppress tics through effort or volition, but suppression leads to rebound intensification afterwards. Tics often lessen or are completely abolished during focused activities; for this reason, stimulant medications can improve tics in children with comorbid ADHD. When anxious, stressed, or tired, a child tics more.

TS is now considered to be a heterogenous disorder. Recently, a range of data reduction statistical techniques (such as factor, cluster, and latent class analyses) have been applied to extract different patterns of TS presentation. Eapen et al. (2018) proposed three distinct subgroups of TS: (1) the first consists of motor and vocal tics only (referred as 'pure TS'); (2) the second with more florid associated features such as coprophenomena and echophenomena ('full-blown TS'); and (3) the third pattern clustered with comorbidities such as OCD, ADHD, and other psychopathologies, including anxiety, depression, and personality disorder ('TS-plus'). Interestingly, about 40% of the 'TS-plus group' displayed coprolalia, contrasting with 0% of the 'pure TS group', whereas OCD in the family history is rare for the 'pure TS group'. Moreover, individuals with complex motor/vocal tics were significantly more likely to report premonitory urges or sensation than those presenting with simple tics or TS (Eapen and Robertson, 2015).

Other factor, cluster, and latent class analyses have also been applied in attempts to parcellate TS phenotypes into discernible and genetically informative grouping; different patterns have emerged, including factor models (with 3- to 5-factor solutions) and latent class models (with 4- to 5-class solutions). Overall, these models suggest the presence of 3–5 subpatterns within the TS construct (Eapen et al., 2018). Briefly, the 3-factor model yielded by a principal component analysis (Robertson and Cavanna, 2007) consists of: (1) a 'pure tics factor'; (2) an 'ADHD–aggressive factor'; and (3) a 'depression–OCS–SIB factor', comprising depression, obsessive-compulsive symptoms (OCS), and self-injurious behaviour (SIB), but also correlating with specific phobias, stuttering, facial grimaces, and abdominal contractions. Alsobrook and Pauls (2002) reported a 4-cluster solution generated by hierarchical agglomerative cluster analysis. A complex 5-factor model has been reported by Robertson et al. (2008). In latent class analysis (LCA), participants are assigned to respective groups according to their symptom profiles, representing a specific categorical version of factor analysis. The first LCA on TS reported a 5-class solution on a mixed sample with TS and chronic tics (Grados et al., 2008). The second LCA (Rodgers et al., 2014) found four subtypes (with sex-related differences). Overall, these findings indicate that TS is a non-unitary syndrome with phenotypic heterogeneity.

In summary, the description of TS has undergone successive changes over time, and ongoing research efforts attempt to parcellate the clinical features into the more genetic informative phenotypes and have revealed phenotypic heterogeneity.

Genetics of TS

TS is a heritable and complex polygenic disorder. In the original case series, Gilles de la Tourette noted the familial expression (Gilles de la Tourette, 1885). However, premillennial pedigree analyses have not detected Mendelian inheritance (Hasstedt et al.,1995; Kurlan et al., 1994), and the precise genetic aetiology to date remains elusive despite intensive genetic research efforts over recent decades.

However, quantitative genetic studies have consistently confirmed significant genetic contributions in the aetiology of TS, based on both twin (Bolton et al., 2007; Lichtenstein et al., 2010) and family studies (Browne et al., 2015; Mataix-Cols et al., 2015). In twin studies, the additive genetic effects have been estimated to be 0.56 for tic disorders in an AE model (i.e. additive genetic (A) and unique environment

(E) effects, but without shared environment (C) effect) (Lichtenstein et al., 2010), and to be 0.5 in an ACE model (Bolton et al., 2007). A recent meta-analysis reported a pooled heritability of 0.45 for tics/tic disorders (Polderman et al., 2015). In a large multigenerational family study conducted using the Swedish National Patient Register (Mataix-Cols et al., 2015), the heritability pattern of TS and chronic tic disorders (CTDs) was found to conform with the ACE model and the additive genetic factors were estimated to be 0.77 (equal for males and females), with non-shared environment at 0.23 and negligible shared environment at 0.03. Interestingly, the familial recurrence risks among relatives increased proportionally to the degree of genetic relatedness—with an odds ratio at 18.69 for first-degree relatives, 4.58 for second-degree relatives, and 3.07 for third-degree relatives. Intriguingly, parents, siblings, and offspring share similar clinical risks for tic disorders as first-degree relatives despite striking differences in life experiences and environmental influences. For children reared together, the odds ratio for recurrence is 17.6 for full siblings (sharing 50% genetic similarity), but 4.4 for maternal half siblings (sharing 25% of genetic similarity). Overall, the findings suggest genetics, rather than the environment, is the primary cause of tic disorder.

Molecular genetic studies have not yielded definitive findings. Despite inconsistent replication, several putative candidate genes have been reported as promising: *NTN4* (Netrin 4) gene (Paschou et al., 2014), *DRD2* gene (Yuan et al., 2015), *DRD4* gene (Liu et al., 2014), AADAC (arylacetamide deacetylase) (Bertelsen et al., 2016) and 5-HT2C (Qi et al., 2017). The *SLITRK1* gene has been implicated in affected individuals within some families (Karagiannidis et al., 2012), indicating that potential rare genetic variants with large effects may play a role in specific TS families. Genome-wide association studies (GWAS) of TS has identified certain genetic signals (Scharf et al., 2013)—with one locus reaching genome-wide significance within the *FLT3* gene (fms-like tyrosine kinase 3) on chromosome 13 (Yu et al., 2019). Epigenetic regulation and mechanisms have also been explored—DNA methylation, histone modifications, and non-coding RNAs as potential mechanisms for variable phenotypic expression (Pagliaroli et al., 2016). To date, the genetic contribution in TS aetiology is well established by quantitative genetics, but molecular genetic studies are yet to reveal the precise molecular genetic architecture, despite some potentially promising results.

Neurobiology of TS

Neuroimaging studies of TS broadly include structural and functional studies. For structural imaging, reduced volumes and abnormal asymmetries of the caudate, putamen, and globus pallidus have been reported; reductions in volume and cortical thickness have also been found in limbic and motor cortices. Functional imaging studies have applied a range of methods—fMRI, PET, SPECT, MEG, and resting-state fMRI—using different probes or conditions, and yielded a range of findings (Debes et al., 2017). Interestingly, premonitory urges have been shown to involve the insula by both PET (Rajagopal et al., 2013) and fMRI (Lerner et al., 2007). Overall, multiple brain regions have been reported to be associated with TS, in particular, for structures within the CSTC circuits.

Indeed, abnormalities in the CSTC circuits have been implicated in the pathogenesis of TS. These circuits involve the projections of the cerebral cortex to the striatum and other basal ganglion structures, then looping back to the cortex via the thalamus. The basal ganglion (BG) comprises the striatrum, the globus pallidus (GP), the substantia nigra (SNr), and the subthalamic nucleus (STN), and the striatum includes the caudate and the putamen, while the GP can be functionally partitioned into the internal part as globus pallidus interna (GPi) and the external part as the globus pallidus externa (GPe). Cortical outputs first travel to the caudate or putamen (the main BG input nuclei), then relay onto the GP and SNr (the main BG output nuclei), which either project down to the brainstem nuclei or project back to the motor cortex via the thalamus. The outputs from the GP/SNr are thought to be primarily inhibitory, as a constant inhibitory control suppressing spontaneous or unwanted movements arising from the thalamus (Graybiel and Canales, 2001).

Normally, to initiate voluntary movements, the cortical excitatory signal travels via the striatum to reach the GPi and inhibit the GPi's inhibition on the thalamus, thereby freeing the thalamus (i.e. reducing the 'default GPi/SNr brake'), thus permitting movement to occur; this is called the 'direct pathway', which is therefore overall excitatory (see Fig. 30.6). The BG also prevents involuntary movements from interfering with goal-directed behaviours through the 'indirect pathway' and 'hyperdirect pathway'. The 'indirect pathway' includes an extra step at the GPe, i.e. the cortical signal travels via the striatum to reach and inhibit the GPe, thereby leading to disinhibition of the GPi (i.e. increasing the 'default GPi/SNr brake', which is the opposite of the 'direct pathway'), and therefore inhibition of the thalamus and thalamocortical neurones. The 'indirect pathway' is therefore overall inhibitory (i.e. reducing unwanted movements). The 'hyperdirect pathway' is also inhibitory and bypasses the striatum (thus its name)—cortical neurones send hyperdirect excitatory signals to the STN, which then stimulates the GPi/SNr and thereby increases inhibition on thalamocortical neurones (i.e. also reducing unwanted movements). Overall, in a healthy brain, the BG modulates behaviour by fine-tuning cortical excitability through its circuits. The 'direct pathway' activates desired motor actions, while both 'indirect' and 'hyperdirect' pathways inhibit unwanted or competing actions.

The direct pathway reduces the 'default brake' on the thalamus and elicits motor movement (green solid in Fig. 30.6). In contrast, the indirect pathway (red solid in Fig. 30.6) increases the 'default brake' via the action of the striatum. The hyperdirect pathway (brown dashed in Fig. 30.6) increases the 'default brake' via the STN, bypassing the striatum. Both the indirect and hyperdirect pathways inhibit and fine-tune movements.

In TS, overactivation of the direct pathway has been proposed as a mechanism, leading to an excess of movements (see Fig. 30.6), i.e. focal aberrations in the striatum cause excessive inhibition of the GPi/SNr within the direct pathway, which leads to disinhibition of thalamocortical neurones, and thus excessive involuntary motor commands arising from the motor cortex (Singer et al., 2016).

PANDAS

In 1998, Swedo and colleagues described 50 cases of acute presentation in prepubertal children of tic disorder with OCD, emotional lability, anxiety, and abrupt decline in school performance; an acronym was coined for this syndrome as 'PANDAS' for 'paediatric autoimmune neuropsychiatric disorders associated with streptococcal infections'. This syndrome was described to present in an episodic manner, following infections with group A β-haemolytic *Streptococcus* (GABHS). According to the 'molecular mimicry' hypothesis, post-streptococcal antibodies are postulated to pass through the blood–brain barrier and react with BG neurones in Sydenham's chorea and PANDAS (Dale, 2013). Sydenham's chorea, historically referred to as St Vitus' dance, is a delayed complication of GABHS (6–9 months) (Swedo et al., 1998) that is typically associated with acute rheumatic fever, while PANDAS is posited to be an earlier (days to weeks) presentation without features of rheumatic fever.

The condition has now been depicted as a continuum of clinical entities (Sigra et al., 2018), ranging from 'PANDAS' (Swedo et al., 1998), 'PANS' (paediatric acute-onset neuropsychiatric syndrome) (Swedo et al., 2012), and 'CANS' (childhood acute neuropsychiatric symptoms) (Singer et al., 2012) to 'PITAND' (paediatric infection-triggered autoimmune neuropsychiatric disorders) (Allen et al., 1995). Within this range, PANDAS is characterized by prepubertal symptom onset, episodic course, and abrupt onset of symptoms or symptom exacerbation, in association with GABHS infection, confirmed by positive throat culture and/or elevated anti-GABHS antibody titres, in the presence of neurological abnormalities. In contrast, PANS, CANS, and PITAND are syndromes mainly based on clinical presentations, rather than signs and laboratory tests of autoimmunity—though there is an assumption of autoimmune aetiology in all of the subtypes (Sigra et al., 2018). It is still disputed whether PANDAS and related variants should be designated as unique clinical categories. They are not formally represented in current diagnostic classification systems. Evidence for the effectiveness of reported treatments with antibiotics, tonsillectomy, corticosteroids, and immunomodulators remains inconsistent and controversial. Further research studies are required to establish the construct validity and predictive validity of these syndromes, their management, and their association with GABHS.

Treatment and management of TS in children

There are important differences in the management of TS between children and adults for both psychopharmacological and psycho-behavioural treatments, due to differences in tolerance of adverse

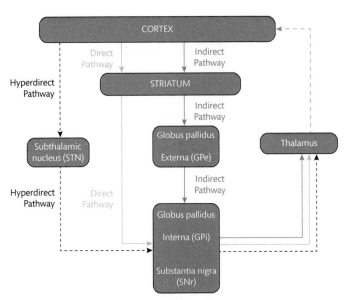

Fig. 30.6 Simplified representation of the direct, indirect, and hyperdirect pathways in the cortico-striato-thalamo-cortical (CSTC) motor circuit.
© 2019 Yulia Furlong & Wai Chen.

reactions and risks to the developing brain and metabolic systems, as well as immaturity in cognitive and metacognitive faculties (Whittington et al., 2016).

For medications, α-2 agonists (i.e. clonidine and guanfacine) are the first-line treatment for children. Atypical neuroleptics are the second-line treatment reserved for cases where α-2 agonists are either ineffective or poorly tolerated. Weight-sparing and metabolically neutral agents should be tried first. For cases with comorbid ADHD, stimulant medications can be used to treat ADHD symptoms, and the evidence now available indicates that ADHD medications neither worsen nor improve tics. However, for some cases, better attention (as optimized by stimulants) can in turn reduce tics—as tics in TS usually subside during focused activities; therefore, ADHD medications can reduce tics indirectly through improved concentration in certain individuals with comorbid ADHD. For cases with comorbid OCD, combined therapy of SSRIs and CBT yields better result.

For psychological treatment, caution should be exercised for young children, as they cannot readily identify premonitory urges and suppress tics. However, for older children and adolescents, habit reversal therapy (HRT) can be effective, teaching an older child to perform a 'competing response'. HRT aims to inhibit a premonitory urge and substitute an alternative and more acceptable behaviour. For example, a premonitory urge for vocal tics can be substituted by whisper reading, and a premonitory urge for motor tics can be substituted by performing 'yo-yo' movements with the affected hand. Furthermore, comprehensive behavioural intervention (CBIT) has been demonstrated to be effective in RCTs, with 45% of responders in the treatment group, compared with 13% in the control therapy (Black, 2017; Piacentini et al., 2010). CBIT is based on HRT and the principle of 'Do Something Else' therapy (instead of 'Stop It' therapy). CBIT combines strategic components, including psychoeducation, self-awareness, relaxation training, and social support; it also makes use of HRT to establish a tic hierarchy and select a target tic and reverse-engineer it, in order to formulate a competing response to the target tic (Cook and Blacher, 2007).

Currently, physical and other therapies, such as use of botulinum toxin, immunoglobulins, deep brain stimulation (DBS), or neurosurgical intervention, are not recommended for tics in children or young people, unless under extreme circumstances.

Summary

TS is a heterogenous condition with a range of phenotypic expression, from very mild tics to a florid full syndrome. The cause for its frequent comorbidity with ADHD and OCD remains elusive, though abnormalities in the CSTC brain circuitry are implicated. Treatment strategies in TS for children and adolescents have to be tailored to meet their special and developmental needs.

Child neuropsychiatry aspects of childhood cranial tumours

Introduction

In this section, we focus on the neuropsychiatric manifestations of a localized brain disorder, as exemplified by childhood cranial tumours. Localizing neurological signs are patterns of clinical features which can aid a clinician to deduce the exact locus of a focal lesion (and in the case of a tumour, a space-occupying lesion), based on knowledge of functional neuroanatomy. The specific neuroanatomical locus of a tumour can also influence the expression of more general higher-order cognitive, psychological, and emotional symptoms, in addition to the localizing neurological signs.

The temporal profile of symptom onset often reveals the underlying brain pathology. Acute (minutes to hours) onset is most likely a vascular event; a subacute (hours to days) course suggests an infectious or immune process, while evolving or chronic progression (days to months) indicates neoplastic growth. The majority of space-occupying tumours affect the functions of specific neural structures and produce localizing neurological and psychiatric symptoms and signs, which can implicate specific spatial loci within the vertical and lateral axes of the CNS. Along the vertical axis, cortical, subcortical, brainstem, and cerebellar tumours cause different patterns of clinical features. Cortical lesions give rise to abnormal mental states, as well as deficits in attention, memory, or executive function, detected by neuropsychological examinations. Subcortical lesions cause emotional, affective, and implicit memory dysregulation, while brainstem and cerebellum lesions are accompanied by cranial nerve signs and coordination neurological signs, respectively. On the horizontal and lateral planes, language deficits suggest pathology in the left hemisphere, while executive function, expressive language, verbal fluency, and encoding deficits are associated with that in the anterior cortex. Attention, planning, organization, inhibition, goal-directed behaviours, and impulse control are more localized to the anterior cingulate and PFC—in particular, the orbitofrontal cortex—which is critical for decision-making, response flexibility, and response selection.

However, cranial tumours can also be associated with psychiatric presentations that are not localizable to the tumour sites, such as psychotic symptoms, TS, OCD, disinhibited behaviours, pathological laughter, emotional lability, flattening or blunting of affect, poor attention, and also with a higher rate of premorbid neurodevelopmental disorders, including autistic spectrum disorders.

Neuropsychiatric presentations and outcomes

Despite being relatively rare, CNS tumours are nevertheless the commonest solid tumours in children, and the second commonest childhood malignancy. More specifically, they comprise 26% of CNS cancers in children aged <14 years (Siegel et al., 2017). At the cellular level, there are several different histological types of brain tumours—with astrocytoma (glioma) being the commonest subtype, accounting for 43% of all childhood CNS tumours, followed by medulloblastoma, a more aggressive and malignant tumour. Anatomically, they can occur in the supratentorial (cerebrum) or infratentorial (cerebellum and brainstem) regions (see Fig. 30.7). Neuropsychiatric presentations are common, both at the point of initial presentation and during the phase of disease progression after diagnosis and treatment.

A systematic literature review (Zyrianova et al., 2015) confirmed that neuropsychiatric presentations are common in children with CNS tumours—with behavioural and psychological symptoms in about 57% of cases (Anderson et al., 2001). Their frequency varies according to age of onset, brain maturation, and time of onset. Although psychiatric symptoms may rarely be the only presenting

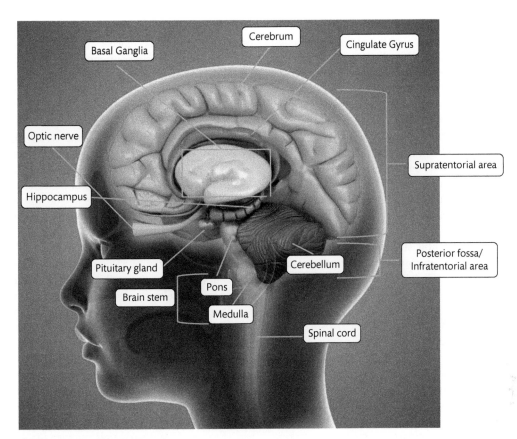

Fig. 30.7 Location of different types of brain tumours.
Science Photo Library / Alamy Stock Photo

features of a brain tumour in children, they remain common 'late effects', i.e. chronic or late-occurring physical or psychosocial outcome persisting or developing well after diagnosis of the tumour, and may occur as a result of treatment due to disruption of developing cognitive processes and the vulnerable immaturity of the brain (Anderson et al., 2001). Neuropsychiatric presentations are variable and include six common patterns of symptoms: (1) emotional under-arousal and internalizing disorders (apathy, poor motivation, and depression); (2) emotional disturbance, over-arousal, and externalizing disorders (irritability, hyperactivity, and aggressiveness); (3) psychosis spectrum disorders; (4) new-onset/worsening of OCD and tic disorders; (5) eating disorders; and (6) memory problems. The precise relationship between the patterns of psychiatric symptoms and the exact anatomical sites of lesions remain elusive, despite intense research efforts that have been made to evaluate their correlation, aiming to develop markers for localizing specific tumours, as well as to extrapolate conceptual models for diagnostic prediction. To date, only 'anorexia without body dysmorphic symptoms' has been found to be significantly associated with hypothalamic tumours; however, other probable associations have been reported, such as psychotic symptoms and pituitary tumours, memory symptoms and thalamic tumours, and mood symptoms and frontal tumours (Madhusoodanan et al., 2010). Lesions of the cerebellar vermis are characteristically associated with dysregulation of affect and, together with supratentorial and right-sided cerebellar lesions, are associated with poorer outcomes (Fuemmeler et al., 2002; Lumsden et al., 2011).

Adjustment disorders are common in patients with CNS tumours, with internalizing symptoms (depression, anxiety) being most prevalent. These symptoms are thought to be caused by a combination of factors, including neurotoxicity caused by the tumour, psychological challenges faced by the children and their families, and treatment side effects. Furthermore, in terms of global outcomes, the most severe cognitive and learning difficulties are associated with being younger at the time of radiotherapy treatment (Kulkarni et al., 2004), due to disruption of developing cognitive processes. In order to avoid damage to the vulnerable immature brain, some treatment protocols modify radiotherapy schedules and postpone treatment in children who are <36 months old (the UK 'Baby Brain' protocol) (Grundy et al., 2007).

Posterior fossa syndrome and post-operative cerebellar mutism

Strikingly, over 50% of child cranial tumours are found in posterior fossa (PF), which houses the cerebellum and brainstem (Fuemmeler et al., 2002). Lesions in this area predispose individuals to two distinct, but related, conditions: posterior fossa syndrome (PFS) and cerebellar mutism (CM). These syndromes are both post-operative phenomena, and a recent call for the introduction of a new term and spectrum disorder entity—'post-operative paediatric cerebellar mutism syndrome'—has been made (Gudrunardottir et al., 2016). CM is defined as a reversible component of a persistent neuropsychiatric syndrome and was first described in 1985 (Rekate et al.,

1985). It is characterized by diminished speech output within 1 week of surgery and often manifesting in the first 1–2 days post-operatively; it is due to dysregulation in voluntary speech production (a higher-order impairment of initiation of language) and is almost always reversible within a short space of time. In contrast, PFS often does not resolve fully after running a course of slow improvement, leaving patients with residual symptoms of ataxia and dysarthric speech (Korah et al., 2010), and its aetiology remains uncertain. Nevertheless, there is a growing consensus on the anatomical substrates involved in the causation of PFS and interruption of the dentato-thalamo-cortical pathway has been attributed to its aetiology (Avula et al., 2016). Around 25% of children develop PFS, while CM affects up to 31% of children undergoing posterior fossa brain tumour resection (Lanier and Abrams, 2017). In these conditions, the mutism component is characterized by absence of speech (verbal mutism), but not absence of non-verbal sounds (i.e. whining, crying, laughter) (Gudrunardottir et al., 2016). The clinical features of PFS include four clusters of symptoms: (1) disruption in motor skills (ataxia, hypotonia); (2) emotional lability; (3) behavioural changes; and (4) variable degrees of mutism (Lanier and Abrams, 2017), as illustrated by the schematic representation in Fig. 30.8.

According to some authors, PFS represents an acute post-operative manifestation of another condition—the cerebellar cognitive affective syndrome (CCAS)—which is characterized by: (1) impairment of executive functions (planning, set shifting, verbal fluency, abstract reasoning, attentional control, and working memory); (2) disruption of spatial cognition; (3) language deficits; (4) personality and 'social skill set' changes (Hopyan et al., 2010; Turkel et al., 2004); and (5) emotional control symptoms. Personality changes manifest as blunting of affect or disinhibited and inappropriate child-like behaviour, and inability to comprehend social boundaries and assign ulterior motives (Schmahmann, 2010).

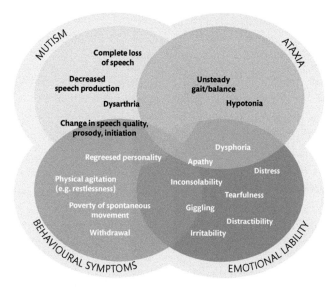

Fig. 30.8 Posterior fossa syndrome.
Reproduced with permission from Lanier, J.C. & Abrams, A.N. Posterior fossa syndrome: Review of the behavioral and emotional aspects in pediatric cancer patients. *Cancer*, 123(4), pp.551–559. Copyright © 2016 American Cancer Society. https://doi.org/10.1002/cncr.30238.

CCAS affects adults and children and can occur as a result of congenital and acquired cerebellar disorders, cerebellar agenesis, dys- and hypoplasias, cerebellar tumour, cerebellar stroke, cerebellitis, trauma and, neurodegenerative diseases (Levisohn et al., 2000).

Levisohn and colleagues (2000) identified a positive correlation between damage to the midline vermis and affective impairment in their study of children with CCAS. The authors proposed that deficits in affect are linked to damage of the vermis and fastigial nuclei, whereas deficits in cognition are linked to damage of the vermis and cerebellar hemispheres. These findings were consistent with earlier results, postulating that the vermis of the cerebellum is responsible for emotional regulation (Heath, 1997) and that the cerebellum plays a key role in cognitive affective processing, acting as a modulator of mental and social functions, and this regulatory role is present and active in early childhood (Hopyan et al., 2010). Wells and colleagues (2008) examined the overlapping relationship between PFS and CCAS in the post-operative child population; they posited that the distinguishing hallmark of PFS is post-operative mutism, beginning 1–2 days post-surgery. It is worth pointing that the exact definitions and boundaries of these conditions remain elusive.

Guidelines

With recent advances in lifesaving treatments, early detection and diagnosis of childhood CNS cancers have become pivotal. Zyrianova and colleagues provided screening and referral guidelines for assisting psychiatrists to recognize paediatric brain tumours as a potential cause of psychiatric presentations (Zyrianova et al., 2015). Furthermore, Hegarty and Furlong reviewed available neuropsychiatric guidelines for identification of brain tumours in primary, secondary, and tertiary health services (Hegarty and Furlong, 2018). Overall, the reviewed guidelines, including the UK's NICE guidelines, recommend an urgent referral (for an appointment within 48 hours) to appropriate specialty guided by local service protocol and resources for cases with *de novo* abnormal cerebellar or other central neurological function in children and young people (National Institute for Health and Care Excellence, 2015).

Recently, novel public awareness campaigns have demonstrated the effectiveness in improving early detection of symptoms by parents, carers, young people, and health professionals. These campaigns disseminate information from the clinical guidelines directly to the public through websites, e-learning, TV advertisements, and digital apps and distributing symptoms cards (i.e. in clinics and waiting rooms) (Shanmugavadivel et al., 2016; Wilne et al., 2006). In the UK, a population-based intervention—'HeadSmart: Be Brain Tumour Aware'—was launched in 2011, as informed by the Royal College of Paediatrics and Child Health guideline (Walker et al., 2016). After this public and professional awareness campaign, a statistically significant reduction was found in the total diagnostic interval in the UK from 14.4 weeks (>3 months) in 2006 to 6.7 weeks (i.e. one of the shortest in the world) (Shanmugavadivel et al., 2016; Walker et al., 2016).

Summary

Here, we highlight the importance of early detection and psychiatric management of childhood CNS cancers. Significantly, in a small number of cases, neuropsychiatric symptoms can be the only presenting complaint—without any neurological symptom or sign. We also recommend routine screening for psychological and psychiatric complications, given their high prevalence, significant morbidity, and salient relevance to clinical management before, during, and after tumour treatments.

In tandem with tumour treatments, neuropsychiatric assessment and management are crucial at all stages of care, as survivors of paediatric brain tumours are at risk of developing immediate, intermediate, and long-term psychiatric morbidities, including cognitive, emotional, and learning difficulties, as well as psychosocial maladjustment.

Post-operative paediatric cerebellar mutism syndromes (CM and PFS) are well recognized and clinically important complications, affecting around 30% of children undergoing PF brain tumour resection. Their aetiology, precise delineation, interrelationship, and management represent rapidly evolving research frontiers—with emerging evidence that both conditions represent a spectrum disorder, rather than being distinct unrelated conditions. Interested readers should keep abreast of developments by consulting research reviews, consensus papers, or published guidance from authoritative bodies, including those from the 'Posterior Fossa Society' and the 'Iceland Delphi Group' (Gudrunardottir et al., 2016).

Fetal alcohol spectrum disorder and psychiatric considerations

Historical background and definitions

Despite historical allusion in art and literature of the eighteenth to nineteenth centuries, the impact of prenatal alcohol exposure on infant development was first explicitly described in the medical literature by Ulleland in 1972 (Ulleland, 1972). The following year, the term fetal alcohol syndrome (FAS) was coined by the dysmorphologists Smith and Jones, who described a case series of children with cognitive impairment, growth deficiencies, and morphological abnormality following prenatal exposure to alcohol in 'Pattern of malformation in offspring of chronic alcoholic mothers' published by *The Lancet* (Jones et al., 1973).

Since then, this central clinical triad of symptoms has been confirmed, with other related conditions described, enriching and extending the conceptualization of FAS, to yield a spectrum of disorders. Around 2000, FASD was proposed as an overarching rubric term to include four separate conditions within the continuum: FAS, partial fetal alcohol syndrome (PFAS), alcohol-related neurodevelopmental disorder (ARND), and alcohol-related birth defects (ARBD). Among these, FAS (signifying the narrowest phenotype) is the only disorder encoded within the ICD-10 as 'Fetal alcohol syndrome (dysmorphic)' Q86.0 (World Health Organization, 1992). In ICD-9, it was coded as 'Alcohol affecting foetus or newborn via placenta or breast milk' (760.71) (Popova et al., 2012). International agreement on diagnostic nomenclature is yet to be reached. Broadly, there are two diagnostic criteria used in the United States (UW 4-digit code, IOM guidelines), one set of criteria used in Canada (Chudley et al., 2005), and one set of criteria used in Australia (Bower et al., 2018). The unifying diagnostic term of FASD represents a commonality encompassing these.

In 2013, the DSM-5 included 'Neurobehavioral Disorder Associated with Prenatal Alcohol Exposure' (ND-PAE), but only in section III which is reserved for disorders 'requiring further study'.

The DSM-5 Task Force found insufficient evidence to warrant inclusion of ND-PAE as a formal mental disorder diagnosis in Section II. The ND-PAE 'diagnostic criteria' were proposed for further study, rather than for clinical use. It is therefore recommended to use instead 'Other Specified Neurodevelopmental Disorder' (code 315.8) with the specifier of 'neurobehavioral disorder associated with prenatal alcohol exposure' (American Psychiatric Association, 2013).

Prevalence and healthcare costs

The estimated rates of FASD vary according to different studies, likely reflecting differences across studies in different countries with regard to methodology, inclusion criteria, and alcohol consumption rates within different populations (and their embedded subpopulations including indigenous communities). In DSM-5, the true prevalence rate of ND-PAE is reported as unknown, with prenatal alcohol exposure estimated at 2–5% in the United States (DSM-5). Alcohol consumption by pregnant women has increased from 7.6% in 2012 to 10% in 2015, with binge drinking (most harmful) rates also on the increase (Tan et al., 2015). Studies assessing the prevalence of FASD in community- and population-based samples (Ospina and Dennett, 2013) reported estimates ranging from 0.02% to 0.5% (which translated to FASD rates of 0.2–5 per 1000 population). Ospina and Dennett (Ospina and Dennett, 2013) highlighted that prevalence estimates were substantially heterogenous for FAS (0.0006–0.3%), as the studies used different methods for case identification, including passive surveillance (e.g. birth certificates and medical chart review), as well as clinic-based studies and active case ascertainment methods. Similar heterogeneity was identified for PFAS (0.0006–0.3%) and both ARND (broad phenotype) and ARBD (narrow phenotype) (1.08% and 0.37%, respectively).

A recent meta-analysis (Popova et al., 2017) estimated the worldwide pooled prevalence of FASD (from 180 countries) as 14.6 per 10,000 people (95% CI: 9.4–23.3). It is also important to note that the rates vary greatly across different regions, highlighting an overrepresentation in certain countries; notably high prevalence rates of FASD were found in Belarus at 69.1 (42.1–103.5), Italy at 82.1 (42.1–134.6), Ireland at 89.7 (50.4–142.8), Croatia at 115.2 (34.8–236.0), and South Africa at 585.3 (430.7–761.7). Furthermore, a growing body of research has now identified high-risk subpopulations, including indigenous communities. For example, May and colleagues (1983) found a much higher rate of FAS in American Indian communities, with 10.3 per 1000 among Plain Indian women, and 25% of all Plain Indian women with one FAS child gave birth to another child with FAS.

A systematic literature review and meta-analysis of original, quantitative studies of service-defined subpopulations globally that were published between 1 November 1973 and 1 December 2018 (Popova et al., 2019) demonstrated that the prevalence of FASD is highly variable and disproportionately impacts some special subpopulations, e.g. in the United States, the prevalence among children in care was 32 times higher (251.5 per 1000; 95% CI = 220.0–281.7), compared to the recently estimated global prevalence of FASD in the general population (7.7 per 1000; 95% CI = 4.9–11.7). Moreover, the prevalence rates of FAS among Australian aboriginal populations, as illustrated by the Lililwan Fitzroy Valley Project (around 12%, i.e. 1200 per 10,000 people), are among the highest reported worldwide (Fitzpatrick et al., 2015).

The prevalence rates are also extremely high among offenders; 36% of detainees had FASD in a Western Australian juvenile prison (Bower et al., 2018). Similarly, the rate of FASD was 65.6% in Canadian aboriginal youths in the criminal justice/forensic psychiatric systems (Rojas and Gretton, 2007).

FASD is associated with increased morbidity and mortality rates, including deaths arising from comorbid psychiatric conditions and suicides (Burd et al., 2008). The associated physical conditions include cardiac malformations (atrial septal defects and ventricular septal defects), enteric neuropathy in GI problems, musculoskeletal and spinal malformations, ophthalmologic problems, hearing deficits, and orofacial and renal malformations, as well as neurological abnormalities including microcephaly, seizure, spinal cord problems, and structural defects in the corpus callosum, cerebellum, caudate, and hippocampus.

FASD is a substantial burden to society due to morbidity and care costs. The healthcare costs associated with FASD are multifaceted, including special education, community social services, juvenile legal services, and law enforcement. High rates of forensic involvement are reflected by high conviction (60%) and incarceration rates (42%) (Streissguth et al., 1996).

Causes

Maternal alcohol consumption during pregnancy is the cornerstone diagnostic criterion of FASD. Alcohol is one of the most potent neurodevelopmental teratogens and the leading cause of functional birth defects in the world. Prenatal alcohol exposure—especially during the first trimester—disrupts organogenesis and organ development, including brain and craniofacial development, during the critical developmental windows.

FASD represents the foremost preventable neurodevelopmental disorder. But there is a complex interplay of genetic factors in FASD expression; these include fetal resistance to alcohol and maternal alcohol dehydrogenase expression. Some of these genetic factors would otherwise be protective in metabolizing and removing alcohol (May and Gossage, 2001). Furthermore, alcohol alters gene expression in key brain regions, likely through the expression of vascular endothelial growth factor A, which regulates blood vessel formation and thus affecting downstream brain development.

Structural and volume reductions have also been reported in multiple brain regions—such as reduction in cortical thickness globally, and reduction in size in the middle frontal lobe, lateral inferior temporal and occipital lobes, left orbitofrontal region, and occipitotemporal and parietal lobes. Reductions in the cortical surface area in the anterior cingulate cortex, right temporal lobe, and other regions have also been found. Cortical folding is also reduced in children (with and without microcephaly) with heavy prenatal alcohol exposure (Hendrickson et al., 2017).

Structural brain abnormalities are the commonest, followed by cardiac (especially septal defects), skeletal, renal, ocular, and auditory abnormalities. However, both the quantity and frequency of alcohol exposure are not directly correlated with FASD caseness or severity. Thus, factors other than just alcohol exposure inevitably play important roles; these include: advanced maternal age, undernutrition, low socio-economic status, frequent binge drinking, psychiatric diagnosis, high gravidity, and high parity (Abel and Hannigan, 1995). High rates of dietary deficiencies have been reported with regard to fibre, calcium, and vitamins D, E, and K in children with FASD, implicating nutrition as potential mediating factors.

Clinical presentation

British (British Medical Association, 2007), Canadian (Chudley et al., 2005), and Australian (Bower and Elliott, 2016) guidelines at large converge in diagnostic practice; children with FASD share common neurodevelopmental difficulties across several domains such as motor function, cognition, language, memory, attention, and executive function. They also experience additional problems with mental health and social interactions such as adaptive behaviour and affect regulation. Both externalizing and internalizing disorders are strongly associated with FASD and prenatal alcohol exposure in children, yet their causal relationship is not well established and two possible mechanisms have been proposed—mental health problems could arise from 'pleiotropic' expressions of a common underlying brain disorder or as secondary complications of FASD and prenatal alcohol exposure syndromes. In terms of common diagnostic categories, recognized comorbidities include ADHD, social communication disorder, PTSD, reactive attachment disorder, and substance misuse disorders, as well as mood, anxiety, and psychotic disorders. However, diagnosis, as based on prototypical phenotypes, can be difficult in some cases, because of the expression of psychological and physical phenotypes changing over the lifespan, as well as bias and unreliability in maternal recall and disclosure of prenatal alcohol consumption.

Fetal exposure to alcohol affects the development of facial features, primarily during the first trimester. The areas most affected are the orbital region (eyes) and the mid face. Affected individuals also display developmental features such as growth delay, small head size, and facial abnormalities, allowing for recognition of the disorder in infancy. Four facial features commonly occur across age, gender, and ethnic groups: (1) small palpebral fissures; (2) short horizontal length of the eye opening, defined as the distance from the endocanthion to the exocanthion; (3) a smooth philtrum (diminished or absent ridges between the upper lip and the nose); and (4) different degrees of thinness in the upper lip. Peripheral stigmata include 'railroad track' ear, clinodactyly, and 'hockey-stick' palmar crease (see Fig. 30.9).

Research has identified phenotypic heterogeneity within FASD, with variable association between facial stigmata and cognitive impairments/outcomes across studies. Overall, the presence or absence of facial dysmorphology does not clinically correlate with neuropsychiatric sequelae or structural brain damage in FASD (Streissguth and O'Malley, 2000).

FASD is not just a childhood disorder, but a lifespan disorder (Stevens et al., 2013), with a predictable developmental trajectory into adulthood, characterized by increased risks for mental health disorders, poor social functioning, and conduct problems. In particular, impulsivity and poor judgement (i.e. inability to stay calm and make rational and considered choices) can lead to reactive, anti-social, and maladaptive behaviours, which are often recalcitrant to mainstay treatments. Significant personal and societal costs are reflected by the over-representation of FASD youths and adults in criminal justice systems.

The heterogeneity of clinical presentation, poor maternal recall, and underestimation of prenatal alcohol consumption, as well as high levels of comorbidities, are among the recognized challenges to successful treatment of FASD (Streissguth et al., 1991).

(a)

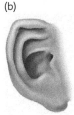

Epicanthal folds

Flat nasal bridge

Small palpebral fissures
"Railroad rack" ears
Upturned nose
Smooth philtrum
Thin upper lip

(b)

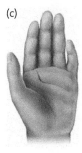

Characteristic features of an ear of a child with fetal alcohol spectrum disorders. Note the underdeveloped upper part of the ear parallel to the ear crease below ('railroad track' apperance).

(c)

Characteristic features of a hand of a child with fetal alcohol spectrum disorders. Note the curved fifth finger (clinodactyly) and the upper palmar crease that widens and ends between the second and third fingers ('hockey stick' crease).

Fig. 30.9 Facial and peripheral features and characteristics of fetal alcohol syndrome.
Darryl Leja / National Human Genome Research Institute.

Management

New insights derived from a better understanding of the neuropsychological and neurobehavioural profiles of FASD offer experts a fresh approach to developing clinical guidelines for interventions that include psychoeducational, psychosocial, pharmacological, and more experimental approaches such as nutritional and physical therapies. Overall, the management preference is for a holistic and individualized approach, tailored around the child and family, in accordance with their individual needs. All treatment programmes should start with *psycho-education* for the family. Interventions addressing the neurocognitive and social aspects of the disorder should utilize a Strengths-Based Model (Rapp and Goscha, 2012) in order to compensate for the identified weaknesses in each individual. Family strategies can focus on resilience-amplifying interventions and working on mobilizing and enhancing family coping strategies (Wilton and Plane, 2006). The *Personal Recovery*

approach (Slade, 2009) also includes empowering the family members to participate in designing intervention plans—which foster hope, self-management, and self-determination, while mobilizing autonomy—rather than remaining as passive recipients of care.

There is no specific pharmacological treatment for FASD, but optimal symptomatic control could be achieved using a range of appropriate psychotropic groups (including stimulants, SSRIs, atypical neuroleptics, and mood stabilizers) in the form of monotherapy or combination therapy. The evidence for psychostimulant use for inattention, hyperactivity, and impulsivity in FAS, PFAS, and ARND was reviewed by O'Malley and Hagerman (O'Malley and Hagerman, 1998) and O'Malley and Nanson (O'Malley and Nanson, 2002). Stimulant response in children with 'ADHD and FASD' can be atypical, as their inattention symptoms are less likely to respond than their hyperactivity and impulsivity symptoms (Oesterheld et al., 1998). Unnecessary polypharmacy should be avoided, including using multiple agents within one class (intra-class) or multiple agents of different classes (inter-class). Benzodiazepines could cause unpredictable and disinhibiting effects—typically worsening (rather than reducing or sedating) aggression in this neurologically compromised population.

Public health implications

FASD is an entirely preventable condition. Therefore, public education is vital in reducing its risks at the population level, in particular among high-risk subpopulations. Notably, UK guidelines have shifted from recommending one/two units of alcohol once/twice a week in 1995 to now recommending complete abstinence (British Medical Association, 2007). Importantly, public health education should dispel the myths around 'safe amount' or 'safe window' of alcohol use during pregnancy. It is now advocated that there is no safe drinking in pregnancy—in quantity or in stage. Preventing FASDs also requires an understanding of why women drink. A Swedish study by Skagerströmet et al. (2015) explored women's attitudes towards alcohol consumption during pregnancy, through focus groups with young, non-pregnant, and non-parous women (Skagerström et al., 2015). They reported that most women were aware of the potential harm to the unborn baby; yet they succumbed to social pressure and factors—these included peer pressure, not wanting to miss out on enjoyment, finding abstinence difficult, not wanting others to suspect they were pregnant, insufficient education, and misinformation that drinking small amounts during pregnancy was harmless. Prevention should target motivations to drinks (i.e. reward), in addition to information on harm (i.e. cost).

Given its high prevalence (and likely rising prevalence worldwide), FASD will continue to exert increasingly high demand for specialist psychiatric and psychological care, especially with now better recognition and detection. Understanding the complexities of FASD and related conditions—especially the interplay between neurobiological, environmental, and adaptive factors—demands highly specialized skills and clinical expertise. No one discipline can meet all aspects of the complex needs of FASD children and youths, especially along the developmental trajectory through the lifespan course, when additional complications emerge.

These clients' needs could only be met by dedicated specialist multidisciplinary teams, for better outcomes. These interventions can only be delivered by both highly resourced specialist centres and more accessible local clinics through a 'shared care arrangement', which allows accessing care through a network of services, in providing a comprehensive package of treatments. In other words, the concept of 'care network' is particularly important for these specialist services.

Summary

The key message here is powerful—at least 10% of women in the general global population, and up to 25% in Europe, continue to expose their unborn babies to alcohol. FASD is entirely preventable, yet in every 10,000 births globally, 15 will suffer from FASD (Popova et al., 2017). Public health education and policies are the cornerstones in prevention. There is no safe amount or safe window for alcohol use during pregnancy. The research in FASD is a rapidly evolving field and our readers are best advised to consult the latest authoritative publications to keep abreast of developments. Our current scientific knowledge of FASD should inform the design and implementation of more effective intervention programmes. Concepts of *care network*, *shared care*, *client-centred*, *strengths-based*, *family-orientated*, and *recovery-orientated* practices should supplement psychopharmacological and conventional management for this highly complex client group.

Conclusion

It is often said that the essence of science is less about obtaining new facts than about discovering new ways of thinking about them. This chapter accordingly focuses on how best to think about known facts and new knowledge in the field of child neuropsychiatry, rather than on particular contents which will inevitably become superseded.

Firstly, we provide a historical perspective through which different past conceptualizations of child neuropsychiatry can be understood and reconciled as a coherent whole. In doing so, we encourage our readers to understand that our current conceptualization is also contingent to, and limited by, the currently available evidence: thus partial and incomplete—rather than superior as 'the state-of-art truth'. Secondly, we provide four specific contrasting conditions to illustrate some key principles in understanding and thinking about clinical diagnoses. We use ADHD to illustrate the limitations of diagnostic criteria stipulated by taxonomic systems, and the neuroscientific model in which the connectivity of the brain is represented as dynamic, and not 'fixed circuits of hard-wiring'. We use TS to illustrate its colourful and heterogenous presentations for a highly heritable neuropsychiatric condition, as a prototypical neuropsychiatric disorder of developmental origin and with its characteristic motor and non-motor features, and provide a description of the CSTC brain circuitry involved, as well as chart the changing identities of TS through the medical discourse over time. The syndrome and its management emphasize the importance and merit in the rapprochement of neurology and psychiatry. We use brain tumours to illustrate how localized brain lesions can present with psychiatric symptoms anatomically related to the sites of tumours, as well as psychiatric syndromes not localizable to the lesion sites. We also highlight the principle of 'evolving taxonomy', as exemplified by how CM, PFS, and CCAS were previously conceived as distinct entities, but now CM and PFS may fuse into a spectrum disorder as new evidence emerges. FASD illustrates how a teratogen can affect the brain and somatic development during different critical exposure windows. It represents an entirely preventable condition, but with regard to public education, we also need to understand why some women continue to drink during pregnancy despite their knowledge of harm. The chapter therefore goes beyond summarizing the current state of facts. It imparts a particular kind of knowledge, which instils a particular kind of self-discipline in 'thinking about our thinking'. If this kind of knowledge could guard against misinformation, misconception, and misclassification, we intend our readers to become formidably armed.

KEY LEARNING POINTS

- Child neuropsychiatry encompasses childhood and adolescent psychiatric syndromes of neurobiological origins. It is an evolving discipline without a consensus on its exact boundary. Given the inconsistencies, we provide a historical perspective through which different conceptualizations of child neuropsychiatry can be understood and reconciled within the coherent whole.
- Four specific contrasting conditions are selected in this chapter to illustrate some key principles: ADHD as 'a diffuse brain disorder'; TS as a prototypical neurodevelopmental disorder of genetic and developmental origin with characteristically florid motor and non-motor features; childhood cranial tumours as 'a localized brain disorder'; and FASD as 'a disorder of a specific cause' represented by toxin exposure.
- ADHD and cranial tumours represent the extremes of the polar divide between 'a childhood neuropsychiatric disorder' and 'the neuropsychiatric manifestation of a childhood neurological disorder'.
- In contrast, FASD and TS illustrate how specific and complex aetiology can present with a wide spectrum of psychiatric disorders. Atypical presentations of psychiatric symptoms, idiosyncratic treatment response, and the effects of interacting comorbidities are also considered.
- We emphasize that child neuropsychiatric conditions are not fixed entities, despite being defined by diagnostic criteria stipulated by authoritative taxonomic systems. Rather, they are the results of the dynamic interplay among environmental factors, developmental maturity, mitigating factors, aberrant neural networks, and innate disease liability.

Acknowledgements

We thank Dr Alex Hegarty and Dr Julia K. Moore for their helpful assistance and comments.

REFERENCES

Abel EL & Hannigan JH. 1995. Maternal risk factors in fetal alcohol syndrome: provocative and permissive influences. *Neurotoxicology and teratology*, 17(4), pp.445–62.

Allen AJ, Leonard HL, & Swedo SE. 1995. Case study: a new infection-triggered, autoimmune subtype of pediatric OCD and Tourette's syndrome. *Journal of the American Academy of Child & Adolescent Psychiatry*, 34(3), pp.307–11.

Alsobrook J, Pauls D. 2002. A Factor Analysis of Tic Symptoms in Gilles de la Tourette's Syndrome. *American Journal of Psychiatry*, 159, pp.291–6.

American Psychiatric Association. 2013. *Diagnostic and Statistical Manual of Mental Disorders: DSM-5*. Washington, DC, American Psychiatric Association.

Anderson DM, et al. 2001. Medical and neurocognitive late effects among survivors of childhood central nervous system tumors. *Cancer*, 92(10), pp.2709–19.

Arnsten AFT. 2009. Stress signalling pathways that impair prefrontal cortex structure and function. *Nature Reviews Neuroscience*, 10(6), pp.410–22.

Arnsten AFT & Rubia K. 2012. Neurobiological Circuits Regulating Attention, Cognitive Control, Motivation, and Emotion: Disruptions in Neurodevelopmental Psychiatric Disorders. *Journal of the American Academy of Child & Adolescent Psychiatry*, 51(4), pp.356–67.

Avula S, et al. 2016. Post-operative pediatric cerebellar mutism syndrome and its association with hypertrophic olivary degeneration. *Quantitative Imaging in Medicine and Surgery*, 6(5), pp.535–44.

Banaschewski T, et al. 2009. *Attention-Deficit Hyperactivity Disorder and Hyperkinetic Disorder*. Oxford, Oxford University Press.

Barkley RA & Fischer M. 2010. The unique contribution of emotional impulsiveness to impairment in major life activities in hyperactive children as adults. *Journal of the American Academy of Child and Adolescent Psychiatry*, 49(5), pp.503–13.

Bertelsen B, Stefánsson H, Jensen LR, et al., 2016. Association of AADAC Deletion and Gilles de la Tourette Syndrome in a Large European Cohort. *Biological Psychiatry*, 79, pp.383–91.

Black KJ. 2017. Tourette syndrome research highlights from 2016. *F1000Res*, 6, pp.1430.

Bolton D, Rijsdijk F, O'Connor TG, et al. 2007. Obsessive-compulsive disorder, tics and anxiety in 6-year-old twins. *Psychological Medicine*, 37(1), pp.39–48.

Bower C, Watkins RE, Mutch RC, et al. 2018. Fetal alcohol spectrum disorder and youth justice: a prevalence study among young people sentenced to detention in Western Australia. *BMJ Open*, 8(2), e019605.

Bower C, Elliott EJ; on behalf of the Steering Group, 2016. *Report to the Australian Government Department of Health: 'Australian Guide to the diagnosis of Fetal Alcohol Spectrum Disorder (FASD)'*. Available at: https://www.fasdhub.org.au/siteassets/pdfs/australian-guide-to-diagnosis-of-fasd_all-appendices.pdf.

British Medical Association. 2007. *Fetal alcohol spectrum disorders: A guide for healthcare professionals*. Available at: http://www.nofas-uk.org/PDF/BMA%20REPORT%204%20JUNE%202007.pdf.

Browne HA, Hansen SN, Buxbaum JD, et al. 2015. Familial clustering of tic disorders and obsessive-compulsive disorder. *JAMA Psychiatry*, 72, pp.359–66.

Buitelaar JK, V.D.G.R., 1998. *Journal of Child Psychology and Psychiatry and Allied Disciplines*, 39, pp.911–19.

Burd L, et al., 2008. Mortality rates in subjects with fetal alcohol spectrum disorders and their siblings. *Birth Defects Research Part A: Clinical and Molecular Teratology*, 82(4), pp.217–23.

Casey BJ, Oliveri ME, Insel T. 2014. A Neurodevelopmental Perspective on the Research Domain Criteria (RDoC) Framework. *Biological Psychiatry*, 76(5), pp.350–3.

Cheung C, Yu K, Fung G, et al. 2010. Autistic Disorders and Schizophrenia: Related or Remote? An Anatomical Likelihood Estimation. *PLoS One*, 5(8), e12233.

Chisholm K, et al. 2015. The association between autism and schizophrenia spectrum disorders: A review of eight alternate models of co-occurrence. *Neuroscience & Biobehavioral Reviews*, 55, pp.173–83.

Chudley AE, et al. 2005. Fetal alcohol spectrum disorder: Canadian guidelines for diagnosis. *Canadian Medical Association Journal*, 172(5 suppl), pp.S1–21.

Cook CR, Blacher J. 2007. Evidence-based psychosocial treatments for tic disorders. *Clin Psychology: Science and Practice*, 14(3), pp.252–67.

Coffey C, Edward B. 2006. *Pediatric Neuropsychiatry*. Lippincott Williams & Wilkins.

Crespi B, Stead P, Elliot M. 2010. Evolution in health and medicine Sackler colloquium: Comparative genomics of autism and schizophrenia. *Proceedings of the National Academy of Sciences of the United States of America*, 107 Suppl(Suppl 1), pp.1736–41.

Cuthbert BN. 2014. The RDoC framework: facilitating transition from ICD/DSM to dimensional approaches that integrate neuroscience and psychopathology. *World Psychiatry*, 13(1), pp.28–35.

Cuthbert BN, Insel TR. 2013. Toward the future of psychiatric diagnosis: the seven pillars of RDoC. *BMC Medicine*, 11(1), p.126.

Dale RC. 2013. Immune-mediated extrapyramidal movement disorders, including Sydenham chorea. *Handbook of Clinical Neurology*, 112, pp.1235–41.

Debes NM, Preel M, Skov L. 2017. Functional neuroimaging in Tourette syndrome: recent perspectives. *Neuroscience and Neuroeconomics*, 6, pp.1–13.

Eapen V, Robertson MM. 2015. Are there distinct subtypes in Tourette syndrome? Pure-Tourette syndrome versus Tourette syndrome-plus, and simple versus complex tics. *Neuropsychiatric Disease and Treatment*, 11, 1431–6.

Eapen V, Walter A, Robertson MM. 2018. Heterogeneity in Tics and Gilles de la Tourette Syndrome. In: Hodes, M, Gau, S, de Vries, PJ, eds. *Understanding Uniqueness and Diversity in Child and Adolescent Mental Health* (pp.57–76). Academic Press.

Fitzpatrick JP, et al. 2015. Prevalence of fetal alcohol syndrome in a population-based sample of children living in remote Australia: The Lililwan Project. *Journal of Paediatrics and Child Health*, 51(4), pp.450–7.

Fuemmeler BF, Elkin TD, Mullins LL. 2002. Survivors of childhood brain tumors: behavioral, emotional, and social adjustment. *Clinical Psychology Review*, 22(4), pp.547–85.

Gillberg C. 1995. *Clinical Child Neuropsychiatry*. Cambridge, Cambridge University Press.

Grados MA, Mathews CA; Tourette Syndrome Association International Consortium for Genetics. 2008. Latent class analysis of Gilles de la Tourette syndrome using comorbidities: clinical and genetic implications. *Biological Psychiatry*, 64(3), pp.219–25.

Graybiel AM, Canales JJ. 2001. The neurobiology of repetitive behaviors: clues to the neurobiology of Tourette syndrome. *Advanced Neurology*, 85, pp.123–31.

Grundy RG, et al. 2007. Primary postoperative chemotherapy without radiotherapy for intracranial ependymoma in children: the UKCCSG/SIOP prospective study. *The Lancet Oncology*, 8(8), pp.696–705.

Gudrunardottir T, et al. 2016. Consensus paper on post-operative pediatric cerebellar mutism syndrome: the Iceland Delphi results. *Child's Nervous System*, 32(7), pp.1195–203.

Harris J. 1995. *Developmental Neuropsychiatry*. New York, NY, Oxford University Press.

Hasstedt SJ, Leppert M, Filloux F, et al. 1995. Intermediate inheritance of Tourette syndrome, assuming assortative mating. *American Journal of Human Genetics*, 57, pp.682–9.

Heath RG. 1997. Foreword. In Schmahmann J, ed. *The Cerebellum and Cognition*. San Diego, CA, Academic Press, pp. xxiii–v.

Hegarty A, Furlong Y. 2018. Neuropsychiatric aspects of childhood cranial tumors. In: Agrawal A, ed. *Brain Tumor: An Update*. InTech Open, Chapter 7.

Hendrickson TJ, et al. 2017. Cortical gyrification is abnormal in children with prenatal alcohol exposure. *NeuroImage: Clinical*, 15, pp.391–400.

Hopyan T, Laughlin S, Dennis M. 2010. Emotions and Their Cognitive Control in Children With Cerebellar Tumors. *Journal of the International Neuropsychological Society*, 16(6), pp.1027–38.

Hulvershorn LA, et al. 2014. Abnormal amygdala functional connectivity associated with emotional lability in children with attention-deficit/hyperactivity disorder. *Journal of the American Academy of Child and Adolescent Psychiatry*, 53(3), pp.351–61.e1.

Huss M, Chen W, Ludolph AG. 2016. Guanfacine Extended Release: A New Pharmacological Treatment Option in Europe. *Clinical Drug Investigation*, 36(1), pp.1–25.

James A, Lai FH, Dahl C. 2004. Attention deficit hyperactivity disorder and suicide: a review of possible associations. *Acta Psychiatrica Scandinavica*, 110(6), pp.408–15.

Jones KL, et al., 1973. Pattern of malformation in offspring of chronic alcoholic mothers. *The Lancet*, 301(7815), pp.1267–71.

Karagiannidis I, Rizzo R, Tarnok Z, et al. 2012. Replication of association between a SLITRK1 haplotype and Tourette Syndrome in a large sample of families. *Molecular Psychiatry*, 17(7), 665.

Korah MP, et al. 2010. Incidence, Risks, and Sequelae of Posterior Fossa Syndrome in Pediatric Medulloblastoma. *International Journal of Radiation Oncology, Biology, Physics*, 77(1), pp.106–12.

Kulkarni AV, Bouffet B, Drake JM. 2004. Ependymal Tumours. In: RA Walker, DA Perinlongo, G Punt, JAG Taylor, eds. *Brain and Spinal Tumours in Childhood*. London, Arnold, pp.331–44.

Kurlan R, Eapen V, Stern J, et al.1994. Bilineal transmission in Tourette's syndrome families. *Neurology*, 44, pp.2336–42.

de Lacy N, King BH. 2013. Revisiting the Relationship Between Autism and Schizophrenia: Toward an Integrated Neurobiology. *Annual Review of Clinical Psychology*, 9(1), pp.555–87.

Lanier JC, Abrams AN. 2017. Posterior fossa syndrome: Review of the behavioral and emotional aspects in pediatric cancer patients. *Cancer*, 123(4), pp.551–9.

Lerner A, Bagic A, Boudreau EA, et al. 2007. Neuroimaging of neuronal circuits involved in tic generation in patients with Tourette syndrome. *Neurology*, 68(23), pp.1979–87.

Levisohn L, Cronin-Golomb A, Schmahmann JD. 2000. Neuropsychological consequences of cerebellar tumour resection in children. *Brain*, 123(5), pp.1041–50.

Lichtenstein P, Carlstrom E, Rastam M, et al. 2010. The genetics of autism spectrum disorders and related neuropsychiatric disorders in childhood. *American Journal of Psychiatry*, 167(11):1357–63.

Liu S, Cui J, Zhang X, et al. 2014. Variable number tandem repeats in dopamine receptor D4 in Tourette's syndrome. *Mov. Disord*, 29(13), pp.1687–91.

Liu L, et al. 2016. Is Emotional Lability Distinct From 'Angry/Irritable Mood,' 'Negative Affect,' or Other Subdimensions of Oppositional Defiant Disorder in Children With ADHD? *Journal of Attention Disorders*, 23, pp. 859–68.

Liu L, Chen W, Sun L, et al. 2017. The characteristics and age effects of emotional lability in ADHD children with and without oppositional defiant disorder. *Journal of Attention Disorders*. Available at: https://doi.org/10.1177/1087054717745594.

Lumsden DE, et al. 2011. Pre-existing neurodevelopmental and neuropsychiatric difficulties in children with brain tumours: implications for future outcome studies. *Developmental Medicine & Child Neurology*, 53(1), p.93.

Madhusoodanan S, et al. 2010. Brain tumor location and psychiatric symptoms: is there any association? A meta-analysis of published case studies. *Expert Review of Neurotherapeutics*, 10(10), pp.1529–36.

Mataix-Cols D, Isomura K, Pérez-Vigil A, et al. 2015. Familial Risks of Tourette Syndrome and Chronic Tic Disorders. *JAMA Psychiatry*, 72, pp.787–93.

May PA, Gossage JP. 2001. Estimating the prevalence of fetal alcohol syndrome. A summary. *Alcohol Research & Health*, 25(3), pp.159–67.

May PA, Hymbaugh KJ, Aase JM. 1983. Epidemiology of fetal alcohol syndrome among American Indians of the Southwest. *Soc Biol*, 30, pp.374–87.

McNaught K. 2010. 125 Years of Tourette Syndrome: The Discovery, Early History and Future of the Disorder. *Quarterly Newsletter of the Tourette Association*, Winter, Vol. 38, No. 3.

Merwood A, et al. 2014. Genetic Associations Between the Symptoms of Attention-Deficit/Hyperactivity Disorder and Emotional Lability in Child and Adolescent Twins. *Journal of the American Academy of Child & Adolescent Psychiatry*, 53(2), pp.209–20.e4.

National Institute for Health and Care Excellence. 2015. *Suspected cancer: recognition and referral*. NICE guideline [NG12]. London, National Institute for Health and Care Excellence.

O'Malley KD, Nanson J. 2002. Clinical Implications of a Link between Fetal Alcohol Spectrum Disorder and Attention-Deficit Hyperactivity Disorder. *Canadian Journal of Psychiatry*, 47(4), pp.349–54.

O'Malley KD, Hagerman RJ. Developing clinical practice guidelines for pharmacological interventions with alcohol-affected children. In: Centers for Disease Control and Prevention, ed. *Intervening with Children Affected by Prenatal Alcohol Exposure: Proceedings of a Special Focus Session of the Interagency Coordinating Committee on Fetal Alcohol Syndrome September 10-11, 1998*. Chevy Chase, MD: National Institute of Alcohol Abuse and Alcoholism; 1999. pp. 145–77.

Oesterheld J, et al. 1998. Effectiveness of Methylphenidate in Native American Children with Fetal Alcohol Syndrome and Attention Deficit/Hyperactivity Disorder: A Controlled Pilot Study. *Journal of Child and Adolescent Psychopharmacology*, 8(1), pp.39–48.

Ospina M, Dennett L. 2013. *Systematic review of the prevalence of fetal alcohol spectrum disorders*. IHE Alberta Canada, Edmonton, April, pp.1–73.

Pagliaroli L, Vető B, Arányi T, et al. 2016. From Genetics to Epigenetics: New Perspectives in Tourette Syndrome Research. *Frontiers in Neuroscience* 10, pp.277.

Paschou P, Yu D, Gerber G, Evans P, et al. 2014. Genetic association signal near NTN4 in Tourette syndrome. *Annals of Neurology*, 76, 310–15.

Piacentini J, Woods DW, Scahill L, et al. 2010. Behavior Therapy for Children With Tourette Disorder: A Randomized Controlled Trial. *JAMA*, 303(19), pp.1929–37.

Polanczyk G, et al. 2007. The Worldwide Prevalence of ADHD: A Systematic Review and Metaregression Analysis. *American Journal of Psychiatry*, 164(6), pp.942–8.

Polderman TJ, Benyamin B, de Leeuw CA, et al. 2015. Meta-analysis of the heritability of human traits based on fifty years of twin studies. *Nature Genetics*, 47(7), pp.702–9.

Popova S, et al. 2017. Estimation of national, regional, and global prevalence of alcohol use during pregnancy and fetal alcohol syndrome: a systematic review and meta-analysis. *The Lancet Global Health*, 5(3), pp. 290–9.

Popova S, et al. 2012. Health Care Burden and Cost Associated with Fetal Alcohol Syndrome: Based on Official Canadian Data S. C. Hausmann-Muela, ed. *PLoS One*, 7.

Popova S, et al. 2019. Prevalence of fetal alcohol spectrum disorder among special subpopulations: a systematic review and meta-analysis. *Addiction*, 114, pp.1150–72.

Purper-Ouakil D. et al. 2011. Neurobiology of Attention Deficit/ Hyperactivity Disorder. *Pediatric Research*, 69(5 Part 2), pp.69R–76R.

Qi Y, Zheng Y, Li Z, Xiong L. 2017. Progress in Genetic Studies of Tourette's Syndrome. *Brain Science*, 7, 134.

Rajagopal S, Seri And S, Cavanna AE. 2013. Premonitory urges and sensorimotor processing in Tourette syndrome. *Behavioral Neurology*, 27(1), pp.65–73.

Randell R, Somerville-Brown L, Chen W. 2019. How relevant is higher-order language deficit (HOLD) to children with complex presentations of attention-deficit hyperactivity disorder?. *ADHD Attention Deficit and Hyperactivity Disorders*, 11, pp. 325–32.

Rapoport J, et al. 2009. Autism spectrum disorders and childhood-onset schizophrenia: clinical and biological contributions to a relation revisited. *Journal of the American Academy of Child and Adolescent Psychiatry*, 48(1), pp.10–18.

Rapp CA, Goscha RJ. 2012. *The Strengths Model : A Recovery-Oriented Approach to Mental Health Services*. Oxford: Oxford University Press.

Rekate HL, et al. 1985. Muteness of cerebellar origin. *Archives of Neurology*, 42(7), pp.697–8.

Robertson MM, Althoff RR, Hafez A, Pauls DL. 2008. Principal components analysis of a large cohort with Tourette syndrome. *British Journal of Psychiatry*, 193(1), pp.31–6.

Robertson MM, Cavanna AE. 2007. The Gilles de la Tourette syndrome: a principal component factor analytic study of a large pedigree. *Psychiatric Genetics*, 17(3), 143–52.

Rodgers S, Müller M, Kawohl W, et al. 2014. Sex-related and non-sex-related comorbidity subtypes of tic disorders: a latent class approach. *European Journal of Neurology*, 21(5), 700–45.

Rojas EY, Gretton HM. 2007. Background, Offence Characteristics, and Criminal Outcomes of Aboriginal Youth Who Sexually Offend: A Closer Look at Aboriginal Youth Intervention Needs. *Sexual Abuse*, 19(3), pp.257–83.

Rutter M. 1984. *Developmental Neuropsychiatry*. Churchill Livingstone.

Scharf JM, Yu D, Mathews CA, et al. 2013. Genome-wide association study of Tourette's syndrome. *Mol Psychiatry*, 18(6), pp.721–8.

Schmahmann JD. 2010. The Role of the Cerebellum in Cognition and Emotion: Personal Reflections Since 1982 on the Dysmetria of Thought Hypothesis, and Its Historical Evolution from Theory to Therapy. *Neuropsychology Review*, 20(3), pp.236–60.

Seymour KE, et al. 2012. Emotion Regulation Mediates the Relationship between ADHD and Depressive Symptoms in Youth. *Journal of Abnormal Child Psychology*, 40(4), pp.595–606.

Shanmugavadivel D, Walker D, Liu, J-F, et al. 2016. HeadSmart: are you brain tumour aware? *Paediatrics and Child Health*, 26(2), pp.81–6.

Shaw P, Stringaris A, Nigg J, Leibenluft E. (2014). Emotion dysregulation in attention deficit hyperactivity disorder. *American Journal of Psychiatry*, 171, pp.276–93.

Siegel RL, Miller KD, Jemal A. 2017. Cancer statistics. *Cancer*, 67(1), pp.7–30.

Sigra S, Hesselmark E, Bejerot S. 2018. Treatment of PANDAS and PANS: a systematic review. *Neuroscience & Biobehavioral Reviews*, 86, 51–65.

Singer HS, Mink JW, Gilbert DL, Jankovic J. 2016. *Movement Disorders in Childhood*, second edition. Philadelphia, PA, Elsevier Inc.

Singer HS, Gilbert DL, Wolf DS, et al. 2012. Moving from PANDAS to CANS. *Journal of Pediatrics*, 160(5), pp.725–31.

Skagerström J, Häggström-Nordin E, Alehagen S. 2015. The voice of non-pregnant women on alcohol consumption during pregnancy: a focus group study among women in Sweden. *BMC Public Health*, 15, p.1193.

Slade M. 2009. *Personal Recovery and Mental Illness: A Guide for Mental Health Professionals*. Cambridge, Cambridge University Press.

Sobanski E, et al. 2010. Emotional lability in children and adolescents with attention deficit/hyperactivity disorder (ADHD): clinical correlates and familial prevalence. *Journal of Child Psychology and Psychiatry*, 51(8), pp.915–23.

Stevens SA, et al. 2013. Towards Identifying a characteristic neuropsychological profile for fetal alcohol spectrum disorders 2. Specific caregiver and teacher rating. *Journal of Population Therapeutics and Clinical Pharmacology*, 20(1), pp.53–62.

Streissguth AP, Barr HM, Kogan J, et al. 1996. *Final report: Understanding the occurrence of secondary disabilities in clients with fetal alcohol syndrome (FAS) and fetal alcohol effects (FAE)*. Seattle, WA.

Streissguth AP, et al. 1991. Fetal alcohol syndrome in adolescents and adults. *JAMA*, 265(15), pp.1961–7.

Streissguth AP, O'Malley K. 2000. Neuropsychiatric implications and long-term consequences of fetal alcohol spectrum disorders. *Seminars in Clinical Neuropsychiatry*, 5(3), pp.177–90.

Sugranyes G, et al. 2011. Autism Spectrum Disorders and Schizophrenia: Meta-Analysis of the Neural Correlates of Social Cognition. *PLoS One*, 6(10).

Swedo SE, Leonard HL, Garvey M, et al. 1998. Pediatric autoimmune neuropsychiatric disorders associated with streptococcal infections: clinical description of the first 50 cases. *American Journal of Psychiatry*, 155(2), 264–71.

Swedo SE, Leckman JF, Rose NR. 2012. From research subgroup to clinical syndrome: modifying the PANDAS criteria to describe PANS (pediatric acute-onset neuropsychiatric syndrome). *Pediatric Therapeutics*, 2(2), 113.

Tan CH, Denny CH, Cheal NE, et al. 2015. Alcohol Use and Binge Drinking Among Women of Childbearing Age—United States, 2011–2013. *MMWR Morbidity and Mortality Weekly Reports*, 64(37), pp.1042–6.

Teicher MH, et al. 2002. Developmental neurobiology of childhood stress and trauma. *Psychiatric Clinics of North America*, 25(2), pp.397–426, vii–viii.

Teicher MH, et al. 2003. The neurobiological consequences of early stress and childhood maltreatment. *Neuroscience and Biobehavioral Reviews*, 27(1–2), pp.33–44.

Tourette G. 1885. Etude sur une affection nerveuse caracterisee par de l'indoordination motrice accompagnee d'echolalie et al copralalie. *Archives of Neurology*, 9, pp.19–42.

Turkel SB, et al., 2004. Case Series: Acute Mood Symptoms Associated With Posterior Fossa Lesions in Children. *Journal of Neuropsychiatry and Clinical Neurosciences*, 16(4), pp.443–5.

Ulleland CN. 1972. The Offspring Of Alcoholic Mothers. *Annals of the New York Academy of Sciences*, 197, pp.167–9.

Walker D, et al. 2016. A new clinical guideline from the Royal College of Paediatrics and Child Health with a national awareness campaign accelerates brain tumor diagnosis in UK children—'HeadSmart: Be Brain Tumour Aware.' *Neuro-Oncology*, 18(3), pp.445–54.

Weinberger DR, Glick ID, Klein DF. 2015. Whither Research Domain Criteria (RDoC)? *JAMA Psychiatry*, 72(12), p.1161.

Wells EM, et al. 2008. The cerebellar mutism syndrome and its relation to cerebellar cognitive function and the cerebellar cognitive affective disorder. *Developmental Disabilities Research Reviews*, 14(3), pp.221–8.

Whittington C, Pennant M, Kendall T, et al. 2016. Practitioner Review: Treatments for Tourette syndrome in children and young people—a systematic review. *Journal of Child Psychology and Psychiatry*, 57(9):988–1004.

William NM, et al. 2010. Rare chromosomal deletions and duplications in attention-deficit hyperactivity disorder: a genome-wide analysis. *The Lancet*, 376, pp.1401–8.

Wilne SH, et al. 2006. The presenting features of brain tumours: a review of 200 cases. *Archives of Disease in Childhood*, 91(6), pp.502–6.

Wilton G, Plane MB. 2006. The Family Empowerment Network: a service model to address the needs of children and families affected by Fetal Alcohol Spectrum Disorders. *Pediatric Nursing*, 32(4), pp.299–306.

World Health Organization. 1992. *ICD-10 Classifications of Mental and Behavioural Disorder: Clinical Descriptions and Diagnostic Guidelines*. Geneva, World Health Organization.

Yu X, et al. 2016. Integrity of Amygdala Subregion-Based Functional Networks and Emotional Lability in Drug-Naïve Boys With ADHD. *Journal of Attention Disorders*, pii: 1087054716661419.

Yu D, Sul JH, Tsetsos F, et al. 2019. Interrogating the Genetic Determinants of Tourette's Syndrome and Other Tic Disorders Through Genome-Wide Association Studies. *American Journal of Psychiatry*, 176(3), pp.217–27.

Yuan A, Su L, Yu S, et al. 2015. Association between DRD2/ANKK1 TaqIA Polymorphism and Susceptibility with Tourette Syndrome: a meta-analysis. *PLoS One*, 10(6), pp.e0131060.

Zyrianova Y, Alexander L, Faruqui R. 2015. Neuropsychiatric presentations and outcomes in children and adolescents with primary brain tumours: Systematic review. *Brain Injury*, 30(1), pp.1–9.

31

Neuropsychiatry of aggression

Shoumitro (Shoumi) Deb and Tanya Deb

Introduction

Diseases that affect the CNS, including trauma, vascular diseases, space-occupying lesions, infectious, metabolic, and degenerative diseases, endocrine deficiency, etc., often lead to neurobehavioural disorders, including impairment of memory, language, emotions/affect, attention, perception, executive functions, and visuospatial skills, among others. One such neurobehavioural symptom is aggression, which is often the reason for referral to neuropsychiatric clinics and is notoriously difficult to treat. Aggression is a major public health concern and often causes distress to patients and their families. It can hinder rehabilitation and cause major disability and impairment for patients and is a source of major stress for family, friends, and carers. It can lead to social isolation and loss of community placements or social and family/friends' support, and may lead to unnecessary use of restraint, hospitalization, and medication. In addition, it has financial implications for patients, their families, and society as a whole.

There is no universal definition of aggression, but one proposed by Baron and Richardson (Baron and Richardson, 1994, p. 7) is 'any form of behavior directed toward the goal of harming or injuring another living being who is motivated to avoid such treatment.' Aggression can be verbal, in the form of abuse or shouting, or physical, directed to other people or property. In some cases, particularly associated with some genetic syndromes of intellectual disabilities (IDs), aggression could be directed to oneself as well [(self-injurious behaviour) (SIB)] (see review by Deb, 1998; Hemmings et al., 2013). Two main types of outwardly directed aggression have been described in the literature and could be observed in clinical practice. Reactive (or affective or defensive) aggression is precipitated by stress-provoking stimuli when a person is frustrated, but the response is out of proportion to the stressor. The behaviour itself is less structured and often associated with emotional and physical signs of anger and arousal. Proactive (or instrumental or predatory) aggression, on the other hand, is led by premeditated, cold-blooded action, is often well structured and goal-directed, and happens in an emotionally calm and concentrated state of mind. Apart from instrumental aggression in the context of certain personality disorders (PDs), reactive aggression is the predominant type of aggression seen in the human race, and also in neuropsychiatric disorders. It is not always easy to distinguish between these two fundamental types of aggression, but different hypotheses have been proposed to explain these two different types. For example, a 'somatic marker' hypothesis—a neurocognitive mechanism—has been proposed to explain affective aggression (Tranel et al., 1999). Conversely, a psychosocial hypothesis—'dysfunctional social learning'—has been proposed as the underlying mechanism for instrumental aggression (Blair, 2001).

Although there is no specific category for aggression, in the new DSM-5 classification (American Psychiatric Association, 2013), intermittent explosive disorder (IED) is the closest diagnosis for reactive aggression and conduct disorder (CD) for proactive aggression. Oppositional defiant disorder (ODD) is described as a milder form of CD, particularly affecting children and adolescents (Deb et al., 2016). In the DSM-5, CD, ODD, and IED are classified within the overall heading 'Disruptive, Impulse Control and Conduct Disorders'.

The DSM-5 provides six criteria for IED, each of which must be present for a diagnosis. These criteria require recurrent impulsive, aggressive behavioural outbursts with a magnitude that is grossly out of proportion to the provocation or to any precipitating psychosocial stressor. Criteria are met only if outbursts are impulsive, rather than premeditated, and must cause significant distress or impairment.

The essential feature of CD is a repetitive and persistent pattern of behaviour that violates the basic rights of others or that breaks major age-appropriate societal norms or rules. Included in the DSM-5 criteria for CD are behaviours that are grouped into four major categories: (1) aggression to people or animals; (2) destruction of property; (3) deceitfulness or theft; and (4) serious violations of rules. The DSM-5 provides a list of 15 symptoms under these four groups. Diagnosis requires the presence of three or more of the symptoms during the preceding 12 months, with at least one symptom being present during the preceding 6 months. As with all psychiatric conditions, the presentation must cause clinically significant impairment in social, academic, or occupational functioning.

The essential feature of ODD is a recurrent pattern of angry/irritable mood, with defiant/disobedient and hostile/vindictive behaviour towards at least one individual who is not a sibling. The DSM-5 provides a list of eight symptoms for ODD across three categories. Diagnosis requires the presence of four or more symptoms lasting at least 6 months. In addition, the disturbance in behaviour has to cause clinically significant impairment in social, academic, or occupational functioning.

In order to provide a diagnostic category for youths with chronic severe irritability and aggression, the DSM-5 has created a new category under 'Depressive Disorders' called 'disruptive mood dysregulation disorders (DMDD)'. Although theoretically, DMDD is distinguishable from ODD and CD on the basis of severity, it is not so easy in practice to apply this distinction. Similarly, whereas IED is supposed to be intermittent, DMDD should have a persistent irritable mood state for a longer duration (over 12 months). DMDD is defined primarily by two features: (1) frequent severe temper outbursts; and (2) persistent irritability evident every day for most of the day. Unlike severe mood dysregulation diagnosis, DMDD excludes hyperarousal (e.g. insomnia, agitation, distractibility, racing thoughts) from the essential criteria.

Of the 12 categories of PDs described in the DSM-5, anti-social PD is a pattern of disregard for, and violation of, the rights of others, which brings this diagnosis close to CD. Similarly, borderline PD (BPD) is a pattern of instability in interpersonal relationships, self-image, and affect, and marked impulsivity, thus bringing this diagnosis close to IED. All the DSM-5 diagnostic categories discussed here have onset before adulthood. In the ICD-11 (World Health Organization, 2018), ODD and CD are included within the category of 'Disruptive Behaviour or Dissocial Disorders', and IED is included within the 'Impulse Control Disorder' category.

Related concepts

There are a number of terms that are related to the concept of aggression. For example, anger is seen as an emotional state which varies in intensity, from mild annoyance or irritability to rage, and is neither necessary nor essential for aggression to occur. Hostility, on the other hand, is conceptualized as an attitudinal or cognitive construct which involves a negative interpretation of stimuli. Behaviours, such as impulsivity, urgency, and sensation-seeking, and cognitive/emotional states, such as irritability and anxiety, could be seen as predisposing, precipitating, and perpetuating factors for aggression. Impulsivity is seen as a swift action without forethought or conscious judgement and could lead to impulsive aggression. Violence, on the other hand, could be seen as an extreme form of aggression. The World Health Organization (WHO) has defined violence as 'The intentional use of physical force or power, threatened or actual, against oneself, another person, or against a group or community that either results in or has a high likelihood of resulting in injury, death, psychological harm, maldevelopment or deprivation' (Krug et al., 2002, p. 1084).

Prevalence

In the UK, 30% of a typical primary care child consultations are for problem behaviours. Childhood CD predisposes to adulthood PD. A meta-analysis reported violence among about 10% of patients with schizophrenia or other psychotic disorders, compared with <2% of the general public, with up to 20 times higher risk of homicide (Fazel et al., 2009, cited in Frogley et al., 2012). In the inpatient setting, aggression is even commoner, with rates of assault

by patients with schizophrenia of between 16% and 28% (Joyal et al., 2008). Although it seems that aggression may be commoner in different psychiatric disorders, such as schizophrenia, bipolar disorder, and depression, their relationship is far from clear. For example, it has been proposed that most of the observed excess risk of violence associated with schizophrenia and other psychoses appears to be mediated by alcohol and substance abuse comorbidity (Fazel et al., 2009). Table 31.1 shows the prevalence of aggression in various neuropsychiatric disorders. As autism spectrum disorder (ASD) and ADHD are both common in ID, the cumulative prevalence rate of aggression in people with ID with comorbid ASD and ADHD is very high (McClintock et al., 2003). Additionally, some recent papers highlighted the possible role of medicinal-induced behaviour disorders (Munjampalli and Davis, 2016) and neuropsychiatric features in primary mitochondrial disease (Marin and Saneto, 2016).

Table 31.1 Prevalence of aggression/agitation in neuropsychiatric disorders

Neuropsychiatric disorder and other populations	Prevalence
US general population (Corrigan and Watson, 2005)	2% (male > female) (age group: 25-34 >15-24 >35-44 >45-54 years)
TBI (Deb et al., 1999; Silver et al., 2005)	37-71% (aggression and agitation)
Dementia (Sadavoy et al., 2008; Zuidema et al., 2007)	48-82% (aggression or agitation) 6-77% (aggression)
ASD (Lai et al., 2014)	16-28% (ODD)
ADHD (Saylor and Aman, 2016)	>50% (problem behaviour)
ID (Hemmings et al., 2013; Sigafoos et al., 1994)	6-60% (problem behaviour) (average: around 30%); 10-15% (aggression)
Psychiatric outpatients (all ages) (Coccaro et al., 2005)	6.3% (lifetime); 3.1% (point prevalence) (IED)
Personality disorder (Johnson et al., 2000)	14.4% (violence)
Schizophrenia (Fazel et al., 2009)	Violent crimes 4-6 times higher than general population
Bipolar disorder II (Corrigan and Watson, 2005)	16% (in manic phase) (aggression)
Schizophrenia (Brekke et al., 2001)	14 times more likely to be a victim than a perpetrator of aggression
Drug and alcohol abuse (Swanson et al., 1990)	12-16 times higher than general population (aggression)
Epilepsy (Brodie et al., 2016)	Aggression can happen in pre-, peri-, and post-ictal stage
Children in the UK (National Institute for Health and Care Excellence, 2013)	8% (boys); 5% (girls) (CD)
MS (Moghadasi et al., 2016)	23% (aggression); 38% (irritability)
Chronic traumatic encephalopathy (punch drunk syndrome) (Antonius et al., 2014)	70% (aggression or violence); 39% (irritability); 24% (agitation)
Parkinson's disease (Zweig et al., 2016)	20% (irritability)
Huntington's disease (Fisher et al., 2014)	22-66% (aggression)

ASD, autism spectrum disorder; ADHD, attention-deficit/hyperactivity disorder; CD, conduct disorder; ID, intellectual disability; IED: intermittent explosive disorder; MS, multiple sclerosis; NICE: National Institute for Health and Care Excellence; ODD, oppositional defiant disorder; TBI, traumatic brain injury.

The relationship between epilepsy and aggression is complex. Overall, people with epilepsy show no more aggression than those without, but some people with complex partial seizures of temporal or frontal lobe origin may show an increased rate of aggression. In any case, the aggressive acts associated with epilepsy are not goal-directed or planned, although inadvertently these actions may cause harm and bodily injuries to other people. Ictal aggression is often associated with automatism, and post-ictal aggression is often part of a confusional state or post-ictal psychosis (Kanemoto et al., 2010). A range of factors may contribute to interictal aggression that include factors related to seizures, brain abnormalities, epilepsy syndrome, medication, and psychosocial issues (Brodie et al., 2016; Deb, 2007; Mula, 2016). The relationship between substance and alcohol abuse and aggression is well established. However, the relationship is complex because of the heterogeneity of the condition and the complicated aetiology (Nestor, 2002). For example, alcohol and certain substances could cause sedation and calmness at the time of use but may precipitate aggression on withdrawal or from chronic use.

Neurobiology of aggression

Neurobiology of aggression is complex, and despite the major advances made in recent years, there are still major gaps in our understanding. Evidence for a neural substrate of aggression comes from the lesion, neuroimaging, neurosurgical, genetic, and peripheral markers, and pharmacological provocation studies in animals and humans.

Neuroanatomy

Our understanding of neural substrates of aggression perhaps starts with the most famous lesion study in the history of cognitive neuroscience, based on the story of Phineas Gage (Harlow, 1868). Gage was a railroad worker in the United States and a tamping rod went through his skull during an accident and damaged his left anterior cingulate gyrus and right ventromedial prefrontal cortex (PFC) (see Fig. 31.1). Before the accident, Gage was a pleasant, friendly man, but after the accident, there was a marked change in his behaviour in that he became irritable, lost his temper easily, and lacked

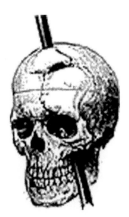

Fig. 31.1 Phineas Gage skull with an inserted iron rod.
Reproduced from John M. Harlow. M.D. (1868) *Recovery from the passage of an iron bar through the head*. Boston: Publications of the Massachusetts Medical Society.

social judgement. His behaviour changed to the extent that his friends stated that Gage is 'no longer Gage'. Interestingly, there were no localizing neurological signs or speech or cognitive abnormalities that one would expect from such a severe brain injury. This is perhaps the first example of our understanding that brain injury could change human behaviour, even in the absence of localizing neurological signs.

The second piece of evidence in support of a neuroanatomical basis for aggression perhaps comes from lesion studies carried out on animals by Klüver and Bucy (1939). They showed that after bilateral ablation of the amygdala, monkeys became placid, less aggressive and fearless, and showed changed sexual behaviour and a tendency to put objects in their mouths. Indeed since then, many reports of Klüver–Bucy syndrome have been described in humans, with a variety of lesions in anterior temporal regions. The role of the amygdala in aggression has been supported further by neurosurgical studies. In a retrospective study of 481 patients who underwent bilateral stereotactic amygdalotomy for intractable aggression, Ramamurthi (1988) reported excellent improvement in 70–76% of patients. In addition, Tonkogony and Geller (1992) reported aggression in patients with temporal lobe tumours. The temporal lobes form part of the paralimbic motivation system, and together with the amygdala, they mediate stimulus–reinforcement learning (Rubia, 2011 cited in Alegria et al., 2016). Also, superior temporal regions modulate attention function (Rubia, 2011); thus, temporal lobe impairment may lead to aggression by affecting attention, motivation, and the decision-making process (Alegria et al., 2016).

A recent meta-analysis of 28 voxel-based morphometry (VBM) studies of adolescents with CD showed reductions in the grey matter in the insula, amygdala, and frontal and temporal regions (Rogers and De Brito, 2016). Positron emission tomography (PET) studies also showed similar findings in psychiatric patients with a history of violence (Volkow et al., 1995). Previous diffusion tensor imaging (DTI) studies showed abnormalities in the uncinate fasciculus, which is a major limbic–prefrontal white matter connection in adolescents with CD (Sarkar et al., 2013). However, recent DTI studies showed impairment across a range of white matter tracts, including the inferior fronto-occipital fasciculus, cingulum, corticospinal tract, thalamic radiations, corpus callosum, and cerebellar areas (Sarkar et al., 2016; Waller et al., 2017).

It is proposed that reduction in the top–down control from the PFC, particularly fronto-medial PFC, or overactivity in the limbic system, particularly the amygdala, hippocampus, and cingulate gyrus, is likely to lead to aggression (Siever, 2008). Structural MRI studies of youths with disruptive behaviour showed abnormalities in the ventral and dorsomedial PFC, anterior cingulate and temporo-limbic regions (Rogers and De Brito, 2016). fMRI studies of youths with disruptive behaviour disorder showed abnormalities in the dorso-rostral anterior cingulate and medial PFC, together with their close connections to the ventral striatum and limbic regions (Alegria et al., 2016). These brain areas lie at the interface between emotion and cognition and form part of the mesolimbic fronto-striatal dopamine pathway modulating reward processing, reward-based decision-making, and motivation control (Alegria et al., 2016). Neuroimaging studies of aggressive and violent behaviour in children and adolescents showed reduced cognitive control from the anterior cingulate cortex, along with reduced reinforcement learning from the ventromedial PFC and reduced emotion regulation by the orbitofrontal cortex that influence the amygdala's activities, leading to impaired emotional recognition (Sterzer and Stadler, 2009). A similar effect is also shown on reduced performance monitoring by the temporo-parietal cortex.

Siever's (2008) schema suggest that potentially provocative stimuli come to our brain through sensory organs like the eyes and ears and are initially processed in the sensory areas such as the visual cortex and auditory cortex. Then they are interpreted in the primary association areas and then the secondary association areas in the brain in the frontal, parietal, and temporal cortices. Ultimately the emotional interpretation of these stimuli takes place in the limbic system. However, before an action is taken through the afferent connections of the limbic area such as the hypothalamus, the PFC will make a logical assessment of the emotional interpretation in order to judge potential threat associated with the potentially provocative stimuli, and depending on past experience stored in the system, the PFC will either allow or inhibit an act of aggression, and things could go wrong at any stage in this pathway.

For example, sensory distortions due to drug and alcohol use or metabolic disturbances, as well as sensory deficits involving hearing and vision, may affect sensory processing of provocative stimuli. Similarly, cultural/social factors influencing perception of aggression, cognitive distortions such as paranoid ideation, and even developmental stress/trauma leading to a negative schema may all affect early information processing and cognitive appraisal of the incoming provocative stimuli, thus leading to misinterpretation of the level of threat and reacting aggressively. In support of this model, resting-state fMRI studies showed that adolescent males with CD exhibited failure of inhibition and restraint due to functional and structural abnormalities in brain regions associated with social cognition and introspective processes (Lu et al., 2015).

Neurochemistry

Given the preponderance of aggression in males, one would expect that testosterone may play a major role in causing aggression. There is some support for this in the literature, but the evidence is not as clear-cut in humans as it is in animal studies (Filley et al., 2001). The three neurotransmitters that have been studied the most in the context of aggression are serotonin, dopamine, and noradrenaline.

Most studies showed an association between low serotonin and aggression. However, some studies failed to do so (Yanowitch and Coccaro, 2011). It has been suggested that a reduction in serotonin activity in emotion-modulating brain areas, such as the PFC and anterior cingulate cortex, leads to a predisposition for impulsive aggressiveness (Seo et al., 2008). It has also been proposed that different 5HT receptors may play a different role in this context. For example, it has been suggested that 5HT2A antagonism, as opposed to 5-HT2C agonism, may be effective in ameliorating aggressive behaviour (Siever, 2008).

However, noradrenaline seems to work in the opposite way than 5HT, in that it is an increase in noradrenaline level in the PFC that is associated with aggression. Noradrenaline acts as a stress hormone and influences the 'fight-or-flight' response. Indirect evidence in support of a role for noradrenaline comes from some genetic and animal studies. For example, people with an underactive *MAO-A* gene have been found to show an increased level of aggression, associated with a reduced volume of the amygdala and anterior cingulate gyrus. An allele of *MAO-A* has also been associated with BPD (Ni et al., 2007).

Both animal and human studies showed evidence that perhaps an increased level of dopaminergic transmission is associated with an increased level of aggression. Greater striatal dopamine transporter density (perhaps indicating increased dopaminergic transmission) was shown to be associated with impulsive violent offenders than with controls (Kuikka et al., 1998). It has been proposed that D2 receptors may be involved in the organization of aggression perhaps by being involved in the general permissive role of arousal than aggression per se. It is suggested that failure of proper interaction between dopamine and serotonin in the PFC may underlie impulsive aggression (Seo et al., 2008, cited in Yanowitch and Coccaro, 2011). Other neuromodulators that have been studied in the context of aggression are GABA, opioid, oxytocin, vasopressin, and acetylcholine (Boy et al., 2011; Deb and Deb, 2016; Kirsch et al., 2005; Steinberg et al., 1997; Wersinger et al., 2007).

Mapping neurochemical abnormalities associated with aggression onto the neuroanatomical impairments is not always straightforward. However, it has been suggested that reduced serotonin and enhanced dopamine and noradrenaline activities in cortical areas, and reduced GABA activity, as opposed to enhanced glutamate activity, as well as increased acetylcholine activity in limbic areas, modulate aggression in humans. Therefore, one would hope that SSRIs (by increasing serotonin), new-generation antipsychotics (by reducing dopamine), and β-blockers (by reducing noradrenaline in the cerebral cortex) will increase cortical inhibition on the limbic system and reduce aggression. Similarly, mood stabilizers by stabilizing the GABA–glutamate imbalance in the limbic system will reduce overactivity, leading to reduced aggression. However, RCT-based evidence does not necessarily support these simple predictions (see Chapter 39). However, the role of any particular neuromodulator in aggression is far from clear at the moment and many of these neurotransmitters may cause aggression by indirect effects, and also there are often interactions among neurotransmitters and they do not always act alone.

Assessment

Management of aggression should start with a thorough assessment of the causes and effects of aggression, taking into account all putative predisposing, precipitating, and perpetuating factors, which should lead to the formulation of an appropriate intervention. The assessment and subsequent intervention have to be person-centred. Broadly speaking, this can be divided into the assessment of symptoms of the behaviour and the associated neuropsychiatric disorder and also the impact of the behaviour on various aspects of the patient's and their family's lives (see Table 31.2). Special attention is required in neuropsychiatry for neurological/physical, cognitive, and behavioural assessment. Cognitive problems, such as memory and attention deficits, can cause frustration and lead to aggression. Similarly, neurological problems, such as paralysis or speech impediment, may lead to frustration and eventual aggressive behaviour. Psychiatric symptoms, such as depression, on the other hand, can lead to attention/memory problems. Similarly, a psychiatric disorder, such as depression, may lead to cognitive deficit, and schizophrenia may lead to executive function impairment. Therefore, it

Table 31.2 Biopsychosocial (BMPPS) model of assessment of aggression

Behaviour (B)	• Past history of aggression • Baseline behaviour prior to onset of current behaviour • Onset of behaviour(s) to describe whether they appeared gradually over time or relatively abruptly, perhaps precipitated by an acute event • Frequency, severity, and duration of behaviour(s) • Nature, content, and context of behaviour, as some behaviours may occur in certain circumstances/settings, but not in others • Associated behaviours (fatigue, lack of motivation, irritability) • Risk factors: predisposing, precipitating, perpetuating • Impact of disabilities/behaviour(s) on the person's life, other's life, and the environment
Medical and organic factors (M)	• Physical symptoms (e.g. bodily pain, headache, paralysis) • Medical conditions (cardiovascular, respiratory, endocrine, gastrointestinal, musculoskeletal, dental, skin, and genitourinary) • Physical disabilities and impairment • Problem with sleep, appetite, weight, bowel, and bladder • Level of arousal, consciousness • Epilepsy and other neurological conditions (e.g. spasticity, movement disorders, multiple sclerosis, brain tumour) • Genetic syndromes (e.g. Lesch–Nyhan, Prader–Willi, fragile X, Smith–Magenis) • Sensory impairment (including hyper-/hyposensitivity) • Communication (including social)/speech problems • Current medication, previous medication, polypharmacy and high-dose medication use, adverse effects including anticholinergic burden • Investigations (e.g. blood, urine, X-rays, EEG, neuroimaging)
Person (P)	• Premorbid personality traits such as impulsivity, adventure-seeking behaviour, aggressive tendency • Substance and alcohol use (pre- and post-development of aggression) • Current accommodation, daytime occupation, employment, finance, friends, family relationship, other family circumstances, leisure activities • Independent living issues • Driving and other self-help skills • Patient's interests, strengths/abilities, likes, dislikes, and preferences, and how they express these • Resources and opportunities available to them • Needs (mental and physical health, educational/occupational/vocational/leisure/social) and service and resource gaps • Daily/weekly routine/diary • Quality of life
Psychological/psychiatric factors (P)	• Psychiatric disorders, e.g. psychoses, bipolar disorder, dementia, depressive disorders, anxiety disorders • Psychological symptoms, e.g. depression, anxiety, obsession, illusion, hallucination, delusion, mood fluctuation, agitation, suicidal ideas • Personality traits • Past history of medical and psychiatric disorders (patient and family) • Dysregulated arousal and affect • Cognition, including attention, different types of memory, executive and visuospatial function
Social/environmental factors (S)	• Crowded/noisy/uncomfortable environment • Demanding activities, lack of interesting activities, too many changes in the activities, etc. • Personalities of other people/staff with whom the patient comes in contact • Need for further support, occupational and vocational rehabilitation, etc. • Change in environment and circumstances • Major life events, including abuse • Carer burden and quality of life • Adequate support for patients and also their carers

may be helpful to keep in mind the schema presented in the form of overlapping circles in Fig. 31.2 when developing a formulation.

The initial assessment can be divided into history taking, examination of both physical and mental health, and investigation. While taking the history from the patient, one should be mindful that impaired consciousness, memory problems, including confabulation, dissociative state, lack of insight to the problem, malingering in the case of compensation, and denial in the form of minimization versus maximization could all distort the information. On the other hand, the patient's inner state and feelings may not be properly appreciated and described by carers, but carers may notice behaviours such as subtle memory problems or even aggressive behaviour, which patients may deny or may not be aware of. Therefore, it is of

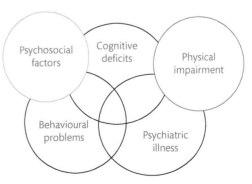

Fig. 31.2 Neuropsychiatric symptoms overlap.

paramount importance, where possible, to gather information from as many sources as possible.

Further information is provided in the following chapters: assessment of neuropsychiatric disorders (see Chapter 2), neurological examination (see Chapter 3), and neuropsychological assessment (see Chapter 11). In neuropsychiatric patients, assessment of executive function is of paramount importance. Commonly used cognitive screening instruments, such as the MMSE (Folstein et al., 1975) and the ACE-R (Mioshi et al., 2006), do not cover assessment of executive functions adequately.

Based on the biopsychosocial model, the assessment could be divided broadly under four headings, namely *Behaviour* itself, *Medical/organic* issues, *Person* showing the behaviour, *Psychiatric/psychological* issues, and *Social/occupational/personal* issues (the BMPPS model) (Deb et al., 2016) (see Table 31.2). A risk assessment is also part of the overall formulation. It is of paramount importance to assess carer burden and the patient's and carer's quality of life (QoL). It is important to use objective measures of outcome as much as possible for generic neuropsychiatric assessment (see Box 31.1) and also specifically for aggression (see Box 31.2) (Parrott et al., 2007).

Assessment of risk, including (1) risk to others, (2) risk to the individual, (3) risk to the environment, and (4) other risks, forms an important part of the formulation. Clinicians should use the right methods of risk assessment, take note of the previous risk assessment, and review risks on a regular basis, and (5) keep records of risk reduction reviews. If necessary, standardized tools, such as the Historical Clinical Risk Management-20 (HCR-20) (Douglas et al., 2013), may be used to measure risk.

Apathy is common after TBI and in many other neuropsychiatric disorders such as dementia and stroke (Marin, 1996; Njomboro and

---

Box 31.2 Scales for assessment of aggression

Self-rated scales

(a) Buss–Durkee Hostility Inventory (BDHI) (Buss and Durkee, 1957) is a 75-item true–false response scale comprising eight subscales: assault, indirect hostility, verbal hostility, irritability, negativism, resentment, suspicion, and guilt.

(b) The Aggression Questionnaire (AQ) is an adaptation of BDHI and has 29 items divided into four subscales: physical aggression, verbal aggression, anger, and hostility (Buss and Perry, 1992).

(c) The Aggression Inventory (AI) (Gladue, 1991) is a 28-item Likert-type scale that includes subtypes of verbal and physical aggression.

(d) Aggressive Acts Questionnaire (AAQ) (Barratt et al., 1999) is a 22-item Likert-type scale that assesses the qualities of the respondent's four most aggressive acts during the past 6 months.

Observational scales

(a) Modified Overt Aggression Scale (MOAS) has four subscales: verbal aggression and physical aggression to others, self, and objects (Ratey and Gutheil, 1991).

(b) Social Dysfunction and Aggression scale (SDAS) (Wistedt et al., 1990).

(c) Staff Observation Aggression Scale (SAOS) (Palmstierna and Wistedt, 1987).

Clinical interviews

(a) Direct and Indirect Aggression Scale (DIAS) (Bjorkqvist et al., 1992).

(b) Life History of Aggression assessment (LHA) (Coccaro et al., 1997).

Deb, 2014). For this reason, patients may appear lazy to their carers, and more and more demands may be placed on them in order to rectify these behaviours. However, the carers may not realize that these behaviours are part of the dysexecutive syndrome caused by the brain insult, and the patients may not therefore have any control over these behaviours. Understanding of this brain–behaviour relationship on the part of the carers and professionals may help immensely in the management of such problem behaviour, the absence of which may lead to conflict with carers and eventually aggressive behaviour. This raises the issue of providing appropriate information/training to family members, as well as paid care staff.

Acute management

Non-pharmacological intervention

Prevention, anticipation, and acting non-confrontationally are key non-pharmacological management strategies at the acute stage of aggression. It is important to recognize early the warning signs when aggression is imminent such as tense facial expressions, prolonged eye contact, restlessness, poor concentration, and withdrawal. Verbal de-escalation measures are the first step of management. Every effort should be made to manage the patient in an open setting or in a designated room or area, which should allow optimum personal space without bright light, noise, and clutter. The room should have routes of safe entry and exit in case of emergency, and arrangements for facilitating observation (National Institute for

---

Box 31.1 Neurobehavioural measures

- P-HIPS/ P-HINAS (Deb et al., 2007a)
- C-HIPS/C-HINAS (Deb et al., 2007b)
- NPI (Cummings et al., 1994)
- NFI (Kreutzer et al., 1996)
- NBRS-R (Levin et al., 1987)
- HoNOS-ABI (Fleminger et al., 2005)
- Apathy scales
  - AES (Marin et al., 1991)
  - LARS (Sockeel et al., 2006)
  - IA (Robert et al., 2002)
  - Apathy Scale (Starkstein et al., 1992)
  +
- Depression scales
  - BDI-II (Beck et al., 1996)
  - HADS (Zigmond and Snaith, 1983)
  +
- ADL + QoL measures (FIM/FAM) (Hall et al., 1993)

P-HIPS, Patient Head Injury Participation Scale; P-HINAS, Patient Head Injury Neurobehavioural Assessment Scale; C-HIPS, Carer-Head Injury Participation Scale; C-HINAS, Carer-Head Injury Neurobehavioural Assessment Scale; NPI, Neuropsychiatry Inventory; NFI, Neurobehavioural Functional Inventory; NBRS-R, Neurobehavioural Rating Scale-Revised; HoNOS-ABI, Health of the Nation Outcome Scale for Acquired Brain Injury; AES, Apathy Evaluation Scale; LARS, Lille Apathy Rating Scale; IA, Apathy Inventory; BDI-II, Beck Depression Inventory, 2nd version; HADS, Hospital Anxiety and Depression Scale; ADL, activities of daily living; FIM/FAM, Functional Independence Measure/Functional Assessment Measure; QoL, quality of life.

Health and Care Excellence, 2015). Where possible, patients should also have easy access to fresh air, daylight, and privacy.

Pharmacological intervention

If prevention and non-pharmacological de-escalation are ineffective, then medication to treat aggression can be used. This should follow the local rapid tranquillization protocol, and oral medication should be tried first before attempting intramuscular (IM) or intravenous (IV) medication (National Institute for Health and Care Excellence, 2015). Both antipsychotics (e.g. olanzapine, risperidone, haloperidol, aripiprazole) and benzodiazepines (e.g. lorazepam 1–2 mg, midazolam IM or unlicensed buccal preparations, clonazepam), either alone or in combination, have been used both as IM or oral preparations (National Institute for Health and Care Excellence, 2015). In cases of benzodiazepine intolerance, IM haloperidol (5 mg) can be combined with IM promethazine (50 mg). There is no definitive evidence to suggest that the combination is more effective than using each medication alone (National Institute for Health and Care Excellence, 2015, 2017). However, if combined, a smaller dose could be used for each medication, thus minimizing the potential for acute extrapyramidal and cardiac adverse effects from antipsychotics and respiratory depression from benzodiazepines. Conversely, if the patient is on regular antipsychotics (or the situation is unclear), lorazepam alone should be used (National Institute for Health and Care Excellence, 2017). Careful consideration is needed if the patient is under the influence of alcohol or any other substance that may interfere with the treatment. If IM/IV routes are used, then it is mandatory to monitor adverse effects, vital signs, hydration level, and consciousness and to intervene rapidly if necessary, e.g. with flumazenil in case of acute respiratory depression (Lonergan et al., 2007; Taylor et al., 2015). In acute confusional states/delirium, the use of benzodiazepines is not recommended, apart from in cases of aggression-associated alcohol withdrawal (Lonergan et al., 2007; National Institute for Health and Care Excellence, 2010). Preliminary evidence supports short-term use of low-dose antipsychotics (e.g. haloperidol, risperidone, olanzapine, or quetiapine) in delirium (Kishi et al., 2016). However, the use of antipsychotics as a preventative measure is not recommended (Kishi, 2016).

Chronic management

Non-pharmacological treatment

Examples of non-pharmacological treatments are psychological therapies, rehabilitation, speech therapy, vocational training, occupational therapy, cognitive retraining, alternative therapy, and social/financial support for patients and their families. Common psychological approaches include cognitive behaviour therapy (CBT), dialectic behaviour therapy (DBT), psychoanalytic psychotherapy (particularly for treatment of PD), modified reasoning and rehabilitation (R&R), anger management, and mindfulness-based relaxation/meditation. Behavioural/environmental management includes functional analysis of behaviour, positive behaviour support, solution-focused therapy, and nidotherapy. Other interventions include music therapy and multi-sensory (snoezelen) therapy (see review by Rampling et al., 2016). Further information on

non-pharmacological management of neuropsychiatric disorders is presented in Chapter 40.

Pharmacological treatment

Different pharmacological options are available for chronic aggression (see the following sections). Here we have outlined the relevant evidence for the efficacy of these medications. Pharmacological intervention must not be used or even be perceived as a 'straitjacket' but should facilitate non-pharmacological approaches to management.

Antipsychotics

There is now reasonable-quality RCT-based evidence available on the efficacy of low-dose risperidone (0.25–4 mg/day) in the management of aggression and agitation in children with ASD and/or ID (Deb, 2016; Unwin and Deb, 2011). However, all these studies were from the United States and mostly supported by pharmaceutical companies. Evidence for the efficacy of risperidone among adults with ID is equivocal; two studies showed risperidone's superiority over placebo (one is a crossover trial), and in another study, no difference between risperidone, haloperidol, and placebo was observed (Deb, 2016; Tyrer et al., 2008). All three studies recruited a small number of participants and therefore lack adequate statistical power. So far, two large-scale RCTs have shown the efficacy of risperidone in treating aggression in patients with schizophrenia (Marder et al., 1997; Peuskens on behalf of the Risperidone Study Group, 1995). Two RCTs have shown the efficacy of aripiprazole in reducing irritability and other problem behaviours in children and adolescents with ASD (Deb et al., 2014). However, both these studies were conducted by the pharmaceutical company that manufactures aripiprazole (Marcus et al., 2009; Owen et al., 2009), and it is not clear whether there was an overlap among the participants recruited in these two studies. The same pharmaceutical company has also published pooled data from five short-term placebo-controlled RCTs on a combined population of 1476 patients with a diagnosis of schizophrenia or schizoaffective disorders that showed aripiprazole's superiority over placebo, but not significantly different from the effect of haloperidol on the hostility subscale score of the Positive and Negative Syndrome Scale (PANSS) (Kay et al., 1987; Volavka et al., 2005). A large number of RCTs established the efficacy of both old- and new-generation antipsychotics in reducing 'behavioural and psychological symptoms of dementia' (BPSD), but the main concern for their use remains in relation to increased rates of cerebrovascular disease and mortality, when compared with placebo (Ballard et al., 2006; Sadavoy et al., 2008). For example, Ballard and colleagues' Cochrane review (Ballard et al., 2006) on the effect of new-generation antipsychotics showed that both risperidone and olanzapine significantly improved aggression, when compared with placebo, in patients with dementia, but both produced significantly higher rates of severe adverse effects, including cerebrovascular (including stroke) and extrapyramidal side effects, along with other severe adverse effects, and a significantly higher dropout rate. Antipsychotics may improve aggression in BPD (Stoffers et al., 2010), but the evidence is not convincing yet. A number of small- and large-scale double-blind, placebo-controlled trials of olanzapine on BPD are available, but the results so far have been equivocal as far as agitation and aggressive symptoms are concerned (Bellino et al., 2013). A few small RCTs on animals and humans showed the efficacy of clozapine in treating aggression in patients with schizophrenia (Frogley et al., 2012). Clozapine was superior to risperidone, haloperidol, and possibly olanzapine in treating aggression in patients with schizophrenia in a head-to-head RCT (Citrome et al., 2001). The anti-aggressive effect seems to be independent of clozapine's antipsychotic and sedative effects (Goedhard et al., 2006). Although this looks promising, at present, not enough robust evidence based on large-scale RCTs exists to draw any definite conclusion about the effectiveness of clozapine for treating aggression.

Mood stabilizers

In a population-based Swedish study of 40,937 men and 41,710 women between 2006 and 2009 who were prescribed antipsychotics and mood stabilizers, Fazel and colleagues (2014) reported that, compared with periods when participants were not on medication, violent crimes fell by 45% among those who received antipsychotics and in 24% of patients who were prescribed mood stabilizers. The effect of mood stabilizers in reducing violent crimes happened in the presence of bipolar disorder, which perhaps indicates that mood stabilizers had an effect on bipolar disorder, rather than on aggression per se. Based on a small number of RCTs, weak evidence exists for the efficacy of antiepileptics in treating aggression in patients with PD, CD, and ASD and in psychiatric outpatients, but not all studies showed superiority of antiepileptic medication, and apart from one study, the rest had included a small number of participants, which did not provide adequate statistical power (Huband et al., 2010; Jones et al., 2011). A small number of older RCTs that included a small number of participants showed the efficacy of phenytoin on aggression, which was well tolerated at 300 mg per day in divided dose, but many of these patients were incarcerated (Lane et al., 2011). A handful of RCTs have shown the efficacy of carbamazepine and valproate in alleviating BPSD, but particularly for valproate, it seems that low doses are ineffective and high doses tend to cause adverse effects, including thrombocytopenia (Sadavoy et al., 2008). Three Cochrane reviews in the UK have shown that valproate is not only ineffective in patients with dementia in treating agitation, but it also has potential for severe adverse effects (Dhindsa, 2019). As a result, in the UK, the National Institute for Health and Care Excellence does not recommend the use of valproate for patients with dementia (National Institute for Health and Care Excellence, 2018). Although a small number of RCTs involving a small number of participants showed weak evidence in support of valproate and carbamazepine, one large-scale RCT of divalproex sodium showed a non-significant result in treating aggression in patients with schizophrenia (Goedhard et al., 2006). Some recent studies have suggested that lithium may have potential neuroprotective properties (Wada et al., 2005). Lithium showed efficacy in some, but not all, old small-scale studies in institutionalized patients (children, prison population, and adults with ID) that did not always use standardized outcome measures (Deb, 2016). Once started, it is difficult to stop lithium treatment, and given its narrow therapeutic window, there is a danger of toxicity. No major large-scale RCT-based evidence exists in support of mood stabilizers, including lithium, for the treatment of aggression, in particular, and problem behaviour in general, in people with ID (Deb et al., 2008).

Antidepressants

Antidepressants are primarily effective in treating depression in dementia, with some possible effects on BPSD, but they have not been shown to be effective in people with ID or ASD, and their adverse effects remain a concern (Deb, 2016; Sadavoy et al., 2008; Sohanpal et al., 2007). However, small-scale RCTs showed the efficacy of fluoxetine, fluvoxamine, and citalopram in treating aggression in patients with PD, which does not allow any definitive conclusion to be drawn (Stoffers et al., 2010). Although SSRIs may have a direct effect on improving stroke symptoms (Mead et al., 2012), there is no evidence to suggest their efficacy in treating aggression in the context of cerebrovascular incidents. The effects of antidepressants on aggression seems to be most prominent when there are anxiety and depressive symptoms present in the background (Deb, 2016). This perhaps indicates that SSRIs work indirectly by treating underlying depression and anxiety, rather than aggression per se. However, there is some debate about whether or not SSRIs increase the risk of aggression and suicide in some patients (Courtet and Lopez-Caströman, 2017; Molero et al., 2015).

Beta-blockers

There is currently no good-quality RCT-based evidence to support the use of β-blockers in ID and/or ASD (Ward et al., 2013), TBI (Deb and Crownshaw, 2004), or BPSD, although a small number of RCTs that included a small number of participants have shown some efficacy in TBI (Fleminger et al., 2006) and BPSD (Sadavoy et al., 2008). There is also weak evidence based on a few small studies showing the efficacy of β-blockers in treating aggression in patients with schizophrenia. However, the dose of β-blockers used in most RCTs is very high, which raises concern about their adverse effects like syncope and bronchospasm (Goedhard et al., 2006).

Psychostimulants

Psychostimulants, such as methylphenidate, work through dopaminergic systems and are known to be effective in treating ADHD symptoms, but a recent meta-analysis has also shown their efficacy on overt and covert aggression when associated with ADHD (Connor et al., 2002). A small number of primarily crossover RCTs showed the efficacy of psychostimulants in enhancing cognition by improving attention and concentration, and also some effect on apathy, but no specific effect on aggression in acquired brain injury patients (Deb and Crownshaw, 2004; Johansson et al., 2015).

Dopaminergic drugs

There are a number of case studies on old-generation dopamine agonist drugs, such as bromocriptine, and a few recent small-scale RCTs on amantadine and rotigotine, showing an equivocal effect on aggression and agitation in acquired brain injury patients (Hammond et al., 2015; Sami et al., 2015). However, now there is concern about serious adverse effects of dopaminergic drugs such as pathological gambling, hypersexuality, and binge eating, all pointing towards an impulse control disorder (Moore et al., 2014).

Other medications

Small-scale primarily crossover trials in children and adults with ID provide weak evidence in support of naltrexone in the treatment of SIB (Roy et al., 2015a, b). Despite a lack of RCT-based evidence, anti-androgen drugs have been used, especially in prison populations and for sexual aggression, particularly in ID populations (Khan et al., 2015). Cholinesterase inhibitors are effective in treating aggression in patients with AD, but there is no definitive evidence for their efficacy in other patient groups (Gauthier et al., 2010; Masanic et al., 2001). Omega-3 has been shown to be effective in patients with BPD, but not specifically on aggression (Stoffers et al., 2010). Similarly, both vasopressin and oxytocin have been used for BPD in the absence of any robust evidence. Other medications may have indirect effects on aggression through effects on, for example, sleep disorders treated with melatonin and pain treated with gabapentin, tiagabine, etc. Benzodiazepines are not recommended for long-term use, and buspirone has shown mixed results from small case studies.

Conclusion

Aggression is prevalent in many psychiatric and neurological disorders and is a common reason for referral to neuropsychiatry clinics. Aggressive behaviour remains a major challenge to manage and causes immense distress to patients and people around them. It can create a major financial burden, may lead to unnecessary hospitalization and use of medication, and leads to exclusion from many social opportunities and loss of support and friends. Aggression is a complex phenomenon and multiple factors influence aggressive behaviour. Both neurobiological and environmental factors play a large role in predisposing to, precipitating, and maintaining aggression, and must be taken into account during an assessment. In addition, comorbidities of physical disorders, psychiatric disorders and symptoms, and drug and alcohol problems can contribute. A biopsychosocial approach to assessment and formulation is essential for successful management. As aggression is multifactorial, its management has to be multifaceted, with multi-professional input in an integrated fashion, with the ultimate goal to improve the patient's and their carers' QoL.

Two primary types of aggression have been described in clinical practice. Reactive aggression results from a disproportional response to a stressful stimulus (part of the 'fight or flight' reaction), whereas instrumental or proactive aggression is often a premeditated, cold-blooded, and goal-directed action. In the DSM-5 classification, IED (and also DMDD) is the closest to a reactive aggression diagnosis, and CD and, to a lesser extent, ODD (and some PDs) to instrumental aggression. It has been proposed that reduction in top–down control from the PFC, particularly fronto-medial PFC, or overactivity in the limbic system is likely to lead to aggression. It has been suggested that reduced serotonin and enhanced dopamine and noradrenaline activities in cortical areas and reduced GABA activity, as opposed to enhanced glutamate activity, as well as increased acetylcholine activity in the limbic areas, modulate aggression in humans.

Although both pharmacological and non-pharmacological managements are available, overall evidence in their support is poor and not always unequivocal. The most commonly used pharmacological interventions for chronic aggression are new-generation antipsychotics for which there is now some RCT-based evidence, particularly among patients with dementia (but there is major concern about serious adverse effects and increased mortality) and ASD children with or without ID. The second most commonly used groups are antiepileptic drugs and SSRIs for which there is no convincing evidence yet, requiring further large-scale well-designed RCTs. In the absence of a robust evidence base to support pharmacological intervention for aggression, guidelines have been developed for good clinical practice (Deb et al., 2009).

In the absence of empirical evidence to support day-to-day clinical practice, clinicians use their own judgement for the choice of drugs to treat aggression and this depends on the exact clinical scenario. On a clinical basis, clinicians tend to use antiepileptic drugs for impulsive outbursts, β-blockers in the presence of restlessness/agitation, and pregabalin or short-term use of benzodiazepine when anxiety is a prominent background feature. However, if there is comorbid depression or anxiety, some clinicians tend to use SSRIs, and where there is severe comorbid agitation, midazolam or lorazepam or low-dose antipsychotics are used. Some neurosurgeons tend to use clonidine for early agitation. Antipsychotics are the obvious choice when there are psychotic symptoms in the background of aggression, but clinicians may choose to use pregabalin or gabapentin if they suspect that pain may be driving the aggression and similarly, associated sleep problems may be treated with melatonin. Pregabalin or some SSRIs or SNRIs may be used if there is a strong element of anxiety in the background of the aggression.

KEY LEARNING POINTS

- Aggression is common in many neuropsychiatric conditions and difficult to manage.
- Multiple factors influence aggressive behaviour.
- Both pharmacological and non-pharmacological managements are available, but overall evidence in their support, particularly for pharmacological intervention, is poor.
- A thorough multidisciplinary assessment and multi-professional input are necessary for a successful outcome.
- The ultimate goal should be to improve the patient's and carer's QoL.

REFERENCES

Alegria, A. A., Radua, J., and Rubia, K. (2016). Meta-analysis of fMRI studies of disruptive behavior disorders. *American Journal of Psychiatry*, **173**, 1119–30.

American Psychiatric Association. (2013). *Diagnostic and Statistical Manual of Mental Disorders*, fifth edition. Arlington, VA: American Psychiatric Publishing.

Antonius, D., Mathew, N., Picano, J., et al. (2014). Behavioral health symptoms associated with chronic traumatic encephalopathy: a critical review of the literature and recommendations for treatment and research. *Journal of Neuropsychiatry and Clinical Neurosciences*, **26**, 313–22.

Ballard, C. G., Waite, J., and Birks, J. (2006). Atypical antipsychotics for aggression and psychosis in Alzheimer's disease (Review). *Cochrane Database of Systematic Reviews*, **1**, CD003476.

Baron, R. A. and Richardson, D. R. (1994). *Human Aggression*, second edition. New York, NY: Plenum Press.

Barratt, E. S., Stanford, M. S., Dowdy, L., Liebman, M. J., and Kent, T. A. (1999). Impulsive and premeditated aggression: a factor analysis of self-reported acts. *Psychiatry Research*, **86**, 163–73.

Beck, A. T., Steer, R. A. Ball, R., and Rainieri, W. F. (1996). Comparison of Beck Depression Inventories-IA and II in psychiatric outpatients. *Journal of Personality Assessment*, **67**(3), 588–97.

Bellino, S., Bozzatello, P., Brignolo, E., and Bogetto, F. (2013). Antipsychotics in the treatment of impulsivity in personality disorders and impulse control disorders. *Current Psychopharmacology*, 2013, **2**, 5–17.

Bjorkqvist, K., Lagerspetz, K. J., and Osterman, K. (1992). *The Direct and Indirect Aggression Scale*. Vasa, Finland, Abo Academic University, Department of Social Sciences.

Blair, R. J. R. (2001). Neurocogntive models of aggression, the antisocial personality disorders, and psychopathy. *Journal of Neurology Neurosurgery and Psychiatry*, **71**, 727–31.

Boy, F., Evans, C. J., Edden, R. A. E., et al. (2011). Dorsolateral prefrontal γ-aminobutyric acid in men predicts individual differences in rash impulsivity. *Biological Psychiatry*, **70**, 866–72.

Brekke, J. S., Prindle, C., Bae, S. W., and Long, J. D. (2001). Risks for individuals with schizophrenia who are living in the community. *Psychiatric Services*, **52**, 1358–66.

Brodie, M. J., Besag, F., Ettinger, A. B., et al. (2016). Epilepsy, antiepileptic drugs, and aggression: an evidence-based review. *Pharmacological Review*, **68**(3), 563–602.

Buss, A. H. and Perry, M. (1992). The aggression questionnaire. *Journal of Personality and Social Psychology*, **63**, 452–9.

Buss, A. H. and Durkee, A. (1957). An inventory for assessing different kinds of hostility. *Journal of Consulting Psychology*, **21**, 343–9.

Citrome, L., Volavka, J., Czobor P., et al. (2001). Effects of clozapine, olanzapine, risperidone, and haloperidol on hostility among patients with schizophrenia. *Psychiatric Services*, **52**, 1510–14.

Coccaro, E. F., Berman, M. W., and Kavoussi, R. J. (1997). Assessment of life history of aggression: development and psychometric characteristics. *Psychiatry Research*, **73**, 147–57.

Coccaro, E. F., Posternak, M. A., and Zimmerman, M. (2005). Prevalence and features of intermittent explosive disorder in a clinical setting. *Journal of Clinical Psychiatry*, **66**, 1221–7.

Connor, D. F., Glatt, S. J., Lopez, I. D., Jackson, D., and Melloni, R. H. (2002). Psychopharmacology and aggression. I: A meta-analysis of stimulant effects on overt/ covert aggression-related behaviors in ADHD. *Journal of American Academy of Child and Adolescent Psychiatry*, **41**(3), 253–61.

Corrigan, P. W. and Watson, A. C. (2005). Findings from the national co-morbidity survey on the frequency of violent behaviour in individuals with psychiatric disorders. *Psychiatry Research*, **136**, 153–62.

Courtet, P. and Lopez-Caströman, J. (2017). Antidepressants and suicide risk in depression. *World Psychiatry*, **16**(3), 317–18.

Cummings, J. L., Mega, M., Gray, K., Rosenberg-Thompson, S., Carusis, D. A., and Gornbein, J. (1994). The neuropsychiatry inventory: comprehensive assessment of psychopathology in dementia. *Neurology*, **44**(12), 2308–414.

Deb, S. (1998). Self-injurious behaviour as part of genetic syndromes. *British Journal of Psychiatry*, **172**, 385–9.

Deb, S. (2007). Mental health and epilepsy among adults with intellectual disabilities. In: Bouras, N. and Holt, G. (eds) *Psychiatric and Behavioural Disorders in Intellectual and Developmental Disabilities*. Cambridge University Press, Cambridge, pp. 238–51.

Deb, S. (2016). Psychopharmacology. In: N. N. Singh (ed) *Handbook of Evidence-Based Practices in Intellectual and Developmental Disabilities, Evidence-Based Practices in Behavioral Health. Springer*, Cham. pp. 347–81.

Deb, S., Bethea, T., Havercamp, S., Rifkin, A., and Underwood, L. (2016). Disruptive, impulse-control, and conduct disorders. In: R. Fletcher, J. Barnhill, and S.-A. Cooper (eds) *Diagnostic Manual–Intellectual Disability: A textbook of diagnosis of mental disorders in persons with intellectual disability*, second edition. NADD Press, Kingston, NY. pp. 521–60.

Deb, S., Bryant, E., Morris, P. G., Prior, L., Lewis, G., and Haque, S. (2007a). Development and psychometric properties of the Patient-Head Injury Participation Scale (P-HIPS) and the Patient-Head Injury Neurobehavioral Assessment Scale (P-HINAS): patient and family determined outcome scales. *Neuropsychiatric Disease and Treatment*, **3**(3), 373–88.

Deb, S., Bryant, E., Morris, P. G., Prior, L., Lewis, G., and Haque, S. (2007b). Development and psychometric properties of the Carer-Head Injury Neurobehavioral Assessment Scale (C-HINAS) and the Carer-Head Injury Participation Scale (C-HIPS): patient and family determined scales. *Neuropsychiatric Disease and Treatment*, **3**(3), 389–408.

Deb, S., Chaplin, R., Sohanpal, S., Unwin, G. Soni, R., and Lenôtre, L. (2008). The effectiveness of mood stabilisers and antiepileptic medication for the management of behaviour problems in adults with intellectual disability: a systematic review. *Journal of Intellectual Disability Research*, **52**(2), 107–13.

Deb, S. and Crownshaw, T. (2004). The role of pharmacotherapy in the management of behaviour disorders in traumatic brain injury patients. *Brain Injury*, **18**(1), 1–31.

Deb, S. and Deb, T. (2016). Neurobiology of aggression. *Neuropsychiatry News*, **12**, 22–6.

Deb, S., Farmah, B. K., Arshad, E., Deb, T., Roy, M., and Unwin, G. L. (2014). The effectiveness of aripiprazole in the management of problem behaviour in people with intellectual disabilities, developmental disabilities and/or autistic spectrum disorder: a systematic review. *Research in Developmental Disabilities*, **35**, 711–25.

Deb, S., Kwok, H., Bertelli, M., et al. (2009). International guide to prescribing psychotropic medication for the management of problem behaviours in adults with intellectual disabilities. *World Psychiatry*, **8**(3), 181–6.

Deb, S., Lyons, I., and Koutzoukis, C. (1999). Neurobehavioural symptoms one year after a head injury. *British Journal of Psychiatry*, **174**, 360–5.

Dhindsa, A. (2019). Valproate in dementia: time to move on? *British Journal of Psychiatry Advances*, **25**, 145–9.

Douglas, K. S., Hart, S. D., Webster, C. D. and Belfrage, H. (2013). *HCR-20V3: Assessing risk of violence: User guide*. Burnaby, Canada: Mental Health, Law, and Policy Institute, Simon Fraser University.

Fazel, S., Gulati, G., Linsell, L., Geddes, J. R., and Grann, M. (2009). Schizophrenia and violence: systematic review and meta-analysis. *PLoS Medicine*, **6**(8), e1000120.

Fazel, S., Zetterqvist, J., Larsson, H., Långström, N., and Lichtenstein, P. (2014). Antipsychotics, mood stabilisers, and risk of violent crime. *The Lancet*, **384**, 1206–14.

Filley, C. M., Price, B. H., Nell, V., et al. (2001). Toward an understanding of violence: neurobehavioral aspects of unwarranted physical aggression: Aspen Neurobehavioral Conference Consensus Statement. *Neuropsychiatry, Neurology, and Behavioral Neurology*, **14**(1), 1–14.

Fisher, C. A., Sewell, K., Brown, A., and Churchyard, A. (2014). Aggression in Huntignton's Disease: a systematic review of rates of aggression and treatment methods. *Journal of Huntington's Disease*, **3**, 319–32.

Fleminger, S., Greenwood, R. R. J., and Oliver, D. L. (2006). Pharmacological management for agitation and aggression in people with acquired brain injury (Review). Issue 4. *The Cochrane Library and the Cochrane Collaboration*.

Fleminger, S., Leigh, E., Eames, P., Langrell, L., Nagraj, R., and Logsdail, S. (2005). HoNOS-ABI: a reliable outcome measure of neuropsychiatric sequelae to brain injury. *Psychiatric Bulletin*, **29**(2), 53–5.

Folstein, M. F., Folstein, S. E., and McHugh, P. R. (1975). 'Mini-Mental State'. A practical method for grading cognitive state of patients for the clinician. *Journal of Psychological Research*, **12**, 189–98.

Frogley, C., Taylor, D., Dickens, G., and Piccioni, M. (2012). A systematic review of the evidence of clozapine's anti-aggressive effects. *International Journal of Neuropsychopharmacology*, **15**, 1351–71.

Gauthier, S., Cummings, J., Ballard, C., et al. (2010). Management of behavioral problems in Alzheimer's disease. *International Psychogeriatrics*, **22**(3), 346–72.

Gladue, B. A. (1991). Aggressive behavioral characteristics, hormones, and sexual orientation in men and women. *Aggressive Baehavior*, **17**, 313–26.

Goedhard, L. E., Stolker, J. J., Heerdink, E. R., Nijman, H. L. I., Oliver, B., and Egberts, T. C. G. (2006). Pharmacotherapy for the treatment of aggressive behavior in general adult psychiatry: a systematic review. *Journal of Clinical Psychiatry*, **67**, 1013–24.

Hall, K. M., Hamilton, B. B., Gordon, W. A., and Zasler, N. D. (1993). Characteristics of functional assessment indices: Disability Rating Scale, Functional Independent Measure, and Functional assessment Measure. *Journal of Head Trauma Rehabilitation*, **8**, 60–74.

Hammond, F. M., Sherer, M., Malec, J. F., et al. (2015). Amantadine effect on perceptions of irritability after traumatic brain injury: Results of the amantadine irritability multisite study. *Journal of Neurotrauma*, **32**, 1230–8.

Harlow, J. M. (1868). Recovery from the passage of an iron bar through the head. *Publications of the Massachusetts Medical Society*, **2**, 237–346.

Hemmings, C., Deb, S., Chaplin, E., Hardy, S., and Mukherjee, R. (2013). Research for people with intellectual disabilities and mental health problems: a view from the UK. *Journal of Mental Health Research in Intellectual Disabilities*, **6**(2), 127–58.

Huband, N., Ferrier, M., Nathan, R., and Jones, H. (2010). Antiepileptics for aggression and associated impulsivity (Review). *The Cochrane Collaboration*, John Willey and Sons Ltd., Oxford.

Johansson, B., Wentzel, A-P., Andréll, P., Mannheimer, C., and Rönnbäck, L. (2015). Methylphenidate reduces mental fatigue and improves processing speed in persons suffered a traumatic brain injury. *Brain Injury*, **29**(6), 758–65.

Johnson, J. G., Cohen, P., Smailes, E., et al. (2000). Adolescent Personality Disorders associated with violence and criminal behaviour during adolescence and early adulthood. *American Journal of Psychiatry*, **157**, 1406–12.

Jones, R. M., Arlidge, J., Gillham, R., Reagu, S., van den Bree, M., and Taylor, P. J. (2011). Efficacy of mood stabilisers in the treatment of impulsive or repetitive aggression: systematic review and meta-analysis. *British Journal of Psychiatry*, **198**, 93–8.

Joyal, C. C., Gendron, C., and Cote, G. (2008). Nature and frequency of aggressive behaviours among long-term inpatients with schizophrenia: a 6-month report using the modified overt aggression scale. *Canadian Journal of Psychiatry*, **53**, 478–81.

Kanemoto, K., Tadokoro, Y., and Oshima, T. (2010). Violence and postictal psychosis: a comparison of postictal psychosis, interictal psychosis, and postictal confusion. *Epilepsy and Behavior*, **19**(2), 62–6.

Kay, S. R., Fiszbein, A., and Opler, L. A. (1987). The Positive and Negative Syndrome Scale for schizophrenia. *Schizophrenia Bulletin*, **13**, 261–76.

Khan, O., Ferriter, M., Huband, N., Powney, M. J., Dennis, J. A., and Duggan, C. (2015). Pharmacological intervention for those who have sexually offended or are at risk of offending. *Cochrane Database of Systematic Reviews*, **2**, CD007989.

Kirsch, P., Esslinger, C., Chen, Q., et al. (2005). Oxytocin modulates neural circuitry for social cognition and fear in humans. *Journal of Neuroscience*, **25**, 11489–93.

Kishi, T. (2016). Routine use of antipsychotics to prevent delirium is not recommended. *Evidence Based Mental Health*, **19**(4), 123.

Kishi, T., Hirota, T., Matsunaga, S., and Iwata, N. (2016). Antipsychotic medications for the treatment of delirium: a systematic review and meta-analysis of randomised controlled trials. *Journal of Neurology Neurosurgery and Psychiatry*, **87**, 767–74.

Klüver, H. and Bucy, P. C. (1939). Preliminary analysis of the functions of the temporal lobes in monkeys. *Archives of Neurology and Psychiatry*, **42**, 979–1000.

Kreutzer, J. S., Marwitz, T., Seel, R., and Serio, C. D. (1996). Validation of a Neurobehavioral Functioning Inventory for adults with traumatic brain injury. *Archives of Physical and Medical Rehabilitation*, **77**(2), 116–24.

Krug, E. G., Mercy, J. A., Dahlberg, L. L., and Zwi, A. B. (2002). The world report on violence and health. *The Lancet*, **360**, 9339.

Kuikka, J. T., Tiihonen, J., Bergstrom, K. A., et al. (1998). Abnormal structure of human striatal dopaminergic re-uptake sites in habitually violent alcoholic offenders: a factor analysis. *Neuroscience Letters*, **253**, 195–7.

Lai, M-C., Lombardo, M. V., and Baron-Cohen, S. (2014). Autism. *The Lancet*, **383**, 896–910.

Lane, S. D., Kjome, K. L., and Moeller, F. G. (2011). Neuropsychiatry of aggression. *Neurology Clinics*, **29**, 49–64.

Levin, H. S., High, W. M., Goethe, K. E., et al. (1987). The neurobehavioral rating scale: assessment of head injury by the clinicians. *Journal of Neurology, Neurosurgery and Psychiatry*, **50**, 183–93.

Lonergan, E., Britton, A. M., and Luxenberg, J. (2007). Antipsychotics for delirium (Review). *Cochrane Database of Systematic Reviews*, **2**, CD005594.

Lu, F-M., Zhou, J-S., Zhang, J., et al. (2015). Functional connectivity estimated from resting-state fMRI reveals selective alterations in male adolescents with pure conduct disorder. *PLoS One*, **10**(12), e0145668.

Marcus, R. N., Owen, R., Kamen, L., et al. (2009). A placebo-controlled, fixed-dose study of aripiprazole in children and adolescents with irritability associated with autistic disorder. *Journal of American Academy of Child & Adolescent Psychiatry*, **48**(11), 1110–19.

Marder, S. R., Davis, J. M., and Chouinard, G. (1997). The effects of risperidone on the five dimensions of schizophrenia derived by factor analysis: combined results of the North American trials. *Journal of Clinical Psychiatry*, **58**, 538–47.

Marin, R. S. (1996). Apathy: concept, syndrome, neural mechanisms, and treatment. *Seminars in Clinical Neuropsychiatry*, **1**, 304–14.

Marin, R.S., Biedrzycki, R.C., and Firinciogullari, S. (1991). Reliability and validity of the Apathy Evaluation Scale. *Psychiatry Research*, **38**, 143–62.

Marin, S. E. and Saneto, R. P. (2016). Neuropsychiatric features in primary mitochondrial disease. *Neurology Clinics*, **34**, 247–94.

Masanic, C., Bailey, M. T., van Reekum, R., and Simard, M. (2001). Open-label study of donepezil in traumatic brain injury. *Archives of Physical Medicine and Rehabilitation*, **82**, 896–901.

Mead, G. E., Hsieh, C. F., Lee, R., et al. (2012). Selective serotonin reuptake inhibitors (SSRIs) for stroke recovery (review). *Cochrane Database of Systematic Reviews*, **11**, CD009286.

Mioshi, E., Dawson, K., Arnold, R., and Hodges, J. R. (2006). A brief cognitive test battery for dementia screening. *International Journal of Geriatric Psychiatry*, **21**, 1078–85.

Moghadasi, A. N., Pourmand, S., Sharifian, M., Minagar, A., and Sahraian, M. A. (2016). Behavioral neurology of Multiple Sclerosis and autoimmune encephalopathies. *Neurology Clinics*, **34**, 17–31.

Molero, Y., Lichtenstein, P., Zetterqvist, J., Gumpert, C. H., and Fazel, S. (2015). Selective Serotonin Uptake Inhibitors and violent crime: a cohort study. *PLoS Medicine*, **12**(9), e1001875.

Moore, T. J., Glenmullen, J., and Mattison, D. R. (2014). Reports of pathological gambling, hypersexuality, and compulsive shopping associated with dopamine receptor agonist drugs. *Journal of American Medical Association Internal Medicine*, **174**(12), 1930–3.

Mula, M. (2016). The butler did it and may be had epilepsy. *Neuropsychiatry News*, **12**, 9–12.

Munjampalli, S. K. J. and Davis, D. E. (2016). Medicinal-induced behavior disorders. *Neurology Clinics*, **34**, 133–69.

McClintock, K., Hall, S., and Oliver, C. (2003). Risk markers associated with challenging behaviours in people with intellectual disability: a meta-analytic study. *Journal of Intellectual Disability Research*, **47**(6), 405–16.

National Institute for Health and Care Excellence. (2010). *Delirium: prevention, diagnosis and management.* National Institute for Health and Care Excellence Clinical Guideline [CG103]. Available at: http://www.nice.org.uk/guidance/cg103.

National Institute for Health and Care Excellence. (2013). *Antisocial behaviour and conduct disorders in children and young people: recognition and management.* Clinical Guideline [CG158]. Available at: http://www.nice.org.uk/guidance/cg158.

National Institute for Health and Care Excellence. (2015). *Violence and aggression: short term management in mental health, health and community settings.* Available at: http://www.nice.org.uk/guidance/ng20.

National Institute for Health and Care Excellence. (2017). *Anticipating, reducing the risk of and preventing violence and aggression in adults.* Available at: http://pathways.nice.org.uk/pathways/violence-and-aggression.

National Institute for Health and Care Excellence. (2018). *Dementia: assessment, management and support for people living with dementia and their carers.* NICE guideline [NG97]. Available at: https://www.nice.org.uk/guidance/ng97.

Nestor, P. G. (2002). Mental disorder and violence: personality dimensions and clinical features. *American Journal of Psychiatry*, **159**(12), 1973–8.

Ni, X., Sicard, T., Bulgin, N., et al. (2007). Monoamine oxidase A gene is associated with borderline personality disorder. *Psychiatric Genetics*, **17**(3),153–7.

Njomboro, P. and Deb, S. (2014). Distinct neuropsychological correlates of cognitive, behavioural, and affective apathy sub-domains in acquired brain injury. *Frontiers in Neurology*, **5**, 1–6.

Owen, R., Sikich, L., Marcus, R. N., et al. (2009). Aripiprazole in the treatment of irritability in children and adolescents with autistic disorder. *Pediatrics*, **124**(6), 1533–40.

Palmstierna, T. and Wistedt, B. (1987). Staff observation scale, SOAS: Presentation and evaluation. *Acta Psychiatrica Scandinavica*, **76**, 657–63.

Parrott, D. J. and Giancola, P. R. (2007). Addressing 'The criterion problem' in the assessment of aggressive behaviour: Development of a new taxonomic system. *Aggression and Violent Behavior*, **12**, 280–99.

Peuskens, J.; on behalf of the Risperidone Study Group. (1995). Risperidone in the treatment of chronic schizophrenia, a multi-national, multi-centre, double-blind, parallel-group study versus haloperidol. Risperidone Study Group. *British Journal of Psychiatry*, **166**, 712–26.

Ramamurthi, B. (1988). Stereotactic operation in behaviour disorders. Amygdalotomy and hypothalamotomy. *Acta Neurochirurgica* Supplement (Wein), **44**, 152–7.

Rampling, J., Furtado, V., Winsper, C., et al. (2016). Non-pharmacological interventions for reducing aggression and violence in serious mental illness: a systematic review and narrative synthesis. *European Psychiatry*, **34**, 17–28.

Ratey, J. J. and Gutheil, C. M. (1991). The measurement of aggressive behaviour: reflections on the use of the Overt Aggression Scale and the Modified Overt Aggression Scale. *Journal of Neuropsychiatry*, **3**, 557–60.

Robert, P. H., Clairet, S., Benoit, M., et al. (2002). The Apathy Inventory: assessment of apathy and awareness in Alzheimer's disease, Parkinson's disease and mild cognitive impairment. *International Journal of Geriatric Psychiatry*, **17**, 1099–105.

Rogers, J. C. and De Brito, S. A. (2016). Cortical and subcortical gray matter volume in youths with conduct problems: a meta-analysis. *Journal of American Medical Association Psychiatry*, **73**(1), 64–72.

Roy, A., Roy, M., Deb, S., Unwin, G., and Roy A. (2015a). Are opioid antagonists effective in attenuating the core symptoms of autism spectrum conditions in children? A systematic review. *Journal of Intellectual Disability Research*, **59**(4), 293–306.

Roy, A., Roy, M., Deb, S., Unwin, G., and Roy, A. (2015b). Are opioid antagonists effective in adults with intellectual disability? A systematic review. *Journal of Intellectual Disability Research*, **59**(1), 55–67.

Rubia, K. (2011). 'Cool' inferior frontostriatal dysfunction in attenton deficit/hyperactivity diosrder versus 'hot' ventromedial orbitofrontal–limbic dysfunction in conduct disorder: A review. *Biological Psychiatry*, **69**, e69–87.

Sadavoy, J., Lanctôt, K. L. and Deb S. (2008). Management of behavioural and psychological symptoms of dementia and acquired brain injury. In: P. Tyrer and K. R. Silk (eds) *Cambridge Textbook of Effective Treatments in Psychiatry*. Cambridge, Cambridge University Press. pp. 187–216.

Sami, M. B. and Faruqui, R. (2015). The effectiveness of dopamine agonists for treatment of neuropsychiatric symptoms post brain injury and stroke. *Acta Neuropsychiatrica*, **27**(6), 317–26.

Sarkar, S., Craig, M. C., Catani, M., et al. (2013). Frontotemporal white-matter microstructural abnormalities in adolescents with conduct disorder: a diffusion tensor imaging study. *Psychological Medicine*, **43**(2), 401–11.

Sarkar, S., Dell'Acqua, F., Walsh, S. F., et al. (2016). A whole-brain investigation of white matter microstructure in adolescents with conduct disorder. *PLoS One*, **11**(6), e0155475, 1–16.

Saylor, K. E. and Aman, B. H. (2016). Impulsive aggression as a comorbidity of Attention-Deficit/Hyperactivity Disorder in children and adolescents. *Journal of Child and Adolescent Psychopharmacology*, **26**(1), 19–25.

Seo, D., Patrick, C. J., and Kenncaly, P. J. (2008). Role of serotonin and dopamine system interaction in the neurobiology of impulsive aggression and its comorbidity with other clinical disorders. *Aggressive and Violent Behavior*, **13**(5), 383–95.

Siever, L. J. (2008). Neurobiology of aggression and violence. *American Journal of Psychiatry*, **165**, 429–42.

Sigafoos, J., Elkins, J., Kerr, M., and Attwood, T. (1994). A survey of aggressive behaviour among a population of persons with intellectual disability in Queensland. *Journal of Intellectual Disability Research*, **38**, 369–81.

Silver, J. M., Yudofsky, S. C. and Anderson, K. E. (2005). Aggressive disorders. In: J. M. Silver, T. W. McAllister, and S. C. Yudofsky (eds) *Textbook of Traumatic Brain Injury*. Washington, DC, American Psychiatric Association Publishing. pp. 259–77.

Sockeel, P., Dujardin, K., Devos, D., Denève, C., Destée, A., and Defebvre, L. (2006). The Lille apathy rating scale (LARS), a new instrument for detecting and quantifying apathy: validation in Parkinson's disease. *Journal of Neurology, Neurosurgery, and Psychiatry*, **77**, 579–84.

Sohanpal, S. K., Deb, S., Thomas, C., Soni, R., Lenôtre, L., and Unwin, G. (2007). The effectiveness of antidepressant medication in the management of behaviour problems in adults with intellectual disabilities: a systematic review. *Journal of Intellectual Disability Research*, **51**(10), 750–65.

Starkstein, S. E., Mayberg, H. S., Preziosi, T. J., Andrezejewski, P., Leiguarda, R., and Robinson, R. G. (1992). Reliability, validity and clinical correlates of apathy in Parkinson's disease. *Journal of Neuropsychiatry and Clinical Neuroscience*, **4**, 134–9.

Steinberg, B. J., Trestman, R., Mitropoulou, V., et al. (1997). Depressive response to physostigmine challenge in borderline personality disorder patients. *Neuropsychopharmacology*, **17**, 264–73.

Sterzer, P. and Stadler, C. (2009). Neuroimaging of aggressive and violent behavior in children and adolescents. *Frontiers in Behavioral Neuroscience*, **3**, 35, 1–8.

Stoffers, J., Völlm, B. A., Rücker, G., Timmer, A., Hubband, N., and Leib, K. (2010). Pharmacological interventions for borderline personality disorder (Review). *The Cochrane Library and the Cochrane Collaboration*. Issue **6**.

Swanson, J. W., Holzer, C. E., Ganju, V. K., and Jono, R. T. (1990). Violence and psychiatric disorder in the community: evidence from the Epidemiologic Catchment area survey. *Hospital and Community Psychiatry*, **41**, 101–37.

Taylor, D., Paton, C., and Kapur, S. (2015). *The Maudsley Prescribing Guidelines in Psychiatry*, twelfth edition. Oxford, John Wiley & Sons Ltd. pp. 611–17.

Tonkonogy, J. M. and Geller, J. L. (1992). Hypothalamic lesions and intermittent explosive disorder. *Journal of Neuropsychiatry and Clinical Neuroscience*, **4**, 45–50.

Tranel, D., Bechara, A., and Damasio, A. R. (1999). Decision making and the somatic marker hypothesis. In: M. S. Gazzaniga (ed) *The New Cognitive Neurosciences*. Cambridge, MA, MIT Press. pp. 1047–61.

Tyrer, P., Oliver-Africano, P. C., Ahmed, Z., et al. (2008). Risperidone, haloperidol, and placebo in the treatment of aggressive challenging behaviour in patients with intellectual disability: a randomised controlled trial. *The Lancet*, **371**, 57–63.

Unwin, G. L. and Deb, S. (2011). Efficacy of atypical antipsychotic medication in the management of behaviour problems in children with intellectual disabilities and borderline intelligence: a systematic review. *Research in Developmental Disabilities*, **32**, 2121–33.

Volavka, J., Czabor, P., Citrome, L., McQuade, R. D., Carson, W. H., and Kostic, D. (2005). Eiificacy of aripiprazole against hostility in sxchizophrenia and schizoaffective disorder: Data from 5 double-blind studies. *Journal of Clinical Psychiatry*, **66**(11), 1362–6.

Volkow, N. D., Tancredi, L. R., Grant, C., et al. (1995). Brain glucose metabolism in violent psychiatric patients: a preliminary study. *Psychiatry Research*, **61**(4), 243–53.

Wada, A., Yokoo, H., Yanagita, T., and Kobayashi, H. (2005). Lithium: potential therapeutics against acute brain injuries and chronic neurodegenerative diseases. *Journal of Pharmacological Sciences*, **99**, 307–21.

Waller, R., Dotterer, H. L., Murray, L., Maxwell, A. M., and Hyde, L. W. (2017). White-matter tract abnormalities and antisocial behavior: A systematic review of diffusion tensor imaging studies across development. *NeuroImage: Clinical*, **14**, 201–15.

Ward, F., Tharian, P., Roy, M., Deb, S., and Unwin, G. L. (2013). Efficacy of beta blockers in the management of problem behaviours in people with intellectual disabilities: A systematic review. *Research in Developmental Disabilities*, **34**, 4293–303.

Wersinger, S. R., Caldwell, H. K., Christiansen, M., and Young, W. S. (2007). Disruption of the vasopressin 1b receptor gene impairs the attack component of aggressive behavior in mice. *Genes Brain and Behavior*, **6**(7), 653–60.

Wistedt, B., Rasmussen, A., Pedersen, L., et al. (1990). The development of an observer-scale for measuring social dysfunction and aggression. *Pharmacopsychiatry*, **23**, 249–52.

World Health Organization. (2018). *International Classification of Diseases 11th revision (ICD-11)*. Geneva, World Health Organization.

Yanowitch, R. and Coccaro, E. F. (2011). The neurochemistry of human aggression. *Advances in Genetics*, **75**, 151–69.

Zweig, R. M., Disbrow, E. A., and Javalkar, V. (2016). Cognitive and psychiatric disturbances in Parkinsonian syndrome. *Neurology Clinics*, **34**, 235–46.

Zigmond, A. S. and Snaith, R. P. (1983). The Hospital Anxiety and Depression Scale. *Acta Psychiatrica Scandinavica*, **67**, 361–70.

Zuidema, S., Koopmans, R., and Verhey, F. (2007). Prevalence and predictors of neuropsychiatric symptoms in cognitively impaired nursing home patients. *Journal of Geriatric Psychiatry and Neurology*, **20**, 41–9.

32

Impulsivity in humans: neurobiology and pathology

Valerie Voon

Introduction

Impulsivity is defined as rash, poorly considered decisions and mistimed and premature behaviours that occur despite negative consequences (Durana and Barnes, 1993; Evenden, 1999). The construct is relevant across our daily decisions and dimensionally across a range of psychiatric symptomatology and behaviours, including pathological food and drug misuse, mania, obsessive–compulsive symptoms, and suicidal behaviours. Impulsivity is not a unitary construct and consists of heterogenous subtypes with discrete, but overlapping, neural substrates (Dalley et al., 2011; Evenden, 1999; Voon et al., 2014). Understanding impulsivity as cognitive endophenotypes allows insight into impairments that might cut across diagnostic categories relevant to the Research Domain Criteria (Insel et al., 2010).

Impulsivity can be broadly divided into motor and decisional subtypes. Motor impulsivity includes: (1) waiting impulsivity or premature anticipatory responding prior to a cue predicting reward; and (2) response inhibition or stopping inhibition of a pre-potent response. Decisional impulsivity includes: (3) delay and probabilistic discounting or the preference for small, immediate rewards over larger, delayed rewards; (4) probabilistic discounting or risk-taking; and (5) reflection impulsivity or the tendency to make rapid decisions without adequate accumulation and consideration of the available evidence. Fig. 32.1 illustrates the mapping of impulsivity constructs onto dissociable resting-state functional connectivity substrates.

Waiting impulsivity

Waiting impulsivity requires action restraint during the waiting period leading up to an expected reward and can be tested using serial reaction time tasks. In the 5-choice serial reaction time task (5CSRTT), rodents are trained to detect brief visual targets and to refrain from responding prior to their onset (Robbins, 2002). High impulsivity predicts the escalation of cocaine and nicotine self-administration (Dalley et al., 2007; Diergaarde et al., 2008) and the

subsequent development of compulsive cocaine self-administration (Belin et al., 2008). As well as being a trait marker for addiction, premature responding can be a secondary consequence of drug exposure.

The neural network underlying premature responding in the 5CSRTT has been extensively mapped in rodents (Dalley et al., 2008; Robbins, 2002). These studies indicate key roles of the infralimbic cortex—probably equivalent to the human subgenual anterior cingulate cortex (ACC)—nucleus accumbens (NAcb), and subthalamic nucleus (STN) (Aleksandrova et al., 2013; Baunez et al., 1995; Baunez and Robbins 1997; Chudasama et al., 2003). Greater premature responding in the human 4-CSRT task is associated with decreased resting-state functional connectivity of the bilateral STN with bilateral subgenual cingulate and the right ventral striatum (Morris et al., 2015) (see Fig. 32.2). These findings provide

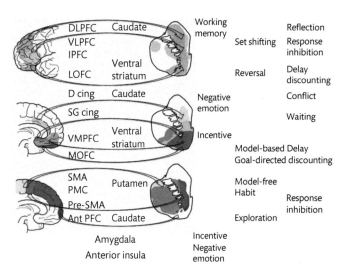

Fig. 32.1 Fronto-striatal substrates of impulsivity and compulsivity.
Adapted from Morris, L.S, Kundu, P., Dowell, N. et al. Fronto-striatal organization: Defining functional and microstructural substrates of behavioural flexibility. *Cortex*, 74: pp. 118–133. Copyright (2015) The Authors. Published by Elsevier Ltd. Distributed under the terms of the Creative Commons Attribution 4.0 International (CC By 4.0) https://creativecommons.org/licenses/by/4.0/.

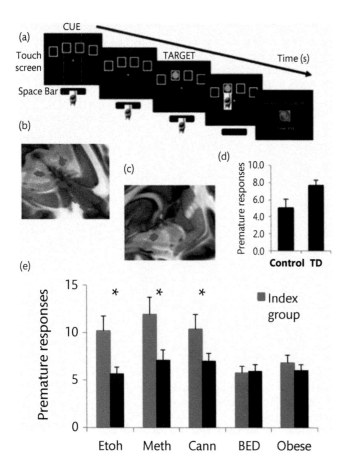

Fig. 32.2 Translational studies of waiting impulsivity in rodents and humans.

translational evidence in humans for a similar network implicated in rodents. Furthermore, this network was shown to be dimensionally relevant across alcohol misuse, with impairment as a function of alcohol severity in social drinkers, binge drinkers, and alcohol use disorders. Using machine-learning techniques, STN connectivity successfully classified those who misused alcohol from healthy volunteers. Central serotonin depletion with tryptophan depletion (Worbe et al., 2014) or acute methylphenidate administration (Voon et al., 2015) increased premature responding, consistent with rodent studies (Economidou et al., 2012; Winstanley et al., 2004b). Thus, human studies converge on rodent studies, implicating a role in substance use disorders, possibly mediated by dopaminergic, noradrenergic, and serotonergic mechanisms and similar underlying neural networks.

In humans, enhanced waiting impulsivity can be assessed using the analogous 4-choice serial reaction time task across multiple substance use disorders (e.g. abstinent methamphetamine and alcohol use disorders), along with current cannabis users and current smokers (Voon et al., 2014). In this task, a premature response was defined as early anticipatory release of the space bar prior to the onset of a target green stimulus within one of four boxes on a touchscreen (Voon, 2014). College-age binge drinkers at elevated risk for the development of later alcohol use disorders also showed enhanced waiting impulsivity, as tested using either the 4-CSRT (Morris et al., 2015) or the Sussex-5-CSRT (Sanchez-Roige et al., 2014). In contrast, obese subjects with and without binge eating

disorder (BED) did not show impaired waiting impulsivity (Voon et al., 2014). This may reflect a diminished sensitivity of obese people to monetary rewards, but further studies (e.g. with food outcomes used instead) would be needed to test this possibility.

Response inhibition

Response inhibition describes the capacity to inhibit a pre-potent response. In human studies, differing subtypes of stopping behaviour have been described, including: fast reactive stopping in response to an external stop signal, proactive stopping in response to a cue predicting a stop signal (Aron, 2011; Jaffard et al., 2008), and stopping in response to an internal signal (Schel et al., 2014). Fast reactive stopping is the most commonly tested form, with extensive translational evidence as action restraint or cancellation, and includes: (1) stopping prior to movement initiation (action restraint), as measured using the Go/NoGo task in which subjects must inhibit responding to an infrequently presented stop signal while responding rapidly to a frequently presented stream of Go signals; and (2) stopping after movement initiation (action cancellation), as measured using the Stop Signal Task (SST) in which subjects inhibit responding to an infrequent stop signal with onset following a delay after the Go signal (Aron, 2011; Chambers et al., 2009; Eagle et al., 2008). In the SST, the stop signal delay changes as a function of successful stopping, such that successful and failed stops occur with a 50% probability. The shorter the delay, the greater likelihood of stopping, while the longer the delay, the lower likelihood of stopping. Whereas the Go/NoGo task measures discrete commission errors, the SST assesses the internal speed of stopping [stop signal reaction time (SSRT)] by assessing the speed at the Go signal and the probability of stopping at the stop signal delay (Logan et al., 1984; Verbruggen and Logan, 2009). This is conceptually based on the Logan's Race model or a race competition between the process of Go and Stop, in which the process that crosses the threshold first is executed.

Another type of inhibitory control, which has been more extensively studied in humans, is that of proactive stopping in which motor control is preparatory and goal-directed (Aron, 2011; Jaffard et al., 2008). This form of stopping has similarities to 'braking' and 'conflict-induced slowing', in which slowing of reaction time may occur in the context of a conflict to prevent impulsive decisions until a decision is made (Frank, 2006, 2007). Proactive stopping can be differentiated from reactive stopping by comparing response inhibition tasks in which either the stop signal is acted upon to countermand the action (proactive condition) or the stop signal is ignored or not present (baseline condition). Proactive inhibition is associated with a decrease in motor-evoked potential, an index of cortical excitability, which is suppressed to a greater extent than at rest when anticipating a stopping response (Cai et al., 2011).

Response inhibition implicates a network across rodent and human studies, including the SMA, right inferior frontal cortex (rIFC), STN, and caudate, and has been extensively reviewed elsewhere (Aron, 2011; Aron et al., 2003b; Dalley et al., 2011; Morris et al., 2015). Studies of proactive inhibition have implicated the same regions as reactive stopping, including the SMA, rIFC, and STN (Ballanger et al., 2009; Jaffard et al., 2008; Obeso et al., 2013; Zandbelt and Vink, 2010). The hyperdirect connections from the

SMA and rIFC to the STN are thought to underlie reactive stopping, whereas the fronto-striatal circuitry via direct and indirect pathways appear to be more important for proactive stopping (Majid et al., 2013; Smittenaar et al., 2013; Zandbelt and Vink, 2010). The neurobiology underlying human and rodent SSRT and Go/NoGo tasks have been extensively discussed (Aron, 2011; Chambers et al., 2009; Eagle et al., 2008).

In rodent studies, the SST appears to be influenced by noradrenergic mechanisms, with a rather more limited influence from DA and 5HT. In humans, methylphenidate improves SST performance in those with impaired SSRT such as cocaine-dependent subjects (Li et al., 2010), as well as children (De Vito et al., 2009; Tannock et al., 1989) and adults (Aron et al., 2003a) with ADHD. In healthy subjects, direct comparisons showed that acute methylphenidate, but not atomoxetine or citalopram, improved response inhibition on the SST (Nandam et al., 2011), although a direct comparison showed efficacy of atomoxetine, but not citalopram, in improving response inhibition on the SST (Chamberlain et al., 2007). However, higher doses of atomoxetine (80 mg versus 40 mg) impaired response inhibition on the Go/NoGo task (Graf et al., 2011). Thus, converging with rodent studies, NA appears to play a role in reactive stopping in humans, with a possible U-shaped dose–response relationship.

Meta-analyses showed deficits in response inhibition, particularly with the SSRT and, to a lesser extent, with Go/NoGo in ADHD (Lipszyc and Schachar, 2010) and across most, but not all, substance use disorders, including stimulants, nicotine, and alcohol, and in pathological gambling and Internet use disorder, but not opioid or cannabis abuse (Smith et al., 2014). Impairments in the SST have also been shown in unaffected siblings of stimulant-dependent subjects, suggesting an endophenotypic risk factor for the development of addiction (Ersche et al., 2012) and predicted adolescent alcohol- and drug-related problems (Nigg et al., 2006) and the progression from heavy alcohol use in adults to alcohol dependence (Rubio et al., 2008). Similarly, both OCD subjects and unaffected family members showed impairments in the SST, suggesting a cognitive endophenotype (Menzies et al., 2007) underlying the development of OCD. However, unlike premature responding, rodent studies have not yet shown that this form of impulsivity predicts compulsive substance use.

Delay discounting

Animals and humans demonstrate an inherent tendency to discount or devalue future outcomes (Ainslie, 1975). Impulsive choice or delay discounting is a form of impulsivity that can be measured using intertemporal choice tasks. In these tasks, subjects choose between a small immediate reward and a larger, but delayed, reward. The devaluation of future reward can be reliably modelled by a hyperbolic function ($V_S = V_A/1 + Kd$) with steeper slopes closer to the time of reward receipt than an exponential function ($V_S = V_A e^{-kd}$) with equal slopes over delay intervals (Ainslie, 1975; Mazur, 1987). With such functions, the subjective value V_S is a modification of the actual value V_A by the delay (d) and a discount constant (K). K represents the steepness of the temporal discounting curve and a measure of impulsivity. A hyperbolic fit implies that when the smaller reward is imminently available, the subjective value of the

smaller immediate reward will be greater than the subjective value of the larger delayed reward, thus resulting in a preference reversal, away from the larger future outcome towards the smaller immediate outcome (Ainslie, 1975).

Rodent studies have implicated a role for DA, 5HT, and NA in delay discounting. In humans, lower D2/3 receptor availability in the ventral striatum appeared to correlate more specifically with greater delay discounting in pathological gambling (Joutsa et al., 2015), methamphetamine dependence (Ballard et al., 2015), and alcohol use disorders (Oberlin et al., 2015). Levodopa, a precursor to DA in healthy humans, increases impulsive choice (Pine et al., 2010) and increases delay aversion in patients with PD (Cools et al., 2003). Prefrontal cortical DA has also been implicated in impulsive choice. Thus, genetic polymorphisms associated with catechol-O-methyltransferase (COMT), an enzyme found in the PFC and responsible for DA breakdown, are associated with a U-shaped relationship between prefrontal dopaminergic function and impulsive choice (Kayser et al., 2012). In humans, the role of 5HT is less clear since tryptophan depletion does not influence delay discounting in healthy controls (Worbe et al., 2014), with and without a family history of alcohol dependence (Crean et al., 2002) or with simulated binging of alcohol (Dougherty et al., 2015).

Rodent lesion studies have implicated the NAcb core, orbitofrontal cortex (OFC), amygdala, and hippocampus in delay discounting (Cardinal et al., 2001; Cardinal et al., 2004; Winstanley et al., 2004a). Human imaging studies have also implicated the ventral striatum, OFC, lateral prefrontal cortex (lPFC), insula, amygdala, posterior cingulate, and parietal cortex in delay discounting for secondary rewards (Ballard and Knutson, 2009; Kable and Glimcher, 2007; McClure et al., 2004; Tanaka et al., 2004) and primary rewards (McClure et al., 2007) (see Fig. 32.3).

The ventral striatum is a key structure implicated in single- and dual-valuation theories of temporal discounting in human studies. In the dual-valuation system, the beta system activates the limbic systems (ventral striatum and medial PFC) and is associated with the choice of the immediate reward, whereas delta regions (lateral prefrontal and parietal cortices) are activated during all decisions (McClure et al., 2004). The beta system is hypothesized to overvalue immediate rewards, while the delta system is considered

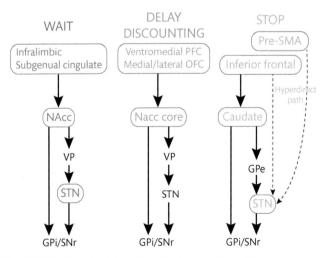

Fig. 32.3 Cortico-striatal circuitry of subtypes of impulsivity.

to discount rewards over a constant rate with time. An alternate dual-valuation system is hypothesized in which delay is coded in the lPFC and magnitude is coded in the ventral striatum (Ballard and Knutson, 2009). The differential involvement of cortico-basal-ganglia loops have been implicated, with the ventro-anterior striatum and insula being preferentially involved in immediate choices and the dorso-posterior striatum and insula being preferentially involved in delayed choices (Tanaka et al., 2004). In contrast, others have argued for a single-valuation system, with the ventral striatum representing the subjective value of the delayed choice (Kable and Glimcher, 2007).

In animal studies, pre-existing impairments in impulsive choice predispose to greater cocaine self-administration and reinstatement of cocaine-seeking behaviour (Perry et al., 2005, 2008) and greater use of alcohol (Mitchell et al., 2006; Poulos et al., 1995) and nicotine (Diergaarde et al., 2008). In humans, delay discounting is a core impairment implicated in ADHD (Noreika et al., 2013) and substance addictions across multiple drug categories and pathological gambling (Bickel et al., 2013, 2014) and in obesity, both with and without BED (Mole et al., 2014; Voon, 2015).

Reflection impulsivity

Reflection impulsivity is predominantly assessed in humans and describes the accumulation of evidence, evaluation of options, and rapid hypothesis testing prior to a decision (Kagan, 1966). This form of impulsivity can be divided into perceptual and probabilistic decisions. Perceptual tasks include the Matching Familiar Figures Task (MFFT) in which subjects decide whether a pattern matches a series of similar patterns of which all but one differ (Kagan, 1966). The impulsivity score captures the core feature of the extent of information sampling or reaction time and accuracy of the decision. Children with ADHD perform more impulsively on the MFFT, which improves with psychostimulant treatment (Brown and Sleator, 1979). MDMA users, but not cannabis users or alcohol-dependent subjects, are also impaired on the MFFT (Morgan et al., 2006; Quednow et al., 2007; Weijers et al., 2001). Other reflection impulsivity tasks assess probabilistic decisions more directly by measuring the extent of information sampling or evidence accumulation, e.g. the Beads-in-a-Jar task ('Beads task') (Volans, 1976) and the Information Sampling Task (IST) (Clark et al., 2006). In the Beads task, subjects must decide from which of two jars beads are being selected, based on known probabilities of the colour ratio of the beads within the jars. Participants are aware of the explicit probabilities of the alternate options, with each piece of evidence accumulated associated with an expected probability of being correct. Using this task, elevated probabilistic reflection impulsivity has been observed in substance use disorders, pathological gamblers (Djamshidian et al., 2012), binge drinkers (Banca et al., 2015), and patients with PD and medication-induced behavioural addictions (Djamshidian et al., 2012). Reflection impulsivity tested using the Beads task is exacerbated by DA receptor agonists, though not by levodopa in studies of PD (Djamshidian et al., 2013). The IST is a similar information sampling paradigm that asks participants to decide which colour is predominant in a 5 × 5 matrix by opening boxes to make a decision (Clark et al., 2006). Current or former amphetamine and opiate users sample less information, compared

to healthy volunteers (Clark et al., 2006). One study has shown an impairment in binge drinkers (Banca et al., 2015), although this was not confirmed in a second study (Townshend et al., 2014).

Volumetric differences between the IST and the Beads task have also been reported (Banca et al., 2015). Greater impulsivity in the Beads task was associated with smaller dorsolateral PFC and left inferior parietal volumes (Banca et al., 2015). The mechanisms underlying evidence accumulation can be subdivided into evidence-seeking or decision-making. The Beads task is associated with parietal activity during evidence-seeking, and dorsolateral PFC activity during both evidence-seeking and decision-making (Furl and Averbeck, 2011). The dorsolateral PFC is important for the resolution of uncertainty (Huettel et al., 2005) and computing differences between costs and benefits (Basten et al., 2010), with the accumulated difference represented in the parietal cortex signalling the final decision and confidence (Kiani and Shadlen 2009; Stern et al., 2010). In contrast, greater impulsivity in the IST was associated with greater left dorsal cingulate and right precuneus volumes (Banca et al., 2015). Similarly, in an fMRI study investigating evidence accumulation, greater uncertainty during evidence accumulation was associated with ACC and precuneus activity, whereas greater uncertainty during decision execution was associated with greater lateral frontal and parietal activity (Stern et al., 2010). The dACC is implicated in error- and conflict-monitoring processes (Botvinick et al., 2001; Scheffers and Coles, 2000) and in coding unexpected and unpredicted outcomes during evidence accumulation (Oliveira et al., 2007; Stern et al., 2010). More recently, enhanced reflection impulsivity was observed when the associative-limbic STN was stimulated in OCD subjects, with parallel findings of decreased functional connectivity observed between the STN and the dorsolateral PFC with greater impulsivity (Voon et al., 2017a).

Clinical implications

Impulsivity can be observed dimensionally across a range of disorders. These can include, but are not limited to, addictions, OCD, ADHD, and bipolar disorder and neurologic disorders such as Parkinson's disease, TS, HS, and FTD.

For the purposes of illustration, a classic neuropsychiatric example of impulsivity related to Parkinson's disease is described. A 54-year-old man with an 8-year history of tremor-dominant Parkinson's disease with marked chorea undergoes bilateral DBS of the STN. He has a premorbid history of gambling disorder with new onset with dopamine agonists, which resolved following a decrease in dose. Following DBS, he develops mild hypomanic symptoms, characterized by impulsive behaviours, including gambling and hypersexuality. The impulsive behaviours may be a function of the underlying neurobiology of Parkinson's disease, individual vulnerability, dopaminergic medications, or subthalamic stimulation (Voon et al., 2017b). Understanding the underlying mechanisms and deconstructing the rationale for the behaviours is critical to behavioural management.

The clinical assessment of impulsivity includes having a high index of suspicion, conducting a careful history, and having an understanding of the pathophysiology of the underlying impulsive behaviours. In this case, inquiring about all known behavioural addictions or impulse control behaviours linked to dopaminergic medications (e.g. gambling, hypersexuality, binge eating, compulsive shopping, punding, and excessive dopaminergic medication use) from both the patient and caregiver is indicated, given the often hidden and shameful nature of the behaviours. A frank, open discussion about the role of medications and their behavioural side effects to normalize the behaviours is useful. To establish the link between the gambling symptoms and DA agonists, a careful history of previous behaviours, including subsyndromal symptoms and family history, the timing of onset of DA agonists and the dose changes in relation to the behaviour, and ongoing subsyndromal symptoms, including ongoing obsessions or craving symptoms, and the means of controlling the behaviours is indicated. Impulse control behaviours related to dopaminergic medications in Parkinson's disease is associated with cognitive impulsivity processes such as greater delay discounting, risk-taking, and impairments in the relative balance of reward and losses (Voon et al., 2017b). The role of executive processes (e.g. working memory, planning) and general cognitive impairment is less clear but should be clinically assessed. The cognitive tasks described in this chapter are predominantly of value on a research basis, and not necessarily on a clinical basis yet, as the clinical value is unclear. Questionnaires focusing on symptoms (e.g the Questionnaire for Impulsive-Compulsive Disorders in Parkinson's disease—QUIP) (Weintraub et al., 2009), which have been validated to assess the presence of impulse control behaviours in Parkinson's disease, and clinical screens, which include executive function processes such as the MoCA or FAB, are clinically useful. Questionnaires on impulsivity, such as the Spielberger State or Trait Anxiety Inventory or Barratts Impulsivity Scale, again may be more useful on a research basis or to track clinical severity of impulsivity over time. More extensive neurobehavioural assessments for executive processes are also useful, particularly if concurrent cognitive impairment is suspected. Management includes decreasing the dose of, or discontinuing, the DA agonist. Impulsivity associated with the pathology of Parkinson's disease itself (e.g. neurodegeneration of noradrenergic or serotonergic cell bodies) may include an assessment of underlying impulsivity constructs, which may help guide possible improvements on serotonergic or noradrenergic agents. For example, atomoxetine has been shown to improve underlying response inhibition in Parkinson's disease as a function of structural and functional fronto-striatal connectivity (Rae et al., 2016; Ye et al., 2015). Using factors such as age, cognitive status, levodopa equivalent dose, and a diffusion-weighted scan, the response to single doses of atomoxetine and citalopram could be predicted with 77–79% accuracy in Parkinson's disease (Ye et al., 2016). Further work to determine the clinical impact and apply these to larger clinical populations and examine the effects of chronic medications is indicated.

Hypomania following DBS of the STN is one of the commonest behavioural side effects, occurring in 4% of patients, that have been shown to be clearly temporally and mechanistically linked to stimulation (Voon et al., 2006). Hypomania can be deconstructed into its component behaviours that include neurovegetative, motor, cognitive, and limbic processes. Critically, a core feature of hypomania is characterized by poor impulse control. The presumed mechanisms underlying hypomania following STN stimulation include stimulation of ventral (limbic and associative) regions of the STN or stimulation within the ventral contacts lying within the substantia nigra, interactions with concurrent dopaminergic medications, and

a possible, but unclear, role for premorbid vulnerability (Chopra et al., 2012). The role of changes in medications pre- and post-operatively following DBS is required to establish any relationship with post-operative hypomania. Management includes decreasing concurrent dopaminergic medication doses, decreasing the stimulation voltage, or changing stimulation contacts from more ventral to dorsal contacts.

Conclusion

These impulsivity constructs map onto distinct fronto-striatal neural and neurochemical systems interacting both at nodal convergent points and as opponent processes, highlighting both the heterogeneity and commonalities of function. We emphasize the relevance of these constructs for understanding dimensional psychiatry. A careful clinical assessment is highlighted to understand the mechanisms underlying the impulsive behaviours, and hence drive appropriate management.

KEY LEARNING POINTS

- Impulsivity refers to premature behaviours and rash, poorly considered decisions, which are made in spite of negative consequences. It is not a singular entity, consisting of a number of sub-categories under the two broad headings of motor and decisional impulsivity.
- The subtypes of motor impulsivity are laid out first, discussing waiting impulsivity, also known as premature responding, which can be a predictor of addiction, and response inhibition impulsivity, which is the capacity to inhibit pre-potent response.
- The chapter then explores the forms of decisional impulsivity, such as delay discounting and reflection impulsivity, along with their relation to ADHD.
- Finally, the prevalence of impulsivity across disorders as wide-ranging as OCD and Huntington's disease is discussed, and a case study of Parkinson's-related impulsivity is presented.

REFERENCES

Ainslie G (1975) Specious reward: a behavioral theory of impulsiveness and impulse control. Psychol Bull 82: 463–96.

Aleksandrova LR, Creed MC, Fletcher PJ, Lobo DS, Hamani C, Nobrega JN (2013) Deep brain stimulation of the subthalamic nucleus increases premature responding in a rat gambling task. Behav Brain Res 245: 76–82.

Aron AR (2011) From reactive to proactive and selective control: developing a richer model for stopping inappropriate responses. Biol Psychiatry 69: e55–68.

Aron AR, Dowson JH, Sahakian BJ, Robbins TW (2003a) Methylphenidate improves response inhibition in adults with attention-deficit/hyperactivity disorder. Biol Psychiatry 54: 1465–68.

Aron AR, Fletcher PC, Bullmore ET, Sahakian BJ, Robbins TW (2003b) Stop-signal inhibition disrupted by damage to right inferior frontal gyrus in humans. Nat Neurosci 6: 115–16.

Ballanger B, van Eimeren T, Moro E, et al. (2009) Stimulation of the subthalamic nucleus and impulsivity: release your horses. Ann Neurol 66: 817–24.

Ballard K, Knutson B (2009) Dissociable neural representations of future reward magnitude and delay during temporal discounting. Neuroimage 45: 143–50.

Ballard ME, Mandelkern MA, Monterosso JR, et al. (2015) Low Dopamine D2/D3 Receptor Availability is Associated with Steep Discounting of Delayed Rewards in Methamphetamine Dependence. Int J Neuropsychopharmacol 18: pyu119.

Banca P, Lange I, Worbe Y, et al. (2015) Reflection impulsivity in binge drinking: behavioural and volumetric correlates. Addict Biol 21: 504–15.

Basten U, Biele G, Heekeren HR, Fiebach CJ (2010) How the brain integrates costs and benefits during decision making. Proc Natl Acad Sci U S A 107: 21767–72.

Baunez C, Nieoullon A, Amalric M (1995) In a rat model of parkinsonism, lesions of the subthalamic nucleus reverse increases of reaction time but induce a dramatic premature responding deficit. J Neurosci 15: 6531–41.

Baunez C, Robbins TW (1997) Bilateral lesions of the subthalamic nucleus induce multiple deficits in an attentional task in rats. Eur J Neurosci 9: 2086–99.

Belin D, Mar AC, Dalley JW, Robbins TW, Everitt BJ (2008) High impulsivity predicts the switch to compulsive cocaine-taking. Science 320: 1352–55.

Bickel WK, Koffarnus MN, Moody L, Wilson AG (2014) The behavioral- and neuro-economic process of temporal discounting: A candidate behavioral marker of addiction. Neuropharmacology 76 Pt B: 518–27.

Botvinick MM, Braver TS, Barch DM, Carter CS, Cohen JD (2001) Conflict monitoring and cognitive control. Psychol Rev 108: 624–52.

Brown RT, Sleator EK (1979) Methylphenidate in hyperkinetic children: differences in dose effects on impulsive behavior. Pediatrics 64: 408–11.

Cai W, Oldenkamp CL, Aron AR (2011) A proactive mechanism for selective suppression of response tendencies. J Neurosci 31: 5965–9.

Cardinal RN, Pennicott DR, Sugathapala CL, Robbins TW, Everitt BJ (2001) Impulsive choice induced in rats by lesions of the nucleus accumbens core. Science 292: 2499–501.

Cardinal RN, Winstanley CA, Robbins TW, Everitt BJ (2004) Limbic corticostriatal systems and delayed reinforcement. Ann N Y Acad Sci 1021: 33–50.

Chamberlain SR, Del Campo N, Dowson J, et al. (2007) Atomoxetine improved response inhibition in adults with attention deficit/hyperactivity disorder. Biol Psychiatry 62: 977–84.

Chambers CD, Garavan H, Bellgrove MA (2009) Insights into the neural basis of response inhibition from cognitive and clinical neuroscience. Neurosci Biobehav Rev 33: 631–46.

Chopra A, Tye SJ, Lee KH, et al. (2012) Underlying neurobiology and clinical correlates of mania status after subthalamic nucleus deep brain stimulation in Parkinson's disease: a review of the literature. J Neuropsychiatry Clin Neurosci 24: 102–10.

Chudasama Y, Passetti F, Rhodes SE, Lopian D, Desai A, Robbins TW (2003) Dissociable aspects of performance on the 5-choice serial reaction time task following lesions of the dorsal anterior cingulate, infralimbic and orbitofrontal cortex in the rat: differential effects on selectivity, impulsivity and compulsivity. Behav Brain Res 146: 105–19.

Clark L, Robbins TW, Ersche KD, Sahakian BJ (2006) Reflection impulsivity in current and former substance users. Biol Psychiatry 60: 515–22.

Cools R, Barker RA, Sahakian BJ, Robbins TW (2003) L-Dopa medication remediates cognitive inflexibility, but increases impulsivity in patients with Parkinson's disease. Neuropsychologia 41: 1431–41.

Crean J, Richards JB, de Wit H (2002) Effect of tryptophan depletion on impulsive behavior in men with or without a family history of alcoholism. Behav Brain Res 136: 349–57.

Dalley JW, Everitt BJ, Robbins TW (2011) Impulsivity, compulsivity, and top-down cognitive control. Neuron 69: 680–94.

Dalley JW, Fryer TD, Brichard L, et al. (2007) Nucleus accumbens D2/3 receptors predict trait impulsivity and cocaine reinforcement. Science 315: 1267–70.

Dalley JW, Mar AC, Economidou D, Robbins TW (2008) Neurobehavioral mechanisms of impulsivity: fronto-striatal systems and functional neurochemistry. Pharmacol Biochem Behav 90: 250–60.

DeVito EE, Blackwell AD, Clark L, et al. (2009) Methylphenidate improves response inhibition but not reflection-impulsivity in children with attention deficit hyperactivity disorder (ADHD). Psychopharmacology (Berl) 202: 531–9.

Diergaarde L, Pattij T, Poortvliet I, et al. (2008) Impulsive choice and impulsive action predict vulnerability to distinct stages of nicotine seeking in rats. Biol Psychiatry 63: 301–8.

Djamshidian A, O'Sullivan SS, Foltynie T, et al. (2013) Dopamine agonists rather than deep brain stimulation cause reflection impulsivity in Parkinson's disease. J Parkinson Dis 3: 139–44.

Djamshidian A, O'Sullivan SS, Sanotsky Y, et al. (2012) Decision making, impulsivity, and addictions: do Parkinson's disease patients jump to conclusions? Mov Disord 27: 1137–45.

Dougherty DM, Mullen J, Hill-Kapturczak N, et al. (2015) Effects of tryptophan depletion and a simulated alcohol binge on impulsivity. Exp Clin Psychopharmacol 23: 109–21.

Durana JH, Barnes PA (1993) A neurodevelopmental view of impulsivity and its relationship to the superfactors of personality. In: McCown WG, Johnson JL, Shure MB (eds) The impulsive Client: Theory, Research and Treatment. American Psychological Association, Washington, DC.

Eagle DM, Bari A, Robbins TW (2008) The neuropsychopharmacology of action inhibition: cross-species translation of the stop-signal and go/no-go tasks. Psychopharmacology (Berl) 199: 439–56.

Economidou D, Theobald DE, Robbins TW, Everitt BJ, Dalley JW (2012) Norepinephrine and dopamine modulate impulsivity on the five-choice serial reaction time task through opponent actions in the shell and core sub-regions of the nucleus accumbens. Neuropsychopharmacology 37: 2057–66.

Ersche KD, Jones PS, Williams GB, Turton AJ, Robbins TW, Bullmore ET (2012) Abnormal brain structure implicated in stimulant drug addiction. Science 335: 601–4.

Evenden JL (1999) Varieties of impulsivity. Psychopharmacology (Berl) 146: 348–61.

Frank MJ (2006) Hold your horses: a dynamic computational role for the subthalamic nucleus in decision making. Neural Networks 19: 1120–36.

Frank MJ, Samanta J, Moustafa AA, Sherman SJ (2007) Hold your horses: impulsivity, deep brain stimulation, and medication in parkinsonism. Science 318: 1309–12.

Furl N, Averbeck BB (2011) Parietal cortex and insula relate to evidence seeking relevant to reward-related decisions. J Neurosci 31: 17572–82.

Graf H, Abler B, Freudenmann R, et al. (2011) Neural correlates of error monitoring modulated by atomoxetine in healthy volunteers. Biol Psychiatry 69: 890–7.

Huettel SA, Song AW, McCarthy G (2005) Decisions under uncertainty: probabilistic context influences activation of prefrontal and parietal cortices. J Neurosci 25: 3304–11.

Insel T, Cuthbert B, Garvey M, et al. (2010) Research domain criteria (RDoC): toward a new classification framework for research on mental disorders. Am J Psychiatry 167: 748–51.

Jaffard M, Longcamp M, Velay JL, et al. (2008) Proactive inhibitory control of movement assessed by event-related fMRI. Neuroimage 42: 1196–206.

Joutsa J, Voon V, Johansson J, Niemela S, Bergman J, Kaasinen V (2015) Dopaminergic function and intertemporal choice. Translational Psychiatry 5: e491.

Kable JW, Glimcher PW (2007) The neural correlates of subjective value during intertemporal choice. Nat Neurosci 10: 1625–33.

Kagan J (1966) Reflection–impulsivity: the generality and dynamics of conceptual tempo. J Abnorm Psychol 71: 17–24.

Kayser AS, Allen DC, Navarro-Cebrian A, Mitchell JM, Fields HL (2012) Dopamine, corticostriatal connectivity, and intertemporal choice. J Neurosci 32: 9402–9.

Kiani R, Shadlen MN (2009) Representation of confidence associated with a decision by neurons in the parietal cortex. Science 324: 759–64.

Li CS, Morgan PT, Matuskey D, et al. (2010) Biological markers of the effects of intravenous methylphenidate on improving inhibitory control in cocaine-dependent patients. Proc Natl Acad Sci U S A 107: 14455–9.

Lipszyc J, Schachar R (2010) Inhibitory control and psychopathology: a meta-analysis of studies using the stop signal task. J Int Neuropsychol Soc 16: 1064–76.

Logan GD, Cowan WB, Davis KA (1984) On the ability to inhibit simple and choice reaction time responses: a model and a method. J Exp Psychol Hum Percept Perform 10: 276–91.

Majid DS, Cai W, Corey-Bloom J, Aron AR (2013) Proactive selective response suppression is implemented via the basal ganglia. J Neurosci 33: 13259–69.

Mazur JE (1987) The effect of delayed and intervening events on reinforcement value. In: Commons ML, Mazur JE, Nevin JA, Rachlin H (eds) An adjustment Procedure for Studying Delayed Reinforcement. Erlbaum, Hillsdale, NJ.

McClure SM, Ericson KM, Laibson DI, Loewenstein G, Cohen JD (2007) Time discounting for primary rewards. J Neurosci 27: 5796–804.

McClure SM, Laibson DI, Loewenstein G, Cohen JD (2004) Separate neural systems value immediate and delayed monetary rewards. Science 306: 503–7.

Menzies L, Achard S, Chamberlain SR, et al. (2007) Neurocognitive endophenotypes of obsessive-compulsive disorder. Brain 130: 3223–36.

Mitchell SH, Reeves JM, Li N, Phillips TJ (2006) Delay discounting predicts behavioral sensitization to ethanol in outbred WSC mice. Alcohol Clin Exp Res 30: 429–37.

Mole TB, Irvine MA, Worbe Y, et al. (2014) Impulsivity in disorders of food and drug misuse. Psychol Med 1–12.

Morgan MJ, Impallomeni LC, Pirona A, Rogers RD (2006) Elevated impulsivity and impaired decision-making in abstinent Ecstasy (MDMA) users compared to polydrug and drug-naive controls. Neuropsychopharmacology 31: 1562–73.

Morris LS, Kundu P, Baek K, et al. (2016) Jumping the Gun: Mapping Neural Correlates of Waiting Impulsivity and Relevance Across Alcohol Misuse. Biol Psychiatry 15: 499–507.

Nandam LS, Hester R, Wagner J, et al. (2011) Methylphenidate but not atomoxetine or citalopram modulates inhibitory control and response time variability. Biol Psychiatry 69: 902–4.

Nigg JT, Wong MM, Martel MM, et al. (2006) Poor response inhibition as a predictor of problem drinking and illicit drug use in adolescents at risk for alcoholism and other substance use disorders. J Am Acad Child Adolesc Psychiatry 45: 468–75.

Noreika V, Falter CM, Rubia K (2013) Timing deficits in attention-deficit/hyperactivity disorder (ADHD): evidence from neurocognitive and neuroimaging studies. Neuropsychologia 51: 235–66.

Oberlin BG, Albrecht DS, Herring CM, et al. (2015) Monetary discounting and ventral striatal dopamine receptor availability in nontreatment-seeking alcoholics and social drinkers. Psychopharmacology (Berl) 232: 2207–16.

Obeso I, Wilkinson L, Rodriguez-Oroz MC, Obeso JA, Jahanshahi M (2013) Bilateral stimulation of the subthalamic nucleus has differential effects on reactive and proactive inhibition and conflict-induced slowing in Parkinson's disease. Exp Brain Res 226: 451–62.

Oliveira FT, McDonald JJ, Goodman D (2007) Performance monitoring in the anterior cingulate is not all error related: expectancy deviation and the representation of action-outcome associations. J Cogn Neurosci 19: 1994–2004.

Perry JL, Larson EB, German JP, Madden GJ, Carroll ME (2005) Impulsivity (delay discounting) as a predictor of acquisition of IV cocaine self-administration in female rats. Psychopharmacology (Berl) 178: 193–201.

Perry JL, Nelson SE, Carroll ME (2008) Impulsive choice as a predictor of acquisition of IV cocaine self- administration and reinstatement of cocaine-seeking behavior in male and female rats. Exp Clin Psychopharmacol 16: 165–77.

Pine A, Shiner T, Seymour B, Dolan RJ (2010) Dopamine, time, and impulsivity in humans. J Neurosci 30: 8888–96.

Poulos CX, Le AD, Parker JL (1995) Impulsivity predicts individual susceptibility to high levels of alcohol self-administration. Behav Pharmacol 6: 810–14.

Quednow BB, Kuhn KU, Hoppe C, et al. (2007) Elevated impulsivity and impaired decision-making cognition in heavy users of MDMA ('Ecstasy'). Psychopharmacology (Berl) 189: 517–30.

Rae CL, Nombela C, Rodriguez PV, et al. (2016) Atomoxetine restores the response inhibition network in Parkinson's disease. Brain 139: 2235–48.

Robbins TW (2002) The 5-choice serial reaction time task: behavioural pharmacology and functional neurochemistry. Psychopharmacology (Berl) 163: 362–80.

Rubio G, Jimenez M, Rodriguez-Jimenez R, et al. (2008) The role of behavioral impulsivity in the development of alcohol dependence: a 4-year follow-up study. Alcohol Clin Exp Res 32: 1681–7.

Sanchez-Roige S, Baro V, Trick L, Pena-Oliver Y, Stephens DN, Duka T (2014) Exaggerated waiting impulsivity associated with human binge drinking, and high alcohol consumption in mice. Neuropsychopharmacology 39: 2919–27.

Scheffers MK, Coles MG (2000) Performance monitoring in a confusing world: error-related brain activity, judgments of response accuracy, and types of errors. Journal of experimental psychology Human perception and performance 26: 141–51.

Schel MA, Kuhn S, Brass M, Haggard P, Ridderinkhof KR, Crone EA (2014) Neural correlates of intentional and stimulus-driven inhibition: a comparison. Front Hum Neurosci 8: 27.

Smith JL, Mattick RP, Jamadar SD, Iredale JM (2014) Deficits in behavioural inhibition in substance abuse and addiction: a meta-analysis. Drug Alcohol Depend 145: 1–33.

Smittenaar P, Guitart-Masip M, Lutti A, Dolan RJ (2013) Preparing for selective inhibition within frontostriatal loops. J Neurosci 33: 18087–97.

Stern ER, Gonzalez R, Welsh RC, Taylor SF (2010) Updating beliefs for a decision: neural correlates of uncertainty and underconfidence. J Neurosci 30: 8032–41.

Tanaka SC, Doya K, Okada G, Ueda K, Okamoto Y, Yamawaki S (2004) Prediction of immediate and future rewards differentially recruits cortico-basal ganglia loops. Nat Neurosci 7: 887–93.

Tannock R, Schachar RJ, Carr RP, Chajczyk D, Logan GD (1989) Effects of methylphenidate on inhibitory control in hyperactive children. J Abnormal Child Psychol 17: 473–91.

Townshend JM, Kambouropoulos N, Griffin A, Hunt FJ, Milani RM (2014) Binge drinking, reflection impulsivity, and unplanned sexual behavior: impaired decision-making in young social drinkers. Alcohol Clin Exp Res 38: 1143–50.

Verbruggen F, Logan GD (2009) Models of response inhibition in the stop-signal and stop-change paradigms. Neurosci Biobehav Rev 33: 647–61.

Volans PJ (1976) Styles of decision-making and probability appraisal in selected obsessional and phobic patients. Br J Soc Clin Psychol 15: 305–17.

Voon V (2014) Models of Impulsivity with a Focus on Waiting Impulsivity: Translational Potential for Neuropsychiatric Disorders. Curr Addiction Rep 1: 281–8.

Voon V (2015) Cognitive biases in binge eating disorder: the hijacking of decision making. CNS Spectrums 20: 566–73.

Voon V, Chang-Webb YC, Morris LS, et al. (2016) Waiting Impulsivity: The Influence of Acute Methylphenidate and Feedback. Int J Neuropsychopharmacol 19: pyv074.

Voon V, Droux F, Morris L, et al. (2017a) Decisional impulsivity and the associative-limbic subthalamic nucleus in obsessive-compulsive disorder: stimulation and connectivity. Brain 140: 442–56.

Voon V, Irvine MA, Derbyshire K, et al. (2014) Measuring 'waiting' impulsivity in substance addictions and binge eating disorder in a novel analogue of rodent serial reaction time task. Biol Psychiatry 75: 148–55.

Voon V, Kubu C, Krack P, Houeto JL, Troster AI (2006) Deep brain stimulation: neuropsychological and neuropsychiatric issues. Mov Disord 21 Suppl 14: S305–27.

Voon V, Napier TC, Frank MJ, et al. (2017b) Impulse control disorders and levodopa-induced dyskinesias in Parkinson's disease: an update. Lancet Neurol 16: 238–50.

Weijers H-G, Wiesbeck GA, Böning J (2001) Reflection–impulsivity, personality and performance: A psychometric and validity study of the Matching Familiar Figures Test in detoxified alcoholics. Personality and Individual Differences 31: 731–54.

Weintraub D, Hoops S, Shea JA, et al. (2009) Validation of the questionnaire for impulsive-compulsive disorders in Parkinson's disease. Mov Disord 24: 1461–7.

Winstanley CA, Theobald DE, Cardinal RN, Robbins TW (2004a) Contrasting roles of basolateral amygdala and orbitofrontal cortex in impulsive choice. J Neurosci 24: 4718–22.

Winstanley CA, Theobald DE, Dalley JW, Glennon JC, Robbins TW (2004b) 5-HT2A and 5-HT2C receptor antagonists have opposing effects on a measure of impulsivity: interactions with global 5-HT depletion. Psychopharmacology (Berl) 176: 376–85.

Worbe Y, Savulich G, Voon V, Fernandez-Egea E, Robbins TW (2014) Serotonin depletion induces 'waiting impulsivity' on the human four-choice serial reaction time task: cross-species translational significance. Neuropsychopharmacology 39: 1519–26.

Ye Z, Altena E, Nombela C, et al. (2015) Improving response inhibition in Parkinson's disease with atomoxetine. Biol Psychiatry 77: 740–8.

Ye Z, Rae CL, Nombela C, et al. (2016) Predicting beneficial effects of atomoxetine and citalopram on response inhibition in Parkinson's disease with clinical and neuroimaging measures. Hum Brain Mapp 37: 1026–37.

Zandbelt BB, Vink M (2010) On the role of the striatum in response inhibition. PLoS One 5: e13848.

33

Neuropsychiatry of nutritional disorders

Nick Medford

Introduction

Globally, an estimated 800 million people are malnourished (Food and Agriculture Organization of the United Nations, 2019). Adding in those with specific nutritional deficiencies swells the number to over 2 billion. Malnutrition is thus a vast global public health problem and often occurs in the setting of other pressures and crises such as poverty, poor sanitation, war, and natural disasters.

There is a clear association between nutritional deficiency and neuropsychiatric disorder. In some cases, this takes the form of well-recognized syndromes such as Wernicke's encephalopathy (WE) in thiamine deficiency or subacute degeneration of the spinal cord in vitamin B12 deficiency. In many cases, however, the findings are of a more general nature—nutritional deficiency appears to be associated with increased rates of a range of neurological and psychiatric conditions, and the neuropsychiatric features described as being associated with some deficiencies are wide-ranging and non-specific.

Nutritional deficiency can arise in several ways, as superimposed upon pre-existing physical or psychiatric illness, or in the context of extreme deprivation, or in the wake of catastrophe such as war or famine. In all these settings, there will inevitably be numerous other variables that may contribute to neuropsychiatric morbidity, and this presents recurring difficulties of interpretation for studies of malnutrition in human populations. These are discussed in detail in this chapter.

Malnutrition

Malnutrition may be defined as 'a state of nutrition in which deficiency or excess of energy, protein, and other nutrients causes measurable adverse effects on tissue and body form and function, and clinical outcome' (Joosten and Hulst, 2008). It arises in two broad ways—through insufficient or inappropriate food intake, or through failure of digestion or metabolism which results in nutrients not being normally processed by the body despite ostensibly adequate intake.

The two major categories of general malnutrition are marasmus, caused by deficiency of calories, and kwashiorkor, caused by severe protein deficiency and marked by oedema, in contrast to thinning and wasting in marasmus. In practice, these overlap, and a mixed category of 'marasmic kwashiorkor' is also recognized. Malnutrition may be acute or chronic, or it may be both—it is not uncommon for acute states to be superimposed on chronic moderate malnutrition.

Early work applied a range of methods for identifying and classifying malnutrition, combining measurements based on weight and height (Gomez et al., 1956; Tanner, et al., 1965), clinical signs (in particular the presence of oedema), and anthropometric measures such as the chest:head ratio and arm circumference. The Waterlow criteria, first published in 1972, simplified matters by suggesting easily calculated measures based on weight and height, compared against population norms (Waterlow, 1972). Since 1999, the most commonly used scheme for classifying malnutrition has been a WHO scheme that uses the number of standard deviations (SDs) between observed and expected values for weight and height. SD scores of −2 and −3 below the mean are the cut-offs for moderate and severe malnutrition (World Health Organization, 1999).

In acute malnutrition due to starvation, changes in the CNS occur as a late consequence, invariably after other organs (e.g. heart, liver, pancreas) have suffered severe damage and compromise. A person who is weak and underfed may, unsurprisingly, exhibit lassitude and mood changes, and in severe acute malnutrition, delirium may occur. Where starvation is fatal, metabolic encephalopathy may precede coma and death. In cases where an individual has survived, and recovered from, a period of malnutrition, identifying specific neuropsychiatric sequelae is difficult for a number of reasons. If malnutrition is illness-related, i.e. it arises through a pre-existing pathology of digestion or metabolism, then it may be hard to disentangle the effects of malnutrition itself from those of the underlying condition. When malnutrition is not illness-related, similar difficulties of interpretation arise—a stark illustration is the fact that studies of World War 2 concentration camp survivors remain some of the largest studies of the long-term sequelae of malnutrition in the Western world. It is unsurprising that people who have lived through protracted horror may develop psychiatric problems in later life; it will be almost impossible to say with certainty how or whether those problems relate to nutrition. Indeed wherever malnutrition arises from forced privation, it is almost inevitable that this will be in a context that provides fertile ground for later psychopathology. Where malnutrition arises not from enforced starvation, but from self-directed behaviours, such as extreme restriction of food intake, then there will almost certainly be pre-existing psychological problems, and these may cloud the picture when trying to assess the eventual neuropsychiatric consequences of lack of nourishment.

There are, however, circumstances that are relatively free of such confounding variables. Klein et al. (1975) studied the sequelae of malnutrition caused by pyloric stenosis in 50 children aged 5–14, observing that this condition 'involves a brief period of starvation in early infancy, is unrelated to socioeconomic conditions, and is easily correctable'. They found that, compared to controls, children who had a history of pyloric stenosis had short-term memory and attentional deficits, and that the severity of these was related to the degree of starvation and weight loss at first presentation. Attentional deficits are also a key theme in the findings from the Barbadian Nutritional Study (BNS), a large 40-year longitudinal study of individuals who had normal birthweight followed by a period of moderate or severe protein–energy malnutrition in the first year of life (Galler, et al., 2012). A series of studies based on BNS data have shown attentional problems, including symptoms of ADHD, persisting into adolescence and middle age in individuals exposed to early childhood malnutrition (Galler & Ramsey 1989; Galler et al., 2012). Inattentive ADHD symptoms were more prominent than hyperactive symptoms, although the latter were nevertheless increased in comparison to controls. Other BNS data suggest a range of neuropsychiatric vulnerabilities in the malnutrition-exposed group—reduction in verbal and performance IQ, an increased rate of specific learning disability, and subtle motor deficits have all been identified in the study cohort (Galler et al., 1983a, 1983b, 1984). Comparable results come from a longitudinal study of Jamaican individuals identified as having growth retardation in the first 2 years of life. At age 17, this group had increased anxiety and depressive symptoms and raised hyperactivity, in comparison to controls (Walker et al., 2007).

These and other findings suggest that early malnutrition is a significant risk factor for long-term cognitive deficit and psychiatric morbidity. The question then arises—in those exposed to malnutrition, is it possible to identify specific patterns of neurological abnormality that relate to the psychological and cognitive features? The brain is apparently spared in all but the most severe malnutrition, with frank macroscopic changes in brain morphology therefore being uncommon. However, there are a number of ways in which malnutrition can compromise the essential processes of CNS development, without causing obvious macroscopic structural changes. Processes such as cortical differentiation, neuronal organization, neurotransmitter metabolism, and synaptic function, among many others, may be adversely affected by protein–energy malnutrition, but the resulting subtle anomalies may not be easy to study in human populations. Data from the BNS and other longitudinal studies suggest that there is a 'critical window' in early life, beginning prenatally and lasting until the end of the second year, when exposure to malnutrition is most likely to lead to later neurocognitive deficits, while malnutrition that occurs later in childhood is much less likely to produce long-term neuropsychiatric sequelae (Galler et al., 2005). However, this does not mean that malnutrition in later life will not affect the CNS. A study examining MRI brain changes in older adults found that malnutrition was associated with core white matter hyperintensities, compared to age-matched controls, but not with an increase in global or local brain atrophy (de van der Schueren et al., 2016). Smoking was associated

with malnutrition, so it seems plausible that at least some of the observed loci of signal hyperintensity reflect compromised cerebrovascular function, and that malnutrition probably acts as one of a number of factors that contribute to microstructural CNS damage in older patients. A recent study of participants in the BNS identified a range of epigenomic changes, many in genes previously linked to neuropsychiatric morbidity, in participants exposed to malnutrition in the first year of life (Peter et al., 2016; Szutorisz and Hurd, 2016). Some of these correlated with measures of attentional deficit in later life, and the authors argued that the long-term effects of early malnutrition are likely to be mediated by subtle, but persisting, epigenetic changes early in life.

Specific deficiencies

The general effects of chronic food shortage and under-nourishment involve deficiency of both macronutrients (proteins, fats, carbohydrates) and micronutrients (vitamins, minerals, trace elements). However, it is possible for more specific deficiencies to arise, either through dietary intake which, while providing adequate energy overall, is deficient in one or more particular nutrients or through pathological processes that compromise the digestion or metabolism of specific components of the diet.

The specific nutritional deficiencies most likely to be seen in neuropsychiatry services are those that result from deficiency of B vitamins, which are considered in the next sections, followed by other micronutrient deficiency (and, in a few cases, toxicity) syndromes.

Vitamin B1 (thiamine) deficiency

Thiamine is an essential factor for several co-enzymes involved in respiration. In the Western world, thiamine deficiency is most commonly seen in the context of alcohol dependence—alcohol compromises the absorption and utilization of thiamine, and many alcoholics also have poor dietary intake. The cumulative effect is a strong association between alcoholism and thiamine deficiency syndromes. It is a consistent finding that around 30% of alcoholics are deficient in thiamine, with some studies finding even higher rates (Abdou and Hazell, 2015). Thiamine deficiency also occurs in contexts other than alcoholism—commonly in malabsorption syndromes associated with malignancy (particularly of the oesophagus and stomach) and other GI conditions. The recent rise in obesity surgery has led to the finding that patients who have undergone bariatric surgery are at particular risk of developing thiamine deficiency in the post-operative period. The deficiency also occurs, but less commonly, in deliberate fasting (severe anorexia nervosa accounts for a subset of these cases), in conditions characterized by protracted vomiting, such as hyperemesis gravidarum, and in patients with severe renal disease who are undergoing dialysis (Latt and Dore, 2014).

Thiamine deficiency is associated with a number of overlapping syndromes, which collectively are known as beriberi. This term was in use at least as long ago as the eighteenth century; its origins remain uncertain (Arnold, 2010; Lanska, 2010). Weakness, lassitude, myalgia, and cardiac irregularities are common, and there are often severe neurological and cardiovascular manifestations. When cardiac failure is severe, oedema is prominent and the syndrome is known as 'wet beriberi', whereas in 'dry beriberi', there is little or no oedema and neurological features predominate. In particular, there is extensive peripheral nerve damage, leading to widespread sensorimotor deficits and muscle wasting. Fatigue and emotional disturbance are common in beriberi, but historical reviews do not identify any particular psychiatric syndrome associated with the condition (Lanska, 2010).

WE is a more specific consequence of thiamine deficiency, in which there is an acute neuropsychiatric crisis, originally said to comprise a triad of confusion, cerebellar ataxia, and ophthalmoplegia. However, it has become clear that the presentation is more variable than the classic description might suggest. Studies showed that only a small minority of cases manifest all three of the triad, and around a fifth have entirely different neuropsychiatric presentations, with none of the classic features (Galvin et al., 2010; Harper et al., 1986). WE pathology can be found in 1–3% of post-mortem brains, with much higher rates among alcoholics (Galvin et al., 2010; Harper, 1983), suggesting that it is far from being an uncommon condition. It seems certain that the diagnosis is often missed, partly due to the heterogeneity of presentation not being widely appreciated and partly because symptoms can mimic those of intoxication—a known habitual heavy drinker appearing drunk is unlikely to be a situation that strikes onlookers as a medical emergency. It is therefore important to maintain a high index of suspicion regarding the possibility of WE whenever acute neurological and/or psychiatric symptoms arise in a patient known to be at risk of thiamine deficiency (Galvin et al., 2010). If untreated, the condition will be fatal in 20–40% of cases (Day et al., 2013, Scalzo et al., 2015), while about 85% of survivors of alcoholic WE will progress to Korsakoff's syndrome (KS). For ease of expression, the two conditions are sometimes grouped together as Wernicke–Korsakoff syndrome (WKS). Outcomes are generally better in non-alcoholic WE, with lower fatality rates and progression to KS in 25–50% of survivors (Scalzo et al., 2015).

Lack of thiamine affects a range of cellular and humoral processes in ways that predispose to neuronal dysfunction and death, accompanied by inflammatory changes and diminished neurogenesis (Abdou and Hazell, 2015; Thomson et al., 2002). In alcoholic patients, these changes may be exacerbated by the effects of alcohol withdrawal. Certain brain areas are particularly vulnerable; the typical neuropathological findings in WE are oedema and microhaemorrhages in periventricular, midbrain, and brainstem structures. The most consistent finding is atrophy of the mammillary bodies, which was present in 75% of a large autopsy sample (Harper, 1983) and is often visible on MRI in living patients. However, normal mammillary body appearances do not necessarily refute the diagnosis, particularly in non-alcoholic WE where sparing is more common. Pathological changes are also often seen in the thalamus, the superior colliculi, the walls of the third ventricle, the pons and medulla, brainstem nuclei, and the cerebellar vermis. Damage to the anterior thalamic nuclei may be critical in the development of the chronic amnestic state seen in KS (Abdou and Hazell, 2015; Harper, 1983). It is likely that in alcoholic WE, there is often a chronic subclinical stage with slow accumulation of neural damage, on which acute WE is then superimposed—perhaps explaining the worse outcomes typically seen in alcoholic WE, compared to non-alcoholic WE.

Thiamine is poorly absorbed when given orally—even in healthy subjects, an oral dose of 100 mg only yields absorption of about 4.5

mg, and in alcoholics or those with malabsorption syndromes, this ratio will be even less favourable. Hence in patients with acute presentations suggestive of WE, parenteral high-dose thiamine should be given early, without waiting for investigations to be completed, although if biochemical testing for blood thiamine levels is available, blood should be taken before thiamine is administered. Dextrose infusion should be avoided in the acute stage, as carbohydrates can precipitate WE in thiamine deficiency. There are a number of published treatment guidelines supporting the use of very high doses of parenteral thiamine (e.g. 600–1500 mg per day, in divided doses)—it appears that creating a steep concentration gradient between plasma and the CNS is necessary to force sufficient thiamine across the BBB to avert permanent brain damage. In the UK, parenteral thiamine is given in the form of Pabrinex®, a combination of high-strength vitamins B and C. Oral thiamine should be prescribed for patients at risk of WE. Lower doses as part of a vitamin B complex preparation may be sufficient. The safety profile of thiamine is very good, so it is reasonable to have a low threshold for prescribing and for using high doses in acute presentations.

KS is the chronic amnestic state which is a frequent sequel of WE, and is presumably caused by damage to the vulnerable brain regions discussed earlier. Unlike WE, administration of thiamine appears to have no effect in treating the symptoms, which are essentially permanent and irreversible. However, it is often appropriate to continue oral thiamine to protect against further episodes of WE, particularly if the patient remains at risk of thiamine deficiency (e.g. if they are an alcoholic who continues to drink). KS is characterized by profound impairment in episodic memory, typically associated with confabulation, a feature that is often provoked by asking patients directly about their personal histories. KS is very difficult to treat, but some patients may make modest improvements over time in slow-stream rehabilitative settings, provided abstinence from alcohol is maintained (Kopelman, 2009). Even so, around a quarter of KS patients eventually require long-term nursing or residential care (Day et al., 2013).

Marchiafava–Bignami disease is a rare disorder that presents with acutely altered mental state and a range of sensorimotor disturbances. Neuroimaging shows characteristic lesions, characterized by demyelination and necrosis, in the corpus callosum. Other subcortical and, more rarely, cortical areas may also be affected. The pathophysiology is unclear, but the condition is probably related to thiamine deficiency. It occurs primarily in alcoholics and is often associated with low serum thiamine, and high-dose parenteral thiamine appears to be the best treatment. Outcomes are often poor. A recent review of published cases found that 15% died and around 40% were left with residual severe disability (Hillbom et al., 2014).

Vitamin B3 (niacin) deficiency

Niacin, or nicotinic acid, is an essential co-factor in many reactions involved in the catabolism of carbohydrates and proteins, and in anabolic reactions important for cell assembly. Deficiency leads to pellagra, a multisystem condition characterized by the 'three Ds': dermatitis, diarrhoea, and dementia. Sometimes a fourth D—death—is added to the list since, untreated, the condition is invariably fatal. It was widespread throughout Europe in the eighteenth and nineteenth centuries, and in the United States in the first decades of the twentieth century where it is estimated to have caused 3 million deaths. It had long been observed to be linked to a diet dependent on maize, which is low in niacin, in comparison to other grains, but for many years, it was thought that the connection with maize might involve some infectious agent. The role of niacin was only uncovered in the 1930s. Niacin fortification of food and changing dietary patterns have rendered it a rare condition in the Western world, although the diagnosis is still occasionally made in chronic alcoholics and others at risk of malnourishment. It can also occur as a complication of conditions affecting tryptophan metabolism (see below). There is some evidence that niacin deficiency is commoner in alcoholics than is generally appreciated. An autopsy series identified the typical neuropathological feature of swollen cells with chromatolysis (disintegration of intraneuronal Nissl bodies) in 20 cases from a sample of 74 chronic alcoholics, with only one case having been diagnosed during life (Ishii and Nishihara, 1981). The diagnosis is hard to make. Many cases lack photosensitive dermatitis, which is the most indicative feature, and the psychiatric features are far more variable than the standard 'dementia' descriptor would suggest, ranging from non-specific fatigue and dysphoria in subacute deficiency to acute psychiatric presentations characterized by confusion, bizarre behaviour, and memory impairment, sometimes accompanied by florid psychosis. Treatment is with high-dose niacin, and while the condition is now rare, it is advisable to prescribe for at-risk groups. In alcoholics presenting with acute alterations in mental state, high-dose vitamin B3 can be given as one of the constituents of Pabrinex® (see Vitamin B1 (thiamine) deficiency, p. 401).

Similar symptoms may occur in conditions where tryptophan metabolism is abnormal, since tryptophan is a precursor of niacin. This occurs most commonly in carcinoid syndrome. Hartnup disease is a rare autosomal recessive condition in which there is an abnormality of the tryptophan transporter gene, leading to a pellagra-like syndrome, often accompanied by cerebellar ataxia (Patel and Prabhu, 2008).

Vitamin B6 (pyridoxine)

Isolated vitamin B6 deficiency is unusual, as pyridoxine and its derivatives are present in many foods and the required daily intake is low, but it may occur in alcoholism, chronic renal failure, and other serious metabolic conditions. It may also occur in patients taking isoniazid or penicillamine. In malnourished children, pyridoxine deficiency is a recognized cause of treatment-refractory epilepsy, and this association has also been described in adults (Gerlach et al., 2011). It is consistently reported that seizures abate within minutes of administration of IV pyridoxine. Low B6 is also associated with polyneuropathy, although this tends to occur in the presence of multiple micronutrient deficiencies and the precise role of pyridoxine is uncertain (Ghavanini and Kimpinski, 2014).

Vitamin B6 has been explored as a possible treatment for tardive dyskinesia and other neurological side effects of antipsychotic medications, with some promising results (Lerner et al., 2007).

Vitamin B12 and folate (B9) deficiency

Vitamin B12 (cobalamin) is an essential co-factor in many metabolic pathways, often acting in concert with folate (vitamin B9). Both are crucial in the conversion of homocysteine to methionine, which is essential for the production of myelin. Cobalamin is also required for the production of tetrahydrofolate, which is involved in purine synthesis. Lack of tetrahydrofolate leads to reduced DNA and RNA synthesis and impaired erythrocyte production, leading to megaloblastic anaemia which is the hallmark of B12 deficiency—pernicious anaemia.

B12 and/or folate deficiency results primarily from a lack of dietary intake, although deficiency may also occur in GI disorders, as gut intrinsic factor is required for B12 absorption. Deficiency remains common, with prevalence studies finding rates in the adult population ranging from 2.7% in the United States to 31% in India. Even in developed countries, there is considerable variation, e.g. prevalence in Germany appears to be around six times that in the United States (McLean et al., 2008). Rates tend to be higher in the elderly, while surveys of women of childbearing age suggest that in the UK, around 12% are deficient in B12 and around 6% are deficient in folate (Sukumar et al., 2016). This is significant because folate deficiency in pregnancy is associated with neural tube defects in the developing fetus, and in many countries, folate supplementation during pregnancy is now recommended as standard.

Pernicious anaemia has been associated with a wide range of neuropsychiatric features. In infants, B12 deficiency may result from an inadequate early diet (including breastfeeding if the mother is herself B12-deficient) and may result in failure to thrive, hepatosplenomegaly, and delayed and disturbed CNS development, with subsequent hypotonia, weakness, and cognitive deficits (Black, 2008). In severe cases, there is brain atrophy.

In adults, particularly the elderly, pernicious anaemia is associated with atherosclerosis and neurological disturbance. Specific psychiatric effects are difficult to disentangle from symptoms of the associated anaemia, but there is evidence for a direct relationship between low B12 and depression, paranoid psychosis, and cognitive impairments (Zucker et al., 1981). Cognitive impairment may be relatively subtle but will tend to improve with appropriate B12 supplementation. Frank dementia is surprisingly rare. Although B12 deficiency is often cited as a cause of reversible dementia, published data suggest that it only accounts for around one in 10,000 cases of dementia (Harrison and Kopelman, 2011; Zucker et al., 1981). However, it is likely that B12 deficiency is under-recognized, particularly in elderly populations where serum cobalamin levels may be normal despite deficient tissue levels.

Neurological symptoms of B12 deficiency are also highly variable, but peripheral sensory changes (numbness and paraesthesiae) are common, and early loss of vibration sense is characteristic. *Subacute combined degeneration of the spinal cord* is a severe neurological manifestation in which there is progressive degeneration of the dorsal and lateral columns of the cord. This results in numbness, tingling, and weakness in the trunk and limbs and, if untreated, can progress to spasticity, paraplegia, and severe ataxia. Symptoms improve with B12 replacement, although more advanced cases may be left with residual symptoms and disability.

The gas nitrous oxide, used medically for pain relief, but also increasingly as a recreational drug, inactivates vitamin B12 and chronic use leads to low serum B12 levels and manifestations of deficiency. Its recent rise in popularity as a 'party drug' has led to a rise in cases, and subacute combined degeneration of the cord has been reported as a consequence of chronic nitrous oxide abuse (Mancke et al., 2016).

Folate deficiency

Folate deficiency in pregnancy is associated with neural tube defects in the developing fetus, such that folate supplementation in pregnancy is now a widespread public health recommendation. The deficiency is, however, commonest in the elderly. One large UK study found folate deficiency in 10% of the over 75s surveyed (Clarke et al., 2004). More generally, the prevalence rate of folate deficiency tends to be around half that of B12 deficiency (see Vitamin B12 and folate (B9) deficiency, p. 404). As folate acts in concert with B12 in many metabolic processes, there is considerable overlap in the clinical features of their deficiencies, although neurological features generally tend to be milder in folate deficiency. Conversely, folate deficiency is more strongly associated with depression, with one study finding deficiency in as many as 71% of elderly depressed adults (Reynolds, 1979). Large population-based surveys of nutritional status, however, have not generally found a close relationship between folate deficiency and depression. It appears that only a subset of folate-deficient patients develop neuropsychiatric symptoms.

The mechanisms by which folate is transported and utilized in the CNS are complex and influenced by genetic variables which are still being elucidated. The finding that genotype variants known to confer an increased risk of psychiatric disorder are associated with folate deficiency (Stover et al., 2017) suggests that genetic susceptibility to some psychiatric conditions may be related to subtle anomalies of folate metabolism in the CNS. Folate deficiency is also common in dementia, particularly in Alzheimer's-type dementia, and while it is unlikely to be the sole cause, it seems probable that it increases the vulnerability to neurodegeneration.

Related to this is the emerging concept of cerebral folate deficiency (CFD), in which there is an abnormally low folate level in the CNS despite normal serum levels. In normal circumstances, CNS folate levels are significantly higher than those in serum, but if the active transport of folate across the BBB malfunctions, the CNS can become folate-deficient without any lowering of serum levels. CFD in early life may result from autoimmunity to CNS folate receptors, and it has been argued that there are distinct autistic, spastic–ataxic, epileptic, and schizophrenic developmental CFD syndromes. This remains an emerging field, but there is evidence that folate supplementation, combined with corticosteroids and a milk-free diet, may be beneficial (Raemekers et al., 2016).

Vitamin A

Retinol (vitamin A) may be considered a prohormone—it is oxidized intracellularly to the active metabolite retinoic acid. In this form, it is important in the embryological development of the CNS. In adult life, it is involved in the regulation of gene transcription and expression, neurogenesis, and cell development and maintenance. It has a particular role in the development and maintenance of the structures of the eye, and globally vitamin A deficiency is the commonest cause of nutritional blindness.

There is evidence that abnormal vitamin A levels, or anomalies in its functions, are linked to neuropsychiatric disorders (Shearer et al., 2012). Low vitamin A is found commonly in AD and MCI, even when patients with evidence of general malnutrition are excluded (Rinaldi et al., 2003). It seems likely that vitamin A deficiency confers an increased vulnerability to Alzheimer's-type pathology. It is also possible to extrapolate findings from molecular neuroscience into a putative link between vitamin A and other conditions such as autism and schizophrenia, although this work remains at an early stage (Shearer et al., 2012). At present, most of the psychiatric literature on vitamin A is in the context of a possible link with depression, particularly in patients taking isotretinoin (an isomer of retinoic acid) for acne. There have been alarming published case reports of previously psychologically healthy patients, typically adolescents or young adults, becoming severely depressed during treatment with isotretinoin, including cases of completed suicide (Bremner et al., 2012). Studies that have investigated an association between isotretinoin and depression have returned mixed findings, but the largest and most rigorous studies have suggested that there is a small, but genuine, increased risk (Bremner et al., 2012). Fatigue is also commonly reported as a side effect of isotretinoin. Psychosis and impulsive aggression have been described, but rarely. Further evidence for a link between exogenous vitamin A and neuropsychiatric illness comes from the unusual condition of 'hypervitaminosis A' where excessive ingestion of the vitamin can lead to alterations in mental state (sometimes very acute) such as mood and sleep changes, lassitude, irritability, and confusion, often accompanied by headache (Silverman et al., 1987).

Vitamin C

Deficiency of vitamin C (ascorbic acid) causes scurvy, a once-dreaded condition characterized by connective tissue degeneration, leading to hyperkeratosis, severe joint and muscle pain, dental avulsion, oedema, and spontaneous haemorrhage. Fatigue and irritability, usually in the early stages, are the most commonly described mental state changes in historical reports. One recent review asserts that fatigue can be considered the first symptom of scurvy (Hirschmann and Raugi, 1999). In the developed world, scurvy is generally only encountered in the context of severe physical or mental illness, e.g. in states of advanced self-neglect associated with dementia. It is likely that vitamin C deficiency is underdiagnosed in these at-risk groups, but when it is identified, the multiple comorbidities make it difficult to attribute symptoms to a lack of vitamin C specifically. However, two recent case reports described patients with multiple health problems, including parkinsonism, which, in both cases, responded rapidly to high-dose parenteral vitamin C given after blood tests had shown low circulating levels (Noble et al., 2013; Wright et al., 2014). The authors argued that, alongside the classic acute presentations of scurvy, there may be a more insidious subacute neuropsychiatric form of the condition, characterized by fatigue, weakness, and extrapyramidal symptoms (Wright et al., 2014).

When vitamin C is administered parenterally, it is advisable to also administer parenteral zinc, as deficiency or abnormal metabolism of zinc often accompanies vitamin C deficiency.

Vitamin D and calcium

Worldwide, lack of vitamin D is the commonest vitamin deficiency. Even in developed countries, prevalence rates of 30–50% of the adult population have been reported, while in some developing countries, the majority have low vitamin D levels, particularly where there is little exposure to sunlight (required for dermal vitamin D synthesis) for climatic or cultural reasons (Holick, 2007). Many of those affected will have no obvious symptoms, but the deficiency is associated with a wide range of mental and physical conditions.

Neuropsychiatric disorders reported to be associated with vitamin D deficiency include schizophrenia, Parkinson's disease, and dementia (Wilkins et al., 2006). The precise relevance of vitamin D to these conditions remains unclear.

Vitamin D deficiency causes hypocalcaemia, and it is plausible that this mediates the CNS effects of the vitamin deficiency. It is of note that hypoparathyroidism, the commonest endocrine cause of hypocalcaemia, is strongly associated with neuropsychiatric disorders, particularly cognitive and intellectual decline. However, it is possible that some of these effects are due to a lack of parathyroid hormone itself, rather than of calcium.

Calcium deficiency can itself arise from poor dietary intake and is common in developing countries where the diet is cereal-based and low in dairy foods. A wide range of neurological symptoms have been reported in connection with hypocalcaemia, but the classic neurological presentation is a state of neuromuscular hyperexcitability characterized by spasm, tetany, and hyperreflexia. Many other symptoms have been reported, but they tend to reflect this same hyperexcitability, e.g. myoclonus, fasciculation. The most commonly reported psychiatric features are confusion and, in less acute cases, depression (Harrison and Kopelman, 2011). Magnesium deficiency (see Magnesium) can cause essentially identical presentations.

Vitamin E

'Vitamin E' is actually an umbrella term for a group of tocotrienol and tocopherol derivatives which are involved in maintaining the integrity of neuronal cell membranes and are thus neuroprotective. Low vitamin E levels have been found in the CSF of patients with AD, and α-tocopherol has been investigated as a possible AD pharmacotherapy, with equivocal results. While there is no evidence of any arrest in the disease process, there is evidence that it may slow some aspects of cognitive decline (Farina et al., 2017). A trial in AD associated with Down's syndrome found no benefit, compared to placebo (Sano et al., 2016). α-tocopherol has also been investigated as a treatment for antipsychotic-induced tardive dyskinesia. One study reporting positive results found that patients given α-tocopherol showed a significant reduction in dyskinetic symptoms, together with increased blood levels of superoxide dismutase (SOD), an enzyme involved in free radical metabolism and much studied in the context of motor neurone disease (Zhang et al., 2004).

Mineral and trace elements

Iron

Reported prevalence rates of iron deficiency (ID) are very high. In developed countries, it affects around 30% or more of the population; in some vulnerable populations, it is almost universal, and worldwide it is probably the commonest of all micronutrient deficiencies. Where psychiatric symptoms are reported, they tend to be symptoms related to microcytic anaemia of ID such as fatigue, weakness, and dysphoria. Like many other deficiencies, however, ID has been shown to be commoner than would be expected by chance in a range of neuropsychiatric conditions. One recent study found it to be associated with mood disorders and neurodevelopmental conditions such as autism and ADHD (Chen et al., 2013). Whether iron

plays any specific role in these disorders is currently unknown, and there are the familiar difficulties of interpretation. It may be that the psychiatric disorder predisposes to poor nutritional intake, rather than the other way round.

Iodine and selenium

Iodine deficiency is a major problem in those parts of the world where diet depends largely on crops grown in low-iodine soils. In adult life, iodine is essential for normal thyroid function and the deficiency usually presents as hypothyroidism with goitre. Iodine deficiency in pregnancy is associated with severe impairment of CNS development in the fetus due to reduced transplacental transfer of maternal thyroid hormone. Prenatal and infant iodine deficiency is the leading worldwide cause of preventable mental retardation and disrupted cognitive and motor development. Severe maternal deficiency leads to a characteristic syndrome in the child of short stature, spasticity, deaf-mutism, and mental retardation, often accompanied by hypothyroidism. Historically this syndrome was known as 'cretinism', a term still in use in some contemporary literature (Zimmermann, 2008). There appear to be two subtypes, dominated by either neurological or myxoedematous features, although these do overlap. Globally there is a major public health programme to combat deficiency by promoting the use of iodized table salt, and a coordinated international effort to monitor iodine availability and intake (Zimmermann, 2012).

Selenium deficiency often co-occurs with iodine deficiency and contributes to the hypothyroid symptoms. Outside this context, there is some evidence that low selenium may be associated with depression and anxiety (Benton, 1991) and a risk factor for the development of dementia (Killin et al., 2016), but the psychiatric associations of this deficiency are little studied.

Magnesium

Magnesium is involved in many metabolic processes. Within the CNS, it has a particular role in regulating the function of cell membrane ion channels. The symptoms of *hypomagnesaemia* mimic those of hypocalcaemia (see Vitamin D and calcium). *Hypermagnesaemia* is rare and usually occurs as an uncommon consequence of chronic kidney disease, rather than through excess nutritional intake. It can cause severe acute encephalopathy, with areflexia, flaccid paralysis, and decreased conscious level.

Zinc

The metabolism of zinc is closely related to that of vitamin C, and effects of zinc deficiency resemble those of scurvy, although the consequences of isolated zinc deficiency do not usually approach the severity of scurvy. Skin lesions, poor wound healing, and increased susceptibility to infectious disease remain the main features. However, a specific neurological syndrome related to zinc deficiency has also been described, dominated by abnormalities of smell and taste; the dysgeusia can become so unpleasant that patients avoid eating, leading to further pathologies. In prolonged zinc deficiency, other neuropsychiatric features, such as ataxia and hallucinations, may emerge (Henkin et al., 1971, 1975). Lack of zinc in infancy is associated with short stature and delayed motor development.

The finding that up to 50% of patients undergoing bariatric surgery for obesity are deficient in zinc preoperatively (Mahawar et al., 2017) suggests that mild, asymptomatic zinc deficiency is probably far commoner than previously realized, especially in patients with GI conditions predisposing to malabsorption.

Recently there has been interest in a possible role for zinc and other trace elements (e.g. copper, manganese, lithium) in anxiety disorders, and studies have reported various deficiencies and excesses found in association with generalized anxiety, panic disorder, and OCD. This research is in its infancy, and current findings are hard to interpret, but this may be an important area for future work (Mlyniec et al., 2017).

Conclusion

Nutritional deficiencies are strongly associated with neuropsychiatric conditions. In many cases, the processes through which these associations arise are far from clear, and the implications for understanding and treating clinical disorders are uncertain. Essential nutrients are involved in a great many vital biochemical pathways. Identifying the precise mechanism by which a particular vitamin or mineral deficiency predisposes to, say, mood disturbance will inevitably require a much greater understanding of the fine-grained molecular and cellular processes of the nervous system than is currently available. It may well be that as this understanding grows, nutritional factors will be seen as ever more central to neuropsychiatry and to other areas of medicine.

There is already a scattered literature suggesting that nutritional supplements can have a positive impact on neuropsychiatric symptoms. One recent meta-analysis concluded that there is now cumulative evidence that administration of B vitamins improves symptoms in schizophrenia (Firth et al., 2017). Currently, nutritional supplements are generally only prescribed when there is a known deficiency or risk thereof, but the widespread neurological and psychiatric associations of micronutrient deficiency suggest that carefully selected and targeted nutritional measures could have a much wider therapeutic role in neurology and psychiatry than is the case at present (Sarris et al., 2016). It seems very likely that the relationship between nutrition and the CNS and the implications of this relationship for neuropsychiatry will be a major field of research in the twenty-first century and have the potential to unlock new insights into the relationships between mind, brain, and body.

KEY LEARNING POINTS

- Malnutrition is a hugely extensive global health issue, with an estimated 800 million affected worldwide and almost 2 billion when those with specific nutritional deficiencies are taken into account.
- This chapter discusses the link between nutritional deficiency and neuropsychiatric disorder. In some cases, this can take the form of a clear cause and effect such as the prevalence of WE in those with thiamine deficiency. However, it is important to develop means to determine the relationship between malnutrition and neuropsychiatric disorders in general.
- It focuses firstly on malnutrition, exploring the cognitive and CNS changes in those who would be found malnourished by the Waterlow criteria, before moving on to specific deficiencies

and their associated neuropsychiatric presentations such as B6 (pyridoxine) and epilepsy or iron and neurodevelopmental disorders such as autism and ADHD.

REFERENCES

Abdou, E. and Hazell, A. S. (2015) Thiamine deficiency: an update of pathophysiologic mechanisms and future therapeutic considerations, *Neurochem Res*, 40(2), pp. 353–61.

Arnold, D. (2010) British India and the 'beriberi problem', 1798–1942, *Med Hist*, 54(3), pp. 295–314.

Benton, D. and Cook, R. (1991) The impact of selenium supplementation on mood, *Biol Psychiatry*, 29(11), pp. 1092–8.

Black, M. M. (2008) Effects of vitamin B12 and folate deficiency on brain development in children, *Food Nutr Bull*, 29(2 Suppl), pp. S126–31.

Bremner, J. D., Shearer, K. D., and McCaffery, P. J. (2012) Retinoic acid and affective disorders: the evidence for an association, *J Clin Psychiatry*, 73(1), pp. 37–50.

Chen, M. H., Su, T. P., Chen, Y. S., et al. (2013) Association between psychiatric disorders and iron deficiency anemia among children and adolescents: a nationwide population-based study, *BMC Psychiatry*, 13, pp. 161.

Clarke, R., Grimley Evans, J., Schneede, J., et al. (2004) Vitamin B12 and folate deficiency in later life, *Age Ageing*, 33(1), pp. 34–41.

De van der Schueren, M., Lonterman-Monasch, S., Wiesje, M., Kramer, M., Maier, A., and Muller, M. (2016) Malnutrition and risk of structural brain changes seen on magnetic resonance imaging of older adults. *J Am Geriatr Soc*, 64(12), pp. 2457–63.

Day, E., Bentham, P. W., Callaghan, R., Kuruvilla, T., and George, S. (2013) Thiamine for prevention and treatment of Wernicke-Korsakoff Syndrome in people who abuse alcohol. *Cochrane Database Syst Rev*, 7, CD004033.

Farina, N., Llewellyn, D., Isaac, M. G., and Tabet, N. (2017) Vitamin E for Alzheimer's dementia and mild cognitive impairment. *Cochrane Database Syst Rev*, 1, CD002854.

Food and Agriculture Organization of the United Nations. 2017. *The State of Food Security and Nutrition in the World 2017*. Available at: http://www.fao.org/state-of-food-security-nutrition/en/

Firth, J., Stubbs, B., Sarris, J., et al. (2017) The effects of vitamin and mineral supplementation on symptoms of schizophrenia: a systematic review and meta-analysis. *Psychol Med*, pp. 1–13.

Galler, J. R., Bryce, C. P., Zichlin, M. L., Fitzmaurice, G., Eaglesfield, G. D., and Waber, D. P. (2012) Infant malnutrition is associated with persisting attention deficits in middle adulthood. *J Nutr*, 142(4), pp. 788–94.

Galler, J. R. and Ramsey, F. (1989) A follow-up study of the influence of early malnutrition on development: behavior at home and at school. *J Am Acad Child Adolesc Psychiatry*, 28(2), pp. 254–61.

Galler, J. R., Ramsey, F., and Solimano, G. (1984) The influence of early malnutrition on subsequent behavioral development III. Learning disabilities as a sequel to malnutrition. *Pediatr Res*, 18(4), pp. 309–13.

Galler, J. R., Ramsey, F., Solimano, G., and Lowell, W. E. (1983a) 'The influence of early malnutrition on subsequent behavioral development. II. Classroom behavior. *J Am Acad Child Psychiatry*, 22(1), pp. 16–22.

Galler, J. R., Ramsey, F., Solimano, G., Lowell, W. E., and Mason, E. (1983b) 'The influence of early malnutrition on subsequent behavioral development. I. Degree of impairment in intellectual performance. *J Am Acad Child Psychiatry,* 22(1), pp. 8–15.

Galler, J. R., Waber, D., Harrison, R., and Ramsey, F. (2005) Behavioral effects of childhood malnutrition. *Am J Psychiatry,* 162(9), pp. 1760–1.

Galvin, R., Bråthen, G., Ivashynka, A., et al. (2010) EFNS guidelines for diagnosis, therapy and prevention of Wernicke encephalopathy. *Eur J Neurol,* 17(12), pp. 1408–18.

Gerlach, A. T., Thomas, S., Stawicki, S. P., Whitmill, M. L., Steinberg, S. M., and Cook, C. H. (2011) Vitamin B6 deficiency: a potential cause of refractory seizures in adults. *J Parenter Enteral Nutr,* 35(2), pp. 272–5.

Ghavanini, A. A. and Kimpinski, K. (2014) Revisiting the evidence for neuropathy caused by pyridoxine deficiency and excess. *J Clin Neuromuscul Dis,* 16(1), pp. 25–31.

Gomez, F., Galvan, R. R., Frenk, S., Munoz, J. C., Chavez, R., and Vazquez, J. (1956) Mortality in second and third degree malnutrition. *J Trop Pediatr (Lond),* 2(2), pp. 77–83.

Harper, C. (1983) The incidence of Wernicke's encephalopathy in Australia--a neuropathological study of 131 cases. *J Neurol Neurosurg Psychiatry,* 46(7), pp. 593–8.

Harper, C. G., Giles, M., and Finlay-Jones, R. (1986) Clinical signs in the Wernicke-Korsakoff complex: a retrospective analysis of 131 cases diagnosed at necropsy. *J Neurol Neurosurg Psychiatry,* 49(4), pp. 341–5.

Harrison, N.A. and Kopelman, M.D (2011) Endocrine diseases and metabolic disorders. In: David A.S, Fleminger, S., Kopelman, M.D., Lovestone, S., Mellers, J. (eds.) *Lishman's Organic Psychiatry,* fourth ed. Wiley-Blackwell.

Henkin, R., Patten, B., Re, P., and Bronzert, D. (1975) A syndrome of acute zinc loss, *Arch Neurol,* 32, pp. 745–51.

Henkin, R., Schechter, P., Hoyle, R., and Mattern, C. (1971) Idiopathic hypogeusia with dysgeusia, hyposmia, and dysosmia. A new syndrome. *JAMA,* 217, pp. 434–40.

Hillbom, M., Saloheimo, P., Fujioka, S., Wszolek, Z., Juvela, S., and Leone, M. (2014) Diagnosis and management of Marchiafava-Bignami disease: a review of CT/MRI confirmed cases. *J Neurol Neurosurg Psychiatry,* 85(2), pp 168–73.

Hirschmann, J. V. and Raugi, G. J. (1999) Adult scurvy, *J Am Acad Dermatol,* 41(6), pp. 895–906.

Holick, M. F. (2007) Vitamin D deficiency. *N Engl J Med,* 357(3), pp. 266–81.

Ishii, N. and Nishihara, Y. (1981) Pellagra among chronic alcoholics: clinical and pathological study of 20 necropsy cases. *J Neurol Neurosurg Psychiatry,* 4(3), pp. 209–15.

Joosten, K. F. and Hulst, J. M. (2008) Prevalence of malnutrition in pediatric hospital patients. *Curr Opin Pediatr,* 20(5), pp. 590–6.

Killin, L. O., Starr, J. M., Shiue, I. J., and Russ, T. C. (2016) Environmental risk factors for dementia: a systematic review. *BMC Geriatr,* 16(1), pp. 175.

Klein, P. S., Forbes, G. B., and Nader, P. R. (1975) Effects of starvation in infancy (pyloric stenosis) on subsequent learning abilities. *J Pediatr,* 87(1), pp. 8–15.

Kopelman, M. D., Thomson, A. D., Guerrini, I., and Marshall, E. J. (2009) The Korsakoff syndrome: clinical aspects, psychology and treatment. *Alcohol Alcohol,* 44(2), pp. 148–54.

Lanska, D. J. (2010) Chapter 30: historical aspects of the major neurological vitamin deficiency disorders: the water-soluble B vitamins. *Handb Clin Neurol,* 95, pp. 445–76.

Latt, N. and Dore, G. (2014) Thiamine in the treatment of Wernicke encephalopathy in patients with alcohol use disorders. *Intern Med J,* 44(9), pp. 911–15.

Lerner, V., Miodownik, C., Kaptsan, A., et al. (2007) Vitamin B6 treatment for tardive dyskinesia: a randomized, double-blind, placebo-controlled, crossover study. *J Clin Psychiatry,* 68(11), pp. 1648–54.

Mahawar K., Bhaskar A., Bindal, V., et al. (2017) Zinc deficiency after gastric bypass for morbid obesity: a systematic review, *Obes Surg,* 27, pp. 522–9.

Mancke, F., Kaklauskaitė, G., Kollmer, J., and Weiler, M. (2016) Psychiatric comorbidities in a young man with subacute myelopathy induced by abusive nitrous oxide consumption: a case report. *Subst Abuse Rehabil,* 7, pp. 155–9.

McLean, E., de Benoist, B., and Allen, L. H. (2008) Review of the magnitude of folate and vitamin B12 deficiencies worldwide. *Food Nutr Bull,* 29(2 Suppl), pp. S38–51.

Młyniec, K., Gaweł, M., Doboszewska, U., Starowicz, G., and Nowak, G. (2017) The Role of Elements in Anxiety. *Vitam Horm,* 103, pp. 295–326.

Noble, M., Healey, C. S., McDougal-Chukwumah, L. D., and Brown, T. M. (2013) Old disease, new look? A first report of parkinsonism due to scurvy, and of refeeding-induced worsening of scurvy. *Psychosomatics,* 54(3), pp. 277–83.

Patel, A., and Prabhu, A. (2008) Hartnup disease, *Indian J Dermatol,* 53(1), pp 31–2.

Peter, C. J., Fischer, L. K., Kundakovic, M., et al. (2016) DNA Methylation Signatures of Early Childhood Malnutrition Associated With Impairments in Attention and Cognition. *Biol Psychiatry,* 80(10), pp. 765–74.

Raemekers, V., Sequeira, J., and Quadros, E (2016). The basis for folinic acid in neuropsychiatric disorders. *Biochimie,* 126, pp. 79–90.

Reynolds, E. H., and Botez, M. I. (1979) *Folic Acid in Neurology, Psychiatry and Internal Medicine.* Raven Press: New York, NY.

Rinaldi, P., Polidori, M., Metastasio, A., et al. (2003). Plasma antioxidants are similarly depleted in mild cognitive impairment and in Alzheimer's disease. *Neurobiol Aging,* 24: 915–19.

Sano, M., Aisen, P. S., Andrews, H. F., et al. (2016) Vitamin E in aging persons with Down syndrome: A randomized, placebo-controlled clinical trial. *Neurology,* 86(22), pp. 2071–6.

Sarris, J., Murphy, J., Mischoulon, D., et al. (2016) Adjunctive Nutraceuticals for Depression: A Systematic Review and Meta-Analyses. *Am J Psychiatry,* 173(6), pp. 575–87.

Scalzo, S. J., Bowden, S. C., Ambrose, M. L., Whelan, G., and Cook, M. J. (2015) Wernicke-Korsakoff syndrome not related to alcohol use: a systematic review, *J Neurol Neurosurg Psychiatry,* 86(12), pp. 1362–8.

Shearer, K. D., Stoney, P. N., Morgan, P. J., and McCaffery, P. J. (2012) A vitamin for the brain. *Trends Neurosci,* 35(12), pp. 733–41.

Silverman, A. K., Ellis, C. N., and Voorhees, J. J. (1987) Hypervitaminosis A syndrome: a paradigm of retinoid side effects. *J Am Acad Dermatol,* 16(5 Pt 1), pp. 1027–39.

Stover, P. J., Durga, J., and Field, M. S. (2017) Folate nutrition and blood-brain barrier dysfunction. *Curr Opin Biotechnol,* 44, pp. 146–52.

Sukumar, N., Adaikalakoteswari, A., Venkataraman, H., Maheswaran, H., and Saravanan, P. (2016) Vitamin B12 status in women of childbearing age in the UK and its relationship with national nutrient intake guidelines: results from two National Diet and Nutrition Surveys. *BMJ Open,* 6(8), pp. e011247.

Szutorisz, H. and Hurd, Y. L. (2016) Feeding the Developing Brain: The Persistent Epigenetic Effects of Early Life Malnutrition. *Biol Psychiatry,* 80(10), pp. 730–2.

Tanner, J. M. (1965) 'Nature and nurture'. In relation to growth and development. *R Inst Public Health Hyg J,* 28(10), pp. 280–1.

Thomson, A. D., Cook, C. C., Touquet, R., and Henry, J. A.; Royal College of Physicians. (2002) The Royal College of Physicians report on alcohol: guidelines for managing Wernicke's encephalopathy in the accident and Emergency Department, *Alcohol Alcohol,* 37(6), pp. 513–21.

Walker, S.P., Chang, S.M., Powell, C.A., Simonoff, E., and Grantham-McGregor, S.M. (2007) Early childhood stunting is associated with poor psychological functioning in late adolescence and effects are reduced by psychosocial stimulation. *J Nutr,* 137, pp. 2464–9.

Waterlow, J. C. (1972) Classification and definition of protein-calorie malnutrition. *Br Med J,* 3(5826), pp. 566–9.

Wilkins, C. H., Sheline, Y. I., Roe, C. M., Birge, S. J., and Morris, J. C. (2006) Vitamin D deficiency is associated with low mood and worse cognitive performance in older adults. *Am J Geriatr Psychiatry,* 14(12), pp. 1032–40.

World Health Organization. (1999) *Management of severe malnutrition: a manual for physicians and other senior health workers.* World Health Organization.

Wright, A.D., Stevens, E., Ali, M., Carroll, D., and Brown, T. (2014) The neuropsychiatry of scurvy. *Psychosomatics* 55, pp. 179–85.

Zhang, X.Y., Zhou, D., Cao, L. Xu, C., and Wu, G. (2004) The effect of vitamin E treatment on tardive dyskinesia and blood superoxide dismutase: a double-blind placebo-controlled trial. *J Clin Psychoparmacol,* 24(1), pp. 83–6.

Zimmermann, M. B. (2008) Research on iodine deficiency and goitre in the 19th and early 20th centuries. *J Nutr,* 138(11), pp. 2060–3.

Zimmermann, M. B. (2012) The effects of iodine deficiency in pregnancy and infancy. *Paediatr Perinat Epidemiol,* 26 Suppl 1, pp. 108–17.

Zucker, D. K., Livingston, R. L., Nakra, R., and Clayton, P. J. (1981) B12 deficiency and psychiatric disorders: case report and literature review. *Biol Psychiatry,* 16(2), pp. 197–205.

34

ADHD in adults

Stefanos Maltezos, Susannah Whitwell, and Philip Asherson

Definition of ADHD

ADHD is a neurodevelopmental disorder characterized by pervasive and impairing levels of inattention and/or hyperactivity–impulsivity. Reliable operationalized diagnostic criteria for ADHD were established in the third edition of the *Diagnostic and Statistical Manual of Mental Disorders* (DSM) in 1980 and have undergone several developments since that time. The condition is currently classified as a neurodevelopmental disorder under both the International Classification of Disease, eleventh revision (ICD-11) (World Health Organization, 2020) and the fifth edition of the DSM (American Psychiatric Association, 2013).

Both DSM and ICD provide diagnostic frameworks for ADHD (see Table 34.1). The DSM classification is more widely used by adult psychiatrists, as it allows for the diagnosis of ADHD in the presence of comorbid disorders and captures a broader group of adults impaired by ADHD symptoms, which fits more closely to clinical practice. The ICD-10 term for ADHD is hyperkinetic disorder, which reflects a more restricted definition, with severe symptoms and impairments in all three domains of inattention, hyperactivity, and impulsivity. Adults meeting hyperkinetic criteria represent a particular severe subgroup of adults with ADHD (National Institute for Health and Care Excellence, 2008).

In the new ICD-11 criteria, ADHD has replaced the term hyperkinetic disorder and has been moved to the grouping of neurodevelopmental disorders because of its developmental onset, characteristic disturbances in intellectual, motor and social functions, and common co-occurrence with other neurodevelopmental disorders (Reed et al., 2019). The criteria are closely similar to DSM-5 but not so clearly operationalized.

The DSM-5 criteria for ADHD recognize the clinical heterogeneity of ADHD by describing three different clinical presentations, depending on the balance of inattentive and hyperactive–impulsive symptoms. Under DSM-IV, these were known as the predominantly inattentive, predominantly hyperactive–impulsive, and combined subtypes. However, under DSM-5, the subtypes are described as clinical presentations in recognition that they are not stable throughout development and can change over time. A typical case of ADHD may present with predominantly hyperactive–impulsive symptoms during infancy, combined symptoms during childhood, and predominantly inattentive symptoms as an adult.

In the development of the DSM-5 criteria, several important changes were made to the previous DSM-IV definition, including a greater focus on the diagnosis in adults. Age-appropriate descriptions of ADHD symptoms were provided that better reflect the expression of the disorder in adults. The age of onset criterion changed from some symptoms and impairments before the age of 7 to several symptoms before the age of 12. The number of symptoms needed to reach the threshold for diagnosis was reduced from six to five in adulthood. The criterion for significant impairment was extended

Table 34.1 Summary of diagnostic criteria in DSM-5 and ICD-10

	DSM-5: attention-deficit/hyperactivity disorder	ICD-10: hyperkinetic disorder
Subtypes or presentations	Combined, predominantly inattentive, or predominantly hyperactive–impulsive presentation. ADHD in partial remission	Inattention and hyperactivity must both be present in two or more situations
Symptoms in adulthood	Five or more inattentive and/or hyperactive/impulsive symptoms	Six or more symptoms of inattention, three or more symptoms of overactivity, and one or more symptoms of impulsivity must all be present
Symptoms in childhood	Several symptoms by age 12	Characteristic behavioural problems present before age 6
Situational pervasiveness	Present in two or more settings	Present in two or more settings
Impairment	Symptoms interfere with, or reduce the quality of, social, academic, or occupational functioning	Impairment in all three symptom domains present in two or more settings
Comorbidity	Symptoms do not occur exclusively during the course of schizophrenia or another psychotic disorder and are not better explained by another mental disorder	Other comorbid conditions, e.g. mood and anxiety disorders, are exclusion criteria

Source data from: *Diagnostic and Statistical Manual of Mental Disorders*, 5th Edition, 2013, American Psychiatric Association; *International Classification of Diseases*, 10th editon. World Health Organization.

from social, occupational, or educational functioning to include reduction in the quality of these activities. Finally, the diagnosis was allowed in the presence of co-occurring autism spectrum disorder (ASD), which was previously an exclusion criterion. This is in line with the reconceptualization of ADHD as a neurodevelopmental disorder, rather than a disruptive behavioural disorder and the recognition that ADHD and ASD commonly co-occur. These changes will increase the prevalence of adult ADHD to some extent, since there is no longer a requirement for impairment from symptoms during childhood, the age of onset has been increased, and the number of symptoms required to reach the threshold has been decreased. However, both the earlier DSM-IV and DSM-5 allowed for the possibility that adult ADHD can be diagnosed in individuals with subthreshold ADHD during childhood.

The rationale for relaxing the age of onset criterion is that individuals giving a retrospective account of childhood behaviour are often unable to provide an accurate account of symptoms and impairments below the age of 12 years. Furthermore, the age of onset criterion was found to have no predictive value in terms of course, outcome, and clinical response. In addition, it is known that children with a high degree of external 'scaffolding', e.g. a highly structured home or school environment, or a high IQ may not experience impairment due to ADHD symptoms until they are older than the previously established age of onset. This led to underdiagnosis of cases reporting significant impairment from ADHD symptoms later in life.

More recently, the possibility of adult-onset forms of ADHD has been raised, with findings from longitudinal population samples suggesting that ADHD symptoms in adults do not always reflect a childhood-onset neurodevelopmental disorder (Agnew-Blais et al., 2016; Caye et al., 2016; Moffitt et al., 2015). A report on 1037 subjects born in Dunedin, New Zealand, revealed that prevalence rates of childhood and adulthood ADHD were in accordance with estimates from the literature—around 6% in children and 3% in adults (Moffitt et al., 2015). However, 87% of those qualifying for a diagnosis of adult ADHD, when the age of onset criterion was ignored, did not meet the criteria for prior childhood ADHD. The childhood- and adulthood-onset groups both had similar levels of symptoms and impairments, indicating that both were equally valid in terms of their need for diagnosis and treatment. However, only the childhood-onset group had cognitive impairments both as children and adults and were predicted by a polygenic risk score derived from a childhood ADHD discovery sample, suggesting that the adult-onset cases might not have the typical neurodevelopmental form of ADHD. However, the interpretation that these studies indicated most adults do not have the typical neurodevelopmental form of ADHD has been challenged (Asherson et al., 2016; Faraone and Biederman, 2016). Although similar findings were reported in further population follow-up samples, these only included follow-up to young adulthood (Agnew-Blais et al., 2016; Caye et al., 2016; Cooper et al., 2018; Sibley et al., 2018). Overall these studies concluded that more than half of young adults meeting the current criteria for ADHD would not have met full criteria as children, although most (but not all) would have had subthreshold symptoms. Furthermore, in most cases, age of onset was between 12 and 16 years. Currently, the status of adult-onset forms of ADHD in clinical practice remains unclear. However, what is certain is that not all cases of ADHD present with above-threshold symptoms and impairments in childhood, in line with the DSM-5 requirement for

'several' symptoms, but not necessarily impairment, before the age of 12 years.

Epidemiology

The estimated prevalence of ADHD from meta-analytic studies of cross-sectional surveys ranges from 2.5% to 3.4% (Fayyad et al., 2007; Simon et al., 2009). In children, the world prevalence is estimated to lie between 5% and 6% (Polanczyk et al., 2007; Willcutt, 2012). Follow-up studies of children with ADHD have given varying rates of persistence in young adulthood, reflecting differences in the baseline characteristics and methods of diagnosis. The most cited study is a meta-analysis based on ten follow-up samples that found that 15% retained the full diagnostic criteria by the age of 25 years, with a further 50% meeting subthreshold criteria with persistence of ADHD symptoms causing continued impairments (Faraone et al., 2006). Recent follow-up studies of European children with DSM-IV combined-type ADHD recruited from child and adolescent mental health services reported far higher persistence rates for the full diagnosis of around 80% (Cheung et al., 2016; Van Lieshout et al., 2016). The predictors of remission and persistence are not well understood. High general cognitive ability appears to be a protective factor, predicting a higher rate of remission, while the severity of ADHD, occurrence of comorbidity, exposure to adversity, and family history of ADHD are risk factors for persistence (Cheung et al., 2016; Faraone et al., 2015). It is also likely that individual differences in brain maturational processes linked to genetic factors play a role (Larsson et al., 2013).

Estimates of prevalence rates are affected by heterogeneity in assessment methods and diagnostic methods adopted in different studies. However, there is no evidence worldwide of an increase in the real prevalence of ADHD over the past three decades or of variability by geographical location (Polanczyk et al., 2007, 2014). In children and adolescents, ADHD predominantly affects males, exhibiting a male-to-female gender ratio in the order of 3–4:1 in epidemiological studies, and 7–8:1 in clinical studies (Biederman et al., 2005). In adults, the differences in prevalence and diagnostic rates according to gender become far less skewed. Recent studies have suggested that despite different symptom profiles and comorbidities, men and women have similar rates of current ADHD and of risky behaviours associated with the disorder (Cortese et al., 2016). The reduction in gender ratio differences with age is likely to reflect, at least in part, referral biases among treatment-seeking patients. Girls may show less disruptive behavioural problems than boys during childhood and are less likely to be referred for this reason, while emotional instability and mood symptoms are common in adults with ADHD and women are more likely to seek help for mental health problems than men.

Aetiology

ADHD tends to run in families, with a 5- to 10-fold increased risk to first-degree relatives of a child or parent with ADHD (Faraone et al., 2000; Mulligan et al., 2008). Heritability is estimated to be around 70–80% in both children and adults (Asherson and Gurling, 2012). Environmental risks reside in the non-shared familial environment or may act through gene–environment interactions (Faraone et al., 2015). Although ADHD is a categorical diagnosis, numerous studies found that ADHD reflects the extreme and impairing tail of one or more heritable quantitative traits (Mulligan et al., 2008). These include inattention, hyperactivity–impulsivity, and emotional dysregulation, which are each likely to reflect the effects of differing underlying neural and cognitive mechanisms.

The disorder is influenced by stable genetic effects that explain the continuity of the disorder throughout the lifespan, as well as new emerging genetic influences at different developmental stages. Genes therefore contribute to the onset, persistence, and remission of ADHD, presumably via stable neurobiological deficits, as well as maturational or compensatory processes influencing development (Faraone et al., 2015). Genetic influences on ADHD are shared with several other psychopathological traits and disorders, explaining their co-occurrence with ADHD, including emotional instability, specific and general learning difficulties, mood disorders, and autism (Asherson and Gurling, 2012). The specific genes involved in risk for ADHD are currently under intense investigation. At the time of writing, candidate gene studies and GWAS have identified several independent genetic loci, including genes involved in neuro-transmission, and neurodevelopmental processes including dopamine, noradrenaline, serotonin, and neurite outgrowth systems.

Environmental risks are also likely to play a role (Banerjee et al., 2007). Acquired risks associated with ADHD include pre- and perinatal factors, such as low birthweight and prematurity, and exposure to environmental toxins such as organophosphate pesticides, polychlorinated biphenyls, and lead. Severe and early deprivation has been shown to increase the risk for ADHD and is related to persistence into adulthood, while hostile parenting style appears to increase the risk for ADHD during childhood (Harold et al., 2013). Recent findings of adult-onset forms of ADHD have raised the possibility that while the commonest forms of ADHD reflect an early-onset neurodevelopmental disorder, there may be later-onset acquired forms of the ADHD syndrome (Asherson et al., 2016). No specific environmental causes of ADHD that can be targeted for the treatment of adult ADHD have been identified. Non-pharmacological treatments therefore currently focus on improved understanding and behavioural adaptations to the disorder.

ADHD is associated with a wide range of cognitive and neural deficits, implicating several underlying neurobiological processes. However, discerning the critical neural systems that lead directly to ADHD symptoms and impairments requires further investigation. Cognitive impairments are seen in multiple domains, including executive function deficits such as visuospatial and verbal working memory, inhibitory control, vigilance, and planning deficits. This has led some to view ADHD as primarily an executive control deficit disorder. However, impairments are also seen in multiple other domains, including processing speed and response variability, arousal/activation, and reward processing deficits. Although most ADHD patients show deficits in one or two domains, some have no deficits and others show deficits in all domains (Coghill et al., 2005; Johnson et al., 2009).

Functional and structural neuroimaging studies reflect the neurobiological heterogeneity of ADHD (Castellanos and Proal, 2012; Posner et al., 2014b). fMRI studies using inhibitory control, working memory, and attentional tasks have documented under-activation of fronto-striatal, frontoparietal, and ventral attention networks, which support goal-directed executive processes and attentional reorienting to external stimuli. Reward-processing

paradigms show reduced activation of the ventral striatum when anticipating rewards. Resting-state MRI studies find that ADHD is associated with reduced or absent anti-correlations between the default mode network (DMN) and the cognitive control network, lower connectivity within the DMN itself, and lower connectivity within the cognitive and motivational loops of the fronto-striatal circuits. Structural brain changes seen in ADHD include delayed maturation of the cerebral cortex, cortical thinning (superior frontal cortex, precentral cortex, inferior and superior parietal cortices, temporal pole, and medial temporal cortex), and cortical thickening (pre-supplementary motor area, somatosensory cortex, and occipital cortex). Basal ganglia volumes are smaller in ADHD, compared to controls, throughout development. In contrast, for ventral striatal surfaces, controls showed surface area expansion with age, whereas ADHD patients experienced progressive contraction of the surface, potentially explaining abnormal processing of reward in ADHD.

The wide range of cognitive and neural impairments associated with ADHD has led to the suggestion that ADHD is a heterogenous neurodevelopmental syndrome, reflecting abnormalities within several different systems. One prominent hypothesis is that two main systems might be involved: executive control and preparation-vigilance systems. ADHD might reflect interactions between these processes through development with persistence and remission reflecting individual differences in maturation processes within these systems. In our own work, we conducted a 6-year follow-up study of 110 young people with childhood DSM-IV combined-type ADHD and 169 controls using cognitive and EEG data. ADHD persisters differed from remitters on preparation-vigilance measures, but not on executive control measures (Cheung et al., 2015), suggesting that the preparation-vigilance measures reflect markers of remission that improve, alongside ADHD symptoms. As such, they might reflect malleable processes that can be targeted for the prevention of long-term persistence of the disorder. High IQ also appeared to play a role in reducing the risk for persistence of ADHD into young adulthood.

Clinical presentation of ADHD in adults

A list of ADHD symptoms with age-appropriate descriptions for adults is listed in Table 34.2. The symptoms of ADHD persist from childhood into adulthood in the majority of cases, either as the full-blown condition or in partial remission with persistence of subthreshold levels of symptoms still leading to impairment (Asherson et al., 2016). There is a general tendency for the hyperactive–impulsive symptoms to reduce, so that for many adults, it is the inattentive problems that cause the greatest levels of impairments. However, when hyperactivity–impulsivity does persist into adulthood, it can be particularly impairing, often being seen in the more severe cases with co-occurring substance abuse or forensic problems. Symptoms of emotional dysregulation, such as frequent irritability, frustration, and anger, are often seen to co-occur in adults with ADHD and are an independent source of impairment (Barkley and Fischer, 2010; Skirrow and Asherson, 2013).

For many adults, inattention is the greatest source of impairment. Common problems include difficulty in sustaining attention on tasks that lack inherent salience or immediate reward. One of the characteristic features of attention control in ADHD is the ability

Table 34.2 Age-appropriate descriptions of ADHD symptoms in adults

Inattention symptoms	Hyperactive-impulsive symptoms
Often fails to give close attention to detail: difficulty remembering where they put things. In work, this may lead to costly errors. Tasks that require detail and are tedious (e.g. income tax returns) become very stressful. This may include overly perfectionistic and rigid behaviour and needing too much time for tasks involving details in order to prevent forgetting any of them	**Fidgets with hands or feet:** this item may be observed, but it is also useful to ask about this. Fidgeting may include picking their fingers, shaking their knees, tapping their hands or feet, and changing position. Fidgeting is most likely to be observed while waiting in the waiting area of the clinic
Often has difficulty sustaining attention: inability to complete tasks such as tidying a room or mowing the lawn, without forgetting the objective and starting something else. Inability to persist with boring jobs. Inability to sustain sufficient attention to read a book that is not of special interest, although there is no reading disorder. Inability to keep accounts, write letters, or pay bills. Attention, however, often can be sustained during exciting, new, or interesting activities like using the Internet, chatting, computer games, etc. This does not exclude the criterion when boring activities are not completed	**Leaves seat in situations in which remaining seated is usual:** adults may be restless. For example, frustrated with dinners out in restaurants, unable to sit during conversations, meetings, and conferences. This may also manifest as a strong internal feeling of restlessness when waiting
Often does not seem to listen when spoken to: adults receive complaints that they do not listen and that it is difficult to gain their attention. Even where they appear to have heard, they forget what was said and follow through. These complaints reflect a sense that they are 'not always in the room', 'not all there', and 'not tuned in'	**Wanders or runs about excessively or frequent subjective feelings of restlessness:** adults may describe their subjective sense of always needing to be 'on the go' or feeling more comfortable with stimulating activities (e.g. skiing) than with more sedentary types of recreation. They may pace during the interview
Fails to follow through on instructions and complete tasks: adults may observe difficulty in following other people's instructions. Inability to read or follow instructions in a manual for appliances. Failure to keep commitments undertaken (e.g. work around the house)	**Difficulty engaging in leisure activities quietly:** adults may describe an unwillingness/dislike to ever just stay home or engage in quiet activities. They may complain that they are workaholics, in which case detailed examples should be given
Difficulty organizing tasks or activities: adults note recurrent errors (e.g. lateness, missed appointments, missing critical deadlines). Sometimes a deficit in this area is seen in the amount of delegation to others such as secretary at work or spouse at home	**Often 'on the go' or acts as if driven by a motor:** significant others may have a sense of the exhausting and frenetic pace of these adults. ADHD adults will often appear to expect the same frenetic pace of others. Holidays may be described as draining since there is no opportunity for rest
Avoids or dislikes sustained mental effort: putting off tasks such as responding to letters, completing tax returns, organizing old papers, paying bills, or establishing a will. One can enquire about specifics, then ask why particular tasks were not attended to. These adults often complain of procrastination	**Talks excessively:** excessive talking makes dialogue difficult. This may interfere with a spouse's sense of 'being heard' or achieving intimacy. This chatter may be experienced as nagging and may interfere with normal social interactions. Clowning, repartee, or other means of dominating conversations may mask an inability to engage in give-and-take conversation
Often loses things needed for tasks: misplacing purse, wallet, keys, and assignments from work, where car is parked, tools, and even children!	**Blurts out answers before questions have been completed:** this will usually be observed during the interview. This may also be experienced by probands, as a subjective sense of other people talking too slowly and of finding it difficult to wait for them to finish. Tendency to say what comes to mind without considering timing or appropriateness
Easily distracted by extraneous stimuli: subjectively experience distractibility and describe ways in which they try to overcome this. This may include listening to white noise, multi-tasking, requiring absolute quiet, or creating an emergency to achieve adequate states of arousal to complete tasks, many projects going simultaneously, and trouble with completion of tasks	**Difficulty waiting in turn:** adults find it difficult to wait for others to finish tasks at their own pace such as children. They may feel irritated waiting in line at bank machines or in a restaurant. They may be aware of their own intense efforts to force themselves to wait. Some adults compensate for this by carrying something to do at all times
Forgetful in daily activities: may complain of memory problems. They head out to the supermarket with a list of things but end up coming home, having failed to complete their tasks or having purchased something else	**Interrupts or intrudes on others:** this is most often experienced by adults as social ineptness at social gatherings or even with close friends. An example might be inability to watch others struggle with a task (such as trying to open a door with a key) without jumping in to try for themselves

to focus well on fast, highly rewarding or novel tasks, whereas it can be extremely difficult to focus on tasks that lack such immediate intrinsic rewards. This can give rise to patchy levels of performance and difficulties in sustaining attention on tasks once the immediate novelty has worn off. Tasks that cause the most problems include reading and writing, completing forms, repetitive work, listening, and following conversations. Some adults with ADHD can hyperfocus on a few things they find particularly interesting, shift their attention from one immediately rewarding activity to another, or spend hours on fast-rewarding activities such as computer games. In this sense, inattention in ADHD should not be seen as a fixed deficit but is dependent to some extent on the context. Other problems related to inattention include difficulties in starting, completing, and organizing tasks; difficulties with holding complex thoughts and concepts in mind; and difficulties with losing things, time keeping, and forgetfulness.

One common feature of the inattentive mental state in adult ADHD is excessive mind wandering, also referred to as mental restlessness (Mowlem et al., 2016). In DSM-5, excessive mind wandering is briefly mentioned as the occurrence of *unrelated thoughts*. Mind wandering in ADHD is characterized by thoughts that are on the go all the time, jump of flit from one topic to another, and multiple lines of thought at the same time.

In ADHD, hyperactivity and impulsivity tend to decline with increasing age. For example, it is unusual for adults with ADHD to run, climb, and jump excessively. However, they may have difficulty remaining seated for long, prefer to walk around, are often fidgety, and frequently describe a feeling of internal restlessness. Impulsivity is often seen in the form of impatience when waiting in queues that is often accompanied by feelings of irritability, and they may avoid situations where they have to wait. Other problems related to impulsivity include saying or doing things without stopping to think, e.g. impulsively getting into arguments or fights, or interrupting people and talking over conversations. Although, in many cases, these problems with hyperactivity–impulsivity may be relatively minor and non-impairing, they are severe in others.

As well as the core features of ADHD, there are other highly characteristic symptoms and impairments that are commonly seen and may be the main presenting complaint (American Psychiatric Association, 2013; Asherson et al., 2016). These are not considered necessary for establishing the diagnosis but are important to recognize in terms of the levels of impairment and to inform management of ADHD. In particular, mood symptoms are common in adults with ADHD. These most frequently consist of emotional dysregulation characterized by excessive emotional reactions, rapid mood swings, and frequent anger, irritability, or frustration. Emotional dysregulation is present in non-comorbid cases of ADHD and can be the most impairing aspect of the disorder (Skirrow and Asherson, 2013).

Another aspect of ADHD is sleep problems, reported by 70% of adults with ADHD. The commonest complaint is of sleep-onset insomnia, which, in some cases, may be a delay in the usual circadian rhythm but may also include broken sleep. The reasons for sleep problems in ADHD are not well understood, but when asked why it is difficult to get to sleep, patients often describe feeling too physically or mentally restless to fall asleep, even though they may feel tired (Van Veen et al., 2010). Sleep deprivation and fatigue may occur in some patients and could exacerbate the symptoms and impairments of ADHD, including sustained attention, mind wandering, and emotional dysregulation.

Another aspect of ADHD is poor behavioural self-regulation, often referred to as executive function deficits (Asherson et al., 2016; Barkley and Fischer, 2011). The use of the term executive function in this context remains controversial because they may not always be secondary to cortical executive control deficits at the neural level. However, at the descriptive level, they are highly characteristic of the difficulties experienced by adults with ADHD.

Differentiating ADHD symptoms from other disorders

One difficulty that can arise is establishing the childhood or adolescent onset and trait-like course of ADHD symptoms. In the absence of a clear detailed account from childhood, questions to elicit the early onset and trait-like nature of ADHD symptoms during clinical interview could include 'When did the symptoms start?' or 'Has there been a time when the symptoms were not present?'. Related to this, one clear distinction from most adult-onset disorders is the typical early-onset and trait-like persistence of ADHD symptoms, which reflect what someone is usually like, rather than a change in premorbid mental state and episodic course (Asherson et al., 2016). This underscores the importance of an extensive assessment, including a full account of the onset and development of mental health symptoms and developmental and psychosocial history. It is important that all patients who present with mental health symptoms and behavioural disturbances of a chronic or trait-like nature are screened for ADHD, and a full diagnostic assessment for ADHD is completed where this is indicated.

Another challenge to the diagnosis of ADHD is that the inattentive, hyperactive, and impulsive symptoms reflect continuous traits, which are present to some degree in the non-ADHD population, rather than reflecting qualitatively distinct symptoms. The categorical disorder is defined by the presence of developmentally inappropriate levels of ADHD symptoms when they lead to significant impairment (American Psychiatric Association, 2013). This is similar to the conceptualization of symptoms of anxiety and depression, and personality traits, as well as hypertension, which also reflect extremes of dimensional traits that occur throughout the population. Although the presence of ADHD symptoms is easy to determine in the most severe cases, difficulties will inevitably arise in determining whether less severe cases meet diagnostic criteria. It is therefore important to determine not only the presence and severity of ADHD symptoms, but also whether they are associated with significant levels of impairment. The degree to which the symptoms are severe and impairing are key discriminating features.

A detailed examination of how ADHD symptoms interfere with day-to-day life is necessary. The UK NICE (National Institute for Health and Care Excellence, 2008) advises that impairment should be established to a degree that, *most people* would consider, requires some form of medical, social, or educational intervention; that without a specialist professional or a higher level of intervention to ameliorate the problems, there is likely to be *long-term adverse* implications for the person affected, as well as problems in the short and medium term. Impairment should be pervasive, occur in multiple settings, and be at least of moderate severity. Significant impairment should not be considered where the impact of ADHD symptoms is restricted to academic/work performance alone, unless there is a moderate to severe impact in other domains. Common impairments in ADHD include reductions in the performance of quality (including excessive mental effort and distress) of functioning in education, work, partner and family relationships, social contacts, free time and hobbies, and self-confidence and self-image.

ADHD therefore presents with a wide range of impairments, from relatively high-functioning individuals to those who are severely impaired and may have considerable difficulties in multiple aspects of their life, leading to considerable personal and social, as well as economic, burdens on society. Examples of common clinical presentations indicating the main areas of impairment are listed in Box 34.1.

Both persistent and subthreshold ADHD have been associated with higher levels of mental health problems and drug use, involvement with the police, and relatively high rates of driving offences, compared to population norms (Kooij et al., 2010). ADHD is associated with work-related problems in adulthood such as poor job performance, lower occupational status, less job stability, and increased absence days, in comparison to adults without ADHD (Adamou et al., 2013; Biederman and Faraone, 2006). Economic evaluation analysis established an important societal cost for ADHD (National Institute for Health and Care Excellence, 2008) resulting from decreased function, comorbidity, or employment problems. ADHD can also have an important influence on the individual's family and personal relationships (Biederman et al., 2006). Parents of young adults with ADHD may experience depression, anxiety, and stress, which has been associated with high levels of family conflict and poor family cohesion.

Box 34.1 Examples of clinical presentations for ADHD in adults

A 26-year-old mother

Disorganized. Ceaseless mental activity. Unable to work and difficulty with completing simple tasks such as shopping. Treated for anxiety/depression but uses cannabis to 'calm thoughts'. Difficulty managing her two children who both have a diagnosis of ADHD.

A 22-year-old male student

Inability to cope at college. Repeated first year of college for third time despite high IQ, high motivation, supportive family, and good education. Robust inattention.

An 18-year-old man with borderline IQ

Low IQ (around 70). Behavioural problems. Lacks insight. Binge drinking. Main presenting complaint was extreme irritability and aggression at home.

A 30-year-old female student

Irritable and volatile moods. Treated for depression. Only retains lecture material by recording and transcribing notes. Managed to pass college examinations but took considerable time and effort to complete studies.

A 25-year-old unemployed man

Unemployed. Sitting around at home. Severe inner restlessness. Unable to focus for more than a few minutes. Grossly distractible and unfocused thought processes.

A 35-year-old man

Extreme impulsiveness. Numerous verbal and physical fights. Very poor attention span and ability to plan ahead, but main problems reported as constant restlessness, severe mood instability, over-reactions to minor setbacks, and impatience.

The risk of impairment shows a linear relationship to the severity of ADHD symptoms in population samples (Kooij et al., 2005). Therefore, careful attention is needed to assess the impact of ADHD symptoms on impairment and QoL, including an understanding of the broader range of problems linked to ADHD, in addition to functional impairments in everyday life. When evaluating impairments, it is important to take into account that even minor levels of symptoms can cause considerable distress to individuals because of the chronic and persistent nature of ADHD symptoms which are experienced by people with ADHD on a daily basis (Asherson et al., 2016).

Comorbidity

Comorbidity is seen in up to 80% of clinic-referred cases with ADHD. This can complicate both the assessment and clinical management of ADHD. Comorbid disorders commonly include anxiety disorders, mood disorders including bipolar affective disorder, personality disorder (particularly emotionally unstable personality disorder), substance use disorders, and other neurodevelopmental disorders. The prevalence of ADHD is also high among individuals presenting with another condition. In one survey, ADHD was seen in around 13% of adults with mood disorders, 10% of adults with anxiety disorders, 11% of adults with substance use disorders, and 12% of adults with impulse control disorders (Kessler, 2007).

Despite the high prevalence of ADHD and the impact on adult psychopathology and functioning, less than one-third of adults with ADHD are diagnosed with the condition (Feifel, 2008). Several

studies point to high rates of undiagnosed ADHD in prisons (~26%) (Young et al., 2014), addiction units (~12%) (Huntley et al., 2012; van de Glind et al., 2013), and general adult mental health services (~16%) (Deberdt et al., 2015). One reason for the underdiagnosis of ADHD by adult mental health services is the nature of the clinical syndrome, which shares characteristics with other common adult mental health disorders (Asherson et al., 2016).

When considering the relationship of ADHD to comorbid symptoms, there are three main categories to consider:

(1) Symptoms of ADHD that mimic other disorders, either because of overlap with core ADHD symptoms, such as impulsivity and poor concentration, or because of characteristic associated features of ADHD such as emotional instability, low self-esteem, and sleep problems. Symptoms that typically overlap between ADHD and comorbid mental health disorders are listed in Table 34.3.

(2) Symptoms of overlapping neurodevelopmental disorders that share aetiological risk factors. These include features of ASD, specific reading difficulties (dyslexia), and developmental coordination disorder (dyspraxia). Family and twin studies have indicated that these result largely from shared genetic factors and likely reflect pleiotropic effects (multiple different outcomes) of genes.

(3) Symptoms of co-occurring mental health conditions which may develop as a complication of ADHD such as anxiety and mood disorders. An example would be an individual with a lifelong history of school failure, who continues to struggle with ADHD-related impairments, presenting with chronic low self-esteem and episodes of depression. Furthermore, children with ADHD may be more sensitive to environmental risk factors for the development of comorbid disorders such as substance abuse and anti-social and emotionally unstable personality disorders.

Comorbid medical conditions are also a concern, with substantial evidence associating adult ADHD with obesity. Recent data have linked ADHD with increased mortality, largely due to serious accidents. Overall, the greater the severity of ADHD, the more likely an individual will develop one or more comorbid disorders.

Table 34.3 Commonly occurring symptoms of ADHD that mimic other conditions

Anxiety	Worrying about performance deficits, excessive mind wandering, feeling overwhelmed, feeling restless, avoidance of situations due to ADHD symptoms such as difficulty waiting in queues or social situations requiring focused attention, sleep problems linked to mental restlessness
Depression	Unstable moods, impatience, irritability, poor concentration, sleep disturbance, low self-esteem
Personality disorder	Chronic trait-like psychopathology linked to behavioural problems, emotional instability, impulsive behaviour, poor social relationships
Bipolar disorder	Restlessness, sleep disturbance, mood instability, ceaseless unfocused mental activity, distractibility

Assessment

ADHD is a clinical and behavioural phenotype and its presence is best evaluated by clinical interview. There are currently no direct biological, cognitive, or neuroimaging tests that are sufficiently accurate for use in clinical practice. Although reproducible cognitive, structural, and functional neuroimaging differences between ADHD cases and controls are well established, these findings lack the sensitivity and specificity to be used in clinical practice. The clinical diagnosis of ADHD in adults can, however, be reliably made using a diagnostic interview approach, particularly if diagnostic assessment tools are used that systematically apply the diagnostic criteria. The approach is similar to that for all other adult mental health disorders, with emphasis on good clinical history taking and an account of the symptoms and impairments of the disorder (Kooij et al., 2010).

The elements of the diagnostic process in adults with suspected ADHD may include the use of screening tools. Rating scales for ADHD are helpful in providing a baseline measure of ADHD symptom severity and can be used to monitor improvement following initiation of treatments. A widely used screening instrument that is free to use is the WHO's Adult ADHD Self Rating Scale (Kessler et al., 2005). This has been validated in primary care populations to inform the decision as to whether an individual should proceed to full assessment. Several other alternative scales consisting of DSM-IV/5 symptom checklists can be used, including those from Barkley, Conners, and Du Paul, among others. However, rating scales are not sufficiently good predictors to ensure a correct clinical diagnosis and should never be used for this purpose.

Diagnostic assessment is based on a full psychiatric review and clinical interview assessment to evaluate each of the diagnostic criteria for ADHD. The main task is to elicit examples for each of the 18 DSM-5 symptoms and ADHD-associated impairments, both currently and during childhood. A key difference from many other adult-onset psychiatric disorders is the need to establish a longitudinal pattern and persistent course of symptoms from childhood to the time of assessment as an adult. Other essential elements of the assessment include a thorough account of the developmental history and a mental health screen for common comorbid conditions that often co-occur with ADHD. Recommended interviews for ADHD include the Conners' Adult ADHD Diagnostic Interview for DSM-IV (Epstein et al., 2001) and the Diagnostic Interview for Adults with ADHD, DIVA 2.0 (Kooij, 2012). The DIVA interview is especially useful being translated in multiple languages, available as a mobile application, and free to use in clinical practice and research (http://www.divacenter.eu). A new diagnostic interview assessment for DSM-5 adult ADHD (ACE +) has recently been developed and is available online at no cost (http://www.psychology-services.uk.com).

Whether or not a structured diagnostic interview is used, the core of the diagnostic process is establishing the longitudinal presence of core and associated ADHD symptoms, associated impairment, and whether the clinical picture is complicated by comorbid disorders. Careful clinical assessment is therefore required to disentangle ADHD symptoms from comorbid presentations, taking into account age of onset and developmental history, evidence of episodic or trait-like symptom pattern, presence of other symptoms suggesting other diagnoses (e.g. elevated mood or unstable self-image and recurrent self-harm may suggest bipolar affective disorder or emotionally unstable personality disorder, respectively), and previous treatment and its effect on symptoms and behaviour.

Whenever possible, it is advised to seek an informant account for both current and retrospective symptoms and impairments. The lack of an informant should not, however, rule out the possibility of establishing diagnostic certainty in individuals who can provide good and reliable descriptions of symptoms and impairments. Informants may include parents or older siblings, partners or friends, school reports, educational psychology reports, child psychiatry or paediatric reports, or adult mental health assessments. With regard to impairment, NICE suggests that assessment should explore the following domains: self-esteem, distress from the symptoms, work function, academic performance, social interactions and relationships, organizing daily activities, behavioural problems, criminal activity, and development of co-occurring psychiatric syndromes.

It should be noted that assessment of the current mental state examination is a necessary part of the clinical interview. Symptoms such as feeling restless and excessive mind wandering are commonly reported by adults with ADHD. However, care needs to be taken in the interpretation of objective signs in an individual with suspected ADHD during the assessment. For many people, ADHD assessment is a novel experience and they may be highly motivated to focus during the assessment. For this reason, usual behaviour, such as fidgeting, restlessness, drifting off during conversations, and irritability, may not be observed, whereas they may be present as common and impairing problems in more everyday situations. The malleable nature of ADHD symptoms and their sensitivity to context is one of the characteristic features of ADHD. For this reason, the assessment should also focus on functioning and ADHD symptoms in normal everyday situations (e.g. normal functioning during a typical week), and not only on how they present during the assessment interview.

As discussed earlier, there is no single cognitive profile for ADHD and great care needs to be taken when interpreting the results of cognitive performance tests. A significant number of false positives and negatives can arise from reliance on cognitive tests. For this reason, we do not currently recommend their use in routine clinical practice. Cognitive testing in adult ADHD would typically include measures of general cognitive ability, sustained attention, working memory, planning abilities, identification of cognitive strengths and weaknesses, and quantification in relation to general population norms. This can aid a comprehensive assessment and can inform management strategies when applied by a specialist in clinical neuropsychology. The cognitive assessment could be used to make recommendations for further referrals for educational support and workplace adjustments and to target psychological treatment, and it can be used to identify particular areas of attention/executive function deficits. The interpretation of cognitive assessment data in ADHD, however, requires considerable expertise and should be conducted by someone with suitable training in both neuropsychology and ADHD.

For these reasons, we do not recommend the use of currently available tests for ADHD in routine clinical practice at this time. However, some test results can be particularly useful and could be applied more widely. It would be helpful to know if someone had very high or low IQ, as this would inform expectations on levels of performance and the ability to develop appropriate coping strategies. Specific reading difficulties (dyslexia) is also commonly seen in ADHD.

Service provision for adult ADHD

Despite wide consensus in national and international guidelines regarding appropriate and evidence-based treatments, in many countries, services remain limited and are often confined to specialist tertiary referral centres. We hope that this chapter will increase awareness and contribute to appropriate diagnosis and treatment of adults with ADHD within generic, as well as specialist, services for adult mental health.

In considering service needs for adults with ADHD, the following factors should be taken into consideration: the rates of undiagnosed ADHD in the adult population, the individual and societal costs of untreated ADHD, and the availability of effective treatments. Undiagnosed and untreated ADHD can lead to persistence, and potentially worsening, of mental health problems over time and should therefore be recognized, so appropriate treatments can be initiated. Since ADHD is prevalent in nearly all adult mental health settings, including community, primary, and secondary care settings, we recommend that all those involved in adult mental health develop the skills to diagnose and treat the disorder.

There is increasing evidence for high rates of untreated ADHD in prisons. Around one in four prisoners are estimated to meet ADHD diagnostic criteria, yet few are ever treated or diagnosed by prison primary or secondary care mental health services (Young et al., 2015). Undiagnosed and untreated ADHD is also seen in 10–15% of patients attending addiction and secondary care adult mental health services (Deberdt et al., 2015; Huntley et al., 2012; van de Glind et al., 2014). ADHD is also common among those with a diagnosis of a personality disorder and chronic mood disorders. Within all of these adult mental health settings, ADHD should be routinely screened for. Rates of adult ADHD in primary care are less well established, but it is likely that a significant group of patients presenting with non-psychotic long-term mental health problems meet diagnostic criteria for ADHD (Faraone et al., 2004). By raising the index of suspicion and awareness of ADHD within adult mental health and forensic services, the opportunity to identify a treatable mental health condition will be increased.

An important area identified as a particular need is to establish transitional arrangements for individuals where ADHD was diagnosed in childhood. Approximately 1–2% of school-age children are currently diagnosed with ADHD in the UK and many will go on to have continued problems as adults. The current situation, however, is that many adolescents with ADHD have difficulty accessing appropriate support and treatment once they enter the late teenage years. This is compounded by the high risk of dropout from medical follow-up, which is a common problem during adolescence across both physical and mental health. Efforts therefore need to be made to establish suitable services and continued support and treatment where this is required. Good practice during the transition period is to provide young people with information about the course of

ADHD and treatment options to help them make decisions about ongoing treatment.

In addition to the management of known cases of ADHD, a significant proportion of adults with ADHD present to services for the first time as adults. This is not surprising since in most (if not all) European countries, few children were diagnosed or treated for ADHD before the mid-1990s, leading to a large pool of undiagnosed adults. Furthermore, even now, ADHD is not always diagnosed and treated during childhood and adolescence. Although diagnosis in boys outnumber that in girls by 4 to 1 in childhood, it is interesting to note that this gender gap narrows in adult ADHD clinics to near-equal rates of male and females. One suggestion is that girls who present with predominantly inattentive symptoms without behavioural disturbance are missed at school. They may be labelled as 'slow learners' and may only present for ADHD in adulthood once impairment in other domains becomes more overt. It also likely reflects the greater propensity for women to seek help for mental health problems than men.

There is increasing awareness of the interaction between criminality and ADHD, with around one-quarter of offenders meeting clinical criteria for ADHD (Young et al., 2011, 2014). Compared to non-ADHD offenders, offenders with ADHD tend to have more convictions and first-time convictions at an earlier age. It is likely that conditions such as addiction or personality disorder mediate some of the increased levels of criminality, but also there is a direct relationship with ADHD-related symptoms and impairments such as inattention and poor educational attainment, impulsivity, low tolerance for frustration, low tolerance for boredom, and problems managing anger and emotional dysregulation. The case for specialist forensic services to routinely diagnose and treat ADHD is strengthened by research which revealed a reduction in criminal behaviour in adults receiving medication for ADHD in a large community sample from Sweden. Periods on ADHD medication, compared to periods off medication, led to a 32% reduction in criminality for men and 41% for women (Lichtenstein and Larsson, 2013). A clinical trial of prisoners with ADHD found very large treatment effects on core ADHD symptoms (Ginsberg and Lindefors, 2012). In the UK, there has been a promising pilot study of methylphenidate for prisoners for ADHD. Her Majesty's Inspectorate of Prisons reporting on the pilot study said that 'some prisoners on the programme to whom we spoke were experiencing some stability of behaviour for the first time in their lives'. They went on to say that 'there should be efforts to ensure continued prescribing of medication and ongoing specialist support for prisoners (who were treated for ADHD) following their release'. This highlights the need for developing care pathways for offenders with ADHD both within prison settings and in the community.

Management of ADHD

Successful management of adult ADHD involves familiarity with the clinical syndrome, its presentation in adults, and good understanding of the effects of treatment. Treatment should follow careful diagnostic assessment of ADHD and associated comorbid disorders. The first-line treatment for adults recommended by national and international guidelines is medication, unless the individual would prefer non-pharmacological treatment or pharmacological treatment is not possible (Bolea-Alamanac et al., 2014; Canadian ADHD Resource Alliance, 2011; Kooij et al., 2010; National Institute for Health and Care Excellence, 2008, 2018). However, all guidelines recommend a multi-modal treatment approach, including psychoeducation and consideration of environmental modification, and medical treatment for ADHD should always form part of a wider treatment plan addressing psychological, educational/occupational, and social needs. Stimulants in the form of methylphenidate and lisdexamfetamine/dexamfetamine are generally recommended as the first-line treatment for ADHD, and the non-stimulant atomoxetine as a second-line treatment. Internationally, there is some variation on the recommended order of these three treatments.

Stimulants

Although both stimulants and atomoxetine show significant evidence for efficacy, stimulants are considered to be more effective (Faraone and Glatt, 2010; Kooij et al., 2010; National Institute for Health and Care Excellence, 2008). For this reason, stimulants continue to be the recommended first-line pharmacological treatment for patients of all ages with ADHD. Both methylphenidate and lisdexamfetamine/dexamfetamine are dopamine and noradrenaline reuptake inhibitors, with additional effects on the release of these transmitters. They provide rapid, short-lived control of ADHD symptoms for a limited period of time—3–4 hours for short-acting formulations, and 6–8 hours for intermediate- and up to 12 hours for longer-acting sustained-release preparations.

Although the efficacy of both classes of stimulants (methylphenidate and dexamfetamine) is similar, some patients preferentially respond to, and tolerate, one over the other. Currently, there are no known reliable predictors of individual patient responses. The dose of stimulants in adults should be individually adjusted, based on response and tolerability, until the patient and clinician feel that an optimal dose has been reached. The goal is to provide the optimal duration of coverage throughout the day according to the needs of the patient, while minimizing any potential adverse effects.

For methylphenidate, a starting dose of 5 mg three times daily (or equivalent for extended-release preparations) is recommended, with weekly increases depending on response and adverse effects. The maximum recommended dose is around 100 mg daily, although, in a small proportion of cases, higher doses are required. Bioavailability varies between formulations, so care must be taken when transferring patients from one preparation to another and caution with use of generic terms such as 'methylphenidate' when writing prescriptions.

The starting dose of dexamfetamine is usually 5 mg twice daily, with a maximum recommended dose of 60 mg daily. Again, a small proportion of cases may need higher doses. The recommended starting dose for lisdexamfetamine is 30 mg once daily and the maximum recommended dose is 70 mg once daily.

A common adverse effect of stimulants is initial insomnia, although it is thought that around 50% of adults with ADHD may actually show improved sleep with stimulants. Decreased appetite is another common complaint, although significant weight loss is rare. The therapeutic use of stimulants is not addictive, contrary to some expressed fears. Studies that investigated links between the treatment of ADHD with stimulants and drug abuse found reductions in drug use (Chang et al., 2014b). In clinical practice, there is no evidence of tolerance developing over time (Asherson et al., 2016), although it remains feasible that this could occur with very long-term use in some patients. As in other areas of medicine and mental health, non-compliance with treatment is a common problem, even in those who have been using stimulants to treat ADHD for many years such as children transitioning from child to adult mental health services for ADHD. This is not the hallmark of an addictive medical treatment. Evidence from controlled trials for the longer-term benefits of pharmacological treatments is largely lacking due to the difficulties in conducting long-term controlled trials. However, pharmaco-epidemiological studies using national registry data highlighted the potential for very significant long-term benefits of treatment, not only on core ADHD symptoms, but also on serious co-occurring problems, including drug use, criminal behaviour, and transport accidents (Chang et al., 2014a, b; Lichtenstein and Larsson, 2013).

Atomoxetine

Atomoxetine is a selective noradrenaline reuptake inhibitor. The mode of action is less well understood than that of stimulants in that its effects are not directly related to transporter blockade or neurotransmitter release and its effects last longer than the half-life and also increase over time, in a similar way to antidepressants. In contrast to stimulants, the effects develop more slowly over several weeks and also take a longer period to decline when stopped.

Atomoxetine is often considered as a first-line treatment where there is a potential for misuse or diversion of stimulants. Another potential first-line indication is ADHD comorbid with anxiety with panic attacks, since stimulants are more likely to exacerbate severe anxiety. Another advantage is the relatively simple dosing regimen which does not require individual titration in the same way as stimulants. When well tolerated, atomoxetine can provide stable control of ADHD symptoms.

The recommended dosing regimen for atomoxetine is a starting dose of 0.5 mg/kg, increasing to 1.2 mg/kg for individuals <70 kg in weight. For those above 70 kg, the recommended starting dose is 40 mg each day, increasing to 80 mg after a minimum of 3 days, with a maximum recommended dose of 100 mg. Due to the common occurrence of minor adverse effects, many practioners prefer to initiate treatment at 20 mg a day, and then increase weekly to the effective dose of 80 mg. Although the majority of individuals respond within the first 2–4 weeks, treatment effects can develop over longer periods of time. It is therefore important to ensure that a period of 12 weeks on the therapeutic dose of atomoxetine has passed before drawing conclusions on the clinical response in individual cases.

Common adverse which can be problematic include gastrointestinal symptoms, such as nausea, and erectile dysfunction. Other common adverse effects are similar to those of stimulants, including effects on pulse and blood pressure. There is a caution regarding rare reports of hepatic disorders and suicidal ideation, with advice that individuals be given specific guidance on reporting symptoms of these promptly if they occur.

Essential checks when prescribing stimulants and atomoxetine

Before commencing treatment with psychostimulants or atomoxetine, it is recommended that a full medical history is taken, with emphasis on cardiac problems in the individual and their family. Blood pressure and heart rate should be checked, as both stimulants and atomoxetine can increase both. While an ECG is not recommended routinely, it is recommended to check the heart for structural defects. Advice from a cardiologist may be needed if there are any concerns. Weight should also be taken and monitored, particularly if there is significant appetite reduction. Risk of potential substance misuse, particularly diversion for cognitive enhancement, should also be considered when prescribing psychostimulants. Use of stimulants as drugs of abuse appears to be rare and can be minimized by the use of formulations such as Concerta˙ XL and lisdexamfetamine.

Treating ADHD and comorbidity

In the case of comorbidity, the integrated treatment plan should address both ADHD and the comorbid condition. The order of pharmacological treatment will depend on the type and severity of the comorbid disorder. The rule of thumb is to address the most serious disorder first. For example, it is recommended that significant anxiety disorders or major depression should be treated with an antidepressant or CBT, before starting treatment for ADHD. However, when the other disorder is appropriately managed, ADHD can then be treated effectively. There is a lack of formal trial data on the use of stimulants and atomoxetine in ADHD cases comorbid with bipolar disorder or schizophrenia, although data have now been generated using pharmaco-epidemiological approaches that support the treatment of such comorbid cases (Chang et al., 2019). These new findings suggest that ADHD can be treated safely in cases with comorbid schizophrenia or bipolar when the mental state is stable and they are maintained on mood stabilizers or antipsychotics as appropriate. Most experts agree that treatment can proceed with due caution and careful monitoring. Stimulants may be safer than atomoxetine in this context because of the very short half-life and short-acting nature of stimulant effects, with rapid withdrawal of the stimulant medication if there is any worsening of the mood or psychotic disorder. However, there are no published data to evaluate the best approach. Combined treatments are therefore frequently used for the management of ADHD in individuals with comorbid disorders.

When making decisions on the order of treatment, attention should be given to the relative balance of ADHD and the comorbid disorder. Symptoms of ADHD often overlap with other conditions and could therefore also result directly from underlying ADHD. Examples include worrying about life problems, low self-esteem, and dysthymia, which are all very common in ADHD and often are directly related to ADHD symptoms and associated impairments. In these cases, it is usual to treat ADHD first. It is essential to be aware that emotional dysregulation commonly accompanies ADHD and also responds to ADHD drug treatments (Posner et al., 2014a). A general algorithm for those presenting with chronic mental health symptoms and comorbid symptoms is presented in Fig. 34.1.

Alternative medical treatments

Other medical treatments, such as long-acting bupropion, guanfacine, and tricyclic antidepressants like desipramine and imipramine, have also been shown to be effective in some studies of adult ADHD. Guanfacine is being introduced as a treatment for ADHD in children and is likely to have similar beneficial effects for

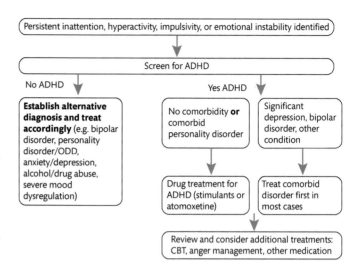

Fig. 34.1 Treatment algorithm for ADHD

adults with ADHD. Bupropion is often used by specialist sin the UK as a third-line option. These medications are generally considered as third- or fourth-line agents due to a smaller evidence base and average effect sizes that are thought to be lower than those of stimulants or atomoxetine. Current studies are investigating the potential use of drugs that target glutamate, GABA, serotonin, and the nicotinic acetylcholine in ADHD (Faraone et al., 2015).

Psychological treatments

Current guidelines recommend psychological therapies are used as an adjunct to medication in adult ADHD (Kooij et al., 2010; National Institute for Health and Care Excellence, 2008). It is recommended that psychological treatments are offered where a patient is titrated to an optimal dosage of medication, but residual symptoms remain; where medication is not an option due to intolerance to medication; where the patient does not wish to take medication; or where symptoms are remitting and targeted psychological intervention alone may be all that is required.

Research on psychological treatments for adults with ADHD remain relatively limited, but the evidence base is growing. Interventions could include specialist CBT, psychoeducation, anger management, daily living skills, family/carer support, and treatment of comorbid disorders. Although several previous studies supported the use of targeted psychological interventions (Philipsen, 2012), these may not target core ADHD symptoms, but rather the broader range of symptoms and impairments that are associated with ADHD. This was one of the conclusions from a recent large-scale study of a psychological intervention targeted at ADHD, compared to medication and treatment as usual (Philipsen et al., 2015). This study found large effects of methylphenidate, but no effects of the psychological intervention, on core ADHD symptoms. However, the targeted psychological intervention was associated with general improvements, captured by the Clinical Global Impression Scale, and long-term improvements over 1 year.

ADHD coaching is another intervention that has gained great popularity among patients with ADHD, providing excellent advice on strategies to manage ADHD and optimize performance in the presence of ongoing ADHD symptoms. Coaching can be very effective when delivered by a trained expert, but as an unregulated branch of treatment, there is a wide range of expertise and no clear standards. Care is therefore required to identify suitably trained professional coaches. There is also emerging evidence for the use of mindfulness-based interventions, with reported effect sizes similar to medical treatments for ADHD on core ADHD symptoms (Cairncross and Miller, 2016; Hepark et al., 2015). Since mindfulness training targets neural processes that are thought to underpin sustained attention deficits in ADHD (Tang et al., 2015), it is feasible that this approach could bring about a reduction in ADHD symptoms in some cases.

Whether psychological interventions reduce the core symptoms of ADHD or rather improve secondary outcomes, such as psychosocial and functional impairments, remains uncertain. Recent studies have suggested that, in many cases, there are no effects on core ADHD, although psychosocial treatments remain an essential part of effective treatment for many adults with ADHD. It should be borne in mind that while medication can reduce symptoms, medication cannot lead to changes in patterns of behaviour or habitual responses that have developed over many years. Therefore, medication, in conjunction with psychoeducation, psychology therapies, and providing problem-solving or organizational strategies, for example, can support individuals to obtain optimum benefit from treatment.

Conclusion and future directions

A diagnosis of ADHD is associated with poor educational, occupational, economic, and social outcomes. Among the more severe outcomes of untreated ADHD are the development of comorbid anti-social and emotionally unstable borderline personality disorders, anxiety and depression, risk of substance use disorders, criminal behaviour, and mortality. Evidence suggests that effective management of ADHD can reduce the level of functional impairment, adult psychopathology, and associated economic and societal burden and costs. Therefore, ADHD should be recognized in the same way as other common adult mental health conditions. Failure to recognize and treat ADHD can be detrimental to the well-being of many patients seeking help for mental health problems. While further research is needed to evaluate the effects of ADHD drug treatments in ADHD complicated by comorbidities, effective clinical management of ADHD should be an essential component of adult mental healthcare.

KEY LEARNING POINTS

- ADHD is a common, highly heritable, heterogenous neurodevelopmental disorder.
- It is associated with significant adult psychopathology and poor educational, occupational, economic, and social outcomes.
- It is often confused with other disorders and is no more difficult to diagnose and treat than other common mental health disorders.
- ADHD is a clinical and behavioural phenotype, and its presence is best evaluated with a full psychiatric review and clinical interview, establishing the longitudinal presence of core and associated ADHD symptoms and associated impairment.

- ADHD is a treatable condition, with evidence-based guidelines. In the case of comorbidity, the integrated treatment plan should address both ADHD and the comorbid condition.
- A comprehensive, holistic shared treatment plan should be provided that addresses psychological, behavioural, and occupational/educational needs and ensure continuity of care for people with ADHD.
- The first-line treatment for adults with ADHD is medication, and psychological therapies are used as an adjunct to medication.
- The efficacy of medication is well established.
- In many countries, services for patients with ADHD remain limited.

REFERENCES

Adamou, M., et al. (2013). Occupational issues of adults with ADHD. *BMC Psychiatry*, 13, 59.

Agnew-Blais, J. C., et al. (2017). Persistence, Remission and Emergence of ADHD in Young Adulthood: Results from a Longitudinal, Prospective Population-Based Cohort. *JAMA Psychiatry*, 73, 713–20.

American Psychiatric Association. (2013). *Diagnostic and Statistical Manual of Mental Disorders—DSM 5—fifth edition*. Washington, DC: American Psychiatric Publishing.

Asherson, P., et al. (2016). Adult attention-deficit hyperactivity disorder: key conceptual issues. *Lancet Psychiatry*, 3, 568–78.

Asherson, P. & Gurling, H. (2012). Quantitative and molecular genetics of ADHD. *Curr Top Behav Neurosci*, 9, 239–72.

Banerjee, T. D., et al. (2007). Environmental risk factors for attention-deficit hyperactivity disorder. *Acta Paediatr*, 96, 1269–74.

Barkley, R. A. & Fischer, M. (2010). The unique contribution of emotional impulsiveness to impairment in major life activities in hyperactive children as adults. *J Am Acad Child Adolesc Psychiatry*, 49, 503–13.

Barkley, R. A. & Fischer, M. (2011). Predicting impairment in major life activities and occupational functioning in hyperactive children as adults: self-reported executive function (EF) deficits versus EF tests. *Dev Neuropsychol*, 36, 137–61.

Biederman, J. & Faraone, S. V. (2006). The effects of attention-deficit/hyperactivity disorder on employment and household income. *MedGenMed*, 8, 12.

Biederman, J., et al. (2006). Functional impairments in adults with self-reports of diagnosed ADHD: A controlled study of 1001 adults in the community. *J Clin Psychiatry*, 67, 524–40.

Biederman, J., et al. (2005). Absence of gender effects on attention deficit hyperactivity disorder: findings in nonreferred subjects. *Am J Psychiatry*, 162, 1083–9.

Bolea-Alamanac, B., et al. (2014). Evidence-based guidelines for the pharmacological management of attention deficit hyperactivity disorder: update on recommendations from the British Association for Psychopharmacology. *J Psychopharmacol*, 28, 179–203.

Cairncross, M. & Miller, C. J. (2016). The Effectiveness of Mindfulness-Based Therapies for ADHD: A Meta-Analytic Review. *J Atten Disord*, 24, 627–43

Canadian ADHD Resource Alliance (CADDRA). (2011). *Canadian ADHD Practice Guidelines (CAP-Guidelines)*, third edition. Toronto, ON.

Castellanos, F. X. & Proal, E. (2012). Large-scale brain systems in ADHD: beyond the prefrontal-striatal model. *Trends Cogn Sci*, 16, 17–26.

Caye, A., et al. (2016). ADHD does not always begin in childhood: Evidence from a large birth cohort. *JAMA Psychiatry*, 73, 705–12.

Chang Z, et al. (2019). Risks and Benefits of Attention-Deficit/Hyperactivity Disorder Medication on Behavioral and Neuropsychiatric Outcomes: A Qualitative Review of Pharmacoepidemiology Studies Using Linked Prescription Databases. *Biol Psychiatry*, 86, 335–43.

Chang, Z., et al. (2014a). Serious transport accidents in adults with attention-deficit/hyperactivity disorder and the effect of medication: a population-based study. *JAMA Psychiatry*, 71, 319–25.

Chang, Z., et al. (2014b). Stimulant ADHD medication and risk for substance abuse. *J Child Psychol Psychiatry*, 55, 878–85.

Cheung, C. H., et al. (2016). Cognitive and neurophysiological markers of ADHD persistence and remission. *Br J Psychiatry*, 208, 548–55.

Cheung, C. H., et al. (2016). Cognitive and neurophysiological markers of ADHD persistence and remission. *Br J Psychiatry*, 208, 548–55.

Coghill, D., et al. (2005). Whither causal models in the neuroscience of ADHD? *Dev Sci*, 8, 105–14.

Cooper, M., et al. (2018). Investigating late-onset ADHD: a population cohort investigation. *J Child Psychol Psychiatry*, 59, 1105–13.

Cortese, S., et al. (2016). Gender differences in adult attention-deficit/hyperactivity disorder: results from the National Epidemiologic Survey on Alcohol and Related Conditions (NESARC). *J Clin Psychiatry*, 77, e421–8.

Deberdt, W., et al. (2015). Prevalence of ADHD in nonpsychotic adult psychiatric care (ADPSYC): A multinational cross-sectional study in Europe. *BMC Psychiatry*, 15, 242.

Epstein, J., et al. (2001). *Conners Adult ADHD Diagnosti Interview for DSM-IV*. North Tonowanda, NY: Multi-Health Systems.

Faraone, S. V., et al. (2015). Attention-deficit/hyperactivity disorder. *Nat Rev Dis Primers*, 1, 15020.

Faraone, S. V. & Biederman, J. (2016). Can Attention-Deficit/Hyperactivity Disorder Onset Occur in Adulthood? *JAMA Psychiatry*, 73, 655–6.

Faraone, S. V., et al. (2006). The age-dependent decline of attention deficit hyperactivity disorder: a meta-analysis of follow-up studies. *Psychol Med*, 36, 159–65.

Faraone, S. V., et al. (2000). Toward guidelines for pedigree selection in genetic studies of attention deficit hyperactivity disorder. *Genet Epidemiol*, 18, 1–16.

Faraone, S. V. & Glatt, S. J. (2010). A comparison of the efficacy of medications for adult attention-deficit/hyperactivity disorder using meta-analysis of effect sizes. *J Clin Psychiatry*, 71, 754–63.

Faraone, S. V., et al. (2004). Attention-deficit/hyperactivity disorder in adults: a survey of current practice in psychiatry and primary care. *Arch Intern Med*, 164, 1221–6.

Fayyad, J., et al. (2007). Cross-national prevalence and correlates of adult attention-deficit hyperactivity disorder. *Br J Psychiatry*, 190, 402–9.

Feifel, D. (2008). Commentary: why diagnose and treat ADHD in adults? *Postgrad Med*, 120, 13–15.

Ginsberg, Y. & Lindefors, N. (2012). Methylphenidate treatment of adult male prison inmates with attention-deficit hyperactivity disorder: randomised double-blind placebo-controlled trial with open-label extension. *Br J Psychiatry*, 200, 68–73.

Harold, G. T., et al. (2013). Biological and rearing mother influences on child ADHD symptoms: revisiting the developmental interface between nature and nurture. *J Child Psychol Psychiatry*, 54, 1038–46.

Hepark, S., et al. (2019). The Efficacy of Adapted MBCT on Core Symptoms and Executive Functioning in Adults With ADHD: A Preliminary Randomized Controlled Trial. *J Atten Disord*, 23, 351–62.

Huntley, Z., et al. (2012). Rates of undiagnosed attention deficit hyperactivity disorder in London drug and alcohol detoxification units. *BMC Psychiatry*, 12, 223.

Johnson, K. A., et al. (2009). What would Karl Popper say? Are current psychological theories of ADHD falsifiable? *Behav Brain Funct*, 5, 15.

Kessler, R. C. (2007). *Comorbidity patterns in a community sample of adults with ADHD: results from the National Comorbidity Survey Replication*. APA 160th Annual Meeting.

Kessler, R. C., et al. (2005). The World Health Organization Adult ADHD Self-Report Scale (ASRS): a short screening scale for use in the general population. *Psychol Med*, 35, 245–56.

Kooij, J. J., et al. (2005). Internal and external validity of attention-deficit hyperactivity disorder in a population-based sample of adults. *Psychol Med*, 35, 817–27.

Kooij, J. J. S. (2012). *Adult ADHD: Diagnostic Assessment and Treatment*, London: Springer Healthcare Ltd.

Kooij, S. J., et al. (2010). European consensus statement on diagnosis and treatment of adult ADHD: The European Network Adult ADHD. *BMC Psychiatry*, 10, 67.

Larsson, H., et al. (2013). Genetic and environmental influences on adult attention deficit hyperactivity disorder symptoms: a large Swedish population-based study of twins. *Psychol Med*, 43, 197–207.

Lichtenstein, P. & Larsson, H. (2013). Medication for attention deficit-hyperactivity disorder and criminality. *N Engl J Med*, 368, 776.

Moffitt, T. E., et al. (2015). Is Adult ADHD a Childhood-Onset Neurodevelopmental Disorder? Evidence From a Four-Decade Longitudinal Cohort Study. *Am J Psychiatry*, 172, 967–77.

Mowlem, F. D., et al. (2016). Validation of the Mind Excessively Wandering Scale and the Relationship of Mind Wandering to Impairment in Adult ADHD. *J Atten Disord*, 23, 624–34

Mulligan, A., et al. (2008). Autism symptoms in Attention-Deficit/Hyperactivity Disorder: A Familial trait which Correlates with Conduct, Oppositional Defiant, Language and Motor Disorders. *J Autism Dev Disord*, 39, 197–209.

National Institute for Health and Care Excellence. (2008). *Attention Deficit Hyperactivity Disorder: The NICE guideline on diagnosis and managment of ADHD in children, young people and adults*. London: National Institute for Health and Care Excellence.

National Institute for Health and Care Excellence. (2018). *Diagnosis and management of ADHD in children, young people and adults*. London: National Institute for Health and Care Excellence.

Philipsen, A. (2012). Psychotherapy in adult attention deficit hyperactivity disorder: implications for treatment and research. *Expert Rev Neurother*, 12, 1217–25.

Philipsen, A., et al. (2015). Effects of Group Psychotherapy, Individual Counseling, Methylphenidate, and Placebo in the Treatment of Adult Attention-Deficit/Hyperactivity Disorder: A Randomized Clinical Trial. *JAMA Psychiatry*, 72, 1199–210.

Polanczyk, G., et al. (2007). The worldwide prevalence of ADHD: a systematic review and metaregression analysis. *Am J Psychiatry*, 164, 942–8.

Polanczyk, G. V., et al. (2014). ADHD prevalence estimates across three decades: an updated systematic review and meta-regression analysis. *Int J Epidemiol*, 43, 434–42.

Posner, J., et al. (2014a). Using stimulants to treat ADHD-related emotional lability. *Curr Psychiatry Rep*, 16, 478.

Posner, J., et al. (2014b). Connecting the dots: a review of resting connectivity MRI studies in attention-deficit/hyperactivity disorder. *Neuropsychol Rev*, 24, 3–15.

Reed, G. M., et al. (2019). Innovations and Changes in the ICD-11 Classification of Mental, Behavioural and Neurodevelopmental Disorders. *World Psychiatry*, 18(1), 3–19.

Sibley, M. H., et al. (2018). Late-Onset ADHD Reconsidered With Comprehensive Repeated Assessments Between Ages 10 and 25. *Am J Psychiatry*, 175, 140–9.

Simon, V., et al. (2009). Prevalence and correlates of adult attention-deficit hyperactivity disorder: meta-analysis. *Br J Psychiatry*, 194, 204–11.

Skirrow, C. & Asherson, P. (2013). Emotional lability, comorbidity and impairment in adults with attention-deficit hyperactivity disorder. *J Affect Disord*, 147, 80–6.

Tang, Y. Y., et al. (2015). The neuroscience of mindfulness meditation. *Nat Rev Neurosci*, 16, 213–25.

Van de Glind, G., et al. (2014). Variability in the prevalence of adult ADHD in treatment seeking substance use disorder patients: results from an international multi-center study exploring DSM-IV and DSM-5 criteria. *Drug Alcohol Depend*, 134, 158–66.

Van de Glind, G., et al. (2013). The International ADHD in Substance Use Disorders Prevalence (IASP) study: background, methods and study population. *Int J Methods Psychiatr Res*, 22, 232–44.

Van Lieshout, M., et al. (2016). A 6-year follow up study of a large European cohort of children with attention-deficit/hyperactivity disorder combined subtype: outcomes in late adolescence and young adulthood. *Eur Child Adolesc Psychiatry*, 25, 1007–17.

Van Veen, M. M., et al. (2010). Delayed circadian rhythm in adults with attention-deficit/hyperactivity disorder and chronic sleep-onset insomnia. *Biol Psychiatry*, 67, 1091–6.

Willcutt, E. G. (2012). The prevalence of DSM-IV attention-deficit/hyperactivity disorder: a meta-analytic review. *Neurotherapeutics*, 9, 490–9.

World Health Organization. (2020). *ICD-11. International Classification of Diseases*, eleventh revision. Available from: https://icd.who.int/en.

Young, S., et al. (2014). A meta-analysis of the prevalence of attention deficit hyperactivity disorder in incarcerated populations. *Psychol Med*, 1–12.

Young, S., et al. (2015). A meta-analysis of the prevalence of attention deficit hyperactivity disorder in incarcerated populations. *Psychol Med*, 45, 247–58.

Young, S. J., et al. (2011). The identification and management of ADHD offenders within the criminal justice system: a consensus statement from the UK Adult ADHD Network and criminal justice agencies. *BMC Psychiatry*, 11, 32.

35

Delirium

David Meagher, Cara Daly, and Dimitrios Adamis

Introduction

Delirium is a major neurocognitive disorder that presents as an acute neuropsychiatric syndrome, characterized by a complex constellation of cognitive impairments and neuropsychiatric disturbances that reflect generalized impairment of brain function. It is common in many clinical settings, occurring in approximately one in five hospitalized patients and with rates of up to 90% reported among patients in palliative and intensive care settings (Ryan et al., 2013). Delirium has a considerable impact on patient outcomes and healthcare costs. Patients with delirium experience more prolonged hospitalizations, more complications, greater costs of care, reduced subsequent functional independence, and increased in-hospital and subsequent mortality (Han et al., 2010; Witlox et al., 2010). Importantly, these adverse health and social outcomes are predicted by the presence of delirium and are relatively independent of confounding factors such as morbidity level, baseline cognition, age, and frailty. In addition, delirium may be an accelerating, and possibly causal, factor in the development of dementia (Davis et al., 2012). No other psychiatric disorder has such penetration across healthcare settings—this frequency, along with the complexity of clinical presentation where typically one half of cases are not detected (O'Hanlon et al., 2014), makes delirium a key target for improved management within our healthcare services.

Definition and diagnosis

Delirium is a complex neuropsychiatric syndrome that occurs in the context of physical insult in the form of illness or drug exposure. The onset is acute or subacute and includes changes to mental state with altered consciousness. Prior to the third edition of the *Diagnostic and Statistical Manual of Mental Disorders* (DSM), acute generalized disturbances of brain function were described with a plethora of labels (e.g. acute confusional state, acute brain failure, toxic encephalopathy, intensive care psychosis) that reflected the setting or population in which they occurred, rather than a scientifically distinct condition. However, the introduction of 'delirium' as an umbrella term subsumed these various synonyms and is the diagnostic term that is used to account for acute global disturbances of brain function. This consistency of definition has promoted a more coherent clinical and research effort.

The current DSM-5 criteria for delirium (American Psychiatric Association, 2013) have further refined the definition to characterize delirium as an acute neurocognitive disorder characterized by prominent disturbance of attention, awareness, and other cognitive and perceptual functions. Although these features are not specific to delirium, the time course and context are distinctive—developing over a short time (hours or days), tending to fluctuate, and with temporal links to medical illness, trauma, or drug effects. A further feature is that these disturbances should not be better attributed to other neurocognitive disorders such as dementia or coma. The concept of subsyndromal delirium (SSD) is classified in DSM-5 as 'attenuated delirium syndrome' in recognition that many patients experience significant delirium symptoms, but without meeting full diagnostic criteria. In many cases, subsyndromal illness occurs during the evolution and/or resolution of a delirious episode. SSD has outcomes that are intermediate between no-delirium and full syndromal delirium (Meagher et al., 2014).

Clinical features

Delirium is a complex neuropsychiatric syndrome that can include a wide range of cognitive and psychiatric disturbances that impact upon consciousness, awareness of the immediate environment, thinking, language, perception, affective regulation, sleep–wake cycle, and motor behaviour. These various disturbances can be grouped into three core domains: cognitive, circadian, and higher-order thinking (see Fig. 35.1) (Franco et al., 2013).

Delirium presents with generalized impairment of cognitive abilities, but with particular disturbance to consciousness and attention. Consciousness can be affected both qualitatively ('clouding') as well as quantitatively in terms of arousal, with both reduced arousal and hyperaroused states possible. Where the level of arousal renders formal testing of cognition not possible, this is considered evidence of severe inattention, and thus consistent with a diagnosis of delirium. The exception is coma, which is considered a separate phenomenon to delirium (European Delirium Association and American Delirium Society, 2014). Disturbances to attention are considered the cardinal cognitive disturbance and are reflected in

The Three Core Domain Phenomenological model of Delirium

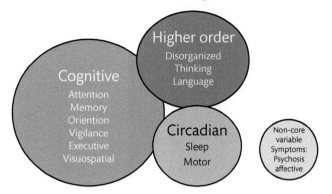

Fig. 35.1 Phenomenological structure of delirium symptoms.

terms of the ability to focus, sustain, and shift attention. This can be demonstrated through the inability to orient to salient stimuli, poor concentration, distractibility, reduced vigilance, and impaired awareness of the immediate environment. Attentional abilities are disproportionately affected, but there are typically discernible disturbances to all other cognitive abilities, including orientation, visuospatial ability, executive function, and short-term memory, which are also commonly impaired and can usually be readily demonstrated with simple bedside tests.

At least one-third of patients have psychotic features. Delusions are typically simple and persecutory and relate to the immediate surroundings (e.g. the hospital is a prison). Perceptual disturbances include illusions and hallucinations and are most commonly visual or tactile. Delirious patients also exhibit affective changes—these usually comprise affective lability (with unpredictable shifts in mood, anger, and/or increased irritability common) but can also present with more sustained lowering of mood that is easily mistaken for depressive illness.

Although delirium is considered as a unitary syndrome of acute generalized cognitive impairment, patients with delirium vary considerably in terms of their neuropsychiatric burden and, in particular, in their patterns of motor activity. Two principal 'hyperactive' and 'hypoactive' presentations are well recognized, as well as an additional 'mixed' category for patients who experience elements of both increased and decreased motor activity within short time frames. Studies that have compared cognitive profiles in these presentations suggest similar levels of disturbance across neuropsychological domains, but with differing patterns in terms of underlying aetiology (hyperactive presentations are commoner in younger patients and substance-related delirium), diagnosis (hypoactive delirium is more frequently missed), and outcomes (hypoactive presentations are linked to poorer prognosis) (Meagher, 2009).

Differential diagnosis

Because delirium encompasses so many potential symptoms, its differential diagnosis is broad and it can be easily mistaken for other neurocognitive and neuropsychiatric disorders such as dementia, depression, or functional psychoses. Accurate diagnosis requires careful consideration of symptoms (including their context) and findings from cognitive assessment and physical investigations.

Importantly, delirium can be the presentation for serious medical illness and, as such. should take diagnostic precedence—i.e. patients experiencing acute changes to mental state in the hospitalized vulnerable should be considered to have delirium until otherwise proven. In practical terms, the clinical rule of thumb is that altered cognition reflects delirium until proven otherwise.

Delirium versus dementia

The most difficult differential diagnosis for delirium is dementia, the other cause of generalized cognitive impairment. While these conditions are classically distinguished by their acuity of onset and temporal course, many dementias (e.g. vascular) can have a relatively acute presentation, while Lewy body dementia can present with a very similar clinical picture to delirium, with fluctuation of symptom severity, visual hallucinations, attentional impairment, alteration of consciousness, and delusions (Gore et al., 2015). Moreover, >50% of cases of delirium occur in the setting of comorbid dementia (Bellelli et al., 2016), which further complicates accurate diagnosis.

However, careful consideration of symptom profile can reliably distinguish delirium and dementia. Abrupt onset and fluctuating course are highly indicative of delirium. In addition, consciousness and attention are invariably disturbed in delirium but remain relatively intact in dementia where memory impairments are cardinal. More recent studies have highlighted bedside tests of attention, vigilance, and visuospatial function which can distinguish delirious (including those with comorbid dementia) from non-delirious patients (Leonard et al., 2016; Meagher et al., 2010). Disorganized or illogical thinking with diminished awareness and grasp of the immediate environment are highly suggestive of delirium. In addition, prominent disruption of the sleep–wake cycle (e.g. severe fragmentation or reversal of cycle) and psychosis are commoner in delirium than in uncomplicated dementia. Where delirium and dementia are comorbid, delirium symptoms tend to dominate the clinical presentation and are thus readily identifiable.

Delirium and mood disorder

Delirium is primarily a neurocognitive disorder, while depressive illness has sustained mood disturbance at its core. However, there is considerable overlap in presentation between hypoactive delirium and depression, with psychomotor retardation characterized by reductions in the amount and speed of activity and speech evident in both conditions. The distinction of delirium and mood disorder is complicated by a range of possible neuropsychiatric presentations, including agitated depression, hyperactive delirium, psychomotor retarded depressive illness, hypoactive delirium, Bell's mania, and depressive pseudodementia, that describe combined mood and cognitive elements. Not surprisingly, delirium and depression are commonly misdiagnosed in clinical practice (O'Sullivan et al., 2014).

Careful assessment of the context of symptoms can facilitate more accurate attribution since delirium is typically more acute in onset and more likely to be linked to acute physical illness, while depressive symptoms typically develop more gradually (weeks) and are linked to psychological stressors. Depressive illness may exhibit diurnal fluctuation in symptom intensity but rarely fluctuates with the intensity of delirium. Disturbances to mood are typically more sustained in depressive illness, while affective lability is more characteristic in delirium. Disturbances of consciousness are more prominent in delirium and underpin the impaired awareness of the immediate environment. The character of psychotic symptoms also differs; in delirium, psychotic features are often simple and persecutory and relate to the immediate environment, while psychotic mood disorders classically include complex mood-congruent psychotic symptoms involving themes of guilt or nihilism.

Overall, the more widespread and profound cognitive changes of delirium, along with the aetiological backdrop and differing clinical course, usually enable a firm distinction from affective disorder.

Delirium and functional psychoses

Although disturbed thinking and perception can occur in both delirium and functional psychoses, such as schizophrenia and psychotic depression, the psychosis of delirium is typically simple, fleeting, and situationally defined, thus contrasting with the often complex and systematized nature of psychosis in primary psychotic illness. Delusional ideas in delirium typically include concerns regarding immediate well-being or perceived danger in the environment. Similarly, in contrast to functional psychoses, hallucinations in delirium tend to be visual, rather than auditory, and so-called Schneiderian features are rare. Consciousness and attention are generally much less impaired in functional psychoses, apart from in the acute stages that can include a 'pseudodelirium' with marked perplexity. However, in such cases, the context of disturbances frequently points towards the correct diagnosis.

Delirium, depression, and dementia

Overall, distinguishing the 3Ds of delirium, depression, and dementia requires careful history taking, augmented by a collateral source where possible, aligned to thorough examination and investigation for acute medical conditions. In more challenging presentations, or where greater diagnostic precision is needed (e.g. in research studies), tools such as the DRS-R98 (Trzepacz et al., 2001) and Cognitive Test for Delirium (CTD) (Hart et al., 1996), can distinguish delirium from other neuropsychiatric presentations. Moreover, the short IQCODE (Jorm, 2004) can reliably identify long-standing disturbances of dementia as long as a reliable informant is available. The Cornell Scale for Depression in dementia (Alexopoulos et al., 1988) can assist in reliably identifying depressive illness in patients with significant cognitive difficulties, including those with dementia. On occasion, the EEG can further assist as the presence of diffuse slowing is more indicative of delirium (81% versus 33%), while the simple 2-lead EEG can also distinguish delirium from non-delirious subjects (Van der Kooi et al., 2015).

The variable clinical course of delirium

The temporal course of a delirium episode characteristically involves an acute onset over hours or days, followed by a fluctuating course where symptoms wax and wane over a 24-hour cycle. Symptoms typically worsen at night and often the patient appears cognitively quite lucid and even recovers in the morning (when assessed on the ward round!).

The onset of delirium is often preceded by a prodromal state in which some delirium symptoms are present, but without full syndromal illness. The patient is often perceived during this period as 'not quite themselves', with non-specific disturbances to concentration, thinking, and energy, with irritability, restlessness, and feelings of malaise (Duppils and Wikblad, 2004). Similarly, resolving delirium also frequently includes a period with lessening intensity of symptoms that is evident as subsyndromal illness (Meagher et al., 2012).

The outcome of delirium is highly variable, ranging from a brief transient episode with full recovery to previous level of cognitive and socioadaptive functioning to a more persistent illness with longer-term cognitive impairment and loss of functional independence. As a consequence, the traditional concept of delirium as a brief, transient, and highly reversible condition is no longer supported by longitudinal studies, as it is estimated that delirium is associated with persistent cognitive problems, including markedly elevated rates of dementia, in around a third of elderly patients with delirium (Davis et al., 2012). Importantly, these difficulties often occur in patients who were assessed as cognitively intact prior to the delirium episode (Maclullich et al., 2009).

Epidemiology

Delirium can occur at any age but is commonest at age extremes. Most epidemiologic studies focus on the elderly, who are at higher risk because of changes that occur in the brain with ageing that increases their vulnerability to delirium. Demographic projections for the general population emphasize increasing agedness over the coming decades and it is expected that delirium rates will increase in parallel with dementia prevalence.

Most studies of the incidence and prevalence of delirium report general hospital populations consisting of either referral samples or consecutive admissions to a given service, with relatively less quality information regarding delirium rates in the general population. Delirium is common across healthcare settings, occurring in 29–64% of medical inpatients (Siddiqi et al., 2006), with even higher rates in medical intensive care units and terminal cancer patients. Delirium is present on admission in half of elderly medicine admissions, while a further third of elderly patients develop delirium during their hospital stay. A clinical rule of thumb seems to be that approximately one in five general hospital patients have delirium some time during hospitalization (Ryan et al., 2013). In long-term residents of care homes, 5–10% typically have delirium at any time.

Prognosis

Delirium is independently associated with adverse outcomes. In a recent meta-analysis of medical, surgical, and ICU studies, delirium was linked with an increased risk of death (2-fold), dementia (12-fold), and new institutionalization (2-fold) (Witlox et al., 2010). Gonzalez et al. (2009), for example, found that mortality was increased by 11% for each additional 48 hours of active delirium. There is also a strong association between delirium and the development of long-term cognitive difficulties (Androsova et al., 2015), including future dementia risk (Davis et al., 2012) and an acceleration in subsequent cognitive decline (Fong et al., 2009). Delirium has also been linked with slow and incomplete recovery of cognitive functioning and persistent cognitive decline after surgery (Saczynski et al., 2012) and in ICU survivors (Pandharipande et al., 2013). Delirium is also associated with subsequent development of PTSD and depression (Davydow, 2009).

Delirious patients are prone to serious complications that include feeding problems, dehydration, pneumonia, urinary incontinence, falls, intravenous line removal, pressure sores, uncooperative behaviour, and problems with consent. However, poor outcomes associated with delirium may relate to a variety of factors, including a consequence of the underlying causes of delirium, complications of active delirium, poor cooperation with medical care, direct neurotoxicity of the delirious state, and toxicity of treatments used to manage delirium. As such, delirium may be linked to poor outcomes by virtue of the functional consequences of the delirious state or direct neurotoxicity or may simply serve as a marker for patients who will do poorly for other reasons. Whatever the mechanism, it is relevant that these poor outcomes correlate with the severity and duration of delirium, such that earlier and more effective symptom reduction is considered a key target within modern healthcare.

Delirium also has significant economic implications since patients with delirium undergo extended hospitalizations that are typically twice as long as non-delirious patients, who have equivalent other morbidity (O'Hanlon et al., 2014).

Pathophysiology

Delirium is considered a unitary syndrome whereby a variety of aetiological insults produce a relatively consistent syndrome of generalized disturbance to brain function, reflecting widespread disturbance of neural networks. This heterogeneity in terms of causation suggests that delirium has many potential underlying mechanisms.

The pathogenesis of delirium is thought to involve interactions between direct brain insults and aberrant stress responses (Maclullich et al., 2008; Maldonado, 2013). Direct brain insults, such as hypoxia, hypoglycaemia, hypercapnia, hyponatraemia, drug effects, stroke, and trauma, directly disrupt brain functioning. However, delirium also occurs due to peripheral disturbances (e.g. urinary tract infection) where there is no obvious direct insult to the brain. In this latter scenario, delirium is thought to represent an abnormal and exaggerated stress response, possibly mediated through cytokines, dysregulation of the hypothalamic–pituitary–adrenal (HPA) axis and glucocorticoid levels, vagal transmission, and communication routes between the periphery and the brain. Such heightened responses are commoner in the ageing or diseased brain, and thus consistent with the two most potent constitutional risk factors for delirium, i.e. older age and pre-existing dementia.

With ageing, for example, higher and more sustained elevation of cortisol occurs in response to acute stressors such as infection. Studies indicate that the delirious state is characterized by elevated cortisol levels, while exogenous glucocorticoids are also known to precipitate delirium. Elevated glucocorticoids may be linked to the delirious state through interactions with monoaminergic neurotransmission, while the longer-term disturbances may reflect the neurotoxic effects of sustained activation of the stress axis that can promote neurodegeneration.

Delirium often occurs in infectious states, and use of cytokines for treatment of medical conditions frequently causes delirium. A number of studies have examined the role of cytokines in delirium, with rather conflicting results. Some reported high levels of pro-inflammatory cytokines (De Rooij et al., 2007), and others (Adamis et al., 2009) low levels of neuroprotective cytokines, to be associated with delirium. Although studies are few to arrive at firm conclusions about the role of cytokines in delirium, a working hypothesis is that deficits in the immunoreactivity of the brain may be associated with delirium. It is possible that high levels or persistence of pro-inflammatory cytokines are not requirements for delirium if there are deficits in the immunoreactivity of the brain (low cerebral reserve). This would explain the observation that delirium occurs more commonly in children and older adults after relatively minor precipitating illnesses, but not in other age groups. Another hypothesis is that, given that cognitive deficits are a strong predictor for delirium, systemic inflammation acts as a stressor that can initiate an acute exacerbation of underling dementia (MacLullich et al., 2008). These hypotheses assume a direct effect of cytokines in the brain. However, it is possible that the relationship between cytokines and delirium is indirect through other mechanism(s) such as cytokine activation of the HPA axis resulting in secretion of glucocorticoids. (MacLullich et al., 2008).

The principal neurochemical disturbances that are linked to delirium involve reduced cholinergic function and hyperdopaminergic drive. Medications with anticholinergic effects can precipitate delirium, while delirium can sometimes be reversed with physostigmine (Dawson and Buckley, 2016). Physiological and structural causes of delirium may act through anticholinergic effects. Age-associated reduction in cholinergic function may underpin the increased delirium incidence with advanced age, while dementia is characterized by reduced brain cholinergic activity. Thiamine deficiency, hypoxia, and hypoglycaemia can all reduce cholinergic function by altering oxidative metabolism of glucose and the production of acetyl coenzyme A (CoA), which is critical as the rate-limiting step in acetylcholine synthesis.

An absolute or relative excess of dopaminergic activity also appears relevant. Intoxication with pro-dopaminergic drugs can cause delirium, while a more direct link is supported by elevation of plasma homovanillic acid levels (a dopaminergic metabolite) during the delirious state (Ramirez-Bermudez et al., 2008). Dopamine-blocking neuroleptic agents remain the most commonly used pharmacological intervention for delirium (Meagher et al., 2013). Of note, these mechanisms are closely linked, whereby D2 receptor activation can inhibit cholinergic activity. Moreover, evidence for involvement of other neurochemical systems (Egberts et al., 2015) suggests that simple pharmacological interventions are unlikely to provide a comprehensive solution in the management of delirious patients.

Studies indicate that localized brain insults are associated with delirium. Neuroimaging studies have demonstrated the involvement of subcortical areas and that white matter hyperintensities may be associated with delirium (Hatano et al., 2013; Omiya et al., 2015). On the other hand, other work have pointed to the involvement of the cortical brain in delirium (Caeiro et al., 2004; Fong et al., 2009). Given that cortical and subcortical areas of the brain are interconnected with long pathways, precise anatomical location of delirium is difficult. Similarly, given that the clinical symptoms of delirium include disturbances of attention, arousal, and thought, cognitive problems, and disruption of the sleep–wake cycle, widespread involvement of both cortical and subcortical structures can be expected. Choi et al. (2012) found that reduction of functional connectivity of subcortical regions with the frontal and prefrontal cortices may underlie the pathophysiology of delirium. An increased duration of delirium has also been associated with smaller frontal lobe and hippocampal volumes and worsening cognitive performance at 3 and 12 months' follow-up (Gunther et al., 2012).

Given that cognitive impairment is a strong risk factor for delirium, Apolipoprotein E (APOE) genotype has been examined as a risk factor for delirium in elderly medical inpatients in ICU, surgery, and other medical settings, with conflicting results. A recent meta-analysis of eight studies (Adamis et al., 2016) indicated no relation of APOE and delirium.

Delirium causation

The occurrence of delirium reflects a dynamic interplay between pre-existing vulnerabilities and precipitating insults, with baseline predisposition especially important. Risk factors for delirium include patient, illness, and treatment factors. The most consistent predictors across patient groups are advanced age, pre-existing cognitive impairment (such as dementia), severe comorbid illness, functional impairment, and psychoactive medication exposure (anticholinergic agents, opioids, and benzodiazepines). Although some risk factors (e.g. age) are non-modifiable, many can be corrected such as uncontrolled pain, anaemia, and infection (see Fig. 35.2) (O'Regan et al., 2013).

The interplay between predisposing and precipitating factors in delirium underlies clinical prediction rules that allow for stratification of patients according to their risk of developing delirium.

This has important implications for preventative practices, as well as the intensity of monitoring effort for emerging delirium. Inouye and Charpentier (1996) developed a model comprising four predisposing factors (cognitive impairment, severe illness, visual impairment, and dehydration), along with five precipitating factors (>3 medications added, catheterization, use of restraints, malnutrition, any iatrogenic event). This model predicted a 17-fold variation in the relative risk of developing delirium and has been validated in subsequent work in other (surgical) populations (Kalisvaart et al., 2005). Similarly, NICE (Young et al., 2010) 2010 guidance on the diagnosis, prevention, and management of delirium highlights four characteristics (i.e. ≥65 years; cognitive impairment or dementia; current hip fracture; severe illness), each of which indicates a need for daily screening.

Prevention of delirium

Improving awareness of delirium through proactive education of staff, combined with risk factor reduction, systematic screening for delirium, and patient-tailored treatment of emergent delirium, can reduce incidence, severity, and duration of incident delirium and delirium-related mortality (Akunne et al., 2012). Delirium is a highly predictable occurrence, such that a variety of patient, illness, and treatment factors can allow for the identification of those who are most at risk (see Fig. 35.1). Many risk factors are modifiable, while others can assist in the assessment of risk–benefit balance of surgical and other interventions in deciding upon optimal care, especially in frail elderly patients with cognitive impairments.

Non-pharmacological interventions

Primary prevention of delirium through non-pharmacological risk reduction strategies has been demonstrated in elderly medical and surgical populations (Siddiqi et al., 2016). Moreover, incident delirium is less severe and of shorter duration when it occurs in the

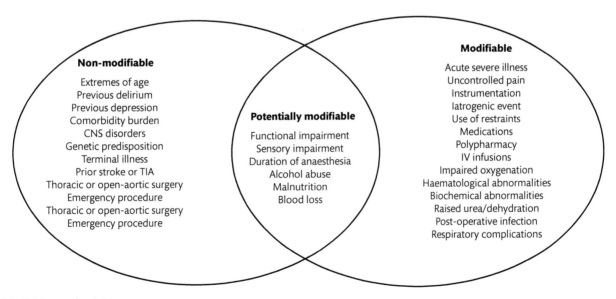

Fig. 35.2 Risk factors for delirium.

setting of active management of delirium proneness. A recent meta-analysis of multifactorial non-pharmacological interventions demonstrated an overall 44% reduction in delirium incidence (Hshieh et al., 2015).

Interventions include many common elements that focus upon assisting orientation, enhancing efficacy (e.g sensory), sleep, pain relief, optimizing physiological parameters (electrolytes, hydration), physical therapy/mobilization, and active review by specialist nurses or geriatricians/geriatric psychiatrists. Many of these represent standard medical and nursing care (e.g. avoiding unnecessary polypharmacy, correcting sensory deficits), but the many competing pressures of modern healthcare environments mean that their protocolization can enhance the standard of care provided in real-world settings. A complex range of factors are involved in delirium causation and, as such, simple interventions (e.g. consensus guidelines, educational interventions) are of limited impact, with better evidence for multifaceted interventions. The success of complex delirium prevention programmes is linked to systems factors that include involvement of clinical leaders, along with support from senior management, integration of activities into everyday routines, and monitoring to promote continued adherence. These interventions are most successful when supported by activities that promote enthusiasm, support implementation, remove barriers, and allow for progress monitoring (Yanamadala et al., 2013).

Notably, these measures appear more effective in preventing delirium in patients at high risk for reasons other than dementia. Moreover, the impact upon longer-term outcomes, such as independence and mortality at 1 year follow-up, is less impressive. In addition, the impact of these programmes is less clear in other settings where risk factors for delirium may differ (e.g. palliative care, community-based settings).

Pharmacological prophylaxis

A series of studies have explored the impact of antipsychotic/anti-dopaminergic and pro-cholinergic agents in the prevention of delirium in high-risk populations. Some prospective work have indicated that prophylactic low-dose use of both typical and atypical antipsychotics may be linked to reduced delirium incidence and/or significantly shorter and less severe delirium where it does occur (Fok et al., 2015). However, a recent review (Inouye et al., 2014) concluded that most evidence suggests limited benefits in terms of hospital length of stay and mortality and, as such, the preventative value of low-dose antipsychotics in high-risk patients remains uncertain. Studies of cholinesterase inhibitors in delirium prevention trials have not demonstrated benefit (van Eijk et al., 2011). Preliminary evidence also supports the use of the α-2 agonist dexmedetomidine as a less deliriogenic means of sedation and melatonin in elderly medical admissions, both of which have been linked with reduced delirium incidence (Djaiani et al., 2016). Careful management of analgesia and/or sedation using protocolized care can also reduce delirium incidence (Dale et al., 2014).

Overall, the evidence for pharmacological prophylaxis is encouraging but does not yet justify routine use, with uncertainties as to the usefulness in high-risk elderly medical inpatients and in those with comorbid dementia. Moreover, optimal dosing and timing of interventions, as well as interaction between pharmacological and non-pharmacological interventions, are unclear.

Diagnostic approach and assessment tools

Assessment

Improving delirium detection in everyday practice is central to reducing the healthcare burden caused by delayed or missed diagnosis of delirium. Studies from across the healthcare spectrum have indicated that typically 50% or more of cases are missed in clinical practice. Lower detection rates occur with hypoactive presentations, comorbid dementia, a history of previous psychiatric problems, and prominent pain, and in the perioperative period (O'Hanlon et al., 2014). A variety of factors underpin this under-identification; 'confusion' in older persons is often trivialized as part of the normal ageing process, leading to under-appreciation of delirium as a clinically important syndrome that warrants thorough investigation and intervention. Similarly, the prevailing stereotype of delirium is of the hyperactive and floridly psychotic clinical picture that characterizes alcohol withdrawal delirium (delirium tremens), but in reality, hypoactive presentations are commoner. Reduced activity is readily overlooked or misattributed to fatigue, senility, and sedation, with the 'good' and 'quiet' patient often presumed to have intact cognition. Importantly, these 'quieter' presentations have a worse prognosis (Meagher, 2009).

A two-step assessment process can promote accurate and efficient delirium detection—an initial simple and brief screening test with high sensitivity, followed by a more detailed and specific assessment for delirium in those who screen positive (Young et al., 2010). This latter stage of assessment is greatly enhanced by an accurate collateral history to clarify the context of symptoms in terms of acuity of onset and normal baseline functioning. Ideally, given its prevalence and seriousness, all high-risk hospitalized patients should undergo daily routine delirium screening.

The initial screening effort should focus upon identifying altered mental status, including cognitive dysfunction. Because delirium includes a disproportionate disturbance of attention, bedside tests that focus upon the ability to focus and sustain attention are advocated for screening. These include reciting the months of the year or days of the week in reverse order, counting backwards from 20, or spelling *WORLD* backwards, with the choice of screening instrument ultimately guided by: (1) the accuracy of the test; (2) the time available; (3) the skillset of the assessor; and (4) the population being assessed. Some tools (e.g. the NuDESC) (Gaudreau et al., 2005) emphasize observable behaviours, instead of formal cognitive testing, and allow accurate screening in healthcare staff who are less familiar with cognitive testing. Sands and colleagues (2010) described a single probe for care staff/relatives—'*Do you think X has been more confused lately*'—in screening for delirium in a palliative care setting and found greater sensitivity (80%), compared to the Confusion Assessment Method (40%)

Delirium testing begins with assessing the level of arousal. Patients who do respond to the clinician's presence but who cannot cooperate with testing should be classed as having severe inattention consistent with delirium (European Delirium Association and American Delirium Society, 2014). This has reduced the use of vague, non-diagnostic terms such as 'stupor' or 'obtundation', with greater use of delirium as a term to describe such patients, thus allowing for more consistent and coherent treatment effort.

The second phase of assessment for delirium focuses upon diagnosis and can be assisted by a variety of approaches. These include tools, such as the CAM (Inouye et al., 1990), the 4As Test (4AT) (Bellelli et al., 2014), the Delirium Observation Screening Scale (DOS) (Schuurmans et al., 2003), or the systematic application of DSM-IV or DSM-5 criteria (Meagher et al., 2014). The CAM is a diagnostic algorithm in which raters perform a cognitive test, such as the MMSE, then seek informant history, then rate the presence or absence of: (1) acute change or fluctuating course; (2) inattention; (3) disorganized thinking; and (4) level of consciousness. The CAM requires specific training and takes 8–10 minutes to complete. The 3D-CAM is a new adaptation of the CAM that is more structured and requires 3 minutes (Marcantonio et al., 2014). The 4AT takes 1–2 minutes to complete and includes items assessing: (1) level of arousal; (2) orientation; (3) attention (months of the year backwards); and (4) acute onset or fluctuating course. No specific training is required. The DOS is designed for nurses to complete at the end of a shift, with 13 features scored as present or absent. It takes 2–3 minutes to complete the scoring sheet. More detailed instruments that require expert assessment include the Delirium Rating Scale–Revised–98 (DRS-R98) (Trzepacz et al., 2001), the Cognitive Test for Delirium (CTD) (Hart et al., 1996), and the Memorial Delirium Assessment Scale (Breitbart et al., 1997), which allow severity grading, as well as differentiation from other neuropsychiatric diagnoses.

Management of delirium

General principles

The optimal management of delirium requires collaboration between primary physicians, nursing staff, family/carers, and delirium specialists. A fundamental challenge is to identify and treat underlying causes, but because delirium (including the severity of its symptoms) predicts poor outcomes independently of underlying morbidities, it is also important to manage delirium symptoms in their own right, rather than relying solely upon addressing the primary aetiological causes as a means of symptom alleviation.

The key principles of management include: (1) ensuring patient and staff safety; (2) minimizing the potential for complications such as falls, self-injury, and hypostasis; (3) simplifying the care environment to avoid excessive sensory stimulation; (4) minimizing the impact of any sensory impediments, while promoting patient autonomy to enhance orientation and functional abilities; (5) promoting healthy sleep–wake patterns, while minimizing pain—all important elements that lay the foundation for recovery. Communication with delirious patients should include simple language expressed in a clearly audible, slow-paced voice. Orienting techniques (e.g. calendars) and familiarizing the environment (e.g. family photographs) are helpful, and engaging family members in care can help to clarify changes from baseline status and is more reassuring for patients who often have a reduced capacity to comprehend their surroundings. Providing an optimal care environment requires careful balancing of the sometimes conflicting needs of minimizing risk versus provision of individualized, patient-focused care that promotes autonomy and dignity. Concerns regarding the safety of delirious patients at risk of falls and wandering can drive restrictive care practices that inhibit re-orientation, mobility, and self-efficacy. Less restrictive care can be facilitated by electronic alarms and pressure mats to monitor patient behaviour and alert staff when vulnerable patients are at risk of wandering or falls

Identifying underlying causes

A fundamental aspect of management is to identify and treat underlying causes of delirium. It is important to remember that single-aetiology delirium is the exception, with typically 3–4 significant causative factors relevant during any single episode, which interact and overlap sequentially to produce or sustain delirium symptoms. Delirium is thus typically multifactorial in aetiology and requires comprehensive assessment for multiple causes. This begins with a thorough history taking and examination, including collateral history from relatives/carers and nursing staff, followed by a careful review of recent medication exposure.

Some of the more commonly performed investigations that should be considered in all delirious patients are shown in Box 35.1, along with other second-line investigations that are guided by clinical assessment and the findings from preliminary tests. The commonest causes are infection, polypharmacy, and metabolic abnormalities (Laurila et al., 2008). No identifiable cause is identified in 10% of cases.

Box 35.1 Work-up of suspected delirium

1 Careful history and physical examination
2 Collateral history:
   – Baseline cognition
   – Presence of sensory impairments
   – Exposure to risk factors
   – Review of medications, procedures, tests, and intraoperative data
3 First-line investigations:
   – Full blood count
   – Electrolytes, magnesium, calcium, phosphate
   – Liver function tests
   – Urinalysis
   – Electrocardiogram
   – Erythrocyte sedimentation rate
   – Blood glucose
   – Chest radiograph
   – Urinalysis
4 Second-line investigations (as indicated):
   – Drug screen
   – Blood cultures
   – Cardiac enzymes
   – Blood gases
   – Serum folate/B12
   – Electroencephalography
   – Cerebrospinal fluid examination
   – Computed tomography of the brain
   – Magnetic resonance imaging of the brain
   – Prolactin level
   – HIV antibodies
   – Syphilis serology
   – Urinary porphyrins

Treatment

Management of an established case of delirium involves the combined efforts of medical, nursing staff, and carers to apply a variety of non-pharmacological and pharmacological strategies, as part of a care plan that should be carefully tailored to the individual needs of each patient. The heterogeneity of causation and symptom profile is such that these needs vary considerably. The lack of good evidence to inform clinical decisions about delirium treatment means that management in everyday practice is guided by expert consensus guidelines (Young et al., 2010). While there is broad agreement regarding most aspects of care, when and how to use medications remains an aspect of delirium care where there is a lack of clear consensus.

Non-pharmacological measures

Management of the care environment for delirious patients is crucial to minimizing complications, while providing a suitable platform for patient recovery. Common strategies are listed in Box 35.2. The complications of delirium can be minimized by careful attention to the potential for falls and avoidance of prolonged hypostasis. Relatives can play an important role in supporting and reorienting patients, but ill-informed, critical, or anxious caregivers can add to the burden of a delirious patient. A non-therapeutic triangle can emerge whereby healthcare providers respond to family distress by medicating patients, which complicates ongoing cognitive assessment. Clarification of the cause and meaning of symptoms, combined with recognition of treatment goals, can allow better management of what is a distressing experience for both patients and loved ones.

The evidence to support the use of non-pharmacological interventions in treating established delirium is less convincing than that for primary prevention. Studies have focused on delirium in frail elderly medical populations where the course of delirium may be less modifiable due to high rates of comorbid dementia. Existing research indicates that non-pharmacological treatments impact modestly upon the duration of delirium and possibly the length of inpatient stay, but longer-term outcomes, such as discharge to independent living and mortality, appear unaltered (Abraha et al., 2015). More recently, efforts have examined the impact of specialist delirium care units in managing prolonged or otherwise challenging cases. Preliminary findings suggest a positive impact on patient and carer experience, but without necessarily impacting upon outcomes such as length of stay (Goldberg et al., 2013).

Box 35.2 Non-pharmacological management of delirium

- Educate patient and family/carer on delirium and prognosis (e.g. information leaflets).
- Involve family/carer in hospital care routine.
- Reorientation and reassurance strategies.
- Normalize sleep patterns.
- Prevent complications, e.g. falls, constipation.
- Ensure adequate hydration.
- Ensure pain relief is adequate.
- Encourage activity—mobility and ADLs.
- Use visual/hearing aids to facilitate communication.
- Nurse with familiar staff in relaxed uncluttered environment.

Pharmacological interventions

Pharmacological management is an aspect of delirium care that remains controversial, with considerable variability in everyday practice. A lack of high-quality evidence to demonstrate benefits in terms of medium- and longer-term outcomes, aligned to the potential for adverse effects, especially in highly morbid and frequently physically frail older patients, mandates that decisions around medication use are made on a case-by-case basis.

Antipsychotics have long been the gold standard pharmacological treatment, based upon their theoretical value, empirical knowledge of their use, and results from over 20 open-label prospective studies. However, antipsychotic agents are associated with a variety of risks, including sedation, hypotension, extrapyramidal effects, cardiotoxicity (e.g. QT interval prolongation), and an increased risk of stroke in patients with dementia.

Conversely, gathering evidence suggests that antipsychotic use can reduce the duration and severity of delirium in older medical and ICU patients. Prospective studies have suggested that around 75% of delirious patients who received short-term low-dose antipsychotic treatment experienced clinical response. Response rates appeared quite consistent across different patient groups and treatment settings (Meagher et al., 2013). Importantly, the extent to which therapeutic effects reflect alleviation of specific symptoms (e.g. sleep or behavioural disturbances) versus a syndromal effect that encompasses both cognitive and non-cognitive symptoms of delirium is not known, but the effectiveness of treatments is not closely related to sedative or antipsychotic effects. Recent NICE guidelines recommend cautious use of olanzapine or haloperidol (Young et al., 2010), particularly where the patient is distressed with severe agitation or psychosis and/or if there is significant risk of physical harm to the patient or others, or delirium symptoms are impeding the ability to provide essential treatments such as oxygen, parenteral fluids, or antibiotics.

Studies have not suggested significant differences in efficacy for haloperidol, compared to atypical agents but reported higher rates of extrapyramidal side effects with haloperidol. Commonly used agents include risperidone (starting dose 0.25 mg), olanzapine (starting dose 2.5 mg), quetiapine (starting dose 12.5 mg), or haloperidol (starting dose 0.5 mg). Of these, quetiapine is relatively more sedative, while haloperidol is readily available both orally or parenterally. Best practice is to 'start low and go slow', with dose titration according to response and adverse effects. Treatment is short term and typically discontinued after 3–5 days.

Benzodiazepines have a limited role in delirium management. They are first-line treatment in withdrawal states or seizures but are otherwise best avoided, as they can perpetuate delirium, cloud ongoing cognitive assessment, and are linked to falls and oversedation. Despite their theoretical appeal, pro-cholinergic treatments do not appear to be effective in the management of acute delirium episodes (van Eijk et al., 2011).

Post-delirium management

The management of delirious patients does not end once the florid phase settles. In many cases, there are persistent or residual cognitive and functional deficits, while delirium is a recurring condition that requires careful consideration of ongoing risk. However, many patients experiencing delirium are discharged before full resolution of symptoms, without adequate arrangements for continued monitoring and management. Further episodes may be prevented by addressing risk factors such as medication exposure and sensory impairments. Also, significant adjustment difficulties, including depression and PTSD, can occur and impact upon subsequent help-seeking. More than half of patients experiencing delirium (O'Malley et al., 2008) recall psychotic symptoms at 6 months' follow-up, many of whom are still distressed by these recollections. Many patients experience lingering concerns that the episode represents a first step towards loss of mental faculties and independence. Explicit discussion of the meaning of delirium can facilitate adjustment and minimize future risk. A follow-up visit soon after hospital discharge can facilitate post-delirium adjustment by clarifying the transient nature of delirium symptoms, in contrast to dementia, as well as providing any ongoing medication adjustments. Moreover, given the frequency of persistent cognitive and functional impairments, such engagements provide an ideal opportunity to plan for ongoing care needs.

Conclusion

Delirium is a common and complex neuropsychiatric syndrome. While it is estimated that approximately one in five hospitalized patients experience delirium at some point, typically 50% or more of cases are missed or misdiagnosed. Delirium is associated with a range of adverse healthcare outcomes, including prolonged hospitalization with elevated costs of care, impaired subsequent socio-adaptive functionality, an increased risk of persistent cognitive difficulties such as dementia, and markedly elevated mortality rates. Importantly, these outcomes are independently predicted by the severity and duration of delirium. The pathophysiology of delirium is not well understood but involves generalized disruption of neural function and is linked to disturbed stress axis function. Key challenges for improving delirium recognition relate to distinguishing it from dementia and depression. Routine systematic cognitive testing aligned to formal screening for delirium in high-risk cases can improve detection in everyday practice. Delirium is highly preventable, with a third of cases avoidable through non-pharmacological strategies that address a variety of patient, illness, and treatment factors. Treatment of incident delirium requires careful consideration of underlying causes and aggravating environmental factors and prudent use of pharmacological strategies. Atypical and typical antipsychotic agents remain the best studied pharmacological intervention, but high-quality evidence to support their safety and effectiveness remains lacking. Careful attention to post-delirium care can minimize functional loss, address any psychological sequelae, and reduce the risk of further episodes.

KEY LEARNING POINTS

- Delirium is a common, complex neuropsychiatric syndrome that occurs in approximately one in five hospitalized patients.
- It is associated with a range of adverse healthcare outcomes that are independently predicted by the severity and duration

of delirium. Typically 50% or more of cases of delirium are missed, misdiagnosed, or diagnosed late in everyday practice. However, routine systematic cognitive testing aligned to formal screening for delirium in high-risk cases can improve detection in everyday practice.

- The relationship between delirium and dementia is complex; dementia is a potent risk factor for delirium and 50% of delirium occurs in the context of a pre-existing dementia, but evidence also indicates that the occurrence of delirium can accelerate the course of dementia and that many cases of delirium are followed by long-term cognitive impairment.
- Delirium is highly preventable, with a third of cases avoidable by addressing a variety of patient, illness, and treatment factors. Treatment of incident delirium requires careful consideration of underlying causes and aggravating environmental factors and prudent use of pharmacological strategies, with antipsychotic agents as the preferred pharmacological intervention. Careful attention to post-delirium care can minimize functional loss, address any psychological sequelae, and reduce the risk of further episodes.

REFERENCES

Abraha, I, Trotta, F, Rimland, J.M., et al. Efficacy of non-pharmacological interventions to prevent and treat delirium in older patients: a systematic overview. The SENATOR project ONTOP Series. *PLoS One* 2015;10(6):e0123090.

Adamis, D., Lunn, M. Martin, F.C., et al. Cytokines and IGF-I in delirious and non-delirious acutely ill older medical inpatients. *Age and Ageing* 2009;38(3):326–32.

Adamis, D., Meagher, D., Williams, J., Mulligan, O., McCarthy, G. A systematic review and meta-analysis of the association between the apolipoprotein E genotype and delirium. *Psychiatric Genetics* 2016; 26(2):53–9.

Akunne, A., Murthy, L., Young, J. Cost-effectiveness of multi-component interventions to prevent delirium in older people admitted to medical wards. *Age and Ageing* 2012;41:285–91.

Alexopoulos, G.S., Abrams, R.C., Young, R.C., Shamoian, C.A. Cornell scale for depression in dementia. *Biological Psychiatry* 1988;23(3):271–84.

American Psychiatric Association. *Diagnostic and Statistical Manual of Mental Disorders (DSM-5®)*. Washington, DC: American Psychiatric Pub; 2013.

Androsova, G., Krause, R., Winterer, G., Schneider, R., Biomarkers of postoperative delirium and cognitive dysfunction. *Frontiers in Aging Neuroscience* 2015;9(7):112.

Bellelli, G., Morandi, A., Davis, D.H., et al. Validation of the 4AT, a new instrument for rapid delirium screening: a study in 234 hospitalised older people. *Age and Ageing* 2014;43(4):496–502.

Bellelli, G., Morandi, A., Di Santo, S.G., et al. 'Delirium Day': a nationwide point prevalence study of delirium in older hospitalized patients using an easy standardized diagnostic tool. *BMC Medicine* 2016;14(1):1.

Breitbart, W., Rosenfeld, B., Roth, A., Smith, M.J., Cohen, K., Passik, S. The memorial delirium assessment scale. *Journal of Pain and Symptom Management* 1997;13(3):128–37.

Caeiro, L., Ferro, J.M., Albuquerque, R., Figueira, M.L., Delirium in the first days of acute stroke. *Journal of Neurology* 2004;251(2):171–8.

Choi, S.H., Lee, H., Chung, T.S., et al. Neural network functional connectivity during and after an episode of delirium. *American Journal of Psychiatry* 2012;169(5):498–507.

Dale, C.R., Kannas, D.A., Fan, V.S., et al. Improved analgesia, sedation, and delirium protocol associated with decreased duration of delirium and mechanical ventilation. *Annals of the American Thoracic Society* 2014;11(3):367–74.

Davis, D.H., Terrera, G.M., Keage, H., et al. Delirium is a strong risk factor for dementia in the oldest-old: a population-based cohort study. *Brain* 2012;135(9):2809–16.

Davydow, D.S., Symptoms of depression and anxiety after delirium. *Psychosomatics* 2009;50(4):309–16.

Dawson, A.H. and Buckley, N.A. Pharmacological management of anticholinergic delirium-theory, evidence and practice. *British Journal of Clinical Pharmacology* 2016; 81(3):516–24.

De Rooij, S.E., Van Munster, B.C., Korevaar, J.C., Levi, M. Cytokines and acute phase response in delirium. *Journal of Psychosomatic Research* 2007;62(5):521–5.

Duppils, G.S. and Wikblad, K. Delirium behavioural changes before and during the prodromal phase. *Journal of Clinical Nursing* 2004;13(5):609–16.

Djaiani, G., Silverton, N., Fedorko, L., et al. Dexmedetomidine versus Propofol Sedation Reduces Delirium after Cardiac Surgery: A Randomized Controlled Trial. *Journal of the American Society of Anesthesiologists* 2016;124(2):362–8.

Egberts, A., Fekkes, D., Wijnbeld, E.H., et al. Disturbed Serotonergic Neurotransmission and Oxidative Stress in Elderly Patients with Delirium. *Dementia and Geriatric Cognitive Disorders Extra* 2015;5(3):450–8.

European Delirium Association. The DSM-5 criteria, level of arousal and delirium diagnosis: inclusiveness is safer. *BMC Medicine* 2014;12(1):141.

Fok, M.C., Sepehry, A.A., Frisch, L., et al. Do antipsychotics prevent postoperative delirium? A systematic review and meta-analysis. *International Journal of Geriatric Psychiatry* 2015;30(4):333–44.

Fong, T.G., Jones, R.N., Shi, P., et al. Delirium accelerates cognitive decline in Alzheimer disease. *Neurology* 2009;72(18):1570–5.

Franco, J.G., Trzepacz, P.T., Meagher, D.J., et al. Three core domains of delirium validated using exploratory and confirmatory factor analyses. *Psychosomatics* 2013;54(3):227–38.

Gaudreau, J.D., Gagnon, P., Harel, F., Tremblay, A., Roy, M.A. Fast, systematic, and continuous delirium assessment in hospitalized patients: the nursing delirium screening scale. *Journal of Pain and Symptom Management* 2005;29(4):368–75.

Goldberg, S.E., Bradshaw, L.E., Kearney, F.C., et al. Care in specialist medical and mental health unit compared with standard care for older people with cognitive impairment admitted to general hospital: randomised controlled trial (NIHR TEAM trial). *BMJ* 2013;347:f4132.

González, M., Martínez, G., Calderón, J., et al. Impact of delirium on short-term mortality in elderly inpatients: a prospective cohort study. *Psychosomatics* 2009;50(3):234–8.

Gore, R.L., Vardy, E.R., T O'Brien, J., Delirium and dementia with Lewy bodies: distinct diagnoses or part of the same spectrum? *Journal of Neurology, Neurosurgery & Psychiatry* 2015;86(1):50–9.

Gunther, M.L., Morandi, A., Krauskopf, E., et al. The association between brain volumes, delirium duration and cognitive outcomes in intensive care unit survivors: a prospective exploratory cohort magnetic resonance imaging study. *Critical Care Medicine* 2012;40(7):2022.

Han, J.H., Shintani, A., Eden, S., et al. Delirium in the emergency department: an independent predictor of death within 6 months. *Annals of Emergency Medicine* 2010;56(3):244–52.

Hart, R.P., Levenson, J.L., Sessler, C.N., Best, A.M., Schwartz, S.M., Rutherford, L.E. Validation of a cognitive test for delirium in medical ICU patients. *Psychosomatics* 1996;37(6):533–46.

Hatano, Y., Narumoto, J., Shibata, K., et al. White-matter hyperintensities predict delirium after cardiac surgery. *American Journal of Geriatric Psychiatry* 2013;21(10):938–45.

Hshieh, T.T., Yue, J., Oh, E., et al. Effectiveness of multicomponent nonpharmacological delirium interventions: a meta-analysis. *JAMA Internal Medicine* 2015;175(4):512–20.

Inouye, S.K., Van Dyck, C.H., Alessi, C.A., Balkin, S., Siegal, A.P., Horwitz, R.I., Clarifying confusion: the confusion assessment method: a new method for detection of delirium. *Annals of Internal Medicine* 1990;113(12):941–8.

Inouye, S.K., Charpentier, P.A., Precipitating factors for delirium in hospitalized elderly persons: predictive model and interrelationship with baseline vulnerability. *JAMA* 1996;275(11);852–7.

Inouye, S.K., Marcantonio, E.R., Metzger, E.D. Doing damage in delirium: The hazards of antipsychotic treatment in elderly persons. *The Lancet Psychiatry* 2014;1(4):312.

Jorm, A.F. The Informant Questionnaire on cognitive decline in the elderly (IQCODE): a review. *International Psychogeriatrics* 2004;16(3):275–93.

Kalisvaart, K.J., De Jonghe, J.F., Bogaards, M.J., et al. Haloperidol Prophylaxis for Elderly Hip-Surgery Patients at Risk for Delirium: A Randomized Placebo-Controlled Study. *Journal of the American Geriatrics Society* 2005;53(10):1658–66.

Laurila, J.V., Laakkonen, M.L., Laurila, J.V., Timo, S.E., Reijo, T.S. Predisposing and precipitating factors for delirium in a frail geriatric population. *Journal of Psychosomatic Research* 2008;65(3):249–54.

Leonard, M., McInerney, S., McFarland, J., et al. Comparison of cognitive and neuropsychiatric profiles in hospitalised elderly medical patients with delirium, dementia and comorbid delirium–dementia. *BMJ Open* 2016;6(3):e009212.

MacLullich, A.M., Ferguson, K.J., Miller, T., de Rooij, S.E., Cunningham, C. Unravelling the pathophysiology of delirium: a focus on the role of aberrant stress responses. *Journal of Psychosomatic Research* 2008;65(3):229–38.

MacLullich, A.M., Beaglehole, A., Hall, R.J., Meagher, D.J. Delirium and long-term cognitive impairment. *International Review of Psychiatry* 2009;21(1):30–42.

Maldonado, J.R. Neuropathogenesis of delirium: review of current etiologic theories and common pathways. *American Journal of Geriatric Psychiatry* 2013;21(12):1190–222.

Marcantonio, E. R., Ngo, L. H., O'Connor, M., et al. 3D-CAM: derivation and validation of a 3-minute diagnostic interview for CAM-defined delirium: a cross-sectional diagnostic test study. *Annals of Internal Medicine* 2014;161:554–61.

Meagher, D. Motor subtypes of delirium: past, present and future. *International Review of Psychiatry* 2009;21(1):59–73.

Meagher, D., Adamis, D., Trzepacz, P., Leonard, M., Features of subsyndromal and persistent delirium. *British Journal of Psychiatry* 2012;200(1):37–44.

Meagher, D., O'Regan, N., Ryan, D., et al. Frequency of delirium and subsyndromal delirium in an adult acute hospital population. *British Journal of Psychiatry* 2014;205(6):478–85.

Meagher, D.J., Leonard, M., Donnelly, S., Conroy, M., Saunders, J., Trzepacz, P.T. A comparison of neuropsychiatric and cognitive profiles in delirium, dementia, comorbid delirium-dementia and cognitively intact controls. *Journal of Neurology, Neurosurgery & Psychiatry* 2010;81(8):876–81.

Meagher, D.J., Morandi, A., Inouye, S.K., et al. Concordance between DSM-IV and DSM-5 criteria for delirium diagnosis in a pooled database of 768 prospectively evaluated patients using the delirium rating scale-revised-98. *BMC Medicine* 2014;12(1):164.

Meagher, D.J., McLoughlin, L., Leonard, M., Hannon, N., Dunne, C., and O'Regan, N. What do we really know about the treatment of delirium with antipsychotics? Ten key issues for delirium pharmacotherapy. *American Journal of Geriatric Psychiatry* 2013;21(12):1223–38.

O'Hanlon, S., O'Regan, N., MacLullich, A.M., et al. Improving delirium care through early intervention: from bench to bedside to boardroom. *Journal of Neurology, Neurosurgery & Psychiatry* 2014;85(2):207–13.

O'Malley, G., Leonard, M., Meagher, D. and O'Keeffe, S.T., The delirium experience: a review. *Journal of Psychosomatic Research* 2008; 65(3):223–8.

Omiya, H., Yoshitani, K., Yamada, N., et al. Preoperative brain magnetic resonance imaging and postoperative delirium after off-pump coronary artery bypass grafting: a prospective cohort study. *Canadian Journal of Anesthesia/Journal Canadien d'Anesthésie* 2015;62(6):595–602.

O'Regan, N.A., Fitzgerald, J., Timmons, S., O'Connell, H., Meagher, D., Delirium: a key challenge for perioperative care. *International Journal of Surgery* 2013;11(2):136–44.

O'Sullivan, R., Inouye, S.K., Meagher, D., Delirium and depression: inter-relationship and clinical overlap in elderly people. *The Lancet Psychiatry* 2014;1(4):303–11.

Pandharipande, P.P., Girard, T.D., Jackson, J.C., et al. Long-term cognitive impairment after critical illness. *New England Journal of Medicine* 2013;369(14):1306–16.

Ramirez-Bermudez, J., Ruiz-Chow, A., Perez-Neri, I., et al. Cerebrospinal fluid homovanillic acid is correlated to psychotic features in neurological patients with delirium. *General Hospital Psychiatry* 2008;30(4):337–43.

Ryan, D.J., O'Regan, N.A., Caoimh, R.Ó., et al. Delirium in an adult acute hospital population: predictors, prevalence and detection. *BMJ Open* 2013;3(1):e001772.

Saczynski, J.S., Marcantonio, E.R., Quach, L., et al. Cognitive trajectories after postoperative delirium. *New England Journal of Medicine* 2012;367(1):30–9.

Sands, M.B., Dantoc, B.P., Hartshorn, A., Ryan, C.J., Lujic, S. Single question in delirium (SQiD): testing its efficacy against psychiatrist interview, the confusion assessment method and the memorial delirium assessment scale. *Palliative Medicine* 2010;24(6):561–5.

Schuurmans, M.J., Shortridge-Baggett, L.M., Duursma, S.A. The Delirium Observation Screening Scale: a screening instrument for delirium. *Research and Theory for Nursing Practice* 2003;17(1):31–50.

Siddiqi, N., House, A.O., Holmes, J.D.,. Occurrence and outcome of delirium in medical in-patients: a systematic literature review. *Age and Ageing* 2006;35(4):350–64.

Siddiqi, N., Harrison, J.K., Clegg, A., et al. Interventions for preventing delirium in hospitalised non-ICU patients. *The Cochrane Library* 2016;3:10.1002/14651858.

Trzepacz, P.T., Mittal, D., Torres, R., Kanary, K., Norton, J., Jimerson, N. Validation of the Delirium Rating Scale-revised-98: comparison with the delirium rating scale and the cognitive test for delirium. *Journal of Neuropsychiatry and Clinical Neurosciences* 2001;13(2):229–42.

Van Der Kooi, A.W., Zaal, I.J., Klijn, F.A., et al. Delirium detection using EEG: what and how to measure. *Chest* 2015;147(1):94–101.

van Eijk, M.M., Roes, K.C., Honing, M.L., et al. Effect of rivastigmine as an adjunct to usual care with haloperidol on duration of delirium and mortality in critically ill patients: a multicentre, double-blind, placebo-controlled randomised trial. *Critical Care* 2011;15(1):1.

Witlox, J., Eurelings, L.S., de Jonghe, J.F., Kalisvaart, K.J., Eikelenboom, P., Van Gool, W.A. Delirium in elderly patients and the risk of postdischarge mortality, institutionalization, and dementia: a meta-analysis. *JAMA* 2010;304(4):443–51.

Yanamadala, M., Wieland, D. and Heflin, M.T. Educational interventions to improve recognition of delirium: a systematic review. *Journal of the American Geriatrics Society* 2013;61(11):1983–93.

Young, J., Murthy, L., Westby, M., Akunne, A., O'Mahony, R. Diagnosis, prevention, and management of delirium: summary of NICE guidance. *BMJ* 2010;341:3704.

36

Catatonia

Max Fink

Introduction

'An unkempt unmoving man, standing silently and stiffly, staring at the ceiling, arms tightly at his sides, paying no heed nor responding to the persons about him.

A child is mute, rocking to and fro, hitting his head against the bed's headboard, requiring restraints to protect him from self-harm.

A distraught and disheveled woman runs through the ward, repeatedly shouting "Don't kill me, don't kill me!" requiring restraint and sedation.

An acutely ill unresponsive young man is brought to the hospital Emergency Room in stupor, febrile, sweating, stiff, and dehydrated.'

Each subject is suffering from catatonia, an acute systemic syndrome that can be effectively treated once it is recognized. For more than a century, catatonia has been cloistered as a marker of the Kraepelin/Bleuler concept of schizophrenia. In the past 40 years, however, catatonia has been divorced from this marriage and is increasingly accepted as an independent, identifiable, and treatable syndrome, distinct from schizophrenia (Fink, 2013; Fink and Taylor, 2003; Shorter and Fink, 2018; Taylor and Fink, 2003).

Before Kraepelin's descriptions of dementia praecox and manic depressive insanity as principal diseases among the chronically ill patients in his university academic hospital, an acute illness of abnormal motor behaviours had been delineated by Karl Kahlbaum in his sanitarium in Görlitz, Germany (Kahlbaum, 1874; Kahlbaum, 1973). In a small book of 110 pages *Die Katatonie oder das Spannungsirresein: eine klinische form psychischer Krankheit*, Kahlbaum presented 26 vignettes of immobile and stuporous patients—some rigid and posturing, others moving and pacing continually, some repeatedly hitting a wall or themselves, or standing and staring, unblinking, repeating words or phrases over and over, sometimes in whispers or repetitive shouts. Many were excited, grandiose, delirious, delusional, or in stupor, but the behaviours that marked them together were their motor behaviours. Some also suffered with syphilis, tuberculosis, or epilepsy.

Kahlbaum delineated his patients so well that many authors quickly recognized the unique syndrome. Kraepelin found Kahlbaum's signs among his long-stay chronically ill. Shuffling index cards in which he had written his patients' histories, he found catatonia most often among those with *dementia praecox*, the life-long illness that progressed slowly to dementia and rarely remitted that he had delineated. In the 6th edition of his textbook in 1899, catatonia became a subtype of dementia praecox (Shorter, 1997).

When the Swiss psychiatrist Eugen Bleuler renamed the illness to *schizophrenia* in 1908, he too described catatonia as an identifying marker. When psychiatric illnesses were formally classified in 1952 by the American Psychiatric Association in the *Diagnostic Statistical Manual of Mental Disorders*, catatonia continued in the Kraepelinian tradition of being cited only as *schizophrenia, catatonic type* (295.2) (American Psychiatric Association, 1952). In subsequent DSM revisions, catatonia continued to be referenced as a singular type of schizophrenia (American Psychiatric Association, 1968, 1980, 1994).

For a century, clinicians could only assign the diagnosis of *schizophrenia, catatonic type* for any patient with catatonia. Following treatment guidelines for schizophrenia, the designation recommended the prescription of potent neuroleptic drugs. Some catatonic subjects developed an acute neurotoxic syndrome with escalating fever, hypertension, tachycardia, sweating, and delirium. Some died. By 1980, the toxic illness was labelled the 'neuroleptic malignant syndrome' (NMS) (Caroff, 1980). Believing NMS to be the result of dopaminergic blockade of neuroleptic drug action, dopamine agonists were prescribed. And erroneously seeing the possibility that muscle weakness was related to malignant hyperthermia, treatment with dantrolene was also prescribed. But these treatments did not relieve NMS. Improvement came when administration of neuroleptics was discontinued.

By the 1980s, benzodiazepines and ECT were accepted as effective treatments.

The connection of catatonia with schizophrenia in the psychiatric classification was partially broken in 1994 in DSM-IV when *catatonia secondary to a medical condition* (293.89) was listed as an identifiable diagnosis. The connection of catatonia with schizophrenia was fully broken in DSM-5 in 2013 with the deletion of the class *catatonia type of schizophrenia* and retention of *catatonia secondary to a medical condition*. Catatonia is now identified as a systemic medical, not as a primary psychiatric, syndrome (Fink et al., 2016a). This designation strengthens the consideration of catatonia in patients referred to modern consultation liaison services.

When to consider catatonia

Catatonia is to be considered in the differential diagnosis of any patient reporting an acute change in motor behaviours—mutism, excitement, delirium, stupor, abnormal speech, posturing, and repetitive rhythmic acts. Alternation of agitation and stupor is characteristic of catatonia. The diagnosis is aided when patients are examined using a Catatonia Rating Scale (CRS), developed at Stony Brook University Hospital and cited as the Bush–Francis CRS, published in 1996 (Bush et al., 1996a, b).

The examination usually requires <5 minutes (see Table 36.1). The instrument lists 23 items, scored on either a 4-point or a 2-point scale (see Box 36.1).

The first 14 items are recommended as a 'screening instrument', to identify subjects with total scores of 2 or more who warrant further testing. In hospital-wide surveys using the CRS, most patients scored 2 or less. Positive catatonia scores range from 4 to 14 on the screening instrument.

Body temperature is the second guide to the diagnosis. Fever and autonomic abnormality mark malignant catatonia, a life-threatening condition. Febrile patients warrant a detailed systemic medical review.

Table 36.1 Examination for catatonia

- The method described here is used to complete the Catatonia Rating Scales.
- Ratings are made based on the observed behaviours during the examination, with the exception of completing the items for 'withdrawal' and 'autonomic abnormality', which may be based upon either observed behaviour and/or chart documentation.
- Rate items only if well defined. If uncertain, rate the item as '0'.

Procedure	Examines
1. Observe patient while trying to engage in a conversation.	Activity level, abnormal movements, abnormal speech
2. Examiner scratches head in exaggerated manner.	Echopraxia
3. Examine arm for cogwheeling. Attempt to reposition, instructing patient to 'keep your arm loose'. Move arm with alternating lighter and heavier force.	Rigidity, negativism, waxy flexibility
4. Ask patient to extend arm. Place one finger beneath hand, and try to raise slowly after stating, 'DO NOT let me raise your arm'.	Passive obedience
5. Extend hand, stating, 'DO NOT shake my hand'.	Ambitendence
6. Reach into your pocket and state, 'Stick out your tongue, I want to stick a pin in it.'	Automatic obedience
7. Examine for the grasp reflex.	Grasp reflex
8. Examine the patient's chart for oral intake, vital signs, and unusual incidents.	
9. Observe the patient indirectly for a brief period each day.	

Box 36.1 Catatonia Rating Scale

- Use the presence or absence of items 1–14 for screening purposes.
- Use the 0–3 scale for items 1–23 to rate severity.

1 Excitement
Extreme hyperactivity, constant motor unrest which is apparently non-purposeful.
Not to be attributed to akathisia or goal-directed agitation.
   0 = Absent
   1 = Excessive motion, intermittent.
   2 = Constant motion, hyperkinetic without rest periods.
   3 = Severe excitement, frenzied motor activity.

2 Immobility/stupor
Extreme hypoactivity, immobility. Minimally responsive to stimuli.
   0 = Absent.
   1 = Sits abnormally still, may interact briefly.
   2 = Virtually no interaction with external world.
   3 = Stuporous, not responsive to painful stimuli.

3 Mutism
Verbally unresponsive or minimally responsive.
   0 = Absent.
   1 = Verbally unresponsive; incomprehensible whisper.
   2 = Speaks <20 words/5 minutes.
   3 = No speech.

4 Staring
Fixed gaze, little or no visual scanning of environment, decreased blinking.
   0 = Absent.
   1 = Poor eye contact. Gazes <20 s before shifting of attention; decreased blinking.
   2 = Gaze held longer than 20 s; occasionally shifts attention.
   3 = Fixed gaze, non-reactive.

5 Posturing/catalepsy
Maintains posture(s), including mundane (e.g. sitting or standing for long periods without reacting).
   0 = Absent.
   1 = <1 minute.
   2 = >1 minute, <15 minutes.
   3 = Bizarre posture, or mundane maintained >15 minutes.

6 Grimacing
Maintenance of odd facial expressions.
   0 = Absent.
   1 = <10 s.
   2 = <1 minute.
   3 = Bizarre expression(s) or maintained >1 minute.

7 Echopraxia/echolalia
Mimicking of examiner's movements/speech.
   0 = Absent.
   1 = Occasional.
   2 = Frequent.
   3 = Continuous.

8 Stereotypy
Repetitive, non-goal-directed motor activity (e.g. finger-play; repeatedly touching, patting, or rubbing self). (Abnormality is not inherent in the act, but in its frequency.)
   0 = Absent.
   1 = Occasional.
   2 = Frequent.
   3 = Continuous.

9 **Mannerisms**

Odd, purposeful movements (hopping or walking tiptoe, saluting passers-by, exaggerated caricatures of mundane movements). (Abnormality is inherent in the act itself.)

0 = Absent.
1 = Occasional.
2 = Frequent.
3 = Continuous.

10 **Verbigeration**

Repetition of phrases or sentences.

0 = Absent.
1 = Occasional.
2 = Frequent, difficult to interrupt.
3 = Continuous.

11 **Rigidity**

Maintenance of a rigid position despite efforts to be moved. (Exclude if cog-wheeling or tremor are present.)

0 = Absent.
1 = Mild resistance.
2 = Moderate.
3 = Severe, cannot be repostured.

12 **Negativism**

Apparently motiveless resistance to instructions or to attempts to move/examine patient. Contrary behaviour, does the opposite of the instruction.

0 = Absent.
1 = Mild resistance and/or occasionally contrary.
2 = Moderate resistance and/or frequently contrary.
3 = Severe resistance and/or continually contrary.

13 **Waxy flexibility**

During reposturing of patient, patient offers initial resistance before allowing himself to be repositioned (similar to that of bending a warm candle).

0 = Absent.
3 = Present.

14 **Withdrawal**

Refusal to eat, drink, and/or make eye contact.

0 = Absent.
1 = Minimal oral intake for <1 day.
2 = Minimal oral intake for >1 day.
3 = No oral intake for 1 day or more.

15 **Impulsivity**

Patient suddenly engages in inappropriate behaviour (e.g. runs down hallway, starts screaming, or takes off clothes) without provocation. Afterwards can give no or an incomplete explanation.

0 = Absent.
1 = Occasional.
2 = Frequent.
3 = Constant or not redirectable.

16 **Automatic obedience**

Exaggerated cooperation with examiner's request, or repeated movements that are requested once.

0 = Absent.
1 = Occasional.
2 = Frequent.
3 = Continuous.

17 **Passive obedience (Mitgehen)**

Raising arm in response to light pressure of finger, despite instructions to the contrary.

0 = Absent.
3 = Present.

18 **Negativism (Gegenhalten)**

Resistance to passive movement that is proportional to strength of the stimulus; response seems automatic, rather than wilful.

0 = Absent.
3 = Present.

19 **Ambitendency**

Patient appears 'stuck' in indecisive, hesitant motor movements.

0 = Absent.
3 = Present.

20 **Grasp reflex**

Strike open palm of patient with two extended fingers of examiner's hand. Automatic closure of patient's hand.

0 = Absent.
3 = Present.

21 **Perseveration**

Repeatedly returns to same topic or persists with same movements.

0 = Absent.
3 = Present.

22 **Combativeness**

Usually in an undirected manner, without explanation.

0 = Absent.
1 = Occasionally strikes out, low potential for injury.
2 = Strikes out frequently, moderate potential for injury.
3 = Danger to others.

23 **Autonomic abnormality**

Circle: Temperature
Blood pressure
Pulse rate
Respiratory rate
Inappropriate sweating.

0 = Absent.
1 = Abnormality of one parameter (exclude pre-existing hypertension).
2 = Abnormality of two parameters.
3 = Abnormality of three or greater parameters.

Reproduced with permission from Bush, G., Fink, M., Petrides, G. et al. Catatonia. I. Rating scale and standardized examination, *Acta Psychiatrica Scandinavica*, 93(2): 129–136. © John Wiley & Sons A/S. Published by John Wiley & Sons Ltd. https://doi.org/10.1111/j.1600-0447.1996.tb09814.x.

Verifying the diagnosis

Catatonia is quickly relieved, albeit temporarily, by the administration of a benzodiazepine (lorazepam, diazepam), a barbiturate (amobarbital), or a GABA agonist (zolpidem). An intravenous injection of 1 or 2 mg of lorazepam or oral administration of 10 mg of zolpidem brings a reduction of catatonia signs within a few minutes. A reduction of the CRS score of 50% or greater verifies the catatonia diagnosis.

Treating catatonia

Catatonia is relieved by high doses of benzodiazepines and induced grand mal seizures (ECT). About 80% of catatonia cases respond to sedative drugs; the remainder recover by inducing seizures.

Benzodiazepines

In 1930, the American physician William Bleckwenn described the rapid relief of catatonia by injections of high doses (0.5–2.0 g) of amobarbital (amytal sodium). Catatonia quickly improved, as he reported and demonstrated in a historic silent black and white film (Bleckwenn, 1930 a, b). Full relief followed the administration of large daily doses.

The favourable response of catatonia to a barbiturate contrasted sharply with the poor response of schizophrenic patients without catatonia to such treatment, raising doubts as to the connection of the two disorders. These doubts led to the separation of catatonia from schizophrenia and its recognition as a systemic disorder (American Psychiatric Association, 2013).

Since Dr Bleckwenn's experience, amobarbital has been replaced by a benzodiazepine, with lorazepam and diazepam being the most frequently used. These compounds are considered safer and less likely to be used in suicide than barbiturates.

For patients with the sedated stuporous form of catatonia marked by mutism, withdrawal, and inhibition of movement, the dosage of lorazepam begins at 1–3 mg orally, progressing rapidly until symptom relief is seen. For severely ill patients, dosages of 15–30 mg/day have been necessary. (Diazepam dosages are calculated as ratios of 5 mg to 1 mg of lorazepam. Zolpidem dosages are quoted up to 40 mg/day.)

Induced seizures (ECT)

In 1934, the Hungarian neuropathologist Ladislas Meduna observed a decreased density of glia in autopsied brains of schizophrenic subjects and a surfeit in those with epilepsy. As some clinical studies had reported an absence of schizophrenia among hospitalized epileptic patients, he conceived of increasing glia in schizophrenic patients by inducing seizures using the chemical pentylenetetrazol (Metrazol, Cardiazol) (Meduna, 1937). Many of his first patients were catatonic and these were the ones who showed the most relief (Gazdag et al., 2009).

Chemically induced seizures were inefficient, however, as many injections failed to elicit a seizure. By 1938, chemical induction was replaced by electricity, a more efficient and more secure method, the modern technique of ECT (Shorter and Healy, 2007). With the benefits of these treatments and increasing use of psychoactive drugs, the sanitaria emptied and catatonia seemed to disappear from psychiatric practices (Mahendra, 1981).

The choice of treatment, whether benzodiazepines or ECT, is determined by the severity of the illness and the degree of fever and autonomic instability. For the more severely ill, who are febrile and exhibiting systemic signs of a malignant illness, ECT is preferred (Fink and Taylor, 2003).

What is an 'effective seizure'?

While we do not understand why or how grand mal seizures have favourable behavioural consequences that permit us, essentially, to 'fight one disease with another', we know that a 'full' grand mal seizure is a necessary marker of effective treatment. Heart rates increase, hypothalamic and pituitary hormones are released into blood and the CSF—most easily measured by serum prolactin levels at 20 minutes post-seizure (Swartz, 1985)—and EEG recordings show patterned seizure rhythms. The seizure, not the currents nor the amounts of electricity nor the effects of the induced motor convulsion, is the basis for a favourable outcome (Fink, 1979, 2009, 2014a) (see Fig. 36.1).

Not all seizures are equal in efficacy. An effective seizure is best determined by the pattern and duration of the seizure EEG. (Modern ECT devices include sophisticated EEG recording instruments.) The electrical stimulus momentarily blocks the recorded brain rhythm, followed by a gradual build-up of ever higher amplitudes and slowing of frequencies (15–25 s), interspersion of spikes and slow waves (10–15 s), and a period of high-amplitude slow waves (10–20 s), ending in a sharp end-point and flattening of energies. For such events to reflect an effective treatment, the minimum overall durations are >30 s, often averaging 40–80 s. Shorter seizure durations are associated with poorer clinical outcomes (Fink, 2000, 2009).

The duration and EEG patterns of the seizure are affected by age, placement of electrodes, energy dosing, types of currents, and pretreatment medications. The protocols for the parameters to induce the seizure vary with the illness being treated. In elderly depressed patients, the common belief that immediate cognitive effects are worsened by electrical energy has encouraged treatment protocols designed to minimize energy dosing, unilateral electrode placement, ultra-brief currents, and 2/week schedules. Such schedules are inefficient in treating catatonia, an illness of greater severity than most mood disorders. To treat catatonia successfully and rapidly, the following guidelines are recommended (Fink et al., 2016b).

1. Bitemporal electrode placement. Treatments are optimized by bitemporal (or bifrontal) electrode placement and dosing by half-age-calculated energies in US-marketed devices (Petrides and Fink, 1996). Since the 1960s, repeated comparisons of the efficacy and safety of unilateral and bilateral electrode placements have compelled the conclusion that treatment efficacy is impaired in unilateral electrode placement (Fink and Taylor, 2007). Considering the mortal risks of dehydration, blood stasis, thrombosis, and death in incompletely treated catatonia patients, there is no justification for the use of right unilateral electrode placements in patients with catatonia.

2. Daily seizures. In patients with malignant catatonia (NMS, delirious mania), daily treatments are useful. Indeed, for patients with high fevers, daily treatments or two seizures a day are lifesaving (Arnold and Stepan, 1952).

3. Flumazenil. Benzodiazepines inhibit seizures, making higher energies necessary for effective treatment. Since catatonic patients are commonly prescribed benzodiazepines before referral for ECT, greater stimulus energies are needed to induce full grand mal seizures. Intravenous administration of the benzodiazepine antagonist flumazenil (0.5 mg) quickly blocks seizure inhibition by the benzodiazepine, encouraging a full seizure to develop. Flumazenil is injected before the seizure, in conjunction with the adjuvants for amnesia, muscle relaxation, and anticholinergic vagal blockade.

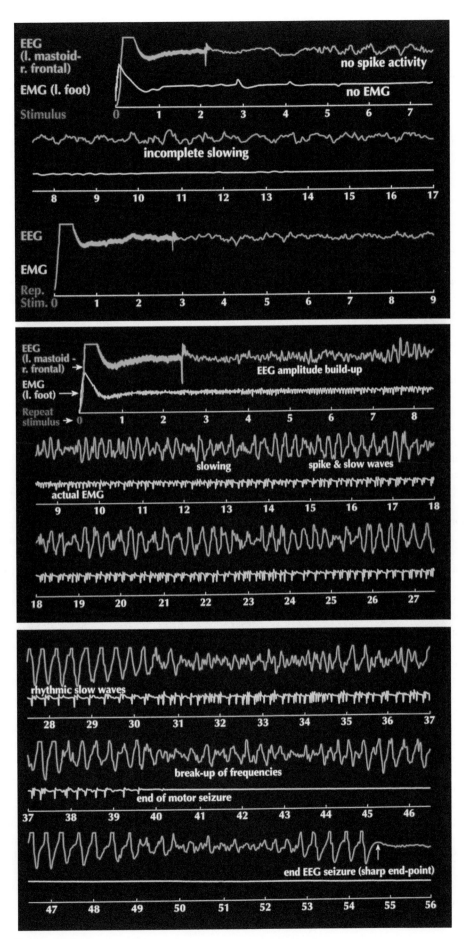

Fig. 36.1 Images of an effective seizure.

4. Ketamine. The commonly used amnesic agents methohexital, thiopental, etomidate, and propofol inhibit both seizure durations and quality. Intramuscular ketamine offers better premedication, especially in excited patients. Ketamine lowers seizure thresholds, enhancing seizure quality, and is a preferred medication (Fink, 2009).

5. Continuation (maintenance) ECT. For historical reasons, many patients are prescribed a fixed limited number of seizures for their treatment course. The number is incorporated into the consent signed by the patient (or by the justice when ECT is endorsed by a court). But such numbers are guesstimates that are founded only on historical averages. The number of seizures, like the dosage of psychoactive medications, varies widely. Since the 1970s, continuation ECT (C-ECT) has been encouraged, and more and more patients are being treated for many months and occasionally for years. (Fink et al., 1996). C-ECT is necessary in sustaining the benefits in treating major depression (Fink, 2014b) and in catatonia (Wachtel and Shorter, 2013).

Accompanying medications and catatonia

Neuroleptics

The prescription of neuroleptics is not recommended in catatonia. Indeed, their use is best interdicted. High-potency neuroleptics like haloperidol precipitate a malignant illness in catatonic patients that is often fatal (Shalev et al., 1989). The widespread use of intramuscular haloperidol in severely agitated and excited patients is too risky to be encouraged; high-dose benzodiazepines are to be preferred to sedate the severely agitated and excited patient. There is little evidence that catatonia is relieved by either typical or atypical neuroleptics. Unfortunately, such use is still common, because of the historical association of catatonia with schizophrenia.

Anticonvulsants

Because many catatonia patients exhibit rhythmic repetitive movements, these have been seen as evidence of seizure disorders and anticonvulsants have been prescribed. Case reports have described carbamazepine, valproate, and lithium as favourable augmenting agents during ECT treatment and during prolonged continuation treatments. We lack evidence of benefit for catatonia by these agents and they are best not used.

The many faces of catatonia

Once catatonia was defined by reliable diagnostic criteria, numerous syndromes were brought into the catatonia tent, firstly by recognition of catatonia signs, and then by the efficacy of catatonia treatments (see Table 36.2). In patients with two or more catatonia signs for 24 hours or longer, quick relief from an acute administration of a benzodiazepine verifies the presence of catatonia, and both induced seizures and high-dose benzodiazepines are clinically effective (Fink and Taylor, 2001, 2003).

A common image of catatonia is the mute, stuporous, posturing, rigid, staring, and negativistic patient. Persistent mutism is described in many different forms, including *selective mutism* and *persistent refusal syndrome*, the latter commonly described in the UK

Table 36.2 The catatonia syndromes and their eponyms

Retarded catatonia Benign stupor	Kahlbaum syndrome (KS)
Excited catatonia	Manic excitement
Delirious mania	Manic delirium Bell's mania
Oneiroid state	*Onirisme,* Oneirophrenia
Malignant catatonia (MC)	Lethal catatonia Pernicious catatonia
Neuroleptic malignant syndrome	NMS; MC/NMS *Syndrome malin* Neuroleptic-induced catatonia
Toxic serotonin syndrome	Serotonin syndrome; TSS
Repetitive syndromes	Tourette's syndrome Post-encephalitic Parkinsonism Self-injurious behaviors Anti-NMDAR encephalitis
Periodic catatonia	
Mixed affective state	Rapid cycling mania
Primary akinetic mutism	Apallic syndrome Stiff man syndrome Locked-in syndrome

Reproduced with permission from Bush, G., Fink, M., Petrides, G. et al. Catatonia. I. Rating scale and standardized examination, *Acta Psychiatrica Scandinavica*, 93(2): 129–136. © John Wiley & Sons A/S. Published by John Wiley & Sons Ltd. https://doi.org/10.1111/j.1600-0447.1996.tb09814.x.

(Fink, 2013). Recognition of catatonia and prescription of catatonia treatments offers rapid effective relief.

A febrile neurotoxic lethal form that follows the administration of high-potency neuroleptic agents, known as the *neuroleptic malignant syndrome* (NMS), was increasingly recognized in the 1980s. The pathophysiology was thought to result from dopaminergic blockade and the agonist bromocriptine was prescribed. Muscular weakness was related to malignant hyperthermia and the muscle relaxant dantrolene was also prescribed (Caroff et al., 2004). But these treatments are ineffective. When the connection to catatonia is seen and benzodiazepines and ECT are prescribed, outcomes are much better. NMS is successfully treated as a form of catatonia (Fink and Taylor, 2003).

The *toxic serotonin syndrome* (TSS) is an acute syndrome with similar motor and vegetative signs as NMS that follows the use of serotonergic agents. It is responsive to catatonia treatments (Fink, 1996).

Malignant (lethal, toxic) *catatonia* was described before the advent of neuroleptic agents, occurring as an acute syndrome with fever, dehydration, and excitement. A life-threatening form labelled *delirious mania* (DM) is identified that is remarkably responsive to daily induced seizures (Fink, 1999).

Self-injurious behaviours (SIBs) are increasingly recognized among adolescents with mental handicap, autism, and ASD (Dhossche et al., 2013; Wachtel and Shorter, 2013). The same repetitive acts are features in Gilles de la Tourette syndrome and OCD. When such patients are seen as ill with catatonia, they have been successfully treated by ECT (Fink, 2013; Trivedi et al., 2003).

Since 2007, an autoimmune encephalitis identified by an abnormality of the NMDA receptor in the serum or CSF is characterized by catatonia. When identified, its treatment as catatonia is successful (Dhossche et al., 2011).

Catatonia is also prominent in patients with melancholia, the severe mood disorder characterized by acute onset, insomnia, anorexia, withdrawal, mutism, agitation, and suicide risk, an illness that is responsive to ECT (Shorter and Fink, 2010; Taylor and Fink, 2006).

Each of these behaviour syndromes is identified by catatonia signs and successful treatment validates the diagnosis of catatonia. The range of behaviours recognized as catatonia, the increasing recognition of catatonia as a systemic medical illness, and the divorce from the century-long association with schizophrenia have moved catatonia from its consideration as a psychiatric disorder to its increasing recognition as a systemic medical disorder (Fink et al., 2016). In surveys of the numbers of patients with catatonia in academic hospitals and emergency rooms, using the CRS, 9–20% of the populations showed two or more catatonia signs (Fink and Taylor, 2003). A review of the prevalence of catatonia reported between 1935 and 2017 found a mean prevalence of 9% (Solmi et al., 2017).

Recognition of such associations with its effective treatments has done much to relieve catatonia in emergency rooms, medical and neurology clinics, and consultation and liaison services. Identifying catatonia as an independent syndrome and its effective relief by available treatments are an unacknowledged successful milestone in the history of medicine.

The biology of catatonia

How are we to envision catatonia among the systemic illnesses that make up the body of medicine? Catatonia is a disorder of posture, movement, and speech, with many patients reporting intense anxiety and fear (Fink, 2013; Shorter and Fink, 2018). It does not result from a structural defect in a single body organ nor is it associated with a physiologic dysfunction. It is not the consequence of a brain lesion. It occurs in the context of general medical illnesses. After catatonia is relieved, we see no residuals; it is as if the blackboard has been erased, with a few smudges left at the corners. It is a behaviour of the whole organism, arising suddenly and vanishing without a trace. It is likened to the inherited behaviours of sleeping, crying, coughing, or sneezing (Fink and Shorter, 2017; Shorter and Fink, 2018).

Catatonia is distinct from other behaviours defined as psychiatric illnesses. It is not a disorder in thought or emotion, although such accompaniments are common. Some authors consider catatonia as an 'end-state' whole-body response to imminent doom, a behaviour inherited from ancestral encounters with carnivores, an adaptation that remains an inherent feature of living (Moskowitz, 2004). This would make catatonia an atavism.

Kahlbaum described his patients as 'astonished' or 'thunderstruck'. Catatonia appeared 'after very severe physical or mental stress … such as a terrifying experience'; 'the patient remains motionless, without speaking, and with a rigid masklike facies, the eyes focused at a distance … devoid of any will to move or to react to any stimulus'. He continues: 'The general impression conveyed … is one of profound mental anguish, or an immobility induced by severe mental shock'[1]

(Kahlbaum, 1973). Citing fear as the central theme of the syndrome, Kahlbaum titled his book *Catatonia, The Tension Insanity*.

An Australian psychiatrist described four patients with systemic physical illness who exhibited catatonia in association with intense fear (Perkins, 1982). Although the patients improved with treatments for catatonia, recovery depended, he believed, on the treatment of the psychological stressors. He regarded catatonia as regression to a primitive state of mind elicited by overwhelming fear.

Georg Northoff and his colleagues in Frankfurt, Germany assessed the experiences 3 weeks after recovery in 24 patients (15 excited, nine inhibited) who met the criteria of four or more catatonia signs (Northoff et al., 1996). The patients' greatest fears were their inability to control intense anxiety. They felt threatened and feared dying. They were less concerned about their lack of control of body movement or of self-care.

Reactions characteristic of catatonia are encountered after immobilization for cardiac surgery. One patient was 'immobilized and almost like a statue'; another 'was frozen and expressionless. She spoke barely audibly in a monotone with long pauses and made no spontaneous comments'. The post-operative reaction has been described as experiencing a catastrophe, the patients resembling 'the photographed faces of survivors of civil disasters, the countenances present staring and vacant expressions of seeming frozen terror. Immobile, apathetic, and completely indifferent to their fate, they respond to inquiries in monosyllables devoid of affect'[2] (Gallup, 1977).

A 'resignation syndrome,' marked by severe stupors and death, is reported among refugee children coming to Sweden from the Syrian wars (Sallin et al., 2016) In the Uganda conflicts, a stuporous, repetitive 'nodding syndrome' progressing to death was reported (Kakooza-Mwesige et al., 2015). Some patients responded to lorazepam.

Are concepts of 'tonic immobility' and 'negative conditioning' in animals relevant? Tonic immobility is the rigid posture elicited by slowly and quietly stroking an animal, gradually releasing, with the animal now remaining immobile with limbs in the unusual postures in which they are placed. The phenomenon was demonstrated in chickens and other fowl, frogs, snakes, guinea pigs, and rabbits (Marx et al., 2008). A tradition of pretending to be dead is described as the behaviour of the Virginia opossum—'playing possum,' as it is described in childhood play (Galliano et al., 1993).

Intense fear is the evolutionary basis for both tonic immobilization and catatonia. Recognition that catatonia is present in 10% of acutely ill psychiatric inpatients, that it is relieved by anxiolytic drugs, and that patients give the appearance of intense anxiety led the psychologist Andrew Moskowitz (2004) to propose that catatonia is '*a relic of ancient defensive strategies, developed during an extended period of evolution in which humans had to face predators in much the same way many animals do today and designed to maximize an individual's chances of surviving a potentially lethal attack.*'

The principal defences of prey animals are flight, fight, and dissimulation. Flight occurs when a predator is at a distance; fight is an option when escape is not possible; and hiding, dissimulation, and absence of movement occur when the predator is at a

---

[1] Reproduced from Kahlbaum KL. *Catatonia*. Translated by G. Mora. Baltimore, MD, US: Johns Hopkins University Press. Copyright © 1973 John Hopkins University Press.

[2] Reproduced with permission from Gallup GG. 1977. Tonic immobility: the role of fear and predation. *Psychol Rec* 1:41–61. Copyright © 1996 Association of Behavior Analysis International. https://doi.org/10.1007/BF03394432.

distance that would permit not seeing an immobile prey. The core catatonic symptoms of stupor, mutism, and immobility can be linked to tonic immobilization, with prominent examples in rape assault and cyber-bullying experiences (Fink, 2013; Shorter and Fink, 2018).

Stupor, rigidity, posturing, and mutism of catatonia are analogous to tonic immobilization. Repetitive words and acts, posturing, and grimacing are dissimulations—attempts to appear other than oneself. Fright and discomfort stimulate crying that brings nursing, cuddling, and relief. Older children develop a repertoire of calls, screams, cries, postures, hiding, throwing, and breaking of objects to bring similar relief. Being mute and not responding brings desired attention. The behaviours may be active or passive, and for each, the caretakers and other children respond, and soon postures, grimaces, repetitive acts, repetitive speech, and withholding of speech become learnt behaviours.

Catatonic behaviours are identified by observation. Changes in movement, posture, and speech are sufficient to identify the syndrome. No damage to the body remains after recovery, indicating that the abnormal behaviour is an exaggeration of a normal state. Catatonia is best viewed as an inherited adaptive syndrome outside the conventional causes of the body's systemic disorders.

After more than a century of being seen as a marker of schizophrenia, catatonia's distinction as a unique motor syndrome was finalized in 2013 in the official DSM-5, published by the APA. Our present understanding is an example of applying the medical model of diagnosis to define a systemic syndrome and effective treatments (Taylor, 2013; Taylor et al., 2010). Populations of catatonia patients are biologically homogenous, characterized by measurable motor behaviours that are relieved by known interventions. By contrast, populations labelled as major depression, bipolar disorder, and schizophrenia are necessarily heterogenous, lacking both verification tests and assured outcomes with the recommended treatments.

Catatonia is a recognizable, verifiable, and treatable behaviour syndrome. It is one of the few recognizable syndromes that meet the medical model of diagnosis, matching neurosyphilis and some vitamin deficiencies. It is commonly found in medical, neurological, and emergency room populations, and is best taught in the body of clinical medicine, rather than its present place in clinical psychiatry.

KEY LEARNING POINTS

- Catatonia is a motor behaviour syndrome of acute onset, recognizable by the presence of two or more behaviours cited in the CRS, for 24 hours or longer.
- It is verified by transient relief with intravenous dosing of a benzodiazepine or barbiturate.
- It has many forms and severity, each relieved by benzodiazepines and barbiturates and, when these fail, by induced seizures.
- It is best viewed within systemic medical teaching, rather than its present position in psychiatry.
- Its biology is the consequence of intense inescapable fears.

REFERENCES

American Psychiatric Association. 1952. *Diagnostic and Statistical Manual of Mental Disorders (DSM-I)*. Washington, DC: American Psychiatric Association.

American Psychiatric Association. 1968. *Diagnostic and Statistical Manual of Mental Disorders*, second edition. Washington, DC: American Psychiatric Association.

American Psychiatric Association. 1980. *Diagnostic and Statistical Manual of Mental Disorders*, third edition. Washington, DC: American Psychiatric Association.

American Psychiatric Association. 1994. *Diagnostic and Statistical Manual of Mental Disorders*, fourth edition. Washington, DC: American Psychiatric Association.

American Psychiatric Association. 2013. *Diagnostic and Statistical Manual of Mental Disorders*, fifth edition. Washington, DC: American Psychiatric Association.

Arnold OH, Stepan H. 1952. Untersuchungen zur Frage der akuten tödliche Katatonie. *Wr Zeitschrift für Nervenheilkunde* 4: 235–87.

Bleckwenn WJ. 1930a. Catatonia cases after IV sodium amytal injection [motion picture]. 1930a. National Library of Medicine, ID 8501040A.

Bleckwenn WJ. 1930b. The production of sleep and rest in psychotic cases. *Arch Neurol Psychiatry* 24:365–72.

Bush G, Fink M, Petrides G, Dowling F, Francis A. 1996a. Catatonia: I: rating scale and standardized examination. *Acta Psychiatr Scand* 93:129–36.

Bush G, Fink M, Petrides G, Dowling F, Francis A. 1996b. Catatonia II: treatment with lorazepam and electroconvulsive therapy. *Acta Psychiatr Scand* 93:137–43.

Caroff SN. 1980. The neuroleptic malignant syndrome. *J Clin Psychiatry* 41:79–83.

Caroff SN, Mann SG, Francis A, Fricchione GL. 2004. *Catatonia: From Psychopathology to Neurobiology*. Washington DC: American Psychiatric Publishing.

Dhossche D, Fink M, Shorter E, Wachtel LE. 2011. Anti-NMDA receptor encephalitis versus pediatric catatonia. *Am J Psychiatry*. 168(7):749–50.

Dhossche D, Wing L, Ohta M, Neumarker K-J. 2007. Catatonia in autism spectrum disorders. *Int Rev Neurobiology* 72:1–314.

Fink M. *Convulsive Therapy: Theory and Practice*. New York, NY: Raven Press, 1979.

Fink M. 1996. Toxic serotonin syndrome or neuroleptic malignant syndrome? Case report. *Pharmacopsychiatry* 29:159–61.

Fink M. 1999. Delirious mania. *Bipolar Disorders* 1:54–60.

Fink M. 2000. Electroshock revisited. *Am Scientist* 88:162–7.

Fink M. 2009. *Electroconvulsive Therapy: A Guide for Professionals and Their Patients*. New York, NY: Oxford University Press.

Fink M. 2013. Rediscovering catatonia *Acta psychiatr Scand* 127 Supplement 447:1–50.

Fink M. 2014a. The seizure, not electricity, is essential in convulsive therapy: The flurothyl experience. *J ECT* 30:91–3.

Fink M. 2014b. What was learned: Studies by the Consortium for Research in ECT (CORE) 1997-2011. *Acta Psychiatrica Scand* 129:417–26.

Fink M, Abrams R, Bailine S, Jaffe R. 1996. Ambulatory Electroconvulsive Therapy: Report of the Task Force of the Association for Convulsive Therapy. *Convulsive Ther* 12(1):42–55.

FINK M. Rediscovering Catatonia: The Biography of a Treatable Syndrome. *Acta Psychiatr Scand* 2013;127 Supplement 441:1–50.

Fink M, Fricchione G, Rummans T, Shorter E. Catatonia is a systemic medical disorder. *Acta Psychiatr Scand* 2016;133(1):250–1.

Fink M, Kellner CH, McCall, WV. Optimizing ECT technique in treating catatonia. *J ECT* 2016;32(3):149–50.

Fink M, Shorter E. Does persisting fear sustain catatonia? *Acta Psychiatr Scand* 2017;136(5):441–4.

Fink M, Taylor MA. The many varieties of catatonia. *Eur Arch Psychiatry Clin Neurosci* 2001;251 Suppl 1:8–13.

Fink M, Taylor MA. 2003. *Catatonia: A Clinician's Guide to Diagnosis and Treatment.* New York, NY: Cambridge University Press.

Fink M, Taylor MA. Electroconvulsive therapy: Evidence and challenges. *JAMA* 2007;298:330–2.

Galliano G, Noble LM, Travis LA, Puechl C. Victim reactions during rape/sexual assault. *J Interpers Violence* 1993;8:109–14.

Gallup GG. Tonic immobility: the role of fear and predation. *Psychol Rec* 1977;1:41–61.

Gazdag, G, Bitter I, Ungvari GS, Baran B, Fink M. László Meduna's pilot studies with camphor induction of seizures: The first 11 patients. *J ECT* 2009;25:3–11.

Kahlbaum KL. 1874. *Die Katatonie oder das Spannungsirresein: eine klinische form psychischer Krankheit.* Berlin: Verlag August Hirshwald.

Kahlbaum KL. 1973. *Catatonia.* Translated by G Mora. Baltimore, MD: Johns Hopkins Press.

Kakooza-Mwesige A, Dhossche DM, Idro R, Akena D, Nalugya J, Opar BT. Catatonia in Ugandan children with nodding syndrome and effects of treatment with lorazepam: a pilot study. *BMC Res Notes* 2015;8:825.

Mahendra B. Where have all the catatonics gone? *Psychol Med* 1981;11:669–71.

Marx BP, Forsyth JP, Lexington JM. Tonic immobility as an evolved predator defense. Implications for sexual assault survivors. *Clin Psychol Sci Prac* 2008;15:74–90.

Meduna L. 1937. *Die Konvulsionstherapie der Schizophrenie.* Halle AS: Carl Marhold Verlagsbuchhandlung, 121 pp.

Moskowitz A. 'Scared Stiff': catatonia as an evolutionary-based fear response. *Psycholog Rev* 2004;111:984–1002.

Northoff G, Krill W, Wenke J, Travers H, Pflug B. The subjective experience in catatonia: systematic study of 24 catatonic patients. *Psychiatr Praxis* 1996;23:69–73.

Perkins RJ. Catatonia:The ultimate response to fear? *Aust NZ J Psychiatry* 1982;16:282–7.

Petrides G, Fink M. The 'half-age' stimulation strategy for ECT dosing. *Convulsive Ther* 1996;12:138–46.

Sallin K, Lagercrantz H, Evers K, Engström I, Anders Hjern A, Predrag Petrovic. Resignation syndrome: Catatonia? Culture Bound? *Front Behav Neurosci* 2016;10:7.

Shalev A, Hermesh H, Munitz H. 1989. Mortality from neuroleptic malignant syndrome. *J Clin Psychiatry* 1989;50:18–25.

Shorter E. 1997. *A History of Psychiatry.* New York, NY: John Wiley and Sons.

Shorter E, Fink M. 2018. *The Madness of Fear: A History of Catatonia.* New York, NY: Oxford University Press.

Shorter E, Healy D. 2007. *Shock Therapy: A History of Electroconvulsive Treatment in Mental Illness.* NJ: Rutgers U Press.

Shorter E, Fink M. 2010. *Endocrine Psychiatry: Solving the Riddle of Melancholia.* New York, NY: Oxford University Press.

Solmi M, Pigato GG, Roiter B, Guaglianone A, et al. 2017. Prevalence of catatonia and its moderators in clinical samples: Results from a meta-analysis and meta-regression analysis. *Schizophr Bull* 2018;44:1133–50.

Swartz C. Characterization of the total amount of prolactin released by electroconvulsive therapy. *Convulsiv Ther* 1985;1(4):252–7.

Taylor MA. 2013. *Hippocrates Cried. The Decline of American Psychiatry.* New York, NY: Oxford University Press.

Taylor MA, Fink M. Catatonia in psychiatric classification: A home of its own. *Am J Psychiatry* 2003;160:1233–41.

Taylor MA, Fink M. 2006. *Melancholia: The Diagnosis, Pathophysiology and Treatment of Depressive Disorders.* New York, NY: Cambridge University Press.

Taylor MA, Shorter E, Vaidya NA, Fink M. The failure of the schizophrenia concept and the argument for its replacement by hebephrenia: applying the medical model for disease recognition. *Acta Psychiatr Scand.* 2010;122:173–83.

Trivedi H, Mendelowitz A, Fink M. A Gilles de la Tourette form of catatonia: Response to ECT. *J ECT* 2003;19(2):115–17.

Wachtel LE, Shorter E. Self-injurious behaviour in children: A treatable catatonic syndrome. *Aust N Z J Psychiatry* 2013;47(12):1113–15.

37

Apathy in neuropsychiatric conditions

Jaime Pahissa and Sergio Starkstein

Introduction

Apathy is a common behavioural disorder in neuropsychiatric conditions. Marin (Marin, 1990) defined apathy as the absence or lack of feeling, emotion, interest, concern, or motivation, not attributable to a decreased level of consciousness, cognitive impairment, or emotional distress. Currently, apathy is conceptualized as a general reduction in motivation and construed as a syndrome consisting of reduced goal-directed behaviour (as manifested by lack of effort, initiative, and productivity), reduced goal-directed cognition (as manifested by decreased interests, lack of plans and goals, and lack of concern about one's own health or functional status), and reduced emotional concomitants of goal-directed behaviours (as manifested by flat affect, emotional indifference, and restricted responses to important life events) (Starkstein and Leentjens, 2008).

This chapter will discuss the diagnosis, clinical correlates, and treatment of apathy in an acute neuropsychiatric condition such as traumatic brain injury (TBI) and a frequent neurodegenerative condition such as Alzheimer's disease (AD).

Diagnosis of apathy in neuropsychiatric disorders

Apathy should be diagnosed only after a thorough psychiatric assessment, including evaluation of the individual's social and physical context, given the wide variety of goals, interests, and pattern of emotional display. After a TBI, important personal and contextual factors, such as role loss, motor and sensory deficits, and cognitive impairments, can all impact on the patient's motivation to engage in work or recreational activities (Kant and Smith-Seemiller, 2002). In AD, it is important to enquire about previous interests and hobbies and the quality of social interaction, and screen for depression.

Assessment for apathy in neuropsychiatry

Apathy is not listed as a specific syndrome or symptom in either the *Diagnostic and Statistical Manual of Mental Disorders*, fifth edition (DSM-5) (American Psychiatric Association, 2013) or the International Classification of Diseases, tenth revision (ICD-10) (World Health Organization, 1993). In the DSM-5, apathy is only listed as a subtype of personality change due to a general medical condition. Nevertheless, relevant phenomenological information

has been collected during the past two decades, and a consensus of experts proposed specific diagnostic criteria for apathy for use in neuropsychiatry (Robert et al., 2009). The core symptom is diminished motivation present for at least 4 weeks, impairment in at least three dimensions of apathy, and exclusion criteria to exclude symptoms and conditions mimicking apathy.

A clinical diagnosis of apathy should be carried out ideally with a semi-structured psychiatric interview. The Structured Clinical Interview for Apathy (SCIA) is the only semi-structured clinical interview validated for use in AD but is yet to be validated in other neurological conditions (Starkstein et al., 2005). Diagnosis should be carried out using the 'inclusive' approach (i.e. all symptoms are scored, regardless of whether they overlap with motor symptoms) to increase diagnostic sensitivity.

There are a number of scales rating the severity of apathy that have been validated for use in AD and TBI. The Apathy Evaluation Scale (AES) is an 18-item instrument that can be administered as a self-rating scale, a caregiver-rating scale, or a clinician-administered test (Marin et al., 1991). This scale has been used in most studies of apathy in TBI. The Apathy Scale is an abridged and modified version of the Marin's AES and can be rated by the patient or an informant. The Children's Motivation Scale is also based on Marin's AES and rates the severity of apathy among children and adolescents. Other scales have been designed for use in specific neurological disorders, such as the Dementia Apathy Interview and Rating (DAIR) (Strauss and Sperry, 2002) to assess apathy among demented individuals, the Apathy Inventory (Robert et al., 2002) which was validated for use in AD, and the Lille Apathy Rating Scale (LARS) (Sockeel et al., 2006) which was validated for use in Parkinson's disease and recently validated for use in patients with very mild to moderate dementia (Fernandez-Matarrubia et al., 2016). The Dimensional Apathy Scale (Radakovic and Abrahams, 2014) is a 24-item scale which may be suitable for use in patients with motor deficits. The Frontal System Behaviour Scale (FrSBe) (Grace et al., 1999) was designed to assess and quantify the domains of disinhibition, apathy, and executive dysfunction. The Neuropsychiatric Inventory (NPI) (Cummings, 1997) is a multidimensional instrument that is administered to a caregiver who is familiar with the patient and includes a specific subscale to rate apathy. Finally, the APADEM-NH is a 26-item scale recently validated for use among institutionalized patients with mild to severe dementia (Aguera-Ortiz et al., 2015).

Lane-Brown and Tane (Lane-Brown and Tate, 2009a), suggested that the use of informants to rate apathy has the limitation of not considering subjective aspects of this dimension and suggested obtaining reports from patients and multiple informants. Radakovic et al. (Radakovic et al., 2015) assessed the psychometric attributes of apathy scales used in AD. They recommended the DAIR and the AES-clinician version for use in dementia.

Ambulatory actigraphy was proposed to help diagnose apathy in a more ecological way (Muller et al., 2006). This technique consists in wearing a wrist device that measures locomotor activity during the daytime. Muller and co-workers (Muller et al., 2006) assessed with ambulatory actigraphy 24 patients with acquired brain damage and 12 healthy controls. Half of the patients met the diagnostic criteria for a personality change due a medical condition (apathetic type), and the other 12 had no or only mild apathy. The main finding was that activity counts were significantly lower and periods with no activity significantly more frequent in the high apathy group, as compared to the no/mild apathy and the healthy control groups. Moreover, patients with high apathy took more frequent naps and had shorter activity episodes mostly in the afternoon. Zeitzer and co-workers (Zeitzer et al., 2013) replicated the finding of a pronounced decline in afternoon activity among AD patients with apathy, which was related to an increase in napping time but was independent from depression, suggesting that actigraphy may be a useful adjunct measure for the diagnosis of apathy in dementia. Chau and co-workers (Chau et al., 2016) investigated visual scanning behaviour as a measure of apathy, independent of the patient's insight, communicative capacities, or caregiver observation. They found that patients with AD and apathy had reduced duration and fixation frequency on social images, as compared to AD patients without apathy.

In conclusion, a diagnosis of apathy requires a formal neuropsychiatric assessment using an appropriate instrument and the use of diagnostic criteria validated for each neurological condition. Rating scales should only be used to rate the severity of apathy, and not to make a diagnosis. There are now reliable and valid scales to rate the severity of apathy in AD, but more instruments should be developed for TBI.

Differential diagnosis

A number of terms have been used to refer to lack of motivation, blunted affect, and flat emotions. Abulia was defined as 'the loss, lack, or impairment of the power of the will to execute what is in mind' (Ribot, 1904). Marin considered abulia as a more severe expression of apathy (Marin, 1990). Psychic akinesia has been described in patients who are fully conscious and able to perform their basic activities of daily living, but only after strong external stimulation (Starkstein et al., 1989). A similar syndrome that can be reversed by external stimulation has been described by Laplane and Dubois (Laplane and Dubois, 2001) and termed the 'autoactivation deficit'. These patients show inertia (i.e. the tendency to stay immobile for relatively long periods), mental emptiness, repetitive and stereotyped activities, flat affect, and blunted emotional responses. Athymormia, from the Greek *thumos* (mood) and *horme* (impulse), was coined by Habib (Habib, 2004) to refer to a major reduction in spontaneous motion and speech. Finally, akinetic mutism is defined as the inability to initiate actions in a patient who appears alert (Sims, 2003). This state is characterized by lack of voluntary movement, mutism, and vigilant gaze (Sims, 2003). Marin and Wilkosz (Marin and Wilkosz, 2005) proposed the term 'disorders of diminished motivation' to include akinetic mutism, abulia, and apathy in a continuum of decreasing severity. Finally, despair and demoralization occur among individuals with no underlying psychiatric disorders when confronted with relevant stressors in their personal and social environment (Marin, 1990).

Frequency and longitudinal evolution of apathy in AD and TBI

In cross-sectional studies, about one-third of patients with AD have comorbid apathy, and about two-thirds of AD patients with apathy had comorbid (major or minor) depression. The progression of apathy in AD was examined by Starkstein and co-workers (Starkstein et al., 2001) who reported an increase in the frequency of apathy, from 14% at the stage of very mild dementia to 61% at the stage of severe dementia, suggesting that most patients with AD suffer from apathy during the course of the illness. A prospective study of apathy that included a series of 491 patients with probable AD showed a prevalence of 21% and a 1-year incidence of 10%. Among those patients with baseline apathy, 61% had apathy at the 1-year follow-up, suggesting that apathy in AD is a reversible phenomenon (Vilalta-Franch et al., 2013).

The frequency of apathy in TBI has been reported to range from 20% (Al-Adawi et al., 2004) to 72% (Lane-Brown and Tate, 2009b). This wide discrepancy may be explained by sampling biases, use of different instruments to rate the severity of apathy, and the lack of standardized diagnostic criteria. Based on prevalence rates studies reported in the literature, van Reekum and co-workers (van Reekum et al., 2005) calculated that 61% of the TBI population have apathy. A recent study by Ciurli and co-workers (Ciurli et al., 2011) included 120 individuals with severe TBI who were assessed with the NPI. Apathy was reported in 42% of the sample but usually coexisted with other neuropsychiatric disorders.

Comorbidities of apathy in AD and TBI

During the past two decades, an increasing number of empirical studies in patients with AD and TBI reported a major overlap between apathy and depression (Starkstein et al., 1992, 1993, 2005, 2009). Marin suggested that apathy should not be diagnosed in the context of moderate or severe cognitive deficits (Marin, 1990). Several studies have demonstrated an increasing frequency of apathy among patients with increasing levels of cognitive decline. Nevertheless, cognitive deficits are not sufficient to produce apathy, since only half of patients with moderate or severe dementia were reported to have no apathy (Starkstein and Merello, 2002, Starkstein et al., 2001).

Apathy is significantly associated with depression in both AD and TBI. One important reason for this overlap is that depression can be diagnosed based on DSM-5 criteria in the absence of depressed mood, provided the symptoms of loss of interest or anhedonia are present. Starkstein reported that apathy can be validly separated from depression in AD (Starkstein, 2000). A major overlap between apathy and depression has been reported in TBI. Kant and co-workers (Kant et al., 1998) assessed 83 consecutive TBI patients who were evaluated at a neuropsychiatric clinic and found that 71% of the patients met the AES cut-off score for apathy, whereas only 11% had apathy without depression. In a study that included 28 patients with TBI, Andersson and co-workers (Andersson et al., 1999) reported that, among non-depressed participants, 28% had apathy, while 59% of patients with mild depression and 80% of those with severe depression had apathy. Glenn and co-workers (Glenn et al., 2002) assessed 45 TBI patients with the AES and BDI and found significant correlations between apathy and depression scales.

Clinical correlates of apathy in AD and TBI

Cross-sectional studies in AD demonstrated that apathy is significantly associated with more severe impairments in activities of daily living (ADLs) and cognitive function, older age, and poor insight (Starkstein et al., 2001). Apathy is a significant predictor of depression, and patients who develop apathy have a greater cognitive and functional decline than those without apathy (Landes et al., 2001). An epidemiological study (Vilalta-Franch et al., 2013) demonstrated that apathy in AD is associated with increased functional disability and increased mortality. A recent study (Jao et al., 2015) found a significant association between increasing levels of stimulation and lower apathy scores, demonstrating the relevance of environmental factors in the association with apathy among elderly individuals with dementia in residential care.

Initial studies found no association between apathy and the severity of TBI (Andersson and Bergedalen, 2002). On the other hand, Ciurli and co-workers (Ciurli et al., 2011) reported that TBI patients with severe disability on the Glasgow Outcome Scale had four times the risk of developing apathetic behaviours than TBI patients with less severe scores. Montenigro and co-workers (Montenigro et al., in press) developed a metric to quantify cumulative repetitive head impacts in 93 American high-school football players. They found a dose–response relationship between their index and cognitive impairment, depression, and apathy at 1-year follow-up. Rao and co-workers (Rao et al., 2013) reported that apathy at baseline was associated with increased sleep disturbance 12 months after the TBI. Andersson and Bergedalen (Andersson and Bergedalen, 2002) found a significant association between more severe apathy and cognitive deficits such as acquisition and recall deficits, executive dysfunction, and psychomotor speed.

Mechanism of apathy in AD and TBI

The mechanism of apathy in neurodegenerative conditions remains unknown, but recent studies have suggested the involvement of subcortical structures and the cholinergic system. Torso and co-workers (Torso et al., 2015) found a significant association between lesions in the anterior thalamic radiations and the severity of apathy. Kim et al. assessed 51 individuals with very mild or mild probable AD using volumetric MRI and DTI (Kim et al., 2011). Volume of interest analyses were performed to compare regional fractional anisotropy (FA) between apathy and apathy-free groups, and to test a linear relationship between regional FA and apathy severity. The

main finding was that the apathy group showed significantly lower FA values than the apathy-free group in the left anterior cingulum (AC), regardless of concomitant depression and psychotropic medication use. Left AC FA values also had significant linear relationship with apathy composite scores as a measure of apathy severity, even after controlling for grey matter density of the ipsilateral AC. The authors suggested that communication failure between the ACC and other brain structures via the AC contributes to the development and aggravation of apathy in AD. Ota et al. (Ota et al., 2012) examined the association between apathy and white matter integrity (based on the FA index) in 21 AD patients. Apathy was found to be associated with impaired white matter integrity in the AC and medial thalamus. The authors proposed that these results lend support to previous findings that implicate limbic dysfunction and related neuronal circuits in the neurobiology of apathy in AD. Tighe et al. (Tighe et al., 2012) examined 22 individuals with MCI and 23 AD patients and found that those within the lowest AC FA tertile were more likely to exhibit irritability, agitation, dysphoria, apathy, and night-time behavioural disturbances, compared to those in the highest tertile. Finally, a recent study by Delrieu and co-workers (Delrieu et al., 2015) showed that apathy in MCI is associated with decreased metabolic activity in the posterior cingulate cortex, as compared to MCI patients without apathy, suggesting that apathy is a prodromal symptom of AD. Theleretis and co-workers (Theleritis et al., 2014) recently suggested that future studies should concentrate on examining potential brain imaging markers in the context of longitudinal studies to help clarify subtypes of apathy in AD.

The mechanism of apathy in TBI remains unknown, but several hypotheses deserve investigation. Goldfine and Schiff (Goldfine and Schiff, 2011) reviewed the role of arousal in motor recovery. They discussed research evidence suggesting an arousal system consisting of glutamatergic and cholinergic neurons in the dorsal tegmentum of the midbrain and pons which activate cortical regions via the basal forebrain bundle and the intralaminar thalamic nuclei. The main cortical regions involved in arousal regulation are the medial frontal and anterior cingulate, as well as the multi-modal parietal regions. The researchers suggested that brain injuries to this system may impair goal-directed behaviour. Knutson and co-workers (Knutson et al., 2014) examined the neural correlates of apathy using voxel-based lesion mapping in a study that included 176 brain-injured male war veterans and 52 uninjured veteran controls. Apathy was diagnosed using the apathy section of the NPI. The main finding was that damage to the left frontal lobe, the supplementary motor region, the AC, the insula, and the white matter in the corona radiata and corpus callosum was significantly associated with more severe apathy. Based on these findings, the researchers suggested that apathy may be caused by reduced motivation from lesions to the AC region. A greater volume of brain loss among participants with apathy, as compared with those without, may have at least partially accounted for the findings.

Treatment of apathy in AD and TBI

There is little evidence that pharmacological or psychotherapeutic treatment may improve apathy in AD. Several retrospective or open-label studies using anticholinesterase inhibitors reported some improvements on NPI apathy scores (Cummings et al., 2001,

2005; Herrmann et al., 2005), but none of them had apathy as the main outcome measure. Rea and co-workers (Rea et al., 2015) presented an interim analysis of a 2-year RCT using donepezil alone or in combination with the cholinergic precursor choline alphoscerate to determine whether increasing the brain levels of acetylcholine may improve apathy in AD. They found that the combination group had significantly lower apathy scores at 12 and 24 months' follow-up than the donepezil alone group.

An RCT in a small sample of AD patients demonstrated that listening to live interactive music may be an effective treatment for apathy (Holmes et al., 2006), and there is preliminary evidence that multi-sensory stimulation, control time, and attention techniques may reduce apathy in late stages of dementia (Politis et al., 2004; Verkaik et al., 2007).

A recent systematic review evaluated the results of four RCTs, nine open-label studies, and one retrospective analysis, examining the efficacy of psychoactive medication to improve apathy in AD. Nine studies examined the efficacy of cholinesterase inhibitors; two trials examined the efficacy of methylphenidate and modafinil, and the efficacy of ginkgo-biloba and citalopram was examined in single studies. One of the RCTs used donepezil (5–10 mg/day) and found no difference with the placebo group after the 24-week treatment period (Seltzer et al., 2004). A small-sample RCT using methylphenidate and apathy as a primary outcome measure showed a significant, but clinically marginal, benefit for the active compound (Herrmann et al., 2008). The design was limited by the short duration and cross-over design, and two patients on methylphenidate developed reversible delusions, agitation, irritability, and insomnia. The efficacy of ginkgo-biloba was assessed in a small-sample 22-week RCT, with apathy, as measured with the NPI, as the secondary outcome measure (Scripnikov et al., 2007). There was a significant improvement in the group on the active compound, but the magnitude of change was not provided. The fourth RCT examined the efficacy of modafinil (200 mg/day) in a small group of AD patients on anticholinesterase inhibitors. The addition of modafinil did not result in additional benefits on apathy treatment (Frakey et al., 2012). Nine studies examined the efficacy of cholinesterase inhibitors (one RCT, eight open-label studies), and only two showed benefits for rivastigmine and donepezil. Of the 7658 patients included in the nine studies, apathy scores improved in only 5% of the sample (Rea et al., 2015). Methylphenidate was successful in two trials, but with important side effects (Rea et al., 2015). A recent study examined the efficacy of methylphenidate in a multi-centre RCT including 60 patients with apathy (Rosenberg et al., 2013). After 6 weeks of treatment, there were significant benefits of methylphenidate over placebo on the Clinical Global Impression scale, but not on the other main outcome measure (the AES). The authors concluded that methylphenidate may be a useful and safe treatment of apathy in AD.

Assessment of behavioural interventions to treat apathy in TBI is still lacking. Kant and Smith-Seemiller (Kant and Smith-Seemiller, 2002) recommended including strategies to help the patient initiate activities such as verbal reminders from caretakers, messaging with audiotapes, or visual cues. Unfortunately, there is a lack of properly designed RCTs for apathy in TBI. While small case series and case reports have suggested some usefulness for psychostimulants, their efficacy and safety have to be properly demonstrated. Psychotherapies 'tailored' to patients' needs may prove a useful option, especially for patients who may not want to take medication or have side effects, but proper studies have yet to be conducted.

Conclusion

Apathy is a frequent behavioural complication of both AD and TBI and may be present in at least half of patients at some stage of AD or in the post-TBI period. Apathy is also highly prevalent in other neurological conditions such as stroke (van Almenkerk et al., 2015), Parkinson's disease (den Brok et al., 2015), HD (Reedeker et al., 2011), and MS (Novo et al., 2016).

One of the most important limitations to diagnosing apathy in TBI is the lack of specific scales to rate the severity of this condition in TBI and the lack of validated diagnostic criteria. Apathy in both AD and TBI is significantly associated with depression and cognitive impairments but may also present as an independent phenomenon in a smaller proportion of patients. One of the major complications of apathy in TBI is its negative impact upon rehabilitation efforts. There are no large RCTs showing clear clinical efficacy of psychotherapy or psychoactive medications to improve apathy in either AD or TBI, and further research in this area is needed.

KEY LEARNING POINTS

- Apathy is a frequent finding in both acute and chronic neurological conditions and is defined as a general reduction in motivation, as manifested by reduced goal-directed behaviours, cognitions, and emotions.
- In this chapter, we review the frequency, diagnostic process, clinical correlates, and treatment of apathy in AD and TBI, as examples of relevant chronic neurodegenerative and acute conditions, respectively.

REFERENCES

Aguera-Ortiz, L., et al. 2015. A novel rating scale for the measurement of apathy in institutionalized persons with dementia: the APADEM-NH. *American Journal of Geriatric Psychiatry,* 23, 149–59.

Al-Adawi, S., et al. 2004. Apathy and depression in cross-cultural survivors of traumatic brain injury. *Journal of Neuropsychiatry and Clinical Neurosciences,* 16, 435–42.

American Psychiatric Association. 2013. *Diagnostic and Statistical Manual of Mental Disorders,* fifth edition. Arlington, VA, American Psychiatric Association.

Andersson, S. & Bergedalen, A. M. 2002. Cognitive correlates of apathy in traumatic brain injury. *Neuropsychiatry, Neuropsychology, & Behavioral Neurology,* 15, 184–91.

Andersson, S., et al. 1999. Apathy and depressed mood in acquired brain damage: relationship to lesion localization and psychophysiological reactivity. *Psychological Medicine,* 29, 447–56.

Chau, S. A., et al. 2016. Apathy and Attentional Biases in Alzheimer's Disease. *Journal of Alzheimer's Disease,* 51, 837–46.

Ciurli, P., et al. 2011. Neuropsychiatric disorders in persons with severe traumatic brain injury: prevalence, phenomenology, and relationship with demographic, clinical, and functional features. *Journal of Head Trauma Rehabilitation,* 26, 116–26.

Cummings, J. L. 1997. The Neuropsychiatric Inventory: Assessing psychopathology in dementia patients. *Neurology*, 48(suppl 6), S10–16.

Cummings, J. L., et al. 2005. Effects of rivastigmine treatment on the neuropsychiatric and behavioral disturbances of nursing home residents with moderate to severe probable Alzheimer's disease: A 26-week, multicenter, open-label study. *American Journal of Geriatric Pharmacotherapy*, 3, 137–48.

Cummings, J. L., et al. 2001. Efficacy of metrifonate in improving the psychiatric and behavioral disturbances of patients with Alzheimer's disease. *Journal of Geriatric Psychiatry & Neurology*, 14, 101–8.

Delrieu, J., et al. 2015. Apathy as a feature of prodromal Alzheimer's disease: an FDG-PET ADNI study. *International Journal of Geriatric Psychiatry*, 30, 470–7.

Den Brok, M. G., et al. 2015. Apathy in Parkinson's disease: A systematic review and meta-analysis. *Movement Disorders*, 30, 759–69.

Fernandez-Matarrubia, M., et al. 2016. Validation of the Lille's Apathy Rating Scale in Very Mild to Moderate Dementia. *American Journal of Geriatric Psychiatry*, 24, 517–27.

Frakey, L. L., et al. 2012. A randomized, double-blind, placebo-controlled trial of modafinil for the treatment of apathy in individuals with mild-to-moderate Alzheimer's disease. *Journal of Clinical Psychiatry*, 73, 796–801.

Glenn, M. B., et al. 2002. Cutoff score on the apathy evaluation scale in subjects with traumatic brain injury. *Brain Injury*, 16, 509–16.

Goldfine, A. M. & Schiff, N. D. 2011. What is the role of brain mechanisms underlying arousal in recovery of motor function after structural brain injuries? *Current Opinion in Neurology*, 24, 564–9.

Grace, J., et al. 1999. Assessing frontal lobe behavioral syndromes with the frontal lobe personality scale. *Assessment*, 6, 269–84.

Habib, M. 2004. Athymhormia and disorders of motivation in Basal Ganglia disease. *Journal of Neuropsychiatry & Clinical Neurosciences*, 16, 509–24.

Herrmann, N., et al. 2005. Galantamine treatment of problematic behavior in Alzheimer disease: post-hoc analysis of pooled data from three large trials. *American Journal of Geriatric Psychiatry*, 13, 527–34.

Herrmann, N., et al. 2008. Methylphenidate for the treatment of apathy in Alzheimer disease: prediction of response using dextroamphetamine challenge. *Journal of Clinical Psychopharmacology*, 28, 296–301.

Holmes, C., et al. 2006. Keep music live: music and the alleviation of apathy in dementia subjects. *International Psychogeriatrics*, 18, 623–30.

Jao, Y. L., et al. 2015. The Association Between Characteristics of Care Environments and Apathy in Residents With Dementia in Long-term Care Facilities. *Gerontologist*, 55 Suppl 1, S27–39.

Kant, R., et al. 1998. Prevalence of apathy following head injury. *Brain Injury*, 12, 87–92.

Kant, R. & Smith-Seemiller, L. 2002. Assessment and treatment of apathy syndrome following head injury. *Neurorehabilitation*, 17, 325–31.

Kim, J. W., et al. 2011. Microstructural alteration of the anterior cingulum is associated with apathy in Alzheimer disease. *American Journal of Geriatric Psychiatry*, 19, 644–53.

Knutson, K. M., et al. 2014. Neural correlates of apathy revealed by lesion mapping in participants with traumatic brain injuries. *Human Brain Mapping*, 35, 943–53.

Landes, A. M., et al. 2001. Apathy in Alzheimer's disease. *Journal of American Geriatric Society*, 49, 1700–7.

Lane-Brown, A. & Tate, R. 2009a. Interventions for apathy after traumatic brain injury. *Cochrane Database of Systematic Reviews*, CD006341.

Lane-Brown, A. & Tate, R. 2009b. Measuring apathy after traumatic brain injury: Psychometric properties of the Apathy Evaluation Scale and the Frontal Systems Behavior Scale. *Brain Injury*, 23, 999–1007.

Laplane, D. & Dubois, B. 2001. Auto-Activation deficit: a basal ganglia related syndrome. *Movement Disorders*, 16, 810–14.

Marin, R. S. 1990. Differential diagnosis and classification of apathy. *American Journal of Psychiatry*, 147, 22–30.

Marin, R. S., et al. 1991. Reliability and validity of the Apathy Evaluation Scale. *Psychiatry Research*, 38, 143–62.

Marin, R. S. & Wilkosz, P. A. 2005. Disorders of diminished motivation. *Journal of Head Trauma Rehabilitation*, 20, 377–88.

Montenigro, P. H., et al. 2017. Cumulative head impact exposure predicts later-life depression, apathy, executive dysfunction, and cognitive impairment in former high school and college football players. *Journal of Neurotrauma*, 34, 328–40.

Muller, U., et al. 2006. Reduced daytime activity in patients with acquired brain damage and apathy: a study with ambulatory actigraphy. *Brain Injury*, 20, 157–60.

Novo, A. M., et al. 2016. Apathy in multiple sclerosis: gender matters. *J Clin Neurosci*, 33, 100–4.

Ota, M., et al. 2012. Relationship between apathy and diffusion tensor imaging metrics of the brain in Alzheimer's disease. *International Journal of Geriatric Psychiatry*, 27, 722–6.

Politis, A. M., et al. 2004. A randomized, controlled, clinical trial of activity therapy for apathy in patients with dementia residing in long-term care. *International Journal of Geriatric Psychiatry*, 19, 1087–94.

Radakovic, R. & Abrahams, S. 2014. Developing a new apathy measurement scale: Dimensional Apathy Scale. *Psychiatry Res*, 219, 658–63.

Radakovic, R., et al. 2015. A systematic review of the validity and reliability of apathy scales in neurodegenerative conditions. *International Psychogeriatrics*, 27, 903–23.

Rao, V., et al. 2013. Correlates of apathy during the first year after traumatic brain injury. *Psychosomatics*, 54, 403–4.

Rea, R., et al. 2015. Apathy Treatment in Alzheimer's Disease: Interim Results of the ASCOMALVA Trial. *Journal of Alzheimer's Disease*, 48, 377–83.

Reedeker, N., et al. 2011. Incidence, course, and predictors of apathy in Huntington's disease: a two-year prospective study. *J Neuropsychiatry Clin Neurosci*, 23, 434–41.

Ribot, T. H. 1904. *Les Malades de la Volonte*. Paris, Alcan.

Robert, P., et al. 2009. Proposed diagnostic criteria for apathy in Alzheimer's disease and other neuropsychiatric disorders. *European Psychiatry*, 24, 98–104.

Robert, P. H., et al. 2002. The apathy inventory: assessment of apathy and awareness in Alzheimer's disease, Parkinson's disease and mild cognitive impairment. *International Journal of Geriatric Psychiatry*, 17, 1099–105.

Rosenberg, P. B., et al. 2013. Safety and efficacy of methylphenidate for apathy in Alzheimer's disease: a randomized, placebo-controlled trial. *J Clin Psychiatry*, 74, 810–16.

Scripnikov, A., et al. 2007. Effects of Ginkgo biloba extract EGb 761 on neuropsychiatric symptoms of dementia: findings from a randomised controlled trial. *Wien Med Wochenschr*, 157, 295–300.

Seltzer, B., et al. 2004. Efficacy of donepezil in early-stage Alzheimer disease: a randomized placebo-controlled trial. *Archives of Neurology*, 61, 1852–6.

Sims, A. 2003. *Symptoms in the Mind*, China, Saunders.

Sockeel, P., et al. 2006. The Lille apathy rating scale (LARS), a new instrument for detecting and quantifying apathy: validation in Parkinson's disease. *Journal of Neurology, Neurosurgery & Psychiatry*, 77, 579–84.

Starkstein, S. E. 2000. Apathy and withdrawal. *International Psychogeriatrics*, 12, 135–8.

Starkstein, S. E., et al. 1989. Psychic akinesia following bilateral pallidal lesions. *International Journal of Psychiatry in Medicine*, 19, 155–64.

Starkstein, S. E., et al. 1993. Apathy following cerebrovascular lesions. *Stroke*, 24, 1625–30.

Starkstein, S. E., et al. 2005. On the overlap between apathy and depression in dementia. *Journal of Neurology, Neurosurgery & Psychiatry*, 76, 1070–4.

Starkstein, S. E. & Leentjens, A. F. 2008. The nosological position of apathy in clinical practice. *Journal of Neurology, Neurosurgery & Psychiatry*, 79, 1088–92.

Starkstein, S. E., et al. 1992. Reliability, validity, and clinical correlates of apathy in Parkinson's disease. *Journal of Neuropsychiatry and Clinical Neurosciences*, 4, 134–9.

Starkstein, S. E. & Merello, M. 2002. *Psychiatric and Cognitive Disorders in Parkinson's Disease*. Cambridge, Cambridge University Press.

Starkstein, S. E., et al. 2009. The Syndromal Validity and Nosological Position of Apathy in Parkinson's Disease. *Movement Disorders*, 24, 1211–16.

Starkstein, S. E., et al. 2001. Syndromic validity of apathy in Alzheimer's disease. *American Journal of Psychiatry*, 158, 872–7.

Strauss, M. E. & Sperry, S. D. 2002. An informant-based assessment of apathy in Alzheimer disease. *Neuropsychiatry, Neuropsychology, & Behavioral Neurology*, 15, 176–83.

Theleritis, C., et al. 2014. A review of neuroimaging findings of apathy in Alzheimer's disease. *International Psychogeriatrics*, 26, 195–207.

Tighe, S. K., et al. 2012. Diffusion tensor imaging of neuropsychiatric symptoms in mild cognitive impairment and Alzheimer's dementia. *Journal of Neuropsychiatry and Clinical Neurosciences*, 24, 484–8.

Torso, M., et al. 2015. Strategic lesions in the anterior thalamic radiation and apathy in early Alzheimer's disease. *PLoS One*, 10, e0124998.

Van Almenkerk, S., et al. 2015. Apathy among institutionalized stroke patients: prevalence and clinical correlates. *American Journal of Geriatric Psychiatry*, 23, 180–8.

Van Reekum, R., et al. 2005. Apathy: why care? *Journal of Neuropsychiatry & Clinical Neurosciences*, 17, 7–19.

Verkaik, R., et al. 2007. The relationship between severity of Alzheimer's disease and prevalence of comorbid depressive symptoms and depression: a systematic review. *International Journal of Geriatric Psychiatry*, 22, 1063–86.

Vilalta-Franch, J., et al. 2013. Apathy syndrome in Alzheimer's disease epidemiology: prevalence, incidence, persistence, and risk and mortality factors. *Journal of Alzheimer's Disease*, 33, 535–43.

World Health Organization. 1993. *The ICD-10 Classification of Mental and Behavioural Disorders*, Geneva, World Health Organization.

Zeitzer, J. M., et al. 2013. Phenotyping apathy in individuals with Alzheimer disease using functional principal component analysis. *American Journal of Geriatric Psychiatry*, 21, 391–7.

38

Focal brain syndromes in neuropsychiatry

Paul Shotbolt

Introduction

The reduction and localization of psychiatric symptoms to focal brain regions are a core concept in neuropsychiatry. The concept of the brain itself, rather than the heart, being the site of thought and intellect is first ascribed to Hippocrates (460–377 BC) and his contemporaries. The subdivision of the brain into different regions with specific functions came much later; the frontal lobes were first described by the French anatomist François Chaussier in the eighteenth century. This was followed by the delineation of the lobes used in modern neurosciences (see Fig. 38.1). In practice, the process of anatomical localization is not always straightforward for psychiatric, as opposed to neurological, symptoms. The difficulty is that lesions to completely different brain areas may be associated with similar or even indistinguishable clusters of psychiatric symptoms. A further complication is that lesions which may appear to be focal are often linked to more disseminated pathology. Truly focal lesions are actually extremely rare; for example, focal brain injury may be associated with damage some distance away from the original site (the classic coup and contrecoup injuries that follow head trauma). Epileptic seizures arising focally can have distinct pathognomonic features; however, in clinical practice, these distinctions often become blurred due to the non-specific nature of epilepsy symptoms and the tendency for seizure activity in one area to spread rapidly to another. Some epilepsy syndromes have an extensive anatomical network basis representing more widespread pathology and consequently may start simultaneously in different, but connected, brain structures. This is particularly true of seizures arising in the limbic system; discussion of the anatomical basis in these seizures represents an oversimplification and is best avoided.

Despite the above caveats, it is clear that there are some focal brain syndromes that are associated with relatively localized brain lesions, although in many cases they can also be seen in pathology that affects the brain more widely. Most of the focal brain syndromes in neuropsychiatry are associated with deficits in cognitive functioning. It is much harder to be certain about the regional basis of psychiatric syndromes such as psychosis or personality

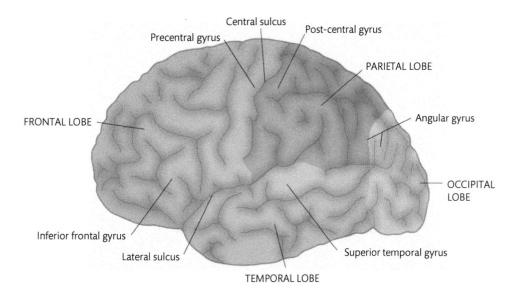

Fig. 38.1 The left cerebral hemisphere, viewed from the lateral aspect.

Reproduced with permission from P. Brodal. Parts of the Nervous System. In *The Central Nervous System*, 5 ed. Oxford, UK: OUP. Copyright 2016, Oxford University Press. DOI: 10.1093/med/9780190228958.001.0001.

changes/disorder. Nevertheless there are some non-cognitive disorders which may be linked to focal lesions. An overview of focal brain syndromes that present with neuropsychiatric features is given below.

Frontal lobes

The frontal lobes are phylogenetically the most recent region of the brain. They occupy more than one-third of the entire cortical area (Damasio and Anderson, 1993). Anatomically, the frontal lobe lies anterior to the central sulcus and is made up of three regions: the dorsolateral, medial, and orbital aspects. The motor cortex comprises the posterior region of both the dorsolateral and prefrontal aspects. The part of the frontal lobe anterior to the motor area is the prefrontal cortex (see Fig. 38.2). Their link to higher mental function has been acknowledged since the eighteenth century. In the mid-nineteenth century, the severe damage suffered by Phineas Gage to his frontal lobes by an iron rod, and the subsequent description of a range of character and behavioural changes, was a major step forward in understanding frontal lobe function. The neuropsychologist Alexander Luria (1902–1977) further investigated the frontal lobes by studying soldiers with penetrating head injuries, as well as patients with tumours and other focal lesions. In his seminal text *Higher Cortical Functions in Man*, first published in 1962, he described the frontal lobes exerting a controlling function in the hierarchy of the brain and operating the planning, executing, and monitoring of mental processes (Luria, 1980). The central role of the dominant frontal lobe in speech was elucidated by Paul Broca, who predicted autopsy findings of lesions in the left frontal lobe in patients with expressive speech disorders. The dramatic behavioural changes of frontotemporal degeneration were first described by Arnold Pick (1851–1924) who reported the classic symptoms of indifference, poor judgement and insight,

diminished creativity, careless dressing, anti-social behaviour, and aphasia (Pick's disease).

Unfortunately some of these clinical and research observations led indirectly to the worst excesses of psychosurgery. It was hypothesized that intentionally damaging the neuronal tracts in the frontal lobes in patients with mental illnesses would lead to clinical improvement (Tierney, 2000). The Portuguese neurosurgeon Egas Moniz received the Nobel Prize for his work in this field in 1949. The American neurologist Walter Freeman took this further with the borehole lobotomy, with >60,000 lobotomies carried out in the United States between 1936 and 1956. However, the high rate of severe complications and the emergence of antipsychotic medications led to frontal lobotomy being abandoned by the 1970s.

In the 1980s, regional specialization within the frontal lobes was increasingly recognized. The prefrontal cortex was further subdivided into the dorsolateral, orbital, and medial prefrontal cortices, as these three prefrontal regions consistently appeared to be correlated with specific neuropsychiatric features, as discussed below. This concept of regional specialization has been extended conceptually to a network model of frontosubcortical circuits, which begin in the prefrontal cortex and then project to the striatum, globus pallidus, and thalamus and back to the cortex again (Cummings, 1993; Damasio and Geschwind, 1985; Masterman and Cummings, 1997).

Dorsolateral prefrontal cortex

Lesions here cause abnormalities in complex psychological functions, leading to the classic dysexecutive syndrome. The patient has difficulties with planning, organization, generation of ideas, inflexibility and poor abstraction skills. The ability to organize events in a temporal sequence is impaired. There are personality, affective, and behavioural changes with indifference, distractibility, emotional instability, diminished anxiety, impulsiveness, and facetiousness. Social and ethical control may be impaired. The patient shows a

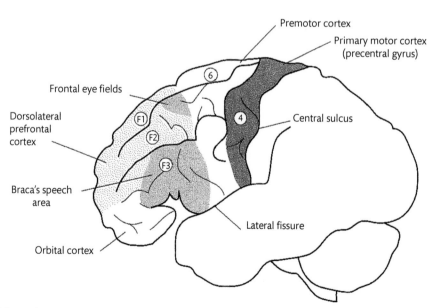

Fig. 38.2 Subdivisions of the prefrontal cortex.

lack of concern for the past or future consequences of their actions. There may be indifference or callous unconcern for the feelings of others. Euphoria, when present, is often empty and fatuous. There may be evidence of an 'environmental dependency syndrome', also termed forced utilization behaviour, whereby the patient will reach out and use objects that are presented to them in a purposeful, yet unintentional, manner (Lhermitte, 1986). Performance on psychometric testing may be well preserved if the patient can be engaged with the process; this is sometimes termed the 'frontal lobe paradox' where patients with apparent dramatic behavioural and executive difficulties in the real world can perform normally on cognitive testing. Typical causes of dorsolateral prefrontal cortex (DLPFC) lesions include tumours, cerebrovascular accidents, and frontal neurodegeneration.

The reduction in verbal fluency seen in patients with Parkinson's disease is thought to be due to impaired dopaminergic projections to the DLPFC. Patients with schizophrenia show abnormal dorsolateral prefrontal activation, particularly in response to tasks that require working memory; there is absence of an increase in blood flow to the DLPFC seen in controls during performance of the Wisconsin Card Sorting Test (Weinberger et al., 1988). Patients with schizophrenia show reduced numbers of D1-like receptors in the prefrontal cortex, which may be the cause of the working memory deficiency, as this function is mediated by the action of dopamine on D1-like receptors (Okubo et al., 1997).

Orbital prefrontal cortex

Lesions here are associated with disinhibition, restlessness, impulsiveness, disinhibition, perseveration, aggression, euphoria, imitation, utilization, compulsive or ritualistic behaviour, inappropriate social behaviour, impaired empathy, and impaired theory of mind (the ability to attribute mental states to others and to oneself). Typical causes include frontal tumours, MS, frontal neurodegeneration, and anterior cerebral artery occlusion, and aneurysm rupture. The orbitofrontal region is close to bony protrusions and, as such, is vulnerable to injury, particularly when rotational forces are applied to the freely moving head. The injury may cause diffuse white matter damage that is not detectable on functional imaging.

Medial prefrontal cortex

Disturbances of the medial prefrontal circuit are associated with apathy and loss of initiative, diminished motor activity, general and emotional indifference, reduced social interest, impaired problem-solving, loss of engagement with ADLs, hyperorality, and loss of insight. Immediately after the onset of the lesion, the patient may exhibit akinetic mutism. Causes include trauma, hydrocephalus, bilateral anterior cerebral artery occlusion, and tumours of the thalamus, third ventricle, hypothalamus, and pituitary.

Frontal lesions which extend to involve the motor cortex lead to contralateral paresis. Initially the affected muscles are flaccid, but subsequently spasticity develops with hyperreflexia and extensor plantar responses (the Babinski sign).

Lesions of Broca's area (inferior frontal gyrus) on the dominant side leads to inability to produce speech, termed expressive aphasia. The patient can still understand the written and spoken word. Lesions to the corresponding area on the non-dominant side result in expressive aprosodia where speech lacks emotional tone.

Frontal lobe seizures can be difficult to diagnose and are sometimes misdiagnosed as a psychiatric disorder or pseudoseizures. The patient may exhibit abnormal body posturing, sensorimotor tics, or other motor abnormalities. There may be short repetitive thrashing, pedalling, thrusting, laughing, screaming, and/or crying. Prolonged behavioural changes may result from non-convulsive frontal lobe status.

A broad range of differential diagnoses should be considered in a patient presenting clinically with a frontal lobe syndrome, including cerebral infarction, haemorrhage, intracerebral or intracranial extracerebral tumours, MS, hydrocephalus, and TBIs. Behavioural variant frontotemporal dementia (bvFTD) is a neurodegenerative disorder that most commonly presents with a pure frontal lobe syndrome. However, Alzheimer's disease (AD), dementia with Lewy bodies, progressive supranuclear palsy, corticobasal degeneration, idiopathic Parkinson's disease, and vascular dementia can all result in similar symptoms. Apathy is commonly found in Parkinson's disease and vascular dementia. Cerebral vasculitides, infectious disorders, or inflammatory brain diseases can also lead to a frontal lobe syndrome. Excessive alcohol use is a common toxic cause.

Functional defects of the frontosubcortical circuits are implicated in psychiatric disorders. The negative symptoms in schizophrenia, depression, dysthymic disorder, or autistic spectrum disorders are likely to involve the same frontosubcortical circuits, resulting in apathy, emotional blunting, and poverty of thought and speech. Similarly, in manic episodes, anxiety disorders, obsessive–compulsive disorder (OCD), or tic syndromes (e.g. Tourette syndrome), other behavioural disturbances associated with frontal lobe lesions, such as stereotypical language, motor stereotypies, or disinhibition, may be seen. In head injury patients, depression has been shown to be a more frequent accompaniment of head injury if there is specific frontal lobe damage (Lishman, 1968) (see Box 38.1).

CASE STUDY 1

A 17-year-old man suffered a severe TBI after his stationary car was hit from behind. His Glasgow Coma Scale score on arrival at hospital was 7/15. A CT scan showed a right frontal subdural haematoma. There was a period of retrograde amnesia of 1 week and of post-traumatic amnesia of 6 weeks. He made an excellent physical recovery but had ongoing executive dysfunction, fatigue, and an organic personality change. He reported difficulty with decision-making and planning. In social situations, he showed poor judgement and disinhibition. He required promoting with self-care and became unconcerned about his appearance. He complained that his sense of taste had changed. His sister reported he had become much less sociable and was argumentative and rigid. He was unable to plan effectively and became profligate with his money. Consequently, he was considered to lack financial capacity. He scored 86/100 on the Addenbrooke's Cognitive Examination. His domain scores were Attention 18/18, Memory 23/26, Verbal fluency 5/14, Language 24/26, and Visuospatial 16/16. His main deficits were clearly in the area of executive function (verbal fluency), with some language and memory problems. His behavioural changes are also consistent with frontal lobe injury.

- Luria's motor sequencing. This tests for the ability to perform and organize rapid-sequence motor tasks. The clinician demonstrates the task by first banging his/her fist, then the edge of the palm, and then the flat palm on the table.
- Desk tap test—for cognitive flexibility. The clinician repeatedly taps the table either once or twice, having asked the patient to copy their action. The clinician then tells the patient that the rule has changed, so that when he/she taps once, they must tap twice, and vice versa. Patients with frontal lobe lesions may perseverate on the old rule.
- Proverb interpretation—asking patients to explain a simple proverb, e.g. 'the grass is always greener on the other side'. This is a useful test of abstract reasoning. Patients will either find this impossible or provide a concrete explanation.
- Similarities/differences. This is another test of abstract reasoning. The patient is asked to describe the differences and similarities between related common objects, e.g. a fence and a wall.
- Verbal fluency. In the phonemic variant, the patient is asked to generate as many words (but not proper nouns, i.e. places/people's names) as they can that begin with a particular letter of the alphabet, e.g. 'p'. They have a minute to perform the task. In the semantic variant, they are asked to do the same task, but for animal names beginning with any letter of the alphabet. Both frontal and temporal lobe areas are implicated in this task, the former being more important in the phonemic variant and the latter in the semantic variant (Lhermitte, 1986). Greater than 11 words/minute is the expected frequency.
- Stroop test. This tests response inhibition, which is particularly impaired in orbitofrontal lesions. The names of several colours are printed in random colours on individual cards (e.g. orange). The patient must suppress the desire to read the name of the colour but instead should say the colour of the writing.
- Cognitive estimates. The patient is asked to estimate a response to a simple numerical question, i.e. 'how tall is a double-decker bus?' or 'how many camels are there in the UK?' Patients with frontal lobe lesions have difficulty producing accurate estimates.

Parietal lobes

The parietal lobe is integral to the perception of external space and body image. Anatomically it underlies the parietal bone of the skull (see Fig. 38.1). Its anterior border is the central sulcus, and it extends medially to the cingulate gyrus. The posterior border is the parieto-occipital fissure. The parietal lobes are differentiated into the dominant (usually the left) and non-dominant (usually the right) lobes. Lesions to the parietal lobes have different effects, depending on whether the dominant or non-dominant lobe is affected. However, lesions of either lobe can lead to visuospatial and/or topographical difficulties. Constructional dyspraxia (inability to copy a simple symmetrical figure) is commoner with non-dominant lesions but may occur with either.

Non-dominant parietal lesions are classically associated with disturbed body image and an impaired sense of position in external space, particularly for the contralateral side. There may be denial of (anosognosia) or indifference (anosodiaphoria) towards the disability. Left-sided limbs may not be recognized or entirely disowned (asomatognosia). Phantom reduplication of body parts can also be seen. Neglect of the left side of external space can occur. This may be seen on drawing, for example, neglecting to complete the left side of a picture. Handwriting may be crowded onto the right side of the paper and left-hand turns may be ignored. Dressing apraxia (confusion when putting on clothes) may be seen as the patient does not recognize the opposite side of his/her body and consequently does not dress it. The patient may also be confused about his/her location in space and yet be unconcerned. Lesions of the dominant parietal lobe are associated with dysphasia and agnosia. Anterior lesions are linked to primary motor dysphasia, while posterior lesions lead to primary sensory dysphasia. The dysphasic patient speaks slowly, makes grammatical errors, and may be mistakenly labelled as confused or uncooperative. Astereoagnosia, whereby the patient cannot name (with eyes closed) a familiar object held in the hand based on the weight and three-dimensional characteristics of the object, may occur. Numbers or letters written on the patient's skin may not be recognized by touch (agraphesthesia). Tactile agnosia, in which the patient cannot name an object by touch alone, may be seen following lesions bordering the post-central gyrus. In addition, autotopagnosia (inability to identify personal body parts, e.g. the fingers) may be seen in dominant lesions. Posterior lesions (parieto-occipital) can cause visual agnosia.

Elements of the Gerstmann's syndrome are seen in dominant inferior parietal lobe lesions, although the complete syndrome is rare. This comprises finger agnosia (difficulty in naming fingers), dyscalculia (difficulty with numbers), dysgraphia (difficulty with writing), and right–left disorientation. The Bálint syndrome is a rare and poorly understood triad of severe neuropsychological impairments, including inability to perceive the visual field as a whole (simultanagnosia), difficulty in fixating the eyes (oculomotor apraxia), and inability to move the hand to a specific object by using vision (optic ataxia). The commonest cause of complete Bálint's syndrome is severe and sudden hypotension, leading to bilateral borderzone infarction in the occipito-parietal region. Cases of Bálint's syndrome have also been found in neurodegenerative disorders and TBIs at the border of the parietal and occipital lobes. Bilateral parietal lesions can also result in movement agnosia (inability to see moving objects), while vision for stationary objects remains intact.

Neurological features of parietal lobe lesions include cortical sensory loss, astereognosis, agraphasthesia, impaired sensory localization, and sensory and visual inattention. Sometimes mild contrateral hemiparesis is seen. There may also be contralateral homonymous lower quadrantanopia (see Box 38.2).

- Drawing a clock face.
- Recognition of a familiar object in the hand (with eyes closed).
- Reading—patients with neglect may ignore the left side of the page.
- Writing—asymmetrical focus.
- Arithmetic—dyscalculia.
- Dressing—apraxia.
- Neurological examination—unilateral deficits in perception.
- Visual field examination—contralateral homonymous lower quadrantanopia.

CASE STUDY 2

A 60-year-old right-handed man suffered a large right hemisphere infarct and developed a dense left-sided hemiparesis. He also noticed that he was unable to perform mental arithmetics, had problems dressing, and had difficulty with navigating his way around his local area. When looking at the newspaper, he had difficulty reading or even recognizing the left-hand side of the page. He would also deny significant aspects of his disability. On examination, his gaze was always directed to the right-hand side of the room. These findings of dyscalculia, geographical and dressing apraxia, neglect, and lack of insight 'anosognosia' are consistent with damage to the right parietal lobe.

Temporal lobes

The temporal lobes are located below the lateral cerebral fissure and are divided into the superior, middle, and inferior gyri on the lateral surface, and the uncus and parahippocampal gyri on the medial surface (see Fig. 38.2). The temporal lobe can be divided into two regions: lateral and ventromedial. The lateral region is categorized as the neocortex and has multiple cognitive functions. The ventromedial region contains major components of the limbic system and contributes to emotional regulation. The temporal lobes are functionally complex; stimulation of the temporal lobes can elicit complex perceptions, memories, and experiences. The neurosurgeon Wilder Penfield showed that stimulation of the lateral surface of the temporal cortex produced re-experiencing of previous memories in awake subjects.

Lesions of the dominant temporal lobe produce more disturbance than lesions of the non-dominant temporal lobe. Dominant lesions may lead to language problems, including receptive dysphasia (Wernicke's aphasia), in which a severe comprehension deficit to spoken language develops. Expressive speech may become hyperfluent with nonsense words. If the lesion extends to the parietal lobe, alexia and agraphia may develop. Lesions of the arcuate fasciculus, which connects Wernicke's area with Broca's area, lead to conduction aphasia, in which the patient has difficulty with repetition.

Non-dominant temporal lesions may be associated with visuospatial difficulties. There can also be impaired learning of non-verbal patterned information such as music. Prosopagnosia may also be present (impaired ability to recognize faces). Receptive aprosody is associated with non-dominant lesions. Patients are unable to comprehend others' intonation and may misinterpret non-verbal social communication. They may also fail to recognize familiar voices (phonagnosia).

Auditory agnosias (cortical deafness) in which patients have difficulty with verbal and non-verbal material are usually the result of bilateral destruction of the primary auditory cortex (Heschl's gyrus). In pure word deafness, patients are entirely unable to understand spoken words, but reading/writing and speech may be relatively preserved. Patients with auditory sound agnosia have difficulty with recognition of non-verbal sounds.

Long-standing temporal lobe lesions are associated with aggression and emotional instability. There is an increased risk of

psychosis and depersonalization. Complex auditory and visual hallucinations may occur.

Epileptic seizures affecting the posterolateral dominant temporal lobe may lead to aphasia. There may also be auditory, visual, and vestibular disturbances. Mesial temporal seizures typically exhibit an aura, followed by staring. Oral automatisms are also common. Seizures affecting the middle and inferior temporal gyri may cause complex hallucinations or aberrant salience attribution to neutral perceptions. Many different emotions can be seen during the course of a temporal lobe seizure, including fear, anxiety, pleasure, depersonalization, depression, déjà vu (familiarity), and jamais vu (unfamiliarity). In a case series of patients with ictal fear, the epileptiform discharges primarily originated in right temporal lobe limbic structures, including the amygdala (Hermann et al., 1992). Ictal activity in this region leads to symptoms similar to functional psychiatric disorders such as aggression, anxiety, and delusions (Mesulam, 1981).

The olfactory cortex is located in the uncus and parahippocampal gyri. Epileptogenic lesions may cause uncinate fits such as those reported in the aura of temporal lobe epilepsy (TLE). The uncus is adjacent to the medial hippocampus and the site of mesial temporal sclerosis, which may explain the association of TLE and olfactory auras.

Patients with bilateral hippocampal lesions typically have severe amnestic syndromes. They are unable to store and recall new information. There may be no other cognitive problems. Projections from the hippocampus form the fornix, and, in turn, many of these fibres terminate in the septal nuclei and mammillary bodies. Lesions in these structures can also produce amnesia (Kopelman, 1995).

The Kluver–Bucy syndrome is caused by bilateral medial temporal lobe lesions. It is characterized by placidity, hypersexuality, hyperorality, altered sexual behaviour, visual agnosia, hypermetamorphosis (compulsive exploration of the environment), and failure to learn from aversive stimuli. Causes include AD, carbon monoxide poisoning, frontotemporal dementia, head injury, herpes encephalitis, temporal lobe stroke, temporal lobectomy, and temporal lobe tumour. The loss of fear in the Kluver–Bucy syndrome is considered to result from bilateral destruction of the amygdala, which has a central role in the assignation of emotional significance to a current percept.

Deeper lesions within the temporal lobe cause contralateral homonymous upper quadrant field defects, due to damage to the visual radiation. There may also be mild contralateral hemiparesis due to corona radiata damage (see Box 38.3).

Box 38.3 Clinical tests for temporal lobe function

- Speech comprehension (test for receptive aphasia and aprosodia).
- Word/sentence repetition (test for conduction aphasia).
- Writing/reading ability.
- Memory:
  - Verbal; short-term recall of address; recall of events in news; knowledge of prime ministers/presidents.
  - Non-verbal: Rey-Osterrieth Complex Figure Test (ROCF); the patient first copies the complex geometrical figure, then 45 minutes later is asked to reproduce the same figure from memory (recall). It is also a test of visuospatial ability (parietal lobe).
- Visual field testing—contralateral homonymous upper quadrantanopia.

CASE STUDY 3

A previously fit and well 35-year-old man presented to Accident and Emergency with severe headaches and nausea/vomiting. He was initially discharged; however, he presented again 36 hours later with photophobia and drowsiness. Herpes simplex virus encephalitis was diagnosed and he was treated with aciclovir. Unfortunately he suffered extensive bilateral damage to the medial temporal lobes, with hippocampal destruction and significant amygdala involvement. Following this episode, he was entirely unable to form new memories and exists in a 'here and now' mental state. He requires several support workers and text reminders to manage his daily routine. He is preoccupied with his previous career as a successful businessman and male model and perseverates on these topics. He also has severe emotional lability and rapidly cycles between elation, despair, and anger.

Occipital lobes

The occipital lobe is distinguished from the parietal lobe on the medial surface by the parieto-occipital sulcus. On the dorsal surface, the border is a line drawn from the parieto-occipital sulcus to the pre-occipital notch (see Fig. 38.1). The occipital lobes are primarily concerned with higher-order visual processing. In order to process visual information from the environment, large numbers of specialized neurons are required in order to process complex information about the form, motion, colour, and depth of perceived objects. There are six layers of the primary visual cortex (in Brodmann area 17) and visual association cortex (prestriate cortex, corresponds with Brodmann areas 18 and 19). Lesions of the occipital lobes are relatively common (posterior cortical artery strokes represent 5% of all territory strokes). Lesions of the primary visual cortex lead to visual blind spots (scotomas) and partial blind spots (amblyopias) in the contralateral visual field.

Bilateral lesions of the occipital cortex lead to visual object agnosia or prosopagnosia. In visual agnosia, patients cannot recognize an object that is presented visually. The object can be seen, but not named. It will be recognizable by the patient on description or touch (Critchley, 1964). Prosopagnosia is the inability to recognize faces. It is due to disconnection of the inferior visual association cortex from the non-dominant temporal cortex (so lesions to either may be causative). These symptoms can co-occur with generalized visual agnosia and field defects. There may also be autoprosopagnosia (inability to recognize self in a mirror). Patients with bilateral occipital lesions may present with Bálint syndrome, consisting of inability to perceive the visual field as a whole (simultanagnosia), difficulty in fixating the eyes (oculomotor apraxia), and inability to move the hand to a specific object by using vision (optic ataxia). Cortical blindness may also be seen with extensive bilateral occipital cortex lesions. In this condition, there is loss of vision, with normal optic fundi and preservation of pupillary light reflexes. Some patients with cortical blindness exhibit the phenomenon of 'blind sight', whereby they can sense nearby objects or even discriminate facial expressions but cannot see (Morris et al., 2001). This results from

| **Box 38.4** Tests of occipital lobe function |

- Visual field testing, including detection of object movement.
- Naming of familiar objects and colours.
- Reading ability.
- Interpretation and description of 'overall meaning' of a complex visual image (test for simultagnosia).

an accessory visual pathway involving the superior colliculus and pulvinar projecting to dorsal visual areas. It may be associated with denial of visual loss (Anton's syndrome).

Lesions of the dominant occipital lobe, particularly at the occipitotemporal junctions, lead to agnosia or pure alexia for written material, colour agnosia, and simultagnosia (where patients can see details of a picture but cannot put it together as a whole). Achromatopsia (loss of colour vision) may result from a lesion in Brodmann area 19. Bilateral occipitoparietal lesions may cause Charcot–Wilbrand syndrome, characterized by loss of ability to create any mental visual images (including revisualization of dream imagery).

Posterior cortical atrophy (PCA) is a neurodegenerative syndrome dominated by deterioration of higher visual function (particularly visuospatial and visuoperceptual abilities) as the pathology predominantly affects the occipital lobe. It is most commonly caused by AD but may also be caused by dementia with Lewy bodies, corticobasal degeneration, or Creutzfeldt–Jakob disease. Patients may present to optometrists, ophthalmologists, or neurologists with non-specific visual complaints. They may exhibit the full Bálint syndrome. The correct diagnosis is often missed, unless clinicians look for the specific visual symptoms and signs of PCA.

Trauma, migraine, and epilepsy affecting the occipital lobe may cause elemental hallucinations (such as flashes of light) and distortion of vision. Visual auras in epilepsy last only seconds, while in migraine, they occur up to an hour before the onset of headache. Complex visual hallucinations occur more commonly with non-dominant hemisphere lesions.

Dysmorphopsias, such as axis shifts, micropsia, macropsia, and movement artefacts, are caused by irritation or damage to the association cortex. In addition, polyopia (visual perseveration precipitated by movement) or after-images (palinopsia) may be apparent. Striate cortex lesions may lead to homonymous defects in the contralateral hemifield (see Box 38.4).

CASE STUDY 4

A 56-year-old lady presented to a memory clinic with decreasing functional ability and some memory complaints. She reported early loss of ability to thread needles. Her inability to read and write was noted as a barrier to occupational therapy interventions. Her daughter reported noticing visual difficulties when she was driving. She was referred to an optometrist, but examination was normal. She was noted to have a fixed gaze and appeared to be looking through people. On one occasion, she asked where the family dog was while she was looking directly at it. CT scan at presentation was normal. She scored 42/100 on the ACR-III (Attention and Orientation 10/18, Memory 9/26, Fluency 4/14, Language 16/26, Visuospatial

3/16). This score was considered to be inconsistent with her functional ability (i.e. worse than expected), and dissociative amnesia was diagnosed. Subsequent testing on the Cortical Vision Screening Test revealed she was unable to name shapes, identify shapes in order of size, or differentiate squares and rectangles. She often appeared to be looking at the wrong place on the stimulus page and had difficulty with right–left orientation. These findings were consistent with bilateral occipital and right parietal lobe dysfunction. An MRI 3 years after presentation showed marked bilateral parietal-occipital loss, consistent with a diagnosis of posterior cortical atrophy.

Corpus callosum

Complete callosal damage may lead to left ideomotor apraxia, right or bilateral constructional apraxia, left agraphia, alexia in the left visual field, and astereognosis in the left hand. Mutism may also occur. Many of these features are caused by the non-dominant hemisphere's lack of access to speech centres in the dominant hemisphere (Geschwind and Galaburda, 1985). There is often left-sided neglect after callosectomy, which has been suggested to be a result of underactivation of the non-dominant hemisphere (Liederman, 1995). Lesions of the anterior corpus callosum can lead to the *alien hand* sign, with loss of control over the non-dominant hand. Lesions in the posterior part of the corpus callosum plus lesions of the left occipital lobe can lead to pure word blindness (alexia with no agraphia).

Lesions of deep midline structures

Lesions of the posterior diencephalon and upper midbrain may lead to somnolence and hypersomnia. Akinetic mutism may be seen in which the patient is immobile and mute but has their eyes open. There may be a frontal lobe syndrome-like picture with disinhibition, carelessness, indifference, and euphoria. Obstructive lesions can lead to intellectual decline secondary to raised intracranial pressure.

Pseudobulbar palsy with extreme emotional lability may be seen in bilateral lesions of the corticobulbar tracts. The outward visible affect may be disconnected from the underlying emotion.

Hypothalamic disturbances may cause polydipsia, polyuria, hyperphagia, obesity, and elevation of temperature. There may be amenorrhoea or impotence in adults, and delayed or precocious puberty in children. If lesions involve the pituitary gland, there may be a wide variety of endocrine changes, a number of which may have psychiatric sequelae.

Lesions of the thalamus are associated with sensory disturbances such as those seen in parietal lobe lesions. In addition, there may be hyperalgesia or analgesia. Neuropathic pain has been treated with deep brain stimulation (DBS) of the ventral thalamic nuclei. Cognitive deficits ('thalamic dementia') may develop with bilateral lesions of the thalamus. Features include amnesia, confusion, affective flattening, and apathy. Personality changes and hallucinations may also be seen.

Basal ganglia

The basal ganglia comprise the caudate, putamen, globus pallidus, substantia nigra, ventral tegmental area, pedunculopontine tegmental nucleus, and subthalamic nucleus (see Fig. 38.2). They are divided into dorsal and ventral divisions (see Fig. 38.3). The term striatum refers to the caudate, putamen, and nucleus accumbens.

Research on the behavioural functions of the basal ganglia was stimulated by the clinical observation that psychiatric and cognitive symptoms are usually present in disorders affecting the basal ganglia. They receive information from the cerebral cortex and send back processed responses to this information to the cerebral cortex. The basic process of action of the basal ganglia is through release of inhibition, hence lesions result in release of behaviour (e.g. the uncontrolled movement of Parkinson's disease). Understanding the mechanism of basal ganglia function and targeting different brain sites may improve motor, cognitive, and motivational aspects of the underlying disease. This knowledge has been used to improve DBS treatment of neurological and neuropsychiatric disorders.

The basal ganglia are susceptible to damage in Huntington's disease, Parkinson's disease, Wilson's disease, heavy metal intoxication, and stroke. Basal ganglia lesions are associated with a wide variety of neuropsychiatric presentations, including Tourette syndrome, dementia, depression, OCD, apathy, aphasia, psychosis, and mania (Bhatia and Marsden, 1994). Lesions of the caudate nucleus produce choreoathetosis on the contralateral side, as well as abulia (apathy with loss of spontaneous thought and emotion). In Huntington's disease, neurons are lost in the caudate, putamen, and ventral tegmental area. Depression commonly antecedes other symptoms of Huntington's disease.

OCD is also linked to basal ganglia pathology such as in myoclonus dystonia syndrome. Patients with this condition often present with severe and disabling OCD, affecting their functioning more significantly than the movement disorder. In Fahr's syndrome,

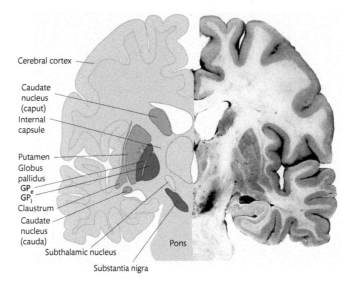

Fig. 38.3 The basal ganglia seen in the frontal plane.
Reproduced with permission from P. Brodal. The Basal Ganglia . In *The Central Nervous System*, 5 ed. Oxford, UK: OUP. Copyright 2016, Oxford University Press. DOI: 10.1093/med/9780190228958.001.0001.

calcification of the basal ganglia occurs, leading to mood disorders, cognitive impairment, OCD, and psychosis. Wilson's disease is caused by an abnormality in copper metabolism, leading to copper deposition in the liver, eyes, and brain. There are both psychiatric and motor manifestations. The neuropsychiatric symptoms include psychosis, cognitive impairment, and affective disorders. As in Huntington's disease, the psychiatric symptoms may be the presenting feature.

Pantothenate kinase-associated neurodegeneration (PKAN) (formerly called Hallervorden–Spatz disease) is an autosomal recessive disorder leading to parkinsonism, dystonia, dementia, and ultimately death. Neurodegeneration in PKAN is accompanied by an excess of iron that progressively builds up in the brain. Radiographic features reflect areas of iron deposition, mainly the globi pallidi, substantia nigra, and red nuclei. T2-weighted MRI images often demonstrate hypointense changes in the globi pallidi and pars reticulata of the substantia nigra. The cortex is usually spared, but caudate atrophy may be seen in more advanced disease. The 'eye of the tiger' sign results from a central T2 relatively hyperintense spot (caused by gliosis) within the hypointense globi pallidi (see Fig. 38.4).

The ventral striatum contains the nucleus accumbens, a structure implicated in goal-directed behaviour and the rewarding effects of carbohydrates, as well as drugs of abuse.

In summary, the basal ganglia have important functions in the regulation of attentional and cognitive functions, and pathology affecting the basal ganglia is increasingly recognized to linking to neuropsychiatric presentations. Understanding the mechanism of basal ganglia function and defining therapeutic targets at different brain sites may improve treatment of the motor, cognitive, and motivational aspects of basal ganglia diseases. This knowledge has been used to improve DBS treatment of neurological and neuropsychiatric disorders.

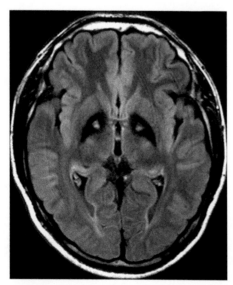

Fig. 38.4 The 'eye of the tiger' sign, seen in pantothenate kinase-associated neurodegeneration.

Reproduced with permission from J.-H. Seo et al. A Novel PANK2 Mutation in a Patient with Atypical Pantothenate-Kinase-Associated Neurodegeneration Presenting with Adult-Onset Parkinsonism. *J Clin Neurol.*, 5(4): 192–194. Copyright © 2009 Korean Neurological Association. https://doi.org/10.3988/jcn.2009.5.4.192.

Cerebellum

The traditional view that the cerebellum is solely responsible for motor function has been challenged since the end of the last century. There is good evidence that it has a role in regulation of both non-motor and motor function. The non-motor symptoms described in the so-called 'cerebellar cognitive affective syndrome' are considered to result from disrupted connections to the cerebral cortex and limbic system (Schmahmann, 2004). New research is expanding our understanding of cerebellar and vestibular involvement in a range of cognitive and affective symptoms in common vestibular disorders (Gurvich et al., 2013; Smith et al., 2005). The features typically described following cerebellar damage include problems with executive function, spatial cognition, language, and affect. Personality changes presenting with blunting of affect or disinhibited and inappropriate behaviour are also reported.

Brainstem

The brainstem has important roles in the regulation of behaviour, cognition, and mood. It is the connection between the spinal cord, cerebellum, and cerebrum, and is the source for the monoamine (noradrenaline, dopamine, and serotonin) neurotransmitter circuits that project cortically to modulate these features. The major subdivisions of the brainstem (from rostral to caudal) are the midbrain, pons, and medulla (see Fig. 38.5). The brainstem serves as a conduit for many ascending and descending pathways, contains most cranial nerve nuclei, and is important for many key integrative functions. The reticular formation is contained in the core of the brainstem. It is phylogenetically one of the oldest components of the brain and is central to modulation of movement, pain, wakefulness, alertness, and arousal. Brainstem regions are at high risk of ischaemic damage because of very limited collateral circulation.

Individuals with brainstem lesions are reported to fail to return to baseline levels of functioning in daily life activities, even after physical and neurological deficits have resolved. The most frequently reported deficits following isolated brainstem lesions are impaired attention and executive functioning (Garrard et al., 2002). Impaired memory and naming ability have also been reported (Bedard et al., 1993; Garrard et al., 2002).

The raphe nuclei positioned along the midline of the medulla, pons, and midbrain all produce serotonin and are implicated in control of sleep, mood/affect, aggression, and other neuroendocrine functions. Pathological crying is often seen after stroke and may be successfully treated with SSRIs, suggesting that this symptom results from damage to the raphe nuclei or their connections to the hemispheres (Andersen, 1995).

Ventral pons injuries can result in locked-in syndrome, characterized by paralysis of all four limbs and paralytic mutism. Cognition has been examined in patients with this condition. While some studies have reported preservation of cognitive functioning, others have suggested impaired attention and memory difficulties, as well as deficits in mental calculation, problem-solving, auditory and visual recognition, and receptive language.

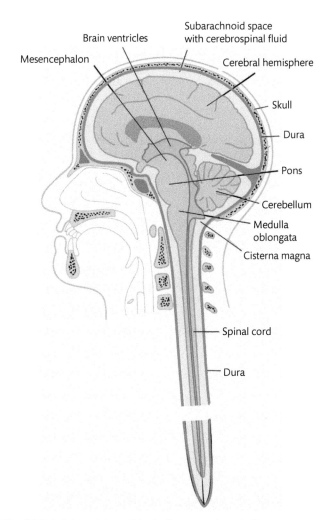

Fig. 38.5 Left lateral view of the brainstem and cerebellum.
Reproduced with permission from P. Brodal. Parts of the Nervous System. In *The Central Nervous System*, 5 ed. Oxford, UK: OUP. Copyright 2016, Oxford University Press. DOI: 10.1093/med/9780190228958.001.0001.

The profile of deficits reported implicates disruption of the frontal–subcortical system, with specific impact on regions involved in attentional and executive functioning. The brain areas usually associated with executive function are the prefrontal and anterior cingulate cortices, as described earlier, and are connected reciprocally with the brainstem. That a similar pattern of deficit is seen in brainstem lesions serves to remind us that particular cognitive functions can be disrupted by injury to areas remote from the cortical areas primarily associated with them.

Conclusion

This chapter aims to provide an overview of focal brain syndromes in neuropsychiatry. The reader should consider this to be purely an introduction to the field; there is clearly much more that can be said about the brain regions and their associated syndromes than can be discussed here. In addition, new research findings ensure that understanding of both normal function and pathology is constantly advancing. However, there are some basic concepts which should be remembered when considering these disorders, as summarized below.

KEY LEARNING POINTS

- Anatomical localization is not always straightforward for psychological, as opposed to neurological, symptoms.
- Specific cognitive functions may be disrupted by injury to areas remote from the cortical areas primarily associated with them.
- Most of the focal brain syndromes in neuropsychiatry are associated with deficits in cognitive functioning.
- Frontal lobe damage leads to dysexecutive syndrome. This clinical syndrome leads to personality, affective, or behavioural changes, working memory problems, indifference, distractibility, emotional instability, diminished anxiety, impulsiveness, facetiousness, euphoria, lack of initiative, and impaired planning ability.
- Parietal lobe damage leads to deficits in processing sensory information from various parts of the body, dyscalculia, visuospatial processing problems, and difficulty with navigation and manipulation of objects in space.
- Temporal lobe lesions cause deficits in language and memory, as well as behavioural changes, including aggression, mood changes, and psychosis.
- Occipital lobe lesions lead to deficits in higher-order visual processing such as visual object agnosia and prosopagnosia. There may also be hallucinations and visual distortions.
- Lesions to brain regions traditionally associated with motor function, such as the basal ganglia, cerebellum, and brainstem, can lead to diverse neuropsychiatric and cognitive symptoms.

REFERENCES

Andersen G. Treatment of uncontrolled crying after stroke. Drugs Aging. 1995;6(2):105–11.

Bedard MA, Montplaisir J, Malo J, Richer F, Rouleau I. Persistent neuropsychological deficits and vigilance impairment in sleep apnea syndrome after treatment with continuous positive airways pressure (CPAP). J Clin Exp Neuropsychol. 1993;15(2):330–41.

Bhatia KP, Marsden CD. The behavioural and motor consequences of focal lesions of the basal ganglia in man. Brain. 1994;117 (Pt 4):859–76.

Critchley M. The problem of visual agnosia. J Neurol Sci. 1964;1(3):274–90.

Cummings JL. Frontal-subcortical circuits and human behavior. Arch Neurol. 1993;50(8):873–80.

Damasio A, Anderson S. The frontal lobes. In: Heilman K, Valenstein E, editors. *Clinical Neuropsychology*, third edition. New York, NY: Oxford University Press; 1993.

Damasio A, Geschwind N. Anatomical localisation in clinical neuropsychology. In: Fredericks AM, editor. *Handbook of Clinical Neurology*. 1985.

Garrard P, Bradshaw D, Jäger HR, Thompson AJ, Losseff N, Playford D. Cognitive dysfunction after isolated brain stem insult. An underdiagnosed cause of long term morbidity. J Neurol Neurosurg Psychiatry. 2002;73(2):191–4.

Geschwind N, Galaburda AM. Cerebral lateralization. Biological mechanisms, associations, and pathology: I. A hypothesis and a program for research. Arch Neurol. 1985;42(5):428–59.

Gurvich C, Maller JJ, Lithgow B, Haghgooie S, Kulkarni J. Vestibular insights into cognition and psychiatry. Brain Res. 2013;1537:244–59.

Hermann BP, Wyler AR, Blumer D, Richey E. Ictal fear: Lateralizing significance and implications for understanding the neurobiology of pathological fear states. Neuropsychiatry, Neuropsychol Behav Neurol. 1992;5(3):205–10.

Kopelman MD. The Korsakoff syndrome. Br J Psychiatry England; 1995;166(2):154–73.

Lhermitte F. Human autonomy and the frontal lobes. Part II: Patient behavior in complex and social situations: the 'environmental dependency syndrome'. Ann Neurol. 1986;19(4):335–43.

Liederman J. A reinterpretation of the split-brain syndrome: implications for the function of the corticocortical fibres. In: Davidson R, Hugdahl K, editors. *Brain Asymmetry*. Cambridge, MA: MIT Press; 1995. pp. 451–90.

Lishman WA. Brain damage in relation to psychiatric disability after head injury. Br J Psychiatry. 1968;114(509):373–410.

Luria AR. *Higher Cortical Functions in Man*, second edition. Springer; 1980.

Masterman DL, Cummings JL. Frontal-subcortical circuits: the anatomic basis of executive, social and motivated behaviors. J Psychopharmacol. 1997;11(2):107–14.

Mesulam MM. Dissociative states with abnormal temporal lobe EEG. Multiple personality and the illusion of possession. Arch Neurol. 1981;38(3):176–81.

Morris JS, DeGelder B, Weiskrantz L, Dolan RJ. Differential extrageniculostriate and amygdala responses to presentation of emotional faces in a cortically blind field. Brain. 2001;124(Pt 6):1241–52.

Okubo Y, Suhara T, Suzuki K, et al. Decreased prefrontal dopamine D1 receptors in schizophrenia revealed by PET. Nature. 1997;385(6617):634–6.

Schmahmann JD. Disorders of the cerebellum: ataxia, dysmetria of thought, and the cerebellar cognitive affective syndrome. J Neuropsychiatry Clin Neurosci. 2004;16(3):367–78.

Smith PF, Zheng Y, Horii A, Darlington CL. Does vestibular damage cause cognitive dysfunction in humans? J Vestib Res. 2005;15:1–9.

Tierney AJ. Egas Moniz and the origins of psychosurgery: a review commemorating the 50th anniversary of Moniz's Nobel Prize. J Hist Neurosci. 2000;9(1):22–36.

Weinberger DR, Berman KF, Chase TN. Mesocortical dopaminergic function and human cognition. Ann N Y Acad Sci. 1988;537:330–8.

SECTION 3
Principles of treatment

39

Psychopharmacotherapy in the neuropsychiatric patient

Joseph J. Cooper, Borna Bonakdarpour, and Fred Ovsiew

Introduction

With pharmacological intervention, the clinician treating neuropsychiatric patients has the opportunity to reduce symptoms and improve functioning and quality of life. Unlike most situations in patients with idiopathic psychiatric illnesses, under some circumstances the neuropsychiatrist can provide a pharmacological intervention that addresses the underlying pathophysiology of the disorder and alters its course. For example, mental symptoms arising from inflammatory brain disease may be relieved by immunomodulatory treatment, and symptoms arising from frequent seizures may be alleviated by improved seizure control. When available, such interventions take precedence over symptom management. Though the two approaches may not be mutually exclusive, the clinician must not get so caught up in addressing symptoms that their possibly treatable cause goes unaddressed.

We do not discuss such disease-modifying interventions in this chapter but confine ourselves to symptomatic treatment. Even in this regard, however, pharmacological management of neuropsychiatric patients differs in some respects from the more familiar psychiatric task of symptom management in idiopathic psychiatric illness. The clinician must be aware that superficially similar symptoms and syndromes in idiopathic states and organic conditions may not derive from the same pathophysiology. There is no guarantee that 'depression' in a young person with a family history of affective disorder is the same condition as *de novo* 'depression' in an elderly person with Alzheimer's disease (AD), even if the symptoms are similar (Chen et al., 2012). It follows that the pharmacological approach familiar to the clinician from idiopathic psychiatric illness cannot be taken for granted in the neuropsychiatric patient. In this chapter, we sketch an approach that derives from the available data in neuropsychiatric illness. Further, the clinician needs to be alert to symptoms or syndromal patterns that are distinctive to neuropsychiatric illness. For example, the syndrome of apathy should be differentiated from depression and call forth specific interventions that address its (relatively well-) known basis in brain disease.

Some tactical aspects of providing pharmacological treatment are not distinctly different from the approach in idiopathic psychiatric illness, but perhaps even more important in a patient population that often has a high rate of coexisting illness and concurrent medication, greater vulnerability to neurotoxicity of medicines, and an impaired capacity to report favourable or adverse responses to treatment. In this regard, the following points are salient:

- First do no harm. Drug toxicity should always be considered as a possible cause of symptoms, and the prescribing clinician should always ask if the potential harm of an intervention outweighs the potential benefit. For example, the use of antipsychotic drugs in dementia is associated with an elevated risk of death; a substantial benefit has to be expected to justify the risk (Maust et al., 2015).
- Obtain a collateral history. A family member's or caregiver's account of the symptom picture and response to treatment is generally required in neuropsychiatric patients.
- 'Start low and go slow.' Dosing should be careful and adjusted for age and coexisting alterations of metabolism. Patients with brain disease may be more sensitive to medicines with potential neurotoxicity. For example, bupropion, often useful in patients with idiopathic depression, is relatively contraindicated in patients with brain diseases that reduce the seizure threshold.
- Do one thing at a time. Dose changes and introduction of new medicines should be done in a way that maximizes the opportunity to recognize what intervention has brought about improvement or caused adverse effects.
- Do not forget psychosocial interventions. Though it may be assumed that symptoms of organic origin require organic treatments, this is not always true, and in some cases the reverse is true. Brain disease, by making a person less capable of independence from the environment, may give rise to symptoms that require environmental management. For example, wandering behaviour and agitation in dementia call for first-line psychosocial interventions.
- Use quantitative scales to measure response when feasible. A wide array of such scales is available.

Cognitive impairment

Management of cognitive impairment is a multidisciplinary task involving both pharmacological and non-pharmacological approaches. A desirable pharmacological intervention would address the underlying aetiology of cognitive impairment. Restorative treatments, however, focus on restoring biochemical pathways that may have been affected by the underlying causative factors.

Aside from stimulants (and related drugs such as atomoxetine and modafinil) which can help with attention disorders, currently only two other groups of medicines are approved by the American Food and Drug Administration (FDA) for management of cognitive impairment: cholinesterase inhibitors and the N-methyl-D-aspartate (NMDA) receptor inhibitor memantine. Recommendations for the use of these agents from the UK's National Institute for Health and Care Excellence are closely similar to American guidelines (National Institute for Health and Care Excellence, 2016).

Cholinesterase inhibitors

Cholinesterase inhibitors (ChEIs) have primarily been studied in individuals with AD. The nucleus basalis of Meynert (NBM) is the major source of brain cholinergic innervation and is a major region affected by Alzheimer pathology (Mesulam, 2013). Cholinergic pathways can also be affected by other diseases of the brain. Lewy body disease (LBD) especially damages the NBM, and ChEIs improve symptoms of dementia with Lewy bodies (DLB) (Knight et al., 2018). In cerebrovascular disease, subcortical cholinergic fibres can be damaged by stroke or white matter disease, and ChEIs have a modest effect in vascular cognitive impairment (Gorelick et al., 2011).

Currently three drugs from this group are FDA-approved for use in AD (donepezil, galantamine, and rivastigmine). No head-to-head clinical trial has compared their efficacy, but meta-analyses have shown small-to-medium effect sizes for all three drugs (Atri et al., 2012; Ballard and Corbett, 2012; Birks, 2006). ChEIs need to be titrated over 4–6 weeks to avoid adverse effects. Common side effects are nausea, diarrhoea, dizziness, and headache. Bradycardia, syncope, and weight loss are more serious side effects, requiring dose adjustment or drug discontinuation.

Higher-dose forms of donepezil (23 mg) and rivastigmine (13.3 mg) have subsequently become available and are associated with slightly greater efficacy (Farlow et al., 2010; Frampton, 2014), but also with a higher rate of side effects (up to 20%).

The term mild cognitive impairment (MCI) applies to patients who have evidence of cognitive decline, but without substantial adverse effects on ADLs. Many of these patients have AD pathology, and treatment with ChEIs may seem reasonable; often patients are eager for some form of treatment. However, available data have failed to show benefit from these agents in MCI in preventing transition to dementia, and no strong evidence supports their use for symptomatic treatment (Petersen et al., 2018; O'Brien et al., 2017).

Though ChEIs are typically considered agents that enhance cognition, inconsistent evidence suggests that non-cognitive symptoms in dementia may improve modestly in response to treatment with ChEIs (Kales et al., 2015; Rodda et al., 2009; Wang et al., 2015). In clinical situations where a ChEI is indicated for cognitive symptoms, a trial for behavioural and mood symptoms is often reasonable.

NMDA receptor antagonists

In animal models of AD, excessive activation of NMDA receptors and the brain glutamatergic pathway, triggered by β-amyloid deposition, leads to calcium-induced neurotoxicity and neurodegeneration (Lewerenz and Maher, 2015). However, whether NMDA antagonists alter this process in clinical AD is not known. Of the NMDA antagonists, only memantine is FDA-approved for treatment of moderate and severe AD (Reisberg et al., 2003). As monotherapy or in combination with ChEIs, memantine has a significant, but small, benefit on cognitive symptoms of moderate to severe AD and is well tolerated (McShane et al., 2019). Therefore, common clinical practice is to add memantine to ChEIs in the moderate stage of AD. As with ChEIs, the drug should be titrated to the full dose over weeks. Mild side effects include constipation, headache, and dizziness. At toxic levels (seen with associated renal disease or administration errors), memantine can cause chorea and dystonia (Borges and Bonakdarpour, 2017). In such cases, with immediate discontinuation, abnormal movements and postures will subside.

Memantine indirectly facilitates dopaminergic function; this can explain its positive effects on attention, information processing, and executive function (Mecocci et al., 2009; Seeman et al., 2008). It also produces some benefit in patients with traumatic brain injury (TBI) (Chew and Zafonte, 2009). A small non-placebo-controlled study in patients with primary progressive aphasia showed lack of progression of cognitive impairment over a 26-week period (Boxer et al., 2009).

Agitation and aggression

Agitated and aggressive behaviours are common features of neuropsychiatric illness and a challenge for practitioners and caregivers. The initial approach to agitation and aggression in neuropsychiatric disorders should be to identify reversible contributors, including general medical conditions (e.g. urinary tract infection), pain, and environmental factors before turning to pharmacotherapy. Environmental management should always be included in the treatment plan and may obviate the need for medication (Kales et al., 2015). Psychotropic drugs can be added to this approach, ideally for a limited time, with attention to the specific behavioural outcome desired and consideration of the risk:benefit ratio of the medicine selected.

The majority of the literature, and controversy, in this area of pharmacotherapy relates to behavioural symptoms of dementia. The use of antipsychotic medicines for agitation and aggression in dementia remains widespread, despite a black-box warning in the United States in 2005 and other calls to curtail such use (Corbett et al., 2014; Greenblatt and Greenblatt, 2016; Kales et al., 2015). The literature should be separated into studies on agitation (restlessness, pacing, fidgeting, hyperactivity, abnormal vocalizations) and studies on aggression (verbal insults, shouting, hitting, biting, throwing objects). Most of the efficacy of antipsychotic medications has been shown in studies of aggression, though agitation is far commoner (Ballard et al., 2009). Data generally support efficacy for short-term (<12 weeks) use of antipsychotic agents for aggression that is severe, persistent, and refractory to other interventions (Ballard et al., 2009;

Greenblatt and Greenblatt, 2016). Safety data show an increased rate of mortality and cardiac events, with odds ratios in the range of 1.5–1.7, though the mechanisms of these associations have not been fully clarified (Ballard et al., 2009; Greenblatt and Greenblatt, 2016). First-generation antipsychotics are associated with less short-term tolerability and at least similar mortality outcomes, and thus are not recommended. Much of the evidence of efficacy has been for risperidone, which remains the best-proven antipsychotic drug for treating aggression in dementia, but the evidence does not indicate it poses lower risk. Avoidance of this risk is advised when possible, but when used, second-generation antipsychotics should be used at the lowest possible dose for the shortest possible duration, with frequent reconsideration of alternative strategies. In our judgement, the elevated mortality risk should be discussed with patients and caregivers; in our experience, some will decline treatment if well informed, though many will accept the risk.

The antidepressants citalopram, sertraline, and trazodone possess some efficacy for agitation in dementia, and though the evidence of efficacy is less than for antipsychotics, particularly regarding clinically significant aggression, the side effect profile is far more favourable (Porsteinsson et al., 2014; Seitz et al., 2011). ChEIs and memantine each have shown some effect in reducing agitation and aggression in large studies where these behaviours were not the main outcome measures (Ballard et al., 2009). A fixed-dose combination of quinidine and dextromethorphan, in use for pseudobulbar affect, showed efficacy for agitation in AD in initial studies (Cummings et al., 2015). Agitation occurring in the evenings, so-called sundowning, may respond to regulation of the sleep/wake cycle by melatonin (Lammers and Ahmed, 2013). This is a particularly attractive intervention, when appropriate, because of the low rate of adverse effects of melatonin. Anticonvulsants and benzodiazepines have not proven useful in this population (Ballard et al., 2009; Defrancesco et al., 2015; Pariente et al., 2016).

Several small, short studies have been conducted on cannabinoids for agitation in dementia (Sherman et al., 2017), some with positive results. However, larger and more rigorous studies are needed before its use can be recommended. In severely refractory cases, electroconvulsive therapy (ECT) has been used, and though it has not been well studied in a prospective manner, a review of 122 published cases found improvement in 88% (van den Berg et al., 2017), with the caveat that this response rate is likely affected by selection and publication bias.

Regarding other neuropsychiatric populations, in patients with TBI, randomized controlled trials for agitation and aggression supported the use of non-selective β-blockers (propranolol and pindolol) (Fleminger et al., 2006), though these findings have not been replicated in large samples and use is limited by cardiovascular intolerance. A recent randomized controlled trial of amantadine showed benefit for aggression, compared to placebo (Hammond et al., 2017). Other options, supported by less evidence, include valproate, carbamazepine, and lamotrigine (Bhatnagar et al., 2016). Use of antipsychotics is common but is not well supported by evidence and raises concern for detrimental effects on cognitive and motor recovery. Use of second-generation agents with less potent D2 receptor blockade (e.g. quetiapine), rather than first-generation agents, has been advocated due to the motor side effect profile (Bhatnagar et al., 2016). Other agents with some reports of utility include sertraline, buspirone, lithium, methylphenidate, and tricyclic antidepressants (Chew and Zafonte, 2009).

When pharmacotherapy is necessary, it is advisable to start with the least harmful options, which typically are serotonergic antidepressants. Escalation to antipsychotics and anticonvulsants may be necessary but should be done with careful regard to the risk:benefit ratio. β-blockers and amantadine can be considered in some populations. Medicines with anticholinergic properties can worsen cognition and should generally be avoided (see Medicines with anticholinergic activity, p.). Benzodiazepines can worsen cognition and paradoxically worsen agitation and should generally be avoided.

Psychosis

Psychosis is an umbrella term for symptoms including hallucinations, delusions, and disordered thoughts or behaviours. The initial steps in management in patients with organic disease include identifying general medical conditions that might contribute to psychosis (such as infection or metabolic derangement) and dose reduction or discontinuation of medicines that might produce psychotoxic effects such as anticholinergics or dopamine agonists in Parkinson's disease (PD).

Hallucinations can occur in any sensory modality. The auditory modality is the commonest presentation of hallucinations in idiopathic psychiatric illness such as schizophrenia or psychosis related to mood disorders. Auditory hallucinations can also occur in organic states, including delirium, drug intoxication, and withdrawal states such as delirium tremens.

Visual hallucinations are classically considered a marker of organic brain disease. Visual hallucinations arise in a variety of focal and diffuse neuropsychiatric conditions. Both visual illusions and visual hallucinations can be seen in delirium and may be more common in paediatric delirium (Leentjens et al., 2008). Visual hallucinations are a core feature of DLB. DLB patients are exquisitely sensitive to dopamine blockers, which should be avoided (Weintraub et al., 2016). This group of medicines include the neuroleptics, but also certain antiemetics such as metoclopramide, promethazine, and prochlorperazine. This risk implies that dopamine blockade should be avoided in demented patients unless LBD can be reasonably excluded as the pathology.

We recommend education as the first-line treatment for visual hallucinations in DLB. Most often patients are untroubled by hallucinations of small children or animals, though families and caregivers may worry. Patients and families should be informed that visual hallucinations are a known part of this type of dementia, do not typically cause distress in the patient, and are not easily treated with pharmacologic agents, whose side effects may be worse than the symptom itself. When these visual hallucinations do become distressing, the first-line treatment should be a ChEI (Stinton et al., 2015). Second-line treatments include gabapentin or the antipsychotics clozapine or quetiapine, which are less likely to worsen parkinsonism. Though quetiapine has not been shown effective in controlled trials, it is relatively safe and commonly used in this setting. Pimavanserin, a novel 5HT2A inverse agonist, has become available as an antipsychotic agent that is well tolerated in PD (Schrag et al., 2015) and is approved by the FDA for hallucinations and delusions in PD. At the time of this writing, pimavanserin has not received approval from the European Medicines Agency. Visual hallucinations as part of the Charles Bonnet syndrome, where hallucinations develop because of pathology of the visual system leading to visual impairment, are another example of the questionable utility of pharmacologic treatment, though no systematic data exist (Hartney et al., 2011).

Tactile hallucinations are most commonly associated with states of intoxication with dopaminergic substances (e.g. cocaine) or withdrawal from alcohol or other sedatives (Berrios, 1982). While antipsychotic medication may be helpful for agitation, treatment is driven by the underlying condition.

Olfactory hallucinations are an uncommon feature of idiopathic psychiatric illness, but a classic feature of organic brain disease near the uncal region of the medial temporal lobe, the location of the primary olfactory cortex. Transient olfactory hallucinations of a foul smell, often impossible for the patient to describe, are a classic feature of seizures arising from this medial temporal location ('uncinate fits'). Diagnosing the underlying aetiology (i.e. seizures) and applying the appropriate pharmacotherapy (i.e. anticonvulsants) are the most appropriate therapeutic response to olfactory hallucinations.

Gustatory hallucinations are rare but, when present, are strongly associated with organic brain disease near the primary gustatory cortex in the insula.

In summary, no substantial evidence supports the treatment of non-auditory hallucinations with antipsychotic drugs. We encourage clinicians to consider the aetiology of such symptoms and employ treatment strategies targeted on the aetiological factors.

Delusions arising in the setting of dementia are typically persecutory and non-specific in nature. Antipsychotic medicines are often tried for such symptoms, but without significant evidence to support their use and with the significant mortality risks referred to above (Greenblatt and Greenblatt, 2016).

Certain types of delusions are more strongly associated with organic brain disease. One such category is the delusional misidentification syndromes (DMS), including Capgras delusion (loved ones have been replaced by imposters) and Fregoli delusion (an unfamiliar person in the environment is actually a familiar person in disguise). Cotard delusion is the belief that one is dead or that part of one's body is dead or dying. Each of these delusions has a significant, though not exclusive, association with organic brain disease (Malloy and Richardson, 1994). There is no systematic evidence for pharmacotherapy of these organic delusional syndromes. However, there are reports of successful antipsychotic use in both DMS and Cotard syndrome (Cipriani et al., 2013; Ramirez-Bermudez et al., 2010).

Catatonia

Catatonia is a state of abnormal movements and affects. Catatonia was classically categorized in psychiatric nosology as a subtype of schizophrenia but is now widely acknowledged to be separate from psychotic symptoms (Fink et al., 2010). Catatonia can arise in a wide variety of neurologic disorders. In particular, anti-NMDA receptor encephalitis (aNMDARE) syndrome presents with catatonic signs in many cases (Dalmau et al., 2008). Phencyclidine intoxication,

systemic lupus erythematous (SLE), seizures, infections, and metabolic disturbances are other organic aetiologies sometimes associated with catatonia (Ovsiew et al., 2009).

The pharmacologic treatment of catatonia is similar for catatonia related to either a psychiatric or an organic condition. The first-line treatment is lorazepam (Hawkins et al., 1995). Other GABA-A agonists, such as zolpidem, also show evidence of efficacy (Sienaert et al., 2014). In catatonia refractory to lorazepam, or if there is evidence of more severe catatonic states, such as malignant catatonia or neuroleptic malignant syndrome (NMS), ECT should be promptly considered (Hawkins et al., 1995). Agents to be considered in refractory cases (or when ECT is unavailable) include amantadine, memantine, bromocriptine, and anticonvulsants such as carbamazepine or valproic acid (Beach et al., 2017, Sienaert et al., 2014). Treatment of the underlying disorder, e.g. by mood stabilizers in bipolar disorder or immunotherapies in aNMDARE, should be initiated concurrently with symptomatic treatment of catatonia. However, treatment with neuroleptics of presumed psychosis in catatonic patients risks evoking malignant features (Berardi et al., 1998) and should be considered only in cases refractory to the above standard measures and administered with concurrent lorazepam (Beach et al., 2017).

Depression and mania

Disturbances of mood are a common feature of organic brain disease. Depression is particularly common and likely multifactorial in origin (Raskind, 2008). Many neurologic diseases involve significant morbidity, functional limitations, unpredictable events (e.g. seizures), or a degenerative course. All of these factors may lead to psychosocial stress, predisposing to depression. Certain organic interventions, such as interferon treatment for hepatitis C, have a particular risk of inducing depressive states (Lucaciu and Dumitrascu, 2015).

Depression likely occurs in more than half of patients with AD (Lee and Lyketsos, 2003), but evidence as to the benefit of pharmacologic treatment remains inadequate. While two earlier meta-analyses indicated a weakly positive class effect of antidepressants (Bains et al., 2002; Thompson et al., 2007), the most recent meta-analysis concluded that the available data were suggestive but did not confirm efficacy (Nelson and Devanand, 2011). Similarly, a systematic review in 2014 found the evidence for an effect to be inconclusive (Leong, 2014). This lack of effect may be related to heterogeneity of the patients, with significant overlap of symptoms of depression with symptoms of the primary dementia process, which are unlikely to respond to antidepressants. Nonetheless, clinicians are often inclined to treat these patients with antidepressants, and a recent study suggested that long-term SSRI use in patients with MCI and past, but not present, depression, compared with other or no antidepressants, was associated with a 3-year delay in progression from MCI to dementia (Bartels et al., 2017). If a trial of antidepressant treatment is undertaken, anticholinergic effects, such as those from tricyclic antidepressants or paroxetine, can worsen cognitive function and should be avoided.

Post-stroke depression (PSD) is a common phenomenon. A mixed literature suggests that depression may be commoner after a left hemisphere stroke, particularly depression within the first

2 months (Robinson and Jorge, 2016). This has been interpreted to indicate that depression is a pathophysiological consequence of a catecholaminergic lesion, not simply a reaction to disability. Pharmacotherapy with antidepressants is supported by a meta-analysis in PSD (Hackett et al., 2008), and some data indicated long-term antidepressant treatment for PSD can improve all-cause mortality years after the stroke (Jorge et al., 2003). Additionally, pooled analysis of available data indicated prophylactic treatment with antidepressants after a stroke can reduce the risk of developing PSD (Salter et al., 2013). However, whether antidepressants contribute to an overall more favourable outcome is less clear (Focus Trial Collaboration, 2019). The majority of PSD evidence favours serotonergic antidepressants. Medicines that may increase blood pressure, such as noradrenergic agents, stimulants, and MAOIs, may confer a higher risk in PSD.

For the majority of neurologic disorders with comorbid depression, there are no evidence-based or theoretical reasons for changing from treatment as usual, with a few exceptions. In PD, there is some evidence for using dopamine agonists to treat depression and anhedonia (Lemke et al., 2006). One trial showed greater efficacy of pramipexole than sertraline, but the sertraline dose was likely too low (Barone et al., 2006). In epilepsy and other neurological conditions that carry an increased risk of seizures, the otherwise first-line antidepressant bupropion should be avoided because of its capacity to provoke seizures. Tricyclic antidepressants also lower the seizure threshold (Cardamone et al., 2013).

ECT may have transient adverse cognitive effects in a cognitively impaired population but has a place in the treatment of depression in neurodegenerative disease, especially in PD, where it may also have favourable motor effects (Moellentine et al., 1998). ECT is not contraindicated in epilepsy and may be delivered safely in a variety of neurological conditions (Ducharme et al., 2015). Neurological conditions considered to be relative contraindications to ECT requiring individual evaluation include unstable vascular malformations or aneurysms, recent stroke, elevated intracranial pressure from masses or hydrocephalus, active exacerbation of MS, intracranial metal devices, and (because of the effect of anaesthetic agents) neuromuscular disease (Baghai and Moller, 2008, Ducharme et al., 2015).

Mania is uncommonly associated with organic brain disease (Schneck, 2002). Most reports in the literature of mania due to structural disease implicate right hemisphere structures, particularly the right temporal and orbitofrontal cortices. Treatments reported to be successful include traditional mood-stabilizing agents such as lithium, divalproex, and carbamazepine. Quetiapine was used successfully in at least two cases of brain injury-related mania (Daniels and Felde, 2008). Certain medicines, particularly corticosteroids, are associated with an increased risk of mania. One case series reported 20 patients who responded to sodium valproate for steroid-induced mania, the largest reported body of evidence to date (Roxanas and Hunt, 2012).

Anxiety

Anxiety symptoms may result directly from organic disease, as is the case in ictal fear (Kanner, 2011) or limbic encephalitis (Tuzun and Dalmau, 2007). More commonly in neuropsychiatry anxiety is the reaction to difficult circumstances of a patient with impaired internal resources for grasping complex situations and modulating affective responses.

First-line pharmacological treatment for chronic anxiety in patients with neurological disease is usually an SSRI. Benzodiazepines must be used with caution in patients with impaired cognition, as discussed previously.

The coexistence of post-traumatic stress disorder (PTSD) in TBI patients complicates the treatment of both disorders (Watson et al., 2016). Failure to address PTSD can lead to avoidance and isolation, impairing the likelihood of pursuing rehabilitation and physical therapy, and the cognitive impairments of TBI may impair the ability to utilize psychotherapeutic treatment. Antidepressants, particularly SSRIs, are the best supported pharmacotherapy in this population. Benzodiazepines should be used with caution, given negative effects cited in the general PTSD literature (Guina et al., 2015) and the additional possibility of worsening cognition. Prazosin has significant support in the PTSD literature for reducing nightmares (De Berardis et al., 2015) but has not been studied in those with comorbid TBI.

Apathy

Apathy is state of diminished motivation and goal-directed behaviour. While the syndrome overlaps with depression, depressive ideation and pervasive low mood are not present in apathy. The subjective experience of the apathetic patient is more suggestive of an overall diminution of emotion. Apathy results from disruption of prefrontal–basal ganglia circuit with a hypodopaminergic state in the cortex (Levy and Dubois, 2006). The terms abulia and akinetic mutism are used to describe more extreme presentations on the apathy spectrum.

Apathy is often not responsive to pharmacotherapy. A first-line approach should be to identify other factors that may be reversible causes of an apathy syndrome, including chronic cannabis use (Volkow et al., 2016), hypothyroidism, or other endocrine abnormalities. Much of the evidence for treatment of apathy comes from the dementia literature (Berman et al., 2012; Rea et al., 2014). In this population, ChEIs are the best studied and are consistently associated with benefit in apathy symptoms, although the benefit is typically mild. One trial found donepezil plus a cholinergic precursor (choline alphoscerate), intended to boost acetylcholine availability, to be a more efficacious treatment of apathy, compared with donepezil alone (Rea et al., 2015). Methylphenidate demonstrated efficacy for apathy in AD in two medium-sized trials (Padala et al., 2017; Rosenberg et al., 2013). Memantine has also been associated with some benefit but is less well studied. Some anecdotal data have reported benefit from second-generation antipsychotics, but there is no strong evidence to support their use. Antidepressants, first-generation antipsychotics, and anticonvulsants do not show evidence of utility.

Other evidence for the treatment of apathy comes from PD (Santangelo et al., 2013), TBI (Starkstein and Pahissa, 2014), and stroke (Jorge et al., 2010). In addition to ChEIs, memantine, and stimulants, dopaminergic medicines including amantadine have some reported benefit, particularly in disorders with dopamine deficit such as PD. Theoretical considerations make dopaminergic treatment appealing, but treatment of apathy with any of these agents lacks strong empirical support. Of these options, stimulants are often the least tolerable, with cardiovascular side effects limiting their use, particularly in the elderly. Additional caution is mandated by the potential behavioural risk of producing increased motivation and goal-directed behaviour in a patient whose judgement may be impaired by brain disease.

Delirium

Delirium, or acute confusional state, is the clinical manifestation of an acute medical condition affecting the brain. First-line interventions include identifying the underlying cause and working to reverse it; a search for potentially exacerbating medicines, including anticholinergics, sedatives, or opiates; and environmental alterations to promote orientation, allow for natural light, help day-night cycle cues, and reduce external stimuli.

Antipsychotics are the first-line pharmacotherapy for the symptomatic treatment of delirium and may be helpful for management of agitation, aggression, and insomnia. However, data from well-designed randomized placebo-controlled trials on episode duration and severity do not support antipsychotic use (Flaherty et al., 2011; Meagher et al., 2013). Additional caution is advised when antipsychotic medicines are used in patients at risk of arrhythmia, particularly those with QTc intervals of >500 ms (Ries and Sayadipour, 2014). Benzodiazepines should generally be avoided in delirium, as they can worsen the confusional state and provoke paradoxical agitation. One crucial exception is withdrawal states from alcohol or other gabaergic substances where benzodiazepines are an essential treatment. Comorbid catatonia—which is seldom recognized in the setting of delirium, though catatonic symptoms occur commonly in confusional states (Grover et al., 2014; Oldham and Lee, 2015)—should be viewed as a reason to utilize a lorazepam challenge and other catatonia treatments, as needed. In fact, ECT is an effective treatment for some cases of delirium, including NMS (Nielsen et al., 2014).

Some evidence supports the use of antipsychotics for prevention of delirium (Siddiqi et al., 2007). In the intensive care unit setting, dexmedetomidine can be considered as a sedative that may offer less incidence of delirium, though bradycardia and hypotension can limit its use (Nelson et al., 2015). Melatonin and melatonin agonists have shown utility for prevention of delirium in several small studies and are quite well tolerated, but the evidence for their efficacy did not hold up as significant in a recent Cochrane review (Friedman et al., 2014; Siddiqi et al., 2007). Suvorexant, an orexin receptor antagonist, approved by the FDA for treatment of insomnia, but currently available only in the United States and Japan, showed positive effects for delirium prevention in medically ill older adults in one study (Hatta et al., 2017).

Cognitive and psychiatric adverse effects of drugs used in neurology

Adverse effects of medication should always be considered in the clinical approach to cognitive impairment and behavioural disturbance. Medicines used to treat epilepsy and PD and medicines with anticholinergic activity will be discussed here.

Antiepileptic drugs

Cognitive impairment in individuals with epilepsy may be due either to epilepsy and its underlying brain abnormality or to the adverse effects of antiepileptic drugs (AEDs) (Hermann et al., 2008, 2010). Adverse cognitive effects of AEDs are usually worst early in therapy and, with time, may subside or be taken for granted. To minimize adverse cognitive effects, AEDs are usually started at low doses and gradually increased to the lowest effective dose. The most sedating AEDs (barbiturates and benzodiazepines) have the most pronounced effect on attention and executive function (Hermann et al., 2010). Valproic acid can cause parkinsonism and cognitive impairment mimicking neurodegenerative disease (Armon et al., 1996; Masmoudi et al., 2006; Tsai et al., 2016). Topiramate produces significant adverse effects on attention, memory, executive function, and verbal fluency (Sommer et al., 2013). Levetiracetam, though apparently safe cognitively, can cause adverse behavioural effects, notably aggression, especially in patients with intellectual disability (Helmstaedter et al., 2008).

In individuals with comorbid epilepsy and psychiatric disorder, the influence of AEDs on psychiatric symptoms needs to be taken into account. Lamotrigine and gabapentin can generally be safely used in patients with depression or psychosis; phenobarbital, primidone, topiramate, and levetiracetam are more likely to have adverse psychiatric effects (Ruiz-Gimenez et al., 2010).

An important consideration in the use of AEDs is the reported increased risk of suicidal thoughts and behaviours (Bagary, 2011). An FDA advisory in 2008 warned about an increased risk of suicidality up to at least 24 weeks after the initiation of any AED, whether its use was for epilepsy or for a different indication (https://www.fda.gov/Drugs/DrugSafety/PostmarketDrugSafetyInformationforPatientsandProviders/ucm100192.htm). However, suicidal thoughts and behaviours occur at an elevated rate in patients with epilepsy, even before the diagnosis of epilepsy (Hesdorffer et al., 2016). The FDA guidance has drawn considerable disagreement (Fountoulakis et al., 2015).

A common issue in the care of patients with epilepsy is drug interactions between AEDs and psychiatric drugs (Patsalos, 2013; Spina et al., 2016). Interactions can have the effect of elevating levels of either the AED or the psychiatric drug, with consequent toxicity, or of reducing the levels of either drug, with consequent ineffective treatment of psychiatric symptoms or failure of seizure control. Some AEDs are relatively free of drug interactions such as lacosamide and levetiracetam; similarly, some psychiatric medicines are less likely to interact with AEDs, such as citalopram and escitalopram. Because of the continuing introduction of new AEDs and new psychopharmacological agents and the varying availability of data on particular combinations of agents, the clinician is faced with a difficult situation. Checking the latest data using online databases of drug interactions before prescribing is a wise precaution.

Parkinson's disease medicines

PD is one clinical phenotype in a larger LBD spectrum that includes PD, PD dementia (PDD), and DLB (Donaghy and McKeith, 2014). Hallucinations and psychosis can occur in the course of PD and can be related to delirium, disease progression, or transition to PDD, or they can be due to medicines used for PD (Grover et al., 2015). Both dopaminergic (levodopa and especially direct-acting dopaminergic) agents and anticholinergic medicines can contribute to PD psychosis; dose adjustment of levodopa and discontinuation of anticholinergics and direct-acting dopamine agonists may be necessary. It is recommended to make dose adjustments in the following order: anticholinergics, selegiline, amantadine, dopamine receptor agonists, catechol-*O*-methyltransferase inhibitors, and finally levodopa (Seppi et al., 2011).

Medicines with anticholinergic activity

Many medicines used in neurology practice have anticholinergic effects that can cause adverse cognitive effects. Anticholinergic medication, especially in the elderly, can exhaust cognitive reserve and contribute to the pathophysiology of degenerative disease (Risacher et al., 2016). Medicines used in neurology practice with substantial anticholinergic effects include the tricyclic antidepressants amitriptyline and nortriptyline and the antihistaminergic drug diphenhydramine. Of the SSRIs, paroxetine is the most anticholinergic (Sanchez et al., 2014). These medicines should be used with caution in the elderly, patients with dementia, and patients who are in a confusional state (delirium).

Conclusion

Pharmacological treatment has much to offer the neuropsychiatric patient, but adverse effects of drugs must always be taken into account. We have emphasized the importance of a search for reversible factors producing psychiatric symptoms, especially drug side effects, and the (perhaps paradoxical) importance of environmental management of these symptoms. In some future edition of this textbook, newer medicines with enhanced benefits and reduced dangers will be recommended—if disease-modifying treatments obviating the need for symptom management have not been developed. For now, however, thoughtful use of available agents must suffice.

KEY LEARNING POINTS

- Patients with brain disease may be more sensitive to neurotoxicity from psychotropic medicines. Lower doses and slow titrations are generally recommended.
- Only few medicines have achieved regulatory agency approvals for neuropsychiatric management in particular, such as ChEIs and memantine for AD and recently pimavanserin for PD psychosis.
- Commonly, medicines approved for idiopathic psychiatric disorders are used for phenotypically similar neuropsychiatric symptoms. However, the evidence for utility of such approaches is mixed.
- Antipsychotic usage may be acutely dangerous in parkinsonian or catatonic states or in undiagnosed DLB, and caution is warranted when antipsychotics are used for lengthy periods in patients with dementia.
- Caution is also warranted in the use of cognitively impairing medications, such as benzodiazepines and anticholinergics, across a wide range of neuropsychiatric conditions.
- Environmental interventions and caregiver education play a large role in the management of neuropsychiatric symptoms and can often obviate, or at least lessen, the need for psychopharmacological intervention.

REFERENCES

Armon, C., et al. 1996. Reversible parkinsonism and cognitive impairment with chronic valproate use. Neurology, 47, 626–35.

Atri, A., et al. 2012. Validity, significance, strengths, limitations, and evidentiary value of real-world clinical data for combination therapy in Alzheimer's disease: comparison of efficacy and effectiveness studies. Neurodegener Dis, 10, 170–4.

Bagary, M. 2011. Epilepsy, antiepileptic drugs and suicidality. Curr Opin Neurol, 24, 177–82.

Baghai, T. C. & Moller, H. J. 2008. Electroconvulsive therapy and its different indications. Dialogues Clin Neurosci, 10, 105–17.

Bains, J., et al. 2002. Antidepressants for treating depression in dementia. Cochrane Database Syst Rev, 4, CD003944.

Ballard, C. & Corbett, A. 2012. Dementia: new guidelines on disorders associated with dementia. Nat Rev Neurol, 8, 663–4.

Ballard, C. G., et al. 2009. Management of agitation and aggression associated with Alzheimer disease. Nat Rev Neurol, 5, 245–55.

Barone, P., et al. 2006. Pramipexole versus sertraline in the treatment of depression in Parkinson's disease: a national multicenter parallel-group randomized study. J Neurol, 253, 601–7.

Bartels, C., et al. 2018. Impact of SSRI therapy on risk of conversion from Mild Cognitive Impairment to Alzheimer's Dementia in individuals with previous depression. Am J Psychiatry, 175, 232–41.

Beach, S. R., et al. 2017. Alternative treatment strategies for catatonia: A systematic review. Gen Hosp Psychiatry, 48, 1–19.

Berardi, D., et al. 1998. Clinical and pharmacologic risk factors for neuroleptic malignant syndrome: a case-control study. Biol Psychiatry, 44, 748–54.

Berman, K., et al. 2012. Pharmacologic treatment of apathy in dementia. Am J Geriatr Psychiatry, 20, 104–22.

Berrios, G. E. 1982. Tactile hallucinations: conceptual and historical aspects. J Neurol Neurosurg Psychiatry, 45, 285–93.

Bhatnagar, S., et al. 2016. Pharmacotherapy in rehabilitation of post-acute traumatic brain injury. Brain Res, 1640, 164–79.

Birks, J. 2006. Cholinesterase inhibitors for Alzheimer's disease. Cochrane Database Syst Rev, 1, CD005593.

Borges, L. G. & Bonakdarpour, B. 2017. Memantine-induced chorea and dystonia. Pract Neurol, 17, 133–4.

Boxer, A. L., et al. 2009. An open-label study of memantine treatment in 3 subtypes of frontotemporal lobar degeneration. Alzheimer Dis Assoc Disord, 23, 211–17.

Cardamone, L., et al. 2013. Antidepressant therapy in epilepsy: can treating the comorbidities affect the underlying disorder? Brit J Pharmacol, 168, 1531–54.

Chen, J. D., et al. 2012. Early and late onset, first-episode, treatment-naive depression: same clinical symptoms, different regional neural activities. J Affect Disord, 143, 56–63.

Chew, E. & Zafonte, R. D. 2009. Pharmacological management of neurobehavioral disorders following traumatic brain injury—a state-of-the-art review. J Rehabil Res Dev, 46, 851–79.

Cipriani, G., et al. 2013. Delusional misidentification syndromes and dementia: a border zone between neurology and psychiatry. American Journal of Alzheimer's Disease and Other Dementias, 28, 671–8.

Corbett, A., et al. 2014. Don't use antipsychotics routinely to treat agitation and aggression in people with dementia. BMJ, 349, g6420.

Cummings, J. L., et al. 2015b. Effect of dextromethorphan-quinidine on agitation in patients with alzheimer disease dementia: A randomized clinical trial. JAMA, 314, 1242–54.

Dalmau, J., et al. 2008. Anti-NMDA-receptor encephalitis: case series and analysis of the effects of antibodies. Lancet Neurol, 7, 1091–8.

Daniels, J. P. & Felde, A. 2008. Quetiapine treatment for mania secondary to brain injury in 2 patients. J Clin Psychiatry, 69, 497–8.

De Berardis, et al. 2015. Targeting the noradrenergic system in posttraumatic stress disorder: a systematic review and meta-analysis of prazosin trials. Curr Drug Targets, 16, 1094–106.

DeFrancesco, M., et al. 2015. Use of benzodiazepines in Alzheimer's Disease: a systematic review of literature. Int J Neuropsychopharmacol, 18, 1–11.

Donaghy, P. C. & McKeith, I. G. 2014. The clinical characteristics of dementia with Lewy bodies and a consideration of prodromal diagnosis. Alzheimers Res Ther, 6, 46.

Ducharme, S., et al. 2015. Retrospective analysis of the short-term safety of ECT in patients with neurological comorbidities: a guide for pre-ECT neurological evaluations. J Neuropsychiatry Clin Neurosci, 27, 311–21.

Farlow, M. R., et al. 2010. Effectiveness and tolerability of high-dose (23 mg/d) versus standard-dose (10 mg/d) donepezil in moderate to severe Alzheimer's disease: A 24-week, randomized, double-blind study. Clin Ther, 32, 1234–51.

Fink, M., et al. 2010. Catatonia is not schizophrenia: Kraepelin's error and the need to recognize catatonia as an independent syndrome in medical nomenclature. Schizophr Bull, 36, 314–20.

Flaherty, J. H., et al. 2011. Antipsychotics in the treatment of delirium in older hospitalized adults: a systematic review. J Am Geriatr Soc, 59 Suppl 2, S269–76.

Fleminger, S., et al. 2006. Pharmacological management for agitation and aggression in people with acquired brain injury. Cochrane Database Syst Rev, 4, CD003299.

Focus Trial Collaboration. 2019. Effects of fluoxetine on functional outcomes after acute stroke (FOCUS): a pragmatic, double-blind, randomised, controlled trial. Lancet, 393, 265–74.

Fountoulakis, K. N., et al. 2015. Report of the WPA section of pharmacopsychiatry on the relationship of antiepileptic drugs with suicidality in epilepsy. Int J Psychiatry Clin Pract, 19, 158–67.

Frampton, J. E. 2014. Rivastigmine transdermal patch 13.3 mg/24 h: a review of its use in the management of mild to moderate Alzheimer's dementia. Drugs Aging, 31, 639–49.

Friedman, J. I., et al. 2014. Pharmacological treatments of non-substance-withdrawal delirium: a systematic review of prospective trials. Am J Psychiatry, 171, 151–9.

Gorelick, P. B., et al. 2011. Vascular contributions to cognitive impairment and dementia: a statement for healthcare professionals from the american heart association/american stroke association. Stroke, 42, 2672–713.

Greenblatt, H. K. & Greenblatt, D. J. 2016. Use of antipsychotics for the treatment of behavioral symptoms of dementia. J Clin Pharmacol, 56, 1048–57.

Grover, S., et al. 2014. Do patients of delirium have catatonic features? An exploratory study. Psychiatry Clin Neurosci, 68, 644–51.

Grover, S., et al. 2015. Psychiatric aspects of Parkinson's disease. J Neurosci Rural Pract, 6, 65–76.

Guina, J., et al. 2015. Benzodiazepines for PTSD: a systematic review and meta-analysis. J Psychiatr Pract, 21, 281–303.

Hackett, M. L., et al. 2008. Interventions for treating depression after stroke. Cochrane Database Syst Rev, 4, CD003437.

Hammond, F. M., et al. 2017. Potential impact of amantadine on aggression in chronic traumatic brain Injury. J Head Trauma Rehabil, 32, 308–18.

Hartney, K. E., et al. 2011. Charles Bonnet syndrome: are medications necessary? J Psychiatr Pract, 17, 137–41.

Hatta, K., et al. 2017. Preventive effects of suvorexant on delirium: a randomized placebo-controlled trial. J Clin Psychiatry, 78, e970–9.

Hawkins, J. M., et al. 1995. Somatic treatment of catatonia. Int J Psychiatry Med, 25, 345–69.

Helmstaedter, C., et al. 2008. Positive and negative psychotropic effects of levetiracetam. Epilepsy Behav, 13, 535–41.

Hermann, B., et al. 2010. Cognition across the lifespan: antiepileptic drugs, epilepsy, or both? Epilepsy Behav, 17, 1–5.

Hermann, B., et al. 2008. The neurobehavioural comorbidities of epilepsy: can a natural history be developed. Lancet Neurol, 7, 151–60.

Hesdorffer, D. C., et al. 2016. Occurrence and recurrence of attempted suicide among people with epilepsy. JAMA Psychiatry, 73, 80–6.

Jorge, R. E., et al. 2003. Mortality and poststroke depression: a placebo-controlled trial of antidepressants. Am J Psychiatry, 160, 1823–9.

Jorge, R. E., et al. 2010. Apathy following stroke. Can J Psychiatry, 55, 350–4.

Kales, H. C., et al. 2015. Assessment and management of behavioral and psychological symptoms of dementia. BMJ, 350, h369.

Kanner, A. M. 2011. Ictal panic and interictal panic attacks: diagnostic and therapeutic principles. Neurol Clin, 29, 163–75, ix.

Knight, R., et al. 2018. A systematic review and meta-analysis of the effectiveness of acetylcholinesterase inhibitors and memantine in treating the cognitive symptoms of dementia. Dement Geriatr Cogn Disord, 45, 131–51.

Lammers, M. & Ahmed, A. I. 2013. Melatonin for sundown syndrome and delirium in dementia: is it effective? J Am Geriatr Soc, 61, 1045–6.

Lee, H. B. & Lyketsos, C. G. 2003. Depression in Alzheimer's disease: heterogeneity and related issues. Biol Psychiatry, 54, 353–62.

Leentjens, A. F. G., et al. 2008. A comparison of the phenomenology of pediatric, adult, and geriatric delirium. J Psychosom Res, 64, 219–23.

Lemke, M. R., et al. 2006. Effects of the dopamine agonist pramipexole on depression, anhedonia and motor functioning in Parkinson's disease. J Neurol Sci, 248, 266–70.

Leong, C. 2014. Antidepressants for depression in patients with dementia: a review of the literature. The Consultant Pharmacist, 29, 254–63.

Levy, R. & Dubois, B. 2006. Apathy and the functional anatomy of the prefrontal cortex-basal ganglia circuits. Cereb Cortex, 16, 916–28.

Lewerenz, J. & Maher, P. 2015. Chronic glutamate toxicity in neurodegenerative diseases—what is the evidence? Front Neurosci, 9, 469.

Lucaciu, L. A. & Dumitrascu, D. L. 2015. Depression and suicide ideation in chronic hepatitis C patients untreated and treated with interferon: prevalence, prevention, and treatment. Ann Gastroenterol, 28, 440–7.

Malloy, P. F. & Richardson, E. D. 1994. The frontal lobes and content-specific delusions. J Neuropsychiatry Clin Neurosci, 6, 455–66.

Masmoudi, K., et al. 2006. Parkinsonism and/or cognitive impairment with valproic acid therapy: a report of ten cases. Pharmacopsychiatry, 39, 9–12.

Maust, D. T., et al. 2015. Antipsychotics, other psychotropics, and the risk of death in patients with dementia: number needed to harm. JAMA Psychiatry, 72, 438–45.

McShane, R., et al. 2019. Memantine for dementia. Cochrane Database Syst Rev, 3, CD003154.

Meagher, D. J., et al. 2013. What do we really know about the treatment of delirium with antipsychotics? Ten key issues for delirium pharmacotherapy. Am J Geriatr Psychiatry, 21, 1223–38.

Mecocci, P., et al. 2009. Effects of memantine on cognition in patients with moderate to severe Alzheimer's disease: post-hoc analyses of ADAS-cog and SIB total and single-item scores from six randomized, double-blind, placebo-controlled studies. Int J Geriatr Psychiatry, 24, 532–8.

Mesulam, M. M. 2013. Cholinergic circuitry of the human nucleus basalis and its fate in Alzheimer's disease. J Comp Neurol, 521, 4124–44.

Moellentine, C., et al. 1998. Effectiveness of ECT in patients with parkinsonism. J Neuropsychiatry Clin Neurosci, 10, 187–93.

Nelson, J. C. & Devanand, D. P. 2011. A systematic review and meta-analysis of placebo-controlled antidepressant studies in people with depression and dementia. J Am Geriatric Soc, 59, 577–85.

Nelson, S., et al. 2015. Defining the role of dexmedetomidine in the prevention of delirium in the intensive care unit. Biomed Res Int, 2015, 635737.

National Institute for Health and Care Excellence. *Donepezil, galantamine, rivastigmine and memantine for the treatment of Alzheimer's disease*. Technology appraisal guidance [TA217]. 2016. Available at: http://www.nice.org.uk/guidance/ta217.

Nielsen, R. M., et al. 2014. Electroconvulsive therapy as a treatment for protracted refractory delirium in the intensive care unit—five cases and a review. J Crit Care, 29, 881 e1–6.

O'Brien, J. T., et al. 2017. Clinical practice with anti-dementia drugs: A revised (third) consensus statement from the British Association for Psychopharmacology. J Psychopharmacol, 31, 147–68.

Oldham, M. A. & Lee, H. B. 2015. Catatonia vis-a-vis delirium: the significance of recognizing catatonia in altered mental status. Gen Hosp Psychiatry, 37, 554–9.

Ovsiew, F., et al. 2009. Neuropsychiatric approach to the psychiatric inpatient. In: Ovsiew, F. & Munich, R. L. (eds.) *Principles of Inpatient Psychiatry*. Philadelphia, PA: Lippincott, Williams & Wilkins; pp. 97–124.

Padala, P. R., et al. 2017. Methylphenidate for apathy in community-dwelling older veterans with mild Alzheimer's Disease: a double-blind, placebo-controlled trial. Am J Psychiatry, 175, 159–68.

Pariente, A., et al. 2016. The benzodiazepine-dementia disorders link: current state of knowledge. CNS Drugs, 30, 1–7.

Patsalos, P. N. 2013. Drug interactions with the newer antiepileptic drugs (AEDs)--Part 2: pharmacokinetic and pharmacodynamic interactions between AEDs and drugs used to treat non-epilepsy disorders. Clin Pharmacokinet, 52, 1045–61.

Petersen, R. C., et al. 2018. Practice guideline update summary: Mild cognitive impairment: Report of the Guideline Development, Dissemination, and Implementation Subcommittee of the American Academy of Neurology. Neurology, 90, 126–35.

Porsteinsson, A. P., et al. 2014. Effect of citalopram on agitation in Alzheimer disease: the CitAD randomized clinical trial. JAMA, 311, 682–91.

Ramirez-Bermudez, J., et al. 2010. Cotard syndrome in neurological and psychiatric patients. J Neuropsychiatry Clin Neurosci, 22, 409–16.

Raskind, M. A. 2008. Diagnosis and treatment of depression comorbid with neurologic disorders. Am J Med, 121, S28–37.

Rea, R., et al. 2014. Apathy in Alzheimer's disease: any effective treatment? ScientificWorld J, 2014, 421385.

Rea, R., et al. 2015. Apathy treatment in Alzheimer's disease: interim results of the ASCOMALVA trial. J Alzheimers Dis, 48, 377–83.

Reisberg, B., et al. 2003. Memantine in moderate-to-severe Alzheimer's disease. N Engl J Med, 348, 1333–41.

Ries, R. & Sayadipour, A. 2014. Management of psychosis and agitation in medical-surgical patients who have or are at risk for prolonged QT interval. J Psychiatr Pract, 20, 338–44.

Risacher, S. L., et al. 2016. Association between anticholinergic medication use and cognition, brain metabolism, and brain atrophy in cognitively normal older adults. JAMA Neurol, 73, 721–32.

Robinson, R. G. & Jorge, R. E. 2016. Post-stroke depression: a review. Am J Psychiatry, 173, 221–31.

Rodda, J., et al. 2009. Are cholinesterase inhibitors effective in the management of the behavioral and psychological symptoms of dementia in Alzheimer's disease? A systematic review of randomized, placebo-controlled trials of donepezil, rivastigmine and galantamine. Int Psychogeriatr, 21, 813–24.

Rosenberg, P. B., et al. 2013. Safety and efficacy of methylphenidate for apathy in Alzheimer's disease: a randomized, placebo-controlled trial. J Clin Psychiatry, 74, 810–16.

Roxanas, M. G. & Hung, G. E. 2012. Rapid reversal of corticosteroid-induced mania with sodium valproate: a case series of 20 patients. Psychosom, 53, 575–81.

Ruiz-Gimenez, J., et al. 2010. Antiepileptic treatment in patients with epilepsy and other comorbidities. Seizure, 19, 375–82.

Salter, K. L., et al. 2013. Prevention of poststroke depression: does prophylactic pharmacotherapy work? J Stroke Cerebrovasc Dis, 22, 1243–51.

Sanchez, C., et al. 2014. A comparative review of escitalopram, paroxetine, and sertraline: are they all alike? Int Clin Psychopharmacol, 29, 185–96.

Santangelo, G., et al. 2013. Apathy in Parkinson's disease: diagnosis, neuropsychological correlates, pathophysiology and treatment. Behav Neurol, 27, 501–13.

Schneck, C. D. 2002. Bipolar disorder in neurologic illness. Curr Treat Options Neurol, 4, 477–86.

Schrag, A., et al. 2015. New clinical trials for nonmotor manifestations of Parkinson's disease. Mov Disord, 30, 1490–504.

Seeman, P., et al. 2008. Memantine agonist action at dopamine D2High receptors. Synapse, 62, 149–53.

Seitz, D. P., et al. 2011. Antidepressants for agitation and psychosis in dementia. Cochrane Database Syst Rev, 2, CD008191.

Seppi, K., et al. 2011. The Movement Disorder Society evidence-based medicine review update: treatments for the non-motor symptoms of Parkinson's disease. Mov Disord, 26 Suppl 3, S42–80.

Sherman, C., et al. 2017. Cannabinoids for the treatment of neuropsychiatric symptoms, pain and weight loss in dementia. Curr Opin Psychiatry, 31, 140–6.

Siddiqi, N., et al. 2007. Interventions for preventing delirium in hospitalised patients. Cochrane Database Syst Rev, 2, CD005563.

Sienaert, P., et al. 2014. A clinical review of the treatment of catatonia. Front Psychiatry, 5, 181.

Sommer, B. R., et al. 2013. Topiramate: Effects on cognition in patients with epilepsy, migraine headache and obesity. Ther Adv Neurol Disord, 6, 211–27.

Spina, E., et al. 2016. Clinically significant pharmacokinetic drug interactions of antiepileptic drugs with new antidepressants and new antipsychotics. Pharmacol Res, 106, 72–86.

Starkstein, S. E. & Pahissa, J. 2014. Apathy following traumatic brain injury. Psychiatr Clin North Am, 37, 103–12.

Stinton, C., et al. 2015. Pharmacological Management of Lewy Body Dementia: A Systematic Review and Meta-Analysis. Am J Psychiatry, 172, 731–42.

Thompson, S., et al. 2007. Efficacy and safety of antidepressants for treatment of depression in Alzheimer's disease: a metaanalysis. Can J Psychiatry, 52, 248–55.

Tsai, P. S., et al. 2016. Effect of valproic acid on dementia onset in patients with bipolar disorder. J Affect Disord, 201, 131–6.

Tuzun, E. & Dalmau, J. 2007. Limbic encephalitis and variants: classification, diagnosis and treatment. Neurologist, 13, 261–71.

Van den Berg, J. F., et al. 2017. Electroconvulsive therapy for agitation and aggression in dementia: a systematic review. Am J Geriatr Psychiatry, 26, 419–34.

Volkow, N. D., et al. 2016. Effects of cannabis use on human behavior, including cognition, motivation, and psychosis: a review. JAMA Psychiatry, 73, 292–7.

Wang, J., et al. 2015. Pharmacological treatment of neuropsychiatric symptoms in Alzheimer's disease: a systematic review and meta-analysis. J Neurol Neurosurg Psychiatry, 86, 101–9.

Watson H. R., et al. 2016. Treatment options for individuals with PTSD and concurrent TBI: a literature review and case presentation. Curr Psychiatry Rep, 18, 63.

Weintraub, D., et al. 2016. Association of antipsychotic use With mortality risk in patients with Parkinson disease. JAMA Neurol, 73, 535–41.

40

Neurobehavioural rehabilitation

Rodger L. Wood, Nick Alderman, and Andrew Worthington

Introduction

Acquired brain injury (ABI) is characterized by a wide range of physical, cognitive, behavioural, and psychosocial disorders, some of which are present in the acute phase, while others emerge at a later time, usually after discharge when individuals are trying to readjust to life in the community. Studies consistently highlight challenging behaviour arising as a more serious long-term impediment to community integration than physical disabilities (Kelly et al., 2008), leading to relationship breakdown, failure to return to work, and a risk of psychiatric disorder. Behaviour is often marked by labile mood, poor impulse control, aggression, and a range of personality changes (Wood, 2001). Impairment of executive functions and disorders of attention lead to problems with insight, awareness, and social judgement. The term 'neurobehavioural disability' (NBD) was introduced to emphasize the role of neurological and neuropsychological factors underpinning many of these post-acute behaviour disorders (Wood, 1987, 1990).

The complex and diverse origins of NBD are mainly attributable to interactions between damaged neural systems, neurocognitive impairment, and premorbid personality traits, exacerbated by post-injury learning as a result of environmental influences (Alderman et al., 2011). Traditional psychiatric syndromal or diagnostic approaches do not readily inform treatment interventions after brain injury. The evidence base for effective pharmacological management of challenging behaviour is limited (Fleminger et al., 2006) and psychological 'talking therapies' are frequently undermined by neurocognitive impairment, disorders of self-awareness, and challenging behaviour (Alderman, 2003; Alderman et al. 2013).

People with ABI and severe challenging behaviour are frequently excluded from neurorehabilitation due to the risks they present, both to themselves and others. They often gravitate to placements where their behaviour can be contained such as secure/forensic psychiatric units and also prison services. ABI is over-represented among offender populations (Williams, 2012), with brain-injured offenders typically offending at a younger age and committing more offences. Increased recidivism rates among offenders with ABI further suggest that prison rehabilitation programmes are ineffective with this population.

The birth of neurobehavioural rehabilitation—the Kemsley Unit

The conceptual basis and current clinical practice of neurobehavioural rehabilitation (NbR) evolved from an innovative approach to the rehabilitation of patients. In 1978, the Kemsley Unit at St Andrews Hospital, Northampton, introduced a radical new rehabilitation programme specifically conceptualized for brain-injured individuals who exhibited challenging behaviour that placed both staff and other patients at risk in existing services. At that time, challenging behaviour effectively excluded such individuals from existing neurorehabilitation services that had been developed primarily to address cognitive and physical disability as a consequence of cerebrovascular accident.

In contrast to prevailing approaches, patient behaviour was the primary treatment goal, and the principal outcome was to change behaviour from disabled, inappropriate, and socially handicapped to adaptive, purposeful, and 'independent'. Helping people with ABI re-adapt to society requires a system that both restores functional skills and provides individuals with opportunities to exercise and apply those skills in a social setting. Rehabilitation goals therefore need to be designated as social, functional, and client-centred (Worthington and Alderman, 2016).

From this conceptual framework, the notion of a 'neurobehavioural' approach emerged (see Wood and Worthington, 2001 and Worthington et al., 2016 for a more detailed exposition of the conceptual origins of this approach to rehabilitation). The 'neuro' prefix emphasized that abnormalities of behaviour were a consequence of damage to the brain, as opposed to a psychological reaction to the injury experience. This focus acknowledges that serious TBI usually implicates prefrontal structures involved in behavioural self-regulation (Damasio et al., 1991; Stuss and Benson, 1987) giving rise to a complex patterns of socially challenging behaviour. The '*behavioural*' suffix represented the aim of rehabilitation—to positively influence disorders of social behaviour, characterized by: (1) labile mood with poor temper control that can escalate into impulsive aggression; (2) impulsivity; (3) inappropriate social or sexual behaviour; (4) lack of tact and discretion during interpersonal activities; (5) diminished self or social awareness; (6) an egocentric attitude, lacking in warmth and empathy towards others; (7) poor attention control, resulting in an inability to maintain goal-directed behaviour; (8) a lack of ability to spontaneously initiate purposeful behaviour; and (9) fatigue, often associated with a lack of drive and motivation. These disorders of behaviour, individually or collectively, became known as 'neurobehavioural disability' (Wood, 1987, 1990, 2001).

NbR differs from other forms of neurorehabilitation in that: (1) it largely addresses problems that emerge at a post-acute stage of recovery; (2) there is no requirement for services to be hospital-based—indeed, most are in community settings; (3) it utilizes methods derived from the learning theory; and (4) where possible, rehabilitation is delivered through a transdisciplinary team (TDT), rather than the more traditional multidisciplinary team (MDT). Consequently, NbR represented a paradigm shift from a medical to a neuropsychological approach to treatment intervention.

Evolution of the neurobehavioural rehabilitation paradigm

NbR must include at least two components (Wood, 1990)—one is behaviour management, in which behaviour is systematically observed, and anti-social or undesirable behaviour contained. The second is a system that promotes learning, making allowances for the cognitive constraints that diminish a person's awareness of environmental cues that normally act as signals for certain behavioural responses. These two components complement each other. The first manages behaviour and creates conditions under which learning can take place. The second provides systematic feedback that increases awareness, improves information processing, and helps refine responses into more purposeful and socially adaptive forms of behaviour. These two components represented the early cornerstones of what became NbR.

Learning theory

Many behaviour disorders are primarily driven by neurocognitive impairment, especially executive function disorders. Reduced initiation, self-monitoring, and an inability to utilize feedback to regulate behaviour result in a lack of 'error awareness', observed as disinhibition, impulsiveness, and poor response to cues. This can result in frustration and aggression because of concurrent difficulties with response inhibition (Alderman, 2003).

Environmental constraints and the demands of community living have an adverse influence on behaviour (Pryor, 2004). Many individuals develop maladaptive coping strategies such as employing aggression as an avoidance/escape function (Alderman, 2001). Alderman (2007) showed how relationships between individual patient characteristics and environmental factors resulted in different types of aggression.

Many disorders of social behaviour are acquired and maintained as a result of associational learning. We make associations between social or environmental stimuli which signal a certain type of event is about to occur and some form of response is needed. We also make associations between a behavioural response and the consequence it produces (either positive or negative). Both forms of association are therefore made on the basis of contingent relationships which occur frequently between stimulus and response, or response

and consequence. This is the essence of the operant conditioning theory.

The optimum condition for associational learning is one in which the person is aware of the connection in a stimulus–response-consequence continuum. However, brain injury often disrupts a person's ability to direct and sustain attention. Neurobehavioural approaches address this problem by providing structured feedback which helps individuals direct attention to the relationship between these elements in order to improve associations, facilitating awareness of the interaction between each component, thereby helping to sequence responses in complex behavioural tasks and promoting learning through repeated practice.

Reinforcement methods have a dual role in associational learning. One is to reward (or withhold reward) in response to increasing or decreasing target behaviours. The reward element can improve motivation and engagement in therapy activities, and generate a sense of achievement in a person struggling with disability. The other role is primarily cognitive. Administration of reinforcement, either in a tangible form or as systematic feedback, improves awareness of relationships between specific aspects of behaviour and their psychosocial consequences. It thereby directs the individual's attention to specific features of behaviour and their consequences, raising awareness of the outcomes of certain actions, increasing the chances that, in a future similar situation, a more appropriate form of behaviour will be exhibited (Wood, 1990; Wood and Burgess, 1988). Another advantage of employing an associational learning paradigm is that it helps individuals learn procedurally, thereby avoiding the impact of cognitive problems that diminish understanding or retention of instructions or experiences that might undermine the efficiency of learning and influence the expression of future behaviour.

Initial experiences at the Kemsley Unit demonstrated how neurocognitive and environmental drivers of challenging behaviour could be positively influenced by methods of associational learning which created and sustained a highly structured environment promoting social learning. These conditions amplified how social learning normally occurs in response to society's rules, which vary in their salience, significance, impact, consistency, and social value. They shape the development of individuals in society by teaching self-restraint, promoting awareness of (and respect for) other people's needs and values, and creating a framework for social interaction (Wood and Worthington, 2001). Those who have sustained injury to the prefrontal cortex and lack the ability to self-regulate behaviour often exhibit diminished awareness of, or concern for, rules of behaviour which reflect social convention. These can, however, be relearnt (at least in part) by the systematic application of feedback via reinforcement contingencies comprising a token economy system and various forms of time-out procedures.

A token economy framework

One way of creating a system to ensure the regular and consistent application of rules is by establishing a 'prosthetic environment' within the framework of a token economy system, which has proven effectiveness when applied to a range of clinical disorders (Kazdin, 1977). The systematic application of tokens, points, or consistent feedback in any form should increase the saliency of environmental cues that call for a change of behaviour, thereby reducing the impact of cognitive deficits which diminish social cognition.

The advantages of a token economy framework in the management of challenging behaviour included:

- Immediate delivery of reinforcement contingencies, following observation of a designated behaviour. The contiguity between the behaviour and reinforcement improved awareness and facilitated learning.
- Provision of explicit feedback through reinforcement, regardless of whether it was delivered immediately or at regular intervals throughout the day. This ensured regular, positive interaction between staff and patients to raise awareness, improve learning, and establish and maintain positive therapeutic relationships.
- Reinforcement being delivered consistently, as well as frequently, to facilitate learning.
- Clear boundaries and enhanced cue saliency regarding what constituted inappropriate behaviour. This not only benefited patients, but also improved communication (and awareness) between staff.
- The administration of reinforcement (in any form) allowing objective measures to be obtained, quantifying the frequency of specific behaviours, or evaluating the quality of a response.

Time-out interventions

In addition to a token economy, time-out methods have further enhanced the clinical effectiveness of early NbR programmes, especially in the management of aggressive behaviour. The goal of implementing a time-out procedure was to decrease future occurrence of challenging behaviour, in favour of more socially constructive behaviour. Time-out has been defined as withdrawal of the opportunity to earn positive reinforcement, or loss of access to positive reinforcement for a specified period of time, contingent on the occurrence of a target behaviour (Cooper et al., 2007), using neither non-exclusion nor exclusion time-out.

Non-exclusion time-out occurs when the person is allowed to remain in the same setting as other patients but is not permitted to engage in any reinforcing activities for a specified period of time. 'Time-out-on-the-spot' (TOOTS) from positive reinforcement (Wood, 1987) has proved invaluable in shaping social behaviour when inappropriate aspects of interaction are maintained by social reinforcement. Once the role of social reinforcement in maintaining inappropriate behaviour has been demonstrated, clinicians and carers are required to systematically ignore, or appear indifferent to, the inappropriate behaviour. This often leads to an initial escalation of the unwanted behaviour, but denying social reinforcement usually leads to a reduction of the behaviour.

Exclusion time-out involves removing a person from a situation that is reinforcing for a specified period of time. Cooper et al. (2007) listed three different methods of implementing an exclusionary time-out: time-out within a specially designated room; partition time-out, when the individual remains in the same room but is screened from staff and other patients; and hallway time-out, in which a person is placed outside the room where a therapy activity is taking place. At the Kemsley Unit, the most frequent form of time-out in response to aggressive behaviour was use of a time-out room. This involved placing a person in a locked room for a brief period of time, usually 5 minutes, or multiples of 5 minutes if the behaviour persisted. Wood (1987) produced a series of case studies which showed that this procedure was effective in eliminating serious forms of aggression at a post-acute stage of recovery. Wood

(2001) presented data on a group of 30 patients who exhibited serious aggressive behaviour after TBI, all of whom made a significant response to a time-out room procedure implemented systematically over a period of 5–10 weeks which was maintained over a 6-month period. The initial outcomes, based on token economy methods in brain injury rehabilitation, were encouraging (Eames and Wood, 1985) and began to be used elsewhere, with reports of improved efficacy over drug treatment (Tate, 1987; Whale et al., 1986). While seclusion time-out is now used less frequently and is carefully controlled by legislative procedures, its original use has to be understood in the context of innovative work being carried out over 30 years ago. When reviewing this approach, Lishman (1984) commented on 'the brave attempts underway to tackle the more disruptive behavioural aftermaths in severely damaged patients by behaviour modification techniques – pioneering work at the rehabilitation unit of St. Andrew's Hospital Northampton.'

Contemporary approaches to neurobehavioural rehabilitation

Improved awareness of factors driving challenging behaviour has resulted in a more individualized programme of rehabilitation that is person-centred and needs-led, instead of procedures orientated to group activities. This requires a detailed assessment of individuals, which has led to a concurrent increase in the number of tools and measures developed specifically for ABI and neurorehabilitation, because tools originally devised for use with psychiatric populations proved unsatisfactory when applied in an ABI context. Together with more sophisticated neuropsychological explanations of challenging behaviour, rehabilitation interventions have evolved to address a broad range of NBD (Alderman 2015, 2017; Alderman et al., 2013).

The rise of individual, multicomponent interventions

The token economy focused on managing contingencies by the deliberate manipulation of consequences to encourage or discourage behaviour. Much has been learnt subsequently about applying contingency management methods on an individual basis, which have a good evidence base for use in NBD, especially when used within a formulation-based approach to intervention (where information about the person, including historical evidence and data from contemporary assessments, is integrated by the clinical team within a conceptual framework, to create a hypothesis regarding what is driving their behaviour—this explanation is used to underpin subsequent treatment (Alderman, 2015). In this respect, differential reinforcement procedures have special relevance, as do response–cost and extinction methods that do not rely on use of a time-out room (see reviews by Alderman and Wood, 2013; Alderman et al., 2013; Wood and Alderman, 2011).

Methods that focus on immediate antecedents to behaviour have also been advocated in the management of children and adults with ABI (see, for example, Ylvisaker et al., 2005, 2007), often referred to as 'positive behaviour supports' (PBS) (Johnston et al., 2006). Approaches falling under this conceptual umbrella endeavour to increase the likelihood that individuals will engage in behaviours that enable them to succeed in their social contexts, and are applicable to many settings, including the community and people's own homes. The chief component of PBS is antecedent control, e.g. avoiding triggers of aggression (Narevic et al., 2011), but a range of other characteristics also apply, including promotion of choice and control, provision of daily routine, setting expectations to ensure success, errorless learning to avoid frustration and optimize skill acquisition, teaching alternative strategies to challenging behaviour to meet needs, increasing positive interaction between staff and recipients of NbR, and increasing cue saliency. This list is by no means exhaustive, but serves to also show there is considerable overlap in programme objectives between methods that primarily aim to manage contingencies to behaviour and those that target antecedents, e.g. increasing the frequency and quality of positive interactions between clinicians and carers with programme participants.

Programmes frequently use several methods concurrently (Ylvisaker et al., 2007); for example, Rothwell et al. (1999) described a case ('Rose') where a variety of methods were used to reduce aggressive behaviour driven by anxiety, low self-esteem, and cognitive impairment. PBS techniques were employed to bring about ecological change (maximizing choice in planning activities, use of a timetable) and apply 'positive programming' (anxiety management training, automated cues to regularly enable this, daily feedback to emphasize strengths and achievements, and counselling regarding the effects of ABI). Contingency management approaches were also used, specifically the use of non-exclusion time-out and a fixed-interval differential reinforcement programme. This drawing together of PBS and contingency management approaches into one overall multicomponent intervention successfully reduced the frequency of verbal and physical aggression over a 17-week period.

This combination of methods is ideally suited to addressing the complex needs of people with NBD, providing they are applied within a structured environment (a *therapeutic milieu*) which generates a social climate that can increase awareness, improve motivation, and create conditions for success by setting expectations about performance and which reinforces appropriate behaviour and skills. Individual fixed-interval reinforcement schemes prompt staff to regularly interact positively with people participating in rehabilitation and, as in Rothwell et al.'s (1999) case, aggression and other challenging behaviours are played down as far as possible. Combined use of PBS and contingency methods creates conditions in which staff are more likely to interact consistently and systematically as a team with individuals, to optimize conditions that support effective learning and reduce the likelihood of behaviours that serve avoidance/escape functions. By setting expectations at an appropriate level, identifying antecedents, equipping people with positive skills and alternative ways to meet their needs, encouraging positive interaction, and directing social reinforcement at desirable behaviour, challenging behaviour can be minimized or eliminated (Alderman, 2003). These 'enriched' environments work by changing behaviour, promoting constructive engagement, and mediating expectations about what can be realistically achieved. This encourages the development of positive social climates that promote therapeutic relationships and good treatment outcomes (Alderman and Groucott, 2012).

A transdisciplinary approach to delivering neurobehavioural rehabilitation

From the beginning, NbR became distinct from traditional neurorehabilitation by its organizational structure which redefined working relationships between different therapy disciplines. In a neurobehavioural context, these needed to be interdisciplinary, rather than multidisciplinary (Wood, 1990, 2003), and ideally should be embraced by a fully transdisciplinary team (TDT). Therapy interventions in every discipline placed emphasis on psychological methods of intervention that recognized how neurocognitive problems undermined many aspects of everyday behaviour, either social or functional, and did not respond to conventional methods of therapy management (e.g. Worthington and Waller, 2009; Worthington et al., 1997).

NbR practitioners therefore needed to have knowledge of learning methods to devise effective rehabilitation interventions (Burgess and Wood, 1990), which is one of the reasons why NbR programmes and services are more often led by psychologists (preferably clinical neuropsychologists), rather that medical doctors (Wood, 2003; Worthington and Merriman, 2008). Rehabilitation extends beyond time-limited formal therapy sessions during the 9-to-5 working day and is seen as a process of enablement, reflected by changes in both functional and social behaviour that needs to be continually reinforced throughout the day. Consequently, the whole staff team need to be empowered to regard their role as that of an agent for behaviour change. In practice, this means that while therapists often conduct assessments and prescribe interventions, the practice of rehabilitation is carried out by a host of therapy care assistants, rehabilitation support workers, and similarly designated groups who work under the guidance of clinicians. Continued evolution and refinement of how the clinical team delivers NbR have resulted in TDT working being an ideal characteristic of contemporary practice in this specialism.

The TDT approach is ideally suited for optimizing service delivery to the complex, heterogenous needs of people with ABI where input is provided from multiple disciplines working together, rather than separately. A TDT shares roles across disciplinary boundaries, so that communication, interaction, and cooperation are maximized among team members. It is characterized by the commitment of its members to teach, learn, and work together to implement coordinated services. This leads to a mutual vision or 'shared meaning' among the team (Davies, 2007) and results in: (1) shared assessment and goal selection; (2) close cooperation and exchange of information, knowledge, and skills across the entire team; and (3) 'role release', characterized by intervention strategies that traditionally were delivered by specific disciplines, being implemented by the entire team, under the supervision of team members whose disciplines are normally accountable for those practices (King et al., 2009). The approach fosters consistency (especially important when behavioural approaches are used), pursuit of functional goals that are meaningful to the recipient, and delivery of rehabilitation 24/7, and encourages generalization of gains.

A move from hospitals to the community

While the Kemsley Unit was located on the campus of a large psychiatric hospital, such settings can be counter-productive for rehabilitation. In part, this is because the needs of the rehabilitation facility are subordinate to those of the larger hospital, with its medical hierarchy, therapists having to work across wards with very different types of patients, and nursing staff often being transferred in and out of the facility at short notice, with neither the time nor inclination to understand the unique NbR approach. The other reason is more endemic—hospitals are for ill people to be cared for; rehabilitation is about learning to do things for yourself. The limitations of hospital-based approaches was noted by Greenwood and McMillan (1993, p. 253): 'The learning difficulties and other neuropsychological deficits that these patients have means that many elements [of rehabilitation] should not be sited at institutions, but in a natural community setting, to emphasise a move towards independence, minimise problems with generalisation to everyday routine and emphasise the educational and training nature of the service.'[1] This awareness has led to greater diversity of units in which NbR is provided. Most notably, a shift in service provision has seen the development of a network of community-based post-acute rehabilitation units in the UK, which, by means of their location, are able to offer a range of opportunities to promote social learning and generalization. Of course, there are some patients for whom delivery of NbR in a hospital setting is appropriate, but the net effect has been the establishment of a much broader care pathway than was originally the case, further optimizing the prospect of good and sustainable long-term outcomes from ABI.

Effectiveness of neurobehavioural rehabilitation

Early evaluation of the initial Kemsley Unit neurobehavioural programme produced results described at the time as surprisingly good (Eames and Wood, 1985). Despite receiving rehabilitation approximately 4 years post-injury, the token economy programme showed clear behavioural gains that were still evident an average of 18 months later at follow-up. Although longer periods of intervention were linked to better outcomes, longer admissions were not necessary to achieve significant improvements. The benefits of NbR were also demonstrated by Eames et al., (1996) in a similar clinical population treated in a separate stand-alone facility not linked to any hospital. Mean time post-injury was almost 29 months and the average length of stay was 11 months. At discharge, 63% had care needs reduced sufficiently to warrant a change of placement (increased to 78% at follow-up) and 55% required professional care, compared with 87% on admission.

An analysis of the outcomes of the first two UK community-based centres was published by Wood et al. (1999), comprising 76 adults, at an average of 6 years post-injury, who underwent at least 6 months' rehabilitation (mean: 14 months) and were followed up 1–5 years after discharge. Improvements were observed in the type of living arrangements upon discharge and significant reductions in hours of care. In addition, 61% were in some form of work placement or education, compared with only 4% before rehabilitation. While gains were greater for people admitted within 2 years of injury, improvement was still evident if rehabilitation began 5 years or more post-injury. The benefits of early admission were corroborated by Worthington (2003) in relation to a community facility developed in close relationship with local hospitals. Whereas only 26% of the cohort in Wood et al.'s study (1999) were admitted for

NbR within 2 years post-injury, Worthington (2003) reported on 50 adults, 70% of whom received treatment within this period. Compared to 38% admitted for >12 months in the Wood et al.'s group (1999), only 10% failed to be discharged within 1 year, with 56% being discharged home with support and 25% to longer-term residential facilities previously inaccessible to them because of their behaviour disorder.

These behavioural and functional gains translate directly into cost savings. Wood et al. (1999) calculated a notional saving in lifetime care costs for each individual of between £0.5 million and £1.1 million, depending on how soon after injury NbR was commenced.

In a larger cohort of 133 adults, Worthington et al. (2006) showed that the high cost of specialist NbR had a negligible effect on overall lifetime cost savings, with sensitivity analysis confirming estimated savings of £0.8–1.1 million for adults admitted within a year of injury and £0.4–£0.5 million for those admitted >2 years after. More recently, Oddy and da Silva Ramos (2013) conducted a similar outcome study but used a more conservative 1.5% discount rate than had previously been employed, due to prevailing economic conditions, and obtained estimated lifetime cost savings of £0.57–1.13 million for those admitted within 12 months of injury. Although it takes longer to recoup costs for those admitted beyond this period, savings in care costs of £0.19–0.86 million were reported. Taking into account the lower discount rate, these figures are comparable with those reported by Worthington et al. (2006).

Conclusion

Neurobehavioural interventions have evolved both theoretically and practically, keeping pace with a changing healthcare system. It is worth noting, however, that the term 'neurobehavioural' had previously been used (Levin et al., 1982), but it lacked any coherence and conceptual validity, being applied either specifically to psychiatric symptoms or in general terms to behaviour without any clear link to underlying brain function. There was no notion of neurobehavioural disability encapsulating diverse functional and behavioural consequences of the breakdown of frontally mediated regulatory control processes, and no theoretical link to intervention.

Financial, social, and political imperatives will always affect how principles are put into practice. However, there is little doubt that NbR is socially and economically beneficial. Recent clinical innovations have seen the development of sophisticated tools for characterizing neurobehavioural disability (Alderman et al., 2011) that have demonstrated cost-effectiveness and the advantage of integrating technology to augment and enhance the work of practitioners. It is very likely that these developments will shape the way neurobehavioural disability is conceptualized and managed in future.

KEY LEARNING POINTS

- Helping brain-injured people re-adapt to society requires a system that provides individuals with opportunities to learn and apply social and functional skills in community settings.
- However, many types of ABI cause damage to prefrontal structures that are central to behavioural self-regulation, giving rise

[1] Reproduced with permission from Greenwood R.J., McMillan T M. Models of rehabilitation programmes for the brain injured adult: I Current provision, efficacy and good practice. *Clinical Rehabilitation*, 7(3): 248–255. Copyright © 1993, SAGE Publications. https://doi.org/10.1177/026921559300700311.

to complex patterns of socially challenging behaviour that can deny access to rehabilitation.

- NbR was initially developed to address long-term problems of challenging behaviour that prevented individuals from engaging meaningfully with the rehabilitation process. However, it has evolved to promote psychosocial recovery more broadly, with the aim of changing behaviour from disabled, inappropriate, and socially handicapped to adaptive, purposeful, and 'independent'.

- It is a paradigm that incorporates methods of associational learning within a structured environment that emphasizes clear feedback to raise awareness of behaviour, in a way that improves social cognition and self-regulation, to promote community independence.

REFERENCES

Alderman N. (2001). Managing challenging behaviour. In: R.L.l. Wood and T. McMillan (eds). *Neurobehavioural Disability and Social Handicap Following Traumatic Brain Injury*. Hove, Psychology Press; pp. 175–203.

Alderman N. (2003). Contemporary Approaches to the Management of Irritability and Aggression Following Traumatic Brain Injury. Neuropsychological Rehabilitation, 13, 211–40.

Alderman N. (2007). Prevalence, characteristics and causes of aggressive behaviour observed within a neurobehavioural rehabilitation service: predictors and implications for management. Brain Injury, 21, 891–911.

Alderman N. (2015). Acquired brain injury, trauma and aggression. In: Dickens G, Picchioni M, and Sugarman P (eds). *Handbook of Specialist Secure Inpatient Mental Healthcare*. London, The Royal College of Psychiatrists.

Alderman N. (2017). Interventions for challenging behaviour. In: McMillan T and Wood RLl (eds). *Neurobehavioural Disability and Social handicap Following Traumatic Brain Injury*, second edition. Psychology Press, Routledge.

Alderman N, Wood RLl, and Williams C. (2011). The development of the St Andrews-Swansea Neurobehavioural Outcome Scale: Validity and reliability of a new measure of neurobehavioural disability and social handicap. *Brain Injury*, 25, 83–100.

Alderman N and Groucott L. (2012). Measurement of social climate within neurobehavioural rehabilitation services using the EssenCES. *Neuropsychological Rehabilitation*, 22, 768–93.

Alderman N and Wood RLl. (2013). Neurobehavioural approaches to the rehabilitation of challenging behaviour. *Neurorehabilitation*, 32, 761–70.

Alderman N, Knight C, and Brooks J. (2013). Rehabilitation approaches to the management of aggressive behaviour disorders after acquired brain injury. *Brain Impairment*, 14, 5–20.

Burgess PW and Wood RLl. (1990). Neuropsychology of behaviour disorders following brain injury. In: Wood RLl (ed). *Neurobehavioural Sequelae of Traumatic Brain Injury*. London: Taylor Francis, pp. 110–33.

Cooper J, Heron T, and Heward W. (2007). *Applied Behaviour Analysis*. New Jersey: Pearson Education.

Damasio AR, Tranel D, Damasio HR. (1991). Somatic markers and the guidance of behavior: theory and preliminary testing. In: Levin HS, Eisenberg HM, Benton AL (eds). *Frontal Lobe Function and Dysfunction*. New York, NY: Oxford University Press, pp. 217–29.

Davies S. (ed) (2007). *Team Around the Child: Working Together in Early Childhood Education*. Wagga Wagga, New South Wales: Kurrajong Early Intervention Service.

Eames P, Wood RLl. (1985). Rehabilitation after severe brain injury: A special unit approach to behaviour disorders. *Disability and Rehabilitation*, 7, 130–3.

Eames P, Cotterill G, Kneale TA, Storrar AL, and Yeomans P. (1996). Outcome of intensive rehabilitation after severe brain injury: A follow-up study. *Brain Injury*, 10, 631–50.

Fleminger S, Greenwood RJ, and Oliver DL. (2006). Pharmacological management for agitation and aggression in people with acquired brain injury. *Cochrane Database of Systematic Reviews*, 4, CD003299.

Greenwood RJ and McMillan TM. (1993). Models of rehabilitation programmes for the brain injured adult: I Current provision, efficacy and good practice. *Clinical Rehabilitation*, 7, 248–55.

Johnston JM, Foxx RM, Jacobson JW, Green G and Mulick JA. (2006). Positive behavior support and applied behavior analysis. *The Behavior Analyst*, 29, 51–74.

Kazdin AE. (1977). *The Token Economy. A Review and Evaluation*. New York, NY: Plenum Press.

Kelly G, Brown S, Todd J, and Kremer P. (2008). Challenging behaviour profiles of people with acquired brain injury living in community settings. *Brain Injury*, 22, 457–70.

King G, Strachan D, Tucker M, Duwyn B, Desserud S, and Shillington M. (2009). The application of a transdisciplinary model for early intervention services. *Infants and Young Children*, 22, 211–23.

Levin HS, Benton AL, and Grossman RG. (1982). *Neurobehavioral Consequences of Closed Head Injury*. New York, NY: Oxford University Press.

Lishman WA. (1984). Book review of Brooks N (ed): Closed head injury: psychological, social and family consequences. *Journal of Neurology Neurosurgery, and Psychiatry*, 47, 1148.

Narevic E, Giles GM, Rajadhyax R, Managuelod E, Monis F, and Diamond F. (2011). The effects of enhanced program review and staff training on the management of aggression among clients in a longterm neurobehavioral rehabilitation program. *Aging and Mental Health*, 15, 103–12.

Oddy M and da Silva Ramos S. (2013a). The clinical and cost-benefits of investing in neurobehavioural rehabilitation: a multi-centre study. *Brain Injury*, 27, 1500–7.

Rothwell NA, LaVigna GW, and Willis TJ. (1999). A non-aversive rehabilitation approach for people with severe behavior problems resulting from brain injury. *Brain Injury*, 13, 521–33.

Stuss DT and Benson FD. (1987). The frontal lobes and control of cognition and memory. In: Perecman E (ed). *The Frontal Lobes Revisited*. New York, NY: The IRBN Press, pp. 141–58.

Tate RL. (1987). Issues in the management of behaviour disturbance as a consequences of severe head injury. *Scandanavian Journal of Rehabilitation Medicine*, 19, 13–17.

Whale AL, Stanford CB, and Pollack IW. (1986). The effects of behaviour modification vs lithium therapy on frontal lobe syndrome. *Journal of Behavior Therapy and Experimental Psychiatry*, 17, 111–15.

Williams H. (2012). *Repairing shattered lives: brain injury and its implications for criminal justice*. Report published by the Barrow Cadbury Trust on behalf of the Transition to Adulthood Alliance.

Available at: http://yss.org.uk/wp-content/uploads/2012/10/Repairing-Shattered-Lives_Report.pdf.

Wood RLl. (1987). *Brain Injury Rehabilitation: A Neurobehavioural Approach*. London: Croom Helm.

Wood RLl. (1990). A neurobehavioural paradigm for brain injury rehabilitation. In: Wood RLl (ed). *Neurobehavioural Sequelae of Traumatic Brain Injury*. London: Taylor and Francis, pp. 3–17.

Wood RLl. (2001). Understanding Neurobehavioural Disability. In: Wood RLl & McMillan TM (eds). *Neurobehavioural Disability and social handicap following traumatic brain injury*. Hove: Psychology Press, pp. 3–29.

Wood RLl. (2003). The rehabilitation team. In: Greenwood RJ, Barnes MP, McMillan TM, Ward CD (eds). Handbook of Neurological Rehabilitation. London: Churchill Livingstone, pp. 41–50.

Wood RLl and Burgess P. (1988). Psychological techniques in the management of behaviour disorders during rehabilitation. In: Fussey I and Giles GM (eds). *A Practical Approach to Head Injury Rehabilitation*.

Wood RLl, McCrea JD, Wood LM, and Merriment RN. (1999). Clinical and cost-effectiveness of post-acute neurobehavioural rehabilitation. *Brain Injury*, 13, 69–88.

Wood RLl and Worthington AD. (2001). Neurobehavioural rehabilitation: a conceptual paradigm. In: Wood RLl and McMillan TM (eds). *Neurobehavioural Disability and Social Handicap Following Traumatic Brain Injury*. Hove: Psychology Press, pp. 107–31.

Wood RL and Alderman N. (2011). Applications of Operant Learning Theory to the Management of Challenging Behavior After Traumatic Brain Injury. *Journal of Head Trauma Rehabilitation*, 26, 202–11.

Worthington A. (2003). Out on a limb? Developing an integrated rehabilitation service for adults with acquired brain injury. *Clinical Psychology*, 23, 14–18.

Worthington AD and Merriman RN. (2008). Residential services. In: Tyerman A and King N (eds). *Psychological Approaches to Rehabilitation After Traumatic Brain Injury*. Oxford: Blackwell, pp. 91–110.

Worthington A and Waller J. (2009). Rehabilitation of everyday living skills in the context of executive disorders. In: Oddy M and Worthington A (eds). *The Rehabilitation of Executive Disorders*. New York, NY: Oxford University Press, pp. 195–210.

Worthington A, Williams C, Young K, and Pownall J. (1997). Retraining gait components for walking in the context of abulia. *Physiotherapy Theory and Practice*, 13, 247–56.

Worthington AD, Matthews S, Melia Y, Oddy M. (2006). Cost-benefits associated with social outcome from neurobehavioural rehabilitation. *Brain Injury*, 20, 947–57.

Worthington A and Alderman N. (2016). Neurobehavioural rehabilitation: an evolving paradigm. In: McMillan T and Wood RLl (eds). *Neurobehavioural Disability and Social Handicap Following Traumatic Brain Injury*, second edition. London: Psychology Press.

Worthington A, Wood RLl, and McMillan TM. (2016). Neurobehavioural disability over the past four decades. In: McMillan T and Wood RLl (eds). *Neurobehavioural Disability and Social Handicap Following Traumatic Brain Injury*, second edition. London: Psychology Press.

Ylvisaker M, Turkstra LS, and Coelho C. (2005). Behavioural and social interventions for individuals with traumatic brain injury: a summary of the research with clinical implications. *Seminars in Speech and Language*, 26, 256–67.

Ylvisaker M, Turkstra L, Coehlo C, et al. (2007). Behavioural interventions for children and adults with behaviour disorders after TBI: A systematic review of the evidence. *Brain Injury*, 21, 769–805.

41

Neurostimulation technologies in neurology and neuropsychiatry

Mayur Bodani and David Wilkinson

Introduction

Neurostimulation technologies comprise distinctive methods for invasively or non-invasively *intervening* in brain function, although defining exactly what *the intervention* is and what the *intervention is doing* at either a neuronal or a cellular level is not obviously clear and awaits the outcome of further current and future research effort.

The broad term 'neurostimulation technologies' encompasses stem cell therapy, tissue engineering, and neural repair and regeneration, but in a brief review such as this, it simply is not possible to cover all these approaches. It is important to note that the terms 'neurostimulation' and 'neuromodulation', though used interchangeably in practice, do not actually mean the same thing. *Neuromodulation* is defined by the International Neuromodulation Society as 'the alteration of nerve activity (*sic firing patterns*) through targeted delivery of a stimulus, such as electrical stimulation or chemical agents, to specific neurological sites' (International Neuromodulation Society, 2016). *Neurostimulation* means induction of these firing patterns (although, of course, it is likely that some neurostimulation techniques have the potential to be neuromodulatory as well). Neurostimulation has generally been the preserve of invasive techniques, but induction of the neural tissue of the central nervous system (CNS), which includes the brain, spinal cord, and peripheral nerves, can now also be done using non-invasive techniques, the most important ones of which will be described in this chapter.

Historical roots and future directions

The history of interest in neurostimulation methods is not new. Records dating to Roman times described the use of electric fish for the treatment of pain by the Roman physician Scribonius Largus (43–48 AD). In later centuries, notable contributions were made by Galvani (1791), Volta (1792), and Aldini (1804) (Utz et al., 2010). Readers are recommended the excellent review by Grabherr et al. (2015) for a detailed historical account.

Since 1995, the number of relevant published articles in major US and UK print media sources related to neurostimulation has seen an exponential increase (Racine et al., 2007). The commercial market in neurostimulation devices is set to reach an estimated $10.8 billion by 2022 (International Neuromodulation Society, 2016).

Although drugs and surgery have been the predominant approach to managing disease since the last century, their limitations are at least one reason driving the current interest in novel neurostimulation technologies. In the field of psychopharmacology, generations of antidepressants, antipsychotics, anxiolytics, and other classes of psychoactive drugs have still left some patients with neuropsychiatric and neurological disorders which are considered resistant to treatment or inadequately responsive. The adverse effects of drugs also limit tolerability for many patients. It is estimated that up to 20% of patients may not respond to treatment or become resistant to treatment over time, particularly in the context of progressive neurodegenerative disease (Danilov et al., 2014).

Further advances in drug treatment are also difficult to predict. New medicines are extremely expensive to research, develop, and deliver, with the time lag from basic research to approved clinical use often lengthy, up to 10–15 years. It is in this context that novel neurostimulation technologies are being seen as important for research and potentially offer a new dawn in neuropsychiatric therapeutics. The need for an understanding of cellular and systems-level processes has enabled researchers from across neuroscience to join the crusade. Hence the field is rapidly changing.

It is important to note that, in parallel with this interest, there has been an ongoing debate on the ethical implications of such new potential treatments (see, for example, Hariz et al., 2015; Heinrichs, 2012). While the ethics of using a new technology in conditions already refractory to treatment (e.g. severe dyskinesia in Parkinson's disease), in which the main motivation is the therapeutic relief of an intolerable condition, seems relatively non-controversial, the possibility of using similar techniques for psychiatric disorders has raised ethical concerns beyond merely adverse effects and side effects. Should, for example, these methods, if effective, be used to treat anti-social behaviour, or for enhancing cognitive abilities (if that proves possible) in healthy individuals? Additionally, would it be ethical to use such techniques for military advantage in training future combat soldiers?

Perhaps understandably, as with any new thing, there seems to be an optimism about this research which is disproportionate to the currently available evidence. There is no doubt a need for in-depth consideration of the potential positive, and also the possible societal consequences, including fair access, and public involvement in shaping policy. Further reading is recommended at the end of the chapter to inform interested readers about this important debate.

As stated, this review cannot cover the whole field of novel neurotechnology, and as the field is rapidly evolving, the principal aim of the chapter will be to enable readers an acquaintance with this subject and an appreciation of its relevance for potential clinical benefits, likely future commercial impact, and possible current and future uses in an expanding range of neurological and psychiatric disorders.

The putative mechanisms of effect of neurostimulation are intriguing (e.g. McIntyre et al., 2004b) but remain speculative, and are a focus of intense research activity. This chapter will consider, albeit briefly, the most recent theories which touch on mechanisms of neural entrainment and immunomodulation.

What is neuronal stimulation?

Neuronal cell membranes consist of a phospholipid bilayer across which selective ion pumps, e.g. sodium (Na^+) and potassium (K^+), work to create a separation of charge, ultimately resulting in a resting cell membrane polarization where the intracellular potential is between 60 and 80 mV below the extracellular fluid and where the bilayer acts as the dielectric of a capacitor. Neuronal stimulation causes depolarization of part of the cell membrane. If this is enough to reduce the transmembrane potential to a threshold level, voltage-gated Na^+ ion channels open, creating a positive feedback loop that amplifies the small depolarization to a full reverse polarization of the membrane, creating an action potential. This, in turn, depolarizes the surrounding membrane and ultimately causes the action potential to propagate along the axon (Luan et al., 2014).

There are several dozen forms of neuronal stimulation currently undergoing research, development, and evaluation as potential interventions in neurological and psychiatric disorders (Danilov et al., 2014). These include electrical or magnetic stimulation, ultrasound, radio waves, and also optical stimulation, all of which can be used to alter the excitability of neural tissue.

This chapter considers neurostimulation technologies either being used or being developed for use in neurological, and psychiatric disorders. Invasive methods (i.e. those involving surgery) include deep brain stimulation (DBS), vagus nerve stimulation (VNS), and spinal cord stimulation. To a lesser extent, peripheral nerve stimulation (PNS) and occipital nerve stimulation (ONS) also involve surgical placement of electrical wires and electrodes subcutaneously.

There are a wide range of non-invasive neurostimulation methods. (*Non-invasive* in this context means non-surgical or non-penetrative through the skin). Examples of non-invasive neurostimulation methods include transcranial direct current stimulation (tDCS), transcranial magnetic stimulation (TMS), transcutaneous electrical nerve stimulation (TENS), motor cortex stimulation (MCS), magnetic seizure therapy (MST), and caloric/galvanic vestibular stimulation (CVS/GVS), but this list is not exhaustive. The two most commonly used non-invasive techniques for neurostimulation are either via a direct current to the surface of the scalp using applied electrodes or via an electrical pulse through a magnetic coil placed over the scalp. The oldest, but not most novel, form of established non-invasive brain stimulation (NIBS)—electroconvulsive therapy (ECT)—merits a brief mention at this point.

In general adult psychiatric practice, the use of ECT is considered effective, even though the public perception of ECT is generally negative. However, in reality, ECT is a safe and efficacious treatment, particularly when treatments for depression (and for other psychiatric disorders, e.g. psychosis) have failed and there is imminent and significant threat to physical and mental health.

Historically, ECT was first investigated by Bini and Cerletti in the 1930s. It remains the 'gold standard' for treatment-resistant depression (TRD). Electrode placement in ECT includes the traditional bilateral and right unilateral placements, and bifrontal and left anterior right temporal (LART) placements. Bitemporal lead placement induces a high level of seizure generalization and hence has high efficacy, but also more side effects, in particular headache and memory loss post-ECT (Akhtar et al., 2016). ECT delivery requires administration of anaesthesia and muscle relaxant to prevent movement. Hence the application of ECT can be a lengthy process, consuming a significant degree of medical and nursing time. Results are slow to appear, and ECT is by no means always successful, hence the need for other options (see Magnetic seizure therapy, p. 488).

Methods employing invasive brain stimulation

Deep brain stimulation

DBS is at present the most widely used form of invasive neurostimulation in neurosurgical practice for nearly all disorders—neurological and psychiatric (Holtzheimer et al., 2011; Kennedy et al., 2011). The procedure, which had its origins in France, around 1987, evolved as a technique for elective ablative and lesional procedures with heat probes applied to small areas of the brain. DBS has now become established as a technique for the implantation of electrode arrays into deep subcortical matter using image-guided stereotactic neurosurgical techniques (Nuffield, 2013). As well as a stereotactic head frame, software may be utilized for determining target coordinates and entry points for safe electrode trajectory to help minimize the risk of brain injury from haemorrhage.

Target placement of electrodes in DBS (unilateral and bilateral) depends on the condition being treated. DBS electrodes are connected to battery-driven stimulus generators placed subcutaneously under the chest wall (see Fig. 41.1). Stimulus parameters are determined by the condition being treated. Stimulation frequency (Hz), pulse width (μs), and voltage (V) are variable parameters. High-frequency DBS of the thalamus, globus pallidus interna (GPi), and subthalamic nucleus (STN) has been widely used as a treatment for motor symptoms of Parkinson's disease, in particular, treatment-resistant dyskinesias, and tremor. STN stimulation can result in immediate improvement of motor symptoms. It has been suggested

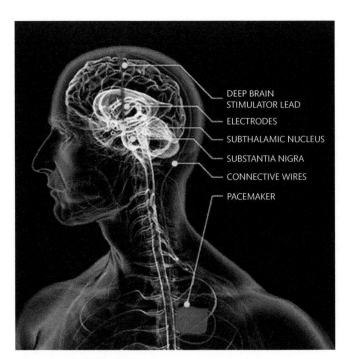

Fig. 41.1 Possible targets for DBS.
Courtesy of The Brain Stimulator, Inc. www.thebrainstimulator.com.

that STN DBS appears to exhibit greater anti-parkinsonian effect than GPi DBS (Goto et al., 2004).

DBS surgery is expensive and invasive, with a risk of serious adverse events which may be anaesthesia- and/or surgery-related. Surgical risk includes intracranial haemorrhage, infection, and seizure. The DBS system may also 'malfunction', e.g. breakage or migration of the implant's wires or electrodes, leading to a possible need for additional surgery. Concerns have been raised about a possible increase in suicide rates after DBS in patients with movement disorders. It is important for preoperative assessment to include an assessment of risk to patients with a pre-existing history of depression (Marangell et al., 2007).

Other reported adverse effects of DBS include mania, cognitive dysfunction, anxiety, and change in personality (Nuffield, 2013, paragraph 2.53). The beneficial and adverse effects most likely depend on where the electrodes are placed but may also include other factors such as intensity and frequency of stimulus pulses.

NICE (UK) recommends that DBS for patients with drug-resistant Parkinson's disease should be assessed by a multidisciplinary team, including a neurologist, a neurosurgeon, and a psychologist, on a case-by-case basis (National Institute for Health and Care Excellence, 2003). DBS has been approved for use in Europe (but not in the UK) to treat chronic severe treatment-resistant obsessive–compulsive disorder (OCD). FDA approval for use in trials on OCD has also been granted (Nuffield, 2013, paragraph 2.44). DBS has also been tried for analgesic treatment-resistant neuropathic pain and is approved for this purpose by NICE, if treatment is assessed and carried out by specialists in chronic pain management. Novel applications of DBS continue to emerge, with case studies suggesting use in obesity, addiction, epilepsy, dementia, headache, and minimally conscious states, among others.

The mechanism of potential benefit of DBS remains speculative, but the most plausible theory relates to excitation (or inhibition) of neuronal cell bodies and axons in the near vicinity of the stimulating electrode, with possible onward effects on brain networks (Nuffield, 2013, paragraph 2.49). High-frequency DBS appears to be the functional equivalent of a brain lesion. DBS is reversible (by switching the current off) and adjustable, but further research studies are clearly needed.

Vagal nerve stimulation

The vagus nerve, or tenth cranial nerve, subserves a number of autonomic regulatory functions, with an anatomical course from the brain to the thorax and abdomen. Constituted within the vagus are a mixture of myelinated and unmyelinated fibres of different sizes. Electrical stimulation of the vagus nerve (VNS) has been used for both neurological (epilepsy) and psychiatric disorders (depression).

VNS involves intermittent repeated stimulation of the left vagus nerve via electrical pulses generated by an implanted neurostimulator to a bipolar lead encircling the nerve in the neck (see Fig. 41.2) (Schlaepfer et al., 2010). Stimulation of the nerve non-invasively, though possible via the skin, had until recently insufficient evidence to support its use in this way for clinical purposes (Huston et al., 2007), but data is now emerging that lends potential promise. VNS is used for treatment-resistant epilepsy adjunctively with antiepileptic medications in tertiary epilepsy treatment centres. VNS for partial seizures has been evaluated as effective and well tolerated when used with one or more antiepileptic drugs in those with treatment-resistant epilepsy (Panebianco et al., 2015).

Complications of VNS surgery appear minimal, and excluding surgical complications (wound infection, rarely left vocal cord paresis, and temporary asystole), the main side effects reported in the acute period are voice alteration, cough, pain, and dyspnoea (in which stimulation intensity is considered a relevant factor after the acute period) (Schlaepfer et al., 2010).

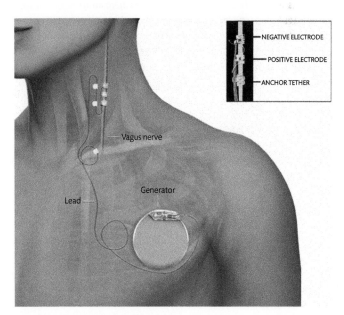

Fig. 41.2 Placement of VNS device.
Reproduced with permission from Verrier, R.L. Baseline elevation and reduction in cardiac electrical instability assessed by quantitative T-wave alternans in patients with drug-resistant epilepsy treated with vagus nerve stimulation in the AspireSR E-36 trial. *Epilepsy & Behavior*, 62: 85–89. © 2016 The Authors. Published by Elsevier Inc. https://doi.org/10.1016/j.yebeh.2016.06.016.

With regard to the use of VNS for TRD, in 2005, the US FDA approved treatment for patients with chronic or recurrent depression (unipolar or bipolar) if there is failed response to at least four antidepressant trials. Hypomania and frank mania have been reported as adverse events, particularly in patients with a prior history of bipolar disorder. Despite having a licensed indication, VNS for depression is rarely used in clinical practice in the UK. NICE only recommends VNS for TRD in rare cases (National Institute for Health and Care Excellence, 2009). Further research is recommended, as evidence on safety and efficacy was considered *inadequate in quality and quantity* by NICE when assessed in 2009.

In TRD outpatients, VNS treatment appears to have improved both depression and sleep (Armitage et al., 2003), as evidenced in sleep EEGs by decreased awake time, decreased stage 1 sleep, and increased stage 2 sleep (although these results did not achieve statistical significance).

Occipital nerve stimulation

A large number of headache syndromes are resistant to treatment with medication alone. For such individuals, there may exist the possibility of relief with invasive stimulation therapy, e.g. ONS.

ONS involves subcutaneous insertion of a stimulating lead in the occipital region of the cranium. Rather than direct contact with the occipital nerve, the lead provides several metallic contact points which generate a 'field' of stimulation. Although the mechanism of effect is not fully understood, research with, for example, PET imaging has suggested brainstem activation in patients treated with ONS (Trentman et al., 2016). Modest benefits have been reported in chronic migraine (Reed et al., 2010) and cluster headache (Walter and Kaube, 2012). However, due to the lack of sufficiently well-designed and powered studies employing a sham condition and randomization, use of ONS is currently limited to the most refractory cases, usually as part of research studies. NICE has stated that ONS for intractable chronic migraine may have short-term efficacy, but evidence for longer-term benefit is lacking. Its clinical use in the UK hence remains limited (National Institute for Health and Care Excellence, 2013). It should be noted, however, that for some sufferers, ONS has been 'life-changing', although predicting beforehand who is likely to benefit the most is unclear.

Methods employing non-invasive neuronal stimulation

Transcranial direct current stimulation

Transcranial electrical stimulation (TES) has evolved into a number of different forms, as newer technologies have become incorporated. The various forms currently include transcranial pulsed current stimulation (tPCS), cranial electrical stimulation (CES), transcerebral electrotherapy (TCET), and neuro-electric therapy (NET), but also many others (Kumar and Sarkar, 2016). Irrespective of the method, the key feature remains, which is electrical stimulation of the brain transcranially using placed electrodes.

In tDCS, a low-intensity, constant current is applied to the cranium via scalp electrodes. The current used typically ranges from 0.5 to 2 mA, and the duration of stimulation between 5 and 40 minutes. The size of the electrodes (which varies from 3 to 100 cm²)

determines the current density (in A/m²) and the total charge applied in coulombs (Tortella et al., 2015). The actual current delivered to the cortex also depends on other factors such as cephalic impedance.

The electric current applied can be subthreshold (i.e. sufficient to modulate neuronal excitability without triggering action potentials) but while still allowing for facilitation or inhibition of spontaneous neural activity, depending on the polarity of the electrodes. Anodal (+) stimulation induces an increase in cortical excitability, whereas cathodal (−) stimulation decreases cortical excitability. This is an oversimplification, as inward current flow at the cortex (or anodal tDCS) generates hyperpolarization of apical dendritic regions of pyramidal cortical neurones and depolarization of somatic regions; and outward current flow (cathodal tDCS) results in somatic hyperpolarization and apical dendrite depolarization of pyramidal cortical neurones (Zaghi et al., 2010, as cited by Tortella et al., 2015). Stimulation effects may last beyond the stimulation period, possibly 30–120 minutes.

EEG studies have demonstrated that stimulation of a specific brain area (e.g. frontal) induces changes to oscillatory activity that synchronizes throughout the brain. Neural changes take place rapidly and persist for several minutes after stimulation has ended. This, however, still does not explain how these effects are transmitted and whether the observed clinical effects are mediated primarily through the area of the cortex being stimulated or secondarily via activation/inhibition of other cortical/subcortical areas. At the molecular level, it is also not known if the mechanism of action of tDCS is via the migration and collection of transmembrane proteins in a prolonged constant electric field or via steric/conformational changes in these proteins inducing functional effects (Zaghi et al., 2010). In addition to modulation of synaptic connectivity, the indications are that tDCS induces neuroplastic changes regulated by several neurotransmitter systems, including dopamine, acetylcholine, serotonin, and brain-derived neurotrophic factor (BDNF). Almost all tissues and cells are sensitive to electric fields, and therefore, tDCS might, in addition to neuronal tissue, elicit changes in non-neuronal brain tissue such as endothelial cells, lymphocytes, or glial cells (Lefaucheur et al., 2017).

Transcranial alternating current stimulation

Transcranial alternating current stimulation (tACS) uses a sine-wave electric field to induce oscillatory activity in stimulated regions. The main difference with tDCS is that the sine-wave field can lead to entrainment of a pattern of oscillatory activity at the frequency of stimulation. Studies using EEG and tACS suggest that stimulating in the alpha frequency band (8–12 Hz) can lead to enhancement at that frequency. The use of tACS has potential for tailoring stimulation, based on an individual's oscillatory activity, as ascertained by EEG. Synchronous neural activity is thought to be a way in which disparate neural regions communicate and are identified as part of the same functional network (Moseley et al., 2016). tACS is an experimental technology. The long-term effects of administering tACS are unknown. The effect of tACS might also be highly dependent on the state of the brain before stimulation. The use of tACS as a treatment for psychiatric disorders is currently extremely limited, but trials of tACS have been suggested for conditions associated with atypical oscillatory activity, e.g. in patients with auditory verbal hallucinations. Entraining or enhancing oscillatory activity in such patients, with scalp electrodes placed over the inferior frontal and superior temporal areas, may enhance gamma synchrony between these areas, which could improve functioning of forward-model systems, which ultimately contributes to experiencing inner speech as self-generated (Moseley et al., 2016).

Transcranial random noise stimulation (tRNS) is a variant of tACS, in which stimulation occurs at a randomly changing frequency (usually between 0.1 and 640 Hz). The therapeutic benefits of tRNS are a focus of further research activity, but studies are limited to single case reports, e.g. trials involving a patient with tinnitus and a patient with schizophrenia with negative symptoms. Moderate effect sizes have been shown, but further studies are clearly needed.

Transcranial magnetic stimulation

The technique of TMS is based on Faraday's principle of electromagnetic induction (1831). Simply stated, a varying magnetic field induces electrical current in a conductor placed within that field. In any nerve (or axon), neuronal activity occurs by movement of action potentials along the axon. Axons hence are electrical conductors.

This principle was exploited by Barker et al. (1985) who connected a wire coil to a source of electric current and placed the coil on the scalp over the motor cortex. They were able to demonstrate a motor action potential following application of a single brief pulse of current through the coil. It was hypothesized (correctly) that neuronal activation was due to current induced in the brain tissue by the rapid, time-varying magnetic field. Subsequent investigation has confirmed that the electrical potential associated with this brain current is sufficient to depolarize neurones in the motor cortex and generate a motor evoked potential (MEP) (Leuchter et al., 2013).

Current methods of TMS employ coil electrodes placed on the scalp regions overlying the areas to be stimulated (see Fig. 41.3). Subjects are conscious; no anaesthetic is required, and serious side effects (e.g. seizure) are uncommon. TMS is delivered in high-frequency bursts for up to 190 s or in low-frequency trains (1 Hz) for up to 30 minutes, with the aim of modulating the activity in underlying brain networks. In general, low-frequency stimulation decreases excitability, and high-frequency stimulation increases neuronal excitability. Magnetic field intensity is in the order of 1–2 tesla.

TMS can be used with a single pulse (single-pulse TMS), as a pair of applied pulses with a variable interval (paired-pulse TMS), or with repeating pulses (repetitive; rTMS). The frequency of stimulation in rTMS can be varied, as with TMS. rTMS is considered to initiate changes to synaptic long-term depression (LTD) and long-potentiating (LTP) mechanisms, activation of feedback loops, and changes in neuronal excitability (Rokyta et al., 2015).

Low-frequency rTMS can induce nausea and painful axial spasms when applied to the premotor cortex in generalized secondary dystonia. Other side effects include induction of epileptic seizures (<1%), which is more likely with high-frequency rTMS (Rokyta et al., 2015).

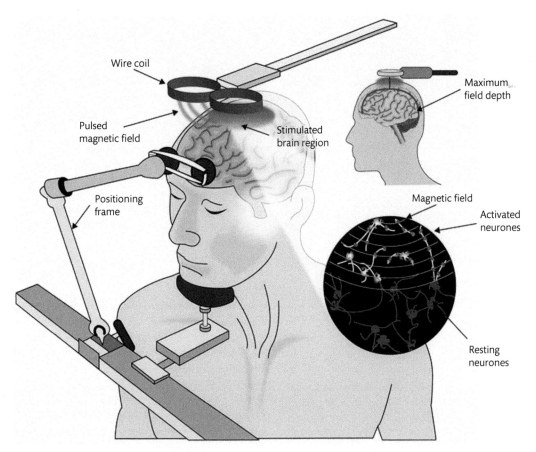

Fig. 41.3 Schematic showing the set-up for generic TMS.
Courtesy of The Brain Stimulator, Inc. www.thebrainstimulator.com.

Magnetic seizure therapy

The need for an electrical stimulus to induce seizures is both the main effect of ECT and its most fundamental limitation. Control over the spatial distribution and magnitude of intracerebral current density is limited by high skull impedance which shunts most of the electrical stimulus through the scalp and cerebrospinal fluid and away from the brain, resulting in widespread stimulation of cortical and subcortical brain regions. Individual differences in skull anatomy result in uncontrolled variation in intracerebral current density. Computer models support the view that current dissipation in ECT is considerable and that the electrode placement associated with the most severe cognitive side effects (bitemporal) is also the placement with higher shunting (Cretaz et al., 2015) and deeper brain stimulation.

Whereas, with ECT, generalized seizures are electrically induced by electrodes focally placed on the scalp, in MST, focal seizure activity is induced by applying TMS. The fact that TMS could induce seizures was initially considered a complication, but eventually the possibility of increasing the magnetic stimulus into the convulsive range as a deliberate action, under controlled conditions, in a patient under anaesthesia, as a treatment came to be explored. Since 2001, there have been several reports of MST in human subjects (Cretaz et al., 2015). The seizure induced by MST is quite different to that produced by ECT. Magnetic pulses, as employed by rTMS and MST, are capable of focusing stimulation to a specific area, since these pass unhindered into the brain without resistance and are not shunted through the scalp and skull, as with ECT. Whereas magnetic pulses penetrate only a few centimetres deep, electrical current can penetrate much deeper structures. Therefore, MST can focus stimulation on superficial regions of the cortex, while with ECT, electrical activity passes deep through the brain. In this way, MST may produce therapeutic benefits in the treatment of depression, as with ECT, but does not induce memory-related side effects, as there is no direct stimulation of medial temporal lobe structures.

Vestibular stimulation

The vestibular system is a target for therapeutic neuromodulation/stimulation. The system detects bodily movement and spatial orientation, and provides an early sensory reference frame for developing systems in the brainstem, cerebellum, and cortex. As a result, signals from the vestibular system have become deeply integrated with processes linked to balance, body schema, mood, well-being, and cognition, most notably memory. The vestibular system is unique among the senses due to the entirely multi-sensory nature of its cortical projections and its overlap with limbic, interoceptive, and cognitive networks.

The inner ear contains receptors for both the auditory and the vestibular systems. The bony labyrinth contains a series of communicating cavities which enclose the cochlea, the vestibule, and the semicircular canals. The three semicircular canals are perpendicular to each other and correspond to the axes of three-dimensional space. They are the lateral or horizontal canal, the superior or anterior canal, and the posterior or vertical canal (see Fig. 41.4). Together the semicircular canals detect head rotation. By contrast, the utricle and saccule detect linear movement of the head, including that associated with gravity.

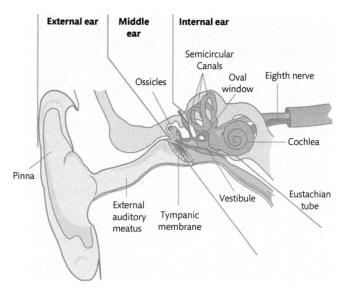

Fig. 41.4 Anatomy of the peripheral audio-vestibular system.
Reproduced with permission from Luxon L.M. Hearing. In *The Oxford Textbook of Medicine*, David A. Warrell D.A., et al. (Eds.). Oxford, UK: OUP. Copyright © 2010, Oxford University Press. DOI: 10.1093/med/9780199204854.001.1. Reproduced with permission of the Licensor through PLSclear.

The vestibular nerve, a division of the vestibulocochlear nerve (cranial nerve VIII), conveys the primary sensory axons of the vestibular system. The central axonal processes enter the brainstem at the cerebellopontine angle, conveying information to the brainstem vestibular nuclei. Pathways from these nuclei project to the thalamus (vestibulothalamocortical pathway) and the cerebral cortex. The dominant vestibular area in man is in the posterior insula, corresponding to the monkey parieto-insular vestibular cortex (PIVC).

Methods of vestibular stimulation

Stimulation of the vestibular organs can be achieved using several different techniques (which include whole-body rotation and optokinetic stimulation). However, CVS and GVS have been the most investigated approaches. Commercial devices are available for GVS, and investigational devices are available for CVS. These devices have been used in patients with a range of disorders, including aphasia after stroke (Wilkinson et al., 2016), conversion disorder (Noll-Hussong et al., 2014), mania (Dodson et al., 2004), balance function (Goel et al., 2015), and many others (mostly as case reports).

Vestibular stimulation alters the release of excitatory and inhibitory neurotransmitters such as glutamate, noradrenaline, serotonin, and acetylcholine (Wilkinson et al., 2013). Neuroimaging studies indicate that vestibular stimulation strongly activates temporal and perisylvian areas, in particular the parieto-insular vestibular cortex (or PIVC, as known in the monkey brain), while deactivating visual areas (Noll-Hussong et al., 2014). The ability of vestibular stimulation to activate so many diffuse, ascending pathways sets it apart from all other pharmacological and neuromodulatory procedures which are non-endogenous and chemically/anatomically localized. A further advantage over other techniques is that the site of stimulation remains unchanged across disease types and individuals. This simplifies administration and makes it especially amenable to home-based and portable use.

Caloric vestibular stimulation

CVS introduces warm or cool temperatures into the external ear canal. Traditionally, ice-cold water has been used to assess brainstem function in unconscious and unresponsive patients, although warmer currents are effective too. Local temperature changes create convection currents in the vestibular endolymph, which deflect the cupula within the ipsilateral horizontal semicircular canal, which, in turn, alters the firing rate of the vestibulocochlear nerve. This, in turn, elicits a widespread haemodynamic response across cortical and subcortical areas of the brain. Unlike tDCS and other forms of TES, patients with electronic implants and certain types of metal plates are not contraindicated.

In the case of expressive and receptive aphasia after a left cerebral stroke, CVS daily for 20 minutes over 4 weeks (20 days) resulted in variable degrees of improved response in three of the four patients investigated by Wilkinson et al., as suggested by outcome measures such as picture naming, sentence repetition, and auditory word discrimination. The speculated mechanism of improvement was suggested as CVS increasing blood flow to left hemispheric language networks, perhaps resulting in increased metabolic activity, with reactivation and reintegration of injured cortical areas (Wilkinson et al., 2013).

In a single case report, by Noll-Hussong , et al. (2014), a patient with a psychogenic movement disorder of 2 years standing, resistant to improvement with conventional treatments, showed immediate and sustained relief from his functional disability following left caloric water irrigation at 30°C for 20 s. The effect lasted several hours, but only at the first trial, and not subsequently. The possibility of 'suggestion' abetting apparent recovery cannot be ruled out, although the authors also speculated on more elaborate vestibular effects such as activation of thalamocortical mechanisms which may reintegrate impaired cortical regions.

The case described by Dodson (2004) has similar intriguing elements. A female patient with long-standing bipolar affective disorder was admitted to a psychiatric ward in a state of manic relapse. Her condition had some history of treatment resistance. Treatment with left caloric water irrigation at 4°C, over 2–3 minutes, resulted in the patient experiencing an immediate improvement in her symptoms of mania which lasted approximately 24 hours, before symptoms returned. Repetition of the procedure resulted in further partial recovery, but still with a gradual return to baseline manic symptoms. Once again, suggestion may have had a role to play in this case, but potential activation of vestibular-activated mood circuits involving the basal ganglia, insula, cingulate gyrus, and prefrontal and parieto-temporal regions has also been speculated.

A study in healthy volunteers assessed the effect of CVS on processing of affective information using a Go/NoGo task, in which participants were given cold left or right ear CVS (20°C) or sham stimulation (37°C). Positive or negative pictures were presented as targets requiring responses to targets (Go) and withholding of responses to distractors (NoGo). Positive mood ratings decreased during left ear CVS, when compared to sham stimulation, with no effect seen after right ear CVS. Affective control improved during right ear CVS when viewing positive stimuli but decreased during

left ear CVS when compared to sham stimulation (Preuss, 2014). The authors concluded that activating left hemispheric vestibular areas by means of right ear CVS may interact with prefrontal emotional networks specifically for emotionally positive stimuli. Asymmetries in the effects of CVS have also been noted in experiments targeting vision, cognition, and attention.

In various other small-scale studies, repeated daily sessions of CVS have been associated with clinically relevant improvements in awareness and voluntary behaviour in patients in minimally conscious states (Vanzan et al., 2017), and in motor and non-motor features of Parkinson's disease (Wilkinson et al., 2016).

Galvanic vestibular stimulation

GVS is transmitted via two electrodes placed over the mastoid processes (see Fig. 41.5). GVS stimulates and/or inhibits all peripheral afferents of both the semicircular canals and the otoliths. The type of stimulation depends on current flow. Modern devices deliver currents in the range of 0–3 mA. The usual maximum current is 5 mA to avoid skin irritation and the risk of burns. The advantage of GVS over CVS is that it allows stimulation to be delivered in brief, more tightly controlled waveforms (Grabherr et al., 2015), and GVS also has been shown to be clinically efficacious at subthreshold levels (typically <0.5 mA) which are well tolerated and possible to experimentally blind.

GVS is applied through very large surface electrodes (60–90 mm²) placed over the mastoids, with care to ensure good, clean skin contact. GVS provides a weak current which acts at the spike trigger zone of vestibular afferents, rather than causing membrane depolarization. Maintained GVS generates a series of action potentials (which adapt) during the course of direct current stimulation (Curthoys et al., 2012). GVS produces complex oculomotor, perceptual, and postural responses, dependent on factors such as the stimulus, electrodes, and context and how responses are measured.

Relatively few RCTs have been conducted with GVS, although in one widely noted example, GVS was applied to patients with stroke

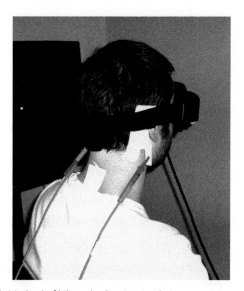

Fig. 41.5 Method of bilateral galvanic stimulation.
Reproduced with permission from Vailleau B., et al. Probing Residual Vestibular Function With Galvanic Stimulation in Vestibular Loss Patients. *Otology & Neurotology*, 32(5): pp.863-871. Copyright © 2011, *Otology & Neurotology*, Inc. doi: 10.1097/MAO.0b013e318213418e.

suffering hemi-spatial neglect (Wilkinson et al., 2014). In this study, 49 patients were randomized to three treatment arms (one active and nine sham treatments versus five active and five sham treatments versus ten active and zero sham treatments) using bipolar (left anodal, right cathodal) binaural GVS administered at a mean noisy current of 0.5–1.5 mA for 25 minutes. As well as the known benefits of GVS improving performance across a range of visuospatial tasks (such as line bisection, figure copying, and target cancellation), in this study, the authors demonstrated a persisting benefit of GVS on the primary outcome measure [Behavioural Inattention Test (BIT)], between baseline and 4 weeks post-GVS, in all treatment arms. This comparable efficacy of a single versus multiple stimulation sessions is notable.

Applications of neurostimulation to specific neurological disorders

Neurostimulation in neurology has been used for a range of conditions, including migraine, movement disorder, and chronic pain. The list of potential conditions being targeted for possible benefit is ever increasing and now also includes Tourette syndrome, dementia, and disorders of consciousness. There is variable evidence of efficacy in most of these potential conditions, due largely to the lack of reliable trial-based data which include sufficiently large cohorts of patients. The evidence is more compelling for treatment of pain and headache.

Neurostimulation for pain

Debilitating chronic pain disorders are common in clinical practice across specialties. Such pain is often poorly responsive to treatment in the form of drugs or pain management employing psychological therapies. Neurostimulation has been trialled for chronic conditions such as failed back surgery syndrome (FBSS) and complex regional pain syndrome (CRPS), as well as for neuropathic pain associated with peripheral neuropathy, post-herpetic neuralgia, and ischaemic pain due to cardiovascular and peripheral vascular disease (Mekhail et al., 2010).

Chronic spinal pain

FBSS is characterized by intractable chronic pain affecting the legs, buttocks, or low back, following spinal surgery that may have successfully corrected the underlying pathology, but without achieving adequate relief. FBSS has been traditionally managed with treatments such as analgesic medication, physiotherapy, nerve root blocks, or epidural steroid injections. Many patients fail to benefit from these approaches, and it is for these that neuromodulation therapy, in the form of spinal cord stimulation (SCS), may offer an alternative way forward. FBSS is now the commonest indication for neurostimulation therapy for chronic spinal pain. The procedure involves placement of one or more multiple contact neurostimulation leads into the posterior epidural space of the spine. The targets for SCS are the dorsal column tracts adjacent to dorsal nerve roots entering the dorsal horn of the spinal cord. When applied, an electric field is created over the cord, resulting in paraesthesiae in the painful regions affected. Pain relief of at least 50% is reported, but

efficacy depends on careful selection of patients, spinal levels targeted, the underlying pathology, and the type of pain generator. Unintentional stimulation of spinal roots can lead to side effects such as dysaesthesia and unpleasant motor responses. SCS has been used to treat pain due to lumbar spinal stenosis and intractable pain originating in the cervical spine. Initial costs of SCS can be substantial, hence limiting its use only to carefully selected patients. A device for SCS was first approved by the FDA in 1989.

Neuropathic pain

In chronic neuropathic pain, the cause of the underlying injury may have resolved, but the pain remains. CRPS is a type of neuropathic pain suitable for treatment with neurostimulation. CRPS is divided into CRPS-I, formerly known as reflex sympathetic dystrophy, and CRPS-II, also known as causalgia. CRPS-I is related to the loss of small-diameter nerve fibres C and A-δ. SCS is reported to have positive benefits in CRPS-I (Mekhail et al., 2010). Early treatment (<4 months from failure of conservative management) is advised.

Nerve stimulation for headache syndromes

The World Health Organization (WHO) estimates headache disorders, including migraine and cluster headache, to be one of the most prevalent conditions affecting man. Ten per cent of the world's population are believed to suffer with migraine. Of these, 50% are self-treating. Only 10% have access to neurology (Armitage et al., 2003). In the United States, 40 million people are estimated to suffer with migraine (World Health Organization, 2011). Chronic migraine affects 2% of the general population in the United States. Treatment-refractory migraine and cluster headache affect approximately 5% of patients attending specialist headache clinics.

Headache conditions can be classified as episodic and chronic. Episodic headache is defined as that occurring <15 days a month for >3 months. Chronic headache is headache occurring >15 days a month for >3 months. Chronic headache sufferers amount to 4% of the global population (Miller et al., 2016). Most chronic headaches are chronic migraine or cluster headache.

The commonest type of migraine is characterized by recurrent episodes of head pain, often throbbing and unilateral, sometimes preceded by aura (Dahlem et al., 2013). Chronic migraine is also defined as the occurrence of >15 headache days per month over a 3-month period, with at least eight of these characterized as migrainous, in the absence of medication overuse. Migraine aura symptoms are most often visual field disturbances but can also involve other sensory modalities or cognitive functions.

Cluster headache is characterized by attacks of severe pain localized orbitally, supraorbitally, or temporally, lasting for 15–180 minutes and occurring from once every other day to eight times daily (Walter and Kaube, 2012). The symptoms of cluster headache include conjunctival injection, lacrimation, nasal congestion, rhinorrhoea, forehead and facial sweating, miosis, ptosis, and eyelid oedema. The usual pattern of occurrence is with remissions (episodic cluster headache), but one in seven sufferers have chronic cluster headache, i.e. no remission periods lasting 1 month or longer.

In a small case series of seven patients, PNS, using wire lead arrays placed at the base of the supraorbital nerve and/or greater occipital nerve, showed a response rate in treating the pain of occipital neuralgia and cervicogenic headache of approximately 88% and 40–50% for primary migraines and cluster headache, respectively

(Reed et al., 2010). Headache with a fronto-temporal distribution appears to be responsive to stimulation of the distant occiput. The authors suggested ONS for occipital pain, supraorbital nerve stimulation (SONS) for frontal pain, and combined ONS-SONS for holocephalic pain. The rationale for combination treatment is suggested by the knowledge that trigeminal and greater occipital nociceptive afferents converge on the same second-order sensory neurones in the trigeminocervical complex, and therefore on a final common pathway to higher structures and nuclei important for pain modulation. (The supraorbital nerve is a branch of the first division of the trigeminal nerve.) Stimulation parameters can be adjusted to control the paraesthesiae achieved.

ONS requires a minor invasive surgical procedure, but this is not widely available and may only be carried out by highly specialized services combining headache and surgical expertise (Miller et al., 2016). The procedure therefore is reserved for those with highly refractory headache syndromes not responsive to all other treatments. ONS has no role in the acute treatment of migraine or cluster headache. When fitted, the occipital nerve stimulator is left on at all times. Adverse events include lead migration (13%), lead fracture (4%), erosion of an electrode through the skin (4%), infection (10%), painful stimulation (17%), and pain over the battery site (18%) (Miller et al., 2016). Although ONS suggests stimulation of the occipital nerve itself, the use of multiple contact points that can be programmed to function as cathodes or anodes (allowing distribution of the locality and intensity of the stimulation) means that the term 'occipital field stimulation' is a more accurate description (Trentman et al., 2016).

Non-invasive neurostimulation for chronic migraine

Transcutaneous electrical nerve stimulation (TENS) modulates neural activity by non-invasive stimulation of peripheral nerves. In migraine, supraorbital transcutaneous stimulation (STS) has been tested, targeting the ophthalmic division of the trigeminal nerve. Using biphasic rectangular alternating current impulses at 60 Hz, Dahlem et al. (2013) reported a therapeutic gain of 26%, similar in efficacy to preventative drug and non-drug treatments.

TMS and TES have also been applied to migraine. These methods target cortical brain regions, rather than peripheral nerves. Early small-scale studies have suggested that TMS may be effective in disrupting cortical spreading depression (SD) in the aura phase, suggesting potential for aborting migraine attacks, but much larger replicated studies are needed.

Two versions of TES are available. In tDCS, cathodal stimulation inhibits neuronal firing and anodal stimulation increases neuronal firing. With tACS, polarity cyclically changes according to the frequency of the alternating current. There is preliminary evidence for a positive, but delayed, response to tDCS applied to motor (anodal) and orbitofrontal (cathodal) cortices in patients with chronic migraine (Dahlem et al., 2013).

CVS has also recently been reported as a potential beneficial adjuvant treatment for the management of episodic migraine. Researchers tested subjects over 3 months using a parallel-arm, block-randomized, placebo-controlled design, with the primary end-point defined as a change in monthly migraine days from baseline to the third-treatment month. Active arm subjects reported immediate and continued steady declines in migraine frequency over the treatment period, with an overall therapeutic gain of 2.8 fewer migraine days (Wilkinson et al., 2017).

Other neurological disorders

Neurostimulation in memory disorders

Patients with AD and other neurodegenerative conditions are set to exponentially increase in number due to ageing populations worldwide surviving to ever longer average lifespans. In the United States alone, an estimated 5.5 million people of all ages have AD. Of these, around 5.3 million are 65 years and older and 200,000 are younger and have early-onset AD. Treatments for AD and other neurodegenerative conditions are currently limited to symptom control, rather than reversal or cure.

Memory impairment is usually the first cognitive manifestation of neurodegenerative processes. rTMS studies have confirmed the role of the prefrontal cortex in encoding and retrieval of verbal or non-verbal material in healthy subjects. Other research has assessed the effect of rTMS on both left and right dorsolateral prefrontal cortices (DLPFCs) on naming and language performance in AD patients using a two-crossover, sham-controlled, single-session study design. Significantly improved accuracy in both action and object naming was found following high-frequency rTMS, an effect seen in both mild AD [Mini-Mental State Examination (MMSE) scores ≥17/30], and moderate to severe AD (MMSE scores <17/30) (Nardone et al., 2015).

tDCS has also been found to be of benefit when applied to patients with AD. Several studies have reported improvements in mild AD using anodal tDCS, particularly recognition memory, but not working memory (Nardone et al., 2015). The initial findings merit replication in much larger sample groups with RCT design and double blinding to confirm whether the effects are definite, the duration of effect (if any), the most optimal stimulation parameters, and patient inclusion criteria.

GVS has also been investigated for effects on cognitive function. In healthy subjects, subsensory anodal stimulation over the left mastoid was found to improve (speed up) visual memory recall of faces (Wilkinson et al., 2008).

Non-invasive neurostimulation for traumatic brain injury

Traumatic brain injury (TBI) is temporary or permanent impairment of brain function, following physical trauma, usually an external force, to the brain. The annual incidence of TBI in the United States is approximately 2000 per million, with an estimated 1.5 million US individuals experiencing a TBI each year (Dhaliwal et al., 2015). There is huge heterogeneity in the type of TBIs suffered, but common themes occur in sufferers' post-TBI neuropsychiatric symptoms such as affective disorder (particularly depression), sleep disturbance, fatigue, anxiety, and varying degrees of cognitive dysfunction (working and episodic memory, cognitive processing speed, executive function, and attentional and concentration difficulties).

After TBI, the side effects of psychotropic medications are less well tolerated and symptoms are more resistant to eradication, leading to chronic disability and societal burden. It is not surprising that, in relation to treatment of any neuropsychiatric consequence of TBI, no medication has to date received approval by the US FDA. Treatments tend to be largely based on clinicians' experience, preferences, and anecdote. This demonstrates the necessity of exploring novel methods of treatment, including NIBS.

A systematic review of studies using NIBS in TBI found evidence in relation to rTMS and tDCS (Dhaliwal et al., 2015). rTMS has been reported mildly beneficial when given to post-TBI inpatients suffering with suicidal thoughts using a protocol of high-frequency rTMS over the left prefrontal cortex administered three times a day (6000 pulses over 30 minutes at 10 Hz and 5-s train duration) for 3 days. The authors (George et al., 2014) found a more rapid rate of recovery in those subjects treated actively, compared to sham, but no other differences between the groups. Case reports have documented improvements in a range of post-TBI symptoms such as hemi-spatial neglect, depression, and executive function, but definite evidence of efficacy remains enigmatic. Similarly, tDCS provides limited evidence of benefit in improvement of various aspects of brain function such as cognition and attention, but studies need to be replicated. The main risk of NIBS in TBI is seizure generation due to increased neural excitability.

Non-invasive neurostimulation for sleep

The sensation of rocking, as in putting a baby to sleep, can also be created by electrical stimulation of the vestibular system, raising the intriguing possibility of vestibular stimulation as a means of addressing disorders of sleep such as insomnia. Physiological evidence of a neuronal basis for connectivity of the vestibular system to sleep mechanisms is suggested by labyrinthine inputs to the pontine reticular formation neurones involved in mediating switching between sleep states, and medial vestibular projections to regions mediating arousal such as the lateral hypothalamus (Krystal et al., 2010).

In a model of transient healthy volunteers measuring polysomnographic latency to persistent sleep in a 4-hour phase advance protocol in normal sleepers, Krystal et al. found that after bilateral electrical stimulation of the vestibular apparatus via electrodes on the skin of the mastoid process at 0.5 Hz (sham-controlled), only a small effect on shortening sleep-onset latency occurred, as compared to sham. More persuasive evidence, however, of an effect of NIBS on sleep architecture has been provided by experiments with TMS which showed that, with appropriate stimulation parameters, TMS pulses at <1 Hz during NREM sleep can evoke slow waves and spindles in sleeping subjects. Evoked slow waves have been shown to lead to a deepening of sleep and an increase in EEG slow-wave activity (0.5–4.5 Hz), which may be associated with 'brain restoration' and memory consolidation (Massimini et al., 2007). The effect has also been reported with tDCS (Bellesi et al., 2014)).

Applications of neurostimulation in psychiatric disorders

An expanding range of psychiatric conditions have been targeted for exploratory 'treatment' with non-invasive neurostimulation methods. These include depression, schizophrenia, anxiety disorders, OCD, addiction, autism, and attention-deficit/hyperactivity

disorder (ADHD) (Baeken et al., 2015; De Melo et al., 2016; Fitzgerald et al., 2012; Hizli et al., 2013; Rajapakse et al., 2013). Possible application to a range of other disorders has also been suggested, including dyslexia, Tourette syndrome, dementia, post-traumatic stress disorder (PTSD), neuroenhancement (i.e. improving cognition in healthy normals), and low awareness states. The evidence for efficacy, however, is often limited to case studies or studies with small samples. Few double-blind, well-powered RCTs have been done, making the case for efficacy of neurostimulation in such a vastly different set of disorders difficult, with as yet no confirmed theory of biological effect at the neuronal level, although various speculative hypotheses are stated.

Depression

That being said, there is still a significant evidence base for the use of tDCS in depressive disorders (e.g. Holtzheimer et al., 2017). The current approach is for enhancement of neural activity in the left DLPFC with anodal stimulation and/or reduction in neural activity in the right DLPFC with cathodal stimulation. tDCS applied in this way also affects deeper brain structures such as the amygdala, hippocampus, and subgenual cortex. The precise changes in resting-state brain networks that produce the antidepressant effects of tDCS remain unknown.

Meta-analyses have suggested that active tDCS is superior to sham treatment and the combination of antidepressant + tDCS is more effective than either alone, suggesting an additive interaction. The possibility of the effect of tDCS being mediated by pharmacological modulation of serotonergic and noradrenergic neurones located in deep brain structures, even though these might not be directly affected by superficial current flow generated by tDCS, has been suggested (Brunoni et al., 2014b, cited in Tortella et al., 2015). Alternatively, or additionally, serotonergic enhancement may boost the neuroplastic effects of anodal tDCS, thus resulting in synergistic effects.

Much research has also investigated the effects of rTMS in depression. Treatment protocols for depression have consisted mostly of 5–25 sessions of high-frequency rTMS to the left DLPFC or low-frequency rTMS applied to the right DLPFC. A meta-analysis of 34 studies comparing rTMS with sham treatment showed a moderate effect size on depressive symptoms, comparable to psychotherapy and pharmacotherapy (de Raedt et al., 2014).

Schizophrenia

Some of the most treatment-resistant symptoms of schizophrenia include persistent auditory hallucinations and negative symptoms such as blunting of affect, poverty of speech and thought, apathy, anhedonia, reduced social drive, loss of motivation, lack of social interest, and inattention to social or cognitive input.

The Repetitive Transcranial Magnetic Stimulation for the Treatment of Negative Symptoms in Schizophrenia (RESIS) trial was conducted from 2007 to 2011. A total of 175 patients were enrolled and randomized to either 10–20 Hz active or sham rTMS applied for 15 sessions to the left DLPFC. Unfortunately, a beneficial effect of active stimulation was not found. However, other treatment studies with different treatment parameters, less strict methodology, and smaller sample sizes have shown positive effects (Hasan et al., 2016).

For the management of auditory hallucinations, inhibitory 1-Hz rTMS applied to the left temporal lobe for 5–20 sessions was found to have been used in 393 patients who had received this protocol in sham-controlled studies, but only half of the studies showed a beneficial effect of the intervention. A significant placebo effect has been reported in one meta-analysis (Hasan et al., 2016). Hence the evidence is equivocal for benefit.

tDCS for persistent auditory hallucinations in schizophrenia has also been studied using a protocol involving stimulation twice a day on five consecutive days, administering 20 minutes of active 2-mA tDCS or sham stimulation to the left temporo-parietal junction (inhibitory cathode), with the excitatory anode placed over the left DLPFC. Active stimulation was found superior to sham stimulation, with a reduction in auditory verbal hallucinations of 31% in a sample of 30 patients with medication-refractory auditory hallucinations. Negative studies, however, have also been reported (Hasan et al., 2016). Hence, in clinical practice, neither tCDS nor rTMS can be recommended, although the evidence for benefit is intriguing. Many other techniques such as tRNS and tACS are also being investigated, but theoretically an infinite number of protocols is possible and there is no consensus yet on what the best parameters or protocol might be. There are also a number of modulating variables, such as cortical architecture, skull thickness, age, sex, genetic factors, and medication in use, which add complexity. The optimal 'therapeutic' dose of stimulation remains uncertain. The underlying physiology of effect (if present) is also unknown.

Anxiety disorders

Anxiety may be a component of a number of common psychiatric disorders such as panic disorder, generalized anxiety, agoraphobia, PTSD, OCD, and others. Herein lies the problem, common to many studies on the efficacy of methods of NIBS in psychiatry, of variable phenomenology and the heterogeneity of psychiatric disorders. There is also the difficulty of providing adequate sham conditions in a population that is difficult to homogenize because of differences in concurrent treatments with psychotropics (e.g. anxiolytics and antidepressants) and behavioural therapies. Hence evidence in this area can, at best, be described as anecdotal, with few systematic, randomized, and blinded controlled trials.

TES is similar in nature to tDCS in that an electrical source is used to stimulate cortical neurones. (Note that TES is also sometimes referred to in the literature as a general term for all modalities of electrostimulation used transcranially with electrodes, with the electrical stimulus often generated by batteries.) When not used as a term in this general way, TES differs from tDCS in the electrodes applied, the current sources used, and the desired effect. TES employs smaller electrodes than tDCS scalp electrodes, leading to much larger stimulating current densities, compared to tDCS. TES actively evokes action potentials from the underlying neural substrate, whereas the effects of tDCS alter the overall excitability of the neural response. Use of TES in awake human subjects is limited due to induced pain from strong activation of skin and scalp pain receptors (Wagner et al., 2007).

TES has been reported (Bystritsky et al., 2008) as effective in generalized anxiety disorder (GAD) using electrical stimulation at 0.5 Hz and 300-µA intensity over 6 weeks (cited by Kumar et al., 2016). The evidence regarding the efficacy of tDCS in GAD, however, is limited.

The evidence supporting the efficacy of NIBS in OCD is more hopeful, with studies using tDCS and rTMS showing benefits. tDCS applied to the DLPFC (anodal left DLPFC, and cathodal right DLPFC) in healthy volunteers reduced anxiety responses to threatening stimuli (Kumar et al., 2016). Meta-analyses of RCTs of rTMS in patients with OCD found active rTMS to be more efficacious than sham rTMS. There is speculation regarding the mechanism of effect, including the possibility that rTMS has a modulating effect on amygdala activity through prefrontal cortical circuitry. Low-frequency rTMS and high-frequency rTMS targeting the right and left medial prefrontal cortices, respectively, for 4 weeks have been reported as effective in social anxiety disorder. It is possible that rTMS in PTSD may be beneficial, but rigorous replicated studies are lacking; hence definite conclusions cannot be drawn. Notably, it has been reported that rTMS at 1 Hz over the right DLPFC, over ten sessions, was better than sham rTMS in improving symptoms of PTSD. A possible mechanism of effect of improvement in PTSD may be disruption of episodic memory recall (of the traumatic memory).

Substance misuse

Substance dependence, whether due to alcohol or other drugs of abuse (e.g. methamphetamines, nicotine, cocaine), represents a significant global burden of disease. Repeated drug or alcohol use is known to lead to neuro-adaptations in the ventral striatum and ventral tegmental areas, which, in turn, results in decreased dopamine secretion (Jansen et al., 2013). Diminished functioning of the DLPFC and anterior cingulate cortex is also noted to be present in addictive disorders, possibly indicating diminished inhibitory control affecting cognitive and behavioural processes. Craving often accompanies addictive behaviours, whether due to food (as in obesity) or substances. Neuroimaging studies have linked craving to reduced prefrontal activation and lower D2 dopamine receptor density in the striatum.

Reducing craving therefore has been seen as an approach suitable for trials of TMS and tDCS. A number of studies have targeted the DLPFC as a stimulation site. The outcomes, though failing replication in other studies with similar study populations, nonetheless, as part of a meta-analysis of only double-blind RCTs, comparing real rTMS/tDCS with sham rTMS/tDCS, suggest a medium effect size favouring non-invasive high-frequency neurostimulation over sham stimulation on craving levels for food and drugs/substances (Jansen et al., 2013). Further research is needed to determine whether these effects are beneficial as stand-alone treatment or should supplement existing treatments.

Neuroenhancement in health

Neuroenhancement describes the use of neuroscience-based techniques for enhancing cognitive function in individuals without a neurological or psychiatric diagnosis. A number of studies have explored direct current stimulation of the brain in healthy adults to enhance attention, learning, and memory (Clark et al., 2014). The results broadly showed reduced performance with cathodal stimulation and increased performance arising from anodal stimulation, but the effect sizes are small. An advantage of tDCS in this setting is that electrode placement may need to be less precise for anatomical targeting, but comparisons between studies is made difficult by the lack of common protocols, common reporting measures of cognitive enhancement, and lack of control conditions.

There are now numerous 'commercial' devices (marketed from a few dollars to several hundreds of dollars), widely available to the public via the Internet, for non-invasive neurostimulation. Sales are not regulated by current legislation which applies to all medical devices, owing to a legal loophole, frequently used in such sales, which often takes the form of a disclaimer to the effect:

> 'The information and devices displayed on this site are not intended to treat, cure, or prevent any medical disease, and this article is not considered to be medical advice. If a reader decides to purchase and use a tDCS machine, it is his or her responsibility to use it correctly and safely and ensure that it works correctly.'

The number of devices actually approved for medical use, e.g. by the US FDA and the Centre for Devices and Radiological Health (CDRH), are, by comparison, very few and usually for indications such as DBS for Parkinson's disease and neurostimulation for epilepsy. Clinical trials that provide data for approval are often restricted in scope and time-limited.

Devices are also undergoing testing in significant numbers in pre-clinical animal work, but with results not always leading to publication, and therefore not available for scrutiny. Researchers have used publicly available US FDA databases to identify pre-market approval (PMA) studies of this type. The results showed that a variety of animals are used in research of this type (e.g. sheep, monkey, dog), with wide variations in stimulation durations (from hours to years) and frequencies of stimulation (from 10 to 10,000 Hz) (Kumsa et al., 2018). The translational value of this research to human subjects is unclear.

Devices used in human trials to study potential for therapeutic benefit, e.g. tDCS for recovery of speech and language after stroke, pain mitigation, etc., also often face the difficulty that, at the end of the trial, patients who have been highly responsive to the intervention may not be able to continue treatment outside of the trial, leading to some patients then seeking alternative 'do-it-yourself' (DIY) devices (Bikson et al., 2016), usually used without any medical supervision.

Putative mechanisms of effect

A variety of putative mechanisms (e.g. Deisseroth et al., 2015; Fertonani et al., 2017; Remue et al., 2016; Tye et al., 2009) have been proposed for the many different stimulation techniques outlined previously, but it is beyond the remit of this chapter to review them in any detail. Instead we comment on just two mechanisms that, partly by virtue of their operation at the systems-level and potential ease of induction, are receiving increasing attention.

Neural stimulation and the immune system

There is increasing evidence of a dynamic and interactive relationship between the nervous system and the immune system. It is only relatively recently that microglial cells, which account for 0.5–16.6% of the total number of cells in the human brain and are a key cellular component of the immune system, have been recognized as having many potentially important functions in the normal development, function, and repair of the central nervous system (CNS) (Gomez-Nicola et al., 2015). Microglia actively 'sense' the microenvironment and activation occurs in response to any disturbance of CNS homeostasis, ranging from infection to acute or chronic brain injury. In neurodegenerative diseases, microglial activation is considered to be a response to inflammation due to disease. Neurones partner with immune cells in the regulation of inflammation. Neurones sense inflammatory products and can mount fast and directed responses to regulate immune function and inflammation (Pavlov and Tracey, 2015). Peripheral immune cell activation, with the release of cytokines and other immune molecules, is communicated to the brain through neural and humoral mechanisms, e.g. via afferent vagus nerve fibres.

Koopman et al. (2016) use the term 'inflammatory reflex' to define the signals that travel in the vagus nerve to inhibit monocyte and macrophage production of tumour necrosis factor (TNF) and other cytokines. Inflammatory reflex signalling, enhanced by electrically stimulating the vagus nerve, significantly reduces cytokine production and attenuates disease severity in experimental models of endotoxaemia, sepsis, colitis, and other models of inflammatory syndromes. Koopman et al. have also shown that VNS delivered once daily for 60 s to a group of rheumatoid arthritis patients with an implanted device could attenuate joint swelling, inhibit cytokine production, and confer significant protection against synovitis and periarticular bone erosions.

In addition to pharmacological interventions, device-generated brain modulation (e.g. tDCS, TMS) not only may have a role in neural modulation, but also could, via this route, influence anti-inflammatory activity in the brain, as a potential mechanism of action for the outcomes being seen in the various disorders in which neuromodulation is being tested.

Brain oscillatory activity and entrainment

A second and important theory of how neuromodulation may be having its effects is via studies of brain EEG activity. The most immediate effect of rTMS on brain function appears to be alterations of the oscillations of the underlying brain tissue. High-frequency stimulation (>5 Hz) leads to synchronization of EEG activity in the alpha and beta bands. Studies have demonstrated that high-frequency rTMS leads to alterations of cortical oscillations not only at the site of stimulation, but also in more distant areas as well, consistent with the idea of linkage of brain regions through corticocortical and thalamocortical loops (Leuchter et al., 2013). rTMS pulses appear to trigger and reset oscillatory mechanisms marked by 'event-related synchronization' (ERS) at the frequency of stimulation in the area stimulated, followed by 'event-related desynchronization' (ERD) and re-emergence of endogenous rhythms. Low-frequency (1 or 5 Hz) stimulation may facilitate emergence of local endogenous rhythms by disrupting persistent low-frequency thalamocortical resonance phenomena. Regardless of frequency of stimulation, enhancement of the re-emergence of endogenous local cortical and thalamocortical rhythms may be central to the mechanism of action of rTMS and other forms of neurostimulation, which can also deliver an entraining stimulus.

Conclusion

In this chapter, a number of neurostimulation technologies, their principles of operation, and potential therapeutic applications have been considered, along with the evidence available for benefit. The technologies continue to evolve and develop. There are emerging theories of how the technologies may be interacting with the nervous and immune systems and the brain's innate oscillatory rhythms. More research is needed to better understand how the technologies work, but also whether the potential therapeutic benefits in neurological, neuropsychiatric, and psychiatric disorders are reproducible in larger, well-designed studies. The twenty-first century is predicted to greatly enhance our understanding of brain systems, brain diseases, and the methods of intervention in health and disease, which may have profound impact on future therapeutic management of neurological and psychiatric conditions. Advanced knowledge of neurophysiology, brain networks, neuroimaging, neuroimmunology, neuroplasticity, and neurogenetics seem certain to be key to enable currently practising and future generations of neuropsychiatrists and neurologists to make the best and most informed use of emergent novel neurotechnologies. There is optimism that these technologies, in due course, will take their deserved place alongside medical approaches based on pharmacotherapy, neurosurgery, and psychological therapy.

KEY LEARNING POINTS

* Current evidence regarding invasive novel neurostimulation technologies favours neurological applications more than psychiatric indications. Invasive technologies are more prone to risk and expense at initiation but are also not without side effects, adverse effects, and limitations. Treatment resistance as an indication, careful patient selection, and multidisciplinary specialist teams are necessary to optimize good outcomes of intervention.

* There are an expanding range of neurotechnologies for non-invasively stimulating the brain for use in neurological, neuropsychiatric, and psychiatric disorders. Research into the clinical efficacy of these technologies has expanded rapidly, particularly in the last decade. Some modalities (e.g. tDCS, TMS, CVS/GVS) have potential to induce clinically relevant improvements in difficult-to-treat patient populations and thus represent possible new tools for intervention in a range of mental disorders. The use of these 'tools' remains in its infancy and much further evidence of efficacy, based on large-scale multi-centre RCTs, is required to progress from research laboratory tools to the clinic.

* The challenges facing researchers include highly variable patient characteristics, differences in concomitant therapies, choice of stimulation parameters and protocols, and study designs. To address these difficulties, sample variability needs to be controlled, and reproducible stimulation parameters defined, to help resolve discrepancies in research findings (Kekic et al., 2016).

* Some neurostimulation technologies have progressed to regulatory approval (e.g. tDCS and rTMS for depression) in clinical populations, but actual provision, particularly in UK-based NHS services, is minimal to nil. Clinical provision is largely via private fee-paying clinics in the UK. This is likely to change as more awareness of these neurotechnologies takes place among clinicians, patients, service commissioners, and other relevant stakeholders.

* The long-term effects of neurostimulation are largely unknown. As commercial 'DIY' devices become increasingly available in larger numbers, at low cost (particularly tDCS stimulators), the perils, as well as the promises, of neurostimulation may become more apparent, with the need to introduce better regulatory protection of consumers.

* There is great need for more translational expertise to move these new technologies from bench to bedside. Grant funders need to show greater willingness to support proof-of-concept studies, where safety risk is lower, as well as mechanism-of-effect studies, which require larger cohorts.

REFERENCES

Akhtar H, et al. (2016) Therapeutic Efficacy of Neurostimulation for Depression: Techniques, Current Modalities, and Future Challenges. Neuroscience Bulletin 32, 115–26.

Armitage R, et al. (2003) The effects of vagus nerve stimulation on sleep EEG on depression: A preliminary report. Journal of Psychosomatic Research 5, 475–82.

Baeken C, et al. (2015). The application of tDCS in psychiatric disorders: a brain imaging view. Socioaffective Neuroscience & Psychology 6, 1–10.

Barker AT, et al. (1985) Non-invasive magnetic stimulation of human motor cortex. The Lancet 1, 1106–7.

Bellesi M, et al. (2014) Enhancement of sleep slow waves: underlying mechanisms and practical consequences. Frontiers in Systems Neuroscience 8, 1–17.

Bikson M, et al. (2016) The off-label use, utility and potential value of tDCS in the clinical; care of particular neuropsychiatric conditions. Journal of Law and Biosciences, 3, 642–6.

Brunoni AR, et al. (2014b) BDNF plasma levels after antidepressant treatment with sertraline and transcranial direct current stimulation: results from a factorial, randomised, sham-controlled trial. European Neuropsychopharmacology 24, 1144–51.

Bystritsky A, et al. (2008) A pilot study of cranial electrotherapy stimulation for generalized anxiety disorder. Journal of Clinical Psychiatry 69, 42–7.

Clark VP and Parasuraman R. (2014) Neuroenhancement: Enhancing brain and mind in health and disease. NeuroImage 85, 889–94.

Cretaz E, et al. (2015) Magnetic seizure therapy for unipolar and bipolar depression: a systematic review. Neural Plasticity 2015, 521398.

Curthoys IS, MacDougall HM. (2012) What galvanic stimulation actually activates Frontiers in Neurology 3, 1–5.

Dahlem MA, et al. (2013) Towards dynamical network biomarkers in neuromodulation of episodic migraine Translational Neuroscience 4, 282–94.

Danilov YP and Kublanov VS. (2014) Emerging Non-invasive Neurostimulation Technologies: CN-NINM and SYMPATOCORECTION. Journal of Behavioral and Brain Science 4, 105–13.

Deisseroth K, et al. (2015) Optogenetics and the circuit dynamics of psychiatric disease JAMA 313, 2019–20.

De Raedt R, et al. (2014) Neurostimulation as an intervention for treatment resistant depression: from research on mechanisms towards targeted neurocognitive strategies Clinical Psychology Review 41, 61–9.

Dhaliwal SK, et al. (2015) Non-invasive brain stimulation for the treatment of symptoms following traumatic brain injury. Frontiers in Psychiatry 6, 1–13.

Dodson MJ. (2004) Vestibular stimulation in mania: a case report. Journal of Neurology, Neurosurgery, and Psychiatry 75, 168–9.

Food and Drug Administration. (2005) *VNS Therapy System for the adjunctive long-term treatment of chronic or recurrent depression.* Available at: https://www.accessdata.fda.gov/cdrh_docs/pdf/P970003S050a.pdf

Felipe RM and Ferrao YA. (2016) Transcranial magnetic stimulation for treatment of major depression during pregnancy: a review. Trends in Psychiatry and Psychotherapy 38, 190–7.

Fertonani A and Miniussi C. (2017) Transcranial Electrical Stimulation: What we know and do not know about mechanisms. The Neuroscientist 23, 109–23.

Fitzgerald PB and Seagrave RA. (2012) Deep brain stimulation in mental health: review of evidence for clinical efficacy. Australian & New Zealand Journal of Psychiatry 49, 979–93.

George MS, et al. (2014) A two-site pilot randomized 3 day trial of high dose left prefrontal repetitive transcranial magnetic stimulation (rTMS) for suicidal inpatients. Brain Stimulation 7, 421–31.

Goel R, et al. (2015) Using low levels of stochastic vestibular stimulation to improve balance function. PLoS One 10, e0136335.

Gomez-Nicola D and Perry VH. (2015) Microglial dynamics and role in the healthy and diseased brain: a paradigm of functional plasticity. The Neuroscientist 21, 169–84.

Goto S, et al. (2004) Subthalamic nucleus stimulation in a parkinsonian patient with previous bilateral thalamotomy. Journal of Neurology, Neurosurgery, and Psychiatry 75, 164–5.

Grabherr L, et al. (2015) The Moving History of Vestibular Stimulation as a Therapeutic Intervention. Multisensory Research 28, 653–87.

Hariz M and Amadio JP. (2015) The new era of neuromodulation. American Medical Association Journal of Ethics 17, 74–81.

Hasan A, et al. (2016) Brain stimulation methods for patients with schizophrenia—new therapies on the horizon? Die Psychiatrie 13, 145–51.

Heinrichs J-H. (2012) The promises and perils of non-invasive brain stimulation. International Journal of Law and Psychiatry 35, 121–9.

Hizli SG, et al. (2014) Transcranial magnetic stimulation during pregnancy. Archives of Women's Mental Health 17, 311–15.

Holtzheimer P and Mayberg H. (2011) Deep brain stimulation for psychiatric disorders. Annual Review of Neuroscience 34, 289–307.

Holtzheimer PE, et al. (2017) *Depression in adults: Overview of neuromodulation procedures.* Available at: https://www.uptodate.com/contents/depression-in-adults-overview-of-neuromodulation-procedures.

Huston JM, et al. (2007) Transcutaneous vagus nerve stimulation reduces serum high mobility group box 1 levels and improves survival in murine sepsis. Critical Care Medicine 35, 2762–8.

International Neuromodulation Society. (2016) Available at: http://www.neuromodulation.com.

Jansen JM, et al. (2013) Effects of non-invasive neurostimulation on craving: a met-analysis. Neuroscience and Biobehavioral Reviews 37, 2472–80.

Kekic M, et al. (2016) A systematic review of the clinical efficacy of transcranial direct current stimulation (tDCS) in psychiatric disorders. Journal of Psychiatric Research 74, 70–86.

Kennedy SH, et al. (2011) Deep brain stimulation for treatment-resistant depression: follow-up after 3 to 6 years. American Journal of Psychiatry 168, 502–10.

Koopman FA, et al. (2016) Vagus nerve stimulation inhibits cytokine production and attenuates disease severity in rheumatoid arthritis. Proceedings of the National Academy of Sciences of the United States of America 113, 8284–9.

Krystal AD, et al. (2010) The effect of vestibular stimulation in four-hour sleep phase advance model of transient insomnia. Journal of Clinical Sleep Medicine 6, 315–21.

Kumar S and Sarkar S. (2016) Neuro-stimulation Techniques for the Management of Anxiety Disorders: An Update. Clinical Psychopharmacology and Neuroscience 14, 330–7.

Kumsa D, et al. (2018) Public regulatory databases as a source of insight for neuromodulation devices stimulation parameters. Neuromodulation 21, 117–25.

Lefaucheur J, et al. (2017) Evidence-based guidelines on the therapeutic uses of transcranial direct current stimulation (tDCS). Clinical Neurophysiology 128, 56–92.

Leuchter AF, et al. (2013) The relationship between brain oscillatory activity and therapeutic effectiveness of transcranial magnetic stimulation in the treatment of major depressive disorder. Frontiers in Human Neuroscience 7, 1–12.

Luan S, et al. (2014) Neuromodulation: present and emerging methods. Frontiers in Neuroengineering 7, 1–9.

Marangell LB, et al. (2007) Neurostimulation therapies in depression: a review of new modalities. Acta Psychiatrica Scandinavica 116, 174–81.

Massimini M, et al. (2007) Triggering sleep slow waves by transcranial magnetic stimulation. Proceedings of the National Academy of Sciences of the United States of America 104, 8496–501.

McIntyre CC, et al. (2004b) How does deep brain stimulation work? Present understanding and future questions. Journal of Clinical Neurophysiology 21, 40–50.

Mekhail NA, et al. (2010) Clinical applications of neurostimulation: forty years later. Pain Practice 10, 103–12.

Miller S, et al. (2016) Neurostimulation in the treatment of primary headaches. Practical Neurology 16, 362–75.

Moseley P, et al. (2016) Non-invasive brain stimulation and auditory verbal hallucinations: new techniques ad future directions. Frontiers in Neuroscience 9, 1–13.

Nardone R, et al. (2015) Neurostimulation in Alzheimer's disease: from basic research to clinical applications. Neurological Sciences 36, 689–700.

National Institute for Health and Care Excellence. (2003) *Deep brain stimulation for Parkinson's disease.* Available at: https://www.nice.org.uk/guidance/ipg19.

National Institute for Health and Care Excellence. (2009) *Vagus nerve stimulation for treatment-resistant depression.* Interventional Procedures Guidance [IPG330]. Available at: https://www.nice.org.uk/guidance/IPG330.

National Institute for Health and Care Excellence. (2013) *Occipital nerve stimulation for intractable chronic migraine.* Interventional Procedures Guidance [IPG452]. Available at: https://www.nice.org.uk/guidance/ipg452.

Noll-Hussong M, et al. (2014) Caloric vestibular stimulation as a treatment for conversion disorder: a case report and medical hypothesis. Frontiers in Psychiatry 5, 1–8.

Nuffield Council on Bioethics. (2013) *Novel Neurotechnologies: intervening in the brain.* London: Nuffield Council on Bioethics.

Panebianco M, et al. (2015) Vagus nerve stimulation for partial seizures. Cochrane Database of Systematic Reviews 4, CD002896.

Pavlov VA and Tracey KJ. (2015) Neural circuitry and immunity. Immunologic Research 63, 38–57.

Preuss N, et al. (2014) Caloric vestibular stimulation modulates affective control and mood. Brain Stimulation 7, 133–40.

Racine E, et al. (2007) Currents of Hope: neurostimulation techniques in US and UK. Cambridge Quarterly of Healthcare Ethics 16, 312–16.

Rajapakse T and Kirton A. (2013) Non-invasive brain stimulation in children: applications and future directions. Translational Neuroscience 4, 217–33.

Reed KL, et al. (2010) Combined occipital and supraorbital neurostimulation for the treatment of chronic migraine headaches: : initial experience. Cephalalgia 30, 260–71.

Remue J, et al. (2016) Does a single neurostimulation really affect mood in healthy individuals? A systematic review. Neuropsychologia 85, 184–98.

Rokyta R and Fricova J. (2015) Noninvasive neuromodulation methods in the treatment of chronic pain. Intech, Chapter 5. Available at: http://dx.doi.org/10.5772/57449.

Schlaepfer TE, et al. (2010) WFSBP Guidelines on Brain Stimulation Treatments in Psychiatry. World Journal of Biological Psychiatry 11, 2–18.

Tortella G, et al. (2015) Transcranial Direct Current Stimulation in Psychiatric Disorders. World Journal of Psychiatry 22, 5, 88–102.

Trentman TL and Schwedt TJ. (2016) Occipital nerve stimulation and beyond: when is invasive peripheral stimulation for headaches appropriate? Expert Review of Neurotherapeutics 16, 237–9.

Tye S, et al. (2009) Disrupting Disordered Neurocircuitry: Treating Refractory Psychiatric Illness with Neuromodulation. Mayo Clinic Proceedings 84, 522–32.

Utz K, et al. (2010) Electrified minds: Transcranial direct current stimulation (tDCS) and Galvanic Vestibular Stimulation (GVS) as methods of non-invasive brain stimulation in neuropsychology—A review of current data and future implications. Neuropsychologia 48, 2789–810.

Vanzan S, et al. (2017). Behavioural improvement in a minimally conscious state after caloric vestibular stimulation: evidence from two single case studies. Clinical Rehabilitation 31, 500–7.

Wagner T, et al. (2007) Noninvasive human brain stimulation. Annual Review of Biomedical Engineering 9, 527–65.

Walter T and Kaube H. (2012) Neurostimulation for chronic cluster headache. Therapeutic Advances in Neurological Disorders 5, 175–80.

Wilkinson D, et al. (2008) Galvanic vestibular stimulation speeds visual memory recall. Experimental Brain Research 189, 241–4.

Wilkinson D, et al. (2014) Galvanic vestibular stimulation in hemispatial neglect Frontiers in Integrative Neuroscience 8, 4.

Wilkinson D, et al. (2013) Caloric vestibular stimulation in aphasic syndrome. Frontiers in Integrative Neuroscience 7, 1–9.

Wilkinson D, et al. (2016). A durable gain in motor and non-motor symptoms of Parkinson's disease following repeated caloric vestibular stimulation: A single-case study. NeuroRehabilitation 38, 179–82.

Wilkinson D, et al. (2017) Preventing episodic migraine with caloric vestibular stimulation: a randomized controlled trial. Headache 57, 1065–87.

World Health Organization. (2011) *Lifting the Burden: Atlas of Headache Disorders and Resources in the World, 2011.* Geneva: World Health Organization.

Zaghi S, et al. (2010) Noninvasive brain stimulation with low-intensity electrical currents: putative mechanisms of action for direct and alternating current stimulation. The Neuroscientist 16, 285–307.

42

Models of neuropsychiatry services and neuropsychiatric care pathways

Rafey Faruqui and George El-Nimr

Introduction and case for specialist neuropsychiatry services

It has been argued that the separation between neurology and psychiatry as two diverse specialist medical disciplines has originated from, or at least has been promoted by, the Cartesian dualism of mind and body in the nineteenth century and the subsequent development of psychoanalysis at the beginning of the twentieth century. We argue that such separation has, by default, placed neuropsychiatry in the 'watershed area' where neither of the two disciplines is fully able to protect it or indeed carry it forward as a distinctive medical sub-specialism. We further argue that this inherent disadvantage also offers growth opportunities by positioning neuropsychiatry as an emerging specialism that is capable of working across complex healthcare pathways and helpful in providing answers to difficult clinical questions related to brain and behaviour.

The scientific advances in neuroimaging, neurophysiological investigations, clinical genetics, and immunology have further strengthened the clinical application of neuropsychiatry by advancing our understanding of the scientific explanation behind a range of health conditions presenting at the brain–behaviour interface. In this context, it could be argued that neuropsychiatry is at the cutting and advancing edge of clinical psychiatric practice across the lifespan.

The first challenge in conceptualizing a neuropsychiatric care pathway is developing a pathway-orientated disease classification model that is able to underpin clinical expertise with knowledge of the patient flow system in a given healthcare system. The next important challenge in this regard is articulating the purpose of a neuropsychiatry service in a given pathway, recognizing that multiple specialist inputs are required in successfully managing these complex care pathways.

It has been proposed that the main role of neuropsychiatry services is to manage psychiatric sequelae of brain disease or injury. Adopting this view, neuropsychiatric conditions can be categorized broadly into progressive neurological conditions (such as Huntington's disease, Parkinson's disease, and various types of dementia) and conditions that involve a degree of acquired brain injury, whether it is traumatic or non-traumatic. However, it is also acknowledged that some neuropsychiatric conditions may not fall neatly within any of these categories. Examples include psychiatric manifestations in the context of epilepsy and sleep disorders and cases of psychosis where an identified organic brain disease is either considered to be causing the condition or contributing towards treatment resistance. The other main function of neuropsychiatry services is caring for patients with unexplained neurological symptoms or functional neurological disorders. Despite the lack of identifiable organic brain pathology in such conditions, neuropsychiatric services do deliver highly regarded services for this patient group. It is also recognized that this patient group could include patients with coexisting neurological and functional presentations such as co-occurrence of epilepsy and non-epileptic attacks in a patient.

In summary, neuropsychiatric services therefore tend to cater broadly for patients with psychiatric effects of neurological disorders, neurological presentation in psychiatric disorders, and coexisting psychiatric and neurological disorders.

We argue that neurology services do traditionally focus on treating the neurological features of the condition, not having the required time, skills, or resources to manage the psychiatric aspects. General psychiatric services, on the other hand, will feel less equipped to look after patients with 'neurological' problems, including evident movement disorders and neuro-disabilities. A specialist neuropsychiatry service provision is therefore clearly required to meet the multifaceted needs of patients with neuropsychiatric disorders and to ensure that they are not being 'discriminated against' or deprived of essential psychiatric care on grounds of case complexity or physical disability. In an acute specialist or a general hospital setting, the patient groups that are most likely to benefit from specialist neuropsychiatry provision are patients stepping down from stroke or trauma pathways and where psychiatric treatment provision needs require clarification due to the presence of an underlying life-threatening brain condition such as brain tumours. Timely neuropsychiatric reviews may also assist in identifying and treating people presenting with suspected or established alcohol-related brain damage (ARBD).

The prevalence of neuropsychiatric problems in common neurological conditions is well documented. This includes brain injury (Deb et al., 1999) and other psychopathology that is identified in other disorders such as epilepsy, Parkinson's disease, Huntington's disease, multiple sclerosis, and stroke (Chemerinski and Robinson, 2000; Feinstein, 2007; Marsh, 2000). There are also data that highlight the prevalence of specific psychiatric problems in neurological populations (e.g. Bridges and Goldberg 1984; Carson et al., 2000; Fink et al., 2003; Jefferies, 2007). Such studies have also indicated that neurologists have a lower rate of recognition for neuropsychiatric conditions and also the low frequency of referring such individuals who have been recognized to have a neuropsychiatric condition. Organic brain conditions in a general psychiatric population are also acknowledged, along with the need for a neuropsychiatric opinion for diagnosis and management. Similarly, conditions like memory disorders, sleep disorders, and developmental neuropsychiatric conditions are traditionally dealt with within a general psychiatry setting and are likely to benefit from a specialist focus provided by neuropsychiatry services.

It is only logical to anticipate that the lack of accessible high-quality neuropsychiatric services would affect patients' quality of life and that of their caregivers and would have an overall impact on disability burden on society (Aarsland et al., 1999; Chipchase and Lincoln 2001; Global Parkinson's Disease Survey Steering Committee, 2002; World Health Organization, 2001).

In the UK, the need for neuropsychiatric care is implied in documents such as the *National Service Framework for Long-term Conditions* (Department of Health, 2005) and disorder-specific documents such as *Rehabilitation Following Acquired Brain Injury: National Clinical Guidelines* (Royal College of Physicians, 2003), *Stepped Care for Functional Neurological Symptoms* (Healthcare Improvement Scotland, 2012), and *Commissioning for Functional Neurological Disorders* (Northern England Strategic Clinical Networks, 2015). It is recognized that despite improvement in the delivery of care for mental health problems in the community, which was supported by a number of important initiatives, such as the National Service Framework (Department of Health, 1999), the current provision of neuropsychiatric services in the UK remains patchy and inadequate (Agrawal et al., 2008).

A model of neuropsychiatry as a bridging discipline spanning neurology, psychiatry, and general medicine

There have been recent attempts to describe the purpose of neuropsychiatry services (Bhattacharya et al., 2015) through broad-based categories, namely:

1. Neuropsychiatric disorder associated with a recognized neurological condition or an organic brain lesion.
2. Neuropsychiatric disorder or mental illness with an as yet unrecognized neurological condition or probable organic aetiology.
3. Functional neurological disorders, excluding primary presentation with general somatoform disorders without prominent neurological symptoms, chronic fatigue, and chronic pain disorders.

4. Other neuropsychiatric conditions—may include specific conditions such as neuropsychiatric sleep disorders, complex neurobehavioural disorders, or neuropsychiatric manifestations of extracranial physical conditions.

A review of the above-mentioned categories identifies a fairly broad-based and overlapping specialist area of practice between a large number of medical specialist disciplines. We argue that neuropsychiatry is a bridging discipline that connects neurology, psychiatry, and general medicine into providing holistic care to a rather complex group of clinical presentations.

Neuropsychiatry as a specialist area of practice has experienced a shifting identity over many decades and across various countries and training schemes. While the term 'neuropsychiatry' refers to a combined approach to the whole of psychiatry and neurology in certain countries, more so in certain historical times, in other countries, it actually refers to a small 'elite' specialism of psychiatry that is practised by a minority of mental health professionals. Furthermore, some behavioural neurologists would use such a term rather loosely to highlight their expertise and area of work. Although this specialty has contributed to a better understanding of mental disorders and has a significant role in formulating an effective management plan, neuropsychiatry service provision remains less appreciated and largely misunderstood.

A number of definitions have been proposed to explain what neuropsychiatry is (Arambepola et al., 2012). These range from being simply an amalgam of neurology and psychiatry, a specialty that deals with disorders that cross the boundaries between these two disciplines, 'a mediator of an artificially created division' to rather simplistically being a specialty that deals with a subsection of psychiatry, namely organic psychiatry. Such definitions are less satisfactory in terms of being able to capture what neuropsychiatry actually is. A more helpful definition is that it is a specialty which 'concerns itself with the complex relationship between human behaviour and brain function, and endeavours to understand abnormal behaviour and behavioural disorders on the basis of an interaction of neurobiological and psychological-social factors' (Sachdev, 2002).

In the above-mentioned context, we propose a functional service model of a bridge with multiple entry and exit points to highlight complex referral pathways and discharge destinations, with a network connecting different medical specialties and professional disciplines. We further propose that such a service model could help align discharge pathways between neurology, psychiatry, elderly care, and neurosurgical departments through the creation of Integrated Managed Clinical Networks working across specialisms and organizational boundaries to look after patients requiring complex case management.

Over recent years, there has been a growing interest in promoting some degree of integration between neurology and psychiatry with regard to clinical practice, as well as training (Eisenberg, 2002; Mitchell and Agrawal, 2005). The nature and scope of specialist training in these two specialist areas have been such that it remains a challenge to provide a universally agreed interface structure for postgraduate training. The educational role of neuropsychiatry services cannot be overemphasized in bridging the curriculum gaps and promoting joint continuous professional development opportunities for neurologists and psychiatrists.

Broad principles for neuropsychiatric service design

Patients with neuropsychiatric disorders should expect comprehensive, person-centred services that are easily accessible and delivered as close to home as possible. Services should have an established and managed interface with social care and physical health services and should be working closely with families, support groups, and relevant voluntary organizations.

Depending on clinical needs and available resources, care could be delivered in various clinical settings, including community care, outpatients, day services, neuroscience liaison (assessing and treating patients on other medical and surgical wards), and specialist inpatient facilities specializing in diagnostics and rehabilitation.

Neuropsychiatric services need to have a clear focus on optimizing functional independence and quality of life, promoting integration within society, maximizing safety, and reducing caregiver burden. It is acknowledged nonetheless that, on occasions, clinicians will have to adopt a rehabilitative model, rather than a curative one, especially in certain irreversible neuropsychiatric conditions. In general terms, patients should expect clinical care that supports assessment, diagnosis, and treatment that employs both curative and rehabilitation models, depending on the nature of the disorder, the clinical presentation, and available treatments.

As a patient group, people with neuropsychiatric conditions tend to require input from a multidisciplinary team to meet their complex clinical needs. Clinical neuropsychiatry practice brings together a number of disciplines, so patients with complex neurological and psychiatric needs related to a brain condition can receive evidence-based treatment that is tailored to meet their complex presentation or disorders.

A competent neuropsychiatrist needs to possess complex case formulation skills, requiring a deep understanding of neurological, psychiatric, neuropsychological, and rehabilitation aspects of the case presentation. It is recommended that a neuropsychiatry multidisciplinary team should include, or have easy access to, the following professional groups:

- Neuropsychiatrist—diagnostic assessments, complex case formulation, brief health education interventions, and medical aspects of care.
- Neuropsychologist—rehabilitation planning, assessment of cognitive functioning, establishing behaviour modification frameworks, and provision of psychological interventions such as cognitive behavioural therapy and cognitive remediation.
- Specialist nursing—referral triage, community case management, group health education interventions.
- Occupational therapist—assessment of functional independence, community rehabilitation, advice on use of assistive technology, and monitoring of daily structure.
- Physiotherapist—mobility and gait assessment, assessment of physical fitness, physical rehabilitation management, use of mechanical aids and robotics.
- Speech and language therapist—swallowing assessment, dysphagia management, assessment of organic and functional speech impairment, speech and voice rehabilitation, use of communication technology.
- Dietician—guiding nutrition management, percutaneous endoscopic gastrostomy (PEG) feeding regimes, management of weight loss, management of significant weight gain, identifying and care planning of organic eating disorders.
- Specialist teacher—post-injury (or disease) literacy and numeracy skills assessment and skills re-acquisition planning, vocational rehabilitation planning.
- Social worker—home life assessment, family liaison, assistance with discharge planning, financial management assistance, work rehabilitation planning.
- Clinical administration staff—handling complex documentation and information flow, service data collection, appointments management.

The above-mentioned list is not exhaustive, and inputs documented against professional staff categories are not mutually exclusive to identified professions. Rehabilitation planning and specific therapy inputs often require co-working between two or more professions. It is important to note in this context that neuropsychiatry multidisciplinary team models are often non-hierarchical in nature in order to promote interdisciplinary or transdisciplinary working.

Challenges in service planning and delivery

Pragmatic issues

While the above-described division between 'organic' and psychiatric services had its historic impact on service planning and delivery, it has been argued that existing neuropsychiatric services will have to justify the significant degree of heterogeneity in their structure and clinical focus. Such variability can range from being tertiary consultation services to 'mainstream' secondary services with dedicated community teams and inpatient facilities.

Given the lack of an agreed framework for neuropsychiatric services, it is difficult to predict what a given service will provide in a given locality and what patients, commissioners, and allied professionals should expect from such services. Certain neuropsychiatric services are more specialist in their focus than others and may only cater for specific disease areas such as tic disorders, sleep disorders, or brain injury; hence the whole service will specifically cater for patients with specific conditions.

It may be argued that the focus of the National Service Framework for mental health on providing comprehensive community services is thought to have placed emphasis in favour of local services, maybe at the expense of regional specialist centres. The closure of Victorian psychiatric hospitals and the move to community treatment at the end of the last century had led to the closure of many of the long-stay wards where neuropsychiatric patients were looked after. The establishment of community centres in a time of economic difficulties had led to neuropsychiatric services being less of a priority, not least with neuropsychiatry not featuring in statutory documents as a specialty that has to be offered by NHS Trusts. In the meantime, with such a gap in the market, the independent sector has quickly 'stepped in' to address such need. In this context, it is noted that four large independent sector organizations are now providing over 500 specialist neuropsychiatric beds in the UK. It is argued that such problems with service provision in neuropsychiatry are at least partly related to the lack of a strategic drive in the public sector. While services for certain disorders (such as acquired brain injury and young-onset dementia) have benefited from a recognizable strategic drive, others are yet to enjoy such privilege. There is indeed a need for a strategic service development drive for the development of coordinated networks of neuropsychiatry services and for recognition of neuropsychiatry as a broad-based specialty.

It is recognized that financial planning and viable business case developments are essential in building a service framework that aligns with the wider health delivery system. It is further recognized that challenges, such as case definition ascertainment and service commissioning, at times hamper the real-life efforts in creating and managing successful service pathways.

Case definition challenges

Agreeing case definitions and case ascertainment is equally difficult to achieve at times. The inadequacy of commonly used classification systems of diseases in addressing and classifying neuropsychiatric conditions does add to the difficulty in undertaking such studies.

As already highlighted, questions like: 'what should be expected from neuropsychiatrists and what should patients expect from neuropsychiatry services?' should certainly be addressed if we are to provide equitable and standardized services for our patients. This should not only improve the quality of care, but also improve communication between stakeholders and establish a common language between clinicians and managers. This should also facilitate the development of quality assurance frameworks.

Commissioning issues

Based on available data, it could be strongly argued that commissioning of neuropsychiatry needs to be streamlined and better integrated. It also needs to be transparent and well identified to ensure equitable access to all patients. An audit (Vhattacharya et al., 2014) indicated that neuropsychiatric service development continues to be negatively affected by the lack of a clear commissioning process. Being at the interface of a number of neuroscience-related disciplines, including neurology and psychiatry, the complex discipline of neuropsychiatry can be at risk of falling between various funding streams. Factors influencing service development could include affiliation to academic institutions, personal influence, leadership, impact of support groups and voluntary organizations, educational and research activities, and support from other stakeholders. This random context of service development has had an impact on national equity of neuropsychiatric service access. Similarly, services could be part of a mental health institution, a neuroscience centre, a rehabilitation unit, or a specialized private unit. At times, patients are therefore left with no alternative but to receive care 'out of area', with a long waiting time and difficult funding battles. This palpable degree of inconsistency in commissioning, along with inequitable access to services, is becoming increasingly concerning. While this is evidenced in the UK, one can assume that it is not too dissimilar in other countries.

Neuropsychiatry continues to receive inadequate and less recognized contribution from a number of funding streams that are 'owned' by other related specialties, including neuro-rehabilitation, old age psychiatry, neurology, neurosurgery, and mental health. Growing knowledge and public expectations place increasing demands on poorly commissioned services to provide equitable, high-quality, and evidence-based care for this patient group.

It is indeed disappointing to see some of the neuropsychiatric services in the UK, for example, having to downsize at a time when a welcome growth of neuroscience and mental health services is witnessed. Ironically, this happens while unrecognized and inadequately treated neuropsychiatric problems in the context of common chronic neurological conditions have been increasingly acknowledged, along with their impact on quality of life, carers' burden, and health economy. The debate of having neuropsychiatry funded by specialist commissioning versus local commissioning is also contributing to the already existing dilemma. While commissioners and providers have felt the lack of 'critical mass' an important barrier in appropriately commissioning neuropsychiatry services, one wonders whether commissioning neuropsychiatric services at a regional level for a larger population would be the way forward or a hub-and-spoke model that incorporates regional specialism with community provision through day hospital-based outreach and the development of sub-specialism of community neuropsychiatry.

Training issues

In some countries, there is considerable uncertainty in relation to the training requirements and core curriculum for trainees who aspire to become neuropsychiatrists. So far there is no specific accreditation system or training pathway that would outline the curricular requirements for a trainee to become a 'recruitable' specialist in this field. In many countries, including the UK, there is a significant degree of variability if one were to scrutinize the quantity and quality of training that existing neuropsychiatrists have received.

It is also worth noting that trainees from related disciplines have repeatedly expressed keenness to access placements and other educational opportunities that would help them shape their career and enhance their knowledge, skills, and attitudes related to their original specialty. There tends to be no agreed process to govern this process and placements are usually organized through personal communications.

Three-tier service model and Managed Care Networks

The broad principles governing good neuropsychiatric care, multidisciplinary team composition, and service structure challenges are covered in the above sections of this chapter. As a general rule, a service structure framework needs to respect the principles of equity, access, and diversity in service provision and planning. It is also important that specific service models should equally be acceptable to all stakeholders and provide evidence-based, efficient, and cost-effective treatment and rehabilitation.

The service models proposed here present a primarily British focus, but in order to keep them meaningful for our international readership, we are not going into details of specialist services commissioning arrangements. It is recognized that service development internationally may follow a local context and also a very different approach to funding, while still benefiting from the British experience in service development and reconfiguration.

We are proposing a three-tier model of neuropsychiatric services connecting neuropsychiatric services located (or co-located) at large neuroscience centres, trauma centres, and stroke units with sub-regional day hospital services (tier-2) integrated with tier-3 community neuropsychiatric services with an outreach function.

We further propose a system of Managed Clinical Networks (MNCs) in health sub-regions to manage access and response systems, in alignment with relevant clinical, social, and voluntary services and ensuring patient flow and cost efficiencies. The MNCs would also ensure that patients are treated close to their homes and, in some cases, by clinicians with a special interest in neuropsychiatry, rather than specialist teams, using a system of outreach clinics and training (Leonard et al., 2002).

Inpatient services

Neuropsychiatric services need connected systems and should have access to a neurology/neuropsychiatry diagnostics unit, neuroradiology and nuclear medicine expertise, and an inpatient rehabilitation unit that is staffed by neuropsychiatry-trained medical, nursing, and therapy staff. Nonetheless, it is acknowledged that some services will only share beds within neuroscience departments or mental health trusts.

It is estimated that 5–10 specialist inpatient beds are needed for a population of 1 million. However, this estimate excludes people with ARBD and those with moderate to severe brain injuries with behavioural difficulties requiring long-stay rehabilitation in locked or secure rehabilitation settings and in complex disability pathways. A number of models have been proposed by various services in an attempt to accommodate the needs of such a heterogenous patient population in a clinically effective and meaningful way. One possibility is that some beds could serve as acute beds—in other words, addressing crisis admissions. Others could serve a neurobehavioural or neuro-rehabilitation function where planned admissions are undertaken. Patients will be admitted to the neurobehavioural unit from acute neuropsychiatry or acute neuroscience services or directly from the community. A dedicated unit for post-traumatic amnesia (post-traumatic brain injury confusion) could be quite valuable; such units will be best placed in close proximity to an acute hospital to ensure adequate medical cover and infrastructure. However, given the practical and financial difficulties in establishing such a unit, these patients can be looked after in an acute neuropsychiatry unit, alongside other acute neuropsychiatric problems. However, special arrangements will be required to ensure effective nursing and therapeutic input for this particular group.

A variation of inpatient neurobehavioural units is provision of residential rehabilitation beds or units in the community, rather than within a psychiatric hospital, which is thought by many patients to be more 'normal' and 'less stigmatizing'. Such provision for relatively less challenging patient groups could achieve significant cost savings through the creation of a less cumbersome governance structure and clinical leadership provided by clinical psychology staff, in collaboration with specialist therapists.

Another potential distinction is to identify a unit or a wing within an inpatient unit where patients with more intense physical health or physical ability needs can be looked after. The other division is to accommodate patients with more behavioural and other mental health needs, including those who are nursed under the Mental Health Act. This is regardless of the underlying disorder.

Disorder-specific units do have their strong advantages in terms of ensuring that patients are looked after by experienced staff that are up-to-date in relation to current evidence. The actual environment and systems will be developed to best suit this specific patient group. Nevertheless, given the great number of neuropsychiatric disorders, most organizations would find it difficult to justify establishing dedicated beds for individual disorders. Moreover, any attempts to do that could obviously lead to the development of 'super-specialist' services, which inadvertently could generate unfavourable heterogeneity among various services at a national level, a position that most neuropsychiatrists would rather avoid. This would also deprive 'mainstream' clinicians of developing specific expertise related to particular disorders. An alternative model is to 'cluster' disorders in a meaningful way that can encompass various disorders with clinical commonalities, e.g. degenerative brain disease versus acquired brain injury or organic versus functional neurological illness.

A decision will have to be made as to where and how patients with severe cognitive impairment and those who are physically frail should be treated.

Regional day services

Day services provide a cost-efficient system of rehabilitation provision, in comparison to costly inpatient units. There are four distinct advantages in establishing a regional day services system:

1. Providing a specialist step-down pathway from inpatient units.
2. Inpatient admission avoidance for people with less intensive rehabilitation needs, thus serving to treat patients close to their home or at their home through outreach work.
3. Promoting specialist practice and retention of staff teams.
4. Acting as a regional training hub.

We argue that the regional location of such services is likely to have higher patient satisfaction and acceptance in accessing assessments and/or rehabilitation without having to be admitted to hospital. Such services can also establish specific therapeutic modules or courses that are time-limited, with a clear agreed set of therapeutic outcomes, and run by a specialist multidisciplinary team. Services, however, should be aware of the risk of being perceived as a day care facility whose primary function is to provide respite to caregivers. This will be quite an unwelcome way of utilizing resources, especially from the view point of healthcare commissioners who will advocate that this should be offered by social care providers.

This aspect of the service is particularly relevant where vocational rehabilitation is considered. Such setting should be able to accommodate equipment and professionals that can deliver various specialist input, including physiotherapy, occupational therapy, speech and language therapy, and neuropsychology. This type of setting will have its difficulties when the service caters for patients who live quite a distance from the service base. An attached outreach team could enhance this aspect of provision through provision of home-based assessments and community follow-ups.

Community neuropsychiatric services

We advocate for establishing community neuropsychiatry teams in every health delivery area. Neuropsychiatric services based in large neuroscience centres have access issues. Once discharged from specialist units, it is difficult for patients to access follow-up despite the often long-term nature of their clinical presentations. In our experience, patients prefer follow-up arrangements and psychology input close to their home areas.

Specialist clinics

Some neuropsychiatric services run specialist clinics for a specific disorder such as Huntington's disease, Tourette syndrome, acquired brain injury, etc. Some of those centres have developed national and international links at various levels, including clinical management, research, and training/education. Nonetheless, it is argued that there is still a place for generic neuropsychiatry clinics to ensure quicker access to clinic and also to ensure that staff continue to utilize generic neuropsychiatry skills.

Referral pathways

The rate of referrals to a neuropsychiatric service is about 20–30 per 100,000 population (Agrawal et al., 2008). Referral pathways vary considerably, depending on several factors. Some services accept referrals only from psychiatrists and neurologists. Such services tend to be tertiary in nature that are run at a regional or national level. Those services can primarily provide consultation services and expect local psychiatry and neurology teams to deliver day-to-day clinical care. Other services tend to accept referrals from general practitioners and other primary care professionals. These services tend to be seen as secondary services where they have their own community teams and inpatient facilities and they deliver care that is comparable to general psychiatry or general neurology services. One drawback of the latter arrangement is that patients tend to be discharged from other psychiatry or neurology services once accepted by neuropsychiatric services. Such complex patients can be disadvantaged by getting deprived from appropriate services/groups that are based in other services. Patients can easily end up receiving less, rather than more, support!

Establishing tertiary services can therefore be a preferred option. Given the expected scarcity of such regional services, the service would primarily accept referrals from secondary services—either mental health or neuroscience specialties. Patients should therefore have had an initial screening by the referring service. Nevertheless, there is an indication from existing literature that the vast majority of referrals to neuropsychiatric services are appropriate, irrespective of the source of referral (Fleminger et al., 2006).

One model is to establish referral pathways that are entirely based on clinical criteria, rather than the source of referral. While generic neuropsychiatry care pathways are welcome, there is a need to also acknowledge the benefit of developing, or at least highlighting, aspects that are specific to individual disorders.

Conclusion

In summary, we advocate a creative understanding of local health integration needs when conceptualizing neuropsychiatric service provision in a defined geographical region. The chapter has provided a critical overview of relevant concepts, challenges, and solutions in establishing neuropsychiatric service pathways. We argue that this is an exciting and rewarding area of service development

that could benefit from integrated service planning and the development of high-standard educational programmes to support work force development needs.

KEY LEARNING POINTS

- This chapter aims to provide the broad principles of service development underpinning good neuropsychiatric care.
- We have utilized our learning from a British service provision context to articulate service design issues relevant to an international health development agenda. The chapter further aims to clarify the purpose and composition of a specialist and multidisciplinary neuropsychiatry team.
- We have advocated for a 'bridging model' for the development of future services in order to embed a holistic care delivery approach into service planning. We have described a three-tier model of service provision and a description of referral pathways in the context of a typical resource-rich health economy.
- However, the key lessons from this chapter could be applied easily to international health contexts where health budgets may be very limited in terms of service provision and human resource development.

REFERENCES

Aarsland D, Larsen JP, Lim NG, et al. Range of neuropsychiatric disturbances in patients with Parkinson's disease. *Journal of Neurology, Neurosurgery & Psychiatry*. 1999;67:492–6.

Agrawal N, Fleminger S, Ring H, Deb S. Neuropsychiatry in the UK: planning the service provision for the 21st century. *Psychiatric Bulletin*. 2008;32:303–6.

Arambepola N, Rickards H, Cavanna A. The evolving discipline and services of neuropsychiatry in the United Kingdom. *Acta Neuropsychiatrica*. 2012;24:191–8.

Bhattacharya R, Rickards H, Agrawal N. Commissioning neuropsychiatry services: barriers and lessons. *BJPsych Bulletin*. 2015;39:291–6.

Bridges K, Goldberg D. Psychiatric illness in inpatients with neurological disorders: patients' views on discussion of emotional problems with neurologists. *BMJ*. 1984;289:656–8.

Carson AJ, Ringbauer B, MacKenzie L, Warlow C, Sharpe M. Neurological disease, emotional disorder, and disability: they are related: a study of 300 consecutive new referrals to a neurology outpatient department. *Journal of Neurology, Neurosurgery & Psychiatry*. 2000;68(2):202–6.

Chemerinski E, Robinson R. The neuropsychiatry of stroke. *Psychosomatics*. 2000;41:5–14.

Chipchase SY, Lincoln NB. Factors associated with carer strain in carers of people with multiple sclerosis. *Disability and Rehabilitation*. 2001;23:768–76.

Deb S, Lyons I, Koutzoukis C, Ali I, McCarthy G. Rate of psychiatric illness 1 year after traumatic brain injury. *American Journal of Psychiatry*. 1999;156:374–8.

Department of Health (1999). *National Service Framework for Mental Health*. Department of Health: London.

Department of Health (2005). *The National Service Framework for Long-Term Conditions*. Department of Health: London.

Eisenberg L. Is it time to integrate neurology and psychiatry? *Neurology Today*. 2002;2(5):4–13.

Feinstein A. Neuropsychiatric syndromes associated with multiple sclerosis. *Journal of Neurology*. 2007;254(S2):II73–6.

Fink P, Hansen MS, Søndergaard L, Frydenberg M. Mental illness in new neurological patients. *Journal of Neurology, Neurosurgery & Psychiatry*. 2003;74(6):817–19.

Fleminger S. The size of demand for specialized neuropsychiatry services: rates of referrals to neuropsychiatric services in the South Thames Region of the United Kingdom. *Journal of Neuropsychiatry*. 2006;18:121–8.

Global Parkinson's Disease Survey (GPDS) Steering Committee. Factors impacting on quality of life in Parkinson's disease: results from an international survey. *Movement Disorders*. 2002;17:60–7.

Healthcare Improvement Scotland (2012). *Stepped Care for Functional Neurological Symptoms*. Healthcare Improvement Scotland: Edinburgh.

Jefferies K, Owino A, Rickards H, Agrawal N. Psychiatric disorders in inpatients on a neurology ward: estimate of prevalence and usefulness of screening questionnaires. *Journal of Neurology, Neurosurgery & Psychiatry*. 2007;78(4):414–16.

Leonard F, Majid S, Sivakumar K, Toone B. Service innovations: a neuropsychiatry outreach clinic. *Psychiatric Bulletin*. 2002;26(3):99–101.

Marsh L. Neuropsychiatric aspects of Parkinson's disease. *Psychosomatics*. 2000;41:15–23.

Mitchell A, Agrawal N. Training in neuropsychiatry: is it time to reintegrate into mainstream psychiatry? *Psychiatric Bulletin*. 2005;29:361–4.

Northern England Strategic Clinical Networks (2015). *Commissioning for Functional Neurological Disorders*. Northern England Strategic Clinical Networks: Newcastle upon Tyne.

Royal College of Physicians (2003). *Rehabilitation Following Acquired Brain Injury*. Royal College of Physicians: London.

Sachdev P. Neuropsychiatry—a discipline for the future. *Journal of Psychosomatic Research*. 2002;53:625–7.

World Health Organization (2001). *The World Health Report (2001): Mental Health: New Understanding, New Hope*. World Health Organization: Geneva.

43

Neuropsychiatry in the criminal courts

Nigel Eastman, Norman A. Poole, and Michael D. Kopelman

Introduction

Forensic psychiatry comprises 'clinical forensic psychiatry', which is concerned with the clinical assessment, treatment, and management of those with mental disorder who have offended or are thought to be at risk of doing so, and 'legal psychiatry', i.e. the law as it relates to all psychiatry. This chapter addresses only the latter, in relation specifically to neuropsychiatry. Further, it addresses only 'criminal legal neuropsychiatry'. Hence, the chapter deals with neuropsychiatric assessment and reporting for the criminal legal process directed at assisting the courts in relation to all stages of the criminal justice process, from police interviewing through trial to sentencing, as well as appeal, but excluding the parole process. Other chapters (see Chapters 2 and 3) offer information relevant to 'clinical forensic neuropsychiatry'.

It will likely assist the reader to be reminded of the nature of criminal legal psychiatric practice generally as a background to considering the interface between specific neuropsychiatric conditions and specific criminal legal questions (beyond the following brief summary, the reader may wish to consult a general forensic psychiatric text such as the *Oxford Specialist Handbook of Forensic Psychiatry* by Eastman et al., 2012).

Law and psychiatry

The purposes of a discipline, and the interests of its practitioners, determine the constructs it uses. Hence, constructs in psychiatry are determined ultimately by its pursuit of human welfare. By contrast, law pursues abstract justice, albeit this may involve balancing the welfare of different parties against one another or that of an individual against societal welfare (Eastman et al., 2012, p. 8).

As a result, there are almost inevitable incongruities inherent in the application of psychiatric evidence towards determining whether criminal defences, or other legal tests, are satisfied (only very rarely does the law 'adopt' a medical construct directly, so as to determine lack of incongruity). Hence differences of purpose almost inevitably determine what amounts to incongruous evidential 'mapping' of medical constructs (e.g. diagnoses or mental state abnormalities) onto any given legal construct (e.g. some specific criminal defence).

More specifically, criminal law is concerned, at trial, solely with responsibility; or, at sentence, with the degree of culpability, the need for punishment, or the risk to others (the only partial exception is sentencing effected by way of mental health legislation). And, in being so, it adopts its own 'mental constructs', e.g. 'confession unreliability' (see Rebutted confessions, p. 512), 'unfitness to plead' (see Unfitness to plead, p. 511), 'insanity' (see Insanity, p. 514), 'diminished responsibility' (see Diminished responsibility, p. 514), and 'automatism' (see Automatism, p. 515), which are alien to medicine.

However, the process of psycho-legal mapping can also be seen as influenced by the degree of 'tightness' of definition of the legal construct in play. Hence, if the mental state is being mapped onto a tight legal definition, then the mapping can be seen as 'focused'; however, where the legal definition concerned is loosely defined, then the mapping is 'blurred'. So highly focused mapping will leave little room for legal discretion (e.g. as with insanity), and blurred mapping will allow much more room for the operation of legal discretion (e.g. as with diminished responsibility).

Thought of in a slightly different way, an attempt to map a medical construct onto a tight legal definition will emphasize any incongruity of the two constructs, whereas mapping onto a loose legal definition will allow room for the application of discretion towards potentially downplaying the significance of the incongruity.

Related to the topic, there is a rich seam of research, both scholarly and increasingly empirical, which comes under the umbrella of 'neuroethics'. This comprises, first, the interface between scientific and ethical constructs; and second, neuroscientific investigation of human ethical decision-making, including, for example, that relevant to 'responsibility'. We deal with neither. However, there are clearly practical medical ethical issues that are inherent to assessing defendants in relation to the criminal legal process, given the great divide between medical and legal purposes and practice, and we do address some of these. Notably, since psychiatry and law operate by applying differing values, or a differing balance of values, for the doctor negotiating the interface between the two is both inherently problematic, and even fraught with ethical danger.

Law and neuropsychiatry

Neuropsychiatry can be relevant to any stage of the criminal legal process. However, issues which commonly arise concern the nature of claimed amnesia for offences and whether this implies automatism (it usually does not); assessment of cognitive impairment (most often dementia) with a view to considering fitness to plead and stand trial; whether there are grounds to support a plea of automatism; and the implications of executive dysfunction, following head trauma or other cause, for a range of legal issues. Moreover, the neuropsychiatrist will often be required to make use of his/her general psychiatric skills in a court case, while being careful not to stray beyond his/her expertise. Neuropsychiatry is, of course, also frequently implicated in civil cases (see Chapter 44).

The forensic neuropsychiatric assessment

Despite the foregoing cautionary text, the neuropsychiatric assessment process (see Chapter 2) is *relatively* well suited to the legal process—given, as it is, to being meticulous, thorough, and often relatively objective. However, the forensic context still poses particular difficulties and complications in regard to both the proper evaluation of subjects* and the presentation of findings in relation to legal issues. Here we describe aspects of optimal assessment, which stand in addition to ordinary clinical neuropsychiatric practice described in other chapters, so as to highlight what may need to be done beyond what would be usual in ordinary clinical practice *and* various potential obstacles to its proper realization within a criminal legal context.

General points concerning assessment

Even before accepting instructions in a case, it is imperative that the lawyer requesting the assessment describes both the legal context, e.g. the alleged offence(s) and 'the prosecution case' (i.e. the narrative), *and* the specific legal questions to which the lawyer considers potential clinical findings may be relevant. This will usually require a dialogue between doctor and lawyer. However, above all, it is imperative never to accept vague instructions to 'provide a medical report'.

In forensic psychiatry, the person being assessed may be a defendant (in criminal or extradition proceedings), or/as well as a litigant (in civil proceedings), and coincidentally s/he may also be a patient. Each role carries, of course, its own particular set of expectations, both clinical and ethical, such that identifying clearly the role involved is crucial. However, for simplicity, we use the noun 'subject' throughout this chapter, unless there is a specific reason for greater precision.

---

* An individual assessed solely for medicolegal purposes is not a 'patient', carrying all that this term implies, ethically, professionally, and legally. Rather s/he may be, for example, a 'suspect' (in relation to 'fitness to be interviewed'), a 'defendant' (in regard to pre-trial, trial, and sentence matters), or an 'appellant' (against conviction or sentence). In order to avoid using multiple such legal terms, we have chosen the generic term 'subject'. We are aware that this seems incongruous with medical practice. However, the term does serve also to emphasize the core message of the chapter, which is that clinico-legal practice is very different from ordinary clinical practice, ethically, legally, and sometimes practically.

Although many, or most, subjects assessed will not be 'patients', but 'defendants', there will still be occasions when the subject is not only a defendant but is already, or previously was, or could in future become, a patient; and this can give rise to major professional ethical concerns and conflicts. We will not address such problems in any detail, since they are inherent to all criminal legal psychiatry. However, it is crucially important to make clear that it is essential explicitly and consciously to think of the subject as a 'defendant', and not a 'patient', with all of the practical and ethical context that goes with that (to many doctors) unfamiliar notion.

Addressing the professional ethical issues in terms of the 'four principles' of 'beneficence', 'non-maleficence', 'autonomy', and 'justice', it is the latter that dominates in all legal psychiatric practice, expressed in terms of 'the primary duty to the court'—this being in clear distinction from the usual dominance of 'beneficence' and 'non-maleficence' within ordinary clinical practice. Indeed, even 'respect for autonomy' can be compromised in some measure within criminal legal psychiatric practice.

Whereas assessment within the clinical setting aims at diagnosis and formulation of the subject's problems with a view to treatment, the forensic neuropsychiatric assessment for a criminal court is fundamentally different in its focus (aside from assessment towards sentencing by way of mental health legislation). Hence, there is likely to be no direct therapeutic benefit offered to the subject; and doctor–patient confidentiality is absent, since the subject is not a 'patient'. Indeed, the subject may even reveal information that is detrimental to his case, yet the assessor must nevertheless include this in his/her report (including, of course, even if instructed by the defence) if it is of any relevance to clinical assessment or to mapping of clinical findings onto a legal test (although, if the report is for the defence, they have the right to withhold it).

It is therefore imperative that the distinct nature of the assessment and the absence of the normal expectations of a clinical consultation are explained to the subject clearly beforehand and that s/he consents to the examination.

In addition, while the core of a forensic neuropsychiatric report is clinical examination and opinion, it should be prepared so as to address the legal question(s) posed by the solicitors and/or court; and again this should be made plain to the subject at the outset. Hence, for example, the focus of clinical assessment may be towards greater emphasis upon the mental state at some time in the past, commonly the time of an alleged offence, than would be appropriate in a purely clinical setting (albeit the latter would be clinically relevant to safe management if he were coincidentally, or were to become, a patient).

It is also important to both bear in mind, and also to make clear to the subject at the outset, that the contemporaneous written notes taken at the time of assessment can be included as part of the current legal proceedings or later in regard to an unrelated legal matter (such as family proceedings, or a mental health tribunal, parole hearing, or a negligence claim).

Finally, bearing in mind that 'psycho-legal mapping' is at the heart of expert evidence, it follows that, even though neuropsychiatric evaluation may reveal evidence of a neurological disorder affecting cognition, emotion, and/or behaviour, this does not necessarily bear upon criminal responsibility or on any other legal issue with which the court is concerned.

The importance of the latter point is emphasized by the fact that psychiatric and legal constructs can often *appear* superficially similar—volition in psychiatry and intention in law, for example—and that this can lead sometimes to miscommunication, and mutual misunderstanding, between expert and court. The competent expert witness must therefore be sufficiently aware of the legal process and relevant tests so as to avoid, or at least minimize, such misunderstanding or miscommunication. Crucially, of course, s/he must aim to assist the court to effect justice (within the ethical principle of 'justice'), and not seek to affect it (within the ethical principle of 'beneficence' or 'non-maleficence').

Sources of information

Clinical assessment

As usual, the subject is interviewed for the purposes of collecting the history and of conducting the mental state and cognitive examinations, while, as the legal case is likely to be a current unresolved stressor, it will be important to consider the effects of this upon the subject's presentation. Furthermore, the subject may well expect a hostile interview or misunderstand the nature and purpose of the assessment, particularly if the prosecution has instructed the psychiatrist. Hence, Rix has described how all subjects, whatever the details of the case and for whom the assessment is being conducted, should be treated with courtesy, respect, sympathetic objectivity, and patience, in order to produce the best possible medicolegal report (Rix, 2011).

If the subject is detained in prison, then permission must be sought from the prison to conduct the assessment, much preferably in the prison's healthcare centre.† It is important to note that failure to access a quiet and confidential environment can adversely affect the quality of the examination and of cognitive testing.

Additional physical investigations and examinations may need to be requested or reviewed. This is especially true of forensic neuropsychiatric assessment in cases where neurological disease is either strongly suspected or already established, albeit its legal relevance may be uncertain. Consenting subjects should therefore undergo a neurological examination, almost certainly conducted in the healthcare centre, plus neuroimaging and blood tests as appropriate. The details and rationales are the same as in the clinical setting. It is worth noting, however, that, in criminal proceedings, the stakes may be extremely high, in a murder trial, for example, so that any suspicion of underlying cerebral pathology that could account for abnormal cognition, emotion, or behaviour, with potential relevance to formulation of the offence, the degree of responsibility, fitness to plead, or sentencing, should be thoroughly pursued. Also, whereas, in clinical practice, it may be appropriate to allow time to reveal the diagnosis, thus saving potentially unnecessary investigations, such luxury is not available in assessment for the court, so that the principles of 'leaving no stone unturned' and of 'doing so now' will likely apply.

The reader should be warned that arranging for specialist investigations is often extremely difficult where a defendant is held on remand in custody, requiring lawyers to negotiate exeats.

Informants

Neuropsychiatrists are accustomed to gaining a good collateral history from informants. Memory impairment, confabulation, difficulties with language comprehension or production, and poor insight, for example, often limit the quality of history obtained from the subject but do, of course, carry implications for the final opinion formed. Ideally, collateral information should be sought from family, friends, colleagues, and professionals (such as a GP or a social worker) who have known the subject for some time. And in some cases, it may be valuable to gain collateral information from witnesses capable of giving information concerning the defendant around the time of the alleged offence beyond what may be available within a witness statement. There may, however, be legal restrictions on doing so, usually where the informant is coincidentally a prosecution witness, so that it is necessary to seek permission from the court or prosecution (giving the assurance that questioning will be restricted to clinical matters). Where the informant is not a prosecution witness, there are few restrictions.

Records

Forensic assessment necessitates fastidious attention to past medical and other records. All medical records must be gained, both NHS (or private) general practice and hospital records, plus inmate medical records (in relation to the current reception into prison and also previous periods in custody), plus the police custody record, in addition to reports previously prepared by psychiatrists or other doctors, including for the legal process, plus social work files—and, if available, school and other educational reports. Where additional material, such as housing or hostel records, is available, that too should also be scrutinized if at all potentially relevant. Letters, diary entries, and other documents produced by the subject can also be used, either with consent or, in its absence, if they form part of the prosecution case. Ideally, these documents should all be reviewed prior to the assessment interview.

Legal papers

Witness statements and police interviews may well be highly relevant to determining both the disorder at the time of the alleged offence and ongoing disorder, as well as to mapping of clinical conclusions onto a given legal definition.

Drawing the information together

All of the foregoing information will be potentially helpful towards forming an opinion concerning the diagnosis plus mental state at the time of the alleged offence, or formulation of the case, including a narrative that incorporates the defendant's disorder in relation to culpability (in relation to the trial) or risk assessment (for sentencing).

A balance sometimes has to be struck between completeness and expediency; the court will have imposed a deadline for the preparation of the report and the Legal Aid Agency is increasingly setting upper limits on the time that can be charged. Yet ethically, and legally, you must be sure that you have had sufficient time, plus access to sufficient sources of information, in order to be able to give

---

† Many doctors insist on assessment in the prison healthcare centre, on the basis that every effort must be made to ensure that the subject feels in as 'safe' a place as possible, so as to minimize the deleterious effect upon assessment that is usually inherent to assessment in prison. Some prisons try to insist on assessment in 'legal visits' (almost always because it is said that the healthcare centre is 'too busy with its NHS work'). Assessment in the healthcare centre is likely to be 'even more crucial' in respect of neuropsychiatric than other psychiatric assessment (see also text).

a confident opinion in regard to all the clinical and legal issues at hand. If you cannot be confident, it is imperative that you inform the court of this and request further time and/or resources. In essence, it is imperative to gain any medical or other records that *could have* a significant bearing upon your current or retrospective clinical assessment or upon mapping of clinical findings onto any legal test or definition.

Neuropsychological assessment

The purpose of a clinical cognitive assessment is to sample various aspects of cognitive function, using tests of graded difficulty (Kopelman, 1994). However, even the better clinical cognitive assessment tools (e.g. Hsieh et al., 2013) are no substitute for a properly structured, quantified, and validated neuropsychological assessment. The latter should be requested (via the lawyers and/or recommended in an interim neuropsychiatric report) whenever putative cognitive impairment may be critical to the legal issues. The findings can then be interpreted in the context of the clinical history and findings, neuroimaging, and other pertinent investigations.

Diagnosis, mental state, and formulation

Diagnosis may be important in establishing the legal relevance of a defendant's condition. However, almost always the devil is in the detail of the mental state, either in relation to the time of the alleged offence (in regard to legal issues relating to culpability) or currently (in regard to 'fitness to plead' or sentencing). Formulation will likely add a suggested 'understanding' of the defendant and offence 'narrative', originating in the diagnosis and mental state, but going beyond these.

Diagnosis

A diagnosis and description of its mental and behavioural manifestations should be stated in the report clearly, with some indication of the level of diagnostic confidence. Include the results of the investigations and psychometric testing that support the diagnosis where relevant, as well as explicitly indicating what information goes against your opinion and the reason(s) for concluding overall as you do.

It is almost always good practice to express diagnosis in terms of one of the two accepted international classification systems. Some experts prefer DSM-5 (American Psychiatric Association, 2013) because it is widely used in research and is expressed in 'required criteria', including the numbers of criteria to be satisfied, and the courts also find such apparent 'precision' fits well the legal model. However, it is important to caution that DSM-5 is not a 'cook book', rather is an aid to, and not a substitute for, clinical diagnosis. Others lean towards the ICD-10 classification scheme (World Health Organization, 1992). However, its looser and prose-like approach may render an opinion more difficult to defend against a hostile and 'adversarial style' cross-examination (either in favour of or against a given diagnosis) than with DSM-5. By contrast, the ICD-10 Diagnostic Criteria for Research (World Health Organization, 1993) uses tighter definitions and can be very valuable in court.

Formulation

Formulation is usually more helpful to the court than the mere diagnosis or mental state description, as it offers an individualized statement about the causal, precipitating, and perpetuating factors relevant to the subject's mental state and behaviour. Such formulation

should include developmental details about early trauma, attachment style, and any early indicators of psychopathy. The latter is especially important where there is uncertainty as to whether antisocial behaviour originates in long-standing personality or has been acquired secondary to brain damage or degeneration. There may be evidence of premorbid impulsivity and risk-taking that contributed to causing, for example, traumatic brain injury, or which has been emphasized by such injury. Hence, the pattern of adult relationships and whether this is relevant to the index offence should also be included within the formulation.

Ideally, a widely adopted model of formulation, such as the biopsychosocial approach, should be presented, and the relevance of any neuropsychiatric disorder to the index offence explained within this. The formulation will also include details of the risk and resilience factors identified on assessment.

Neuropsychiatric findings in relation to specific legal issues‡

'Mapping' clinical findings onto legal definitions and questions

The report provided to lawyers or the court should distinguish clearly between 'facts' and 'opinion', and there should also be a clear distinction between different 'sources of facts', as well as between 'clinical opinion' and 'legal implications' (Eastman et al., 2012, pp. 296–301) (in other words, first describe the relevant clinical opinion and then approach the 'mapping' of this onto any legal definitions indicated as relevant to the legal questions posed). Each legal issue to be addressed in the report should be dealt with under a separate heading in the opinion section of the report.

The opinions expressed should be supported by, and not go beyond, the facts contained within the body of the report, although they must obviously not amount to mere repetition of facts. The reasons for forming the opinions should be provided, and the expert must also be candid about matters that serve to weaken the opinions or that support an alternative opinion, plus the reasons for preferring the opinions expressed.

The rest of the chapter will now address legal issues and definitions to which neuropsychiatric findings are commonly, or sometimes problematically (even if not frequently), relevant. And here it will be important to bear in mind throughout that legal definitions are not only determined by their 'justice' context but are also specific to a particular justice issue. For example, the legal definition of 'fitness to plead' bears no necessary legal relation to 'insanity' as a defence. In regard to each legal issue addressed, we both describe the relevant legal definition(s) and also consider how particular neuropsychiatric findings may (or may not) 'map' onto it/them.

Fitness to be interviewed

The psychiatrist can be asked to assess a subject's fitness to be interviewed by the police at the time of interview or (much more usually)

---

‡ Unless otherwise made plain, we use definitions from the law of England and Wales, though the mapping principles will be similar for similar tests found in other legal jurisdictions (for UK domestic jurisdictions, the alternative tests can be found in the Oxford Specialist Handbook of Forensic Psychiatry, Eastman et al., 1992).

retrospectively, in relation to the admissibility of the interview as evidence or the weight that should be attached to aspects of it.

Determination at the time of interview is usually made by the local forensic medical examiner (FME) or, in more complex cases, by a general psychiatrist (rarely by a forensic psychiatrist). Yet it is very commonly organic brain states that are potentially at issue, e.g. severe intoxication or withdrawal, or learning disability. In addition to considering fitness per se, at the time of the interviews, the clinician will likely also provide an opinion on whether interviewing could be significantly detrimental to the subject's health. However, again, a neuropsychiatrist is unlikely to be consulted at this stage.

Judicial consideration of the admissibility of interview evidence may still require neuropsychiatric expertise where underlying neurological disease or disorder is suspected or established. Often there will have been only a cursory assessment by an FME and notes that offer little detailed clinical information, and this emphasizes the importance of having access to the full custody record. While fitness to be interviewed is not anywhere clearly defined legally, despite its potential profound importance, the Police and Criminal Evidence Act 1984 (PACE) and its Codes of Practice ('the Codes') (Home Office, 2005) imply that it is fundamentally a capacity test (so that it is not the diagnosis that is usually crucial).

The majority of the case law on inadmissibility of interview evidence pertains to subjects with learning difficulties or below-normal intelligence (see Ventress et al., 2008 for a helpful review on this area).

The expert witness must consider the specific effect the condition likely had upon the subject's capacity to deal with the questioning to which he was subjected, since in order to be relevant to determining inadmissibility, it is necessary to demonstrate that the disorder likely led to some unreliability in the evidence given. In order to offer some (not exhaustive) examples, *disorientation to time and place* will likely impact upon a subject's capacity to understand the nature and purpose of the interview; *confabulation* will offer erroneous (or at least unfounded) assertions, which can be either provoked by questioning or spontaneous (the latter resulting from specific brain pathology) (Kopelman, 2010); while *memory impairment* may give rise to apparently incompatible claims that might be taken erroneously as evidence of dissimulation.

Unfitness to plead

Criminal trials proceed on the assumption that the defendant is 'fit to plead', unless s/he is proven not to be so.

The legal test for a finding of 'unfitness' is evidently outdated in scientific terms. Based upon *R v Pritchard* (1836), albeit somewhat extended in *R v M (John)* (2003), the defendant will be found unfit only on what amount to restrictively 'cognitive' bases (the test is exclusive to English law, although similar tests are found in Scotland and the Republic of Ireland).

Specifically, s/he will be found unfit if unable to do one (or more) of the following:

1. understand the nature of the charge(s);
2. decide whether to plead guilty or not;
3. exercise the right to challenge jurors;
4. instruct solicitors and counsel;
5. follow the course of the proceedings;
6. give evidence in his own defence.§

Once the issue is raised (which can be by the defence, the prosecution, or the court), two medical practitioners are required to assess the defendant, and, by convention, they are invited to offer not only a clinical opinion, but also an opinion on whether the legal test is satisfied**; the judge determines whether or not the test is indeed met. When raised by the prosecution or by the court, unfitness must be proved 'beyond reasonable doubt', whereas the lower test of 'on the balance of probabilities' is applied if the issue is raised by the defence.

Once a defendant has been found 'Pritchard unfit', there must then be a 'trial of the facts' before a jury, in order to determine whether the defendant committed the *actus reus* (i.e. the behavioural element of the crime; see The mental element of an offence, p. 514), and only if he is found to have done so will he then be found 'unfit to plead'.

If the defendant is likely to be found unfit to plead due to a treatable condition, then the expert should recommend that the trial be delayed until their mental state can be improved sufficiently, or even optimally, to engage in the trial process. Only if the defendant is unlikely to regain 'fitness' within a reasonable timescale ought a formal hearing against the Pritchard test be recommended.

The bar for a finding of unfitness to plead is set very high by the Pritchard test, even with the addition of the test in *R v M (John)* (2003) requiring fitness to give evidence, resulting in few successful claims; while the recent Law Commission report into fitness to plead also identified that psychiatrists and the courts understood and applied the tests inconsistently. Thus, some defendants are likely to be unfit to be tried and yet remain unidentified as such by the courts. More fundamentally, the Law Commission has recommended that a capacity-based test be enacted, in order to determine that the defendant is capable of 'effective participation' in the trial *and* in order to apply a test which is more congruent with the medical notions of 'disability'.

Beyond the Pritchard test clearly being highly cognitive in nature, even the requirement of the ability to apply normal 'judgement' is eschewed. Hence, in *R v Robertson* (1968), in which the defendant was deluded about the very circumstances of the alleged offence, he was still deemed 'fit', in that 'mere failure of a defendant to decide how to plead in his own best interest does not make him unfit'.

For perhaps obvious reasons of public policy, apparent inability to recall the facts surrounding the alleged offence, arising from anterograde amnesia, has been ruled out as a basis for a finding of unfitness. Specifically, in *R v Podola* (1960), 'hysterical' amnesia for the alleged killing was considered not to make the defendant unfit, in that it did not undermine his ability to follow the trial process or instruct counsel. In *R v M (John)* (2003), the Court of Appeal dismissed a claim that the defendant, found guilty of sexually abusing his granddaughter, should have been considered unfit to plead as a consequence of alcohol-related brain damage, resulting in severe amnesia, in that,

---

§ This was the addition to the test which arose from *R v M (John)* [2003] EWCA Crim 3452.

** This amounts to contravention of the usual rule that experts may not express an opinion upon the 'ultimate (legal) issue'; albeit there is protection against 'trial by expert' by way of the decision being taken by the trial judge (until recently it was a specially empanelled jury that decided).

while he may have been unable to remember evidence soon after it was given, he was considered still able to follow the proceedings with assistance and to make notes of what evidence had been given.

Beyond amnesia, it remains less than clear in many respects what nature and degree of psychiatric and/or cognitive pathology the courts consider capable of undermining fitness to plead, and there remains a lack of rigorous research comparing those considered 'fit' versus those found 'unfit'.

Specifically, as regards the test of 'fitness to give evidence', in *R v M (John)* (2003), it was held that, in order to be fit, a defendant must be able to understand the questions put to him/her, apply his/her mind to answering them, and convey intelligibly to the jury the answers s/he wishes to give. It is not necessary, however, for fitness to be retained that a witness's answers should be plausible, believable, or reliable, or that they should be seen as such by the witness, although failure in any such regard might give rise to separate concerns about the reliability of the evidence s/he might give, and therefore its admissibility, or at least the weight that should be applied to it (see Sentencing, p. 516) (Eastman et al., 2012, pp. 474–7).

Problems with the Pritchard/M test also include that it may well not allow for subtleties of disability. For example, in regard to unfitness to give evidence, the bar seems set at a higher level than is applied, e.g. in respect of finding unreliability in respect of police interviews (see Rebutted confessions), wherein suggestibility or compliance may make answers unreliable and inadmissible or properly carrying of lesser weight. Hence, there is arguably greater protection provided in regard to vulnerable individuals being interrogated by the police than when being cross-examined in court. Also, the individual criteria for finding unfitness to give evidence are liable to differing interpretations (about how to assess and how to define) between experts.

More specifically, conditions such as dysexecutive syndrome or mild Asperger's syndrome (or indeed being from a very different cultural background) might not prevent a witness from meeting the above criteria but might still lead to them being unable to stand up robustly, as would an ordinary defendant, to the sometimes rapid, nuanced, or slanted cross-examination pursued by a barrister intent upon discrediting their evidence.

The evidential impact of such a defendant's relative vulnerability can sometimes be properly limited by allowing expert evidence describing to the jury the nature of his/her mental disorder and how this may influence his/her answers to questions and their body language. However, this may not always amount to adequate counterbalancing. Also, special measures may at least assist in counteracting vulnerability, such as allowing frequent breaks for the witness to regain their composure, about which the expert may properly advise the court.

Unfitness to attend court

Unfitness to attend court bears no necessary relationship to fitness to plead, in that it amounts simply to 'not being in a fit state to attend' (related to either a physical or a psychological disability). Hence, clearly a defendant may be unfit to plead and yet still be fit to attend a hearing, e.g. where s/he, though unfit to plead, may properly be required to attend court for the purposes of some aspect of proceedings, including an 'unfitness hearing'. Or a defendant may be fit to plead yet not be fit to attend court.

There are no specific criteria for unfitness to attend, but in general, it relates to either physical incapacitation or, in the case of mental disorder, the safety of the defendant or others, were they to attend. Psychiatrically, this is more likely to be an issue with inpatients where severe psychotic or other symptoms, or suicidal ideation, determine risk to self or others. And a psychiatrist reporting to the court will clearly be required to consider whether adaptions to the court proceedings, such as allowing a nurse escort or shortened sessions, would facilitate attendance.

As the number of historical child abuse prosecutions rises, there is likely to be an increasing need for neuropsychiatric and old age psychiatric expertise concerning not only fitness to stand trial, but also fitness to attend court. Attendance at court by a defendant with moderate dementia could precipitate a catastrophic reaction, arising from an over-stimulating and/or a disorientating environment, placing themselves and/or others at risk, so that the court may seek an estimate of the likelihood of this occurring, plus advice on how best to manage such an occurrence (a challenge, given the paucity of relevant studies). If you consider that the foregoing applies to one of your subjects, it is important to communicate this voluntarily to the Clerk of the court in good time, as some hearings will have to be adjourned if the defendant cannot be present, whereas others may still be able to proceed. If you report that a defendant is unfit to attend court, it is very helpful to give an indication of how soon the defendant may become fit, if at all, in order to allow proceedings to be rescheduled appropriately.

Fitness of witnesses

Whereas fitness to plead is obviously relevant only to defendants, all witnesses must be fit to give evidence. And again, the issue is one for the judge to determine, based upon expert evidence from psychiatrists. Many witnesses for the prosecution are vulnerable people, such as children, the frail and elderly, or learning disabled, in circumstances where the prosecution case may rely exclusively upon their testimony in order to secure a conviction. Therefore, if they are unfit to give evidence, the trial may have to be abandoned, although, based upon expert advice, special measures can often be applied by the court in order to avoid the trial being lost.

No specific test of fitness of witnesses to give evidence has been developed, although the judge in *R v M (John)* (see Unfitness to plead, p. 513) ruled that a witness must be capable of giving evidence in the same terms as a defendant. Fitness to give evidence is, of course, distinct from consideration of the reliability of the evidence given, which is for the jury to ascertain, potentially including aided by expert evidence.

Rebutted confessions

In England and Wales (but not Scotland), a defendant can be convicted on the sole basis of confession (i.e. in the absence of 'corroborating' evidence). And a psychiatrist, usually combined with a clinical psychologist, may become involved where that confession is later retracted or where other aspects of police interviews that might contribute to a jury finding the defendant guilty, are retracted or otherwise considered to be unreliable.[††]

†† It is important to emphasize that the proper term to use in this context is not 'false confessions' but 'rebutted confessions', since it cannot be known, without trial, whether a confession is false.

There are three types of confession open to rebuttal (Wrightsman and Kassin, 1993). The first is a 'voluntary confession' where the confession was provided willingly, knowing it to be false, in order to achieve some ulterior motive such as protecting a loved one from prosecution or financial gain. This accounts for around half of all rebutted confessions and is particularly common among women protecting their partners and, to a lesser degree, men under 21 years of age shielding peers (Gudjonsson, 2009). The second type is the 'coerced-compliant confession' wherein again the confessor knows the statement to be false but makes it as a result of external or internal pressure. For instance, the defendant may willingly confess in order to end a forceful interrogation, to bolster self-esteem, or to please the interviewer. This may be commoner in those with learning disability, anxiety disorders, and depressive conditions, as they are more likely to comply with others' statements, especially in highly pressured environments. The third form of confession open to rebuttal is the 'coerced-internalized' type. Here the confessor actually believes that the confession is indeed true. Psychologically, this is associated with the trait of 'suggestibility'‡‡, expressed by way of accepting information embedded within questions asked ('yield') and pliability following criticism of answers given ('shift'). The interviewee thus comes to believe the content of the confession, although s/he may later retract it once removed from the interrogative situation. Interrogative suggestibility may be of particular relevance to neuropsychiatrists, as it is associated with poor memory recall, confabulation§§, low intelligence, anxiety, and lack of assertiveness (Gudjonsson et al., 1999).

In regard to each source of giving information to the police which is later rebutted, expert evidence may be applied within a *voir dire* (a 'trial within a trial', in the absence of the jury) wherein the defence seeks to exclude the relevant interviews, or parts thereof. If the defence fails in this regard, so that the interviews, or parts thereof, remain as 'evidence', the same experts may then be asked to give similar evidence in front of the jury, in order for the jury to be properly assisted in determining what weight should be attached to the evidence, reflective of some degree of alleged (un)reliability.

When assessing in relation to a rebutted confession, it is necessary to request the full interview transcripts and/or tapes, since the assessment is not solely of whether the defendant can be shown to exhibit the traits of 'compliance' and/or 'suggestibility', for example, but also whether such traits likely operated in the context of the police interview(s) in question. These should therefore be carefully reviewed for evidence of leading or closed questions to which the defendant responded positively, pressure from the interviewer and/or the interviewee apparently incorporating into subsequent answers information provided within questions, plus whether there was an 'appropriate adult' present and the extent to which that appeared to influence the defendant's responses. Ofshe and Leo (1997) have emphasized that the post-admission narrative must be analysed thoroughly, in that a poor fit between specific statements and particulars of the crime casts doubt upon the reliability of a confession. They described three ways to evaluate the reliability of a confession, in terms of whether: (1) it leads to new evidence; (2) it includes unusual features of the crime not made public; and (3) it includes accurate mundane details of the crime scene.

In many of the circumstances just described, neuropsychological testing of memory and intelligence should be undertaken also by a clinical psychologist, plus psychological testing for the specific traits of 'suggestibility' and 'compliance'. Gudjonsson's validated scales—Gudjonsson Suggestibility Scale 1 (GSS1), GSS2, Gudjonsson Compliance Scale (GCS)—for assessing these are particularly helpful. However, as already emphasized, the presence of these traits merely lays the foundation for the possibility of unreliability, since it must be shown that they operated so as likely to have resulted in unreliable statements.

Suggestibility, as measured by GSS1 and GSS2, has been shown to correlate negatively with both memory function and general tests of intelligence (Gudjonsson, 2009, pp. 360–414). Also, confabulatory responses may be found in those with frontal lobe impairment and intellectual disability, albeit they can also be found in those with a heightened capacity for vivid imagination (Gudjonsson and Young, 2010).

All of the foregoing said, psychiatrists should be mindful that they have no special ability or training towards evaluating the truth or falsity of claims (Halligan et al., 2003), and so they should restrict their reports to giving objective evidence and to statements about likely 'reliability', rather than 'validity'.

Malingering

Defendants may, of course, seek to malinger cognitive deficits, particularly relating to memory for events surrounding the alleged offence, in the hope of evading conviction or minimizing responsibility or punishment.

Malingering is suggested where there are gross discrepancies between observed behaviour or functional abilities *and* performance on tests of cognitive function. It is also suggested where test scores are at odds with known patterns of cognitive impairment or suggest severe impairment across all domains, or where underperformance is suggested (which could be caused by malingering). Caution is required, however, as depression and apathy can also lead to underperformance, particularly on tests requiring effort, and both are common in neuropsychiatric disorders. Differentiating malingered and dissociative amnesia is also difficult.

Psychometric tests, such as the Test of Memory Malingering (TOMM), have been developed that attempt to differentiate between malingered amnesia and true amnestic states. All such tests are based on the principle that malingerers will underperform (e.g. scoring below chance) on tasks that appear onerous but are actually performed satisfactorily by those with an amnestic syndrome. A test that examines the possibility of malingering across a broader range of psychopathological symptoms is the Structured Inventory of Reported Symptoms (SIRS). All such tests, however, require careful interpretation and should only be used by those trained and experienced in neuropsychological assessment of offenders. Also, finding malingering based upon such tests does not rule out mental disorder, since odd patterns of test responses may themselves be determined by disorder, and so reporting of test results alone as relevant to whether a defendant is malingering can be dangerous (Rix and Tracy, 2017; Tracy and Rix, 2017).

---

‡‡ Suggestibility must be distinguished from 'compliance' (going along with propositions) and 'acquiescence' (answering affirmatively to questions), each of which can be assessed by way of psychological instruments.

§§ It is worth noting that Gudjonsson uses confabulation to refer primarily to those memory distortions provoked by questioning, rather than the more florid spontaneous confabulations familiar to neuropsychiatrists.

The mental element of an offence

For most offences, except for crimes of 'strict liability' (such as unlawful parking and indecent exposure), guilt requires coincidence of the *actus reusi* (guilty act) and *mens rea* (guilty mind) where the latter is defined in different ways for different offences (e.g. 'intention' or 'recklessness').

A psychiatrist can be called upon to comment upon the defendant's capacity to have formed the required intent for the offence, at the time of commission of the *actus reus*, i.e. whether he was capable of forming the *mens rea* for the offence (notably the reason, or motive, for committing the *actus* is irrelevant—albeit motive may suggest intention). S/he cannot, however, properly comment upon whether the defendant did form the relevant *mens rea* (since that would contravene the rule that no expert can comment on 'the ultimate issue').

Some crimes require only (what is termed) 'basic intent', while others require 'specific intent'. For example, 'arson with intent to endanger life' requires the specific intent to do so, whereas 'simple arson' is a crime requiring only 'basic intent'. However, there are no consistent and robust criteria whereby particular crimes are determined to require basic or specific intent.

Most commonly the distinction is relevant where the defendant was severely intoxicated at the time of committing the *actus*, such that he *may* (extremely rarely) be able to plead that he lacked the capacity to form specific intent*** (*DPP v Majewski*, 1977). Where the offence charged is one only requiring 'basic intent', even the 'Majewski defence' is not available to a defendant, irrespective of how intoxicated he was (see also Intoxication, p. 516).

Where it cannot be demonstrated that an intoxicated defendant formed the required intent to cause the relevant outcome coincidental with committing the *actus*, but that outcome would have been 'reasonably foreseeable' to such a defendant in an intoxicated state before he became so (whether or not he formed such foresight), then the doctrine of 'presumed prior foresight' operates so to allow his guilt to be established.

In regard to some offences, the required mental element is not 'intention', but 'recklessness' or 'negligence', so that, for example, again it is merely required that a 'reasonable person' would, or should have foreseen the likely harm consequent upon the act.

Application of an 'objective' test in relation to *mens rea*, requiring only that the defendant should have foreseen the likely consequences of his actions, clearly favours the victim and public safety. However, a defendant with a mental disorder may, depending upon the disorder, properly be judged, not as would be the 'reasonable person', and expert evidence (which is rebuttable) may therefore be called by the defence in order to assist the jury towards viewing the defendant according to his particular disordered nature.

As an example, those with frontal lobe impairment are likely to engage in reckless behaviour, given their tendency towards impulsivity, impaired planning, and decreased empathy. The court may regard them as lacking the subjective element necessary to secure conviction or consider the impairment as a mitigating factor in sentencing, although such impairment might serve merely to demonstrate the likelihood that the defendant was, indeed, 'reckless'. The forensic neuropsychiatrist may therefore be required to assess carefully executive function and its relation to the mental element of the crime.

Insanity

Defendants are presumed by the courts to be 'sane', and hence responsible for their actions, so that the burden of proving 'insanity' falls upon the defence, to the proof standard of 'the balance of probability' (not 'beyond reasonable doubt'). The legal threshold is both defined very narrowly and set very high (as with 'unfitness to plead', the issue can be raised also by the prosecution or the court, but with the higher standard of proof of 'beyond reasonable doubt' being required).

The McNaughton rules, 1843, state that, 'to establish a defence on the ground of insanity, it must be clearly proved that, at the time of committing the act, the party accused was labouring under such a *defect of reason*, from *disease of the mind*, as *not to know the nature and quality of the act* he was doing; or, if he did know it, that *he did not know that what he was doing was wrong*' (emphases added).

Clearly, the phrase 'defect of reason' does the bulk of the work in these rules, and notably it is reasoning specifically, rather than cognitive functioning per se, that is crucial. Hence, neither impulsivity nor disinhibited urges can constitute a defect of reason—there might have been distorted reasoning present, but there was likely crudely to have been 'reasoning'. However, in insanity, neuropsychiatric evidence may still be important in assisting whether the defence is made out.

Diminished responsibility

Diminished responsibility is a partial defence, and to murder only, so that successfully pleading the defence leads to a conviction of manslaughter, thereby avoiding the mandatory life sentence for murder.

Section 52, Coroners and Justice Act 2009, amending S.2 Homicide Act 1957, is applicable in England and Wales and Northern Ireland to killings committed after 4 October, 2010. It is detailed and attempts to pay regard to the quasi-medical notion of 'substantial mental impairment arising from a recognised medical condition' (i.e. it offers less incongruousness with medicine than previously).

Hence, in order to succeed in the defence, it must be shown that the defendant was: (1) suffering from an 'abnormality of mental functioning' (in terms of 'substantial impairment' of the defendant's ability to 'understand the nature of his/her own conduct' or 'to form a rational judgement' or 'to exercise self-control') *and* which both (2) 'arose from a recognized medical condition' and (3) 'provides an explanation for the (killing)', meaning it 'was a significant contributory factor'.

The unamended defence was much simpler, being expressed in terms solely of a lay notion of 'abnormality of mind', meaning 'a state so different from that of ordinary human beings that the reasonable man would term it abnormal' *and* with (resultant) 'substantial impairment of mental responsibility' (*R v Byrne*, 1960). However, it was because it was so 'lay' in its definition, albeit depending upon expert evidence for its proof, that amendment was pursued in order to make the defence both more congruent with the medical notion of 'disability' and dependent upon explicit medical diagnosis.

*** Public policy is strongly reflected in the law's attitude that 'self-induced intoxication' shall not be an excuse, unless the defendant was so intoxicated that he was incapable of forming the specific intent required within the offence.

The defence can be established in regard to any type of mental state abnormality ('the mind in all its aspects'; see *R v Byrne*, 1960). Hence, altered consciousness, perception, cognition, mood, and volition are all relevant, except where caused by voluntary or involuntary intoxication. The exception to the foregoing caveat is where addiction is such that, in simple terms, there was 'an irresistible impulse to take the first drink/drug of the day' (*R v Tandy*, 1989), the test being somewhat softened in *R v Stewart* (2010) and *R v Wood* (2008) whereby the addiction can then amount to the relevant 'recognised medical condition'. However, the threshold is set very high, in terms of 'irresistible impulse'.

While medical evidence establishing diminished responsibility is clearly necessary, it is not sufficient, in that there may be conflicting expert evidence, and the decision is ultimately one for the jury (however, the jury may not convict of murder in the face of uncontested expert testimony on medical matters; see *R v Brennan*, 2015).

Similar tests exist for a range of common law jurisdictions; however, the expert should seek clarification from appropriate local resources and the instructing solicitors (all UK jurisdictions are addressed in Eastman et al., 2012).

Automatism

Automatism is defined legally as 'lack of a willed action', so that there cannot have been an *actus reus* (although some scholars suggest the defence is that there was absence of '*mens*', and so there cannot have been '*mens rea*'). In any event, a finding of automatism results formally in acquittal (but if the automatism satisfies the definition of insanity, then the latter determines the legal disposal; see also Sentencing, p. 516). Hence, medically, any condition that determines a total lack of control over one's actions, due to physical or mental disorder, is capable of laying the foundation for a legal automatism. Merely *impaired* control is insufficient for a successful defence; rather, the action must have been both unconscious and wholly involuntary. Yet, as Fenwick (1990) has observed, both adjectives are frustratingly difficult to define. Kopelman (2013) has attempted a pragmatic (rather than philosophically sound) medical definition of 'automatism', i.e. 'an abrupt change of behaviour, in the absence of conscious awareness or memory formation, associated with certain specific clinical disorders, such as epilepsy, parasomnia, hypoglycaemia, and head injury'.

Rather arbitrarily, and perhaps with little medical justification, the law distinguishes between 'sane' and 'insane' automatisms, according to whether or not the cause of the automatism was a legal 'disease of the mind', so that if it was, then necessarily the rest of the insanity defence will also be satisfied. Whether or not the cause will be deemed a 'disease of the mind' has been adjudicated upon two different bases—first, and most usually, whether the cause of the action was 'internal' (disease of the mind) or 'external' (not disease of the mind) (see *R v Quick*, 1973); and second, whether the condition made the defendant violent and is 'prone to recur' (see *Bratty v Attorney-General for Northern Ireland*, 1963).

Causes considered external are psychological and physical trauma, drugs or alcohol taken involuntarily (see earlier concerning voluntary intoxication), and externally induced hypnosis. Internal causation may arise, for example, from epilepsy, stroke, or diabetic hyperglycaemia. This rule has led, however, to the drawing of some very fine distinctions. For example, a hypoglycaemic automatism, induced by administration of insulin, constitutes grounds for a sane automatism (*R v Quick*, 1973), but behaviour in diabetic hyperglycaemia counts as insane automatism (*R v Hennessy*, 1989). A dissociative fugue, or trance state, induced by an unusual and extreme external stressor, such as rape (e.g. in *R v T*, 1990), is considered to be a sane automatism in law, although some doctors would argue that it is not a '*medical* automatism', and so it should not be deemed *to be* a legal automatism. Whereas a dissociative fugue, if not triggered by a major external factor, legally would imply an insane automatism. Thus, 'ordinary stresses and disappointments' of life, such as unrequited love, which cause dissociation, are viewed as internal to the defendant.

Perhaps the archetypal defence of automatism concerns an act carried out during an epileptic seizure, which amounts to an insane automatism. However, a thorough review found only 13 cases of epileptic automatism in the years 1975–2001 (Reuber and Mackay, 2008). It is likely that automatisms involving parasomnias have become more frequently run as a defence, but this rapidly evolving, scientifically and legally somewhat problematic field is beyond the scope of this chapter. Fenwick has helpfully articulated six criteria that should be fulfilled in order for a defence of epileptic automatism to be potentially successfully run, as paraphrased below:

1. The person should be a known epileptic. A claim that the act occurred during a first seizure should be rejected, unless there is overwhelming evidence for this. The case for epileptic automatism is strengthened if there is evidence that the person has experienced ictal or post-ictal automatisms previously and that behaviour during the criminal act is consistent with previous automatisms.

2. The act should be out of character for the individual and inappropriate to the circumstances. A violent act resulting from an automatism during a fight is less likely to persuade the court than one which occurs during a Sunday stroll.

3. There should be no evidence of premeditation or concealment. Evidence of preplanning before the act precludes automatism, and concealment afterwards makes it improbable.

4. On regaining consciousness after an epileptic automatism, a person is unlikely to register the full meaning of the events which have occurred. His natural response to such a situation is immediately to seek help, and not to conceal the evidence of any crime.

5. A witness to the act would be expected to discern an abnormality of consciousness. Features to enquire about include: staring, vacant state, stereotyped movements, disorientation to surroundings, plus inappropriate/incoherent speech.

6. Memory for the act, but not events preceding the automatism, should be impaired.

7. The diagnoses of automatism and epilepsy are based on clinical grounds alone. While investigations such as EEG and neuroimaging can support the diagnosis of epilepsy, they must not be relied upon in court to make the diagnosis. Neurological opinion should be sought where necessary.

The distinction between sane and insane automatism is crucially important in terms of disposal. A sane automatism results in acquittal, because the person did not carry out a willed *actus*. Insane automatism, on the other hand, leads to a finding of 'not guilty by reason of insanity' and, as such, potentially lays the foundation for a mental health disposal under Criminal Procedure (Insanity and Unfitness to Plead) Act (1964, amended 1991).

Intoxication

Automatism cannot be invoked as a defence in the context of voluntary intoxication where the behaviour was a 'natural and probable' consequence of being intoxicated, since the defendant is held responsible via the doctrine of 'presumed foresight'. Neither, again via the doctrine of 'foresight', can voluntary intoxication be used to suggest lack of the required intention for the offence, except in a very particular circumstance. Hence, if the offence requires only 'basic intent' (see The mental element of an offence, p. 514), then no matter how incapacitated the defendant might have been, there is no defence available via voluntary intoxication. Only if the offence requires 'specific intent' and the defendant was so intoxicated that he was incapable of forming the intention for the offence, can voluntary intoxication be pleaded as a defence (see *DPP v Majewski* , 1977 and above), and the level of incapacity required is so high that it is hardly ever pleaded or successfully pleaded. Advice should always be sought from the instructing solicitor as to the mental element required for the alleged crime and the specific test of capacity required.

Nevertheless, voluntary intoxication *can* be used as a defence where the intoxication led to the defendant forming a mistaken belief and, where this had direct relevance, the mental element of a crime. For instance, erroneously believing oneself in danger of a serious assault is a valid defence as, were it to have been true, self-defence can be a complete defence (assuming other aspects of the defence are satisfied). Involuntary intoxication is, however, a defence, as the defendant is deemed to be not responsible for the intoxication or subsequent behaviour. However, there must be clear evidence that the defendant was unaware of the likely intoxication, such as where a drink has been 'spiked' with alcohol or through voluntary use of a drug not 'normally' considered intoxicating or via a side effect from prescribed medications.

Sentencing

If required to do so by Parliament, the judge will apply a mandatory (in the case of murder, for example, that of a 'life sentence'), or an automatic, sentence. In the latter case, the judge has some discretion, in 'exceptional' circumstances. Otherwise, within 'sentencing guidelines' applicable to the offence concerned, the judge will consider the seriousness of the offence, aggravating factors (e.g. hate crimes), mitigating factors (including sometimes mental disorder, genuine remorse, a guilty plea), past convictions, and the perceived risk of re-offending. Sentences may be custodial or 'community'-based, while there can also be orders made ancillary to the sentence (e.g. fines or banning orders). The forensic neuropsychiatrist may be asked to submit a pre-sentence report addressing mitigating factors, future risk, and any possible mental health disposal (but never addressing the appropriate severity of punishment per se). The risk of further offending can have a major impact upon the sentence imposed, towards an increased or even indeterminate sentence. And the neuropsychiatrist may be asked to offer an opinion on risk, placing him/her in an ethically difficult position, the escape from which relies upon application of the duty to assist 'justice', rather than 'to do no harm'.

A neuropsychiatric pre-sentence or sentence report should address specifically whether admission to hospital is warranted. This may be appropriate, for example, in the context of frontotemporal dementia, Huntington's disease, or traumatic brain injury, where appropriate inpatient treatment could ameliorate manifestations of the condition or the risk of future offending (assuming it is deemed the risks cannot be safely managed by community services). However, a report written towards recommending a 'hospital order' may then be used, in fact, by the judge towards imposition of an even lengthier prison sentence than would otherwise have been given, because of the impact of the opinion offered upon the perception of risk to the public. An example of the latter is a well-publicized homicide case where the offender had suffered some degree of personality change as a result of being beaten on the head with a hammer some time before committing the offence.

Conclusion

Assessing defendants for criminal trial or sentencing, as with assessment towards civil legal proceedings, should not be undertaken without training or mentorship and developing experience. The context of assessing for a wholly non-therapeutic purpose (except where recommending a mental health disposal on conviction) is inherently 'alien' to clinicians unused to providing medical evidence directed towards answering wholly non-medical questions, while, in terms of medical ethics, acting in a manner underpinned not by 'beneficence' and 'non-maleficence', but by 'justice', requires a wholly different mindset from that applied within ordinary clinical practice. Even thinking of the subject of assessment always not as a 'patient', but as a 'defendant', requires a conscious effort, but an effort that is crucially important to expend in order to think within the correct paradigm. And this applies as much to forensic neuroscience as to any other forensic psychiatric practice.

Put simply, there is 'expertise in being an expert', in terms of both ethics and practice per se, because the adversarial legal process of common law jurisdictions renders the unwitting clinician vulnerable both to failing to explain his opinion adequately to the court, when giving evidence in chief, and to attack under cross-examination. This is not the usual game of 'cricket' to which the clinician is used. Rather, it is 'rugby–cricket', a game invented and practised by others, and played with 'a small rugby ball', which bounces oddly and in ways that the unwitting medical batsman will be hard-pressed to predict. Playing such a game requires practice, as well as, crucially, a developing and real understanding of the relationship between law and medicine.

KEY LEARNING POINTS

- Medical constructs are distinct from legal constructs, and providing expert medical evidence requires 'mapping' of the former onto one or more of the latter.
- Neuropsychiatric expertise can be requested at each stage of the criminal legal process (from consideration of fitness of a suspect to be interviewed to fitness of a defendant to plead and stand trial, through to issues relating to criminal responsibility and sentencing), and there is therefore a range of criminal legal constructs in relation to which an expert may be asked

to offer an opinion. Each is distinct and implies a particular mapping exercise.

- Discuss the case first with the instructing lawyer, and be clear on the legal questions and tests that the medical evidence is required to address.
- You should have available to you all of the legal papers and medical records, plus a detailed letter of instruction, before examining the defendant or interviewing any informant.
- An individualized formulation addressing the causal, including precipitating and perpetuating, factors linking any mental disorder to relevant legal tests is often required by the court, beyond simply giving details of the diagnosis or of the likely mental state at a particular time.
- You may be asked incorrectly to address 'the ultimate issue' in a case, such as not only whether the defendant was capable of forming the *mens rea* for the particular offence (which it is permissible to answer), but also whether s/he did, in fact, form the required *mens rea*. This must be resisted.
- Attention to the possibility of malingering or exaggeration is particularly important in a legal context, and the 'validity' basis of any opinion should be explicitly addressed in the report.
- Of course a doctor offering a 'neuropsychiatric' opinion should have appropriate training and expertise relating to the topic at hand, such as is covered elsewhere in this volume. However, s/he should also have clinico-legal training and experience in regard to the application of clinical findings to the legal process.
- Your primary duty is to the court, and not to the side that has instructed you.

LAW REPORTS

Bratty v Attorney-General for Northern Ireland [1963] 1 AC 386.
R v Brennan [2015] 1 Cr App R 14.
R v Byrne [1960] 2 QB 396.
R v Hennessy [1989] EWCA Crim 1.
R v M (John) [2003] EWCA Crim 3452.
DPP v Majewski [1977] AC 443.
R v Podola [1960] 1 QB 325.
R v Pritchard [1836] 7 CP 303.
R v Quick [1973] 1 QB 910.
R v Robertson [1968] 3 AllER 557.
R v Stewart [2010] EWCA Crim 2159
R v T [1990] CrimLR 256
R v Tandy [1989] 1 WLR 350.
R v Wood [2008] EWCA Crim 1305.

REFERENCES

American Psychiatric Association. (2013). *Diagnostic and Statistical Manual of Mental Disorders* (fifth edition). Arlington, VA: American Psychiatric Publishing.

Eastman, N., Adshead, G., Fox, S., Latham, R., and Whyte, S. (2012). *Oxford Specialist Handbooks in Psychiatry: Forensic Psychiatry*. Oxford: Oxford University Press.

Fenwick, P. (1990). Automatism, medicine and the law. *Psychological Medicine. Monograph Supplement*, S17, 1–27.

Gudjonsson, G.H. (2009). *The Psychology of Interrogations and Confessions: A Handbook*. Chichester: John Wiley & Sons.

Gudjonsson, G.H., Kopelman, M.D., and MacKeith, J.A.C. (1999). Unreliable admissions to homicide: A case of misdiagnosis of amnesia and misuse of abreaction technique. *British Journal of Psychiatry*, 174, 455–9.

Gudjonsson, G. H. and Young, S. (2010). Does confabulation in memory predict suggestibility beyond IQ and memory? *Personality and Individual Differences*, 49, 65–7.

Halligan, P.W., Bass, C., and Oakley, D.A. (2003). Wilful deception as illness behaviour. In: Halligan, P.W., Bass, C., and Oakley, D.A. (editors). *Malingering and Illness Deception*. Oxford: Oxford University Press, pp. 3–30.

Home Office. (2005). *Police and Criminal Evidence Act 1984* (s.60(1)(a), s.60A(1), and s.66(1)). Codes of Practice A–G, 2005 edition. London: The Stationery Office.

Hsieh, S., Schuberta, S., Hoona, C., Mioshia, E., and Hodges, J.H. (2013). Validation of the Addenbrooke's Cognitive Examination III in Frontotemporal Dementia and Alzheimer's Disease. *Dementia and Geriatric Cognitive Disorders*, 36, 242–50.

Kopelman, M.D. (1994). Structured psychiatric interview: assessment of the cognitive state. *British Journal of Hospital Medicine*, 52, 277–81.

Kopelman, M.D. (2010). Varieties of confabulation and delusion. *Cognitive Neuropsychiatry*, 15, 14–37.

Kopelman, M. (2013). Memory disorders in the law courts. *Medico-Legal Journal*, 81, 18–28.

Ofshe, R.J. and Leo, R.A. (1997). The decision to confess falsely: rational choice and irrational action. *Denver University Law Review*, 74, 976–1122.

Reuber, M. and Mackay, R.D. (2008). Epileptic automatisms in the criminal courts: 13 cases tried in England and Wales between 1975 and 2001. *Epilespia*, 49, 138–45.

Rix, K. (2011). The medico-legal consultation. In: *Expert Psychiatric Evidence*. London: RCPsych Publications, pp. 26–34.

Rix, K.J.B. and Tracy, D.K. (2017). Malingering mental disorders: Medicolegal reporting. *Advances in Psychiatric Treatment*, 23, 115–22.

Tracy, D.K. and Rix, J.B. (2017). Malingering mental disorders: Clinical assessment. *Advances in Psychiatric Treatment*, 23, 27–35.

Ventress, M.A., Rix, K.J.B., and Kent, J.H. (2008). Keeping PACE: fitness to be interviewed by the police. *Advances in Psychiatric Treatment*, 14, 369–81.

World Health Organization. (1992). *The ICD-10 classification of mental and behavioural disorders: clinical descriptions and diagnostic guidelines*. Geneva: World Health Organization.

World Health Organization. (1993). *The ICD-10 classification of mental and behavioural disorders: diagnostic criteria for research*. Geneva: World Health Organization.

Wrightsman, L. S. and Kassin, S. M. (1993). *Confessions in the Courtroom*. Newbury Park, CA: SAGE Publications.

Guidelines for the Assessment of General Damages in Personal Injury Cases. These are updated frequently and neuropsychiatrists should be familiar with the categories and degrees of severity of 'brain and head injury' and 'psychiatric and psychological damage'.

Secondly, 'special damages' are awarded for direct financial loss such as loss of earnings, care costs, and therapy costs. Before any compensation can be awarded, it has to be decided or agreed (between the parties) whether D is 100% liable for the injuries or whether there has been some 'contributory negligence' on the part of C (such as not wearing a seatbelt). In the event of a substantial degree of contributory negligence, this will have a significant effect on the final amount in compensation and, since legal costs will generally be paid out of the compensation first, then this may significantly affect whether C or their legal team will be prepared to go on with the claim.

Other financial aspects which the medical expert may wish to understand in greater detail include periodical payments, in which compensation is paid to C at regular intervals, rather than in a single lump sum, and the financial significance of finding C to lack mental capacity either to conduct the litigation or to manage the compensation awarded, or both.

Finally, in understanding the motivations of lawyers when 'settling' cases, it behoves the expert to be aware that if, when a case comes to court, C is awarded a smaller sum than D had already offered and which C had rejected, then C will have to pay D's legal costs, as well as their own, from the date of C's rejected offer.

Such considerations add spice to the difficult calculations which the legal teams will need to make. It is, of course, not any part of the medical expert's job to be involved in such calculations, but understanding them at a basic level will assist the expert in understanding the outcome of their cases, the great majority of which will be settled out of court and sometimes in apparent disregard of the expert's opinion as to the level of damage and how it has been occasioned.

Preparation of the expert

It is very important, before embarking on any medicolegal work, that the expert trains and develops skills as an expert. A clinician can be pre-eminent in their own clinical field, but of very little use to the court as an expert if they have not accepted that the law often works in a fundamentally different way from the way in which clinical work proceeds. A lack of proper awareness of these differences can result in bruised egos or worse. The medical expert should attend training courses in the writing of medicolegal reports and oral testimony as a minimum. Continuing professional education should be undertaken so as to keep up-to-date with important medicolegal cases and judgements. An active medicolegal expert would generally be expected to join one or more expert witness organizations and to read their publications. Experts, in addition to attending continuing professional development and belonging to a peer group relating to their clinical work, should also do so, if necessary separately, in relation to their medicolegal work and this should include case-based discussion of their medicolegal work (Rix, 2011, p. 232).

Training must include an understanding of how the law of negligence operates and what the tests are for negligence. The tort of negligence has three components: (1) a duty of care owed by D to C; (2) a breach of the duty by D; and (3) damage resulting from the breach of duty. The tests for negligence are set out in Box 44.2.

> **Box 44.2** The legal tests for medical negligence
>
> 'The true test for establishing negligence in diagnosis or treatment ... is whether he has been proved guilty of such failure as no doctor of ordinary skill would be guilty or if acting with ordinary care'.[1]
>
> 'The test is the standard of the ordinary skilled man exercising and professing to have that special skill ... it is sufficient if he exercises the ordinary skill of an ordinary competent man exercising that particular art ... he is not guilty of negligence if he has acted in accordance with a practice accepted as proper by a responsible body of medical men skilled in that particular art'.[2]
>
> 'The use of these adjectives ('responsible', 'reasonable', 'respectable') all show that the court has to be satisfied that the exponents of the body of opinion relied upon can demonstrate that such opinion has a logical basis ... the judge before accepting a body of opinion as being responsible, reasonable or respectable, will need to be satisfied that, in forming their views, the experts have directed their minds to the comparative risks and benefits and have reached a defensible conclusion on the matter'.[3]
>
> [1] Hunter v Hanley [1955] SLT 213.
> [2] Bolam v Friern Hospital Management Committee [1957] 1 WLR 582.
> [3] Bolitho v City and Hackney Health Authority [1998] AC 232.

However, where consent is an issue, the *Bolam* test does not apply and the test is one of informed consent (*Montgomery v Lanarkshire Health Board (Scotland)*, 2015). The doctor's duty is to provide comprehensible information sufficient for the patient to exercise choice having regard to what the prudent patient, in the patient's circumstances and with the patient's characteristics, would want to know (Rix, 2017).

In practice, an expert may be expected to advise as to whether there was a breach of duty (the 'liability' issue) and whether damage resulted from the breach (the 'causation' issue). Was the neuropsychiatrist under a duty to carry out a cognitive examination and, in failing to do so, did they do what no neuropsychiatrist of ordinary skill and acting with ordinary care would have done having regard to a responsible, reasonable, or respectable body of neuropsychiatric opinion? Did the delay in carrying out a CT scan make any difference to the outcome and, if it did, what injury would not have occurred but for that delay?

Of vital importance for the medical expert is that they can reasonably claim expertise in the area or areas about which they have been asked to provide opinions. This expertise is usually by way of training, study, and sufficient experience in that particular field and nurtured by a process of continuing professional development. It would be inappropriate, for instance, for a psychiatrist, or even a neuropsychiatrist, who had no real experience of the assessment and management of the long-term complications of severe head injuries, to become involved in such cases where these are the issues. All experts will have to prepare a medicolegal curriculum vitae. Lengthy experience of looking after, for example, people who have suffered from head injuries will often outweigh a long list of scientific works in a vaguely related field. In general, the neuropsychiatrist will cover the effects, organic and psychological, of head injuries (from minor to severe), anoxic and metabolic brain injury, and sometimes the late effects of perinatal injury (although children must only be assessed by those with neuropaediatric expertise), and, if they have the experience, they may reasonably be asked to deal with somatic symptom disorders, post-traumatic stress disorder, and, nearly always, the psychiatric effects of injury, including depression and anxiety.

It is the responsibility of the expert to limit their evidence to matters of which they have sufficient knowledge or experience. This was demonstrated in the cases of *Meadow v General Medical Council* (2006) and *Pool v General Medical Council* (2014). Rather than being deterred by the Meadow and Pool judgements, experts who assist the court in neuropsychiatric cases may take some comfort in the case of *Huntley v Simmons* (2010). In this case, it was argued that, where the issue was the community treatment and prognosis of someone with brain damage, the principally relevant expertise was not neuropsychiatric or neurological, but neuropsychological. The judge was not persuaded that the issue was one on which a neuropsychiatrist or neurologist was unable to express a valid opinion and added 'clinicians do not operate in impermeable boxes'.

What matters are the expert's training and experience and their relevance to the issues in the case. The psychiatrist who sets out what they believe to be their relevant training and experience and is explicit about any relevant gaps before they accept instructions and who then confines their evidence to their field of expertise ought to have no fear of criticism.

When dealing with the question of whether it is within the expert's area of expertise, it may be helpful for the expert to ask themselves whether they would feel happy to assess and treat such a case in their clinical practice. Indeed they should be prepared to answer in cross-examination a question as to when they last did so. If the answer will be that they have not, or have not done so for a long time, then the expert would be well advised to decline instructions.

Once the expert is properly prepared for the job, they must then become aware of the likely process and progress of any particular case in which they are reporting. They must be aware of the timescale within which an assessment and report are expected by the court. The court will set precise dates by which expert reports, joint statements, and other such matters must be finalized. Therefore, if the expert is to do a proper job, they may well have to clear their desk of other matters or refuse instructions which could not be completed in time.

The sequence of events in relation to any particular medicolegal instruction usually starts with an instruction letter which should provide a clear outline of the issues, the timescale, and an agreement to pay the expert's reasonable fees. The expert is often reminded of the CPR declaration and of the requirement for the appropriate statement of truth. The expert, unless this is a 'desktop' report, should then arrange to interview C and any relevant others. Adequate time for the consultation must be given. All relevant documentation must be reviewed by the expert and if important pieces of information are missing (e.g. an MRI scan report or school and work records), then this must be pointed out and the opinions given may be only preliminary. Following this, the report will be prepared and sent to the instructing solicitor, who will then generally discuss it with their client (D or C). The solicitor may then seek further clarification or may even attempt to put pressure on the expert to change their opinion. Any such pressure should be resisted unless the expert is persuaded, on the basis of their own assessment or consideration, for example, of new evidence or argument about their reasoning, that a change of opinion is justified. Following payment, the instructing party owns the report, but the expert still owns, and must be able to justify, the opinion. Following

the preparation and receipt of what may be a draft report, there is then often a conference with counsel to test the evidence that the expert is giving and possibly to attempt to influence the expert to shift from their independent and unbiased position, or at least to reconsider it. Reports will then usually be exchanged with the 'other side' and the expert will often be asked questions ('Part 35 questions'). Further 'clarification' may be sought from the expert from time to time over ensuing months or years and new information may be sent for comment.

The next step will generally be the preparation of a joint statement between experts of like discipline (at times a contentious issue). For over 20 years, but put on a formal basis in the 1999 Civil Procedure Rules, there have been provisions for experts' discussions and a joint statement of matters agreed and disagreed. A recent case (*Siegel v Pummell*, 2015) illustrates, for the benefit of all experts, what can go wrong. It is of particular relevance because one expert was a neuropsychiatrist. The judge was critical of 'the attitude of, respectively, (the neuropsychiatrist) and (the psychologist) who were incapable of approaching the exercise in anything like the cooperative spirit which it requires' and said that 'it was obvious that the joint statement process was no longer contributing to an effective and proportionate disposal of the litigation. That circumstance had arisen out of the mutual intransigence and disrespect between (the neuropsychiatrist) and (the psychologist) and their mutual unwillingness to cooperate with one another.' Experts must concentrate on the issues relevant to their specialism. They are there to help the judge resolve these issues. The judge is ultimately likely to be far more interested in the underlying issues than the level of qualification of the experts. An expert demonstrates expertise by doing their best to help the tribunal in a fair, transparent, and independent way, not by belittling their opposite number.

It is important to cooperate (and to be seen to cooperate) with the opposing expert as far as possible. The role of an expert is to provide an expert opinion, and not to act as an advocate for the instructing party.

If the case goes to court, which only occurs in some 5% of civil cases, then the expert's opinion will be tested as to its reasoned logic, impartiality, and objective basis. The expert should be aware that, at any time in the process, a 'Part 36 offer' of settlement from D can be made, including when the case is actually being heard in court. Further discussion will take place, sometimes with the expert witness being asked for additional expert opinion about such matters as current prognosis and future care and therapy needs at this time. Subject to the court's approval, the case may then be settled.

Preparation of the neuropsychiatric report

The expert's approach to C at interview is very important. There is generally no use at all in alienating C, for instance by frequent interruptions or expressions of opinion during the interview. Claimants are increasingly recording the consultation; if that happens, then it is sensible for the expert to do likewise. At the start of the consultation, the expert should explain to C the purpose of the examination, the expert's impartiality, what will happen to the information given by the claimant, how confidentiality is missing from the medicolegal process (i.e. there is nothing off the record), the likely course of the consultation, and the time it will take. A written consent form can assist (Rix, 2011, pp. 250–1). Claimants will usually report back to their solicitor on the demeanour of the expert. The expert should be aware that adverse comments from C may be heard in court. It is sensible to have read at least the medical documentation before the interview and it is often helpful to refer C to previous records in order to give C a chance to explain matters. However, the expert must not refer to any documentation which has not yet been 'disclosed' to the opponents (such as so far undisclosed expert reports). Since the expert usually has only one interview with C, a considerable amount of 'diplomacy' may be needed in order to obtain a full history, whereas in clinical practice, the secrets may emerge over a period of time.

Having interviewed and examined C, usually at length, along with relevant others, and having read all of the documentation available (pleadings as to the claim and its defence, witness statements, every medical record available, educational records, occupational records, criminal records, care records, other expert reports, and any other documentation), the expert's opinion can be prepared.

An expert report should be understandable to the intelligent, educated, but non-medical person. Every word and concept in the report should be considered carefully. Any opinion expressed should take account of all the information available and should encompass a reasonable range of opinion. Any opinion must be defendable in court where, if heard, it should stand up to hostile scrutiny.

The use of scientific literature should probably be sparing and closely to the point. If and when scientific papers are used, they should be part of the accepted and established medical and informed view; 'cherry-picking' of findings is to be avoided. It is often preferable to use an authoritative scientific review than to quote a series of scientific papers dealing with small and specific issues. It is also important to realize that any scientific literature produced for the court will be scrutinized in full and there may well be various caveats written in the paper itself, such is the nature of scientific papers. These may throw doubt upon the results and such doubts will be pounced upon by opposing counsel (and probably by experts for the 'other side').

In *Mitchell v Allianz Cornhill* (2008), the judge was critical of experts whose 'evidence paid either insufficient or no attention' to a WHO report which concluded that it was clear that there were no long-term residual effects of mild traumatic brain injury in children and of which the other party's expert said, 'You cannot get any better evidence'. Indeed one expert was not even aware of the WHO report. The judge castigated C's experts for not subjecting the methodology and conclusions in the report to critical comment.

The report must be set out in a logical and clearly structured way. Different experts use different structures, but all reports must contain a summary of the substance of all material instructions and details of the consultation (date, duration, place of interview, and the presence of others), complying where appropriate with the *Guidance*. The report will need to include a summary of the conclusions, which is often most helpfully placed at the beginning of the report, having been prepared once the report has been completed. It is then sensible to include a short paragraph about what the claimant was told about the consultation process or to refer to an appended copy of the consent form.

The neuropsychiatric expert will then generally want to set out the content of the interview with the claimant. It is important to remember that court reports should be clear, cogent, and engaging.

They are generally the presentation of an inherently complex narrative which is a rational distillation of the individual's story. It will therefore include relevant aspects of family history, early and more recent life experiences, important relationships, use of alcohol and other drugs, medical history, and psychiatric history. It is generally best to have a template for the history-taking which can then be dictated or typed straight into the report. It is important to include as much verbatim content as is possible. The expert may well be referred back to their notes, either in conference with counsel or in court, and for which they must be retained.

The expert should always be aware that almost any C's narrative will contain what have been referred to as 'contextual lies'. These include such things as leaving out details (e.g. to protect the claimant's dignity or family secrets), a degree of embellishment and emphasis, family myths, as well as biased tone, and emotional evasion. Whereas the goal is, of course, for both C and the expert to tell the truth, as well as to give a persuasive narrative, what the expert sets out as facts are only assumed facts and the court will decide what facts form the basis for its decision. The expert must therefore not leave out the 'difficult' bits of the history and must enquire about them with C.

Neuropsychiatrists should set out the examination of C's mental state, which will include relevant negatives (such as that the patient was not depressed). The neuropsychiatric expert will often need to carry out a clinical cognitive examination, preferably using an accepted methodology (such as the Addenbrooke's Cognitive Examination—ACE III). However, this may not be necessary or could be confounding if C has recently undergone a full neuropsychological examination or is about to do so.

The account of the examination is then followed by the documentary 'factual' basis (statements, records) and then other opinion (expert reports), but being careful not to duplicate unnecessarily what is already available to the court.

The author's opinion section will, of course, be the most important part of the report. This should be set out in a logical and reasoned fashion, and it should address each one of the identified issues in the case. If it appears that there are other issues which ought to be addressed, this will need the approval of the instructing solicitors as they may be issues already agreed or which it has been decided not to address.

It would be usual to start with a description of the neuropsychiatric injuries and some comment about other injuries. In a head injury case, for instance, the severity of the head injury should be discussed, or in a case of psychological injury, the nature of the potentially traumatizing experience should be set out.

There should then be a very important section relating to pre-accident vulnerabilities of health or personality and any newly intervening factors of relevance which have occurred since the time of the accident so as to inform the opinion as to causation.

There should then be a section relating to the current neuropsychiatric condition, perhaps initially without any presumption as to the causation of any ongoing problems. This should take into account not only the assessment of C's condition on examination, but also other evidence such as witness statements. In *C v Dixon* (2009), there was an issue as to the impact of frontal lobe difficulties or organic personality disorder on the claimant's day-to-day functioning. It was the evidence of a general psychiatrist that the claimant's disabilities were far less than the professionals believed, but the court rejected this on the basis that it was not borne out by the lay evidence.

Following this, there will generally be a section relating to the likely causation of any such problems. Here, the expert may be creeping into legal territory, and so extra care is required. The court needs to build up a view as to what would have happened to the claimant 'but for' the accident or allegedly negligent treatment. There may be complex matters such as whether the problems arising were reasonably foreseeable, the 'eggshell skull' issue as to the unforeseen effects of some predisposition, additive effects, and whether the failure of reasonable care ('the tort wrong') likely resulted in all or some of the adverse condition. There may well be no single cause of the adverse condition, in which case the expert will need to consider whether the index event has made a 'material contribution' to the condition. All these are very subtle matters which will be helped by wide reading of the medicolegal literature, as well as by seeking appropriate advice about the law from instructing solicitors and listening to it.

The expert must remember that any agreed failure of care may not actually have been the, or the only, cause of the claimed damage. The understandable human presumption that if something happens after some specific event, then that event must have caused that thing to happen must be examined carefully, as it may be wrong for a variety of reasons. However, the legal dictum '*res ipsa loquitur*' (the thing speaks for itself) may appear persuasive. A balance of logic and reasoning must be achieved in which the expert, as far as is possible, comes to a carefully argued, independent conclusion about causation ('on the balance of probabilities').

Following the 'condition and causation' part of the report, there should then usually be a section as to the likely prognosis and the need for case management and care (unless only a 'liability and causation' report has been requested).

The opinion section must not introduce new facts. The expert should almost never write 'always' or 'never'. The expert must remember that saying that something is 'possible' or 'may be the case' is of very little use to the court. The expert should avoid using such terms as 'clearly' and 'obviously'. The expert is generally better advised not to use legal terms in the report. The expert must avoid even codified personal attacks on other experts when commenting upon their reports.

The report should be very carefully drafted and checked, so that the precise use of words can assist the court. It should be checked not only for readability, typographic errors, and solecisms, but also that a reasonable range of opinion has been set out, whether the opinions expressed can logically be drawn from the facts and assumed facts, and whether any inconsistencies (for instance, between interview content and the medical records or any surveillance) have been carefully addressed. It is not for the expert to tell the court that the claimant is lying nor to give opinions on matters of fact other than where expert opinion can inform the court's findings as to the facts. However, the expert must assess C's clinical plausibility. Only the neuropsychiatrist will be able to assist the court as to whether C's presentation is consistent with what is encountered in ordinary clinical neuropsychiatric practice.

Just as too much scientific evidence and medical detail may overwhelm or underimpress the court, the opinion should not contain too much 'heart-searching' and repetitive reasoning. The court will have a great deal of reading to do and will generally be much more appreciative of a concise, reasoned argument than a lengthy exposition, either of the experts' established views or of the experts' quavering uncertainty.

It may be appropriate for a neuropsychiatric expert to recommend, either in the report itself or in a supplementary letter, that additional expertise needs to be obtained. For instance, C may have said that they are troubled with hearing or balance problems which have not emerged elsewhere and the expert may wish, if appropriate, to draw the solicitor's attention to the need for an expert opinion on this matter. However, the courts also require that any such recommendations should be proportional to the likely value of the case.

In a complex case, the expert will need to acknowledge the difficulties and the potential range of opinion on a matter, and if in truth, the expert cannot make up their mind, then they will have to express the honest opinion that, on the basis of the current evidence, an opinion ('on balance') cannot be expressed. In that event, the expert will need to identify the factors which are important and which need to be resolved. Every case, until it arrives at a settlement or a court ruling, is an ongoing process. An individual complex case often cannot rely upon epidemiological evidence from large populations or on specific scientific studies and must therefore rely upon 'clinical expertise' and experience. If there is no single clear causation, the expert may need, if that is their opinion, to state that the original event has made a 'material contribution' (which must be 'more than minimal') to the adverse condition. It is generally best for the expert to avoid giving precise percentages of attribution, as these can nearly always be challenged, but it helps the court to offer some general indication as to proportion. In *Smith v LC Window Fashions Ltd* (2009), albeit that the issue was prognosis, rather than causation, the neuropsychiatrists were asked to estimate the risk of the seriously brain-injured claimant's marriage breaking down as this would have implications for his care needs. C's neuropsychiatrist estimated the likelihood as 10–15% and D's neuropsychiatrist simply said that it was unlikely. The judge decided it was 10%.

Finally, it is important that the expert does not, other than exceptionally, offer an opinion on what is called the 'ultimate issue', for instance compensation. An exception is in a case of alleged medical negligence where the judge wants to know, for example, if the neuropsychiatrist exercised the ordinary skill of an ordinary, competent neuropsychiatrist. In such cases, as the judge stated in *Routestone Ltd v Minories Finance Ltd* (1977), there is no need to 'simply creep up to the opinion without giving it'.

Some key issues in personal injury cases

Constitutional or traumatic?

In many cases, there is an issue as to whether or not the head injury is the cause of subsequent behavioural change. *Mitchell v Allianz Cornhill* (2008) is the case of a boy who was 7 years old when he was injured in a road traffic accident and is illustrative of how the court may approach this issue. The judge rejected the evidence called on his behalf to the effect that the serious behavioural problems which he manifested were the result of brain injury. He found that, as a matter of fact, the boy had not been rendered unconscious and that 'the evidence … to the effect that he suffered a brain injury in the accident was essentially inferential in nature.' Also the neuropsychological test results were inconsistent with acquired brain injury and

Box 44.3 Criteria by which to test whether a particular behaviour has been caused by a brain injury

(a) The severity of the brain injury (mild, moderate, or severe, assessed by the duration of loss of consciousness at the time of the accident);

(b) The epidemiological evidence about the effects, if any, of brain injury on the severity suffered by the subject;

(c) Whether the injury suffered was focal or diffuse; and, if there is any doubt about whether brain injury of a particular severity can cause particular neurological deficits;

(d) Whether neuropsychological test results show deficits in those areas of brain functioning that accord with the behaviour which is suggested to be a consequence of the brain injury.

(*Mitchell v Allianz Cornhill*, 2008, ScotCS CSOH 132)

the mental state examination findings of three experts were not consistent with diffuse axonal brain injury. This led the judge to set out the scientific criteria against which any hypothesis that that particular behaviour has been caused by a brain injury has to be tested (see Box 44.3). The judge found that the evidence of C's experts failed to satisfy these criteria and failed to establish any brain injury with neurological consequences.

Organic or psychogenic?

A number of contentious cases involving neuropsychiatric evidence have been contentious because there has been disagreement as to whether symptomatology is organic or psychogenic. Although these distinctions may have implications for treatment and prognosis, the court found in *Telles v South West SHA* (2008), where it was not possible to separate the organic cognitive impairment from any non-organic impairment, that C was entitled in law to recover as against D for her reasonable needs flowing from both (once the court, as it did, had excluded malingering for financial gain).

Care

Another contentious issue in head injury cases is often care and, in particular, whether the actual level of care being provided is more than the claimant needs. In *Edwards v Martin* (2010), the court found a wide gulf between the neuropsychiatrists. The neuropsychiatrist instructed by C identified a lifelong need for a carer or support worker and a case manager, but the neuropsychiatrist instructed by D argued that this would lead to C continuing to depend on others when he could do much more for himself. The judge found for C on this issue and in doing so enunciated a principle, which is fundamental to the law of tort and to which heed should be paid in other similar cases:

'The principle which I must apply is to endeavour to place the Claimant, as far as reasonably possible, into the position he would have been in but for the injuries he sustained as a result of the tort. I interpret the word "need" in this wider context rather than in the narrower context which might justify the withdrawal of regular weekly support and case manager input. Just as I am satisfied that the Claimant would be unable to manage his financial affairs, I am satisfied that to maintain a reasonable quality of life he needs regular professional support.'[4]

Capacity issues

In head injury cases and other cases of organic brain disease, neuropsychiatrists may be asked for their opinion on capacity. The specific issues are often capacity to litigate and capacity to manage property and financial affairs (Rix, 2011, Chapter 8), but other types of decision-making, such as testamentary capacity, may also arise. The precise examination of this issue in the light of the Mental Capacity Act 2005 should be set out. This will often be a very complex matter in which, for instance, C's impulsivity in 'real life' must be taken into account and a balance achieved between overprotective recommendation of the removal of liberties which are 'presumed' in the Act on the one hand and reasonable protection from vulnerabilities due to disorder of brain or mind on the other.

In *Verlander v Rahman* (2012), the neuropsychiatrists agreed that the C's 'impulsivity prevents her from properly weighing the necessary information to make a decision about her money'. However, in *V v R* (2011), although it was the contention of the neuropsychiatrist that C, who had sustained a closed head injury and exhibited impulsivity, lacked litigation capacity, the judge concluded that this evidence went only so far as to prove that C would have difficulties, and not that she would be unable to weigh the evidence and make the relevant decisions.

In a number of the contentious capacity cases, the disagreements between the psychiatrists have often had more to do with the weight they have attached to evidence in the case than with aspects of neuropsychiatry. The courts recognize, as, for example, in *Loughlin v Singh & Ors* (2013), that 'many of the points cut in both directions'.

Cases involving frontal lobe injury seem particularly contentious. One reason seems to be because there is a difference between the artificial environment, as it were, of the consulting room and the real world. As was put in *Loughlin*:

'... it is very well recognised that folk with frontal lobe brain injuries say one thing and do another. And it's the unpredictability of the real world that renders them vulnerable. So with all the best intentions he may have wished to do something, but in certain circumstances, given unpredictable conditions, he could easily do the opposite. And that's my concern, that he would be vulnerable in an unpredicted and unmanaged environment.'[5]

Malingering

It is for the judge to make an assessment of the reliability of the witnesses, including C. As the fundamental feature of malingering is dishonesty, an opinion to the effect that C is malingering will come so close to usurping the role of the judge in assessing their honesty that it is best avoided.

Rix and Tracy (2017) have suggested a framework for use in reports where malingering is suspected. This includes consideration of diagnostic evidence from the history and mental state examination, including discrepancies and C's response to exploration of their previous medical history, particularly a relevant documented history which is not mentioned or about which concealment is attempted; diagnostic evidence from psychometric testing (Tracy, 2014) such as clinical scales used to support a diagnosis and scales utilized to assess malingering; and diagnostic evidence from any collateral and

---

[4] Edwards v Martin [2010] EWHC 570 (QB). © Crown copyright.

[5] Loughlin v Singh & Ors [2013] EWHC 1641 (QB).

secondary information sources. These all lead to a balanced objective summary account of those factors that are in favour of and those against the illness or diagnosis and their relative strengths, an active consideration of the likely effect of possible diagnostic confounders and biases, and expert opinion on the plausibility of C's difficulties being fully accounted for by psychiatric, neurological, or developmental factors. These are put forward in a straightforward, logical sequence, so as to assist the court in determining C's credibility.

In *Ali v Caton & Motor Insurers Bureau* (2013), C suffered a very severe brain injury as a result of a road traffic accident. D submitted that C had been consistently malingering and relied on the fact that after the accident, C attended a further education college where he demonstrated a level of cognitive functioning and motivation inconsistent with his case; there was evidence of deliberate exaggeration on psychometric tests, including symptom validity tests; his performance was worse than it had been during months of residential rehabilitation, and of his own volition and initiative, he had taken and passed the UK citizenship test. Although the court found that C had knowingly underperformed in medicolegal examinations, it found in his favour and rejected D's submission. The judgement in this case reveals how expert evidence is used and tested in cases where malingering is an issue.

The case of *Edwards v Martin* (2010), where it was agreed that C suffered an organic personality disorder, went to trial because there was an issue as to the severity of C's neuropsychiatric problems. Evidence included covert surveillance and neuropsychological testing. Although D's psychologist argued that there was no genuine neuropsychological explanation for C's performance on some of the tests, C's neuropsychologist would not accept that a finding of deliberate exaggeration could be justified on the strength of psychometric testing alone. He stressed the importance of taking into account the lay evidence and other professionals' evidence as to the nature and extent of C's disability. He argued that there could be other explanations for the inconsistencies. The judge found that there had been no conscious exaggeration on C's part and commented on D's expert's reliance on effort testing and how she stood alone in expressing the view that C consciously exaggerated his disability and did so solely on the strength of these tests.

Some practical advice

The medical expert should remember that, unlike clinical practice, the civil courts are essentially all about money. The expert, although always remaining a medical professional, will need to consider the level of financial remuneration which they would expect from this level of work. It is always preferable to have a prepared contract to send to solicitors for them to sign before the expert does any work. The expert should have a method for checking that these have been signed and returned. In most medicolegal practice, it is essential to have an efficient PA/secretary who, sooner or later, becomes an experienced medicolegal PA. The expert will need to decide where the consultations are to take place and, if on NHS premises, would need to discuss this with line managers. They will need to consider their hourly rate, their rate for days in court, and the issue of cancellation/non-attendance fees. The expert will need to deal with the question of solicitors who say that they are only willing to pay at the end of the litigation, in which case an appropriate percentage uplift should

reflect their payment of income tax on fees not yet received and the risk of non-payment. Experts are firmly advised against 'conditional fees' (fees conditional upon whether the case is successful or not), not least because only extremely exceptionally will the courts accept them. A medical expert who is considering doing more than a minimal amount of medicolegal work will need to think about their professional profile, marketing of their expertise, the tax situation, and their professional indemnity. They will particularly need to consider how they will fit this into their clinical work (and indeed their leisure time).

The medical expert should remember that he or she is generally only thought of as being as good as their last court appearance. Instructing lawyers rarely comment upon the expert's competence, but they rarely forget their cases and how the expert has performed. The only way that the expert may find out about this is because they have not been instructed again. In view of the fact that fewer and fewer court appearances are taking place, such opinions are often formed when experts attend conferences with counsel and therefore careful preparation, as if for a court appearance, should be undertaken before such conferences.

This chapter has dealt very little with appearance in court, partly because it is relatively rare now, but also because the advice about report writing applies equally to appearances in court. If the report has been properly prepared and cogently argued, and if the expert has considered the whole range of opinion and can deal with it in what might be a hostile (although always polite) debate, then the expert should really have no problem, as long as he or she does not become upset, fearful, or angry.

KEY LEARNING POINTS

- Acting as an expert neuropsychiatric witness requires training as an expert witness, as well as competence in neuropsychiatry as evidenced by training or experience.
- If the expert is to do a proper job, they may well have to clear their desk of other matters or refuse instructions which cannot be completed in time.
- Civil litigation can only offer monetary redress in the form of financial compensation for the effects of the wrongful act on the part of the defendant.
- It is the responsibility of the expert to limit their evidence to matters of which they have sufficient knowledge or experience.
- Any pressure to change an opinion should be resisted, unless the expert is persuaded, on the basis of their own assessment or consideration, for example, of new evidence or argument about their reasoning, that a change of opinion is justified.
- It is important to cooperate (and to be seen to cooperate) with the opposing expert as far as possible.
- The opinion section will be the most important part of the report.
- The opinion should be set out in a logical and reasoned fashion, and it should address each of the identified issues in the case.
- The court will generally be much more appreciative of a concise, reasoned argument than a lengthy exposition.
- The expert is generally only thought of as being as good as their last court appearance, their last conference with counsel, or their last report.

LAW REPORTS

AC v Omar Farooq, The Motor Insurers Bureau (2012) EWHC 1484 (QB).

Ahmad v Cleasby (2006) EWHC 3687 (QB)

Ali v Caton & Motor Insurers Bureau (2013) *EWHC* 1730 (QB).

Bolam v Friern Hospital Management Committee (1957) 1 WLR 582.

Bolitho v City and Hackney Health Authority (1998) AC 232.

C v Dixon (2009) EWHC 708 (QB).

DPP v Kilbourne (1973) AC 729.

Edwards v Martin (2010) EWHC 570 (QB).

Hunter v Hanley (1955) SLT 213.

Huntley v Simmons (2010) EWCA Civ 54.

Kerr v Stiell Facilities Limited (2009) CSOH 67.

LN v Surrey NHS Primary Care Trust (2011) UKUT 76 (AAC).

Loughlin v Singh & Ors (2013) EWHC 1641 (QB).

Meadow v General Medical Council (2006) 1 WLR 1452, C.

Mitchell v Allianz Cornhill (2008) ScotCS CSOH 132.

Montgomery v Lanarkshire Health Board (Scotland) (2015) UKSC 11.

Pool v General Medical Council (2014) EWHC 3791 (Admin).

R v Bunnis (1964) *50* WWR, 422.

R v Turner (1975) *1* All ER 70.

Routestone Ltd v Minories Finance Ltd (1977) BCC 180.

Siegel v Pummell (2015) EWHC 195 (QB).

Smith v LC Window Fashions Ltd (2009) EWHC 1532 QB.

Telles v South West SHA (2008) EWHC 292 (QB).

V v R (2011) EWHC 822 (QB).

Verlander v Rahman (2012) EWHC 1026 (QB).

REFERENCES

Civil Justice Council (2014) *Guidance for the instruction of experts in civil claims.*

Judicial College (2015) *Guidelines for the Assessment of General Damages in Personal Injury Cases.*

Malek HM (editor) (2013) *Phipson on Evidence* (18th edition). London: Sweet and Maxwell.

Rix K, Eastman N, Adshead G (2015) *Responsibilities of psychiatrists who provide expert opinion to courts and tribunals.* College Report CR193. London: Royal College of Psychiatrists.

Rix KJB (2011) *Expert Psychiatric Evidence.* London: RCPsych Publications,

Rix KJB (2017) After a prolonged gestation and difficult labour, informed consent is safely delivered into English and Scottish law. *BJPsych Advances* **23**:63–72.

Rix KJB, Tracy DK (2017) Malingering mental disorders: medicolegal reporting. *BJPsych Advances* **23**:115–22.

Tracy DK (2014) Evaluating malingering in cognitive and memory examinations: a guide for clinicians. *Advances in Psychiatric Treatment* **20**:405–12.

SECTION 4

Perspectives of neuropsychiatry worldwide

45

Neuropsychiatric services in Australia and New Zealand

Greg Finucane, Adith Mohan, and Perminder S. Sachdev

Introduction

This chapter will focus on neuropsychiatric services offered within the public health sector in Australia and New Zealand for the adult population, while recognizing that there are a number of psychiatrists in Australasia who offer largely outpatient neuropsychiatric care in the private sector. Paediatric and adolescent services are outside its scope, although some services, such as the Alfred Health Neuropsychiatry Clinic in Caulfield, Melbourne extend their adolescent service to age 24 years. The scope also excludes intellectual disability services, while acknowledging that neuropsychiatrists do assist with the care of adults with developmental disorders, such as attention-deficit/hyperactivity disorder (ADHD) and autism spectrum disorders (Taylor et al., 2016), and some, such as the Department of Developmental Disability Neuropsychiatry at The Prince of Wales Hospital in Sydney, have this as their exclusive focus.

In Australia, which has a federal system of government, the Federal Minister of Health administers the national health policy, and the state and territory governments manage healthcare resources within their jurisdictions, including the operation of public hospitals and particular healthcare services. The overall healthcare expenditure in 2015–2016, according to the Australian Institute of Health and Welfare (2016) was A$170.4 billion for a population of 24 million, representing 10.3% of the gross domestic product. Of this, A$9 billion (5.2%) was spent on mental health. In New Zealand, the Ministry of Health controls public funding, and services are provided and managed through a system of 20 District Health Boards. The New Zealand Treasury indicates that NZ$15.6 billion was the core Crown health spending in New Zealand in the 2015/16 financial year (Government of New Zealand, 2016) for a population of 4.5 million. There is no centralized guidance or contracting to ensure access to neuropsychiatry services in the Australian or New Zealand healthcare systems. However, in Australia, a National Mental Health Service Planning Framework is now online (https://nmhspf.org.au), and the draft of the Fifth National Mental Health Plan intends supporting integrated planning and service delivery at the regional level, steered by data, to reduce service gaps and duplication and to target areas of highest need. While in the past, individuals with neuropsychiatric disorders, such as those with psychiatric

sequelae of traumatic brain injury, epilepsy, and Huntington's disease, were often managed in state institutions, there has now been an almost complete shift to treatment in short-stay general hospital inpatient units and management in the community, but often with inadequate resources and bedevilled by a highly variable population density and large geographical distances (see Fig. 45.1).

New South Wales

New South Wales (NSW) is the most populous state in Australia, with 7.7 million residents, roughly 4.6 million of whom live in the greater Sydney area (Australian Bureau of Statistics, 2016). There are two tertiary neuropsychiatry services in the state based in the coastal cities of Sydney and Newcastle. These are the Neuropsychiatric Institute (NPI) in Sydney and the Neuropsychiatry Service in Newcastle. These units operate within a tertiary consultation framework receiving referrals primarily from psychiatry and clinical neuroscience (neurology and neurosurgery) in both public and private sectors, but additionally are referred patients by other medical specialties, such as rheumatology, immunology, infectious diseases, anaesthesia, and pain services, as well as primary care providers. The services provided may be categorized broadly as outpatient clinics and consultation–liaison and inpatient services, consistent with services across the globe (Agrawal et al., 2008, 2015; Fleminger et al., 2006).

The clinical team within each NSW service comprises two neuropsychiatrists, two neuropsychologists, and up to two postgraduate trainees, in addition to administrative and research staff. The respective local health districts' mental health programmes host the neuropsychiatry services, providing the operational and governance structures, while commissioning the services from their centralized mental health budgets. Additional funding from specific streams within neurology support both services, increasing available neuropsychiatrist time. At the NPI, this is directed towards running a specialist epilepsy-neuropsychiatry clinic and an epilepsy consultation service, assisting in the care and management of patients with neuropsychiatric morbidity in epilepsy, as well as those undergoing surgical intervention for treatment-refractory epilepsy. In the Newcastle

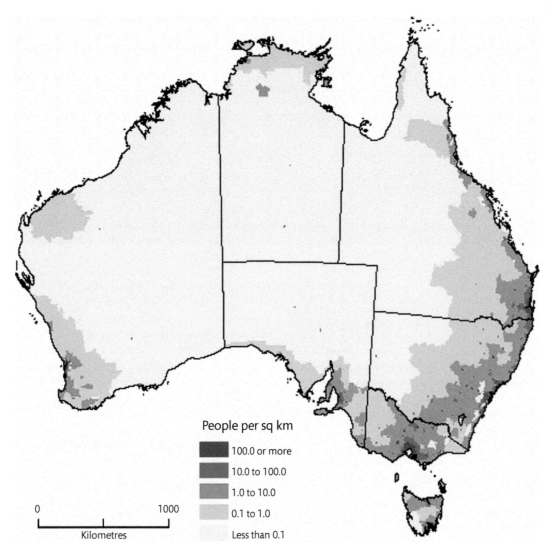

Fig. 45.1 Map of Australian population density, June 2017.

Reproduced from the Australian Bureau of Statistics. Population Density by SA2, Australia – June 2017. In: *3218.0 - Regional Population Growth, Australia, 2016–17*. www.abs. gov.au. Distributed under the terms of the Creative Commons Attribution 4.0 International (CC BY 4.0). https://creativecommons.org/licenses/by/4.0/.

People per sq km

- 100.0 or more
- 10.0 to 100.0
- 1.0 to 10.0
- 0.1 to 1.0
- Less than 0.1

0 — 1000
Kilometres

Neuropsychiatry Service, the director of the service (a behavioural neurologist by training) remains on staff within the general hospital neurology department. Core disorders are catered for to span the care and treatment of patients with psychiatric morbidity in neurological disorders, neurological presentations in psychiatric disorders, disorders characterized by neurological morbidity putatively driven by psychological factors, and coexisting psychiatric and neurological morbidity. There is some variability in the specific disorders for which each service caters, with greater numbers of patients with epilepsy and neurodevelopmental and tic disorders being seen at the NPI, for example, while the Newcastle unit has links with the local traumatic brain injury (TBI) and Huntington's disease services.

With inpatient services, the NPI has been subject to considerable downsizing over the last two decades, and currently the service offers two tertiary beds fulfilling a primarily diagnostic function. Being sited within a major tertiary metropolitan teaching hospital in Sydney, the inpatient arm of the NPI does, however, benefit from easy access to specialist neurology, neurosurgery, and immunology consultations within the general hospital, as well as a video-EEG

telemetry unit, functional neuroimaging facilities, and academic clinics in complex mood disorders, frontotemporal and young-onset dementias, and neurostimulation, among others. Such access is critical to complex patients referred to the NPI for diagnosis. By contrast, the Newcastle Neuropsychiatry Service retains a 12-bed specialized neuropsychiatry unit for assessment, treatment, and rehabilitation inpatient services for people aged 18 years or older with behavioural, psychiatric, and/or cognitive disturbances due to brain injury or disease. Being located on site at a regional hospital location, the unit offers a more generous median length of stay, relative to the average 1- to 2-week duration at the NPI, allowing for a more multidisciplinary interventional focus. Given the regional location of the unit, on-site access to specialist medical input is, however, limited.

Each service also functions as a regional 'hub' fulfilling key teaching and research functions, these being key facets of neuropsychiatry as a clinical academic discipline (Sachdev and Mohan, 2013). The NPI has an impressive track record of research in neuropsychiatry, having actively established research programmes on drug-induced movement disorders, neurocognitive disorders, and tic disorders, to name but a few, in addition to having a clinical and research focus on neurostimulation in neuropsychiatric disorders. In Newcastle, clinicians and infrastructure related to neurostimulation services are soon to merge with the current Neuropsychiatry Service to jointly form a Centre for Neuropsychiatry, Neuropsychology, and Neurostimulation, considerably expanding the potential for research in this area.

Victoria

Victoria is the second most populous state with 5.9 million residents, with Melbourne as the state capital. The premier tertiary neuropsychiatric service is the Royal Melbourne Hospital (RMH) Neuropsychiatry Unit. The Neuropsychiatry Unit is the clinical arm of the Melbourne Neuropsychiatry Centre (MNC), a research centre jointly funded by the University of Melbourne and Melbourne Health. The MNC is directed by a scientific director and a clinical director. The RMH Neuropsychiatry Unit provides a state-wide service for neuropsychiatric assessment and advice, taking referrals from public and private specialists working in mental health services, general medical and neurological services, and general practitioners. Referrals are primarily from Victoria but may be accepted from outside the state in appropriate circumstances. The Neuropsychiatry Unit approach is multidisciplinary, with neuropsychology, occupational therapy, social work, neurology, speech therapy, art therapy, and nursing components, in addition to the neuropsychiatric component. The 8-bed inpatient unit and outpatient clinics are supplemented by telemedicine capability and a consultation–liaison service to the RMH Comprehensive Epilepsy Program. The average length of stay in the inpatient unit is 10 days.

Medical staffing includes four neuropsychiatrists (one full-time, three part-time), a neurologist [0.2 equivalent full-time (EFT)], four senior registrars, and a half-time resident medical officer. This provides considerable scope for training opportunities and has contributed to the training of several neuropsychiatrists now practising elsewhere in Australia and New Zealand. The registrar positions are divided across four areas of the service: inpatient, young-onset dementia, neuropsychiatry of epilepsy, and neuropsychiatry neuroimaging.

The inpatient and general neuropsychiatry outpatient services provide inpatient multidisciplinary diagnostic assessments. Half of the referrals will be diagnosed with younger-onset dementia; about one-third have an established mental illness (schizophrenia, bipolar) with comorbidity, and the remainder have a broad range of neuropsychiatric conditions. The service has access to neuroimaging and neurogenetic, neuropathological, and biochemical testing, including CSF, autoimmune, and metabolic testing. This broad range of conditions and exposure to investigational techniques provides an excellent foundation for neuropsychiatric training.

The Younger Onset Dementia (YOD) Service accepts patients under the age of 65 with established or suspected dementing illnesses, including Huntington's disease, Alzheimer's disease, and frontotemporal dementia. The Huntington's Clinic and predictive testing clinic works in collaboration with Genetic Health Services Victoria and Huntington's Victoria. A recent innovation is the

funding of a telehealth service to provide services locally and nationally. The registrar position has been part-funded through Dementia Australia to provide tertiary consultation to the YOD Key Worker Program.

The Neuropsychiatry Neuroimaging Fellow is involved in reporting of imaging with neuroradiology and coordination of regular clinical neuroimaging rounds, and has an inpatient patient role. The fourth training position is the Neuropsychiatry Epilepsy Fellow position with the Comprehensive Epilepsy Programme at RMH. This full-time position includes half-time neuropsychiatry consultation to the 4-bed telemetry unit and participation in epilepsy and first-episode seizure clinics. Finally, the Neuropsychiatry Unit oversees a Deep Brain Stimulation in OCD programme, with 11 patients having received this treatment to date.

The RMH service has an active research programme, ranging widely across most neuropsychiatric topics, but with a particular focus on degenerative aspects of schizophrenia, younger-onset dementia, and rare neuropsychiatric disorders, including phenylketonuria and Niemann–Pick disease type C (NPC). Recent treatment trials have included miglustat and intrathecal cyclodextrin for NPC. The Neuropsychiatry Unit is an international site for intrathecal antisense oligonucleotide trials for Huntington's disease, which began in 2019.

The Brain Disorders Program at the Royal Talbot Rehabilitation Centre in Melbourne is a state-wide specialist service providing community- and inpatient-based neuropsychiatric rehabilitation. Referrals are accepted from all sources, including consumers and caregivers. The service is designed to meet the needs of individuals aged 16–64 years with cognitive and psychiatric disability, and it has a rehabilitation focus that aims to assist people in regaining function and independence where possible.

The four core components of the service are:

- A 30-bed inpatient unit (Mary Guthrie House), consisting of a 10-bed unit with a psychiatric focus and the possibility of involuntary treatment, and a 20-bed unit with a stronger physical rehabilitation focus.
- A 3-bed community re-integration house (step 2).
- A community-based state-wide team [Community Brain Disorders Assessment and Treatment Service (CBDATS) and ABI Behaviour Consultancy (ABIBC)].
- A neuropsychiatric outpatient clinic (Neurobehaviour Clinic) staffed by two psychiatrists, a psychiatric registrar, and a neuropsychologist. Some assessments are undertaken in collaboration with a Neurology Movement Disorders Clinic.

Since 2013, Austin Hospital in Melbourne has provided Australia's first dedicated Functional Neurology Clinic, staffed by a consultant psychiatrist and a psychiatric registrar, working closely with hospital services and private providers and offering diagnosis and management of conversion disorder. It accepts specialist referrals from across Australia and supports an extensive research programme.

The Austin Hospital Neurology Service also includes neuropsychiatry service provision for inpatients, as well as an outpatient epilepsy clinic, staffed by two part-time psychiatrists and one full-time psychiatry registrar. The clinic commenced in 2014 under a co-located model with a neuropsychiatrist in one of the rooms within the epilepsy clinic. The inpatient service was developed to provide neuropsychiatric opinion for those admitted under the Comprehensive Epilepsy Service but has expanded to cover neurology, stroke, and neurosurgery as well.

The Neurology Department at St Vincent's Hospital, also in Melbourne, includes two neuropsychiatrists, who see patients with a range of neuropsychiatric conditions, primarily as outpatients. The department also includes a Cognitive Disorders Clinic. Inpatient consultations are available on request.

A new neuropsychiatry service has been established at the Alfred Hospital in South Melbourne. This serves the Comprehensive Epilepsy Programme, including a 6-bed video-EEG monitoring unit and a Non-Epileptic Seizures Clinic; a Movement Disorders Programme, including deep brain stimulation; an inpatient Acquired Brain Injury Unit and a Cognitive Disorders/Memory Service. It also provides general neurology liaison.

Queensland

Queensland is next in the population stakes at 4.8 million, with Brisbane as the state capital. The Director of Neurosciences at St Vincent's Hospital, Brisbane, is an academic and a clinical neuropsychiatrist who works clinically with the Northern Brain Injury Rehabilitation Service. There is a Huntington's Disease Clinic and also epilepsy surgery work undertaken at the Royal Brisbane and Women's Hospital by a neuropsychiatrist and a nurse, with an associated STP-funded neuropsychiatry fellowship. At the Mater Centre for Neurosciences, a private hospital that is contracted to also provide public services, there are three psychiatrists providing liaison to the Advanced Epilepsy Unit, the Functional Neurology Disorders Unit, and other inpatients, with some outpatient clinics. There is an associated Neuropsychiatry Certificate delivered by Mater Education, covering the care of patients with epilepsy, Parkinson's disease, and FND. This has been very popular with trainees in psychiatry.

Northern Queensland is served by a Neuropsychiatry Clinic at Townsville Hospital. The director of the 30-bed Townsville Community Care and Acquired Brain Injury Unit at the Kirwan Health Campus in Townsville is a psychiatrist, with a full multidisciplinary team, including a registrar, psychiatric nurses, a neuropsychologist, clinical psychologists, an occupational therapist, a social worker, an indigenous mental health worker, and administration staff. There is an associated Community Outreach Programme at the Princess Alexandra Hospital in Townsville.

New Zealand

The capital of New Zealand is Wellington, but Auckland is the largest city, with about one-third of the national population of 4.5 million residing in the greater Auckland region. The service landscape in New Zealand is affected by the activity of the Accident Compensation Corporation, which funds care for patients who have sustained accidental brain injury, including TBI, but also anoxia resulting from medical misadventure or drowning, etc., and this is provided outside of the public mental health system for the most part.

There are no specific neuropsychiatric services outside the Auckland metro region where about one-third of the overall New Zealand population lives, and there are similar issues in Australia regarding population density and geographical distance, on a smaller scale (see Fig. 45.2).

There was previously a specific brain injury service in Christchurch directed by a neuropsychiatrist, with inpatient beds located at the Burwood Hospital, but after restructuring, there is no longer a neuropsychiatry component to this. However, there is neuropsychiatry liaison to the Huntington's Disease Clinic in that city.

In Auckland, the Community Neurobehavioural Service for managing challenging behaviour after acquired brain injury was operational from 1996 to 2015, but it closed after the reallocation of a Ministry of Health contract. A Regional Huntington's Disease Service was established within the Auckland DHB Mental Health Directorate in 2014 and this is ongoing, with 0.4 psychiatrist, and one nursing EFT, with access to a neuropsychologist. Service provision covers all aspects, from predictive testing to palliative care, with close collaboration with Genetics and Neurology, but there is no specific access to inpatient beds. Outpatient clinics are provided in all three Auckland metro District Health Board (DHB) areas, as well as Whangarei in Northland.

Also in Auckland, there is neuropsychiatrist liaison to the Auckland DHB General and Acquired Brain Injury Rehabilitation Facility at Rehab Plus, the National Epilepsy Surgery Programme, and the National Deep Brain Stimulation Programme. Assessments for the latter are now also done locally in Christchurch for South Island patients by a psychogeriatrician.

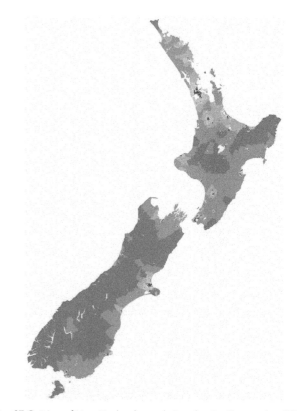

Fig. 45.2 Map of New Zealand population density, Census data 2006. Reproduced from Stats NZ. https://www.stats.govt.nz/. Distributed under the terms of the Creatice Commons Attribution 4.0 International (CC BY 4.0).

Other Australian states (Western Australia, South Australia, Tasmania, and Australian Capital Territory)

Western Australia has a number of groups undertaking neuropsychiatry-related research, and in 2015, the state presented a plan for the development of neuropsychiatric services and beds as part of the Western Australia Mental Health, Alcohol and Other Drug Services Plan 2015–2025. This includes the intention to develop specialized state-wide inpatient services for neuropsychiatric disorders. Current clinical services include a consultant neuropsychiatrist working in the Consultation Liaison Department at the Fiona Stanley Hospital, who also provides services at the Huntington's Disease Outpatient Clinic in the State Neurosciences Unit at the Graylands Hospital and the Neuropsychiatry Unit at the downsized Fremantle Hospital.

There is a Neuropsychiatry Unit with a primarily consultation-liaison-based model, but no dedicated inpatient facility, at the Royal Adelaide Hospital (South Australia), with provision for a senior psychiatry registrar. The Huntington's Disease Service at the Flinders Medical Centre in South Australia is provided by the Social Work and Counselling Service.

Neuropsychiatric consultations in Canberra Australian Capital Territory are primarily carried out through the Old Age Psychiatry service, with some outpatient service through the private sector. Medical staffing in the ACT includes one clinical academic neuropsychiatrist who is currently the head of the Academic Unit of Psychiatry and Addiction Medicine, Australian National University Medical School. Training in old age/liaison neuropsychiatry is available, in conjunction with academic psychiatry/research training. There is an active neuropsychiatric and neuroimaging research programme focused on neurodegenerative disease, also based at the Academic Unit of Psychiatry and Addiction Medicine, Australian National University Medical School, in collaboration with the Neuropsychiatry Unit at the RMH.

In Tasmania, a Huntington's Disease Clinic is provided (in Hobart) for the Southern half of the population by an old age psychiatrist, although it may prove possible to dedicate a specific neuropsychiatry role in the near future. The brain injury rehabilitation service does not have specific neuropsychiatry liaison.

Clinics for individuals with Huntington's disease have been established in most regions, and this perhaps reflects an appreciation by both neurology and psychiatry colleagues of the value of a neuropsychiatric skill set in this clinical setting. The prevalence of Huntington's disease in Australia and New Zealand has been estimated at around six in 100,000 (except in Tasmania where it is double that figure, attributed to one large kindred with a single ancestor from Somerset, UK). This may be a serious underestimate, as the Auckland Huntington's Disease Service is aware of over 300 local patients, indicating a local prevalence of 20 in 100,000. Even so, by contrast, the provision of neuropsychiatric expertise to cases of TBI seems patchy, given how commonly they are encountered. A recent New Zealand study of the prevalence of TBI (Feigin et al., 2013) estimated a figure of 790 in 100,000, inclusive of mild TBI. The strategic driver might be the combination of complexity (neurological and psychosocial) and acuity.

Neuropsychiatric services have tended to adopt flexible referral pathways to maximize access. Audit data from such services in the South of England confirmed the overall appropriateness of referrals made for consultation and input (Fleminger et al., 2006). Equally, given recent neuropsychiatric referral rate estimates of 20–30 referrals per 100,000 of the population (Agrawal et al., 2015), it is likely that there remains significant unmet need, despite accessible models of care being implemented.

There are large geographical distances between population centres in Australasia, which is very obvious in Australia, but even in New Zealand, the Southern DHB cares for a population of about 319,000 in an area almost half the size of England. Attempts to meet the needs for rural and remote populations include the piecemeal development of telemedicine facilities, as well as outreach clinics, but much more is required.

Postgraduate trainees in psychiatry and neurology seeking to sub-specialize in neuropsychiatry continue to rely on a period of training within tertiary units such as those in Victoria and NSW, following an apprenticeship model of training characteristic of advanced training in the field across the world (Agrawal et al., 2015). These sub-specialist training experiences constitute a key component of the service agenda for the two major Australian units and attract high-quality trainees from across Australia and New Zealand. There is clearly sufficient clinical activity to allow sustainable workforce development.

Discussion

As a clinical discipline, neuropsychiatry has, in many ways, been marked by constantly shifting boundaries and diagnostic territory, while retaining a fundamental approach that focuses on 'the complex relationship between human behaviour and brain function' and attempts to understand behaviour disorders 'on the basis of an interaction of neurobiological and psychological-social factors' (Sachdev, 2002). This inconsistency has indeed been replicated in the Australasian service context. The current distribution of neuropsychiatric services in Australia and New Zealand is, in part, dictated by their proximity to nationally and internationally important neurological and neurosurgical centres, but this does not explain there being relatively well-resourced centres at Newcastle and Townsville or which disorders are catered for at which locations.

Conclusion

To sum up, there are several centres in Australasia capable of acting as regional 'hubs' within the 'hub and spoke model' that is recommended for implemention as part of neuropsychiatry services worldwide (Sachdev, 2005). Indeed, there are dedicated clinical neuropsychiatry posts, although not necessarily full-time, in all cities with a population of over 1 million, and these centres all serve a large enough outlying population to achieve critical mass, and hence sustainability of services.

However, it is recognized that the 'spokes' of such a model remain underdeveloped within Australasia. Elements of the necessary infrastructure do exist, including critical links to local medical and psychiatric services and affiliations to local universities, but further partnerships between state-based public sector services, private healthcare providers, and non-governmental sector organizations need development.

As in the UK, neuropsychiatry commissioning remains disjointed and variable (Bhattacharya et al., 2015).

National service frameworks for neuropsychiatry services in both Australia and New Zealand are a priority. Providing adequate care to these patients with combined neurological and psychiatric disadvantages requires such initiatives to be developed and implemented over the coming years, to avoid the 'postcode lottery' which currently exists.

KEY LEARNING POINTS

- Neuropsychiatry service provision in Australia and New Zealand is patchy, with no guiding national service planning frameworks in place.
- This is especially so with regard to inpatient neuropsychiatry beds.
- Services for younger-onset dementia and Huntington's disease are better developed than those for acquired brain injury.
- The major training opportunities in Australasia are in Sydney and Melbourne, and the same two centres produce world-class research.

REFERENCES

Agrawal, N., Bhattacharya, R., & Rickards, H. (2015). Provision of neuropsychiatry services: variability and unmet need. BJPsych Bull, 39(6), 297–301.

Agrawal, N., Fleminger, S., Ring, H., & Deb, S. (2008). Neuropsychiatry in the UK: planning the service provision for the 21st century. The Psychiatrist, 32, 303–6.

Australian Bureau of Statistics (2016). 3101.0 – Australian Demographic Statistics, Jun 2016. Available at: http://www.abs.gov.au/ausstats/abs@.nsf/mf/3101.0/.

Australian Institute of Health and Welfare. *Health expenditure Australia 2014–15*. Health and welfare expenditure series no 57. Cat no HWE 67. Canberra: Australian Institute of Health and Welfare, 2016.

Bhattacharya, R., Rickards, H., & Agrawal, N. (2015). Commissioning Neuropsychiatry Services: barriers and lessons. BJPsych Bull, 39, 291–6.

Feigin, V.L., et al. (2013). Incidence of Traumatic Brain Injury in New Zealand. The Lancet Neurology, 12, 53–64.

Fleminger, S., Leigh, E., & McCarthy, C. (2006). The size of demand for specialized neuropsychiatry services: rates of referrals to neuropsychiatric services in the South Thames region of the United Kingdom. Journal of Neuropsychiatry and Clinical Neurosciences, 18, 121–8.

Government of New Zealand (2016). *Vote Health—Supplementary Estimates 2015/16*. 22 May 2016. Government of New Zealand.

Sachdev, P.S. (2002). Neuropsychiatry—a discipline for the future. Journal of Psychosomatic Research, 53, 625–7.

Sachdev, P.S. (2005). Whither neuropsychiatry? Journal of Neuropsychiatry and Clinical Neurosciences, 17, 140–1.

Sachdev, P.S. and Mohan, A. (2013). Neuropsychiatry: Where are we and where do we go from here? Mens Sana monographs, 11, 4.

Taylor, L.J., Eapen, V., Maybery, M.T., et al. (2016). Diagnostic evaluation for Autism Spectrum Disorder: a survey of health professionals in Australia. BMJ Open, 6, e012517.

46

Neuropsychiatry services in Japan

Koho Miyoshi

Introduction

Nowadays, neuropsychiatry is faced with the serious problem of an ageing society. The elderly population in industrial countries is increasing rapidly, and the prevalence of neuropsychiatric disorders, including dementia, is rising continuously. Japan is one of the countries with the highest aged population in the world. Consequently, neuropsychiatry in Japan is most seriously faced with the issues of an ageing society. The needs for neuropsychiatric services are increasing in Japan. To cope with this problem, a large number of specialists in the field of neuropsychiatry are required to participate in the provision of neuropsychiatric services. However, at present, the number of neuropsychiatry specialists is quite limited. Therefore, it is an urgent issue for Japanese neuropsychiatry to establish a specialist training pathway and to encourage psychiatrists and neurologists to participate in providing neuropsychiatric services.

For better understanding of the present situation, this chapter deals mainly with current status, service provision, training and career opportunities, brief history, and scientific activities in the field of neuropsychiatry in Japan.

What are neuropsychiatric services?

Neuropsychiatric services are provided for patients with neuropsychiatric symptoms in neuropsychiatric disorders. 'Neuropsychiatric symptoms' are psychiatric manifestations due to organic cerebral disorders, namely, dementia, mild cognitive disorder, amnestic syndrome, delirium, hallucinations, delusion, catatonia, mood disorder, apathy, anxiety, obsession–compulsion, dissociation, personality change, and behavioural disorders (Miyoshi and Morimura, 2010). 'Neuropsychiatric disorders' are neurological diseases causing psychiatric symptoms, including Alzheimer's disease, frontotemporal lobar degeneration, Lewy body disease, Parkinson's disease, Huntington's disease, prion disease, cerebrovascular disorders, encephalitis, multiple sclerosis, metabolic encephalopathy, thiamine deficiency, traumatic brain injury, alcoholism, and chemical intoxication (David et al., 2012; Miyoshi and Morimura, 2010). Epilepsy is also encompassed in

neuropsychiatric disorders. In fact, neurological diseases are, for the most part, neuropsychiatric diseases (Lyketsos, 2006).

Neurological disorders are commonly accompanied by psychiatric symptoms. For example, depression and delusion in Alzheimer's disease (Lyketsos and Odin, 2002), visual hallucination and disturbance of consciousness in Lewy body disease (Kosaka, 1990; McKeith et al., 2005), depression in Parkinson's disease (Cummings, 1992; Miyoshi et al., 1996), and depression in cerebrovascular disorders (Alexopoulos et al., 1997) are common neuropsychiatric manifestations. Neurocognitive impairment is frequently accompanied by agitation, namely 'behavioural and psychological symptom of dementia' (Finkel, 1996), especially in patients with neurodegenerative disorders and cerebrovascular diseases.

Neuropsychiatric services are provided to these patients in general hospitals, as well as in psychiatric hospitals. The services provide the clinical diagnosis based on psychological, physical, and neuroradiological examinations, and treatment for psychiatric symptoms of neurological disorders.

Neuropsychiatric disorders should be carefully diagnosed, because occasionally they can mimic functional psychoses, like depression, delusion, and hallucination (Lyketsos, 2006). The principles of pharmacological treatment of organic psychoses are essentially similar to, although not necessarily the same as, medical treatment of functional psychoses. The Japanese government recently issued warning about cautious use of SSRIs and SNRIs for the treatment of organic depressive symptoms, because of particular risks associated with unexpected excitation. Use of antipsychotic drugs is not recommended for the treatment of agitation in demented patients because of a significant increase in mortality risk (Schneider et al., 2005; Steinberg and Lyketsos, 2012; Trifiro et al., 2009). The neurobiological basis of psychiatric symptoms should be carefully considered in the treatment of neuropsychiatric disorders.

Increased needs for neuropsychiatry services

According to a governmental survey, the number of patients with neuropsychiatric disorders, including Alzheimer's disease and vascular dementia, is rapidly increasing in Japan (see Table 46.1). In

Table 46.1 Estimated number of patients with neuropsychiatric disorders in psychiatric hospitals in Japan

Year	1996	1999	2002	2005	2008	2011	2017
Organic mental disorders							
Alzheimer's disease	20	29	89	176	240	366	562
Vascular and unspecified dementia	91	121	138	145	143	146	142
Mental and behavioural disorders							
Schizophrenia, schizotypal, and delusional disorders	721	666	734	757	797	731	792
Mood disorders	433	441	711	924	1,041	958	1276

All units are in thousands.

Source data from Governmental report: Ministry of Health,Labour & Welfare. Total number of patients with major disorders (in Japanese).

psychiatric hospitals, the proportion of organic mental disorders has increased significantly in the last two decades.

Reports by the Japan Intractable Diseases Information Center on the number of patients with neurological disorders indicate an upward trend in the prevalence of major neuropsychiatric disorders. According to the organization's statistical information, the number of patients with neurological disorders, including Parkinson's disease, multiple system atrophy, amyotrophic lateral sclerosis, and multiple sclerosis, has increased consistently over the last decade (see Table 46.2).

Who should provide neuropsychiatric services?

Specialists in neuropsychiatry

Only few studies have reported on neuropsychiatric service provision in various countries, presumably because of difficulties with obtaining epidemiological data at a national level (Agrawal et al., 2008a, b). The same difficulty exists when overviewing the provision of neuropsychiatric services in Japan.

Ideally, neuropsychiatric services should be provided by neuropsychiatry specialists, because comprehensive neurology and psychiatry knowledge and professional skills are required for the medical care of neuropsychiatric disorders. Therefore, clinical diagnosis and medical treatment of neuropsychiatric symptoms should be the tasks of specialists.

However, in reality, neuropsychiatric services in Japan are provided mainly by general psychiatrists, and less frequently by clinical neurologists, who have an interest in the psychiatric aspects of cerebral disorders. Geriatric psychiatrists are also involved in providing

medical treatment of psychiatric symptoms of brain disorders, especially dementia.

Psychiatrists in Japan

Traditionally, the term 'neuropsychiatry' is synonymous with 'psychiatry' in Japan. Until now, the majority of psychiatric departments in medical schools were called 'Department of Neuropsychiatry' and usually have facilities for neurobiological research, as well as for clinical psychiatry.

The Japanese Society of Psychiatry and Neurology (JSPN) is the oldest and most influencial psychiatry society. It was established originally as the Japanese Society of Neurology in 1902, and its name was changed to JSPN in 1935 (Nakane and Radford, 1999). There are currently approximately 17,000 members, including 10,104 certified psychiatrists (see Table 46.3). Therefore, the majority of Japanese psychiatrists might also more or less consider themselves to be 'neuropsychiatrists'.

The Japanese Psychogeriatric Society was founded in 1986 (see Table 46.3). Its membership comprises 2772 psychiatrists, including 906 certified geriatric psychiatrists who provide treatment for elderly patients with organic mental disorders. As a matter of fact, many geriatric psychiatrists are enthusiastic to be involved in the treatment of psychiatric symptoms of organic brain disorders, as well as functional psychoses.

Neurologists in Japan

In the 1950s, neurologists, who were mainly based in departments of internal medicine in medical schools and general hospitals, worked actively towards the creation of a new professional society, which culminated in 1960 in the establishment of the Japanese Society of

Table 46.2 Number of recipients of medical treatment of intractable neurological diseases

Year	2004	2006	2008	2010	2012	2014
Parkinson's disease	75,026	86,425	98,356	106,637	120,406	136,559
Huntington's disease	672	705	762	798	851	933
Prion disease	341	332	575	492	475	584
Amyotrophic lateral sclerosis	7007	7695	8285	8406	9096	9950
Multiple system atrophy	8885	9779	10,937	11,096	11,733	12,741
Spinocerebellar degeneration	17,947	19,948	22,239	23,290	25,447	27,582
Multiple sclerosis	10,759	11,938	13,435	14,492	17,073	19,389

Source data from the annual report of Japan Intractable Disease Information Center.

Table 46.3 Membership of academic societies in Japan

Society	Membership	Year
Psychiatry		
Japanese Society of Psychiatry and Neurology	Approximately 17,000	2018
Certified psychiatrists	10,104	2016
Neurology		
Japanese Society of Neurology	9003	2018
Certified neurologists	5505	2018
Societies related to neuropsychiatry		
Japanese Neuropsychiatric Association	Approximately 700	2018
Japanese Society for Dementia Research	3200	2013
Certified specialists	1034	2016
Japanese Psychogeriatric Society	2772	2017
Certified geriatric psychiatrists	906	2016

Source data from the homepages of societies as well as Governmental report. www.mhlw.go.jp/toukei/saikin/hw/iryosd/14/dl/1-4.pdf

Neurology (JSN) as a separate body from JSPN. The society now has 9003 members, including 5505 certified neurologists.

The Japanese Society for Dementia Research is an academic society that was established in 1982. The majority of its members include neurologists who are involved in the provision of neuropsychiatric services. Currently the society has approximately 3200 members, including 1034 certified specialists.

Neuropsychiatrists in Japan

Following the separation of neurology from psychiatry, there was decreased interest in psychiatric symptoms of cerebral disease among most neurologists. Added to this, the neurological skills of general psychiatrists occasionally seemed inadequate in the provision of appropriate treatment of brain disorders. This serious situation prompted the realization that a close collaboration between psychiatrists and neurologists is necessary for the treatment of organic mental disorders.

This led to the establishment of the Japanese Neuropsychiatric Association (JNA) in 1996 to foster collaboration among professionals in clinical neurosciences. Since then, the JNA has held its annual congress as a platform for the exchange of scientific findings among researchers in neuropsychiatry. Although there are currently no more than 700 members, the annual congress attracts an attendance of approximately 1000 delegates every year.

For the last two decades, the topics covered in the annual congress have included discussion of clinical, biological, and radiological aspects of organic mental disorders. For example, a recent JNA's annual congress included the following topics: (1) neuropsychiatric symptoms of anti-NMDA receptor encephalitis, which could be misdiagnosed as functional psychoses; (2) mechanism and treatment of neuropsychiatric symptoms of Alzheimer's disease; and (3) pathophysiology and treatment of hallucination and delusional symptoms in neuropsychiatric disorders.

Training and career opportunities

Training in neuropsychiatry

At present, specialists in psychiatry are certified following passing relevant examinations set by the academic society, with 5 years' experience in clinical practice, including completing 3-year training in a hospital approved by the academic society for postgraduate clinical education. In addition, psychiatrists in Japan should learn and be competent in the medicolegal aspects of patient care, which includes the Act on Mental Health and Welfare for the Disabled—this would lead to the trained psychiatrist to be certified as a 'Designated Mental Health Doctor'. Thus, overall, certification in psychiatry requires a total of 5 years as a medical doctor, including 3 years in psychiatry.

Board certification in neurology requires 6 years' clinical experience in general medicine and neurology, as well as passing relevant examinations.

Although there is no training curriculum or certification system for specialists in neuropsychiatry, training for this sub-specialty can be obtained in medical schools, general hospitals, and psychiatric hospitals under the guidance of experts. The training curriculum should essentially be the same as that set by the International Neuropsychiatric Association (INA) (Sachdev, 2010)—which includes obtaining first-hand experience in common neuropsychiatric disorders and developing competency in recognition and management of common psychiatric and neurological disorders. Concurrent training in developing skills in critical evaluation of research evidence is important, as well as developing expertise in the use and interpretation of specialized neuropsychiatric investigations. Another training objective is to develop specialized skills in physical treatment of neuropsychiatric patients (Sachdev, 2010).

Because of a limited number of neuropsychiatry specialists in Japan, there is urgency in establishing an appropriate training and certification system in order to address the issue. Importantly, this issue of shortage of neuropsychiatry specialists not only affects Japan, but also exists in other countries across the world (Mitchell and Agrawal, 2005). For now, all general psychiatrists should be trained to build knowledge in neurological disorders, while all clinical neurologists should gain experience in the treatment of psychiatric symptoms of neuropsychiatric disorders. In this way, all neurologists and psychiatrists will be able to provide appropriate neuropsychiatry services.

Career opportunities in neuropsychiatry

What is the current situation of career opportunities for specialists in neuropsychiatry? There is no specified institution for neuropsychiatry in Japan. However, there are openings available for neuropsychiatrists to work in medical schools, psychiatric hospitals, and general hospitals. All medical schools (a total of 81) have a department of psychiatry, as well as a department of neurology, involved in education, research, and clinical practice. Therefore, neuropsychiatrists have the option of working in medical education, as well as in clinical practice, in medical schools.

To date, there are 1059 psychiatric hospitals in Japan (see Table 46.4). In addition, a large number of general hospitals have a psychiatric department (a total of 1740).

Table 46.4 Medical care institutions in psychiatry and neurology in Japan (2017)

	Number
Psychiatry	
Medical schools (departments of psychiatry)	81
Psychiatric hospitals	1059
General hospitals	1740
Private clinics	6864
Neurology	
Medical schools (departments of neurology)	81
General hospitals	2512
Private clinics	3120

Source data from the Governmental report. Ministry of Health, Labour and Welfare.

Neurologists in Japan work mainly in general hospitals and medical school hospitals. In this setting, psychiatric symptoms of brain disorders are treated by neurologists with the assistance of psychiatrists.

Particular issues of neuropsychiatric services in Japan

Rising population of elderly with dementia

Japan's proportion of people aged 65 years and older was the highest in the world in 2006 at 21.0%, surpassing Italy's 20%. There has since been a persistent increase in the elderly population in Japan, with a current estimation of 28.0% (n = 3,550,800) of the total population (n = 126,443,000). In addition, the proportions of old-old people aged 75 years and over and those aged 85 years and over are estimated to be 14.1% (n = 1,787,000) and 4.5% (n = 569,600), respectively.

Recent studies in Japan (Ikejima et al., 2012) (19) showed that the increase in the elderly population, in particular the 'oldest old' group, contributed to an increased prevalence of dementia. According to a governmental survey of recipients of long-term insurance services, the estimated number of elderly persons who met the diagnostic criteria of dementia (i.e. 'major neurocognitive disorder' according to the DSM-5) was 2.80 million (9.5%) in 2010, and 3.45 million (10.2%) in 2015. According to the Japanese government, the number of elderly people with dementia is predicted to increase to 4.10 million (11.3%) by 2020 and to 4.70 million (12.8%) by 2025 (see Fig. 46.1).

Governmental measures to cope with dementia issue

In 1989, the Japanese Ministry of Health and Welfare, in anticipation of the growing problem of the ageing Japanese society, launched a comprehensive 10-year project, called the Gold Plan, to tackle the issues associated with its ageing population. Minor amendments to the Gold Plan were subsequently made in 2001.

In 2000, a mandatory insurance scheme for the elderly, called 'Long-Term Care Insurance', was implemented (Tsutsui and Muramatsu, 2007), whereby all persons aged over 40 years should pay an insurance premium. Resulting from this, elderly people aged 65 years and over are eligible to receive care services or financial support. Since implementation of the scheme, there has been significant improvement in institutions' capacities to deliver residential care, namely 'Intensive Care Home for the Elderly' (*Tokuyo*), 'Long-term Care Health Facility' (*Rohken*), and 'Sanatorium Medical Facility for the Elderly requiring Long-term Care'. Moreover, provision of 'Home Help Services', 'Home Nursing', 'Day Respite Care', and 'Short Stay' has also started for the elderly people who need home care.

Recently, the Japanese government introduced a comprehensive plan, called the Orange Plan, to cope with issues associated with

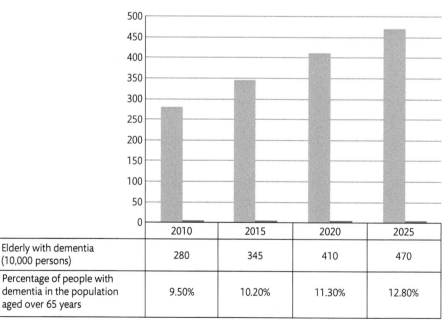

	2010	2015	2020	2025
Elderly with dementia (10,000 persons)	280	345	410	470
Percentage of people with dementia in the population aged over 65 years	9.50%	10.20%	11.30%	12.80%

Fig. 46.1 Number of the elderly people with dementia in Japan.
Source data from governmental report: Ministry of Health, Labour & Welfare. (2012).

dementia care (Nakanishi and Nakashima, 2014). The objective of the Orange Plan is to create a society where people with dementia are respected and can continue to live in a good environment in a familiar community.

The role of specialists

Dementia, i.e. major neurocognitive disorder (according to the DSM-5), commonly causes psychiatric symptoms, including agitation, behavioural change, depression, hallucination, and delusion. Therefore, appropriate neuropsychiatric services are required for patients with dementia.

Neuropsychiatry specialists, as well as those in related neurosciences, should play a leading role in providing neuropsychiatric services in a clinical setting. One of the most important duties of these specialists should be to accept referrals from mental health professionals, as well as from general physicians.

Names and affiliations of certified specialists who are members of the Japanese Society for Dementia Research, as well as of the Japanese Psychogeriatric Society, are available from the academic societies' website—which helps patients and their families find a specialist for medical treatment. The same setup for finding neuropsychiatry specialists is desirable.

Neuropsychiatry in Japan

Research

At the dawn of modern Japanese medicine, many scientists who studied in western countries contributed to neuropsychiatry. Miyake (1906) and Fisher (1907) discovered neuritic plaques in the aged brain in 1906, prior to the famous Alzheimer's report. In 1913, Noguchi and his co-worker (Noguchi and Moore, 1913) made a tremendous contribution when they found *Treponema pallidum* in the brain of patients with general paralysis. Onari and his German colleague (Onari and Spatz, 1926) established the concept of Pick disease in 1926. Hayashi (1931) described, in 1931, the neuropathology of a particular type of acute encephalitis—encephalitis epidemica japonica. The effects of nuclear radiation on the brain of Hiroshima and Nagasaki casualties were reported by Shiraki and his co-workers (Shiraki et al., 1958) in 1958.

Neuropsychiatry contributed to solving some problems of enigmatic endemic of neuropsychiatric disorders, which attracted public attention. The cause of a neuropsychiatric disorder epidemic in Minamata city in Kyushu since the 1950s was revealed, using intensive investigations by psychiatrists and neurologists, to be organic methylmercury intoxication as a result of contaminated wastewater from a chemical factory released into the sea (Ekino et al., 2007; Harada, 1995; Shiraki and Takeuchi, 1971). Further, in the late 1960s, a peculiar neuropsychiatric disorder, called subacute myelino-optico-neuropathy (SMON), which was accompanied by abdominal symptoms, was proved by neurologists and psychiatrists to be an intoxication caused by persistent and excessive administration of the anti-diarrhoeal drug clioquinol (Igata, 2010; Igata and Toyokura, 1970; Shiraki, 1975; Tateishi, 2000). These unpredictable tragedies caused by chemical intoxication shocked the Japanese people at the time.

In recent years, Japanese scientists have made significant contributions to neuropsychiatry research, especially on dementia. Ihara and co-workers (Ihara et al., 1986) discovered phosphorylated tau protein in neurofibrillary tangles in Alzheimer's disease. Kosaka (1978, 1990) contributed to establishing the concept of Lewy body disease by reporting clinico-pathological cases, especially in Japan. Iwatsubo's group (Baba et al., 1998) described the role of α-synuclein aggregates in the formation of Lewy bodies. Mitsuyama and Takamatsu (1979) reported the first cases of what is now known as frontotemporal lobar degeneration with motor neurone disease (FTLD-MND) from their post-mortem examinations.

International activities

The INA (Miyoshi, 2010) was first established in Seville in 1996 as the International Organization of Neuropsychiatry (ION). The JNA has been affiliated with the INA since the beginning and hosted the Third International Congress of Neuropsychiatry in Kyoto in 2001 where approximately 700 participants gathered from 31 countries. The Congress proceedings entitled *Contemporary Neuropsychiatry* were published subsequently (Miyoshi et al., 2001). The INA's 2009 conference was held in Kobe, and papers from the conference were published in a monograph entitled *Neuropsychiatric Disorders* (Miyoshi et al., 2010).

International collaboration is essential in order to tackle neuropsychiatric issues, especially in relation to dementia. In 2008, neurologists and psychiatrists in China established an academic association called the Chinese Neuropsychiatry Summit which holds annual meetings gathering hundreds of medical professionals. Thus, the future looks promising in terms of establishing close ties among neuropsychiatric organizations in East Asia, including the JNA.

Conclusion

The elderly population is steadily increasing in Japan, while the number of people with neuropsychiatric disorders is also rising rapidly. In this setting, specialists in neuropsychiatry and related neurosciences should play a leading role in the provision of neuropsychiatric services. In reality, however, neuropsychiatric services are provided mainly by general psychiatrists and, less frequently, by clinical neurologists. In an attempt to remediate the lack of neuropsychiatrists, there is urgency for the JNA to set up an appropriate training system to encourage more young doctors to enter the field of neuropsychiatry.

This chapter gives an overview of the current status of neuropsychiatry in Japan, particularly in terms of service provision, training, career opportunities, and relevant academic societies and scientific activities.

KEY LEARNING POINTS

* Japan is one of the countries with the oldest population in the world. Consequently, neuropsychiatry in Japan is faced most seriously with the issues of an ageing society. The number of patients with neuropsychiatric disorders, including Alzheimer's disease, vascular dementia, and Parkinson's disease, have been increasing consistently over the last decade in

Japan. The increase in the elderly population has contributed to an increased prevalence of these disorders.

• Neuropsychiatric services in Japan are provided mainly by general psychiatrists or by clinical neurologists who have an interest in the psychiatric aspects of cerebral disorders. The Japanese Neuropsychiatric Association was established in 1996 to foster collaboration among professionals in clinical neurosciences.

• In 2000, a mandatory insurance scheme for the elderly, called 'Long-Term Care Insurance', was implemented by the Government. Since then, there has been significant improvement in institutions' capacities to deliver residential care. In relation to this, provision of home care services has also started for the elderly people. Neuropsychiatry specialists, as well as those in related neurosciences, play a leading role in providing neuropsychiatric services in this setting.

REFERENCES

Agrawal, N., Fleminger, S., Ring, H., et al. (2008a). Neuropsychiatry in the UK. National survey of existing service provision. *Psychiatric Bulletin*, **32**, 288–91.

Agrawal, N., Fleminger, S., Ring, H., and Deb, S. (2008b). Neuropsychiatry in the UK. Planning the service provision for the 21st century. *Psychiatric Bulletin*, **32**, 303–6.

Alexopoulos, G.S., Meyers, B.S., Young, R.C., et al. (1997). Vascular depression hypothesis. *Archives of General Psychiatry*, **54**, 915–22.

Baba, M., Nakajo, S., Tu, P.H., et al. (1998). Aggregation of α-synuclein in Lewy bodies of sporadic Parkinson's disease and dementia with Lewy bodies. *American Journal of Pathology*, **152**, 879–84.

Cummings, J.L. (1992). Depression and Parkinson's disease. A review. *American Journal of Psychiatry*, **149**, 443–54.

David, A., Fleminger, S., Kopelman, M., et al. (2012). *Lishman's Organic Psychiatry: A Textbook of Neuropsychiatry*, fourth edition. London: Wiley-Blackwell.

Ekino, S., Susa, M., Ninomiya, T., et al. (2007). Minamata disease revisited. An update on the acute and chronic manifestations of methyl mercury poisoning. *Journal of Neurological Sciences*, **262**, 131–44.

Finkel, S.I. (1996). New focus on behavioral and psychological signs and symptoms of dementia. *International Psychogeriatrics*, **8** (suppl 3), 215–16.

Harada, M. (1995). Minamata disease. Methylmercury poisoning in Japan caused by environmental pollution. *Critical Reviews in Toxicology*, **25**, 1–24.

Hayashi, M. (1931). Encephalitis epidemica japonica. *Allgemeine Zeitschrift fuer Psychiatrie*, **95**, 55–8.

Igata, A. (2010). Clinical studies on rising and re-rising neurological diseases in Japan. A personal contribution. *Proceedings of the Japan Academy Series B*, **86**, 366–77.

Ihara, Y., Nukina, N., Miura, R., et al. (1986). Phosphorylated tau protein in integrated into paired helical filaments in Alzheimer's disease. *Journal of Biochemistry*, **99**, 1807–10.

Igata, A. and Toyokura, Y. (1970). SMON in Japan. Zur Frage der Chinnoform Vergiftung. *Muenchener Medizinishe Wochenschrift*, **113**, 1062–5.

Ikejima, C., Hisanaga, A., Meguro, K., et al. (2012). Multicentre population-based dementia prevalence survey in Japan. *Psychogeriatrics*, **12**, 120–3.

Kosaka. K. (1978). Lewy bodies in cerebral cortex. Report of three cases. *Acta Neuropathologica*, **42**, 127–34.

Kosaka, K. (1990). Diffuse Lewy body disease in Japan. *Journal of Neurology*, **237**, 197–207.

Lyketsos, C.G. (2006). Lessons from neuropsychiatry. *Journal of Neuropsychiatry and Clinical Neurosciences*, **18**, 445–9.

Lyketsos, C. G. and Olin, J. (2002). Depression in Alzheimer's disease. Overview and treatment. *Biological Psychiatry*, **52**, 243–52.

McKeith, I.G., Dickson, D.W., Lowe, J., et al. (2005). Diagnosis and management of dementia with Lewy bodies. Third report of the DLB consortium. *Neurology*, **65**, 1863–72.

Mitchell, A. and Agrawal, N. (2005). Training in neuropsychiatry. Is it time to reintegrate into mainstream psychiatry? *Psychiatric Bulletin*, **29**, 361–4.

Mitsuyama, Y. and Takamatsu, S. (1979). Presenile dementia with motor neuron disease in Japan. A new entity? *Archives of Neurology*, **36**, 592–9.

Miyake, K. (1906). Beitrag zur Kenntnis der Altersveraenderung der menschlichen Hirnrinde. *Obersteiners Arbeiten*. BdXIII. (cited from: 'Early Story of Alzheimer's Disease' (1987). Bick, K., Amaducci, L., Peperu, G. (editors), pp. 5–18, Raven Press).

Miyoshi, K. (2010). Brief history and current status of the International Neuropsychiatric Association. In: Miyoshi, K., Morimura, Y., Maeda, K. (editors). *Neuropsychiatric Disorders*. pp. 301–15. Tokyo: Springer.

Miyoshi, K. and Morimura, Y. (2010). Clinical manifestations of neuropsychiatric disorders. In: Miyoshi, K., Morimura, Y., Maeda, K. (editors). *Neuropsychiatric Disorders*. pp. 3–15. Tokyo: Springer.

Miyoshi, K., Morimura, Y., and Maeda, K. (editors) (2010). *Neuropsychiatric Disorders*, Tokyo: Springer.

Miyoshi, K., Shapiro, C., Gaviria, M., and Morita, Y. (editors) (2001). *Contemporary Neuropsychiatry*. Tokyo: Springer.

Miyoshi, K., Ueki, A., and Nagano, O. (1996). Management of psychiatric symptoms of Parkinson's disease. *European Neurology*, **36**(suppl1), 49–54.

Nakane, Y. and Radford, M. (editors) (1999). *Images in Psychiatry: Japan*. Paris: World Psychiatric Association.

Nakanishi, M. and Nakashima, T. (2014). Features of Japanese national dementia strategy in comparison with international dementia policies. How should a national dementia policy interact with the public health- and social-care system? *Alzheimer's & Dementia*, **10**, 468–76.

Noguchi, H. and Moore, J.W. (1913). A demonstration of *Treponema pallidum* in the brain of cases of general paralysis. *Journal of Experimental Medicine*, **17**, 232–8.

Onari, K. and Spatz, H. (1926). Anatomische Beitraege zur Lehre von Pickschen umschriebenen Grosshirnrindenatrophie (Picksche Krankheit). *Zeitschrift fuer gesamtes Neurologie*, **101**, 470–511.

Sachdev, P. (2010). Core curriculum in neuropsychiatry of the International Neuropsychiatric Association. In: Miyoshi, K., Morimura, Y., Maeda, K. (editors). *Neuropsychiatric Disorders*. pp. 317–46. Tokyo: Springer.

Schneider, L.S., Dagerman, K., and Insel, P. (2005). Risk of death with atypical antipsychotic drug treatment for dementia. meta-analysis of randomized placebo-controlled trials. *JAMA*, **294**, 1934–43.

Shiraki, H. (1975). The neuropatholgy of subacute myelo-optico-neuropathy, 'SMON', in humans: with special reference to the quinoform intoxication. *Japanese Journal of Medical Science and Biology,* **28**(suppl), 101–64.

Shiraki, H. and Takeuchi, T. (1971). Minamata disease. In: *Pathology of the Nervous System (II).* New York, NY: McGraw-Hill.

Shiraki, H., Uchimura, Y., Matsuoka, S., et al. (1958). Effects of atomic radiation on the brain in man a study of the brains of forty-nine Hiroshima and Nagasaki casualties. *Journal of Neuropathology & Experimental Neurology,* **17**,79–137.

Steinberg, M. and Lyketosos, C.G. (2012). Atypical antipsychotic use in patients with dementia. Managing safety concerns. *American Journal of Psychiatry,* **169**, 900–6.

Tateishi, J. (2000). Subacute myelo-optico-neuropathy. Clioquinol Intoxication in humans and animals. *Neuropathology,* **20**(Suppl), 20–4.

Trifiro, G., Spina, E., and Gambassi, G. (2009). Use of antipsychotics in elderly patients with dementia. Do atypical conventional agents have similar safety profile? *Pharmacological Research,* **59**, 1–12.

Tsutsui, T. and Muramatsu, N. (2007). Japan's universal long-term care reform of 2005: containing costs and realizing a vision. *Journal of American Geriatric Society,* **55**, 1458–63.

47

Neuropsychiatry service provision in India and South Asia

Ennapadam S. Krishnamoorthy and Vivek Misra

Introduction

Neuropsychiatry as a specialty barely exists in India and South Asia. Indeed, in many countries in the region, neurology and psychiatry are like chalk and cheese, the interface largely ignored. There are no fellowship training programmes of note, even in the more developed countries in the region, with neuropsychiatry being an area of 'special interest' to some psychiatrists and the occasional neurologist (often more focused on the sister specialties of cognitive and behavioural neurology). However, specific conditions like dementia and, to a lesser extent, epilepsy, have prompted the specialties to merge, at least in clinical work. Indeed, one outcome of this clinical merger is the evolution of home-grown best practice models, mostly focused on caregiving and psychosocial support. In this chapter, we will review the neuropsychiatric service organization, as published in the literature, examine what comprehensive care in neuropsychiatry entails, and use a case study to describe the evolution of best practice model in India.

Neuropsychiatric service organization in India and South Asia

Worldwide there are about 450 million individuals across all societies who, during their lifetime, will suffer from a neuropsychiatric disorder that will exact a high toll on individual productivity and costs and present serious health challenges (including death). With the global burden of disease attributable to neuropsychiatric disorders expected to rise from 12.3% in 2000 to 14.7% in 2020, the situation is set to worsen (Murray and Lopez, 1997). Further, with rapidly changing socio-demographic profiles in South East Asia, we are witnessing an unprecedented increase in both the incidence and the prevalence of neuropsychiatric disorders in the region.

In India, neuropsychiatric disorders account for about 10.8% of the global burden of disorders (Whiteford et al., 2013). As per the government of India's National Commission on Economics and Health Report of 2005, the prevalence of serious mental illness in the Indian population is at least 6.5%, which, by a rough estimate, would be 71 million people (National Commission on Macroeconomics and Health, 2005). Recent community-based research from Chennai, has suggested a prevalence of memory impairment close to 43% (Samuel et al., 2016), whereas our group reported a prevalence of common mental disorder close to 48% (Srivatsa, 2016).

The treatment gap, as measured by the absolute difference between the true prevalence of a disorder and the proportion of treated individuals affected by the disorder, has also been found to be very high. As per WHO's multi-country survey, approximately 76–85% of people with serious mental disorder have received no treatment in the previous 12 months in less developed countries. One of the major reasons attributed to such a wide treatment gap is the problem of inadequate resources, which is more apparent in developing countries like India. Indeed, inadequacy exists not just in terms of infrastructure, but also in terms of human resources, a fact made apparent by statistical data provided by the WHO Mental Health Atlas, as summarized in Table 47.1. Whereas the ideal ratio should be one professional per 10,000 population (Thirunavukarasu and Thirunavukarasu, 2010), in India, we have a ratio of 0.20 per 100,000 population (World Health Organization, 2005).

Training and accreditation

Neuropsychiatric practice was said to encompass 'Janus-faced-like realms of care delivery in clinical neurosciences—the diagnosis and treatment of psychiatric disorders from the perspective of their

Table 47.1 Mental healthcare resources in India

Total psychiatric beds per 10,000 population	0.25
Number of psychiatrists per 100,000 population	0.20
Number of psychiatric nurses per 100,000 population	0.05
Number of psychologists per 100,000 population	0.03
Number of social workers per 100,000 population	0.03

Data accessed from the *WHO Mental Health Atlas*, 2005.

neurological basis, and the clinical care of neurological patients with concomitant mood or behaviour disturbances' (Schiffer and Rogel, 1996).

Clinical practice and treatment in neuropsychiatry require strong neuroscientific foundations with emphasis on research. Unlike in developed countries where some jurisdictions already have well-established neuropsychiatry training programmes, accreditation and training in neuropsychiatry in India and South East Asia are non-existent and largely non-regulated. In the Indian context, exposure to neuropsychiatry training follows a model where a larger tertiary university-affiliated centre offers more structured training through cross-placement of postgraduate trainees in neurology and psychiatry for limited periods of time.

However, there are few published postdoctoral programmes in neuropsychiatry available on the Indian subcontinent. Large national institutes like the National Institute of Mental Health and Neurosciences (NIMHANS) in Bengaluru, the All India Institute of Medical Sciences (AIIMS) in New Delhi, and the Post-Graduate Instiute of Medical Sciences & Research (PGIMER) in Chandigargh all have advanced programmes in neurology and psychiatry, with research at the interface. In addition, the Indian Institute of Science (IIS) in Bengaluru, the National Center for Biological Sciences (NCBS) also in Bengaluru, and the National Brain Research Centre (NBRC) in Manesar all have active neuroscience research programmes at the interface. The Institute of Neurological Sciences at VHS Multispecialty Hospital and Research Institute offers a PhD programme in neuropsychiatry affiliated to the Tamil Nadu Dr. M.G.R. Medical University (State Medical University). The centre focuses upon epilepsy, dementia, neurodevelopmental disorders in childhood, and epidemiology and health outcomes research.

Eligibility criteria for programmes include completion of 3–5 years of training in neurology and/or psychiatry. Programmes in neuropsychiatry are aimed at developing a sound knowledge base in the neuroscientific principles underlying neuropsychiatric practice, in relation to neurophysiology, neuropharmacology, epidemiology, and public health. They also must enable trainees to gain first-hand experience of common neuropsychiatric disorders and become competent in their diagnosis and management; develop expertise in the use and interpretation of specialized neuropsychiatric investigations, particularly neurophysiology, neuroimaging, and neuropsychology; and develop specialized skills in physical treatments in neuropsychiatry, but without ignoring the principles of psychotherapeutic and rehabilitative approaches.

Beyond the clinical training component, training programmes must help to develop skills in the critical evaluation of research evidence in the pathophysiology, phenomenology, and treatment of neuropsychiatric disorders, and conduct research to improve the empirical basis of neuropsychiatric knowledge and practice. Finally, all neuropsychiatrists must be trained to act as advocates for sufferers of neuropsychiatric illnesses and to contribute to the development of the profession.

Table 47.2 describes service provision for dementia in some parts of South East Asia and rural Australia (Krishnamoorthy et al., 2010).

Comprehensive care for neuropsychiatry: 5W1H (who, what, why, when, where, and how)

What is a Comprehensive Care Programme?

A Comprehensive Neuropsychiatry Programme (CNP) links intervention in the narrower medical sense (drugs or surgery) with non-medical interventions (counselling, psychosocial assistance, rehabilitation), thus implying multi-professional structures in diagnosis and treatment. It enquires into every treatment goals, while including the patient's (and their relatives') subjective evaluations and perspectives. The CNP explores functional and cultural aspects of treatment and provides a framework for intervention and quality of life-related outcome.

What constitutes a Comprehensive Neuropsychiatry Programme?

Targeting patients, caregivers, healthcare professionals, and society at large, with a focus on helping the person with a neuropsychiatric disorder, minimizes stigma and achieves optimal levels of participation in activities of daily living (ADLs), health-related quality of life (HRQoL), and social, educational, and occupational milestones. The CNP includes:

- Information and education about the disorder and living with it, delivered in a goal-directed and structured manner.
- Medical and nursing interventions that can help improve outcomes.
- Psychosocial interventions: psychological support and counselling—educational support, cognitive enhancement, and behavioural modification; social empowerment—identification of special needs and benefits.
- Advocacy: governmental understanding, legislation, and civil rights such as driving and insurance.
- Engendering research into neuropsychiatric outcomes.
- Support groups, knowledge forums, other community-engendered activities.

Why Comprehensive Care?

For those with severe or difficult-to-treat conditions, the central concern is to adapt the patient to her/his environment, to a life with symptoms. Beyond this, however, even patients with treatable conditions struggle with stigma and a range of other psychosocial issues, for which the CNP may well be the solution.

Where should Comprehensive Care be delivered?

The CNP requires a multidisciplinary team that works in tandem. It is often seen as a solution that is restricted to state-of-the-art centres that boast of such teams. However, several distributed and community-based models of care have emerged over time, especially for conditions like epilepsy (Birbeck, 2010) and dementia.

Neuropsychiatric services should be community-based and it is important to integrate these services into the primary healthcare structure to ensure sustainability. The Indian model of epilepsy care (Krishnamoorthy and Misra, 2017) is one such example where epilepsy care has been incorporated into programmes for poverty alleviation. Public–private partnerships and non-governmental

Table 47.2 Mental health service provision in South East Asia and Australia

Country	Location (s)	Best practice	Learning point	Reported by
Australia	Rural and remote services	• Multimedia education of community and professionals • Practical workshops addressing day-to-day issues like BPSD • Volunteer recruitment • Clear pathways and access to care: referral protocols • Service partnership agreements • Technology: telemedicine for consultations, case conferences • 24-hour helplines • Outreach clinics	• Close links between staff members • Transdisciplinary principle: going beyond narrow professional boundaries in establishing and delivering services • Pivotal role for primary care practitioners and nurses • Community cohesion—knowledge of, and respect for, persons with dementia	Sadanand Rajkumar, Rural Medical School. Orange, Sydney (Rajkumar and Lane, 2010) 10
China	Hong Kong Special Administrative Region, China	• Adopting and adapting established Western models (e.g. in Hong Kong—the Nottingham model, 1991) • Focus on specialty development: psychogeriatricians for dementia care • Community teams of psychiatrists and nurses for designated catchment areas • Community support services: daycare centres, home help, and home rehabilitation, with NGO support • Guardianship Board to appoint guardians who make decisions for the mentally incapacitated • Public education and advocacy (Alzheimer's Disease China)	• Role for geriatric psychiatrist, neurologist, and traditional Chinese medicine (TCM) doctors • Improved medical resources in rural areas via establishing a 3-tiered service network consolidating county, township, and village • Establishing nursing homes that can cater for the needs of the person with dementia: role of NGOs • Provision of community support: a family bed system providing medical and nursing care at home • Role of nursemaids (paid caregivers)	Helen Chiu, Department of Psychiatry, Chinese University of Hong Kong (Chiu et al., 2011) (11)
Malaysia	Johor Bahru	• Establishment of a multidisciplinary team led by a psychiatrist with nurses, physical therapist, occupational therapist, social worker, pharmacist, and dietician: meets every month • Nurses in charge of overseeing care for patients with dementia living at home (30 patients each) • Establishing a consumer support group—Johor Bahru Alzheimer's Disease Association Support Group (JOBADA)—provides care support and organizes caregiver meetings and counselling	• Family remains the main provider of care • Most affected persons choose home help and home support care • Few dedicated teams offer psychogeriatric services • Few daycare centres mainly in the urban areas • Only two government-run nursing homes—not specific to dementia care • Patients prefer care at home and enjoy better quality of life when cared for at home	Suraya Yusoff, Ministry of Health, Johor, Malaysia (Yusoff et al., 2013) (12)
Japan	Tokyo	• Provision of long-term care insurance • Establishment of an integrated community care system that has five pillars: medical care, long-term care, prevention of long-term care, livelihood support service, and housing. It should be available within 30 minutes of each individual • Community Support Coordinator on Dementia Care (CSC-DC) in order to enhance implementation of dementia care policies, including creating a connection between medical and long-term care facilities/organizations • Initial-Phase Intensive Support Team (IPIST) in charged of organizing the support system for early detection and early diagnosis. Members of IPIST include a certified doctor and medical and long-term care specialists, and the team is set in the integrated community care support centre. Focuses on people living alone with BPSD	• The problem of super-ageing population (25% of people are aged over 65 years) • Increasing elderly population with decreasing population of younger people—shortage of caregivers • Need for elderly to continue to reside in their own communities and enjoy a good quality of life • Many elderly live on their own and suffer from: 1. Lack of a proper diagnosis 2. Lack of continuing medical services 3. Lack of proper welfare services 4. Discontinuous services despite a proper diagnosis	Akira Homma, The Center for Dementia Research & Practices, Tokyo (Homma, 2011) (13)

Source data from Krishnamoorthy ES, Prince MJ, Cummings JL. *Dementia: A global approach*: Cambridge University Press; 2010.

organizations (NGOs) are also important components of the Indian model.

Who needs the CNP?

All people with a neuropsychiatric disorder will potentially benefit from the CNP. There is considerable evidence to suggest that information, education, and understanding help people deal with their condition better. There is also evidence in epilepsy (Pramuka et al., 2007) and dementia that psychosocial interventions improve outcomes. Those who especially will benefit from the CNP are people with intractable or difficult-to-treat conditions, those with comorbidities and complications, etc.

Who should participate in the CNP?

Participants in the CNP should be necessarily multidisciplinary. Thus, apart from physicians (neurologists/paediatricians/geriatricians, as appropriate for the target audience), mental health professionals (psychiatrists/psychologists), nurses, paramedical professionals (physical and occupational therapists, special educators, speech therapists), clinical pharmacologists, and a range of other professionals make up such a team. In addition, apart from patients and caregivers, teachers, various members of legislative, social, and judicial bodies, as appropriate, those working with NGOs and service organizations for the disabled, and others who feel the desire to help can all participate in the CNP.

When should Comprehensive Care commence?

There is no perfect time for the CNP to commence. Ideally, the CNP should be initiated when there is the earliest suggestion of physical, cognitive, or psychosocial impairment in a person with epilepsy.

How should Comprehensive Care be delivered?

Given the diversity of clinical settings and patient expectations around the globe, there is no single preferred model of CNP delivery. Each of the settings reviewed in a textbook on Comprehensive Care in epilepsy published in 2001 (Pfäfflin et al., 2001) had a unique approach to Comprehensive Care. So too did each of the caregiving models reviewed in the World Health Organization Report on dementia in 2012 (World Health Organization, 2012). We present below a best practice model that we have developed and implemented for a range of neuropsychiatric disorders in India. Beginning in a secondary–tertiary care hospital, this model has been now established across a network of four primary (family) healthcare centres in Chennai as a model of chronic disease management.

A novel service delivery model for developing nations

The multidisciplinary team managing this programme is led by a neuropsychiatrist (team leader) supported by a team of 40 professionals and healthcare workers (doctors, clinical psychologists and neuropsychologists, psychiatric social workers, physical and occupational therapists, special educators and child guidance counsellors, nurses, paramedical staff, research and support staff). The team provides a gamut of services, including a range of physical, occupational, and psychological therapies, as well as counselling and advocacy services (see Fig. 47.1). The team has developed its own multidisciplinary electronic medical record (EMR) system which integrates the entire care delivery process, enhancing the healthcare experience for patients and the treatment team, while ensuring continuous quality data collection with inputs from several disciplines.

In this service delivery model, the counselling psychologist/social worker serves as the case manager, and hence the first port of call for patients with neuropsychiatric disorders, including epilepsy. They provide counselling, liaison, and advocacy services, directing the patient to appropriate members of the clinical team. In this way, the case manager establishes a link between themselves and the patient and his/her family. In the Indian context, the family plays a significant role and is closely involved with the medical management team of the individual. By being the link between the patient and their family and the medical team, the social worker as the case manager can optimize the delivery of care and support services. The effort is to leverage individual, family, and community support systems to the best extent possible that would ensure rehabilitation needs are met and quality of life optimized. This model of teamwork with a case manager taking the lead has, in our

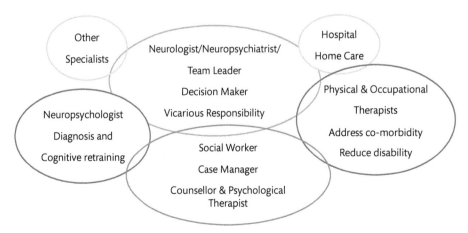

Fig. 47.1 An ideal model for neuropsychiatry and psychosocial service delivery and rehabilitation for people with neuropsychiatric disorders in India.

Typical Workflow

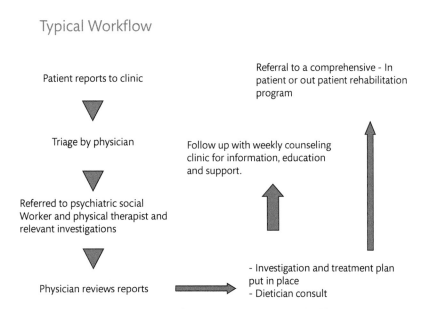

Fig. 47.2 A working model of multidisciplinary case management for neuropsychiatry across the lifespan.

view, considerable potential in the developing nation setting, as it reduces dependence on the doctor and allows scarce medical skill resources to be used optimally. Fig. 47.2 depicts the working of this model of multidisciplinary case management for neuropsychiatry across the lifespan.

More recently, the team has managed to integrate traditional medical systems into its approach—Ayurveda, acupuncture, acupressure, reflexology, naturopathy, and yoga (Misra et al., 2019)—thus enhancing the cultural relevance of the programme and lowering the 4A barriers to healthcare delivery, namely availability, accessibility, accountability, and acceptability.

CASE STUDY

Miss V, a 14-year old with a childhood history of febrile seizures, suffered from repeated episodes of jerking and being 'absent' that tended to cluster around her menstrual periods. She also had falling academic grades, mood swings, anxiety, disturbed digestion, and poor sleep. A good student whose childhood epilepsy had been well controlled, she was bemused by the sudden outbreak of symptoms around menarche that had, over a year, substantially reduced her quality of life.

Consultations with an array of specialists and close observation by her intelligent and attentive parents led to the understanding that the problem was not easily responsive to conventional medication; was closely linked to stress, both academic and familial; clustered around her menstrual periods; was unpredictable and at times subtle (a jerk or two while at the dining table that could otherwise pass off as a teenage mannerism); and could affect her on several days in a month. Indeed, her father, a diligent record-keeper, could identify as many as 50–60 events in each month, occurring in 5–6 clusters. Interesting also, she had a narrow therapeutic window within which AEDs appeared to be efficacious, beyond which there was rapid worsening of symptoms.

A Comprehensive Care approach for such a patient in our setting would comprise detailed neuropsychiatric history documentation encompassing general medical, neurological, psychiatric, developmental, social, familial, gynaecological, and nutritional history. A detailed treatment history would include drugs, doses, side effects, and impact of treatment. History taking would be followed by biochemical and imaging investigations to exclude comorbidities and complications. Upon clinical consensus on the diagnosis, a therapeutic alliance would be established with the family, focusing upon a firm commitment to work together, with transparency, mutual respect, and common goals.

An interdisciplinary therapeutic programme was planned which included nutritional, psychological counselling, yoga therapy, and naturopathic and Ayurveda therapies for digestion, sleep, and perimenstrual symptoms. A carefully graded approach to drug treatment of epilepsy was taken, with the aim to identify the ideal drug combination and the therapeutic window thereof.

After adopting a similar approach for Miss V over a 1-year period, with her attending periodic sessions of therapy, as her symptoms demanded and school schedule permitted, and stabilizing her on a two-AED (lamotrigine and topiramate) combination at relatively low doses, we observed several gains. The frequency and severity of seizure episodes improved, with a reduction in the number of episodes from 50 to 2–3 a month, with brief and limited impact, which only lasted a couple of hours at best. Mood swings and anxiety had remitted, while sleep and appetite had improved significantly. Miss V's stress levels had fallen and peri-menstrual periods had become bearable. At the end of the therapy programme, Miss V was compliant with the medications and tolerated her drug doses well.

A therapeutic alliance and an interdisciplinary approach—a recommended global best practice model of epilepsy care (Krishnamoorthy and Gillam, 2009)—appear to have worked for Miss V, who is firmly on the road to recovery.

Conclusion

There is a crucial need for Comprehensive Care programmes, which focus on biopsychosocial well-being of people with neuropsychiatric illness and their caregivers. A multidisciplinary approach or, even better, an interdisciplinary approach (where team members are in active and dynamic engagement with patients) not only focusing upon symptoms, but also aiming to improve quality of life, while addressing comorbid biopsychosocial outcomes, is the need of the hour. Many resource-poor countries are manpower-rich and may benefit substantially from such a model. If the programme is to have a lasting impact, it would be essential to work with, and educate, the local professionals and public about the recent advances in neuropsychiatric care and choice of treatment.

KEY LEARNING POINTS

- Neuropsychiatry as a specialty is significantly underrepresented in India, with neurology and psychiatry giving each other a wide berth in many of the country's regions.
- This chapter reviews the state of the neuropsychiatric services in India and South Asia, before moving on to explore what constitutes a Comprehensive Neuropsychiatry Programme (CNP).
- This encompasses education and research on neuropsychiatric outcomes, advocacy at a governmental level, and community-engendered activities, all with a view to attaining optimal levels of participation in activities of daily living (ADLs), health-related quality of life (HRQoL), and various social and educational milestones.
- The model employed by a multidisciplinary team for use in developing nations is then described, along with a case study to demonstrate best practice.

REFERENCES

Birbeck GL. Epilepsy care in developing countries: part I of II. Epilepsy Currents. 2010;10(4):75–9.

Chiu H, Tsoh J, Yu X. Care arrangement for patients with dementia: China. In: Krishnamoorthy ES, Prince MJ, Cummings JL, editors. *Dementia: A Global Approach*. Cambridge: Cambridge University Press; 2010. pp. 107–12.

Homma A. Non-pharmacological approaches: patient-centered approached: Japan. In: Krishnamoorthy ES, Prince MJ, Cummings JL, editors. *Dementia: A Global Approach*. Cambridge: Cambridge University Press; 2011. pp. 141–6.

Krishnamoorthy ES, Gilliam F. Best clinical and research practice in adult epileptology. Epilepsy & Behavior. 2009;15(2):S55–9.

Krishnamoorthy ES, Misra V. Comprehensive epilepsy care: transcultural issues and the development of a best-practice model In India. In: Krishnamoorthy ES, Shorvon SD, Schachter SC, editors. *Epilepsy—A Global Approach*. Cambridge: Cambridge University Press; 2017. pp. 77–82.

Krishnamoorthy ES, Prince MJ, Cummings JL. *Dementia: A Global Approach*. Cambridge: Cambridge University Press; 2010.

Misra V, Srivatsa VG, Krishnamoorthy ES. Epilepsy and behavior: response to an integrative treatment paradigm highlighting complementary and alternative medicine. In: Hauptman AJ, Salpekar JA, editors. *Pediatric Neuropsychiatry*. Cham: Springer; 2019. pp. 189–204.

Murray CJ, Lopez AD. Alternative projections of mortality and disability by cause 1990–2020: Global Burden of Disease Study. The Lancet. 1997;349(9064):1498–504.

National Commission of Macroeconomics and Health. *Burden of diseases in India*. New Delhi: National Commission of Macroeconomics and Health; 2005.

Pfäfflin M, Fraser RT, Thorbecke R, Specht U, Wolf P. *Comprehensive Care for People With Epilepsy*. London: John Libbey; 2001.

Pramuka M, Hendrickson R, Zinski A, Van Cott AC. A psychosocial self-management program for epilepsy: a randomized pilot study in adults. Epilepsy & Behavior. 2007;11(4):533–45.

Rajkumar S, Lane J. Service delivery and management. In: Krishnamoorthy ES, Prince MJ, Cummings JL, editors. *Dementia: A Global Approach*. Cambridge: Cambridge University Press; 2010. p. 113.

Samuel R, McLachlan CS, Mahadevan U, Isaac V. Cognitive impairment and reduced quality of life among old-age groups in Southern Urban India: home-based community residents, free and paid old-age home residents. QJM. 2016;109(10):653–9.

Schiffer R, Fogel B. Evolution of neuropsychiatric ideas in the United States and United Kingdom—1800–2000. Neuropsychiatry. 1996:1–10.

Srivatsa VG. *Determinants of BPS in an urban elderly population* [Dissertation]. Chennai: Tamil Nadu Dr. M.G.R. Medical University; 2016.

Thirunavukarasu M, Thirunavukarasu P. Training and National deficit of psychiatrists in India—A critical analysis. Indian J Psychiatry. 2010;52(Suppl 1):S83–8.

Whiteford HA, Degenhardt L, Rehm J, et al. Global burden of disease attributable to mental and substance use disorders: findings from the Global Burden of Disease Study 2010. The Lancet. 2013;382(9904):1575–86.

World Health Organization. *Mental Health Atlas 2005*. Geneva: World Health Organization; 2005.

World Health Organization. *Dementia: A Public Health Priority*. Geneva: World Health Organization; 2012.

Yusoff S, Koh CT, Mohd Aminuddin MY, Krishnasamy M, Suhaila MZ. Initial evaluation of the training programme for health care professionals on the use of Malaysian clinical practice guidelines for management of dementia. East Asian Archives of Psychiatry. 2013;23(3):91.

48

Neuropsychiatry services in Central, Southern, and Eastern Europe

Martín L. Vargas, Alla Guekht, and Josef Priller

Development of neuropsychiatry services worldwide

Development of neuropsychiatry services worldwide is an objective for consolidating the discipline (Agrawal, 2012). The nature and range of the essential skill sets required by neuropsychiatrists are well defined. It must include basic skills in psychiatry and neurology, as well as expertise in neuroimaging, neuropsychology, and neurophysiology (Sachdev, 2005). These attributes constitute the core of the 'neuropsychiatric approach' that can be complemented with skills in neuropsychological counselling, cognitive rehabilitation, and physical treatments. The World Health Assembly's Resolution on epilepsy is a good example of the inter-professional and international perspective needed in the achievement of optimal care for neuropsychiatric diseases (Covanis et al., 2015).

Most scientific work in neuropsychiatry scientific production relates to the clinical aspects of the discipline, whereas only 6.4% of the publications during the last years dealt with service evaluation, classification, and the history of neuropsychiatry (Srirathan and Cavanna, 2015). Provision of neuropsychiatry services has been mainly studied in the UK. Using standardized questionnaires for commissioners and service providers, the provision of neuropsychiatry services was examined in London (Agrawal et al., 2015). The study concluded that a huge variability exists across different parts of London, with a 25-fold variation in incidence across the 30 referring geographical units. Among the factors accounting for this variation, different grades of awareness of neuropsychiatry among commissioners and providers were noted. Another study, specifically designed for service commissioners, observed that the perception of what constitutes neuropsychiatry varied significantly between commissioners and providers (Bhattacharya et al., 2015). There is a consensus in the neuropsychiatric community that defining neuropsychiatry constitutes a priority for consolidation of the discipline.

In Central, Southern, and Eastern Europe, the implementation of neuropsychiatric services has not been carefully studied, but it can be expected that a similar degree of variability to that in the UK exists. Additional variability in continental Europe may derive from differences in the theoretical background of neuropsychiatry in continental Europe, compared with the Anglo-Saxon tradition. Thus, in order to promote international homogeneity of services and practices, local historical perspectives need to be considered.

Historical perspectives in Central, Southern, and Eastern European neuropsychiatry

The origins in Central Europe

Neuropsychiatry is one of the oldest medical disciplines. Many brain disorders had been known from ancient times, but for centuries, mostly empirical data about neuropsychiatric diseases were accumulated. Even in ancient times, there were remarkable discoveries, among which was the understanding of epilepsy as a disease of the brain that was declared by Hippocrates. However, 'the history of neuropsychiatry is yet to be written', as Berrios and Marková reminded us when reviewing the historical roots of the concept (Berrios and Marková, 2002). The history of neuropsychiatry is closely related to that of other disciplines such as phenomenology (Trimble, 2016a).

The major initial contributions towards a better characterization of neuropsychiatric disorders in continental Europe were made in France during the first decades of the nineteenth century. This concurs with the epistemological context of positivism and autonomy. Among the most important achievements was the evolution from restriction to treatment, which was made by Philippe Pinel (1745–1826), who removed the 'chains' from the mentally ill. In 1860, the first neurological department was founded in the Pitié-Salpêtrière Hospital under the leadership of Jean-Martin Charcot (1825–1893). Many neurological diseases were described in Charcot's school. He was an outstanding mentor and many physicians from other countries completed their internships in the Pitié-Salpêtrière Hospital. The French school was complemented in the first decades of the twentieth century with neuropathological studies coming from Germany, beginning with Griesinger half a century before Kraepelin (Hoff, 2015). Under the common discipline of 'Nervenheilkunde', German-speaking regions maintained the unity of neurology and psychiatry for a long time with a neuropathology-based perspective. The 'Deutsche Forschungsanstalt für Psychiatrie' represents this period very well (Weber, 2000). In Spain and Italy, Cajal's and Golgi's laboratories markedly contributed to this classical period of European continental neuropsychiatry where a positivist, naturalistic, and integrated vision prevailed.

The period between the two World Wars was associated with a weakening of the unified concept of neuropsychiatry. Notably, the psychoanalytic movement was divisive, exemplified by the different approaches that Meynert, Freud, and Wagner-Jauregg took towards the emergent problem of psychoneuroses during the Great War (Bogousslavsky and Tatu, 2013). Another important factor for the decline of neuropsychiatry in the middle of the twentieth century was the devastating impact of nazism and fascism in continental Europe. It resulted in the emigration of many German-speaking Jewish neuropsychiatrists, mainly to North America (Arzy and Danziger, 2014; Peiffer, 1991).

The European neuropsychiatric tradition broke with the Second World War, and the division between neurology and psychiatry became explicit at the end of the 1940s (Arzy and Danziger, 2014; Stahnisch and Russell, 2016). The proclamation that 'there is no neuropathology of schizophrenia', which was made during the First International Congress of Neuropathology in Rome in 1952, finally tore the ties between neurology and psychiatry. One might say that schizophrenia was not only a 'graveyard for neuropathologists', but also a 'graveyard for neuropsychiatry'.

During the second half of the twentieth century, the continuity of the German neuropsychiatric tradition was preserved in Frankfurt (Main) and Berlin by the Wernicke–Kleist–Leonhard school (Neumarker and Bartsch, 2003). New neuropsychiatric perspectives, which incorporated phenomenological elements, emerged in the second half of the century in the Gerd Huber school (Rzesnitzek, 2013).

Other roots were important in European neuropsychiatry, such as the hierarchical model of John Hughlings Jackson, who was a major figure, besides Charcot, of the 'heroic age of neuropsychiatry' (Trimble, 2016b). Jackson's model inspired the 'dynamical perspective' of neuropsychiatry practised in France by Henry Ey. The 'organodynamic' model of Ey represented an important opportunity to develop a monistic model of neuropsychiatry, integrating both psychoanalysis and neurobiology (Chebili, 2016). However, differences in interpretation of the teaching coming from Gaëtan Gatian de Clérambault by Henry Ey and Jacques Lacan impeded the consolidation of the organodynamic theory in France. The end of monistic neuropsychiatry in France began with the disappearance of accreditation in neuropsychiatry in 1968, substituted by accreditation in either neurology or psychiatry (Pinel, 2005).

In the UK, the hierarchical model of Jackson inspired neurologists more than psychiatrists. In the middle of the twentieth century, the Anglo-American tradition represented by the teaching of Adolf Meyer and William Mayer-Gross laid the foundation for a perspective later consolidated by Alwyn Lishman (Lishman, 1992). According to Sachdev's approach of delineating the territory of neuropsychiatry (Sachdev, 2005), it may be called a 'clinical territorial perspective'. In this perspective, emphasis was placed on the set of diseases to be treated by neuropsychiatrists. Given the well-defined differentiation between neurology and psychiatry in the English-speaking tradition, the focus was on the 'frontier territory'.

Historical perspectives of neuropsychiatry in Southern Europe (Spain)

Different countries in Mediterranean Europe have their own traditions. As examples, we note here the child neuropsychiatry tradition in Italy, the research of Egas Moniz in Portugal, the long tradition of the Pula Congress in Croatia (Barac and Demarin, 2015), or the celebration of the Fifth International Congress of Neuropsychiatry in Athens in Greece in 2004.

Historically, psychiatry in Spain has been focusing on providing healthcare. This was accomplished by religious congregations, in collaboration with the state administration, who have been maintaining psychiatric hospitals since 1410, when 'Padre Jofre' founded in Valencia the 'Hospital d'Innocents, Follcs i Orats', which has been suggested to be the first psychiatric hospital in the world (Lopez-Ibor, 2008). The contemporary precursor of psychiatry in Spain was Pere Mata i Fontanet (1811–1877) who introduced the discipline from legal medicine. After him, Joan Giné i Partagás (1836–1903) in Barcelona and José María Esquerdo Zaragoza (1842–1912) in Madrid prepared the social, political, and scientific environment in the last third of the nineteenth century for the subsequent work of Cajal and his neuropsychiatric school during the beginning of the twentieth century. The former organized the first Spanish Congress of Psychiatry ('Certamen Frenopático Español') in Barcelona in 1883 (Villasante Armas, 1997), while Esquerdo is considered to be the person who introduced the anatomo-clinical method to Spanish psychiatry (Huertas, 2003).

The Spanish history of psychopathology in the twentieth century can be divided into three epochs (Lázaro, 2003). The first one, until the Civil War (1936–1939), was influenced by French psychopathology. With regard to neuropsychiatry, the concession of the Nobel Prize to Santiago Ramón y Cajal in 1906 enhanced the diffusion of the neurone theory and influenced the teaching in Germany and other European countries. A new generation of Spanish neuropsychiatrists emerged who were encouraged by Cajal's prestige and supported by the government institution 'Junta de Ampliación de Estudios e Investigaciones Científicas', which was founded in 1907 and presided by Cajal himself. In 1911, the first Spanish society for clinical neurosciences—the 'Sociedad de Psiquiatría y Neurología de Barcelona'—was created. The foundation in 1920 of the journal *Archivos de Neurobiología* and the constitution in Barcelona in 1924 of the 'Asociación Española de Neuropsiquiatras' (Lázaro, 2000) constituted the scientific framework into which Spanish neuropsychiatry was born around Santiago Ramón y Cajal (1852–1934). Psychiatrists, neurologists, and neuropathologists, including Luis Simarro (1851–1921), Luis Barraquer I Roviralta (1855–1928), Nicolás Achúcarro (1880–1918), Pío del Río Hortega (1882–1945), and Gonzalo Rodríguez Lafora (1886–1971), led this movement (Valenciano Gayá, 1977). On the stele of Lafora, considered the pioneer of Spanish neuropsychiatry (López-Muñoz et al., 2007), a neuropsychiatric group grew in the area of Murcia in the middle of the twentieth century, with authors such as Bartolomé Llopis Lloret (Llopis, 2001), Román Alberca, and Luis Valenciano Gaya.

During Franco's rule (1939–1975), psychiatry was influenced by the German tradition. In 1949 the 'Sociedad Española de Neurología', in 1958 the 'Sociedad Española de Psiquiatría', and in 1974 the 'Sociedad Española de Psiquiatría Biológica' were founded. Since the democratic period, Spanish psychiatry has been mainly under

Anglo-Saxon influence. Juan José López Ibor, Juan José López-Ibor Aliño, and Carlos Castilla del Pino were the main leaders in the second half of the twentieth century, when phenomenology, existentialism, psychoanalysis, and social psychiatry replaced neuropsychiatry as theoretical frameworks. Julián de Ajuriaguerra, who was born in Bilbao but developed his scientific work close to Hécaen in France and in Geneva, remained close to neuropsychiatry. In the twenty-first century, Spanish psychiatry achieved an international perspective, independent of schools.

Since 1977, after the separation of neurology and psychiatry in the middle of the twentieth century, the 'Asociación Española de Neuropsiquiatría' (AEN) turned its priority to the political aspects of psychiatry. As a result, the field of neuropsychiatry had a low degree of development, with some exceptions like the work of Demetrio Barcia and others. The points of view of biological psychiatry took over the area of classical neuropsychiatry. In 2012, the section of Clinical Neuroscience of the AEN was created, in an attempt to provide new impulses for neuropsychiatry in Spain from a cognitive neuroscience point of view. Nowadays, psychiatry and neurology in Spain do not share any specific area of training in neuropsychiatry.

Historical perspectives of neuropsychiatry in Eastern Europe (Russia)

The first department of psychiatry in Russia was organized in 1857 at the Saint Petersburg Medicosurgical Academy by Ivan Balinsky (1827–1902). Ten years later, he created a European-level clinic of psychiatry in the Academy with a theatre, a greenhouse, and separate occupational therapy premises (Krasnov and Gurovich, 2012).

The founder of Russian neurology Aleksey Kozhevnikov (1836–1902) (Valko and Bassetti, 2006) was a trainee of Charcot and a mentor to many world-renowned Russian psychiatrists and neurologists: Sergei Korsakov (1853–1900), Grigory Rossolimo (1860–1928), Liverij Darkshevich (1858–1925), Vladimir Roth (1848–1916), Lazar Minor (1855–1942), and others. Aleksey Kozhevnikov triggered the establishment of new departments and hospitals for neurologically and mentally ill people in Russia; he founded the Russian Society of Neurologists and Psychiatrists and the *Korsakov's Journal of Neurology and Psychiatry* that is currently the leading Russian journal in the area of brain diseases (Valko and Bassetti, 2006).

One of the most famous Russian neurologists and psychiatrists at the end of nineteenth and the beginning of the twentieth century was Vladimir Bekhterev (1857–1927) (Lerner et al., 2006). He began his career in the city of Kazan where he founded the Psychophysiology Laboratory and the professional Society of Psychiatrists and Neurologists. In 1881, he had completed his doctoral thesis on '*Clinical studies of temperature in some forms of mental disorders*'. In 1884, he got an internship in Germany where he learnt from Westphal, Mendel, and Dubois-Reymond; he also visited psychiatric clinics in Paris, Munich, and Vienna. Later, Bekhterev returned to Saint Petersburg where he founded the first Russian Institute of Neuropsychiatry in 1907, which became the centre of research and education in psychology, psychiatry, neurology, and neurosurgery. Bekhterev's contribution to the understanding of the nuclei and pathways of the brain was outstanding; for instance, he was the first to mention the role that the hippocampus plays in memory. Bekhterev paid special attention to neurophysiology and psychology. He tried to understand the biological,

psychological, and philosophical causes of nervous and mental disorders and their aetiology and pathogenesis; among his areas of interest were hypnosis and suicidality and its prevention. He published more than 600 papers and many books, among which included *Suggestion and its Role in Social Life, Consciousness and its Borders, Psyche and Life, Objective Psychology, The Pathways of the Brain and the Spinal Cord, Subject Matter and Tasks of Social Psychology as an Objective Science*, and *General Principles of Human Reflexology*. He founded several journals, including *Archives of Psychiatry, Neurology and Experimental Psychology, Bulletin of Psychology, Criminal Anthropology and Hypnotism*, and *The Bulletin of Neurology and Psychiatry* (now named after him), as well as the Institute of Neuropsychiatry in Saint Petersburg.

From the beginning of the twentieth century, neurology and psychiatry in Russia increasingly separated and developed as different fields of medicine. Neurologists studied organic (structural) lesions of the brain such as stroke, Parkinson's disease, multiple sclerosis, and others, whereas psychiatrists focused on diseases without organic signs—schizophrenia, depression, and personality disorders.

One of the most famous Russian psychiatrists was Sergey Korsakov (1854–1900) (Ovsyannikov and Ovsyannikov, 2007), who greatly contributed to the understanding and classification of psychoses. One of his merits was the system of non-restriction of mentally ill patients; he was against surgical castration of psychotic patients. The psychiatric clinic of First Moscow Medical University and the *Neurology and Psychiatry Journal* were named after him.

Peter Gannushkin (1875–1933) was a follower of Korsakov. Gannushkin completed fellowships in the Munich clinic of E Kraepelin and St Anne Clinic in Paris. Being very interested in psychoanalysis, he was the creator of the 'small psychiatry' concept. He studied pathologic characters, and the monograph *The Clinic of Psychopathies: Statics, Dynamics and Systematics* made him famous all over the world.

Another outstanding Russian psychiatrist was Vasily Gilyarovsky (1876–1959). For approximately 40 years, he was the head of the psychiatry department of the Second Moscow Medical University and the head of one of the largest psychiatric hospitals (N8). His work was devoted to the fundamental aspects of clinical psychiatry—the role of exogenous factors in the genesis of schizophrenia and neuroses. He did much for the development of the outpatient medical services and psychiatric aid for children. The hospital N8 became the Moscow Research and Clinical Centre for Neuropsychiatry—one of the leading Russian research centres and clinics where neurology and psychiatry are closely interrelated.

Since the beginning of the twenty-first century, the trend to merge neurology and psychiatry is becoming more obvious. The comorbidity of many neurological and psychiatric diseases is apparent. Both disciplines use the same methods, including neuroimaging, neurochemistry, and psychological scaling, and both centre around prevention, diagnosis, and treatment of brain diseases.

Historical perspectives of neuropsychiatry in Central Europe (Germany)

In contrast to the Anglo-American tradition, the discipline of 'Nervenheilkunde' in Germany has traditionally encompassed neurology and psychiatry. Many of the pioneers worked in Berlin. Moritz Heinrich Romberg (1795–1873) was director of the Department for

Internal Medicine at the Charité and the founder of clinical neurology in Germany. Inspired by English and French colleagues, he wrote the first textbook of nervous diseases in humans (*Lehrbuch der Nervenkrankheiten des Menschen*). Romberg classified organic disorders ('neuroses') based on careful clinical description, pathoanatomical findings, and the results of animal experiments. His successor at the Charité, Wilhelm Griesinger (1817–1868), held chairs in internal medicine, neurology, and psychiatry during his career. He strongly advocated the integration of neurology and psychiatry. Griesinger opposed the practice of 'Anstaltspsychiatrie' in insane asylums, which separated psychiatry from the more prestigious field of general medicine. Together with Ludwig Meyer (1827–1900) in Göttingen, he founded the journal *Archiv für Psychiatrie und Nervenheilkunde*, which can be regarded as the beginning of academic psychiatry in Germany. Griesinger's approach to mental health was materialistic and he considered the brain to be the primary organ responsible for psychosis in his famous textbook of psychiatry *Die Pathologie und Therapie der psychischen Krankheiten, für Aerzte und Studirende dargestellt* (1845). Inspired by Marshall Hall's work on the spinal reflex arc, he postulated that a dysfunction of mental reflexes was at the origin of mental disorders, whose different forms were considered to reflect different stages of a unitary disease process ('Einheitspsychose'). Griesinger's assistant Carl Friedrich Otto Westphal (1833–1890) was appointed full Professor of Psychiatry at the Charité in 1874. His seminal contributions to neurosciences, including the description of a deep tendon reflex anomaly in tabes dorsalis, 'pseudosclerosis', narcolepsy, agoraphobia, and an accessory nucleus of the oculomotor nerve, inspired subsequent generations of eminent 'Nervenärzte', including Hermann Oppenheim (1833–1890), Karl Wernicke (1848–1905), and Arnold Pick (1851–1924). It should be pointed out that the institutional dominance of psychiatry in the newly formed university departments called 'Psychiatrische und Nervenkliniken' in Berlin, Breslau, Erlangen, Göttingen, Halle, and Leipzig could not conceal the strong influence of neurology on psychiatry at the time (Shterenshis, 1999). This can be nicely exemplified by the work of the psychiatrist Wernicke on encephalopathy and aphasia. It was not until Wilhelm Erb (1840–1921), a specialist in internal medicine like Romberg, that neurology separated from general medicine and psychiatry to become an independent discipline in Germany. In 1880, Erb was appointed director of the Department of Internal Medicine at the University of Leipzig, and he was supported by Adolf Strümpell (1853–1925) in his endeavour to liberate neurology from the influence of psychiatrists (Martin et al., 2016). Following Erb's recommendation, Hermann Oppenheim founded the association 'Gesellschaft Deutscher Nervenärzte (GDN)' in 1907 to specifically reflect the interests of neurologists. Finally, in 1919, Max Nonne (1861–1959) was appointed to the first Clinical Chair of Neurology at the University of Hamburg. The schism between neurology and psychiatry was promoted by the revolutionary influence that the psychodynamic theory and psychoanalysis had on German-speaking psychiatrists. Trained as a neuroanatomist and a neurologist, the Austrian Sigmund Freud (1856–1939) was an expert on cerebral paralysis and aphasia and was the first to introduce the term of 'agnosia', before he developed psychoanalysis with Josef Breuer (1842–1925) under the influence of Charcot's studies on hysteria (Miller and Katz, 1989). In contrast to Freud, Emil Kraepelin (1856–1926), the other influential psychiatrist at the beginning of the twentieth century, was more inclined to follow the 'degeneration' theory of mental illnesses. Kraepelin worked in Leipzig, Dorpat (Estonia), Heidelberg, and Munich. He was strongly inspired by experimental psychology and introduced the nosological dichotomy of endogenous psychoses, which differentiated 'manic depression' from 'dementia praecox' [later called 'schizophrenias' by the Swiss psychiatrist Paul Eugen Bleuler (1857–1939)]. Kraepelin also pioneered psychopharmacological research. Together with Aloysius (Alois) Alzheimer (1864–1915), he introduced 'presenile dementia' as a disease entity. During the First World War, neuropsychiatry continued to flourish in Germany, with seminal contributions by Karl Kleist (1879–1960), Kurt Goldstein (1878–1965), and many others. In 1924, the psychiatrist Hans Berger (1873–1941) performed the first human electrocorticogram recording in Jena. With the advent of national socialism in Germany, the golden age of neuropsychiatry was abruptly terminated. The Nazis squashed the emerging autonomy of neurology and merged the GDN into the 'Gesellschaft deutscher Neurologen und Psychiater (GDNP)', in order to facilitate their eugenics programme ('Aktion T4') and human experimentation. Jewish neuropsychiatrists were dismissed from their positions and replaced by 'Aryan' physicians who supported the new regime. Among the clinical subjects, neurology and psychiatry had the highest percentage of dismissed academics (65%) (Martin et al., 2016). Those who could fled the country and promoted neuroscience in England—Max Bielschowsky (1869–1940), Felix Plaut (1877–1940); the United States—Kurt Goldstein, Alfred Albert Quadfasel (1902–1981), Friedrich Heinrich Lewy (1885–1950), Leo Alexander (1905–1985)); and Israel—Kurt Löwenstein (1883–1956). Many committed suicide or were killed, as for example Ludwig Pick (1886–1944). German neuropsychiatry never recovered from the disaster. After the Second World War, Karl Leonhard (1904–1988) in East Berlin and Karl Kleist (1879–1960) in Frankfurt established a classification system of psychosis in Wernicke's tradition. Today, medical specialization in 'Nervenheilkunde' has been formally abolished in Germany. Although prospective neurologists still need to spend a rotational year in psychiatry during their 5-year residency training, and vice versa, this regulation has been called into question by the German Neurological Society (DGN). The integration of psychiatric services into general medicine is provided by two independent disciplines in Germany—psychiatry and psychotherapy, as well as by psychosomatics and psychotherapeutic medicine (Diefenbacher, 2004). As a result of the increasing fragmentation, the discipline of neuropsychiatry has witnessed a renaissance in Germany (Priller et al., 2011). In 2008, the first independent academic clinical department of neuropsychiatry was established at the Charité in Berlin. Three years later, the German Association for Psychiatry, Psychotherapy, and Psychosomatics (DGPPN) recognized the field of neuropsychiatry by establishing a dedicated committee.

Clinical neurosciences as an encompassing discipline in the twenty-first century

Despite the long history of neuropsychiatry in Europe, the 'Internet era' and globalization determine the present and future of science. While the past may help us to understand the present, it tells us little about the future. The future of neuropsychiatry probably depends more on the rational consensus of international scientific and medical communities than on geographical, cultural, or historical perspectives.

The topic of the 'territory' seems to be pivotal for the definition of neuropsychiatry and its consolidation as a solid scientific paradigm. Neuropsychiatry is currently experiencing a renaissance (Arambepola et al., 2012), and it is therefore important to remember Sachdev's warning: 'Neuropsychiatry cannot afford to be expansive on the back of a neuroscientific juggernaut, as psychiatry and neurology have tickets for the same ride' (Sachdev, 2005).

Systems and molecular neurosciences are beginning to elucidate brain functions, which are linked to the pathogenesis of many neuropsychiatric diseases. A change of paradigm is necessary in research and education (Rubin and Zorumski, 2012; Taylor et al., 2015). Clinical neurosciences may drive this change, opening a window of opportunity to integrate neurology, psychiatry, clinical neurophysiology, neuropsychology, and other clinical disciplines related to brain diseases into a comprehensive, transcultural, and systematic field of practice. Drawing on an epistemological, scientific, and clinically coherent framework (Vargas, 2017; Vargas Aragón, 2012), the comprehensive paradigm of clinical neurosciences may be defined by the following three principles:

1. Epistemological: clinical neurosciences must adopt a monist response to the brain–mind problem (Sachdev, 2002). Emergentist (e.g. Bunge, 2010), integrative (e.g. Northoff, 2008), or any other epistemological monist model is compatible with clinical neurosciences. As, by definition, science is realistic and materialistic, any idealist monist model (e.g. some conceptions of phenomenology or psychoanalysis) and any dualist model (e.g. nineteenth-century neurology–psychiatry separation) are incompatible with scientific ontological materialism. Clinical neurosciences are rooted in science, more specifically in neurosciences, which, as cognitive neurosciences overcome a mere neurobiological perspective.

2. Medical: the medical model is necessary and sufficient to any brain-related medical discipline. The model is characterized by evidence-based definition of disease, prevention, diagnosis, therapy, and rehabilitation. The medical model is compatible with other models applied in health sciences and service provision such as the 'disorder' orientation proposed by the DSM.

3. Operational: high-quality attendance to complex clinical problems requires clinical services and medical specialties with a definite and narrow territory of intervention. 'Ars longa, vita brevis,' Seneca wrote. The family of medical, psychological, and basic science disciplines related to brain diseases and behavioural disorders should develop synergistically, based on the above-mentioned shared epistemological and medical principles.

Under the paradigm of clinical neurosciences, some new integrative perspectives in psychiatry, such as neurophenomenology (Olivares et al., 2015), neuropsychoanalysis (Johnson and Flores Mosri, 2016), or 'neuronal integration' models (Northoff, 2008), can be easily accomodated. In the same way, new classification schemes, such as the Research Domain Criteria (RDoCs) (Casey et al., 2013) or 'data mining' clustering methods (Fontaine et al., 2015), can be applied.

KEY LEARNING POINTS

- Neuropsychiatry is an old and heterogenous discipline that is becoming a well-defined clinical specialty in the twenty-first century. Despite different historical roots, implementation of neuropsychiatry services in continental Europe is closely linked with developments in the UK, North America, and thoughout the world.

- An international perspective is required for the evolving discipline in the era of globalization. The paradigm of clinical neurosciences defined by epistemological, medical, and operational principles may be helpful for the consolidation of neuropsychiatry and the establishment of services in Central, Southern, and Eastern Europe.

REFERENCES

Agrawal, N. (2012). Editorial: Development of neuropsychiatry services worldwide. Acta Neuropsychiatrica 24: 189–90.

Agrawal, N., et al. (2015). Provision of neuropsychiatry services: variability and unmet need. BJPsych Bull 39(6): 297–301.

Arambepola, N., et al. (2012). The evolving discipline and services of neuropsychiatry in the United Kingdom. Acta Neuropsychiatrica 24: 191–8.

Arzy, S. and S. Danziger (2014). The science of neuropsychiatry: past, present, and future. J Neuropsychiatry Clin Neurosci 26(4): 392–5.

Barac, B. and V. Demarin (2015). Six Decades of the Pula Neuropsychiatric Meetings—from Neuropsychiatry to Borderlands of Neurology and Psychiatry Brain and Mind. Acta Clin Croat 54(4): 500–8.

Berrios, G. E. and I. S. Markova (2002). The concept of neuropsychiatry: a historical overview. J Psychosom Res 53(2): 629–38.

Bhattacharya, R., et al. (2015). Commissioning neuropsychiatry services: barriers and lessons. BJPsych Bull 39(6): 291–6.

Bogousslavsky, J. and L. Tatu (2013). French neuropsychiatry in the Great War: between moral support and electricity. J Hist Neurosci 22(2): 144–54.

Bunge, M. (2010). Mater and Mind. A philosophical Inquiry. Dordrecht, Heidelberg, London, New York: Springer.

Casey, B. J., et al. (2013). DSM-5 and RDoC: progress in psychiatry research? Nat Rev Neurosci 14(11): 810–14.

Chebili, S. (2016). [Malaise in psychiatry and its history]. Encephale 42(2): 185–90.

Covanis, A., et al. (2015). From global campaign to global commitment: The World Health Assembly's Resolution on epilepsy. Epilepsia 56(11): 1651–7.

Diefenbacher, A. (2004) Consultation-liaison psychiatry and psychosomatics in Germany: futile dispute or lesson to be learned? Adv Psychosom Med 26:177–80.

Fontaine, J. F., et al. (2015). Assessment of curated phenotype mining in neuropsychiatric disorder literature. Methods 74: 90–6.

Hoff, P. (2015). The Kraepelinian tradition. Dialogues Clin Neurosci 17(1): 31–41.

Huertas, R. (2003). Elaborando doctrina: Teoría y retórica en la obra de José María Esquerdo (1842–1912). Frenia 3(2): 81–109.

Johnson, B. and D. Flores Mosri (2016). The Neuropsychoanalytic Approach: Using Neuroscience as the Basic Science of Psychoanalysis. Front Psychol 7: 1459.

Krasnov, V. N. and I. Gurovich (2012). History and current condition of Russian psychiatry. Int Rev Psychiatry 24(4): 328–33.

Lázaro, J. (2000). Historia de la Asociación Española de Neuropsiquiatría (1924–1999). Revista de la Asociación española de Neuropsiquiatría 20(75): 397–515.

Lázaro, J. (2003). L'évolution de la psychopathologie espagnole du XXe siècle. Annales Médico Psychologiques 161: 510–20.

Lerner, V., et al. (2006). Vladimir Mikhailovich Bekhterev (1857–1927). J Neurol 253(11): 1518–19.

Lishman, W. A. (1992). What is neuropsychiatry? J Neurol Neurosurg Psychiatry 55(11): 983–5.

Llopis, B. Single psychosis. In: J. López-Ibor, C. Carbonell, and J. Garrabé (editors) Anthology of Spanish Psychiatric Texts. Saint-Amand-Montrond: World Psychiatric Association; 2001. pp. 344–401.

Lopez-Ibor, J. J. (2008). The founding of the first psychiatric hospital in the World in Valencia. Actas Esp Psiquiatr 36(1): 1–9.

López-Muñoz, F., et al. (2007). Lafora y el origen de la neuropsiquiatría biológica española. Psiquiatría Biológica 14(3): 108–20.

Martin, M., A. Karenberg, and H. Fangerau (2016). German neurology and neurologists during the Third Reich: Preconditions and general framework before and after 1933. Nervenarzt 87 Suppl 1: 5–17.

Miller, N. S. and J. L. Katz (1989). The neurological legacy of psychoanalysis: Freud as a neurologist. Compr Psychiatry 30(2): 128–34.

Neumarker, K. J. and A. J. Bartsch (2003). Karl Kleist (1879–1960)—a pioneer of neuropsychiatry. Hist Psychiatry 14(56 Pt 4): 411–58.

Northoff, G. (2008). Neuropsychiatry. An old discipline in a new gestalt bridging biological psychiatry, neuropsychology, and cognitive neurology. Eur Arch Psychiatry Clin Neurosci 258(4): 226–38.

Olivares, F. A., et al. (2015). Neurophenomenology revisited: second-person methods for the study of human consciousness. Front Psychol 6: 673.

Ovsyannikov, S. A. and A. S. Ovsyannikov (2007). Sergey S. Korsakov and the beginning of Russian psychiatry. J Hist Neurosci 16(1–2): 58–64.

Peiffer, J. (1991). Neuropathology in the Third Reich. [Memorial to those victims of National-Socialist atrocities in Germany who were used by medical science]. Brain Pathol 1(2): 125–31.

Pinel, P. (2005). La normalisation de la psychiatrie française. Regards Sociologiques 29: 3–21.

Priller, J., Gelderblom, H., and A. Heinz (2011) Neuropsychiatrie als Spezialisierung. Die Psychiatrie 8: 241–5.

Rubin, E. H. and C. F. Zorumski (2012). Perspective: Upcoming paradigm shifts for psychiatry in clinical care, research, and education. Acad Med 87(3): 261–5.

Rzesnitzek, L. (2013). 'Early Psychosis' as a mirror of biologist controversies in post-war German, Anglo-Saxon, and Soviet Psychiatry. Front Psychol 4: 481.

Sachdev, P. S. (2002). Neuropsychiatry—a discipline for the future. J Psychosom Res 53: 625–7.

Sachdev, P. S. (2005). Whither neuropsychiatry? J Neuropsychiatry Clin Neurosci 17(2): 140–4.

Srirathan, H. and A. E. Cavanna (2015). Research Trends in the Neuropsychiatry Literature Since the New Millennium. J Neuropsychiatry Clin Neurosci 27(4): 354–61.

Stahnisch, F. W. and G. Russell (2016). New perspectives on forced migration in the history of twentieth-century neuroscience. J Hist Neurosci 25(3): 219–26.

Shterenshis, M. V. (1999). The position of nervous diseases between internal medicine and psychiatry in the XIXth century. Vesalius, V, 2: 67–71.

Taylor, J. J., et al. (2015). Beyond neural cubism: promoting a multidimensional view of brain disorders by enhancing the integration of neurology and psychiatry in education. Acad Med 90(5): 581–6.

Trimble, M. (2016a). The intentional brain—a short history of neuropsychiatry. CNS Spectr 21(3): 223–9.

Trimble, M. (2016b). The Intentional Brain: motion, emotion, and the development of modern neuropsychiatry. Baltimore, MD: Johns Hopkins University Press.

Valenciano Gayá, L. (1977). El Doctor Lafora y su época. Madrid: Morata.

Valko, P. and C. L. Bassetti (2006). Aleksej Yakovlevich Kozhevnikov (1836–1902). J Neurol 253(4): 537–8.

Vargas Aragón, M. (2012). Ni neurología desalmada, ni psiquiatría descerebrada: Neurociencia clínica. Kranion 9: 11–15.

Vargas, M. (2017). Neurosciences and philosophy: what is new in the 21st century? Neurosciences and History 5(1): 38–46.

Villasante Armas, O. (1997). Primer certamen frenopático español (1883): Estructura asistencial y aspectos administrativos. Asclepio 49(1): 79–93.

Weber, M. M. (2000). Psychiatric research and science policy in Germany: the history of the Deutsche Forschungsanstalt fur Psychiatrie (German Institute for Psychiatric Research) in Munich from 1917 to 1945. Hist Psychiatry 11(43 Pt 3): 235–58.

49

Neuropsychiatric services in South America

Gilberto Slud Brofman and Luis Ignacio Brusco

Introduction

The South American continent consists of 12 countries. Nine of these are Spanish-speaking countries—Argentina, Bolivia, Chile, Colombia, Ecuador, Paraguay, Peru, Uruguay, and Venezuela—home to approximately 202 million people in total. One is a Portuguese-speaking country—Brazil—which by itself shelters almost the same number of inhabitants of 201 million. There are also two small countries—English-speaking Guyana and Dutch-speaking Suriname—and the French territory French Guiana, each of which has a population of around half a million inhabitants.

In this chapter, we will outline the historical evolution of neuropsychiatry in Brazil and Argentina and the situation of neuropsychiatry services in these countries. We will also highlight some data from Peru and, concluding the chapter, we will attempt to shed some light on what may be expected for the future of this branch of medicine on the South American continent.

Historical context

In order to better understand the status quo of neuropsychiatry and the institutions dedicated to it in South America, it is important that we know the history of neuropsychiatry development on this continent. This history is specific to Brazil; nonetheless it reflects, to a greater or lesser degree, what happened in most countries of South America, which, in turn, also reflects the landscape of neuropsychiatry in Europe, notably in France and Germany (Bogousslavsky and Moulin, 2007).

Neuropsychiatry is a sub-speciality of psychiatry which deals with psychological and behavioural manifestations of brain diseases; however, unlike what it may seem at first glance, neuropsychiatry did not derive from psychiatry, but rather, it gave rise to psychiatry and neurology as different medical specialties. The pioneers in these two medical specialties were what today we would call neuropsychiatrists.

José Martins da Cruz Jobim (1802–1878) is considered the first Brazilian neuropsychiatrist. His studies were focused on the connection between infectious diseases, poverty, and mental illness. He also became interested in the poor living conditions of patients in their housing institutions, about which the physician made a number of public complaints. In 1831, Jobim wrote the first article about mental illness in Brazil called *Insânia Loquaz* (Loquations Insanity), based on clinical and pathological data consistent with tuberculous meningitis. He also wrote about hydrophobia (1831), another pathology of what was then labelled as 'infectious psychiatry' (Gomes et al., 2013).

Up to the second third of the nineteenth century, mentally ill people in the main urban areas of Brazil were kept in dreadful living conditions, either in the basements of the *Santas Casas de Misericórdia* (Holy Houses of Mercy, which were charity hospitals derived from the Portuguese tradition and organized by the Catholic Church), in chains, or, in case they were not aggressive, abandoned on the streets. Between 1854 and 1895, with the support of the Emperor Dom Pedro II, a principle of a mental patient assistance policy was created, which resulted in the opening of five major institutions, then called hospices. Such institutions were located in major cities and aimed to host the patients, care for them, and provide them with an occupation. The oldest institution is the NHI—*Hospício Nacional dos Alienados Dom Pedro II* (Dom Pedro II National Hospice for the Insane) (see Fig. 49.1) founded in the city of Rio de Janeiro in 1854. Other examples are the *Hospício São Pedro* (São Pedro Hospice) (1884) (see Fig. 49.2) in Porto Alegre (Piccinini, 2000) and the *Asilo de Alienados do Juqueri* (Juqueri Asylum for the Insane) (1895) in São Paulo.

The medicine then practised in these hospices was modelled on what today corresponds to neuropsychiatry, i.e. it sought the diagnosis of organic conditions, whether infectious or not, which should be responsible for the aetiology of the mental and behavioural disorders presented by the patients. The first professorships in psychiatry were created around these asylums by the end of the nineteenth century and the beginning of the twentieth century, and the neurology professorships followed a few years later. Rio de Janeiro, the then capital of the Brazilian Empire, had its First Psychiatry Cathedra founded in 1883 at the NHI, and its holder was Dr João Carlos Teixeira Brandão. The First Neurology Cathedra was founded in 1912, with classes taught at the Santa Casa de Misericórdia and with Dr Austregésilo Rodrigues de Lima as its first holder. Thus, starting from a common root at the beginning

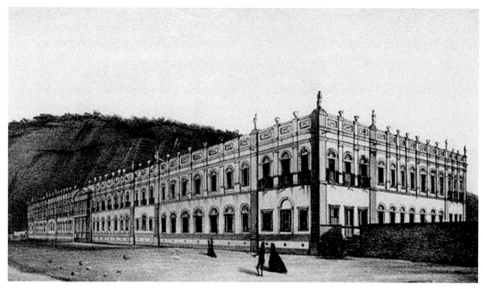

Fig. 49.1 Picture of the Hospício Nacional dos Alienados Dom Pedro II (Rio de Janeiro), today part of a campus of the Federal University of Rio de Janeiro.

of the twentieth century, with its pioneers working in the same mental institutions, with no boundary defined between the pathologies later classified as neurological or psychiatric, these two medical specialties began their individual paths, keeping a constant distance between them (Gomes and Cavalcanti, 2013; Gomes and Engelhardt, 2013).

Similar to what occurred in the majority of the countries, while neurology was setting its roots in general hospitals, along with other medical specialties, psychiatry remained isolated in its hospices and living with a growing dilemma with regard to its pathologies—organic basis versus socio-psychogenic basis, or brain versus mind.

During the decades of 1910s and 1920s, while psychiatry and neurology were establishing themselves as distinct specialties, South America started to receive the first contributions of the new field of psychoanalysis, initiated by Freud in Vienna. Psychoanalysis was introduced in Brazil around 1912, by the hands of Juliano Moreira, founder of modern Brazilian psychiatry (Piccinini, 2002).

In 1927, the first psychoanalysis society of South America was founded in São Paulo—the *Sociedade Brasileira de Psicanálise* (Brazilian Society of Psychoanalysis). From this moment on, psychoanalytic theories were quickly disseminated on the South American continent where they were met with great enthusiasm,

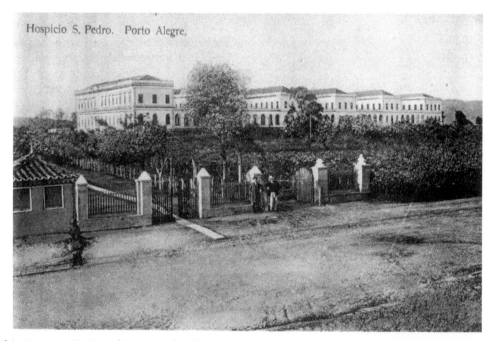

Fig. 49.2 Picture of the Hospício São Pedro (Porto Alegre), still in operation today and now renamed as Hospital Psiquiatríco São Pedro (São Pedro Psychiatric Hospital).

especially in Argentina and Brazil. Societies and official centres linked to the International Psychoanalytic Association (IPA) were founded in most of the large cities (Salim, 2010).

In the following decades (the 1930s, 1940s, 1950s), psychoanalytic theories become predominant in psychiatry, both as an explanation for the aetiology of psychiatric disorders and for clinical practice, mainly through analytical-based psychotherapies. The popularity and pervasiveness of this strong trend led psychiatry to move even further away from its neuropsychiatric roots, reinforcing, to a great extent, the aetiological, social, psychogenic branch.

Yet the growing contribution of the neurosciences and the beginning of modern psychopharmacotherapy (1960s, 1970s, 1980s) gradually made the pendulum of the 'aetiological equation' swing back to the organic side (brain). In South America, this movement developed in a considerably slower fashion than in Europe and North America. This intense adherence of South American psychiatrists to the psychoanalytic theories is, among others, the main reason for the little interest shown by them for a field such as neuropsychiatry, which, while not neglecting the use of psychotherapeutic techniques, deals with the so-called organic processes. Moreover, it is important to note the lack of habit of these physicians to work within multidisciplinary teams, which is how the neuropsychiatry services are organized.

There was, and there still is, a common view that the overall care of pathologies concerned with neuropsychiatry belongs to the neurology sphere.

This historical perspective aids us in understanding the reasons for this still incipient and little diffused development of neuropsychiatry, particularly in Brazil, when compared to other countries. As shown in Figs. 49.3 and 49.4, it is possible to visualize the moments in which this distance differs in Brazil and in the rest of the world.

Neuropsychiatry services in Brazil

The deficiency of the neuropsychiatry services in Brazil is also linked to another set of situations that are described in the following paragraphs.

Relevant medical education system and training pathway in neuropsychiatry are virtually non-existent. There are neither residencies nor internships in this area. There is only one Brazilian university that offers a graduate programme with the title of 'Neuropsychiatry'. Nearly all medical colleges and universities are still training professionals in a closed and stiff manner, i.e. either in neurology or in psychiatry. The term neuropsychiatry is not included in the syllabus. In the neurology sphere, some attention is placed on behavioural neurology, which is the counterpart of neuropsychiatry in psychiatry. In the field of psychiatry, we can find the term geriatric psychiatry, which comes closer to neuropsychiatry.

Likewise, in the medical societies, there are no neuropsychiatry departments. That is the case of both the Brazilian Association of Psychiatry and the Brazilian Academy of Neurology.

The Federal Council of Medicine, which is the body that regulates and supervises the practice of medicine in Brazil, does not consider, from a legal point of view, and therefore does not regulate, neuropsychiatry as a medical specialty.

This same distance that psychiatrists keep from neuropsychiatry is replicated among Brazilian psychologists—only recently have we begun to see some interest in neuropsychology, which deals with

important tools for the diagnosis of neuropsychiatric disorders. In recent years, however, numerous psychometric test batteries have been validated for use in Brazil; furthermore, several tests have also been developed in the country, such as the '*Instrumento de Avaliação Neuropsicológica Breve—Neupsilin*' (Brief Neuropsychological Assessment Tool—Neupsilin), taking into account the cultural and educational levels of the local population.

In Brazil, there is only one publication whose title refers to neuropsychiatry, which is the journal of the Brazilian Academy of Neurology—*Arquivos de Neuro-Psiquiatria* (*Archives of Neuropsychiatry*). Despite its title, the journal addresses predominantly neurology topics. Argentina, Chile, and Peru also have publications devoted to neuropsychiatry that are issued regularly. The *Revista de Neuro-Psiquiatría do Peru* (*Peru's Neuropsychiatry Journal*) is the oldest in South America and continues to be published up to the present date. It was launched in 1938 by the psychiatrist Honorio Delgado and the neurologist Oscar Trelles who also founded, in that same year, the *Sociedad Peruana de Neuro-Psiquiatría* (Peruvian Neuro-Psychiatry Society) that no longer exists.

The practice of neuropsychiatry, albeit timid, is different among the various segments of healthcare in Brazil.

The Brazilian health system is composed of three segments: the *Sistema Único de Saúde* (Unified Health System, or SUS), which is supported by the government and serves, free of charge, most of the Brazilian population (71%), predominantly the low-income population. Another segment (23%) concerns private healthcare plans, paid for by the user, and a smaller portion of the population (6%) makes use of private medical services.

In the SUS segment, there are virtually no neuropsychiatry services, the only exceptions being the newly created Neuropsychiatric Outpatient Clinic at the Hospital Psiquiátrico São Pedro in Porto Alegre and some neurology services at university hospitals for the diagnosis of dementias. The population is served either by primary care physicians or specialists, psychiatrists, or neurologists, in an isolated manner. Eventually, a larger hospital provides a consultation–liaison psychiatry system. For users of private healthcare plans and private medical services, the situation is a little better, particularly in the most recent years. Several hospitals, especially in large cities, offer, for instance, diagnosis and treatment services for dementia while working with a neuropsychiatry vision, i.e. integrating neurologists, psychiatrists, neuropsychologists, radiologists, and other professionals. The ageing of the Brazilian population and the subsequent marked increase in the incidence of neuropsychiatric pathologies have been the drivers for the advent of these neuropsychiatry services.

To sum up the foregoing, it can be said that, even though neuropsychiatry was the shared root of psychiatry and neurology in Brazil, psychiatrists and neurologists continue to work, with rare exceptions, without acknowledging the vast common and overlying border that these two specialties share.

The lack of a 'neuropsychiatry vision', which is still in its infancy, is reflected in a number of consequences—relevant medical education system and training pathway in this field are rare; the national medical societies related to these two specialties do not have a neuropsychiatry component, and therefore do not promote scientific events in the field; there is no legal nor academic acknowledgement and recognition of neuropsychiatry as a specialty or sub-specialty. The most serious implication of these is the lack of medical care services focused

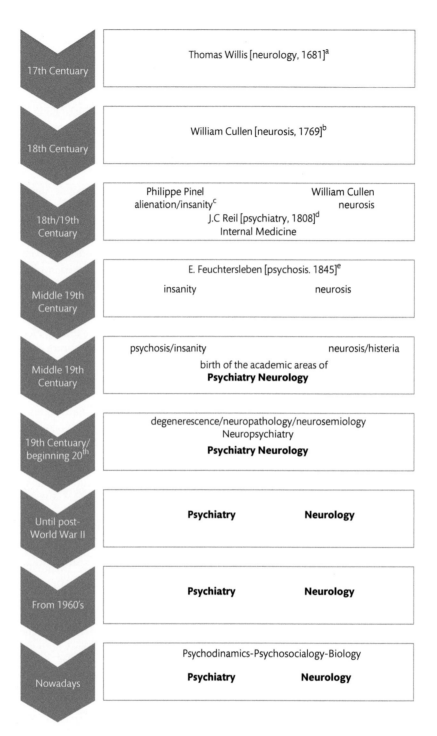

17th Century

Thomas Willis [neurology, 1681][a]

18th Century

William Cullen [neurosis, 1769][b]

18th/19th Century

| Philippe Pinel alienation/insanity[c] | William Cullen neurosis |

J.C Reil [psychiatry, 1808][d]
Internal Medicine

Middle 19th Century

E. Feuchtersleben [psychosis. 1845][e]

insanity   neurosis

Middle 19th Century

psychosis/insanity   neurosis/histeria

birth of the academic areas of
Psychiatry Neurology

19th Century/ beginning 20th

degenerescence/neuropathology/neurosemiology
Neuropsychiatry
Psychiatry Neurology

Until post-World War II

Psychiatry   Neurology

From 1960's

Psychiatry   Neurology

Nowadays

Psychodinamics-Psychosocialogy-Biology

Psychiatry   Neurology

I: In Cerebri Anatome (1664), a neuroanatomy text, Thomas Willis (1621–1675)coined the term neurology, but in its English edition (1681). II: Other term, for a time dubious, was neurosis (1784) presented by William Cullen (1710–1790) to refer to "disorders of sense and motion" caused by a "general affection of the nervous system". It denotes all diseases of the nerves and muscles, and it suggests a physical cause. III: Philippe Pinel (1745–1826) published "Medicophilosophical treatise on mental alienation or mania" (1801). IV: Johann Christian Reil (1808) coined the term psychiatry: "medical treatment of the soul". V: The term psychosis was coined by Ernst Feuchtersleben in 1845 to denote "mental disorder which affected the personality as a whole" and was a subcategory of the then much wider category of neurosis. The insanities, by contrast, were viewed as diseases of the mind and not generally of physical origin.

Fig. 49.3 Critical points in the parallel historical evolution of neurology and psychiatry.

Courtesy of *Arquivos de Neuro-Psiquiatria* Dr. Oswaldo Lange, from Gomes, Marleide da Mota and Engelhardt, Eliasz Historical sketches of the beginnings of the academic 'Mental and Nervous Diseases' in Brazil, and European influences. *Arq. Neuro-Psiquiatr.*, Aug 2013, vol.71, no.8, p.562–565. ISSN 0004-282X, with permission.

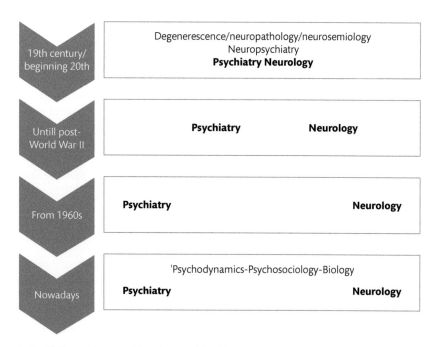

In Brazil, the gap between Neurology and Psychiatry was even greater, and they remain as two distinct areas, with little integration between them.

Fig. 49.4 Critical points in the parallel historical evolution of neurology and psychiatry in Brazil.

on neuropsychiatry. Neurologists pay slightly greater attention to this field, whereas psychiatrists remain as showing little interest, still keeping themselves isolated from other medical specialties.

Neuropsychiatric services in Argentina

Neuropsychiatry, considered as a discipline that studies the cognitive, mental, and behavioural disorders associated with an alteration of the nervous system, is a relatively new sub-speciality in Argentina, recognized and accredited since 2007 by the University of Buenos Aires School of Medicine under the title of '*Carrera de Médico Especialista en Neurología Cognitiva y Neuropsiquiatría*' (Specialist Physician in Cognitive Neurology and Neuropsychiatry).

The origins of neuropsychiatry in Argentina date back to the birth of neurology in the late nineteenth century, influenced by the European mainstream with the work of Jean-Martin Charcot at the Salpêtrière (France), which, in turn, was closely related to psychiatry from its beginnings, barely setting itself apart from it (Besada, 2010, p. 74).

In Argentina, psychiatry emerged with the physician Lucio Meléndez (1844–1901) from La Rioja province, who, following the teachings of JE Esquirol and P Pinel, introduced the specialty in the country and was the first director of the Hospicio de las Mercedes (Mercedes' Hospice), nowadays the Neuropsychiatric Hospital José T Borda. There, Meléndez devoted himself to the study of mental conditions, seeking improvements in the quality of life of the State's patients (publicly funded healthcare), in the sphere of public health (Alarcón, 1990).

Meanwhile, the Ministry of Foreign Affairs, during the office of Julio A Roca in 1899, hired Dr Christfried Jakob (German) to take charge of the Neurological and Psychiatric Clinic Laboratory of the Hospicio de las Mercedes where he carried out his work with human brains (Orlando, 1966). Different phylo-ontogenetic, neuroanatomical, and microscopy studies were focused on establishing clinical correlations between neurological syndromes and neuropathological changes (De Robertis, 1891). His work set the basis for the neurobiological concepts of current Argentinian neuropsychiatry, which was followed by his disciples, including Braulio Moyano, José Borda, Jacinto Orlando, and Diego Outes, who, in turn, also gave rise to important scientific discoveries.

During the twentieth century, a revolution of the psychoanalytical theory took place, heavily influenced by the Freudian and Lacanian schools which are oriented towards the reflection of the clinical experience focusing primarily on subjective aspects through the understanding of immaterial external forces, being introduced in Argentina by Enrique Pichon–Rivière (1907–1977). On the other hand, following the German branch, characters such as Jose Ramos Mejia, Francisco de Veyga, and Jose Ingenieros boosted forensic psychiatry through the study of the relationship between insanity and crime (Fernández Labriola and Kalina, 2001).

Subsequently, the advances in psychopharmacology post-1950, with the advent of chlorpromazine in France, led to a major change in psychiatric therapy. Personalities such as Edmund Fischer (1904–1974), a Hungarian psychiatrist nationalized in Argentina, notably influenced this field, being one of the first to postulate the hypothesis of phenylethylamine being linked to depression, as well as to consider that the symptoms of schizophrenia could be caused by an abnormal formation of bufotenin, a strongly hallucinogenic substance derived from serotonin. There are several publications on the topic: *Farmacoterapia de las Enfermedades Nerviosas y Mentales* (*Pharmacotherapy of Nervous and Mental Disease*) in 1971, *Introducción a la Psiquiatría Biológica* (*Introduction to Biological Psychiatry*) in 1974, and *Esquizofrenia, Depresión, Toxicomanías*

(*Schizophrenia, Depression, Addiction*) in 1977 (López-Muñoz and Álamo González, 2006). Similarly, despite not being a psychiatrist and working independently, Eduardo De Robertis (1913–1988), a physician and biologist at the University of Buenos Aires, was the discoverer of the synaptic vesicles in the axon terminals as the site for accumulation of neurotransmitters, a discovery which has had major implications for neuropsychopharmacological research (De Robertis, 1891).

Neurophysiology, in the 1970s, was another important milestone in the development of neuropsychiatry, with Bernardo Houssay (1887–1971), a physician, pharmacist, and Nobel Prize Winner in Medicine, as the champion of physiology, who made it a medical discipline of greater vigour and development in Argentina. In the same field, Daniel P Cardinali, Head of Physiology at the University of Buenos Aires School of Medicine, investigated the mechanisms of action of melatonin and its association with circadian rhythms, light, and sleep disorders (Brusco, 2012; Cardinali, 2015).

Towards the end of the twentieth century, in the 1990s, other areas of importance that contributed to the understanding of diseases from the neuropsychiatric point of view were developed, such as neuropsychology, neuroendocrinology, neuroimaging, and, in particular, developments regarding the decryption, analysis, and understanding of the genetic basis (Marquez and Brusco, 1999).

In 1998, Luis Ignacio Brusco, alongside Guillermo Tórtora, created the Asociación Neuropsiquiátríca Argentina (Argentinian Neuropsychiatric Association), following a worldwide trend for the development of associations of neuropsychiatry. Two years later, Brusco joined the International Neuropsychiatric Association, creating one of the busiest annual conferences of Latin America and, in 2003, he also created the Instituto de Posgrado CECYS (Postgraduate Institute 'Centre of Cognitive and Social Studies').

Clearly, various scientific advances have shown that the combination of neurology and psychiatry is essential in order to understand how a brain disease leads to a mental disorder.

The Centro de Neuropsiquiatría y Neurología de la Conducta (Centre Neuropsychiatry and Behavioural Neurology) (CENECON) was established at the University of Buenos Aires School of Medicine, operating at the Clinical Hospital and the Lanari Institute of the university.

An institution dedicated specifically to neurological pathologies has also been created at the Fundación para la Lucha Contra las Enfermedades Infantiles del Niño (Foundation for the Fight Against Childhood Diseases), as well as a rehabilitation centre for highly complex diseases of the nervous system.

Within the Department of Public Health of the University of Buenos Aires, a National Data and Research Program for Alzheimer's Disease was set up, with an epidemiological and statistical database on dementias and, specifically, a genetic databank for dementias, the first in Latin America (http://www.pronadial.org.ar) (Brusco, 2016).

It also features basic research groups in neuropsychiatry, among which we can highlight the Leloir Institute that carries out extensive research in genetics using animal models of Alzheimer's disease. In the province of Córdoba, there is a similar initiative where the Ferreira Institute is developing different research in metabolomics and cellular reprogramming in order to better understand the neurological mechanisms by which a disease occurs.

This Ferreira Institute has also created a Masters course in translational science, which is a graduate programme that focuses on how basic science can be derived from, and used in, applied science.

The Ferreira Institute, together with the Leloir Institute and the University of Buenos Aires' CENECON, has been awarded a grant from the World Bank and the Ministry of Science and Technology for the translational study of Alzheimer's disease. This work is carried out at the Eva Peron Hospital, a public hospital in the Province of Buenos Aires. The Eva Peron Hospital has also received a substantial donation in aid of building a unit for education and prevention of dementia and other neurocognitive disorders.

Future prospects

The portrait of neuropsychiatry presented in this chapter shows, despite some recent advances, a difficult prospect for a greater and more substantial expression of a 'neuropsychiatric vision' (and therefore a neuropsychiatric approach) on the South American continent. This follows a global trend and stems from a basic core problem, namely the arbitrary division, without any scientific basis whatsoever, of diseases which are considered either psychiatric or neurological, perhaps mainly due to an expression of the old conflict of *neurological = organic and psychiatric = functional or brain × mind*, noting that, in their early days, there was no such detachment between the specialties (Crespo de Souza, 2003; Martin, 2002).

This segregation (Yudofsky and Hales, 2002) promoted an agglutination of complex brain disorders in simplistic categories which are based on a single symptom—for instance, Parkinson's disease, which shows a high prevalence of psychosis, depression, and dementia, as a 'movement disorder'; or schizophrenia, in which patients suffer from cognitive, mood, and motivation disorders, as a 'psychotic disorder'. This accounts for the scenery in which neurologists undervalue psychiatric consequences and, likewise, psychiatrists underestimate the neurological consequences in patients with neuropsychiatric disorders.

This original sin arisen from the individualization of psychiatry and neurology continues to cause damage and remains in need of an evolution that may set it right, which can occur through the theoretical–practical integration and approach of both specialties (Pies, 2005, p. 304). From a practical point of view, in order to have prospects of a future in which we can offer neuropsychiatric patients a fast diagnosis and the best treatment possible, using all the tools in an integrated and comprehensive way, two attitudes are fundamental: incentives for educational processes (residencies, graduate courses) and integration of neuropsychiatry departments in medical societies and fostering scientific events in neuropsychiatry (Meyer and Chemali, 2013).

In this sense, it is worth quoting the efforts made by Dr Moises Gaviria, a Peruvian psychiatrist based in the United States, who, since 1990, welcomed South-American physicians at the University of Illinois at Chicago (UIC)'s Department of Neuropsychiatry for training in the field. Dr Gaviria was one of the founders, in 1996, of the International Neuropsychiatric Association (INA), a scientific organization that has promoted and/or supported numerous conferences in various countries on the continent and continues to do so. In addition to the events, the INA aims to promote scientific exchanges with other medical associations, such as the cooperation agreement signed in 2014 with the Associação Brasileira de Psiquiatria (Brazilian Psychiatric Association) (ABP) and, since 2000, with the Asociación Neuropsiquiátrica Argentina (Neuropsychiatric Association of Argentina) (ANA).

Examples such as these have certainly contributed to the promotion and dissemination of the 'neuropsychiatric vision' and knowledge, stimulating the creation of new services in this area and attracting the interest of new generations of physicians. It is our responsibility to break down the barriers that today hinder the process of full collaboration between psychiatry and neurology, noting that nowadays we have a common language that unites these two specialties—the neurosciences.

We owe it to the physician's *raison d'être*—our patient.

KEY LEARNING POINTS

- This chapter examines the historical evolution of neuropsychiatry in Brazil and Argentina, with a view to understanding what the future may hold for the field in South America.
- A brief historical context is given, before the limitations of neuropsychiatric services in Brazil are discussed, with reference to the lack of attention afforded in education and training and the absence of long-established links between the psychiatric and neurology communities.
- Although neuropsychiatry only gained official recognition and accreditation in Argentina in 2007, there is a precedent of neuropsychiatric study in the country dating back to Charcot's theories in the nineteenth century, and carried forward by expatriate psychiatrists such as Edmundo Fischer in the twentieth century.
- The future development of neuropsychiatry in South America remains uncertain due to the unscientific distinction between psychiatry and neurology, leading to simplistic diagnoses such as classifying Parkinson's disease as simply a 'movement disorder' or schizophrenia as purely 'psychotic'.

REFERENCES

Alarcón, R. (1990). *Identidad de la Psiquiatría Latinoamericana*, Siglo XXI Editores, México.

Besada, C.H. (2010). Dr. Christofredo Jakob: Historia de la Escuela Neurobiológica Germano-argentina. *Revista Argentina de Radiología*, 74(2), 133–9.

Bogousslavsky, J. and Moulin, T. (2009). From Alienism to the Birth of Modern Psychiatry: A Neurological Story? *European Neurology*, 62, 257–63.

Brusco, L.I. (2012). *Trastornos del sueño y de los ritmos biológicos en la enfermedad de Alzheimer*. Editorial Salerno, Buenos Aires.

Brusco, L.I. (2016). *Conciencia intersubjetiva del tiempo y la cuestión de la temporalidad*. Editorial Universidad de Morón, Buenos Aires.

Cardinali, D.P. (2015). *Cincuenta años con la piedra de la locura: apuntes autobiográficos de un científico argentino*, Editorial AAPC, Buenos Aires.

Crespo de Souza, C. (2003). Quem deve tratar transtornos psiquiátricos em pacientes neurológicos? *Psychiatry On-line Brazil*, 8(5). Available at: http://www.polbr.med.br/ano03/artigo0503_2.php.

Gomes, Mda, M. and Cavalcanti, J. (2013). The Brazilian Neurology centenary (1912–2012) and the common origin of the fields of Neurology and Psychiatry. *Arquivos de Neuro-Psiquiatria*, 71(1), 63–5.

Gomes, Mda, M. and Engelhardt, E. (2013). Historical sketches of the beginnings of the academic 'Mental and Nervous Diseases' in Brazil, and European influences. *Arquivos de Neuro-Psiquiatria*, 71(8), 562–5.

Gomes, Mda, M., Engelhardt, E., and Chimelli, L. (2013). The first Brazilian neuropsychiatrist, José Martins da Cruz Jobim, tuberculous meningitis and mental disease. *Arquivos de Neuro-Psiquiatria*, 71(3), 191–3.

De Robertis, E. (1891). *Biología Celular y Molecular*. El Ateneo, Buenos Aires.

Fernández Labriola, R. and Kalina, E. (2001). *Psiquiatría Biológica Argentina*. Cangrejal, Buenos Aires.

López-Muñoz, F. and Álamo González, C. (2006). *Historia de la psicofarmacología*, Vol. 3. Editorial Medica Panamericana, Buenos Aires.

Martin, J. (2002). The Integration of Neurology, Psychiatry, and Neuroscience in the 21st Century. *American Journal of Psychiatry*, 159(5), 695–704.

Marquez, M.A. and Brusco, L.I. (1999). *Funciones cognitivas. Fisiología Humana*, second edition. Editores: J. Tresguerres, McGraw-Hill-Interamericana, Madrid.

Meyer, F. and Chemali, Z. (2013). On Education: Teaching the Neurology-Psychiatry interface using a flexible quadrant model. *Clinical Neuropsychiatry*, 10, 171–3.

Orlando, J.C. (1966). *Christofedo Jakob: su vida y obra*. Mundi, Buenos Aires.

Piccinini, W. (2000). Breve História da Psiquiatria do Rio Grande do Sul à Luz das suas Publicações. *Psychiatry On-line Brazil*, 5(11). Available at: http://www.polbr.med.br/ano00/wal1100.php.

Piccinini, W. (2002). Juliano Moreira—Um brasileiro extraordinário. *Psychiatry On-line Brazil*, 7(7). Available at: http://www.polbr.med.br/ano02/wal0702.php.

Pies, R. (2005). Why Psychiatry and Neurology Cannot Simply Merge. *Journal of Neuropsychiatry and Clinical Neurosciences*, 17(3), 304–9.

Salim, S.A. (2010). A História da Psicanálise no Brasil e em Minas Gerais. *Mental*, 8(14). Available at: http://pepsic.bvsalud.org/scielo.php?script=sci_arttext&pid=S1679-44272010000100009.

Yudofsky, S. and Hales, R. (2002). Neuropsychiatry and the Future of Psychiatry and Neurology. *American Journal of Psychiatry*, 159(8), 1261.

Index